Y0-DVQ-137

Handbook of Experimental Pharmacology

Volume 104/I

Opioids I

Contributors

H. Akil, S. Archer, A. Beaumont, M. Blum, D. Bronstein, S.R. Childers
A.D. Corbett, B.M. Cox, V. Dauge, R. Day, S. Dermer, J. Donnerer
A.W. Duggan, R. Elde, S.M. Fleetwood-Walker, L.D. Fricker
M.-C. Fournié-Zaluski, T.L. Gioannini, A. Goldstein, T. Hökfelt
V. Höllt, J.W. Holaday, H. Khachaturian, N. Kley, C.M. Knapp
H.W. Kosterlitz, N.M. Lee, F.M. Leslie, N. Levin, M.E. Lewis
J.P. Loeffler, H.H. Loh, D. Lorang, J.R. Lundblad, A. Mansour
A.H. Mulder, R.A. North, S.J. Paterson, D.E. Pellegrini-Giampietro
J.E. Pintar, F. Porreca, P.S. Portoghese, J.L. Roberts, B.R. Roques
J. Rossier, R.B. Rothman, M.K.H. Schäfer, P.W. Schiller
A.N.M. Schoffelmeer, R.E.M. Scott, E.J. Simon, A.P. Smith
J.A.M. Smith, S. Spector, A. Tempel, H. Teschemacher, K.A. Trujillo
E. Young, S.J. Watson, P.L. Wood, R.S. Zukin

Editor: Albert Herz

Section Editors: H. Akil and E.J. Simon

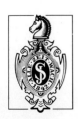

Springer-Verlag
Berlin Heidelberg New York London Paris
Tokyo Hong Kong Barcelona Budapest

Professor Dr.med. ALBERT HERZ
Max-Planck-Institut für Psychiatrie
Abteilung Neuropharmakologie
Am Klopferspitz 18
W-8033 Martinsried, FRG

Section Editors

Dr. med. HUDA AKIL
Mental Health Research Institute
School of Medicine
University of Michigan
205 Zina Pitcher
Ann Arbor, MI 48109, USA

Dr. med. ERIC J. SIMON
New York University
Medical Center
School of Medicine
550 First Avenue
New York, NY 10016, USA

With 74 Figures and 52 Tables

ISBN 3-540-55397-5 Springer-Verlag Berlin Heidelberg New York
ISBN 0-387-55397-5 Springer-Verlag New York Berlin Heidelberg

Library of Congress Cataloging-in-Publication Data. Opioids I / contributors, H. Akil . . . [et al.]; editor, Albert Herz; (H. Akil and E.J. Simon, section editors). p. cm. – (Handbook of experimental pharmacology; v. 104) Includes bibliographical references and index. ISBN 3-540-55397-5 (pt. 1: alk. paper). – ISBN 0-387-55397-5 (pt. 1: alk. paper) 1. Opioids. 2. Opioids – Receptors. I. Akil, H. (Huda) II. Herz, Albert, 1921– . III. Simon, Eric J. IV. Title: Opioids 1. V. Series. [DNLM: 1. Endorphins. 2. Receptors, Endorphin. W1 HA51L v. 104 / QU 68 O603] QP905.H3 vol. 104 [RM328] 615′.1 s – dc20 [615′.78] DNLM/DLC for Library of Congress   92-2325 CIP

Typesetting: Best-set Typesetter Ltd., Hong Kong
27/3130 – 5 4 3 2 1 0 – Printed on acid-free paper

List of Contributors

AKIL, H., Mental Health Research Institute, School of Medicine, University of Michigan, 205 Zina Pitcher, Ann Arbor, MI 48109, USA

ARCHER, S., Department of Chemistry, Cogswell Laboratory, Rensselaer Polytechnic Institute, Troy, NY 12180-3590, USA

BEAUMONT, A., Département de Chimie Organique, U 266 INSERM, UA 498 CNRS, UFR des Sciences Pharmaceutiques et Biologiques, 4, avenue de l'Observatoire, F-75006 Paris, France

BLUM, M., The Fishberg Research Center in Neurobiology, Mount Sinai School of Medicine, One Gustave L. Levy Place, New York, NY 10029, USA

BRONSTEIN, D., Laboratory of Molecular Integrative Neuroscience, National Institute of Environmental Health Sciences, Research Triangle, Park, NC 27709, USA

CHILDERS, S.R., Department of Physiology and Pharmacology, Bowman Gray School of Medicine, Medical Center Boulevard, Winston-Salem, NC 27157-1083, USA

CORBETT, A.D., Department of Biomedical Sciences, University of Aberdeen, Marischal College, Aberdeen AB9 1AS, Great Britain

COX, B.M., Department of Pharmacology, Uniformed Services University of the Health Sciences, 4301 Jones Bridge Road, Bethesda, MD 20814-4799, USA

DAUGE, V., Département de Chimie Organique, U 266 INSERM, UA 498 CNRS, UFR des Sciences Pharmaceutiques et Biologiques, 4, avenue de l'Observatoire, F-75006 Paris, France

DAY, R., J.A. DeSève Laboratory of Biochemical and Molecular Neuroendocrinology, Clinical Research Institute of Montreal, 110 Pine Avenue West, Montreal, Quebec, Canada H2W 1R7

DERMER, S., The Fishberg Research Center in Neurobiology, Mount Sinai School of Medicine, One Gustave L. Levy Place, New York, NY 10029, USA

DONNERER, J., Department of Experimental and Clinical Pharmacology, University of Graz, A-8010 Graz, Austria

DUGGAN, A.W., Department of Preclinical Veterinary Sciences, Royal (Dick) School of Veterinary Studies, University of Edinburgh, Summerhall, Edinburgh EH9 1QH, Great Britain

ELDE, R., University of Minnesota, Department of Cell Biology and Neuroanatomy, 321 Church Street SE, Minneapolis, MN 55455, USA

FLEETWOOD-WALKER, S.M., Department of Preclinical Veterinary Sciences, Royal (Dick) School of Veterinary Studies, University of Edinburgh, Summerhall, Edinburgh EH9 1QH, Great Britain

FRICKER, L.D., Department of Molecular Pharmacology, Albert Einstein College of Medicine, 1300 Morris Park Avenue, Bronx, NY 10461, USA

FOURNIÉ-ZALUSKI, M.-C., Département de Chimie Organique, U 266 INSERM, UA 498 CNRS, UFR des Sciences Pharmaceutiques et Biologiques, 4, avenue de l'Observatoire, F-75006 Paris, France

GIOANNINI, T.L., Department of Psychiatry, New York University Medical Center, 550 First Avenue, New York, NY 10016, and Baruch College, CUNY, New York, NY 10010, USA

GOLDSTEIN, AVRAM, Stanford University, 735 Dolores, Stanford, CA 94305, USA

HÖKFELT, T., Karolinska Institute, Department of Histology and Neuro-biology, P.O. Box 60 400, S-104 01 Stockholm, Sweden

HÖLLT, V., Physiologisches Institut, Universität München, Pettenkoferstraße 12, W-8000 München, FRG

HOLADAY, J.W., Medicis Corporation, 100 East 42nd Street, 15th Floor, New York, NY 10017, USA

KHACHATURIAN, H., Molecular and Cellular Neuroscience Research Branch, National Institute of Mental Health, Room 11C-05, Parklawn Building, Rockville, MD 20857, USA

KLEY, N., Molecular Neurooncology Laboratory, Massachusetts General Hospital, Harvard Medical School, 149 13th Street, Charlestown, MA 02129-9142, USA

KNAPP, C.M., Department of Pharmacy, Veterans Admin. Hospital, 130 W. Kingsbridge Road, Bronx, NY 10468, USA

KOSTERLITZ, H.W., Unit for Research on Addictive Drugs, Marischal College, University of Aberdeen, Aberdeen AB9 1AS, Great Britain

LEE, N.M., Department of Pharmacology, University of Minnesota Twin Cities, Medical School, 3-249 Millard Hall, 435 Delaware Street, S.E., Minneapolis, MN 55455, USA

LESLIE, F.M., Department of Pharmacology, California College of Medicine, University of California, Irvine, CA 92717, USA

LEVIN, N., The Fishberg Research Center in Neurobiology, Mount Sinai School of Medicine, One Gustave L. Levy Place, New York, NY 10029, USA

LEWIS, M.E., Cephalon, Inc., 145 Brandywine Parkway, West Chester, PA 19380, USA

LOEFFLER, J.P., Laboratoire de Physiologie Générale, IPCB, 21, rue René Descartes, F-67100 Strasbourg Cedex, France

LOH, H.H., Department of Pharmacology, University of Minnesota Twin Cities, Medical School, 3-249 Millard Hall, 435 Delaware Street, S.E., Minneapolis, MN 55455, USA

LORANG, D., The Fishberg Research Center in Neurobiology, Mount Sinai School of Medicine, One Gustave L. Levy Place, New York, NY 10029, USA

LUNDBLAD, J.R., The Fishberg Research Center in Neurobiology, Mount Sinai School of Medicine, One Gustave L. Levy Place, New York, NY 10029, USA

MANSOUR, A., Mental Health Research Institute, University of Michigan, 205 Zina Pitcher Place, Ann Arbor, MI 48109-0720, USA

MULDER, A.H., Department of Pharmacology, Free University Medical Faculty, Van der Boechorststraat 7, NL-1081 BT Amsterdam, The Netherlands

NORTH, R.A., Vollum Institute, Oregon Health Sciences University, 3181 SW Sam Jackson Park Road, Portland, OR 97201, USA

PATERSON, S.J., U.M.D.S., Guy's and St. Thomas's Medical and Dental School, Department of Pharmacology, Lambeth Palace Road, London SE1 7EH, Great Britain

PELLEGRINI-GIAMPIETRO, D.E., Department of Neuroscience, Albert Einstein College of Medicine, 1300 Morris Park Avenue, Bronx, NY 10461-1988, USA

PINTAR, J.E., Department of Anatomy and Cell Biology, Columbia College of Physicians and Surgeons, 630 W. 168th Street, New York, NY 10032, USA

PORRECA, F., Department of Pharmacology, College of Medicine, University of Arizona, Tucson, AZ 85724, USA

PORTOGHESE, P.S., Department of Medicinal Chemistry, College of Pharmacy, University of Minnesota, 308 Harvard Street, S.E., Minneapolis, MN 55455, USA

ROBERTS, J.L., The Fishberg Research Center in Neurobiology, Mount Sinai School of Medicine, One Gustave L. Levy Place, New York, NY 10029, USA

ROQUES, B.R., Département de Chimie Organique, U 266 INSERM, UA 498 CNRS, UFR des Sciences Pharmaceutiques et Biologiques, 4, avenue de l'Observatoire, F-75006 Paris, France

ROSSIER, J., Institut Alfred Fessard, Centre National de la Recherche Scientifique, F-91198 Gif-sur-Yvette Cedex, France

ROTHMAN, R.B., Laboratory of Clinical Psychopharmacology, NIDA Addiction Research Center, P.O. Box 5180, Baltimore, MD 21224, USA

SCHÄFER, M.K.H., Anatomisches Institut, Johannes-Gutenberg-Universität, Saarstraße 21, W-6500 Mainz, FRG

SCHILLER, P.W., Laboratory of Chemical Biology and Peptide Research, Clinical Research Institute of Montreal, 110, avenue des Pins Ouest, Montréal, Québec, Canada H2W 1R7

SCHOFFELMEER, A.N.M., Department of Pharmacology, Free University Medical Faculty, Van der Boechorststraat 7, NL-1081 BT, Amsterdam, The Netherlands

SCOTT, R.E.M., Department of Anatomy and Cell Biology, Columbia College of Physicians and Surgeons, 630 W. 168th Street, New York, NY 10032, USA

SIMON, E.J., Departments of Psychiatry and Pharmacology, New York University Medical Center, 550 First Avenue, New York, NY 10016, USA

SMITH, A.P., Department of Pharmacology, University of Minnesota Twin Cities, Medical School, 3-249 Millard Hall, 435 Delaware Street, S.E., Minneapolis, MN 55455, USA

SMITH, J.A.M., Department of Pharmacology, California College of Medicine, University of California, Irvine, CA 92717, USA

SPECTOR, S., Vanderbilt University Medical School, Department of Psychiatry and Pharmacology, Nashville, TN 37232, USA

TEMPEL, A., Department of Psychiatry, Hillside Hospital, Division of L.I.J.M.C., 266th Street and 16th Street Avenue, Glen Oaks, NY 11004, USA

TESCHEMACHER, H., Rudolf-Buchheim-Institut für Pharmakologie der Justus-Liebig-Universität, Frankfurter Straße 107, W-6300 Gießen, FRG

TRUJILLO, K.A., Mental Health Research Institute, University of Michigan, 205 Zina Pitcher Place, Ann Arbor, MI 48109-0720, USA

YOUNG, E., Mental Health Research Institute, University of Michigan, 205 Zina Pitcher Place, Ann Arbor, MI 48109-0720, USA

WATSON, S.J., Mental Health Research Institute, University of Michigan, 205 Washtenaw Place, Ann Arbor, MI 48109-0720, USA

WOOD, P.L., Mayo Clinic Jacksonville, 4500 San Pablo Road, Research Building 3, Jacksonville, FL 32224, USA

ZUKIN, R.S., Department of Neuroscience, Albert Einstein College of Medicine, 1300 Morris Park Avenue, Bronx, NY 10461-1988, USA

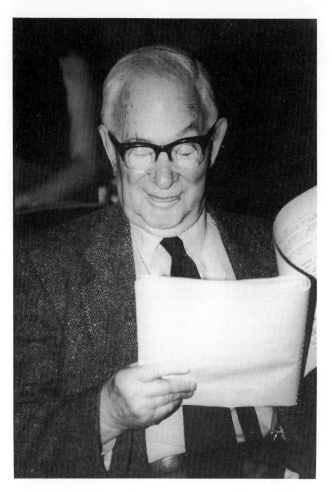

HANS KOSTERLITZ

Dedication

It is a great pleasure to dedicate this volume to Professor HANS KOSTERLITZ, of the University of Aberdeen, Scotland. Professor KOSTERLITZ is undoubtedly one of the leaders in the opioid field, whose scientific vision has exerted a significant impact on the development of this field of research. His career represents a lifetime of successful and important research, which culminated after his official retirement, when he and his colleague, Dr. JOHN HUGHES, along with a dynamic scientific team, discovered the first endogenous opioid peptides, the enkephalins.

Dr. KOSTERLITZ received his M.D. degree in 1928 from the University of Berlin and worked in that medical school until 1933. He then decided to leave Germany and took a position in the Physiology Department at the University of Aberdeen, where Nobel laureate J.J.R. MACLEOD held the chair. His research on carbohydrate metabolism bore fruit in 1937 when he isolated galactose-1-phosphate, an important intermediate in the conversion of galactose to glucose in the liver. In 1968, Dr. KOSTERLITZ was appointed to the newly created chair of pharmacology. In 1973, he retired at the age of 70 and became professor emeritus. The same year he was named director of a new laboratory established at the University of Aberdeen, called the Unit for Research on Addictive Drugs.

Starting in the 1940s his research increasingly began to reflect his interest in neuroscience and particularly in the mode of action of morphine and related narcotic analgesics. In the early 1950s, he demonstrated that the isolated guinea pig ileum is an excellent bioassay system for these drugs. In spite of ridicule by scientists who felt that any work not directly concerned with the central nervous system was irrelevant, he persisted. In extensive and thorough research, he clearly demonstrated the usefulness of in vitro bioassay systems for the study of opiates. His laboratory has developed several bioassay systems in addition to the guinea pig ileum. These include the mouse vas deferens and, more recently, the hamster and rat vas deferens systems, all of which are now used throughout the world for the assay and differentiation of the various types of opioid receptors.

It was also the use of the in vitro systems that permitted HANS KOSTERLITZ and his young collaborators, most notably JOHN HUGHES, to isolate from pig brain the first endogenous peptides with opiate-like activity in 1975, which they named methionine- and leucine enkephalin. This was a major discovery which catalyzed major advances in the field of neuropeptide research, an area which has since become one of the most active in neuroscience. It is of interest that this discovery was made two years after Dr. KOSTERLITZ' official retirement.

Professor KOSTERLITZ continued his work on opioids, focusing on the mechanism of release of enkephalins and on the multiplicity of opioid receptors. His wide ranging interests have encompassed almost every level of study of endogenous opioids, from physical structure, pharmacology, regulation, to overall physiological functions. It is, therefore, fitting that this volume, which attempts to cover the multiple levels of discourse in the study of endogenous opioids, be dedicated to him.

Looking back at Professor KOSTERLITZ' career, one is struck by two remarkable characteristics: First, he has changed his areas of scientific interest more than once, and the changes have not been minor (e.g. from carbohydrate metabolism to endogenous opioids), and second, he made significant and lasting contributions in each of these fields.

To have altered the course of research in one area is a feat and an honor, yet to have done so repeatedly is a sign of true scientific genius. Interestingly, Professor KOSTERLITZ attributes[1] his success to the very fact that he changed his research interests during the course of his career, a process which he says suited him "temperamentally." Dr. KOSTERLITZ asserts that "such a change creates a challenge to become familiar with new concepts and then try to compete as a newcomer." While this may create "worrisome complications," he believes that the difficulties "are helpful in postponing the inevitable losses in flexibility and adaptability."

We can think of no one who better exemplifies these characteristics than Professor KOSTERLITZ. We hope that this volume will inspire similarly fresh and novel ideas among its readers.

                                                                                    The Editors

---

[1] From H.W. KOSTERLITZ (1979) The best laid schemes o' mice an' men gang aft agley. Ann Rev Pharmacol Toxicol 19:1–12.

Preface

In 1957 Otto SCHAUMANN, one of the pionieers in pharmacological research on morphine and the first to prepare synthetic opiates, presented a monograph entitled "Morphin und morphinähnliche Verbindungen" as Volume 12 of the *Handbook of Experimental Pharmacology*. Now, 35 years later, we are publishing in the same series a new comprehensive volume covering the present status of opioid research. Since that time the topic has expanded enormously. The identification of opioid receptors and the detection of their endogenous ligands were landmarks which opened a new era in opioid research and fertilized the entire field of neurobiology. The rapid development of this field is illustrated in the figure, which represents the number of papers published on opioid research since 1970 (searches performed on the MEDLINE data base).

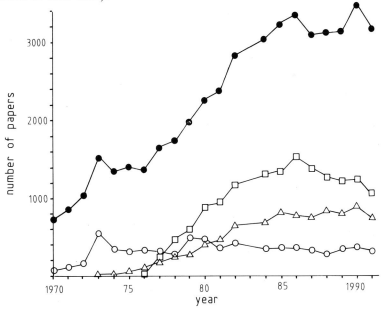

Fig. 1. The number of papers published on opioids between 1970–1991 (Medline data base). *Key,* □—□ endorphins, ○—○ opiate/opioid receptors, △—△ narcotic dependence, ●—● opioids (total, includes morphine, morphine derivatives, endorphins, opiate/opioid receptors, and narcotic dependence)

Attempts to bring out a similar state-of-the-art volume some 10–12 years ago had to be abandoned due to the logarithmic escalation in the amount of opioid research being performed at that time. Highly stimulating and often important papers on opioid research continue to appear in large numbers, but the growth phase seems to have reached a plateau. Although our knowledge on the molecular structure of opioid receptors is still very preliminary, this seems to be an appropriate time to summarize the current status of this most stimulating research domain.

Given the immense amount of literature which has accumulated on opioids during recent years and the limited space available in this publication, we were faced with the difficult task of selecting what we considered to be the most important topics of current and earlier research. We hope that our judgement was fair.

Part I deals with the multiplicity of opioid receptors (characterization, distribution, regulation etc.), the chemistry of opiates and the biochemistry and molecular biology of opioid peptides (gene expression, biosynthesis, inactivation, receptor selectivity of ligands, etc.), and the neurophysiology of opioids and their moleclular actions. Part II reviews a broad spectrum of physiological and behavioral functions and pharmacological actions of opioids. In addition, the neuroendocrinology of opioids as well as opioid tolerance and dependence are discussed in a series of chapters. The final part deals with the pathophysiology and clinical uses of opioids. Some unavoidable overlap occurs between several chapters, but the detailed subject index should help orient readers.

We would like to express our sincere thanks to the authors, who wrote their chapters without too much delay, enabling us to present up-to-date accounts. We are indepted to Prof. H. HERKEN, who initially suggested the writing of this treatise. Finally, we would like to express our gratitude to Mrs. DORIS WALKER and the other staff at Springer-Verlag as well as to our secretaries for their efforts in bringing this work to fruition.

Contents

CHAPTER 5

Anatomical Distribution of Opioid Receptors in Mammalians:
An Overview
A. Mansour and S.J. Watson. With 6 Figures

CHAPTER 6

Opioid Receptor Regulation
R.S. Zukin, D.E. Pellegrini-Giampietro, C.M. Knapp,
and A. Tempel

CHAPTER 7

Multiple Opioid Receptors and Presynaptic Modulation
of Neurotransmitter Release in the Brain

CHAPTER 8

Opioid Receptor-G Protein Interactions:
Acute and Chronic Effects of Opioids

CHAPTER 10

Allosteric Coupling Among Opioid Receptors:
Evidence for an Opioid Receptor Complex
R.B. Rothman, J.W. Holaday, and F. Porreca. With 4 Figures 217

Section B: Chemistry of Opioids with Alkaloid Structure

CHAPTER 11

Chemistry of Nonpeptide Opioids
S. Archer 241

CHAPTER 15

Regulation of Pituitary Proopiomelanocortin Gene Expression
J.L. ROBERTS, N. LEVIN, D. LORANG, J.R. LUNDBLAD, S. DERMER,
and M. BLUM. With 2 Figures 347

CHAPTER 16

Molecular Mechanisms in Proenkephalin Gene Regulation
N. KLEY and J.P. LOEFFLER 379

CHAPTER 17

**Proopiomelanocortin Biosynthesis, Processing and Secretion:
Functional Implications**
E. YOUNG, D. BRONSTEIN, and H. AKIL. With 1 Figure 393

CHAPTER 18

Biosynthesis of Enkephalins and Proenkephalin-Derived Peptides

CHAPTER 19

Prodynorphin Biosynthesis and Posttranslational Processing

CHAPTER 22

Opioid Peptide Processing Enzymes

L.D. FRICKER 529

CHAPTER 23

Peptidase Inactivation of Enkephalins:
Design of Inhibitors and Biochemical, Pharmacological
and Clinical Applications
B.P. ROQUES, A. BEAUMONT, V. DAUGE, and M.-C. FOURNIÉ-ZALUSKI.

CHAPTER 24

Coexistence of Opioid Peptides with Other Neurotransmitters
R. ELDE and T. HÖKFELT. With 6 Figures 585

CHAPTER 25

**Interrelationships of Opioid, Dopaminergic, Cholinergic
and GABAergic Pathways in the Central Nervous System**
P.L. WOOD. With 2 Figures 625

CHAPTER 26

Selectivity of Ligands for Opioid Receptors
A.D. Corbett, S.J. Paterson, and H.W. Kosterlitz 645

Section D: Neurophysiology

CHAPTER 29

Opioids and Sensory Processing in the Central Nervous System
A.W. Duggan and S.M. Fleetwood-Walker. With 4 Figures 731

CHAPTER 30

Opioid Actions on Membrane Ion Channels
R.A. North. With 4 Figures 773

Contents of Companion Volume 104, Part II

Section A: Opioid Receptors/Multiplicity

CHAPTER 1

Opioid Receptor Multiplicity: Isolation, Purification, and Chemical Characterization of Binding Sites

E.J. SIMON and T.L. GIOANNINI

A. Introduction

This chapter will deal primarily with what researchers have been able to learn about the properties of opioid receptors, or more precisely, of opioid binding sites, by isolating and purifying them. In order to do this with clarity it is necessary to present first some introductory comments about the different types of opioid receptors currently known, or at least postulated, and about their properties based on studies other than chemical isolation and separation.

B. Opioid Receptors Exist in Multiple Types

When opioid binding sites were first demonstrated (SIMON et al. 1973; PERT and SNYDER 1973; TERENIUS 1973) it was generally thought that opioid receptors represent a homogeneous group. This simplistic idea was quickly dispelled when it was realized that there are multiple opioid peptides each of which could have its own receptor. Moreover, it is a general finding that every neurotransmitter tends to have more than are receptor and some, if not all, opioid peptides seem to be neurotransmitters or modulators.

The first definitive pharmacological evidence for multiple opioid receptors was published by MARTIN and colleagues (GILBERT and MARTIN 1976; MARTIN et al. 1976). They performed pharmacological studies in chronic spinal dogs and found that morphine and several of its analogs differed in their pharmacological profiles. Moreover, these drugs were unable to substitute for each other in the prevention of withdrawal symptoms in animals made dependent on one of them. These results led MARTIN and coworkers to postulate the existence of three types of opioid receptors, which they named for the prototypic drugs used in their studies: μ for morphine, κ for ketocyclazocine, and σ for SKF 10047 (N-allylnormetazocine). The existence of these three types of receptors has been confirmed in many laboratories by behavioral and in vitro binding studies.

After the discovery of the enkephalins, Kosterlitz and coworkers (LORD et al. 1977) obtained evidence that these opioid peptides seem to bind to yet another type of opioid receptor. This receptor was the predominant type in the isolated mouse vas deferens, while it was virtually absent in the isolated guinea pig ileum. They named this site the δ-receptor (for deferens). Since then many other types of receptors have been postulated and these will be discussed briefly.

It was found (Lemaire et al. 1978; Schulz et al. 1979) that contractions of the isolated rat vas deferens (RVD) were highly sensitive to inhibition by β-endorphin but not by the enkephalins nor by morphine and related opiate alkaloids. It was suggested that this tissue contains an opioid receptor specific for β-endorphin and different from μ, δ, κ, or σ. This receptor was called ε (Wuester et al. 1978). Further support for its existence was obtained from the observation (Schulz et al. 1981b) that when the RVD was made highly tolerant to etorphine, there was only moderate tolerance to β-endorphin. The high degree of tolerance to etorphine was assumed to be the result of the presence of small quantities of μ-opioid receptors. For high-affinity binding at the ε-receptor at least the sequence β-endorphin 1–21 was found to be required. The question whether this receptor type is present in other tissues, such as the central nervous system, is still not resolved. Chang et al. (1984) have suggested that the benzomorphan-binding site characterized by them in rat brain may be the ε-receptor, while Nock et al. (1990) have recently reported that a binding site, previously characterized by them as a κ-receptor subtype, may be the ε-receptor.

Yet another novel type of opioid receptor was found in rabbit ileum (Oka 1980). Enkephalins and their analogs had high affinity whereas opiate alkaloids were without effect. This characteristic and the finding that the tissue is more sensitive to enkephalins than to β-endorphin suggested that this receptor is quite different from the δ-receptor. The receptor was named the iota (intestinal) opioid receptor by the authors, who suggest that it may be present in intestinal tissues of other species.

A binding site with high selectivity for 4,5-epoxymorphinans was called lamda (laudanum) (Grevel and Sadee 1983). The site was found in freshly prepared rat brain homogenates in which the classical opioid binding sites were blocked by diprenorphine (300 nM). Neither alkaloids lacking the epoxy group nor opioid peptides had significant affinity for this site. The site is highly unstable in vitro, being converted to a low-affinity state with a half-life of <2 min at 20°C. Naloxone, the best ligand for this receptor, has an affinity of 6 nM to the high-affinity lamda site.

Finally, it has been reported (Zagon et al. 1989) that opioids have growth inhibitory effects in neuroblastomas and in cell cultures derived from neural tumors. Evidence was presented that this effect is mediated via yet another opioid receptor type, which they have called zeta (for *zoe*, Greek for life). This receptor, characterized in S20Y murine neuroblastoma cells, has high affinity for most peptides derived from proenkephalin A and for some derived from prodynorphin. Naltrexone binds about ten-fold better than (-)-naloxone. Alkaloids and selective ligands for μ, δ, κ, σ, or ε receptors exhibit low affinity for the zeta site. S20Y cells appear to have few opioid receptors of the other varieties.

There is also evidence for the existence of subtypes of the major types of opioid receptors, such as μ_1 and μ_2 (WOLOZIN and PASTERNAK 1981; PASTERNAK and WOOD 1986) and κ_1 and κ_2 (see, for example, ATTALI et al. 1982; SU 1985; ZUKIN et al. 1988).

This review will concentrate on the three most studied and best established receptor types, μ, δ, and κ. The σ-receptor has also been widely studied, but it appears to be the binding site for another class of abused drugs, phencyclidine (PCP) and its analogs (VINCENT et al. 1979; ZUKIN and ZUKIN 1979). Effects mediated via this receptor are not reversed by even very high concentrations of opioid antagonists, such as naloxone. It is, therefore, not an opioid receptor in the strict sense and is not included in the present discussion.

C. Selective Ligands for the Major Types of Opioid Receptors

The naturally occurring opioid peptides tend to show a preference but are not highly specific for any one opioid receptor type. There was therefore a need to develop highly specific ligands that would permit clear distinction between the various receptor types. Such highly specific ligands have now become available through synthesis and in a few interesting cases through isolation of natural peptides from such unexpected sources as casein hydrolysate and frog skin (see also Chap. 26).

For μ-receptors, an analog of enkephalin, D-Ala^2-MePhe^4-Glyol^5-enkephalin (DAGO), was the first highly selective ligand synthesized (HANDA et al. 1981) and is still the most widely used. Others include morphiceptin (CHANG et al. 1981), a peptide isolated from casein hydrolysate and its analog PL017 (CHANG et al. 1983). All of them have at least 100-fold selectivity for μ- over δ- and even more when compared to κ-receptors. A new class of opioid peptides isolated from frog skin (BROCCARDO et al. 1981), named appropriately dermorphins, was found to be quite selective for μ-opioid receptors.

For δ-receptors two analogs of enkephalin with D-penicillamine in position 2 and D- or L-penicillamine in position 5, DPen^2,DPen^5- and DPen^2,LPen^5-enkephalin (DPDPE and DPLPE), respectively (MOSBERG et al. 1983), have proved highly selective. A disulfide bridge between the SH-groups of the penicillamine residues, which gives rigidity to the peptide structure, seems to be an essential feature. Tyr-DSer-Gly-Phe-Leu-Thr (DSLET) and an analog with an *O-tert*-butyl group on the serine (DSBuLET), synthesized by Gacel et al. (1980) and DELAY-GOYET et al. (1988), are also highly selective for δ-opioid receptors. Finally, several peptide analogs of the enkephalins isolated from frog skin (ERSPAMER et al. 1989) were found to be highly selective ligands of δ-opioid receptors. They have been named deltorphins.

A number of highly selective κ-ligands have also been synthesized. These include the nonpeptide compounds, U 50,488H and U 69,593 synthesized at Upjohn (VON VOIGTLANDER et al. 1983; LATHI et al. 1985) and PD 117302 made at Park-Davis (CLARK et al. 1988). Others were made by modification of dynorphin A, including Tyr-Gly-Gly-Phe-Leu-Arg-Arg-Ile-Arg-Pro-Arg-Leu-Arg-Gly-NH(CH$_2$)$_5$-NH$_2$ (DAKLI), made by A. Goldstein in collaboration with Syntex Corp. (GOLDSTEIN et al. 1988) and D-Pro^{10}-dynorphin 1–11 synthesized by GAIRIN et al. (1986) in Toulouse.

Very recently highly selective antagonists have also become available. Cyclic analogs of somatostatin have proved to be highly selective antagonists at μ-receptors (GULYA et al. 1986). For δ-receptors the peptide ICI 174,864 (COTTON et al. 1984) and a derivative of naltrexone, naltrindole (PORTOGHESE et al. 1988), are selective antagonists, while a "double-headed" analog of naltrexone, nor-binaltorphimine (PORTOGHESE et al. 1987), proved to be an effective and selective κ-antagonist. All of these compounds were synthesized more or less empirically. The structural features responsible for their selectivity are not well understood (for details on nonpeptide antagonists see Chap. 11).

A number of affinity ligands for different types of opioid receptors have also been synthesized as well as opioids coupled to solid supports for affinity chromatography. The most useful of these derivatives will be discussed under the purification procedures in which they have been utilized. They will be discussed in detail in the chapter by ARCHER.

D. Characterization of Membrane-Bound Opioid Receptor Types

Early evidence supporting the existence of separate μ- and δ-receptors came from a comparison of the relative binding of various ligands. Thus, LORD et al. (1977) found that opiate alkaloids bound to guinea pig ileum membranes with higher affinity than enkephalins, whereas the opposite was true for the mouse vas deferens (MVD). Functional studies have also been very useful in this regard. Thus, in these studies the enkephalins were found to be more effective in inhibiting contractions of the MVD than opiate alkaloids, whereas the opposite was true for the guinea pig ileum. The two in vitro bioassay systems also differed in their sensitivity to reversal of opioid inhibition by naloxone, the guinea pig ileum (largely μ) being about tenfold more sensitive than the MVD (largely δ).

While the existence of κ-receptors was readily demonstrable in behavioral experiments, early attempts to do so by in vitro binding studies proved negative (HILLER and SIMON 1980; HARRIS and SETHY 1980). The reasons for this are now known. Ethylketocyclazocine and bremazocine, both κ-type drugs in animals, had almost equally high affinities for μ-, δ-, and κ-sites. Moreover, the rat brain used in these studies proved to have a very low level of high-affinity κ-sites. The use of guinea pig brain, relatively rich in κ-sites, and the addition of saturating concentrations of selective μ- and δ-ligands to block these sites, permitted KOSTERLITZ and his group (KOSTERLITZ et al. 1981; MAGNAN et al. 1982) to demonstrate the existence of κ-sites.

It should be pointed out that one of the difficulties in these early studies was the absence of highly selective ligands. As mentioned earlier, the natural opioid peptides, though they may have a preference for a given type of receptor, e.g., enkephalins for δ-receptors, are by no means highly selective for the preferred receptor. Thus, enkephalins react with μ-receptors with only about four to sixfold less affinity than for δ, β-endorphin reacts with equal affinity to μ-and δ-sites, and the dynorphins, though selective for κ-sites, have significant affinity for the other opioid sites.

The availability of highly selective ligands for each of the three major opioid receptor types has permitted a variety of new approaches to the characterization of membrane-associated opioid receptor types, a few of which will be mentioned here.

It has been shown that selective tolerance can be produced to a given type of opioid receptor. The clearest demonstration of selective tolerance of μ- or δ-receptors was the work of the Herz group (SCHULZ et al. 1980) in the mouse vas deferens from animals treated chronically with selective ligands. In vitro addition of selective opioids to the isolated MVD gave similar results. Studies done by this group (SCHULZ et al. 1981b) on the ilea of chronically treated guinea pigs gave clear differentiation between tolerance of μ- and κ-receptors but no selective tolerance of δ-receptors. It is now established that the guinea pig ileum contains very low levels of δ-sites. SCHULZ et al. (1981a) reported selective tolerance to μ- and δ-opioids in the brain of intact rats using catatonia and analgesia as the responses tested.

Ontogenetic studies by several laboratories have resulted in the finding that the development of the major opioid receptor types differs (for a review of such work up to 1986 see MCDOWELL and KITCHEN 1987; for more recent work see OETTING et al. 1987; KORNBLUM et al. 1987; MAGNAN and TIBERI 1989; DE VRIES et al. 1990). In the rat, the μ-receptor develops quite early and is readily detectable at birth, the δ-receptor tends to develop later and becomes measurable at about 10–12 days of age. The κ-receptor develops rather early but its increase to adult level is much slower than that of μ.

There has been a great deal of work done on the detailed mapping of μ-, δ-, and κ-receptors in the various regions of rat brain (see Chap. 4). The results of these autoradiographic studies also suggest that the three types of receptor are different, since, though there is overlap, their distributions are quite distinct.

Finally, there have been studies on the selective inhibition or inactivation of different receptor types. Inactivation of opioid receptors is readily achieved by such reagents as N-ethyl-maleimide (NEM) and phenoxybenzamine, which are thought to alkylate SH groups essential for ligand binding. It was found that such inactivation can be made type specific by including selective ligands which protect the receptor type other than the ones to be inactivated. This was shown for phenoxybenzamine by Kosterlitz's laboratory (Robson and Kosterlitz 1979) and for NEM in our laboratory (Smith and Simon 1980). More recently, James and Goldstein (1984) improved this selective protection procedure for enrichment of a tissue in one particular receptor type. They used β-chlornaltrexamine (β-CNA), which is specific for opioid receptors and therefore much less toxic to the tissues than nonspecific agents like NEM. They found that inclusion of a selective ligand for a given type of receptor permitted significant enrichment of the tissue in that receptor type.

In our laboratory (Hiller et al. 1984) it was found that aliphatic alcohols, such as ethanol and butanol, selectively inhibit δ-receptors. Significantly higher concentrations are required to inhibit μ- and κ-receptors. The inhibition is totally reversible and is, as expected, not competitive. The evidence obtained suggests that the effect of the alcohols is on the fluidity of the membrane and that the δ-receptor is more sensitive to this environmental change for reasons not yet understood.

Another difference between the three major types of opioid receptors is in their sensitivity to reducing agents, such as DTT and mercaptoethanol (Gioannini et al. 1989). The binding of opioid ligands is inhibited by DTT in a reversible manner, with μ-ligands the most sensitive, δ-ligands somewhat less, and κ-ligands exhibiting very little sensitivity. Our evidence indicates that the effect is due to the breakage of disulfide bridges, essential for binding and receptor activation.

Very recently this laboratory has found yet another difference between opioid receptor types (Hiller et al. 1990). The reagent cyanogen bromide is used frequently for breaking peptide bonds at methionine residues. It was found to inhibit binding to the three major opioid binding sites, with κ-sites again the most resistant. An interesting difference was found between μ- and δ-sites. Inhibition at μ-sites was due to a reduction in receptor number (B_{max}), whereas the effect at δ-sites was a reduction of binding affinity. We have postulated that a critical methionine occurs within the binding site of μ-receptors, where cleavage would lead to destruction of the binding site. The methionine on δ-receptors is thought to be well outside the binding site and hydrolysis at this site may reduce binding affinity by altering receptor conformation.

All of these results clearly suggest that the three types of opioid receptor are different. The question whether they are different molecular entities or different conformations of a single molecule can only be proven by their separation and purification. Even if, as these results seem to suggest, they are distinct molecules, only complete amino acid sequencing of the receptor types will tell us whether the difference is in the protein molecule (primary gene product) or in a posttranslational modification, such as glycosylation or phosphorylation.

Evidence that the three major opioid receptor types are separable molecules will be discussed in a subsequent section. Since cloning and full amino acid sequencing has not been accomplished at the time this chapter is being written, progress toward this important goal will also be summarized.

E. Putative Endogenous Ligands

Before describing the separation and purification of opioid binding sites, a word should be said about the putative endogenous ligands for the three major opioid receptors. The δ-receptor remains the putative major receptor for the enkephalins, while the κ-receptor seems most likely to be the receptor for the peptides derived from prodynorphin, namely dynorphin A and B and the neoendorphins. A number of candidates have been suggested as endogenous ligands for the μ-receptor. These include β-endorphin, morphine, recently found to be present in animal tissues (see Chap. 13), as well as the enkephalins, for which the μ-receptor could be a lower affinity "isoreceptor." At the present time there is no way to distinguish between these possibilities.

F. Separation and Purification of Opioid Binding Sites

I. Solubilization

The first step in any purification of a receptor which is an integral membrane protein is its removal from the membrane by solubilization. This step is seldom trivial and took in the case of the opioid receptors several years to achieve. Attempts as early as 1974 to solubilize opioid binding sites led to initial success in 1975, when we succeeded in solubilizing a binding site prebound with [^{3}H]etorphine using the detergent BRIJ 37 (SIMON et al. 1975). The solubilized receptor was, however, inactive with respect to ligand binding, i.e., it could neither exchange bound ligand for free nor rebind ligand after dissociation of the prebound etorphine. Since then a number of detergents have been found to be useful in the solubilization of prebound opioid binding sites, of which digitonin and lysophosphatidylcholine were the most effective (70%–75% yield). Bee venom phospholipase A_2 together with the synergistically acting peptide melittin caused up to 80% solubilization of prebound opioid receptors (RUEGG et al. 1982).

The first solubilization of an active binding site, i.e., one which was able to bind ligands in solution, was achieved in 1980 in our laboratory (RUEGG et al. 1981), when digitonin was found to solubilize opioid binding sites from toad or frog brain in very good yield (40%–50%). This method was later adapted to mammalian brain (Gioannini et al. 1982b; Howells et al. 1982) by the inclusion of high concentrations of sodium chloride (0.5–1 M) in the extraction medium. It is of interest that this requirement for salt is not an effect of ionic strength but a specific action of sodium ions, mimicked only partly by lithium but by no other cations so far examined. It is thought that sodium may be required to preserve a stable conformation of the receptor. It should be mentioned that this procedure, most often used by us for extraction of receptors from cow striatal membranes, gives very good yields of antagonist binding (35%–45%), but does not permit high-affinity agonist binding in solution. Some agonist binding can be preserved by solubilizing in the presence of a protective ligand and removing most of the digitonin from the soluble receptor by precipitation of the protein with polyethylene glycol (PEG). A preliminary report on this work was presented at the 1986 meeting of INRC (Crema et al. 1986). A modification that seems to preserve agonist binding was reported by Demoliou-Mason and Barnard (1984). Digitonin solubilization was done in TES buffer supplemented with magnesium.

At about the same time Bidlack and Abood (1980) and Loh and coworkers (Cho et al. 1981) had success with the nonionic detergent Triton X100, a detergent that had worked only with prebound receptors in our laboratory (Ruegg et al. 1982).

The solubilization of opioid binding sites from NG108-15 cells with the then newly developed synthetic detergent CHAPS, a zwitterionic derivative of desoxycholate, {3-[(3-cholamidopropyl)dimethylammonio]-1-propanesulfonate}, was reported by Klee and coworkers (Simonds et al. 1980). We have recently found that this detergent can be adapted to solubilize binding sites in good yield from mammalian tissues by the inclusion, as with digitonin, of high concentrations of sodium chloride (Ofri et al. 1992). It has the advantage over digitonin that agonist binding is readily restored by simple procedures such as precipitation of solubilized receptor protein with PEG. Thus, the binding of the selective μ-ligand, DAGO, undetectable in the unprocessed CHAPS extract, is recovered after PEG precipitation and resuspension in buffer in 35%–40% yield based on binding in the striatal membranes.

II. Physical Separation

One way to test the hypothesis that the different types of opioid binding sites are separate molecular entities rather than conformational variants of a single molecule is to demonstrate that they can be separated physically. There has been progress in the separation of native κ-receptors from other types by simple one-step procedures, which will be summarized here. The separation of native μ- and δ-sites required more sophisticated means and will be discussed under affinity cross-linking and purification of opioid binding sites.

In our laboratory (ITZHAK et al. 1984) the separation of κ-receptors was accomplished as follows. A digitonin extract (see Sect. F.I) of guinea pig brain was layered on top of a sucrose density gradient devoid of sodium and containing only a low concentration of digitonin (0.02%). After centrifugation, fractions were collected and assayed for binding with the universal ligand [^{3}H]bremazocine. Two peaks of binding were observed. Detailed characterization of the binding properties revealed that peak 1 contained virtually pure κ-sites, whereas the properties of peak 2 suggested that it contained a mixture of μ- and δ-sites.

A similar separation of κ-sites was achieved by CHOW and ZUKIN (1983), who used molecular exclusion chromatography. CHAPS-solubilized rat brain membranes were passed through a column of Sepharose CL-6B. A small peak capable of binding [^{3}H]bremazocine in the presence of saturating concentrations of μ- and δ-ligands was found to elute corresponding to a Stokes radius of 50 Å, while the major peak of [^{3}H]dihydromorphine binding eluted corresponding to a Stokes radius of 70 Å.

These studies provide evidence that κ-sites can be separated from other opioid receptor types and suggest that they are distinct molecules.

III. Affinity Cross-Linking

A technique that has proved very successful in our laboratory (HOWARD et al. 1985, 1986), and more recently in others (HELMESTE et al. 1986; ZIPSER et al. 1988; McLEAN et al. 1989), is affinity cross-linking and separation of the labeled proteins to demonstrate differences in their apparent molecular weights.

The characterization of μ- and δ-binding proteins by this method was carried out with human [^{125}I]β-endorphin (β-End$_h$), which has a tyrosine in position 27. The molecule specifically radioiodinated in this position (TOOGOOD et al. 1986) had just become commercially available and, in contrast to Tyr^1-iodinated β-endorphin, retains its high affinity for both μ- and δ-sites (it has negligible affinity for κ-sites), permitting the study of both receptors in the same tissue. Membrane-bound opioid receptors were labeled with [^{125}I]β-End$_h$ and washed to remove free or loosely bound ligand. Cross-linking was achieved by treatment with a commercially available bifunctional reagent. The reagent, bis[2-(succinimidooxycarbonyloxy)-ethyl]sulfone (BSCOES), which forms bridges between amino groups in ligand and receptor, worked most effectively. The cross-linked membranes were solubilized in SDS and submitted to SDS-polyacrylamide gel electrophoresis (SDS-PAGE) followed by autoradiography. As shown in Fig. 1, this procedure (HOWARD et al. 1985) revealed the presence of two to four labeled bands, depending on the tissue used, all of which were eliminated when the binding was done in the presence of excess opiates, such as naloxone or bremazocine (not shown), and are therefore opioid receptor

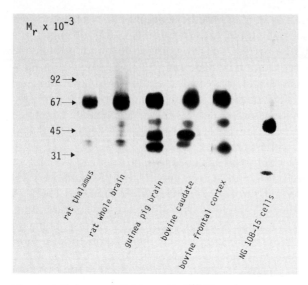

$M_r \times 10^{-3}$

92 →
67 →
45 →
31 →

rat thalamus
rat whole brain
guinea pig brain
bovine caudate
bovine frontal cortex
NG 108-15 cells

Fig. 1. Affinity cross-linking with $[^{125}I]\beta$-endorphin of opioid receptors in tissues and cells arranged in descending order of $\mu:\delta$ ratios. Cross-linking of membrane fractions, solubilization, SDS-PAGE, and autoradiography were carried out as described in Howard et al. (1985)

related. The most important finding was the presence of a band at apparent M_r of ca. 65 kDa in all tissues known to contain μ-receptors and a band at 53 kDa in all tissues and cells known to contain δ-receptors. There was correlation between $\mu:\delta$ ratios in the tissues or cells and the relative intensity of the bands. At the extremes were rat thalamus (largely μ) which exhibited only the 65-kDa band and NG 108-15 cells (only δ-sites), which exhibited the 53-kDa band but not the 65-kDa band. The identity of the smaller bands has not yet been established.

Further and more convincing evidence that these proteins of different apparent size are subunits of μ- and δ-binding sites was obtained by competition with selective ligands (Howard et al. 1986). Figure 2 shows typical results obtained in bovine frontal cortex. When the binding of $[^{125}I]\beta$-end$_h$ to membranes was carried out in the presence of the highly selective μ-ligand, DAGO, followed by affinity cross-linking, the radioactive band usually seen at 65 kDa was greatly diminished or eliminated, while the 53-kDa band was essentially unchanged. When similar experiments were done with the highly selective δ-ligand, DPDPE, the 53-kDa band was selectively reduced. These results provide strong evidence that the binding proteins of μ- and δ-receptors differ in molecular size. Cross-linking experiments in two cell lines, one high in μ-receptors (SK-N-SH), the other containing only δ-receptors (NG108-15), gave similar results (Keren et al. 1988).

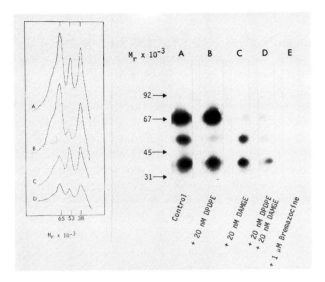

Fig. 2. Affinity cross-linking of bovine frontal cortical membranes with $[^{125}I]\beta$-endorphin in the presence of highly selective ligands for μ- and δ-opioid binding sites. DAMGE is DAla^2-gly-ol^5-enkephalin, abbreviated DAGO in text. (From HOWARD et al. 1986)

Recently we have carried out cross-linking studies on κ-receptors (YAO et al. 1989). For this purpose we obtained the selective κ-ligand, D-Pro^{10}-dynorphin (1–11) (DPDYN) from Dr. Gairin, Toulouse, France. Radio-iodination of this peptide was performed as described by him and his coworkers (GAIRIN et al. 1986). Guinea pig cerebellum, shown to contain at least 80% κ-receptors (ROBSON et al. 1984), was used for the cross-linking experiments. The $[^{125}I]$DPDYN was allowed to bind to a membrane fraction from this tissue, in the presence and absence of excess unlabeled bremazocine (to determine nonspecific binding). Cross-linking and visualization by auto-radiography revealed two protein bands of apparent M_r of 55 and 35 kDa, displaceable by unlabeled bremazocine. Neither band was significantly reduced when the binding was carried out in the presence of μ- or δ-ligands at a concentration of 100 nM. However, when the binding was done in the presence of a similar concentration of the κ-selective ligand, U50 488, the 55-kDa band was completely suppressed, while the density of the 35-kDa band was reduced but not eliminated. When competition was done with DPDYN, significant reduction of the 55-kDa band was seen at concentrations as low as 0.5 nM. It is therefore postulated that the 55-kDa band represents a high-affinity κ-receptor. The nature of the 35-kDa band is not clear. It may be a low-affinity κ-site, perhaps the κ_2 postulated by several investigators, or a mixture of a relatively high affinity κ-site with another (nonopioid) protein of the same size.

IV. Partial Purification

Before discussing purification to homogeneity of the three major opioid
receptor-binding sites, we shall review briefly the earlier results of a number
of laboratories concerning partial purification, which formed the basis for
the more recent success in total purification.

The earliest report of partial purification came from the laboratory of
Bidlack et al. (1981). Opioid binding sites were solubilized with Triton
X-100 and purified on an affinity column prepared by coupling 14-β-
bromoacetamido-morphine to Sepharose-AH, which has side arms that
terminate in amino groups. Elution of binding sites was accomplished with
opioid ligands, such as levorphanol or etorphine at micromolar concentrations. The purified receptor bound dihydromorphine with high affinity
($K_d = 3.8\,nM$) and a B_{max} of 40 pmol/mg protein. This represents a purification of 200- to 400-fold. In spite of this relatively modest purification,
SDS-PAGE of this material showed only three protein bands at apparent M_r
of 43, 35, and 23 kDa.

Partial purifications by two methods were reported from our laboratory.
The first, based on our finding (Gioannini et al. 1982a) that opioid receptors
are glycoproteins, utilized wheat germ agglutinin (WGA) agarose, which
retained about 40% of applied binding sites from a crude soluble preparation. Elution with N-acetylglucosamine resulted in 25- to 30-fold purification, as determined by the specific binding of [^{3}H]diprenorphine.

A more effective purification was achieved with affinity chromatography
(Gioannini et al. 1984). A newly synthesized derivative of naltrexone,
β-naltrexyl-6-ethylenediamine (NED), was coupled to CH-Sepharose, which
possesses a six carbon spacer ending in a carboxyl residue. Opioid receptors
derived from cow, rat, or toad brain were retained by this column (50%–
75%) and eluted with micromolar concentrations of naloxone in yields of
20%–30% of receptor applied. The purification we reported was 300- to
500-fold, as determined by the specific binding of [^{3}H]diprenorphine.
However, improved washing procedures and better protein determinations
revealed that a single pass through the affinity column resulted in 3000- to
5000-fold purification of the applied opioid binding sites (see below).

Cho et al. (1983) utilized an affinity gel constructed by coupling 6-
succinylmorphine to aminohexyl agarose as described earlier by us (Simon
et al. 1972). Attempts to elute the receptor with opioids were unsuccessful
and it became necessary to elute with high salt. The partially purified
receptor was inactive unless combined with an acidic lipid fraction eluted in
a later peak from the same column. In a more recent report from this group
(Cho et al. 1985) it was found that an active binding fraction containing both
protein and acidic lipid could be eluted in a single peak by using TRIS
buffer containing naloxone, NaCl, and CHAPS. Binding of high affinity,
primarily with μ-ligands, was obtained and the purification was estimated to
be 3200-fold.

Two other reports of partial purification should be mentioned. MANECKJEE et al. (1985) used an affinity matrix constructed from Hybromet, a morphine analog synthesized by ARCHER et al. (1985), coupled to an agarose containing SH groups, Affigel 401. Elution with normorphine yielded binding sites that appeared to be primarily μ in their binding properties. The overall yield was only 0.6% and the receptor was highly unstable, making estimation of purification difficult. It was estimated to be about 500-fold. On SDS-PAGE this preparation showed a major band at $M_r = 94$ kDa and minor bands at 44 and 35 kDa.

Finally, FUJIOKA et al. (1985) constructed an affinity matrix by coupling the peptide D-Ala²-leu-enkephalin (DALE) to AH-Sepharose. Digitonin-solubilized binding sites were retained by this affinity gel and eluted with 0.1 mM DALE. The eluate was concentrated and fractionated on Sephadex G-75. The purification reported was 450-fold based on [³H]DADLE binding (K_d of 34 nM and B_{max} of 200 pmol/mg protein).

V. Purification to Homogeneity

The first report of purification of an active opioid binding protein to apparent homogeneity came from our laboratory (GIOANNINI et al. 1985). From bovine striatal membranes a protein was purified which has an apparent M_r of 65 kDa on SDS-PAGE. The purification scheme is shown in Fig. 3. Digitonin-solubilization of opioid binding sites was followed by two purification steps: affinity chromatography on NED-agarose and lectin-affinity chromatography on WGA-agarose. As shown in Table 1, the affinity chromatographic step gave 3000- to 5000-fold purification in a single pass. Further purification on the WGA-agarose gave an overall yield of 4%–6% and a total purification of about 65 000-fold, based on the specific binding of [³H]bremazocine (K_d of 2–3 nM and B_{max} of ca. 13 000 pmol/mg protein). This is in good agreement with the theoretical purification assuming a single binding site per 65 kDa. A single band of apparent M_r of 65 kDa was observed on SDS-PAGE, visualized by silver staining or by autoradiography of radioiodinated purified protein. This protein binds antagonists, such as naloxone, naltrexone, bremazocine, and diprenorphine, with high affinity but binds agonists with very low affinity. Nevertheless, considerable evidence has been accumulated indicating that the isolated protein is the binding component of μ-receptors.

Since then purification to homogeneity of μ-binding sites has been reported by CHO et al. (1986), UEDA et al. (1987, 1988), and DEMOLIOU-MASON and BARNARD, though the latter work was presented only in oral communications but never published. CHO et al. (1986) purified receptors, solubilized from rat brain with Triton X-100, by chromatography on the affinity matrix succinylmorphine-agarose (see above), followed by gel filtration on AcA 34, lectin chromatography on WGA-agarose, and iso-

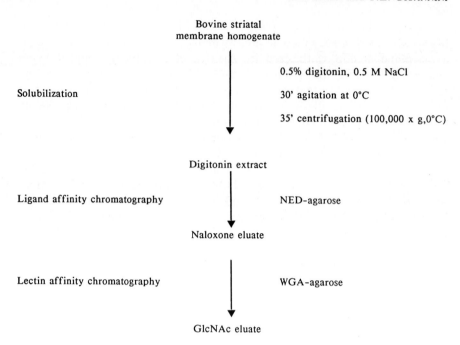

Fig. 3. Scheme for purification to homogeneity of μ-opioid binding sites from bovine striatal membranes

electric focussing. This provided material that has a pI of 4.4 and a molecular weight on SDS-PAGE of 58 kDa. To obtain high-affinity specific binding a mixture of acidic lipids had to be added to the purified protein. It is not clear why this requirement for lipids does not appear in the purification used by others. It may reflect a more complete delipidation of the receptor by the procedures used by Cho et al. (1986). Ueda et al. (1987, 1988) used a very similar scheme involving affinity chromatography on succinylmorphine-agarose and isoelectric focussing. They report a protein of the same molecular weight but the pI was higher, about 5.6. Demoliou-Mason and Barnard used two affinity columns, the first involved the ligand D-Ala^2-leu-enkephalin chloromethylketone (DALECK) (Newman and Barnard 1984), the second a derivative of codeinone, both immobilized on agarose beads.

The purification to apparent homogeneity of an affinity-labeled δ-receptor from NG 108–15 cell membranes was reported from Klee's laboratory (Simonds et al. 1985). The membranes were covalently labeled with tritiated 3-methylfentanyl-isothiocyanate ("superFIT"). The labeled receptors were extracted with a mixture of Lubrol and CHAPS. The purification involved three steps, lectin chromatography on WGA-agarose, immunoaffinity chromatography on a column of anti-FIT antibodies coupled to agarose and preparative SDS-PAGE. The resulting protein was purified

Table 1. Purification of an opioid binding protein from bovine striatum[a]. (From GIOIANNINI et al. 1985)

Preparation	Protein (mg)	Activity[b] (pmol)	Step yield %		Overall yield %		Specific activity (B_{max}) pmol·mg^{-1}	Purification factor x-fold
			Protein	Activity	Protein	Activity		
Membrane homogenate	3270	667	100	100	100	100	0.20	1
Digitonin extract	1308	258	40	38	40	38	0.19	
Eluate from NED-Sepharose	0.070[c]	64	<0.001	24.8	<0.001	9.6	914	4570
Eluate from WGA-Agarose	0.003[d]	39	4.3	60.9	<0.001	5.8	13 000	65 000

[a] Data are from a typical experiment in which ~50 g tissue was homogenized and solubilized with digitonin.
[b] Measured by [3H]bremazocine binding at 1.5 nM and B_{max} calculated from saturation curves at identical conditions (0.5 M NaCl, 0.05% digitonin). Values shown represent specific binding at saturation.
[c] Determined by densitometric scanning of Coomassie blue-stained SDS-PAGE gels using bovine serum albumin and carbonic anhydrase as calibration standards.
[d] Determined by amino acid analysis.

about 30000-fold in an overall yield of 1%–2% and contained 21000 pmol superFIT/mg protein, in agreement with total purification of a glycoprotein of M_r of 58 kDa containing one binding site per molecule.

Very recently, there has been a preliminary report of the purification to homogeneity of active δ-opioid receptors from rat brain (LOUKAS et al. 1990). Affinity chromatography on a column of N,N-diallyl-Tyr-DLeu-Gly-Tyr-leucyl-ω-aminododecylagarose was followed by chromatography on lentil-lectin-agarose. If upheld by a more detailed report, this will be the first purification of an active δ-opioid binding site.

Reports of κ-opioid receptor purification from two sources have appeared. SIMON et al. (1987) reported the purification of κ-sites from the brain of the frog, *Rana esculenta*. The receptors present in the brain of toads and frogs had previously been shown by us (SIMON et al. 1982) to resemble mammalian κ-receptors. Affinity chromatography on a matrix of DADLE coupled to epoxy-activated Sepharose 4B gave a purification of 4300-fold and was followed by gel permeation chromatography on Sepharose 6B. This gave an apparently pure protein with binding properties similar to those of mammalian κ-receptors. A similar purification of κ-receptors from frog brain (*Rana ridibunda*) was carried out in Meunier's laboratory (MOLLEREAU et al. 1988). These workers used affinity chromatography on a dynorphin-agarose column as their major purification step. It is of interest that these investigators suggest that their evidence indicates that the receptor in the frog is different from any of the three major types of mammalian opioid receptors. This difference between the results of the Hungarian and French laboratories need to be resolved. They could be due to the different species of frogs employed, though this appears unlikely to this reviewer.

κ-Receptors have also been purified from human placenta (AHMED et al. 1989). The authors do not claim homogeneity, but the specific binding activity is about 50% of the theoretical value. This result is remarkable in view of the fact that no biospecific purification step was used. The purification involved covalent chromatography on an SH-containing Sepharose column followed by a WGA-agarose column, neither of which is specific for opioid receptors.

G. Recent Studies on Purified μ-Opioid Binding Protein

I. Antibodies Generated Against Peptide Sequences

We will briefly summarize recent studies on the μ-opioid binding protein (OBP) purified in our laboratory from bovine striatal membranes as described above. These studies are unpublished except for a preliminary report presented at the 1990 meeting of INRC (GIOANNINI et al. 1990). The purified OBP was found to be blocked at its amino terminal, necessitating chemical fragmentation of the protein and reisolation of peptides for sequencing. In collaboration with Dr. C. Strader at Merck Sharp and Dohme, we succeeded in isolating and sequencing two peptides from fragmentation of the purified protein with cyanogen bromide. Peptide 1 had 20 amino acids and peptide 2 had 13 amino acids. Neither peptide was found to have significant homology with any peptide sequences found in protein structure data bases. In collaboration with Drs. H. Akil, S. Watson, and L. Taylor at the University of Michigan, six antibodies were prepared to two regions of peptide 1 and to the N-terminal ten amino acids of peptide 2. All of the antibodies were able to immunoprecipitate up to 65% of radioiodinated purified OBP at dilutions of 1:200. The antibodies also gave immunoblots at the appropriate apparent M_r of 65 kDa with purified OBP.

A signal on immunoblots at the same M_r was also observed with crude digitonin and CHAPS extracts of cow striatal membranes. This observation led to further experiments, which indicated good correlation between tissue levels of opioid receptors and intensity of signals on immunoblots. Thus, extracts of membranes from striatum, frontal cortex, and hippocampus gave strong signals at M_r 65 kDa, while extracts from cerebellum and pons gave very weak signals and white matter was completely negative. Such correlation was also seen with cell cultures, where NG108-15 and SK-N-SH cells, both rich in opioid receptors, gave positive signals, while HeLa and C-6 cells, known to be devoid of opioid receptors, gave no detectable signals. The result with NG108-15 cells is of interest, since this culture has been reported to have only δ-receptors. A positive result with our antibody suggests either cross-reactivity with δ-receptors or the presence of a small number of μ-receptors in these cells, not previously detected by less sensitive measures. The fact that the band seen in immunoblots of NG 108-15 cell extracts is consistently slightly smaller than that seen with other tissues and the SK-N-SH cell line favors the notion of cross-reactivity with δ-receptors.

Our experiments are highly supportive of our previous reports that the protein we purified is, in fact, an opioid binding protein. They also provide evidence that the two peptides sequenced are derived from the same protein. Thus, the same M_r is observed on immunoblots with antisera against either peptide and immunoprecipitation by antibodies against one peptide results in no further precipitation by the other.

II. Rhodopsin Antibodies React with Purified OBP

Based on the hypothesis that opioid receptors belong to the family of G protein-coupled receptors, we obtained from Drs. E. Weiss and G. Johnson six antibodies generated against bovine rhodopsin, or peptide sequences present in this protein, the prototype of G protein-coupled receptors. Some of these antibodies had previously been shown to cross-react with the β-adrenergic receptor (WEISS et al. 1987). Our studies (GIOANNINI et al. 1990; 1992) showed that some rhodopsin antibodies produced bands at

65 kDa with our purified OBP. More importantly, the antibodies that reacted positively with OBP were the same that had been found to cross-react with the β-adrenergic receptor protein. The conditions and dilutions of antisera used were the same in both instances. This represents strong experimental support for the notion that opioid receptors, at least the μ-type, belong to the family of G protein-coupled receptors, which exhibit the rhodopsin-like structure, i.e., seven transmembrane domains.

III. Attempts to Clone the cDNA of Purified OBP

Efforts to clone opioid receptor genes or cDNA to derive the total amino acid sequence have to date led to the sequencing of only one protein with opioid binding activity. This protein called OBCAM is discussed in detail in Chap. 3. It is not a typical G protein-coupled receptor and its significance is still under investigation. We shall summarize here the present status of our attempts to clone cDNA corresponding to our purified OBP.

Briefly stated, in collaboration with workers at Merck and more recently at Neurex Corp., oligonucleotides corresponding to the two peptides, sequenced from the OBP purified in our laboratory, have been prepared and used to screen bovine striatal cDNA libraries. Because of the considerable degeneracy in our amino acid sequences (many amino acids coded by four or six codons), a number of false-positive clones have been isolated and partially sequenced. Screening is continuing with other oligonucleotides and new libraries. Attempts to use PCR and expression cloning using our antipeptide antibodies are also in progress.

H. Concluding Comments

This chapter and others in this section provide the reader with summaries of the current stage of our knowledge about the structure and function of opioid receptors. It is evident that a lot of important information has been accumulated in the past two decades. The observation that these receptors exist in a number of different types and perhaps subtypes is of great importance to our understanding of their functions. The finding that tolerance can be developed to a specific receptor type requires a careful reinvestigation of the role of the endogenous opioid system in the development of tolerance to and dependence on opiate narcotic analgesic drugs. The recognition that several types of opioid receptors act via second messenger systems involving coupling to G proteins is another important advance and this has become a very active area of investigation.

One very significant advance discussed in this chapter is the ability to separate and purify the major receptor types. This has provided evidence that μ-, δ-, and κ-receptors are different molecules, separable from each other by physical methods. As stated earlier, this work does not tell us that the differences reside in the polypeptide chains (primary gene products). Rather than being the product of different genes they could be coded for by the same gene but differ in posttranslational modifications. The work on other neurotransmitter receptors has resulted in the finding that to date all of the types and subtypes of receptors discovered are products of separate genes. This may also prove to be the case for the different types of opioid receptors, but this question can be resolved only once their complete amino acid sequences are known.

It was hoped that the total amino acid sequence would be available for one or more types of opioid receptor by the time this chapter was written. The cloning of these receptors has proved to be extraordinarily recalcitrant for reasons that are not clear. It has led some investigators to suggest that opioid receptors may be somehow different from receptors of the G protein coupled superfamily. The authors of this review have made it clear that they do not share this view and have cited recent results which support the idea that opioid receptors do belong to this receptor family. It should be noted that opioid receptors are not alone in resisting cloning for long periods and that considerable difficulty was encountered even with many proteins that have now been successfully cloned and sequenced. There is little doubt that a knowledge of the amino acid sequence of opioid receptors and availability of cDNA probes for their messenger RNAs would represent a very significant step forward in this important research area and would permit the kind of precise and meaningful dissection of receptor structure and function already carried out in an elegant manner with some other receptors, such as with the adrenergic and nicotinic acetylcholine receptors.

References

Ahmed MS, Zhon D-H, Cavinato AG, Maulik D (1989) Opioid binding properties of the purified kappa receptor from human placenta. Life Sci 44:861–871

Archer S, Michael J, Osei-Gyimah P, Seyed-Mozaffari A, Zukin S, Maneckjee R, Simon EJ, Gioannini TL (1985) Hybromet: a ligand for purifying opioid receptors. J Med Chem 28:1950–1953

Attali B, Gouarderes C, Mazarguil H, Audigier Y, Cros J (1982) Evidence for multiple "kappa" binding sites by use of opioid peptides in the guinea pig lumbo-sacral spinal cord. Neuropeptides 3:53–64

Bidlack JM, Abood LG (1980) Solubilization of the opiate receptor. Life Sci 27: 331–340

Bidlack JM, Abood LG, Osei-Gyimah P, Archer S (1981) Purification of the opiate receptor from rat brain. Proc Natl Acad Sci USA 78:636–639

Broccardo M, Erspamer V, Falconieri-Erspamer G, Improta G, Linari G, Melchiorri P, Montecucchi PC (1981) Pharmacological data on dermorphins, a new class of potent opioid peptides from amphibian skin. Br J Pharmacol 73:625–631

Chang K-J, Killian S, Hazum E, Cuatrecasas P, Chang J-K (1981) Morphiceptin: a potent and specific agonist for morphine (mu) receptors. Science 212:75–77

Chang K-J, Wei ET, Killian A, Chang J-K (1983) Potent morphiceptin analogs: structure activity relatilonships and morphine-like activities. J Pharmacol Exp Ther 227:403–408

Chang K-J, Blanchard SG, Cuatrecasas P (1984) Benzomorphan sites are ligand recognition sites of putative epsilon receptors. Mol Pharmacol 26:484–488

Cho TM, Yamato C, Cho JS, Loh HH (1981) Solubilization of membrane-bound opiate receptors from rat brain. Life Sci 28:2651–2657

Cho TM, Ge BL, Yamato C, Smith AP, Loh HH (1983) Isolation of opiate binding components by affinity chromatography and reconstitution of binding affinities. Proc Natl Acad Sci USA 80:5176–5180

Cho TM, Ge B-L, Loh HH (1985) Isolation and purification of morphine receptor by affinity chromatography. Life Sci 36:1075–1085

Cho TM, Hasegawa J-T, Ge BL, Loh HH (1986) Purification to apparent homogeneity of a mu-type opioid receptor from rat brain. Proc Natl Acad Sci USA 83:4138–4142

Chow T, Zukin RS (1983) Solubilization and preliminary characterization of mu and kappa opiate receptor subtypes from rat brain. Mol Pharmacol 24:203–212

Clark CR, Birchmore B, Sharif NA, Hunter JC, Hill RG, Hughes J (1988) PD117302: a selective agonist at the kappa opioid receptor. Br J Pharmacol 9:618–626

Cotton R, Giles MG, Miller L, Shaw JS, Timms D (1984) ICI 174864: a highly selective antagonist for the opioid delta receptor. Eur J Pharmacol 97:331–332

Crema G, Gioannini TL, Hiller JM, Simon EJ (1986) The direct demonstration of binding of mu, delta and kappa agonists to digitonin-solubilized opioid receptors from bovine striatum. NIDA Res Monogr 75:9–12

De Vries TJ, Hogenboom F, Mulder AH, Schoffelmeer ANM (1990) Ontogeny of mu-, delta- and kappa-opioid receptors mediating inhibition of neurotransmitter release and adenylate cyclase activity in rat brain. Brain Res Dev Brain Res 54:63–69

Delay-Goyet P, Seguin C, Gacel G, Roques BP (1988) ^{3}H-[D-Ser^2(O-tert-butyl), Leu^5]enkephalyl-Thr^6 and [D-Ser^2(O-tert-butyl), Leu^5]enkephalyl-Thr^6(O-tert-butyl), two new enkephalin analogs with both a good selectivity and a high affinity toward delta-opioid binding sites. J Biol Chem 263:4124–4130

Demoliou-Mason CD, Barnard EA (1984) Solubilization in high yield of opioid receptors retaining high-affinity delta, mu and kappa binding sites. FEBS Lett 170:378–382

Erspamer V, Melchiorri P, Falconieri-Erspamer G, Negri L, Corsi R, Severini C, Barra D, Simmaco M, Kreil G (1989) Deltorphins: a family of naturally occurring peptides with high affinity and selectivity for delta opioid binding sites. Proc Natl Acad Sci USA 86:5188–5192

Fujioka T, Inoue F, Kurujama M (1985) Purification of opioid binding materials from rat brain. Biochem Biophys Res Commun 131:640–646

Gacel G, Fournie-Zaluskie M-C, Roques BP (1980) Tyr-DSer-Gly-Phe-Leu-Thr, a highly preferential ligand for delta-opiate receptors. FEBS Lett 118:245–247

Gairin JE, Jomary C, Pradayrol L, Cros J, Meunier J-C (1986) ^{125}I-DPDYN, monoiodo[D-Pro^{10}]dynorphin (1–11): a highly radioactive and selective probe for the study of kappa opioid receptors. Biochem Biophys Res Commun 134:1142–1150

Gilbert PE, Martin WR (1976) The effects of morphine- and nalorphine-like drugs in the nondependent morphine-dependent and cyclazocine-dependent chronic spinal dog. J Pharmacol Exp Ther 198:66–82

Gioannini TL, Foucaud B, Hiller JM, Hatten ME, Simon EJ (1982a) Lectin binding of solubilized opiate receptors: evidence for their glycoprotein nature. Biochem Biophys Res Commun 105:1128–1134

Gioannini TL, Howells RD, Hiller JM, Simon EJ (1982b) Solubilization in good yield of active opiate binding sites from mammalian brain. Life Sci 31:1315–1318

Gioannini TL, Howard AD, Hiller JM, Simon EJ (1984) Affinity chromatography of solubilized opioid binding sites using CH-Sepharose modified with a new naltrexone derivative. Biochem Biophys Res Commun 119:624–629

Gioannini TL, Howard AD, Hiller JM, Simon EJ (1985) Purification of an active opioid binding protein from bovine striatum. J Biol Chem 260:15117–15121

Gioannini TL, Liu YF, Park YH, Hiller JM, Simon EJ (1989) Evidence for the presence of disulfide bridges in opioid receptors essential for ligand binding. Possible role in receptor activation. J Mol Recognit 2:44–48

Gioannini TL, Yao Y-H, Hiller JM, Simon EJ, Strader CD, Taylor L, Akil H, Watson S, Weiss ER, Johnson GL (1990) Studies using antibodies generated against peptide sequences from opioid binding protein and antibodies against rhodopsin. In: Van Ree JM, Mulder AH, Wiegant VM, Van Wimersma Greidanus TB (eds) New leads in opioid research. Excerpta Medica, Amsterdam, pp 168–169

Gioannini TL, Weiss ER, Johnson GL, Hiller JM, Simon EJ (1992) Immunoblots with rhodopsin antisera suggest that a purified μ opioid binding protein has structural characteristics of a G-proootein-coupled receptor. Proc Natl Acad Sci USA 89:52–55

Goldstein A, Nestor JJ Jr, Naidu A, Newmann SR (1988) "DAKLI": a multipurpose ligand with a high affinity and selectivity for dynorphin (kappa opioid) binding sites. Proc Natl Acad Sci USA 85:7375–7379

Grevel J, Sadee W (1983) An opiate binding site in the rat brain is highly selective for 4,5-epoxymorphinans. Science 221:1198–1200

Gulya K, Pelton JT, Hruby VJ, Yamamura HI (1986) Cyclic somatostatin octapeptide analogues with high affinity and selectivity toward mu opioid receptors. Life Sci 30:2221–2229

Handa BK, Lane AC, Lord JAH, Morgan BA, Rance MJ, Smith CFC (1981) Analogues of beta-LPH 61–64 possessing selective agonist activity at mu opiate receptors. Eur J Pharmacol 70:531–540

Harris DW, Sethy VH (1980) High affinity binding of [^{3}H]-ethylketocyclazocine to rat brain homogenate. Eur J Pharmacol 66:121–123

Helmeste DM, Hammonds RGH Jr Li CH (1986) Preparation of [^{125}I-Tyr^{27}, Leu^5]beta$_h$-endorphin and its use for crosslinking of opioid binding sites in human striatum and NG108-15 neuroblastoma-glioma cells. Proc Natl Acad Sci USA 83:4622–4625

Hiller JM, Simon EJ (1980) Specific high affinity ^{3}H-ethylketocyclazocine binding in rat central nervous system: lack of evidence for kappa receptors. J Pharmacol Exp Ther 214:516–519

Hiller JM, Angel LM, Simon EJ (1984) Characterization of the selective inhibition of the delta sub-class of opioid binding sites by alcohols. Mol Pharmacol 25:249–255

Hiller JM, Fan LQ, Simon EJ (1990) Differential effects of cyanogen bromide on ligand binding by mu, delta and kappa opioid receptors. In: Van Ree JM, Mulder AH, Wiegant VM, Van Wimersma Greidanus TB (eds) New leads in opioid research. Excerpta Medica, Amsterdam, pp 166–167

Howard AD, de la Baume S, Gioannini TL, Hiller JM, Simon EJ (1985) Covalent labeling of opioid receptors with radioiodinated human beta-endorphin. J Biol Chem 260:10833–10839

Howard AD, Gioannini TL, Hiller JM, Simon EJ (1986) Identification of distinct binding site subunits of mu and delta opiate receptors. Biochemistry 25:357–360

Howells RD, Gioannini TL, Hiller JM, Simon EJ (1982) Solubilization and characterization of active opiate binding sites from mammalian brain. J Pharmacol Exp Ther 222:629–634

Itzhak Y, Hiller JM, Simon EJ (1984) Solubilization and characterization of mu, delta and kappa opioid binding sites from guinea pig brain: physical separation of kappa receptors. Proc Natl Acad Sci USA 81:4217–4221

James IF, Goldstein A (1984) Site-directed alkylation of multiple opioid receptors: binding selectivity. Mol Pharmacol 25:337–342

Keren O, Gioannini TL, Hiller JM, Simon EJ (1988) Affinity cross-linking of
    ^{125}I-labeled human beta-endorphin to cell lines possessing either mu- or delta
    type opioid binding sites. Brain Res 440:280–284
Kornblum HI, Hurlbut DE, Leslie FM (1987) Postnatal development of multiple
    opioid receptors in rat brain. Brain Res Dev Brain Res 37:21–41
Kosterlitz HW, Paterson SJ, Robson LE (1981) Characterization of the kappa-
    subtype of the opiate receptor in the guinea pig brain. Br J Pharmacol 73:939–
    949
Lahti RA, Mickelson MM, McCall JM, von Voigtlander PF (1985) ^{3}H-U-69,593 a
    highly selective ligand for the opioid κ receptor. Eur J Pharmacol 109:281–284
Lemaire S, Magnan J, Regoli D (1978) Rat vas deferens: a specific bioassay for
    endogenous opioid peptides. Br J Pharmacol 64:327–329
Lord JAH, Waterfield AA, Hughes J, Kosterlitz HW (1977) Endogenous opioid
    peptides: multiple agonists and receptors. Nature 267:495–499
Loukas S, Panetsos F, Merkouris M, Zioudrou C (1990) Purification of a 58 kDa
    protein from rat brain membranes which binds selectively delta opioid agonists.
    In: Van Ree JM, Mulder AH, Wiegant VM, Van Wimersma Greidanus TB
    (eds) New leads in opioid research. Excerpta Medica, Amsterdam, pp 173–175
Magnan J, Tiberi M (1989) Evidence for the presence of mu- and kappa- but not
    delta-opioid sites in the human fetal brain. Brain Res Dev Brain Res 45:275–281
Magnan J, Paterson SJ, Tavani A, Kosterlitz HW (1982) The binding spectrum of
    narcotic analgesic drugs with different agonist and antagonist properties.
    Naunyn Schmiedebergs Arch Pharmacol 319:197–205
Maneckjee R, Zukin RS, Archer S, Michael J, Osei-Gyimah P (1985) Purification
    and characterization of the mu opiate receptor from rat brain using affinity
    chromatography. Proc Natl Acad Sci USA 82:594–598
Martin WR, Eades CG, Thompson JA, Huppler RE, Gilbert PE (1976) The effects
    of morphine- and nalorphine-like drugs in the nondependent and morphine-
    dependent chronic spinal dog. J Pharmacol Exp Ther 197:517–532
McDowell J, Kitchen I (1987) Development of opioid systems: peptides, receptors
    and pharmacology. Brain Res Rev 12:397–421
McLean S, Rothman RB, Chuang DM, Rice KC, Spain JW, Coscia CJ, Roth RB
    (1989) Cross-linking of [125I]beta-endorphin to mu opioid receptors during
    development. Brain Res Dev Brain Res 45:283–289
Mollereau C, Pascaud A, Baillat G, Mazarguil H, Puget A, Meunier J-C (1988)
    Evidence for a new type of opioid binding site in the brain of the frog *Rana
    ridibunda*. Eur J Pharmacol 20:75–84
Mosberg HI, Hurst R, Hruby VJ, Gee K, Yamamura HI, Galligan JJ, Burks TF
    (1983) Bis-penicillamine enkephalins possess highly improved specificity toward
    delta opioid receptors. Proc Natl Acad Sci USA 80:5871–5874
Newman EL, Barnard EA (1984) Identification of an opioid receptor subunit
    carrying the μ binding site. Biochemistry 23:5385–5389
Nock B, Giodano AL, Cicero TJ, O'Connor LH (1990) Affinity of drugs and
    peptides for U-69,593-sensitive and -insensitive kappa opiate binding sites: the
    U-69,593-sensitive site appears to be the beta endorphin-specific epsilon
    receptor. J Pharmacol Exp Ther 254:412–419
Oetting GM, Szucs M, Coscia CJ (1987) Differential ontogeny of divalent cation
    effects on rat brain delta-, mu- and kappa-opioid receptor binding. Brain Res
    Dev Brain Res 31:223–227
Ofri D, Ritter AM, Liu Y, Gioannini TL, Hiller JM, Simon EJ (1992) Charac-
    terization of solubilized opioid receptors: reconstitution and uncoupling of
    guanine-nucleotide-sensitive agonist binding. J Neurochem 58:6628–6635
Oka T (1980) Enkephalin receptor in the rabbit ileum. Br J Pharmacol 68:198–195
Pasternak GW, Wood PL (1986) Multiple mu opiate receptors. Life Sci 38:1889–
    1898

Pert CB, Snyder SH (1973) Opiate receptor; demonstration in nervous tissue. Science 179:1011–1014

Portoghese PS, Lipowski AW, Takemori AE (1987) Binaltorphimine and nor-binaltorphimine, potent and selective κ-opioid receptor antagonists. Life Sci 40:1287–1292

Portoghese PS, Sultana M, Takemori AE (1988) Natrindole, a highly selective and potent non-peptide delta opioid receptor agonist. Eur J Pharmacol 146:185–186

Robson LE, Kosterlitz HW (1979) Specific protection of the binding site of D-Ala^2-D-Leu^5-enkephalin (delta receptors) and dihydromorphine (mu-receptors). Proc R Soc Lond [Biol] 205:425–432

Robson LE, Foote R, Maurer R, Kosterlitz HW (1984) Opioid binding sites of the kappa-type in guinea pig cerebellum. Neuroscience 12:621–627

Ruegg UT, Cuenod S, Hiller JM, Gioannini TL, Howells RD, Simon EJ (1981) Characterization and partial purification of solubilized active opiate receptors from toad brain. Proc Natl Acad Sci USA 78:4635–4638

Ruegg UT, Cuenoud S, Fulpius BW, Simon EJ (1982) Inactivation and solubilization of opiate receptors by phospholipase A$_2$. Biochim Biophys Acta 685:241–248

Schulz R, Faase E, Wüster M, Herz A (1979) Selective receptors for beta-endorphin on the rat vas deferens. Life Sci 24:843–850

Schulz R, Wüster M, Krenss H, Herz A (1980) Lack of cross-tolerance on multiple opiate receptors in the mouse vas deferences. Mol Pharmacol 18:395–401

Schulz R, Wüster M, Herz A (1981a) Differentiation of opiate receptors in the brain by the selective development of tolerance. Pharmacol Biochem Behav 14:75–79

Schulz R, Wüster M, Rubini P, Herz A (1981b) Functional opiate receptors in the guinea pig illeum: their differentiation by means of selective tolerance development. J Pharmacol Exp Ther 219:547–550

Simon EJ, Dole WP, Hiller JM (1972) Coupling of a new active morphine derivative to Sepharose for affinity chromatography. Proc Natl Acad Sci USA 69:1835–1837

Simon EJ, Hiller JM, Edelman I (1973) Stereospecific binding of the potent narcotic analgesic ^{3}H-etorphine to rat brain homogenate. Proc Natl Acad Sci USA 70:1947–1949

Simon EJ, Hiller JM, Edelman I (1975) Solubilization of a stereospecific opiate-macromolecular complex from rat brain. Science 190:389–390

Simon EJ, Hiller JM, Groth J, Itzhak Y, Holland MJ, Beck SG (1982) The nature of the opiate receptors in toad brain. Life Sci 31:1367–1370

Simon J, Benye S, Hepp J, Khan A, Borsodi A, Szucs M, Mezihradszky, K, Wolleman K (1987) Purification of a kappa-opioid receptor subtype from frog brain. Neuropeptides 101:19–28

Simonds WF, Koski G, Streaty RA, Hjemlmeland LM, Klee WA (1980) Solubilization of active opiate receptors. Proc Natl Acad Sci USA 77:4632–4627

Simonds WF, Burke TR Jr, Rice KC, Jacobson AE, Klee WA (1985) Purification of the opiate receptor of NG 108-15 neuroblastoma glioma hybrid cells. Proc Natl Acad Sci USA 82:4974–4978

Smith JR, Simon EJ (1980) Selective protection of stereospecific enkephalin and opiate binding against inactivation by N-ethylmaleimide: evidence for two classes of opiate receptors. Proc Natl Acad Sci USA 77:281–284

Su TP (1985) Further demonstration of kappa opioid binding sites in the brain: evidence for heterogeneity. J Pharmacol Exp Ther 232:144–148

Terenius L (1973) Stereospecific interaction between narcotic analgesics and a synaptic plasma membrane fraction of rat brain cortex. Acta Pharmacol Toxicol (Copenh) 32:317–320

Toogood CIA, McFarthing KG, Hulme EC, Smyth DG (1986) Use of ^{125}I-Tyr^{27}-beta-endorphin for the study of beta-endorphin binding sites in rat cortex. Neuroendocrinology 43:629–634

Ueda H, Harada H, Misawa H, Nozaki M, Takagi H (1987) Purified opioid mu receptor is of a different molecular size than delta and kappa receptors. Neurosci Lett 75:339–344

Ueda H, Harada H, Nozaki M, Katada T, Ui M, Satoh M, Takagi H (1988) Reconstitution of rat brain mu opioid receptors with purified guanine nucleotide-binding regulatory protein Gi and Go. Proc Natl Acad Sci USA 85:7013–7018

Vincent JP, Kartolovski B, Geneste P, Kamemka JM, Lazdunski M (1979) Interaction of phencyclidene (angle dust) with a specific receptor in rat brain membranes. Proc Natl Acad Sci USA 76:4578–4582

Von Voigtlander PF, Lathi RA, Lundens JH (1983) U 50,488H; a selective and structurally novel non-mu (kappa) opioid agonist. J Pharmacol Exp Ther 224:7–12

Weiss ER, Hadcock JR, Johnson GL, Malbon CC (1987) Antipeptide antibodies directed against cytoplasmic rhodopsin sequences recognize the beta-adrenergic receptor. J Biol Chem 262:4319–4323

Wolozin BL, Pasternak GW (1981) Classification of multiple morphine and enkephalin binding sites in the central nervous system. Proc Natl Acad Sci USA 78:6181–6185

Wüster M, Schulz R, Herz A (1978) Specificity of opioids towards the mu, delta and epsilon-opiate receptors. Neurosci Lett 15:193–198

Yao Y-H, Gairin J, Meunier J-C, Hiller JM, Gioannini TL, Cros J, Simon EJ (1989) Crosslinking of kappa receptors in the guinea pig cerebellum with D-pro[10] dynorphin (1–11). In: Cros J, Meunier J-C, Hamon M (eds) Progress in opioid research. Pergamon, Oxford, pp 21–24

Zagon IS, Goodman SR, McLaughlin PJ (1989) Characterization of zeta: a new opioid receptor involved in growth. Brain Res 482:297–305

Zipser B, Ruff MR, O'Neill JB, Smith CC, Higgins WJ, Pert CB (1988) The opiate receptor: a single 110 kDa recognition molecule appears to be conserved in *Tetrahymena*, leech, and rat. Brain Res 463:296–304

Zukin, RS, Eghbali M, Olive D, Unterwald EM, Tempel A (1988) Characterization and visualization of rat and guinea pig brain kappa opioid receptors: evidence for kappa$_1$ and kappa$_2$ opioid receptors. Proc Natl Acad Sci USA 85:4061–4065

Zukin SR, Zukin RS (1979) Specific ^{3}H-phencyclidine binding in rat central nervous system. Proc Natl Acad Sci USA 76:5372–5376

CHAPTER 2
Expression Cloning of cDNA Encoding a Putative Opioid Receptor

AVRAM GOLDSTEIN

A. Project History

The first demonstration of stereospecific opioid binding to brain membranes was reported 20 years ago (GOLDSTEIN et al. 1971), and the decisive demonstration of opioid receptors by ligand binding followed 2 years later (TERENIUS 1973; PERT and SNYDER 1973; SIMON et al. 1973; see also Chap. 1, this volume). The first membrane receptor to be cloned was the nicotinic acetylcholine receptor (COLD SPRING HARBOR SYMPOSIUM 1983) from the specialized electric organs of electric fish – an extraordinarily rich source compared with ordinary skeletal muscle.

The challenge of cloning an opioid receptor has confronted everyone in the opioid field since those early days. I recall a discussion 10 years ago with Jean-Pierre Changeux about the prospects of success if the classical method – so successful with the acetylcholine receptor – were followed. "Classical method" means purification to homogeneity, fragmentation by partial proteolysis (because a free NH_2-terminus is required for sequencing, and the NH_2-terminus of many receptors is blocked), purification of the proteolytic fragments, determination of partial sequence by stepwise Edman degradation, construction of corresponding oligonucleotide probes, and then "fishing" in an appropriate cDNA library made from tissues in which the desired receptor is known to be expressed. Changeux said (I paraphrase): "If you don't have the opioid equivalent of an electric fish, forget it!"

Elementary computations reinforced that pessimistic view. We knew that opioid receptors of a given type were present in brain at about 1 pmol/g wet weight tissue. Ten years ago, to determine a sequence of 15–20 amino acids by the Edman procedure required about 1 nmol pure material (sensitivity has improved since then). My own experience with dynorphin made a profound impression; it took my group 4 years to obtain the necessary 1 nmol (about 2 µg), pure, for Lee Hood's laboratory to sequence the first 13 residues (GOLDSTEIN et al. 1979), and another couple of years to obtain enough further material to complete the 17 residues of dynorphin A (GOLDSTEIN et al. 1981). I learned how poor the overall yields in protein purification can be. If we assumed 1% overall yield of pure receptor protein from tissue extracts, and again a few percent yield in purifying fragments (e.g., after cyanogen bromide treatment), it was evident we might need as much as a ton of beef brain to start with.

The intrinsic difficulty of the problem seems to have frustrated several skillful and committed groups who pursued the classical approach for years. Although several have reported purifying one or another protein to homogeneity, none has succeeded in the cloning (SIMON 1991). Horace Loh's group is an exception (SCHOFLELD et al. 1989). After purifying a μ-opioid binding protein to homogeneity, they prepared oligonucleotide probes and obtained a cDNA that encodes a protein they called *OBCAM* (see Chap. 3). This deduced protein, however, has no transmembrane domain and therefore is unlikely to be an opioid receptor. Moreover, it has not yet been expressed in cells to confirm that it encodes a protein capable of binding opioid ligands.

B. Expression Cloning

I. Methodology

In 1983 I persuaded Paul Berg to lecture at our Gordon Research Conference on Opiates about the new method called *expression cloning* that he had just developed for mammalian cells (OKAYAMA and BERG 1983). This novel approach seemed a way around the problems associated with the classical method, because no purification was required. All one needed was a reliable method of detecting the desired receptor on cells that expressed it, i.e., on cells transfected with a plasmid containing the right cDNA insert, however rare that message might be in the tissue mRNA pool.

Detection of a receptor could be by means of an antibody, as in the expression cloning of the NGF receptor (RADEKE et al. 1987). Or detection could be by ligand binding. It seemed to me that, in view of the rich literature on binding of multiple opioid ligands to the multiple opioid receptors, ligand binding would be the most foolproof approach. It is interesting, in this connection, that the NGF receptor detected by the antibody procedure turned out not to have typical high-affinity binding characteristics except in association with another protein, the *trk* proto-oncogene (HEMPSTEAD et al. 1991).

Because of my fatherly relationship to the dynorphin peptides, and the fact that these are κ-selective opioid ligands, I decided to focus our efforts on cloning a κ-receptor. We first devoted effort to developing novel κ-ligands as tools for the expression cloning project. Dynorphin A is difficult to derivatize without destroying its κ-selectivity. In addition to the essential NH_2-terminal free NH_2 group, it has two reactive lysine ε amino groups, which are both important for optimal recognition by the κ-receptor. It is especially difficult to radioiodinate, because tyrosine-1 is absolutely essential for interaction with the receptor, and iodination interferes. To obtain a more useful κ-ligand, we collaborated with John Nestor (Syntex) (GOLDSTEIN et al. 1988), preparing a dynorphin A-(1–13) derivative in which both lysine-11 and lysine-13 were substituted by arginine. Our assumption that this would make no difference to the affinity and selectivity proved to be correct. We also knew that it would be safe to extend the peptide at its C-terminus, inasmuch as the full-length dynorphin A [with WDNQ (single-letter code) as residues 14–17] had the same activity as the 13-residue peptide, and inasmuch as even dynorphin-32 (FISCHLI et al. 1982), with a C-terminal extension of 15 residues beyond dynorphin A, also had high affinity and κ-selectivity. By extending the C-terminus with glycine followed by diaminopentane, and leaving the t-Boc blocking group on the NH_2 of tyrosine-1 after removal of the peptide from the resin, we obtained a multipurpose dynorphin pro-ligand, DAKLI, in which the only reactive NH_2 group was at the C-terminus. Here we could couple Bolton-Hunter reagent to obtain [125I]-labeled peptide of specific radioactivity 4000 Ci/mmol. Alternatively, we could couple biotin or activated fluorescein, or prepare a dynorphin affinity resin.

My Chinese colleague Guo-xi Xie is central to subsequent developments. He trained with Jisheng Han in physiology and neuroscience at the Beijing Medical University, earning one of the first PhD degrees in a medical science in the People's Republic of China. He came to me as a postdoctoral fellow for a couple of years, and then, when I closed my Stanford laboratory, he moved to the DNAX Research Institute nearby. That institution, with close ties to Stanford, is one of the world's leading centers for molecular biologic research in immunology. I owe a debt of gratitude to J. Allan Waitz, president of DNAX, for accepting Xie and allowing us to pursue our expression cloning project for the subsequent 4 years, under the expert guidance of DNAX senior scientists, especially Atsushi Miyajima and Ken-Ichi Arai.

All the experimental work to be described below was carried out with extraordinary skill, hard work, and perseverance by Dr. Xie, in spite of my frequent interference.

II. Attempt by Stable Transfection

We began by constructing a guinea pig brain cDNA library, using the poly(A)$^+$ RNA from this tissue because of its well-known and well-studied content of κ-receptors. Incorporating the cDNA into a pCD expression vector (improved from the original Okayama-Berg vector), we transfected mouse fibroblasts (L cells, A9 clone). To detect any transfected cell that might be expressing κ-binding sites, we plated at a density sufficiently low to permit replication of each cell to a miniclone of about 1000 cells in the final confluent monolayer. We then tried a direct approach to detection by a method that was novel at that time. We flooded the dish with [125I]DAKLI, incubated, then washed away unbound radioligand, and simply set the dish on a X-ray film in the dark, allowing any positive clone to "take its own picture" by means of high-energy γ-radiation penetrating through the bottom of the dish. We had calculated, from a reasonable estimate of the number of receptors per cell, and knowing the specific radioactivity and the spotting of test samples of radioactive DAKLI on a dish, that a clone of 1000 cells ought to be detectable. And so it was. We found a few strong spots, at a frequency of about one per million transfected cells. Unfortunately, the positive fibroblast clones proved not to be viable; the cells had evidently been killed by the intense ^{125}I radioactivity. This problem was readily solved, however, by making replicas of the confluent growth on nylon membrane screens before exposing the master plates to DAKLI. Then positive clones could be rescued from the appropriate locations on the replica screens.

In this kind of stable transfection, the circular plasmid is opened and incorporated into the recipient cell genome. It can be recovered by forming hybrid cells with COS-7, a monkey kidney cell line that contains the appropriate replication machinery (T-antigen), which will recognize the SV40 promoter in the plasmid, and will replicate flanking sequences in both directions. In this way, by amplifying the recovered cDNA in *Escherichia coli*, and selecting single colonies, we were able eventually to obtain a single plasmid that induced opioid binding in COS-7 cells. This binding, using either [3H]bremazocine (BREM) or [125I]DAKLI as radioligand, had affinity in the low nanomolar range and also typical κ-selectivity – U50,488 or dynorphin peptides competed well; DAGO and DPDPE did not; nor did 3H-labeled DAGO or DPDPE bind.

I reported this encouraging progress in an oral presentation (unpublished) at the International Narcotic Research Conference in Albi the summer of 1988. It seemed that final success was just around the corner. However, when we sequenced the insert in the effective plasmid (which we call *P9*), we found that the longest open reading frame would only encode 72 amino acids, certainly not long enough for a receptor; and there was no strong sequence similarity to any known nucleic acid in the data base. Further investigation, the details of which I shall skip here, showed us that the original cDNA insert from the guinea pig brain library had been drastically rearranged in the mouse fibroblast genome. Thus, even though *P9* effectively and specifically induced the expression of κ-binding sites, only fragments of it corresponded to anything in the original library; the remainder presumably consisted of mouse sequences. Whatever *P9* really is, it does contain enough information to induce typical κ-opioid binding sites. Whether it does this by encoding a sufficient portion of a κ-receptor (e.g., the binding site alone), or whether it is a κ-receptor gene activator, *P9* is obviously of great interest. For the moment, however, we put it on the shelf and began again.

III. Transient Transfection, Panning

Our second attempt was by transient transfection of COS-7 cells, affinity enrichment by panning, and isolation of an effective plasmid by the method of pools. The successful outcome of this work was published recently (XIE et al. 1992).

To produce tools for this approach, Xie synthesized an entire set of chimeric peptides (XIE et al. 1990), which all shared the C-terminal sequence of dynorphin-32 (recognized by monoclonal antibody 17.M developed in my laboratory) (BARRETT and GOLDSTEIN, 1985), but had various NH$_2$-terminal sequences derived from different type-selective opioid peptides such as DAGO, DPDPE, dermorphin, and deltorphin. The utility of these chimeric peptides is considerable, for one can, in principle, select any single one according to the receptor type of interest, yet be able to interact with the same antibody, e.g., in affinity enrichment procedures, as described below. This approach generalizes the DAKLI principle – that the C-terminal domain of dynorphin peptides can be manipulated or bound without affecting the critical N-terminal domain essential for opioid binding affinity and κ-selectivity.

We began with a human placenta cDNA library, as this tissue is an abundant source of κ-receptors. Plasmid pME18S, developed at DNAX, was a novel high-copy-number small plasmid with a strong promoter, suitable for constructing unidirectional cDNA libraries and for expression in mammalian systems. The library was size-fractionated to exclude inserts less than 1.5 kb in size. Cells were transfected, then about 2 days later they were panned, using the chimeric peptide technique described above, as follows. The population of transfected cells was exposed to dynorphin-32 and then placed in a dish coated with monoclonal antibody 17.M. Ideally, only cells binding the opioid peptide would attach to the antibody-coated dishes. Gentle washing removed unattached cells. The remaining cells were lysed to recover the plasmids, and those were amplified in *E. coli*. Repeated panning cycles, each taking about a week, enriched for cells expressing sites capable of binding the free N-terminal portion of dynorphin-32 (the C-terminus being bound to antibody). We tested the degree of enrichment by competition with U50,488 in the panning procedure itself. Initially, U50,488 had no effect on the number of cells observed per microscope field, but after four rounds of panning, the number of cells remaining on a dish increased, and the competitor could then reduce the number of attached cells by 80%. Moreover, the positive result at the fourth cycle required the presence of both dynorphin-32 and the antibody.

There is a limit to what panning can achieve because a single COS-7 cell takes up more than a hundred plasmids. Thus, even if 100% of the cells expressed κ-binding sites, there would still be a mixture of plasmids. The next step, therefore, was to select individual *E. coli* colonies (each bacterial cell contains only a single clonal population of plasmids), recover plasmid from each, and transfer to separate wells of 96-well ELISA plates. Then fresh transfections of COS-7 populations were carried out, using pools of 96 plasmids initially. We tested which were effective by [^{3}H]BREM binding and U50,488 competition. Then, forming a smaller pool from each effective pool, we tested again, and eventually in this manner obtained a single effective plasmid, which we call *K1R*. Thus, our overall procedure selected for cells that could bind a κ-selective opioid peptide (dynorphin, at the panning stage) and that could also bind nonpeptide κ-selective ligands (BREM and U50,488 at the testing stage).

C. Ligand Binding by the Expressed Receptor

Unfortunately, COS-7 cells bind [^{3}H]BREM nonspecifically (i.e., not competed by U50,488), so that in our experiments specific binding by transfected cells was only about 30%–40% of total binding. Besides, the transfection efficiency, as one might expect, was variable between experiments. Consequently, a great many experiments were required to establish the properties of the binding sites in a quantitative manner. We used mock transfection as our negative control, i.e., actual transfection by the same vector, but lacking any cDNA insert. The increment in binding produced by transfection, as compared with mock transfection, corresponded well with specific binding in transfected cells as defined by U50,488 competition. In some experiments, we used as positive control the H187 cell line (which expresses both κ- and μ-sites) (MANECKJEE and MINNA 1990).

There were two unexpected and disturbing features of the expressed binding sites. First, the K_d of BREM, from the saturation isotherm, was 87 nM, about two orders of magnitude greater than for typical κ-sites in brain. K_i values for such competitors as U50,488 and dynorphin A-(1–13) were in the same range of modest rather than high affinities.

Accompanying the unexpectedly low affinity was a lack of κ-selectivity. Thus, the μ-selective DAGO and the δ-selective DPDPE competed about as well as U50,488. Likewise, U63,639 (μ-selective) competed as well as U63,640 (κ-selective).

On the other hand, two properties of the binding sites were typically opioid. First, it is well known that opioid peptides of the enkephalin, endorphin, and dynorphin families require free NH$_2$-terminal tyrosine for receptor binding. We considered it very significant, therefore, that the binding sites induced on transfected cells by *K1R* were competed for by dynorphin A-(1–13) but not by [desTyr]dynorphin A-(1–13).

Second, stereoselectivity is a defining characteristic of opioid binding sites. We considered it very significant, therefore, that the binding sites induced by *K1R* were competed for by (−)levorphanol but not by its (+)enantiomer dextrorphan.

D. Sequence Analysis, Structure of the Receptor

The *K1R* insert was exceptionally long, 4.9 kb. Sequencing was unusually difficult because of a remarkably high GC content in the 5′ domain, as high as 80% in some regions. To establish the sequence unequivocally we used the dideoxy method in both double-strand and single-strand procedures, always with multiple redundant overlaps in both directions, 5′ to 3′ and 3′ to 5′; for some regions we used Taq polymerase at high temperature, and sometimes we used ITP or deaza-GTP. The final result was satisfying, in that a long open reading frame encoded a 440-residue protein with seven unmistakable hydrophobic transmembrane segments. That we obtained a receptor belonging to the 7-helix family was reassuring, because a mass of evidence over the years – with respect to both ligand binding and function – has made it clear that the opioid receptors are coupled to G proteins, probably G_i and/or G_o.

Several possible reasons for reduced affinity and poor selectivity come to mind, and these will have to be explored over the coming months. For one thing, nearly 3.5 kb of sequence is in the 3′ untranslated region, so that despite the length of the insert, it may be incomplete at its 5′ end. The first methionine is encoded in a sequence CCCATGG, which does not conform to the most frequent consensus, which is ACCATGG. But more important, the reading frame remains open upstream of that methionine, i.e., there is no in-frame stop codon between ATG and the beginning of the insert. It is quite likely, therefore, that we are missing a 5′ coding sequence, so that the NH_2-terminal domain of the deduced protein is actually longer than presently appears. If the NH_2-terminal extracellular domain plays a role in the recognition and binding of peptide ligands, the deficiency here could be the cause of the anomalous binding properties.

Another plausible reason could be absence of the correct G protein in the COS-7 cells. There is a recent precedent with the secretin receptor (also in the 7-helix family), which did not bind with high affinity until the correct G protein was cotransfected (ISHIHARA et al. 1991). The G protein requirement for high-affinity binding is related to the well-known effect of GTP in reducing ligand binding affinity of agonists in membrane preparations by one or two orders of magnitude, through its action in favoring G-protein dissociation from the receptor.

There are other possible reasons. For example, there are two putative N-glycosylation sites in the extracellular NH_2-terminal domain. These could be improperly glycosylated by COS-7 cells, and that could affect ligand binding.

Finally, a search of the data base revealed an astonishing degree of similarity between K1R and the rat neuromedin K receptor (rNKR) (SHIGEMOTO et al. 1990). It is as though K1R were a chimeric receptor, which contains virtually the entire transmembrane domain of rNKR (greater than 90% identity), linked to a much less similar C-terminal cytoplasmic domain (70% identity) and a quite different extracellular NH_2-terminal domain. The "snake" cartoon (Fig. 1) shows this clearly.

Naturally, we were concerned that K1R might simply be human NKR (hNKR). Professor Nakanishi (Kyoto University), however, was kind enough to communicate the sequence of hNKR prior to its publication

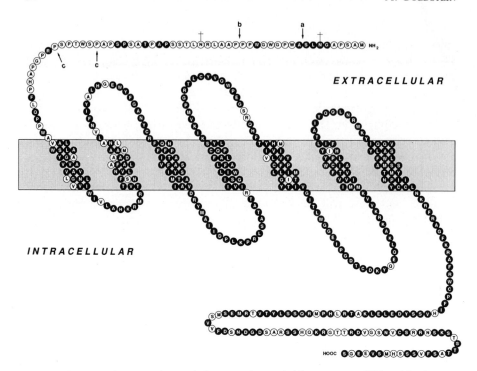

Fig. 1. Structural comparison of the putative opioid receptor, *K1R*, with the rat neuromedin receptor, *rNKR*. *Letters in circles* are amino acids (single-letter code) of the *K1R* sequence. *Rectangular-shaded block* represents membrane bilayer. Transmembrane segments are assigned according to *rNKR* (SHIGEMOTO et al. 1990), in general (but not exact) agreement with Kyte-Doolittle hydropathy analysis of *K1R*. *Dark circles* indicate identical residues in the two receptors. *Crosses* indicate potential glycosylation sites in the NH$_2$-terminal domain of *K1R*. *Arrows* marked *a* and *b* show where gaps (one and two residues, respectively) in *K1R* are required for optimal matching of the two sequences. *Arrows* marked *c* show where a seven-residue gap in *rNKR* is required opposite the sequence PSWTPSP of *K1R*. As can be seen, these gap placements (from the Wisconsin program) do not produce many matches; the entire NH$_2$-terminal extracellular sequence of *K1R* could be regarded as but little related to that of *rNKR*

(TAKAHASHI et al. 1992); it is not *K1R*, although the sequence similarity of its transmembrane domain is slightly greater than that of *rNKR*, as one would expect.

The critical experiments were made possible by Professor Nakanishi's willingness to share his *rNKR* clone, which Dr. Robert C. Thompson (University of Michigan) kindly helped us prepare for use. We transfected COS-7 cells side by side with *K1R* and *rNKR*, and carried out extensive binding assays with both opioid and tachykinin ligands. I can summarize these experiments as follows: Cells transfected with *rNKR* behaved as expected, binding a tachykinin radioligand (eledoisin, ELED), which was competed against most potently by neuromedin K, less effectively by substance P or substance K. Those cells showed no specific binding of

[^{3}H]BREM (no competition by U50,488) and [^{3}H]ELED binding was not affected by U50,488. On the other hand, cells transfected by *KIR* did not bind [^{3}H]ELED, nor did tachykinins compete with [^{3}H]BREM for the binding sites.

E. Conclusions

These results show that – as has been observed with some other receptors – one may have a very high degree of sequence similarity, yet have very different ligand binding properties. We know, from the beautiful work of Lefkowitz and his colleagues on adrenergic receptor chimeras (DOHLMAN et al. 1991), that single amino acid changes by site-directed mutagenesis at critical positions can have profound effects on ligand affinity and selectivity. Our results seem to indicate that, in contrast to the inference drawn from such studies with compact nonpeptide ligands – that they bind exclusively in a pocket formed within the membrane by the seven helixes – peptide ligands of the opioid family may be recognized also by a part of the receptor lying outside the membrane. Considering the message-and-address concept, which I adopted years ago from Schwyzer and applied to dynorphin peptides (GOLDSTEIN 1982), it may be that the compact YGGF message binds in a membrane pocket, while the extended address (LRRIRPKLK . . .), which determines κ-selectivity, is recognized by the NH$_2$-terminal extracellular domain of the receptor.

In summary, we believe the preponderance of the evidence suggests that *KIR* encodes an opioid receptor (or most of an opioid receptor), perhaps κ$_1$, in view of the panning procedure employing a dynorphin ligand, and the competition by U50,488. If this proves to be true, it reveals a remarkably close evolutionary relationship of an opioid receptor to the tachykinin receptor family. The conclusive proof will rest, of course, on a reconstitution of the full high-affinity and κ-selectivity. That is the next goal, which Dr. Xie will be pursuing in the laboratory of Huda Akil and Stanley Watson, to which he has just moved.

Acknowledgements. I thank Dr. Guo-xi Xie for the major role he played in this project and for his thoughtful comments on this manuscript, and Dr. Lee F. Allen (Duke University) for the construction of Fig. 1.

References

Barrett RW, Goldstein A (1985) A monoclonal antibody specific for a dynorphin precursor. Neuropeptides 6:113–120

Cold Spring Harbor Symposia in Quantitative Biology (1983) Acetylcholine receptor and its channel. In: Watson JD, McKay R (eds) Molecular Neurobiology, vol. 48, pp 1–146

Dohlman HG, Thorner J, Caron MG, Lefkowitz RJ (1991) Model systems for the study of seven-transmembrane-segment receptors. Annu Rev Biochem 60:653–688

Fischli W, Goldstein A, Hunkapiller MW, Hood LE (1982) Isolation and amino acid sequence of a 4000-dalton dynorphin from porcine pituitary. Proc Natl Acad Sci USA 79:5435–5437

Goldstein A, Lowney LI, Pal BK (1971) Stereospecific and nonspecific interactions of the morphine congener levorphanol in subcellular fractions of mouse brain. Proc Natl Acad Sci USA 68:1742–1747

Goldstein A, Tachibana S, Lowney LI, Hunkapiller M, Hood L (1979) Dynorphin-(1–13), an extraordinarily potent opioid peptide. Proc Natl Acad Sci USA 76:6666–6670

Goldstein A, Fischli W, Lowney LI, Hunkapiller M, Hood L (1981) Porcine pituitary dynorphin: complete amino acid sequence of the biologically active heptadecapeptide. Proc Natl Acad Sci USA 78:7219–7223

Goldstein A (1982) Dynorphin and the dynorphin receptor: some implications of gene duplication of the opioid message. In: Schmitt FO, Bird SJ, Bloom FE (eds) Molecular genetic neuroscience. Raven, New York, pp 249–262

Goldstein A, Nestor JJ Jr, Naidu A, Newman SR (1988) DAKLI: A multipurpose ligand with high affinity and selectivity for dynorphin (kappa opioid) binding sites. Proc Natl Acad Sci USA 85:7375–7379

Hempstead BL, Martin-Zanca D, Kaplan DR, Parada LF, Chao MV (1991) High-affinity NGF binding requires coexpression of the trk proto-oncogene and the low-affinity NGF receptor. Nature 350:678–683

Ishihara T, Nakamura S, Kaziro Y, Takahashi T, Takahashi K, Nagata S (1991) Molecular cloning and expression of a cDNA encoding the secretin receptor. EMBO J 10:1635–1641

Maneckjee R, Minna JD (1990) Opioid and nicotine receptors affect growth regulation of human lung cancer cell lines. Proc Natl Acad Sci USA 87:3294–3298

Okayama H, Berg P (1983) A cDNA cloning vector that permits expression of cDNA inserts in mammalian cells. Mol Cell Biol 3:280–289

Pert CB, Snyder SH (1973) Opiate receptor: demonstration in nervous tissue. Science 179:1011–1014

Radeke MJ, Misko TP, Hsu C, Herzenberg LA, Shooter EM (1987) Gene transfer and molecular cloning of the rat nerve growth factor receptor. Nature 325:593–597

Schofield PR, McFarland KC, Hayflick JS, Wilcox JN, Cho TM, Roy S, Lee NM, Loh IIII, Seeburg PH (1989) Molecular characterization of a new immuno-globulin superfamily protein with potential roles in opioid binding and cell contact. EMBO J 8:489–495

Shigemoto R, Yokota Y, Tsuchida K, Nakanishi S (1990) Cloning and expression of a rat neuromedin K receptor cDNA. J Biol Chem 265:623–628

Simon EJ (1991) Opioid receptors and endogenous opioid peptides. Med Res Rev 2:357–374

Simon EJ, Hiller JM, Edelman I (1973) Stereospecific binding of the potent narcotic analgesic [3H] etorphine to rat-brain homogenate. Proc Natl Acad Sci USA 70:1947–1949

Takahashi K, Tanaka A, Hara M, Nakanishi S (1992) The primary structures and gene organizations of human substance P and neuromedin K receptors. Eur J Biochem 204:1025–1033

Terenius L (1973) Stereospecific interaction between narcotic analgesics and a synaptic plasma membrane fraction of rat cerebral cortex. Acta Pharmacol Toxicol 32:317–320

Xie G, Miyajima A, Yokota T, Arai K, Goldstein A (1990) Chimeric opioid peptides: tools for identifying opioid receptor types. Proc Natl Acad Sci USA 87:3180–3184

Xie G-X, Miyajima A, Goldstein A (1992) Expression cloning of cDNA encoding a seven-helix receptor from human placenta with affinity for opioid ligands. Proc Natl Acad Sci USA 89:4124–4128

Characterization of Opioid-Binding Proteins and Other Molecules Related to Opioid Function

A.P. SMITH, H.H. LOH, and N.M. LEE

A. Introduction

Nearly 2 decades after their discovery in mammalian brain, opioid receptors remain largely uncharacterized structurally and functionally. While a great body of pharmacological and biochemical information has accumulated from studies of membrane-bound opioid receptors, continued difficulties in purifying these receptors has precluded investigators from obtaining such standard knowledge as the receptor's amino acid sequence, its overall conformation in the cell membrane, the location of its ligand-binding site, and the identity of functional molecules associated with it.

Though there are several aspects of opioid receptors that might be expected to make them more difficult to isolate than other cell surface receptors, including their heterogeneity, sensitivity to detergents, and lack of a simple functional assay (LOH and SMITH 1990), it is not entirely clear why methods that have worked well for so many other receptors have failed in this case. Fortunately, however, the conventional approach of purification is no longer the only option available for characterization of receptors. Recent developments in molecular biology, immunology, and cell biology have provided investigators with a number of powerful tools that can be used not only to achieve the same aim, but, indeed, to extend knowledge about a receptor's structure and function.

In this article, we review the work that has been done in applying these new approaches to understanding opioid receptors and associated molecules that may contribute to their functional effects. While the conventional approach of attempting to purify opioid receptors continues to be a major focus of several laboratories, including our own, we believe that these newer methods hold great promise for revealing at last details of the structure and function of opioid receptors.

B. cDNA Cloning

The development of modern molecular biological techniques has made it possible to obtain or infer a great deal of information about proteins indirectly, from the sequences of the DNA coding for them. The DNA sequence determines the amino acid sequence, and, from this information alone, the investigator may be able to gain insights into the conformation of the protein, the way it interacts with the cell membrane, and even the second messengers that mediate its cellular effects. For example, all the cell surface receptors known to have their functions mediated by GTP-binding proteins (G proteins) have seven hydrophobic regions of conserved amino acid sequences that are presumed to span the membrane (Dohlman et al. 1987). Two other large receptor families, effects of which are mediated by tyrosine kinase (Yarden and Ullrich 1988) and tyrosine phosphatase (Streuli et al. 1989), have conserved intracellular domains possessing the catalytic activity as well as conserved extracellular domains that are presumed to be involved in ligand binding.

Having available the receptor's DNA and amino acid sequence also opens up numerous possibilities for further studies. Antibodies to peptides corresponding to portions of the amino acid sequence can be raised, and used to pinpoint functional regions of the receptor, to localize it in biological tissues, and to purify it by affinity chromatography. Oligonucleotide probes consisting of portions of the cDNA sequence can be used to determine the localization and regulation of the receptor's mRNA, and to probe the genomic organization of the receptor code. Antisense cDNA, cDNA complementary to the coding strand of the receptor cDNA, can be used to inactivate selectively a single mRNA species, confirming its functions and perhaps illuminating more subtle ones.

DNA sequences for receptors, in turn, can be obtained in several ways. If even small quantitites of purified receptor are available, the most straightforward way is by partially sequencing the receptor, synthesizing oligonucleotide probes that correspond to the coding region of this sequence, and using these probes to screen a cDNA library, constructed from all the mRNAs present in the tissue containing the receptor. In theory, the probes should hybridize with a unique sequence (sometimes present in several different cDNAs) corresponding to that coding the receptor. An additional benefit of this procedure, though, is that, under sufficiently relaxed conditions of hybridization, the probes may also recognize other, highly related sequences, providing evidence for a family of proteins closely related to the receptor of interest.

If purified receptor is not available, it is still possible to isolate its cDNA, if there is a rapid and reliable way to measure receptor activity, such as ligand binding or ligand-mediated alteration of some biochemical process. In this case, the cDNA library, or mRNA itself, is introduced into cells that normally do not express the receptor, and the cells screened for receptor activity. This step may be carried out by transfection of cDNA by phage vectors into mammalian cell lines, or by direct injection of mRNA into large cells such as oocytes.

While this approach has now been successfully used for dozens of receptors, and can in principle be applied to any receptor of interest, for several reasons it may present difficulties in individual cases. First, in order for the screening process to work, the receptor must be expressed in the transfected or injected cells in a form capable of recognizing ligand. For such full functional expression, however, the successful translation of the appropriate message into a polypeptide may not be sufficient. For one thing, posttranslational processing is frequently necessary to convert polypeptides into functional receptors – for example, the addition of specific carbohydrate groups to specific portions of the protein molecule – and any cells that normally do not express these receptors may be incapable of carrying out these additional steps with the required specificity. In addition, a receptor may consist of more than one polypeptide chain, each of which is necessary to form the high-affinity binding site; this is the case for the interleukin-2 receptor (SMITH 1987).

A second major disadvantage of approaches based on receptor expression is that, even if cells are capable of synthesizing fully functional molecules, the screening process is quite laborious; typically, one is looking for one or a few receptor-containing clones out of millions. Thus this approach may need to be combined with others that are capable of a priori limiting the number of clones that need to be examined. Two such techniques that have been used successfully to clone some receptors and other functional molecules are subtractive hybridization and the use of consensus sequences.

Subtractive hybridization takes advantage of those situatins in which two tissues contain nearly identical complements of proteins and their mRNAs, but differ in that only one contains the receptor or other protein of interest. In this case, mRNA is isolated from both tissues, and cDNA prepared from the mRNA that includes the receptor transcripts. This cDNA is then hybridized with the other population of mRNA, which, in theory, should "subtract" all the common messages between the two tissues, leaving cDNA highly enriched in receptor-encoding sequences. This relatively small library can then be transfected into cells and screened for receptor function.

While the principle of subtractive hybridization is very simple, in practice it can be very difficult to apply. One reason for this is that there are relatively few (if, indeed, any) situations in which only a single molecule of interest, and no other, is differentially expressed in two tissues. It is much more likely that differences will be observed with respect to several, perhaps many, molecules. In our own work with the opioid receptor, for example, based on downregulation of the receptors in response to chronic exposure to opioid agonist (discussed in more detail below), we have identified more than a dozen different, apparently unrelated proteins. While all of these proteins may in some way play a role in the downregulation process, and thus be of some relevance to our understanding of opioid receptors, their presence greatly complicates the task of identifying the receptor itself.

A second difficulty with subtractive hybridization is that, even in an ideal case, where only a single protein is differentially expressed, this protein may not be detected unless it is relatively abundant in one tissue, and either absent or greatly reduced in the other tissue. This is because even large changes in a relatively rare message would be smaller, in absolute value, than small, statistically insignificant changes in highly abundant messages. Thus, contamination of genuinely altered messages with messages from nonaltered but abundant proteins is to be expected.

Despite these difficulties, subtractive hybridization has been used successfully to clone several proteins. KAVATHAS et al. (1984) cloned the gene coding the human T lymphocyte differentiation antigen Leu-2 by preparing mRNA from two sets of L cells, those expressing and not expressing this antigen. FORNACE and MITCHELL (1986) identified several transcripts involved in the response of Chinese hamster cells to heat shock, by subtraction of sequences from shocked and nonshocked cells. Subtractive hybridization has also been used to enrich transcripts specific for certain brain regions, by subtracting messages from other brain regions (RHYNER et al. 1986). These investigators estimated that transcripts comprising only 0.0005% of the total cellular mRNA could be identified in this way.

In addition to subtractive hybridization, the search for a specific cDNA can also be greatly accelerated by the use of consensus sequences. The rationale underlying this approach is that most cell surface receptors belong to a well-defined family of proteins that share significant homologies in their amino acid sequence. By designing oligonucleotide probes that correspond to the most commonly shared or consensus portions of these sequences, one can preferentially screen for members of this family.

The use of oligonucleotide probes based on consensus sequences has been successfully applied to the isolation of new members of the G protein-coupled receptors (HERSHEY and KRAUSE 1990; PARMENTIER et al. 1989). This is a family of cell surface receptors that is coupled to second messengers by G proteins, and members of which each possess seven putative trans-membrane sequences. These sequences show a relatively high degree of conservation among members of this family, and so can be used to screen cDNA libraries for new members.

In summary, there are two general procedures for cloning the cDNA of a receptor of interest: (1) oligonucleotide probes are designed from a partially sequenced receptor, and used to screen a cDNA library prepared from a tissue containing the receptor; and (2) introduction of cDNA or mRNA into cells that are subsequently screened for their expression of the receptor. The latter approach, despite its associated difficulties, is of greater interest and relevance to opioid receptor investigators, as it does not require purified receptor. However, several laboratories, including our own, have reported purification of opioid receptors (CHO et al. 1986; GIOANNINI et al. 1985; MANECKJEE et al. 1987; SIMONDS et al. 1985), thus making available small quantities of material that could in principle be used to obtain cDNA by the direct approach. Our own work with a purified opioid-binding protein illustrates how this is done.

I. Molecular Cloning of OBCAM

Several years ago, we reported purification from bovine brain of a 58-kDa protein selective for opioid alkaloid ligands, using a combination of affinity chromatography, lectin chromatography, and gel filtration (CHO et al. 1986). A novel feature of this protein was that it required acidic lipids possessing unsaturated fatty acids in order to manifest binding activity; neither the protein nor the lipids alone possessed significant opioid binding (HASEGAWA et al. 1987). The binding affinities of ligands to this reconstituted material were lower than the corresponding values for binding to brain membranes, but the rank order of binding affinities to the two preparations were highly correlated (CHO et al. 1986; HASEGAWA et al. 1987).

In an attempt to characterize this protein more thoroughly, and to obtain further evidence for its role as an opioid receptor, we partially sequenced it, synthesized oligonucleotide probes, and were able to identify a unique cDNA clone (SCHOFIELD et al. 1989). The predicted amino acid sequence contained 345 amino acids, with a search of the NBRF-PIR data base revealing significant sequence homologies with several members of the immunoglobulin superfamily (SCHOFIELD et al. 1989). This is a group of proteins characterized by repeating domains flanked by cysteine residues (WILLIAMS 1987; WILLIAMS and BARCLAY 1988). The highest degree of homology was to molecules involved in cell adhesion or cell recognition, including the vertebrate proteins neural cell adhesion molecule (N-CAM) and myelin-associated glycoprotein (MAG), and the invertebrate proteins amalgam, neuroglian, and fasciclin II. The sequence of each of these proteins is 20%–25% homologous with that of the opioid binding protein. Somewhat lower significance values, also suggestive of an evolutionary relationship, were found for several peptide receptors, including those for interleukin-6 (IL-6) and platelet-derived growth factor (PDGF).

Sequence analysis is therefore consistent with the notion that this protein functions as a neuropeptide receptor, while suggesting that it could also play a role in cell adhesion. Accordingly, it has been named OBCAM, or opioid binding cell adhesion molecule. Interestingly, a recent study has shown that opioids can modulate cell-cell interactions of monocytes (STEFANO et al. 1989). Moreover, the homologies of OBCAM with immunoglobulins and immune cell receptors such as the T-cell receptor and the IL-6 receptor are consistent with a growing body of evidence indicating links between opioids and the immune system (SIBINGA and GOLDSTEIN 1988).

The homologies of OBCAM with members of the Ig superfamily may also provide some clues as to how the receptor functions. Several members of this superfamily, including the PDGF receptor and the colony stimulating factor-1 (CSF-1) receptor, possess a single transmembrane domain with an extended cytoplasmic region; the latter region contains a tyrosine kinase domain (YARDEN and ULLRICH 1988). Peptide ligand binding to the extra-cellular portion of these receptors induces a conformational change that activates the intracellular kinase, which in turn phosphorylates a number of intracellular proteins. These phosphorylated proteins in turn alter the metabolism of the cell in specific ways.

Very recently, another single transmembrane receptor family possessing extracellular Ig domains has been described (Streuli et al. 1989). These are protein tyrosine phosphatases (PTPases), which have been isolated from human placenta and from *Drosophila* embryos. As with the tyrosine kinases, the catalytic activity of these proteins is manifested by an intracellular domain that shows a high degree of conservation among different members of the family, as well as with several other proteins that have no extracellular domains, or extracellular domains that are not Ig in nature. Though ligands for these membrane-bound molecules have not yet been identified, it is presumed that they are receptors that mediate effects opposite those of tyrosine kinases, and which thus may work in concert with the latter. Moreover, because Ig domains are found in many cell adhesion molecules that regulate cell-cell interactions, it has been hypothesized that these tyrosine phosphatases may act as suppressors of tumors and other malignancies that arise from uncontrolled cell growth.

The amino acid sequence of OBCAM indicates that it lacks an intracellular domain. It possess only a short hydrophobic sequence at its C-terminus, which presumably anchors the protein to the cell membrane. Recently, however, it has been found that a number of cell surface receptors with single transmembrane domains exist in multiple forms, with or without the cytoplasmic region, including the cell adhesion molecules N-CAM, neuroglian, fasciclin II and fasciclin III, growth hormone receptor, insulin-like growth factor (IGF) receptor, and a tyrosine kinase receptor (Baumbach et al. 1989; Cunningham et al. 1987; Czech 1989; Klein et al. 1990; Grenningloh et al. 1990). The existence of these different forms of cell surface receptors has been shown in some cases to result from alternative splicing of mRNA, so that a message originally containing both extracellular and cytoplasmic domains can be translated either intact, or only with the extracellular domain. This raises the possibility that the clone we obtained for OBCAM may represent a truncated form of a larger sequence, which contains an intracellular domain.

The single transmembrane structure of OBCAM is somewhat surprising, because at least some opioid receptors, namely the δ-type in NG108-15 neuroblastoma $\times$ glioma hybrid cells and in mammalian striate, are coupled via a G protein to adenylate cyclase (Koski et al. 1982; Sharma et al. 1975a). This has suggested that these receptors are structurally and functionally related to a group of cell surface receptors that are associated with G proteins, including the $\beta 1$-, $\beta 2$-, and α_2-adrenergic, m1, m2 and m3 muscarinic, serotonin 1_a, and 1_c, dopamine D_2, substance K and P, thyrotropin and luteinizing hormone receptors (Bunzow et al. 1988; Dixon et al. 1986; Julius et al. 1988; Kobilka et al. 1987; Kubo et al. 1986; Loosfelt et al. 1989; Parmentier et al. 1989; Peralta et al. 1987). All of these receptors have seven hydrophobic regions in their interior, which are thought to span the membrane.

Very recent studies, however, suggest that some receptors with a single transmembrane domain and an intracellular tyrosine kinase domain may also interact with G proteins. Much of this evidence indicates an indirect interaction, mediated by phosphorylation. Both the insulin receptor (ZICK et al. 1986) and the EGF receptor (VALENTINE-BRAUN et al. 1986) have been shown to phosphorylate G proteins, which in turn results in the inhibition of adenylate cyclase; other protein kinases have also been shown to be capable of phosphorylating G proteins (KATADA et al. 1985; RESNICK and RACKER 1988). In addition, however, a direct interaction between the IGF-II receptor and a G protein has been demonstrated in reconstitution experiments (NISHIMOTO et al. 1989). Thus it appears that receptors containing seven transmembrane domains not necessarily the only kind that may mediate their effects through G proteins.

An additional possibility is that OBCAM may be part of a larger receptor complex, with the other subunits providing the interaction with G proteins. Recently, it has been proposed that the IgE receptor may be constructed in this way (BLANK et al. 1989). This contains three subunits. The α-subunit is a typical Ig superfamily member, with several Ig domains and a single hydrophobic domain. Thus it is largely extracellular, and is presumably anchored to the cell membrane by a single transmembrane sequence. However, the other two subunits, β- and γ-, contain several hydrophobic regions. Thus the complex together could conceivably possess seven transmembrane regions.

In conclusion, the amino acid sequence of OBCAM clearly establishes it as a member of the immunoglobulin superfamily, most closely related with several cell adhesion molecules and with several peptide receptors. The biochemical functions of OBCAM, however, are not clear from this sequence, though the most attractive possibility at present is that an extended form of the molecule exists that possesses catalytic activity, such as tyrosine kinase or tyrosine phosphatase.

II. Molecular Cloning and Characterization of Gene Products Downregulated by Chronic Opioid Treatment of NG108-15 Cells

Because of the difficulty in purifying opioid receptors, alternative methods of cloning receptor cDNA are attractive. As discussed earlier, one method of reducing the laborious screening this normally entails is to use subtractive hybridization. This approach is particularly feasible with cultured NG108-15 neuroblastoma × glioma hybrid cells, a relatively simple system that has been widely used to study opioid receptors. Introduced by SHARMA et al. (1975a), these hybrid cells retain many neuronal properties, including excitable membrane, light and dense core vesicles, ability to synthesize acetylcholine, and the ability to grow neurites. They also contain a homogenous population of opioid receptors, consisting of only the δ-type, which are coupled to a well-studied effector molecule, adenylate cyclase.

SHARMA et al. (1975a) originally showed that opioid agonists administered to NG108-15 cells inhibited both basal and prostaglandin E1 (PGE1)-stimulated adenylate cyclase. This inhibition was dose dependent and naloxone antagonizable, and the inhibitory potencies of a series of opioid agonists correlated well with their binding affinities to these cells. Subsequently, this group found that chronic opioid agonist treatment resulted in a gradual loss of opioid inhibition of cyclase, with cyclic AMP levels returning to normal (SHARMA et al. 1975b). Furthermore, withdrawal of agonist at this time resulted in increased adenylate cyclase activity, above that of control level. These effects of chronic opioid agonist are at least superficially analogous to the state of opioid tolerance/dependence, suggesting that NG108-15 hybrid cells might be a suitable model system for investigating the molecular basis of these phenomena.

The chronic effects of opioids in NG108-15 cells are also similar to those of other ligands that affect adenylate cyclase (LEFKOWITZ et al. 1980; SU et al. 1980). Subsequent studies in our laboratory as well as by other groups have shown that the chronic opioid treatment of NG108-15 cells induces three distinct adaptation processes: (1) desensitization, manifested in a reduction of agonist affinity and an uncoupling of receptors from adenylate cyclase (LAW et al. 1982, 1983); (2) downregulation, a loss of receptor number, manifested as a decrease in B_{max} of ligand binding (CHANG et al. 1982; LAW et al. 1983); and (3) an increase in adenylate cyclase, observed upon withdrawal of opioid (SHARMA et al. 1977).

The dramatic loss of opioid receptors occurring during downregulation suggests that the subtractive hybridization technique could also be applied to clone the opioid receptor present in these cells, by hybridizing cDNA prepared from untreated cells to mRNA from downregulated cells. To date, several laboratories, including our own, have used this approach to clone proteins that do appear to be specifically downregulated by opioid agonist. However, none of these proteins has been shown to bind opioids, and in several cases data base searches have revealed that these sequences are identical or highly similar to known, nonreceptor proteins. Since these proteins generally are relatively abundant constituents of the cell, it is possible that they have been isolated as contaminants.

In addition, however, our laboratory has isolated by subtractive hybridization a cDNA that has no significant homology to any previously published sequence. This clone, NGD5, codes for a predicted amino acid sequence of about 350 amino acids, with a single putative transmembrane region, consistent with its being a cell surface receptor. Though we have not yet expressed NGD5, to determine whether it codes for an opioid binding molecule, we have shown that antisense cDNA to NGD5 results in serious alterations in cell morphology (see below). Thus NGD5 appears to play a vital role in the cell.

III. Use of Consensus Sequences in cDNA Cloning of Opioid Receptors

As discussed above, a receptor that is known or believed to belong to a particular superfamily can be screened for in a cDNA library by using oligonucleotide probes corresponding to conserved regions common to members of this family. Successful application of this procedure to cloning opioid receptors, of course, depends on knowing what superfamily of receptors they belong to. As discussed earlier, most investigators believe that opioid receptors are members of the G protein coupled superfamily, which contain seven putative transmembrane regions of fairly highly conserved sequences. This assumption is based on the observation that opioid receptors are coupled to G proteins in NG108-15 cells, as well as in several regions of the mammalian CNS.

To date, this approach, like subtractive hybridization, has not been successful in obtaining a protein with opioid binding activity. However, as discussed earlier, there is now some evidence that not all G protein-coupled receptors contain the seven transmembrane structure. Thus while the use of these sequences as probes for opioid receptor cDNA is a reasonable approach, it is not certain that it will work.

C. Use of Antibodies to Characterize Opioid Receptors

As mentioned earlier, the availability of antibodies to a receptor or other functional protein makes possible many inquiries into its structure and function. While it is simplest to raise antibodies against a purified receptor, they can also be prepared against preparations that are only partially pure. Moreover, the receptor need not bind ligand. Antibodies can be made to denatured receptors, such as those identified by covalent labeling with a tritiated ligand, and partially purified by SDS gel electrophoresis. Antibodies to receptors can even be prepared in the absence of receptors, by preparing antibodies to ligand, then using these antibodies as antigen to prepare anti-idiotypic antibodies. Once such antibodies are available, they can be efficiently screened by their ability to inhibit opioid binding in vitro.

Several recent reports illustrate the potential of this approach in purifying opioid receptors. SIMONDS et al. (1985) covalently labeled δ-receptors on NG108-15 neuroblastoma-glioma cells with tritiated N-phenyl-N-[1-(2-(4-isothiocyanato) phenylethyl)-4-piperidinyl] pro-panamide (FIT), which served as a marker to follow the receptors in subsequent purification steps. Then antibodies to protein-conjugated FIT were prepared, and used to construct an affinity column. When detergent-solubilized hybrid cell membranes were applied to this column, the FIT-receptor complex was preferentially bound, thus effecting a major purification step. When this step was combined with an additional lectin affinity column elution, the receptor-

FIT complex was purified to essentially homogeneity. It had a molecular weight of 58 kDa.

An alternative immunological approach, which has the considerable advantage of requiring no receptor preparation to begin with, is to prepare anti-idiotypic antibodies. Antibodies are first raised to an opioid ligand, which in principle should contain a site similar to the ligand binding site of the receptor. These antibodies are then used as an antigen to raise anti-antibodies, which should be directed against this binding site.

Using β-endorphin as the original opioid ligand, GRAMSCH et al. (1988) prepared a monoclonal antibody that exhibited binding characteristics similar to opioid receptors. They then used this as an antigen to prepare monoclonal anti-idiotypic antibodies; the resulting hybridoma clones were screened using Fab fragments of the anti-β-endorphin antibody. Two of the positive clones secreted monoclonal antibodies that were able to displace μ- and δ-, but not κ-, opioid ligands from rat brain membranes. This profile matches the selectivity of β-endorphin. Both antibodies also inhibited opioid inhibition of adenylate cyclase in NG108-15 neuroblastomaglioma cells.

Another group reported the presence of anti-idiotypic antibodies to β-endorphin in serum of patients suffering from major depressive disorder (B.F. ROY et al. 1988). Binding of the antibodies to brain membranes was inhibited by several opioid ligands. In addition, the anti-idiotype bound to a 60-kDa peptide in Western immunoblots.

Several groups have now prepared antibodies to opioid receptor preparations that were previously purified in their laboratory. BIDLACK et al. (1981) reported purification of an opioid receptor from Triton-solubilized rat brain membranes, using affinity chromatography. Subsequently, this group prepared a monoclonal antibody to this material, which proved to be directed against the 35-kDa band observed on SDS gels. This mab was capable of partially inhibiting opioid to the solubilized preparation (BIDLACK and DENTON 1985), though long incubation periods were required. Moreover, Fab fragments prepared from the antibody rapidly and completely inhibited binding of μ- and δ-opioid ligands to brain membranes (BIDLACK and O'MALLEY 1986).

MANECKJEE et al. (1987) prepared a polyclonal antibody to a highly purified opioid binding protein they had previously isolated from bovine striatum. This antibody inhibited selectively the binding of μ-opioids to rat brain membranes, and also selectively precipitated a 94K band from detergent-solubilized striatal membranes.

As discussed earlier, we recently purified to homogeneity an opioid binding protein (OBCAM) from bovine brain (CHO et al. 1986), and isolated the cDNA coding for this protein (SCHOFIELD et al. 1989). Both monoclonal and polyclonal antibodies have been prepared to this protein, as well as polyclonal antibodies to peptides corresponding to portions of the predicted amino acid sequence of the cDNA (S. ROY et al. 1988a,b; SCHOFIELD et al. 1989). The monoclonal antibodies, or Fab fragments derivèd from them, inhibit opioid binding to both the purified protein and to brain membranes, with binding of μ-, δ-, and κ-ligands all affected (S. ROY et al. 1988b). The polyclonal antibodies to the purified protein also inhibit opioid binding to brain membranes (S. ROY et al. 1988a).

Although OBCAM shows some selectivity toward μ-alkaloid ligands, the ability of the monoclonal Fab fragments to inhibit δ- and κ-opioid binding brain membranes suggests that these other receptors may contain common antigentic epitopes. Furthermore, the monoclonal Fabs also inhibit opioid binding to NG108-15 cell membranes, which contain exclusively δ-opioid receptors. Western blot analysis revealed that the antibodies interacted with a 39-kDa band as well as a 58-kDa band in NG108-15 cells. In addition, a polyclonal antibody, raised to a peptide corresponding to a portion of OBCAM's predicted amino acid sequence, specifically absorbed proteins of 39 and 58 kDa from detergent-solubilized NG108-15 cell membranes (S. ROY, unpublished data). It is of interest to note that, while OBCAM has a molecular weight of 58 kDa, the amino acid content of OBCAM gives a theoretical molecular weight of just 38 kDa (SCHOfiELD et al. 1989); thus the differences in molecular weights between the two NG108-15 species reacitve with the OBCAM antibodies could possibly be due to differences in glycosylation.

To determine whether either of the two bands recognized by polyclonal antibodies to OBCAM in NG108-15 cells are involved in opioid receptor function, the cells were treated with 100 nM DADLE for 24 h, to downregulate the opioid receptors in these cells. Under these conditions, both bands were decreased, in a time-dependent, naloxone-reversible fashion. However, the 39-kDa band proved to be much more sensitive to this treatment.

Selective downregulation was also demonstrated by first labeling NG108-15 cells with [^{35}S]methionine, isolating and solubilizing their surface membranes, and passing the solubilized material down an affinity column constructed from the antibodies. As expected, a portion of the solubilized radioactivity was specifically absorbed, which could be eluted with high salt, and this radioactivity was reduced in downregulated cells. However, the extent of reduction was about 50%. This was more than expected on the basis of gel experiments, as the 58-kDa band that was not downregulated was of greater intensity than the 39-kDa band, and the latter was reduced in intensity by only about half in downregulated cells. When the material specifically absorbed to the antibody column was analyzed by SDS gels and ^{35}S-autoradiography, only the 39-kDa band was present; however, if this material was iodinated, a 58-kDa band also appeared. This suggests that either this latter species does not contain cysteine and methione residues, or that it turns over relatively slowly. We are currently carrying out studies to distinguish between these possibilities.

We have also demonstrated a role of OBCAM-like material in downregulation using immunofluorescence. In these studies, NG108-15 cells were incubated with a peptide antibody, MN-3, followed by a fluorescent goat anti-Ig. Fluorescent material on the surface of these cells clearly indicated the presence of OBCAM or an OBCAM-like protein. Moreover, treatment of the cells for 24 h with opioid agonist resulted in a marked decrease in the immunofluorescence. That this disappearance was specifically related to opioid receptor downregulation was indicated by two observations. First, the ligand selectivity of the downregulation of the antibody-reactive material closely paralleled that of opioid receptor downregulation. Thus incubation of cells for 24 h with 125 nM DADLE, etorphine, or β-endorphin resulted in 60%–95% downregulation, while DAGO and morphine had little effect. Naloxone was able to prevent or reverse the downregulation. Second, chronic treatment of the NG cells with carbachol, a muscarinic agonist, had no effect on immunofluorescence.

D. Antisense cDNA

Any receptor or other cell protein is coded for by a specific nucleotide sequence contained on one of the two strands of DNA in the chromosomes, which is transcribed into an equivalent mRNA sequence. The sequence on the other strand is antiparallel or "antisense" to the coding strand, and, in theory, mRNA containing this sequence should bind to the sense strand, forming a duplex, just as occurs with genetic DNA. Since mRNA is translated in a single-strand form, such duplex formation should inhibit translation of the sense mRNA, thus selectively preventing expression of that gene product.

Several studies have now demonstrated the power of the antisense technique to block the expression of selective genes of known function, suggesting that it could ultimately have very valuable clinical applications. For example, antisense RNA injected into cultured cells can prevent infection of those cells by certain viruses (AGRAWAL et al. 1989; KABANOV et al. 1990; SANKAR et al. 1989; VON RUDEN and GILBOA 1989), while injection of antisense cDNA into mouse embryos resulted in their development into adults resembling those with specific genetic mutations (KATSUKI et al. 1988). But for the present, antisense oligonucleotides are an elegant tool for confirming or elucidating the functions of newly cloned proteins. Thus the role of the recently discovered cell protein cyclin in cell growth and cell division was confirmed by demonstrating that its antisense mRNA blocked these processes in cultured cells (JASKULSKI et al. 1988; MINSHULL et al. 1989), while antisense RNA to the transcriptional regulator c-*fos* was shown to inhibit differentiation of endodermal precursor cells (EDWARDS et al. 1988).

Incorporation of an antisense message into cells can be achieved either in a transient fashion, by adding antisense mRNA directly to the cell, or in a stable or permanent fashion, by incorporating antisense cDNA into the genome, which may either block transcription of a specific gene, or stimulate synthesis of antisense mRNA. We have stably transfected NG108–15 cells with a relatively short antisense cDNA sequence to NGD5, designed to bind to the region surrounding the initiation site for transcription. The morphological appearance of these cells indicated that their normal functioning had been seriously compromised. Thus it is clear that the NGD5 gene product plays an important role in cell function, though the nature of that role in opioid receptor function or opioid tolerance remains to be elucidated.

Acknowledgements. Our laboratory's research that was discussed in the article was supported by National Institute of Drug Abuse grants DA00564, DA01583, DA02643, and DA05695, and Research Scientist Awards K05-DA70554 (HHL) and K05-DA00020 (NML).

References

Agrawal S, Ikeuchi T, Sun D, Sarin PS, Konopka A, Maizel J, Zamecnik PC (1989) Inhibition of human immunodeficiency virus in early infected and chronically infected cells by antisense oligodeoxynucleotides and their phosphorothioate analogues. Proc Natl Acad Sci USA 86:7790–7794

Baumbach WR, Horner DL, Logan JS (1989) The growth hormone-binding protein in rat serum is an alternatively spliced form of the rat growth hormone receptor. Genes Dev 3:1199–1205

Bidlack JM, Denton RR (1985) A monoclonal antibody capable of inhibiting opioid binding to rat neural membranes. J Biol Chem 260:15655–15661

Bidlack JM, O'Malley WE (1986) Inhibition of mu and delta but not kappa opioid binding to membranes by Fab fragments from a monoclonal antibody directed against the opioid receptor. J Biol Chem 261:15844–15849

Bidlack JM, Abood LG, Osei-Gyimah P, Archer S (1981) Purification of the opiate receptor from rat brain. Proc Natl Acad Sci USA 78:636–639

Blank U, Ra C, Miller L, White K, Metzger H, Kinet J-P (1989) Complete structure and expression in transfected cells of high affinity IgE Receptor. Nature 337:187–189

Bunzow JR, VanTol HHM, Grandy DK, Albert P, Salon J, Christie M, Machida CA, Neve KA, Civelli O (1988) Cloning and expression of a rat D_2 dopamine receptor cDNA. Nature 336:783–787

Chang KJ, Eckel RW, Blanchard SG (1982) Opioid peptides induce reduction of enkephalin receptors in cultured neuroblastoma cells. Nature 296:446–448

Cho TM, Hasegawa J, Ge BL, Loh HH (1986) Purification to apparent homogeneity of a mu-specific opioid receptor from rat brain. Proc Natl Acad Sci USA 83:4138–4142

Cunningham BA, Hemperly JJ, Murray BA, Predeiger EA, Brackenbury R, Edelman GM (1987) Neural cell adhesion molecule: structure, immunoglobulin-like domains, cell surface modulation, and alternative RNA splicing. Science 236:709–806

Czech MP (1989) Signal transmission by the insulin-like growth factors. Cell 59:235–238

Dixon RAF, Kobilka BK, Strader DJ, Benovic JL, Dohlman HG, Frielle T, Bolanowski MA, Bennett CD, Rands E, Diehl RE, Mumford RA, Slater EE, Sigal IS, Caron MG, Lefkowitz RJ, Strader CD (1986) Cloning of the gene and cDNA for mammalian β-adrenergic receptor and homology with rhodopsin. Nature 321:75–79

Dohlman HG, Caron MG, Lefkowitz RJ (1987) A family of receptors coupled to guanine nucleotide regulatory proteins. Biochemistry 26:2657–2664

Edwards S, Rundell AY, Adamson ED (1988) Expression of c-*fos* antisense RNA inhibits the differentiation of F9 cells to parietal endoderm. Dev Biol 129: 91–102

Fornace AJ Jr, Mitchell JB (1986) Induction of B2 RNA polymerase III transcription by heat shock: enrichment for heat shock induced sequences in rodent cells by hybridization subtraction. Nucleic Acids Res 14:5793–5811

Gioannini TL, Howard AD, Hiller JM, Simon EJ (1985) Purification of an active opioid-binding protein from bovine striatum. J Biol Chem 260:15117–15121

Gramsch C, Schulz R, Kosin S, Herz A (1988) Monoclonal anti-idiotypic antibodies to opioid receptors. J Biol Chem 263:5853–5859

Grenningloh G, Rehm EJ, Goodman CS (1991) Genetic analysis of growth cone guidance in *Drosophila*: Fascidin II functions as a neuronal recognition molecule. Cell 67:45–57

Hasegawa J-I, Loh HH, Lee NM (1987) Lipid requirement for mu opioid receptor binding. J Neurochem 49:1007–1012

Hershey AD, Krause JE (1990) Molecular characterization of a functional cDNA encoding the rat substance P receptor. Science 247:958–961

Jaskulski D, deRiel JK, Mercer WE, Calabretta B, Baserga R (1988) Inhibition of cellular proliferation by Antisense Oligodeoxynucleotides to PCNA cyclin. Science 240:1544–1546

Julius D, MacDermott AB, Axel R, Jessell TM (1988) Molecular characterization of a functional cDNA encoding the serotonin 1c receptor. Science 241:558–564

Kabanov AV, Vinogradov SV, Ovcharenko AV, Krivonos AV, Melik-Nubarou NS, Kiseler VI, Severin ES (1990) A new class of antivirals: antisense oligonucleotides combined with a hydrophobic substituent effectively inhbit influenza virus reproduction and synthesis of virus-specific proteins in MDCK cells. FEBS Lett 259:327–330

Katada T, Gilman AG, Watanabe Y, Bauer S, Jakobs KH (1985) Protein kinase C phosphorylates the inhibitory guanine-nucleotide-binding regulatory component and apparently suppresses its function in hormonal inhibition of adenylate cyclase. Eur J Biochem 151:431–437

Katsuki M, Sato M, Kimura M, Yokoyama M, Kobayashi K, Nomura T (1988) Conversion of normal behavior to shiverer by myelin basic protein antisense cDNA in transgenic mice. Science 241:593–595

Kavathas P, Sukhatme VP, Herzenberg LA, Parnes JR (1984) Isolation of the gene encoding the human T-lymphocyte differentiation antigen Leu2 (T8) by gene transfer and cDNA subtraction. Proc Natl Acad Sci USA 81:7688–7692

Klein R, Conway D, Parada LF, Barbacid M (1990) The *trkB* tyrosine protein kinase gene codes for a second neurogenic receptor that lacks the catalytic kinase domain. Cell 61:647–656

Kobilka BK, Matsui H, Kobilka TS, Yang-Feng TL, Francke U, Caron MG, Lefkowitz RJ, Regan JW (1987) Cloning, sequencing, and expression of the gene coding for the human platelet α-adrenergic receptor. Science 238:650–656

Koski G, Streaty RA, Klee WA (1982) Modulation of sodium-sensitive GTPase by partial opiate agonist: an explanation for the dual requirement for Na^+ and GTP in inhibitory regulation of adenylate cyclase. J Biol Chem 257: 14035–14040

Kubo T, Fukuda K, Mikami A, Maeda A, Takahashi H, Mishina M, Haga T, Haga K, Ichiyama A, Kangawa K, Kojima M, Matsuo H, Hirose T, Numa S (1986) Cloning, sequencing and expression of complementary DNA encoding the muscarinic acetylcholine receptor. Nature 323:411–416

Law PY, Hom DS, Loh HH (1982) Loss of opiate receptor activity in neuroblastoma × glioma NG108-15 hybrid cells after chronic opiate treatment: a multiple step process. Mol Pharmacol 22:1–4

Law PY, Hom DS, Loh HH (1983) Opiate receptor down-regulation and desensitization in neuroblastoma × glioma NG108-15 hybrid cells are two separate cellular adaptation processes. Mol Pharmacol 24:413–424

Lefkowitz RJ, Wessels MR, Stadel JM (1980) Hormones, receptors and cyclic AMP; their roles in target cell refractoriness. Curr Top Cell Regul 17:205–230

Loh HH, Smith AP (1990) Molecular characterization of opioid receptors. Annu Rev Pharmacol Toxicol 30:123–147

Loosfelt H, Misrahi M, Atger M, Salesse R, Hai-Luu Thi MTV, Jolivet A, Guiochon-Mantel A, Sar S, Jallal B, Garnier J, Milgrom E (1989) Cloning and sequencing of porcine LH-hCG receptor cDNA: variants lacking transmembrane domain. Science 245:525–528

Maneckjee R, Archer S, Zukin RS (1987) Characterization of a polyclonal antibody to the mu opioid Receptor. J Neuroimmunol 17:199–208

Minshull J, Blow JJ, Hunt T (1989) Translation of cyclin mRNA is necessary for extracts of activated Xenopus eggs to enter mitosis. Cell 56:947–956

Nishimoto I, Murayama Y, Katada T, Ui M, Ogata E (1989) Possible direct linkage of insulin-like growth factor-II receptor with guanine nucleotide-binding proteins. J Biol Chem 264:14029–14038

Parmentier M, Libert F, Maenhaut C, Lefort A, Gerard C, Perret J, van Sande J, Dumont JE, Vassart G (1989) Molecular cloning of the thyrotropin receptor. Science 246:1620–1622

Peralta EG, Winslow JW, Peterson GL, Smith DH, Ashkenazi A, Ramachandran J, Schimerlik MI, Capon DJ (1987) Primary structure and biochemical properties of an M2 muscarine receptor. Science 236:600–605

Resnick RJ, Racker E (1988) Phosphorylation of the RAS2 gene product by protein kinase A inhibits the activation of yeast adenylyl cyclase. Proc Natl Acad Sci USA 85:2474–2478

Rhyner TA, Biguet NF, Berrard S, Borbely AA, Mallet J (1986) An efficient approach for the selective isolation of specific transcripts from complex brain mRNA populations. J Neurosci Res 16:167–181

Roy BF, Bowen WD, Frazier JS, Rose JW, McFarland HF, McFarlin DE, Murphy DL, Morihasa JM (1988) Human antiidiotypic antibody against opiate receptors. Ann Neurol 24:57–63

Roy S, Zhu YX, Lee NM, Loh HH (1988a) Different molecular weight forms of opioid receptors revealed by polyclonal antibodies. Biochem Biophys Res Commun 150:237–244

Roy S, Zhu YX, Loh HH, Lee NM (1988b) A monoclonal antibody that inhibits opioid binding to rat brain membranes. Biochem Biophys Res Commun 154:688–693

Sankar S, Cheah KC, Porter AG (1989) Antisense oligonucleotide inhibition of encephalomyocarditis virus mRNA translation. Eur J Biochem 184:39–45

Schofield PR, McFarland KC, Hayflick JS, Wilcox JN, Cho TM, Roy S, Lee NM, Loh HH, Seeburg PH (1989) Molecular characterization of a new immunoglobin superfamily protein with potential roles in opioid binding and cell contact. EMBO J 8:489–495

Sharma SK, Nirenberg M, Klee WA (1975a) Morphine receptors are regulators of adenylate cyclase activity. Proc Natl Acad Sci USA 72:590–594

Sharma SK, Klee WA, Nirenberg M (1975b) Dual regulation of adenylate cyclase accounts for narcotic dependence and tolerance. Proc Natl Acad Sci USA 72:3092–3096

Sharma SK, Klee WA, Nirenberg M (1977) Opiate-dependent modulation of adenylate cyclase. Proc Natl Acad Sci USA 74:3365–3369

Sibinga NES, Goldstein A (1988) Opioid peptides and opioid receptors in cells of the immune system. Annu Rev Immunol 6:219–249

Simonds WF, Burke TR, Rice KC, Jacobson AE, Klee WA (1985) Purification of the opioid receptor of NG108-15 neuroblastoma × glioma hybrid cells. Proc Natl Acad Sci USA 82:4774–4778

Smith KA (1987) The two-chain structure of high affinity IL-2 receptors. Immunol Today 8:11–13

Stefano GB, Leung MK, Zhao X, Scharrer B (1989) Evidence for the involvement of opioid neuropeptides in the adherence and migration of immunocompetent invertebrate hemocytes. Proc Natl Acad Sci USA 86:626–630

Streuli M, Krueger NX, Tsai AYM, Saito H (1989) A family of receptor-linked protein tyrosine phosphatases in humans and *Drosophila*. Proc Natl Acad Sci USA 86:8698–8702

Su YF, Harden TK, Perkins JP (1980) Catecholamine-specific desensitization of adenylate cyclase: evidence for a multi-step process. J Biol Chem 255: 7410–7419

Valentine-Braun KA, Northrup JK, Hollenberg MD (1986) Epidermal growth factor (urogastrone)-mediated phosphorylation of a 35 kDa substrate in human placental membranes: relationship to the β subunit of the guanine nucleotide regulatory complex. Proc Natl Acad Sci USA 83:236–240

Von Ruden T, Gilboa E (1989) Inhibition of human T-cell leukemia virus type I replication in primary human T cells that express antisense RNA. J Virol 63:677–682

Williams AF (1987) A year in the life of the immunoglobin superfamily. Immunol Today 8:298–303

Williams AF, Barclay AN (1988) The immunoglobin superfamily – domains for cell surface recognition. Annu Rev Immunol 6:381–405

Yarden Y, Ullrich A (1988) Growth factor receptor tyrosine kinases. Annu Rev Biochem 57:443–478

Zick Y, Sagi-Eisenberg R, Pines M, Gierschik P, Spiegel AM (1986) Multisite phosphorylation of the alpha subunit of transducin by the insulin receptor kinase and protein kinase C. Proc Natl Acad Sci USA 83:9294–9297

CHAPTER 4

Use of Organ Systems for Opioid Bioassay

J.A.M. SMITH and F.M. LESLIE

A. Introduction

I. Rationale for the Use of Isolated Organ Systems

The fundamental principle of bioassay is that interaction of an agonist drug with a specific cellular receptor leads to the production of a biological response. Since this involves a physiological endpoint, receptors can be examined in their native, functional state. This contrasts to radioligand binding assays, which are often carried out under nonphysiological conditions, and can only provide information about the receptor ligand recognition site.

Bioassay systems for measurement of opioid activity range in complexity from single cells to behavioral measures in intact animals (see LESLIE 1987, for review). However, isolated organs are the system of maximal complexity in which accurate measurements of pharmacological constants can be made. Provided that adequate precautions are taken in experimental design, as will be discussed in more detail in Sect. B.II, the primary effects of drugs may be determined in isolated preparations without the problems of pharmacokinetics and reflex mechanisms which are associated with in vivo experimentation. To date, isolated organs have been favored over other in vitro systems for bioassay of opioid activity for reasons of simplicity, convenience, reliability, and cost-effectiveness.

II. Tissue Preparations

Since it was first shown that opioids inhibit the peristaltic reflex of isolated intestinal muscle (TRENDELENBURG 1917), a wide variety of peripheral tissues have been shown to be sensitive to the actions of opioids (see HUGHES 1981; LESLIE 1987; COX 1988 for review). The predominant effect of opioid receptor activation in the periphery is to inhibit smooth muscle contraction, in most cases via decreased release of neurotransmitter from excitatory neuronal inputs (for review see LESLIE 1987).

Although many isolated organs have been shown to be sensitive to the pharmacological actions of opioids, few are used routinely for opioid bioassay. Those which have been used extensively include guinea pig ileum

(GPI) and the vasa deferentia of a number of species, particularly mouse. Many of these preparations exhibit differences in their opioid receptor populations (see Sect. C). Whereas some express multiple types of opioid receptor, more precise analyses may be possible in those which contain homogeneous receptor populations (see Sect. B.I for further discussion).

III. Applications of Peripheral Tissue Bioassay

As will be described in detail in a later chapter (Chap. 26), isolated organs have been used extensively for determination of structure-activity relationships of related drugs. Characterization of opioid agonist or antagonist activity in different isolated tissues can facilitate identification of important pharmacophores in drug molecules and, hence, provide information critical to the development of therapeutic agents with increased receptor selectivity and/or affinity. Such structure-activity analyses have also been used to elucidate the structural nature of opioid receptors, particularly the ligand recognition domains (Chavkin and Goldstein 1981a; Schiller 1982; Portoghese 1990).

The biochemical processes underlying opioid receptor-mediated effects have been examined in isolated peripheral tissues, using electrophysiological activity, second messenger production, transmitter release, or muscle contraction as a physiological endpoint (recently reviewed by Johnson and Fleming 1989). These preparations have also served as useful models for analysis of the mechanisms underlying the phenomena of opioid tolerance and dependence (see Chap. 54, this volume, part II).

The use of isolated organ systems has played a crucial role in the isolation and identification of endogenous opioids in tissue extracts or biological fluids. While some investigators have used membrane binding assays to characterize endogenous opioid activities (Pasternak et al. 1975; Terenius and Wahlstrom 1975), this approach is hampered by an inability to distinguish between opioid-mediated inhibition of radioligand binding and nonspecific effects of other tissue components. Using muscle contraction as a physiological endpoint, however, an opioid-mediated action can be easily identified through the use of specific antagonists, such as naloxone (Hughes 1975). Both GPI and mouse vas deferens (MVD) have been used as bioassay preparations for purification of endogenous opioid peptides (Hughes et al. 1975b; Goldstein et al. 1979; Broccardo et al. 1981). GPI longitudinal muscle-myenteric plexus, which expresses primarily μ- and κ-receptors (see Sect. C.I), was used for the isolation of the κ-selective peptide dynorphin from pituitary extracts (Goldstein et al. 1979) and of the μ-selective peptide dermorphin from frog skin extracts (Broccardo et al. 1981). In contrast, met- and leu-enkephalin, which have high affinity for δ-receptors (Lord et al. 1977), were purified using MVD (Hughes et al. 1975b).

B. Measurement of Pharmacological Constants

I. Theoretical Considerations

1. Determination of Agonist Affinity

In contrast to radioligand binding assay, isolated tissue bioassay cannot provide a direct measure of the affinity of an agonist for a receptor. The measured potency of an agonist in a bioassay preparation is a function of both the affinity of the agonist-receptor complex *and* the efficacy of receptor-effector coupling (KENAKIN 1984; LESLIE 1987). Thus, two drugs which have similar affinities for the same receptor, but different efficacies, will exhibit differences in agonist potency in a given tissue preparation (Fig. 1). Indeed, a drug will behave as a partial agonist or a full antagonist, rather than as an agonist, if its efficacy is very low.

It is important to note that the efficacy of receptor-effector coupling is a function not only of the drug under investigation but also of the tissue in which drug response is measured (Fig. 2). As a result, the potency of an agonist and its agonist/antagonist profile will vary from tissue to tissue, even when interacting with the same receptor type (see Sect. C). Even within a single tissue, drug efficacy is dependent upon experimental con-

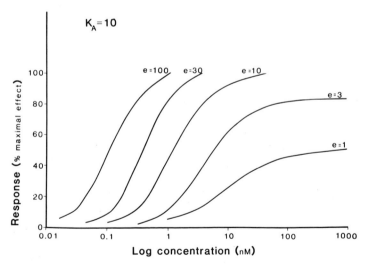

Fig. 1. Relationship between agonist response and concentration, for agonists which have the same dissociation constant ($K_A = 10\,\mathrm{n}M$) but different values of efficacy ($e = 1$–100). Data represent theoretical curves derived from the equation describing the relationship between biological response and stimulus (STEPHENSON 1956). (From LESLIE 1987)

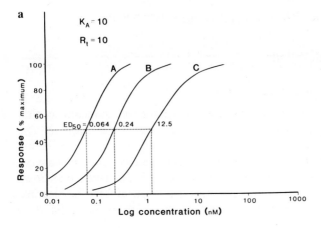

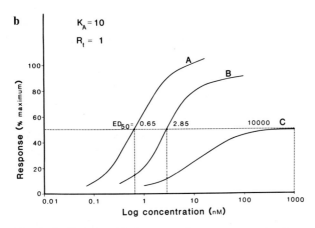

Fig. 2a,b. Relationship between tissue receptor density and agonist response. **a** and **b** compare the response of three agonists (*A*, *B*, *C*) which have the same dissociation constant ($K_A = 10\,nM$) in two different tissues in which the receptor density (R_t) is tenfold different. Data represent theoretical curves derived from the equation describing the relationship between response and stimulus (STEPHENSON 1956) and that for intrinsic efficacy (FURCHGOTT 1966). (From LESLIE 1987)

ditions. Alterations in the extracellular concentration of calcium in the bathing medium, for example, have been shown to influence the potency of opioid agonists in a number of isolated tissue preparations (DOUGALL and LEFF 1987; SHEEHAN et al. 1988; BUDAI and DUCKLES 1989). Such calcium-induced potency changes have been ascribed to alterations in receptor-effector coupling, rather than to differences in receptor affinity and/or number (DOUGALL and LEFF 1987). Similarly, the decreased potencies of μ-agonists in morphine-tolerant GPI appear to result from an alteration in the efficiency of stimulus-response mechanisms in this preparation, rather than in the ligand-binding properties of the receptor (Cox and PADHYA 1977; PORRECA and BURKS 1983; CHAVKIN and GOLDSTEIN 1984).

Given these considerations, it is clear that the concentration of agonist which produces a half-maximal response (IC_{50}) in an isolated tissue preparation does not necessarily correspond with the equilibrium dissociation constant (K_A), i.e., the concentration of drug which occupies 50% of the available receptors. Furthermore, because of possible differences in the effective receptor reserve, agonist potency is dependent upon the tissue in which it is measured and on the assay conditions which are used. In order to characterize ligand selectivities and receptor populations in isolated tissues it is therefore preferable to consider agonist K_A values, which are comparatively constant for a given type of receptor in different preparations (KENAKIN 1984). Measurements of the K_A values of full agonists are frequently made using the method of FURCHGOTT (1966), which compares equiactive agonist concentrations before and after irreversible inactivation of a fraction of the receptor population. Alternatively, an operational model-fitting procedure for analysis of agonist concentration-effect curves can be used (BLACK and LEFF 1983; DOUGALL and LEFF 1987).

The Furchgott method assumes drug interaction with a single receptor type (KENAKIN 1984). However, several of the most widely used bioassay preparations contain heterogeneous populations of opioid receptors (see Sect. C). In tissues with mixed opioid receptor populations, valid K_A estimates will only be obtained if the agonist is sufficiently selective to interact with a single receptor type, even at the high concentrations necessary to elicit a response following irreversible antagonist blockade.

2. Determination of Antagonist Affinity

Pharmacological characterization of opioid receptors in isolated tissues has generally relied upon determination of equilibrium dissociation constants (K_B) of competitive antagonists. K_B or pA_2 (-log K_B) values are calculated by comparing agonist potencies before and after treatment with one or more concentrations of a competitive antagonist. Since comparison of equal responses should represent conditions of equal receptor occupancy for the agonist, this technique requires no assumptions as to the tissue mechanisms which translate drug-receptor stimulus into response.

The antagonist pA_2 has served as the primary means of classification of opioid receptors because it is characteristic of a particular antagonist and receptor type, and is independent of the agonist used or tissue-related parameters (KENAKIN 1984; LESLIE 1987). Although it has recently been suggested that differences in antagonist pA_2 values may occur when agonists interact with the same receptor in different tissues (RAFFA et al. 1989), it has generally been well accepted that differences in antagonist pA_2 values reflect drug interaction at different receptors (FURCHGOTT 1972; SCHILD 1957; KENAKIN 1984). The converse is not true, however. Similar pA_2 or K_B values may result from antagonist interaction at distinct receptor sites (Table 1).

Table 1. Naloxone antagonist potency against μ-, δ-, and κ-agonists in different isolated tissue preparations

Drug	Naloxone K_B (nM)					Refs.
	GPI	MVD	RVD	HVD	LVD	
μ-Agonists						
DAGOL	1.3	3.7	3.9			e
Normorphine	1.9	3.1				c
δ-Agonists						
DADLE	2.6	27.3		34.5		b, d
DSLET	2.3	23.2		29.3		a, d
κ-Agonists						
EKC	15.4	15.8			18.8	e
U50488	28.3	19.4			34.5	e

DAGOL, [D-Ala^2,MePhe^4,gly-ol^5]enkephalin; DADLE,[D-Ala^2,D-Leu^5]enkephalin; DSLET, [D-Ser^2,D-Leu^5]enkephalin-Thr^6; EKC, ethylketocyclazocine.
References: a) Hurlbut et al. (1987); b) Leslie et al. (1980); c) Lord et al. (1977); d) McKnight et al. (1985); e) Miller et al. (1986).

The most rigorous method of determining antagonist affinity in an isolated tissue preparation is by Schild regression analysis (Arunlakshana and Schild 1959). In this approach, agonist concentration-response curves are constructed before and after tissue exposure to several concentrations of antagonist. The ratio of IC$_{50}$ values in the presence and absence of each concentration of antagonist (B), the dose ratio (DR), is calculated and a plot of log (DR-1) vs. log B constructed. Provided that simple, competitive kinetics occur, this Schild plot should be linear and have a slope of unity, with an intercept at the abscissa of -log K_B or pA$_2$.

The Schild analysis assumes that agonist activity reflects drug interaction with a single receptor type. In tissues with heterogeneous opioid receptor populations, such as GPI and MVD, an artifactual pA$_2$ value may be calculated which reflects drug interaction at multiple sites (James et al. 1984). When pA$_2$ values are used as a primary means of receptor classification, the measurement of "intermediate" values may lead to the erroneous identification of novel receptor types. It is important, when constructing Schild plots, to identify deviations from linearity which may indicate interaction with a heterogeneous population of receptors. However, since such deviations may not always be easily detected (Furchgott 1972; Kenakin 1984), these problems may be avoided by the use of highly selective agonists which interact with a single receptor type, even at the high concentrations required to overcome competitive antagonist blockade. It should be noted that nonlinear Schild plots may also be related to nonequilibrium conditions resulting from inappropriate assay methodology (Furchgott 1972; see Sect. B.II).

An alternative method for measurement of antagonist K_B values is the rapid "single-dose" method of KOSTERLITZ and WATT (1968), in which equiactive doses of agonist are determined in the presence and absence of one concentration of antagonist. This method is useful for determination of the affinities of antagonists which have agonist activity, or in tissues which are not viable for prolonged periods or which undergo rapid desensitization. However, this approach assumes competitive antagonism, receptor homogeneity, and equilibrium experimental conditions and, therefore, is not as rigorous as the Schild analysis.

II. Methodological Considerations

1. Choice of Tissue Preparation

Although numerous peripheral organs are sensitive to the actions of opioids (LESLIE 1987; COX 1988), very few are suitable for routine use as bioassay preparations. Various factors, such as expense, ease of dissection, stability of response, and lack of spontaneous activity must all be considered in determining the suitability of a particular tissue. The choice of species is also an important consideration, since peripheral tissues exhibit marked species variability in their responses to administration of opioid agonists (see Sect. C). Even within a single species, strain differences in receptor density and stimulus-response mechanisms may be apparent (BERTI et al. 1978; WATERFIELD et al. 1978; MILLER et al. 1986; SHEEHAN et al. 1988). Thus, in order to ensure reproducibility in isolated tissue experiments, age-, weight-, sex-, and strain-matched animals should be used (KENAKIN 1984).

2. Tissue Preparation and Setup

There are numerous methods to prepare smooth muscle preparations. During dissection, attention should be paid to the anatomical differentiation of the tissue. Thus, for example, the longitudinal muscle-myenteric plexus is advantageous over the intact GPI for isolated tissue work (RANG 1964). The anatomical location of the tissue should be kept constant in order to avoid possible variations in responsiveness, such as has been observed between the prostatic and epididymal portions of the rabbit vas deferens (LVD; OKA et al. 1980). Where drug access to receptors may be limited by a connective tissue sheath, this should be removed prior to tissue setup.

Following dissection, isolated organs are perfused, superfused, or incubated in appropriate nutrient solutions which maintain them in a viable state. The ionic concentration and composition of the bathing medium can influence the basal activity of tissues and their responsiveness to drugs. Calcium concentration, in particular, can be a critical determinant of the sensitivity of isolated preparations to opioids (OPMEER and VAN REE 1979; DOUGALL and LEFF 1987; SHEEHAN et al. 1988; BUDAI and DUCKLES 1989).

Other factors which affect tissue viability and responsiveness include oxygen delivery, and the pH and temperature of the bathing medium. The influence of such factors on tissue responses has been extensively reviewed (Kenakin 1984).

In the majority of bioassay preparations, opioids do not directly affect smooth muscle contractility but, rather, inhibit the electrically stimulated release of an excitatory neurotransmitter (see Leslie 1987, for review). Variations in the intensity of the electrical stimulus can profoundly influence opioid actions (Lees et al. 1972). In general, transmitter release mechanisms are most sensitive to inhibition by opioids at low stimulus frequencies or short train durations (Henderson and Hughes 1976; Cowie et al. 1978; Budai and Duckles 1989). Increases in stimulus frequency or train duration result in decreased potencies of opioid agonists and, in some cases, the manifestation of partial agonist characteristics (Smith 1984).

3. Optimization of Equilibrium Conditions

The equations from which pharmacological constants are derived assume that a drug interacts with a single receptor under equilibrium conditions (Furchgott 1972; Kenakin 1984). If equilibrium conditions do not pertain, the assumptions which underlie the derivation of pharmacological constants are not valid, resulting in serious errors in their estimation. Several factors must be considered in the optimization of equilibrium conditions. These include:

a) Tissue Stability

Pharmacological null procedures, such as the Schild and Furchgott analyses, are based on tests of tissue responsiveness before and after experimental manipulations (see Sect. B.I). In order to obtain valid measures of pharmacological constants using such procedures, it is critical that the sensitivity of the preparation does not change throughout the course of the experiment. Alterations in tissue responsiveness are most apparent in the initial phase of an experiment during equilibration in the novel environment, but may also be observed during the final stages as a tissue undergoes physiological deterioration (Leslie 1987). Systematic decreases in tissue sensitivity may also occur as a result of frequent or prolonged tissue exposure to an agonist. Such desensitization may be receptor mediated, i.e., an agonist-induced conformational change of the receptor, or may reflect a non-selective process such as tissue fatigue.

Controls should be undertaken to confirm that the basal state of a tissue and its sensitivity to drugs do not change during the course of an experiment. In some tissues, such as GPI, it may be necessary to expose the tissue to several concentrations of drug before starting the experiment in order to allow for equilibration (Gyang and Kosterlitz 1966). In other tissues, such as LVD continuous changes in tissue sensitivity may be observed throughout the course of an experiment (OKA et al. 1980; CORBETT et al. 1985). Such changes may be controlled for by continuously monitoring the sensitivity of a matched preparation which is not exposed to the test drug and, from this, calculating correction factors for application to the experimental tissue. Alternatively, a "bracketing" procedure may be used, in which changes in tissue sensitivity are monitored by constructing concentration-response curves to a standard agonist before and after exposure to the test drug.

b) Equilibrium Conditions

The methods of analysis of pharmacological constants assume that, for reversible ligands, the concentration of drug in the vicinity of the receptor is constant and in diffusion equilibrium with the external bathing solution (FURCHGOTT 1972). It is critical to know the true concentration of drug at the receptor, since this is the independent variable from which all calculations of affinity and efficacy are made.

Under ideal conditions, in which there is no active process of removal of the drug from the bathing solution, a finite time is required for the concentration of drug at the receptor to reach equilibrium. It is therefore essential that measurements of agonist and antagonist potency are made only after complete equilibration of the drug within the receptor compartment (FURCHGOTT 1972; KENAKIN 1984). In both GPI and MVD, the rate of onset of drug action has been shown to be inversely related to lipid solubility, probably as a consequence of drug binding at lipid-rich secondary binding sites (KOSTERLITZ et al. 1975). In these isolated tissues, the rate of onset of drug action is also directly correlated with drug concentration (KOSTERLITZ et al. 1975). For certain drugs, such as the κ-selective antagonist norbinaltorphimine (norBNI) an equilibration period of 30 min or more may be required (BIRCH et al. 1987).

A number of factors can result in continuous removal of the drug from the bathing medium, such that equilibrium with the receptor is not achieved (FURCHGOTT 1972; LESLIE 1987). Important considerations include chemical degradative processes, such as oxidation, and nonspecific adsorption to the surface of the organ bath. Probably the most significant factor when using opioid peptides, however, is enzymatic degradation. Peptidase inactivation has long been recognized as a source of error in radioliogand binding assays (LESLIE and GOLDSTEIN 1982; and references therein), but was not initially considered to be as significant in bioassay because of the shorter duration of drug exposure to the tissue. More recently, a number of studies have demonstrated an increase in the activity of opioid peptide agonists in several isolated organ systems following inhibition of endogenous peptidase activity (CORBETT et al. 1982; McKNIGHT et al. 1983; KUNO et al. 1986). Enzymatic degradation of exogenously applied peptides has been confirmed using biochemical methods (MILLER et al. 1985; DIXON and TRAYNOR 1990). All opioid agonists are not equally sensitive to the degradative actions of endogenous peptidases. Whereas the potencies of short-chain endogenous peptides, such as enkephalin, are markedly enhanced by peptidase inhibition, those of longer-chain endogenous peptides, stable peptide analogs, and alkaloids are unaffected (McKnight et al. 1983).

Peptidase degradation of exogenously administered drugs may not only result in underestimation of agonist potency, but also in erroneous assessment of receptor selectivities. Inclusion of peptidase inhibitors in the bathing medium has been reported to increase the agonist potencies of dynorphin and its analogs in GPI, and to alter pA_2 values for naloxone antagonism of their agonist actions (James et al. 1984; Dixon and Traynor 1990). These data suggest that the products of enzymatic degradation have selectivities which differ from those of the parent compounds.

c) Agonist Interaction at More Than One Site

Many peripheral tissues, including GPI and MVD, contain heterogeneous opioid receptor populations, all of which mediate the same response (see Sect. C). When both agonist and antagonist recognize more than one receptor within a tissue preparation, measurement of pharmacological constants can be confounded, as discussed in Sect. B.I2. Such problems may be circumvented by using agonists and/or antagonists which exhibit a high degree of receptor selectivity. Alternatively, isolated tissues with homogeneous receptor populations, such as LVD or hamster vas deferens (HVD), may be used (see Sect. C.III). If neither of these approaches is feasible, preparations with mixed receptor populations may be enriched in a particular receptor type using a "selective protection" protocol, in which the tissue is incubated with the nonselective, irreversible antagonist β-chlornaltrexamine (β-CNA) in the presence of a competing drug which has high affinity and selectivity for a single receptor (Goldstein and James 1984; Sheehan et al. 1986a; Takemori et al. 1986).

In addition to their interactions with opioid receptors, agonist and antagonist drugs may have nonopioid actions which confound measurement of pharmacological constants. Nonopioid actions, defined as those which do not exhibit appropriate stereospecificity and which are not antagonized by naloxone, have been described for both peptides and alkaloids (Kosterlitz and Waterfield 1975a; Walker et al. 1982; Leff and Dougall 1989). Such nonopioid interactions are of particular significance when they induce a functional interaction in the tissue preparation which is being used. Thus, anticholinesterase actions, such as have been described for morphine and meptazinol (Kosterlitz and Waterfield, 1975a; Bill et al. 1983; Galli 1985), will produce functional antagonism in the GPI. In MVD, which has an excitatory sympathetic innervation, nonopioid actions on adrenergic function may obscure opioid inhibitory effects (Leslie 1977). A method for estimating affinity constants of mixed competitive antagonists and functional antagonists has been reported (Hughes and Mackay 1985). Analytical methods to determine the affinity constants of drugs which act as both opioid agonists and functional interactants have also been described (GOODALL et al. 1986).

C. Assay Preparations

As has been described in detail elsewhere (HUGHES 1981; LESLIE 1987; COX 1988), a wide range of peripheral tissues are sensitive to the inhibitory actions of opioid drugs. Few of these tissues have been well characterized, however, in terms of the pharmacology of their opioid receptor populations. The following discussion of opioid receptor properties will be limited to those preparations which have been used most frequently for opioid bioassay.

I. Guinea Pig Ileum

Since the first demonstration that the GPI myenteric plexus-longitudinal muscle is sensitive to morphine (PATON 1957), this tissue has become the "classical" preparation for bioassay of opioids. The specific action of opioids in this tissue is to inhibit electrically stimulated longitudinal muscle contraction, via inhibition of release of the excitatory neurotransmitter acetylcholine (PATON 1957; COX and WEINSTOCK 1966; COWIE et al. 1968; PATON and ZAR 1968). As is described below, pharmacological analysis of opioid actions in GPI is complex, since more than one opioid receptor type is localized on cholinergic nerves in this tissue.

1. μ-Receptors

There is a good correlation between the relative potencies of morphine-like agonists as inhibitors of GPI twitch and as analgesics in man (KOSTERLITZ and WATERFIELD 1975b; Fig. 3). This suggests that GPI contains a μ-receptor with properties similar to that of brain. Radioligand binding studies, in which comparable pharmacological profiles of μ-binding sites in GPI and brain membranes have been observed, lend further support to this view (CREESE and SNYDER 1975; LESLIE et al. 1980; however, see below).

Inactivation studies with the irreversible antagonists, β-funaltrexamine (β-FNA) and β-CNA, have shown that, for many agonists, there is a considerable μ-receptor reserve in GPI, such that IC_{50} is less than K_A (PORRECCA and BURKS 1983; CHAVKIN and GOLDSTEIN 1984; CARROLL et al. 1988; PORRECA et al. 1990). K_A values for twitch inhibition in GPI correlate well with K_I values for inhibition of [³H]naloxone binding to brain membranes in sodium-containing buffer, but not with [³H]DAGOL binding in low ionic strength buffer (CARROLL et al. 1988; Fig. 4). Such findings confirm the similarities between μ-receptors in brain and GPI, and further suggest that the low-affinity state of the receptor is that which is functionally relevant.

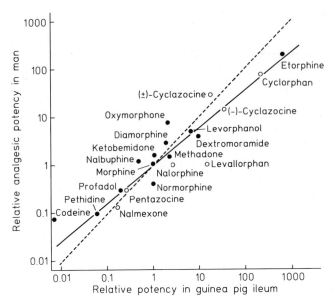

Fig. 3. Correlation between the relative agonist potencies of narcotic analgesics in guinea pig ileum and in analgesia in man (morphine = 1). The values are plotted on a logarithmic scale. Correlation coefficient without codeine, $r = 0.926$ ($n = 19$). The *solid line* has been drawn from log $y = 0.79$ log $x - 0.03$, the slope being different from unity ($P < 0.02$); the *interrupted line* has a slope of unity. The slopes for the compounds with (*open circles*) and without (*closed circles*) antagonist activity do not differ, and the apparent shift of the values of the drugs with antagonist acitivity is not statistically significant. (From Kosterlitz and Waterfield 1975b)

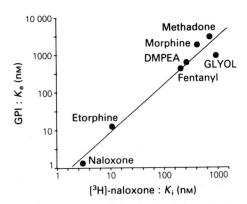

Fig. 4. Relationship between agonist affinity (K_A) determined in the GPI and K_I values for inhibition of [³H]naloxone binding to rat whole brain homogenates for a range of opioid standards. Regression line by least squares analysis, $r = 0.98$; *slope* = 1.25. *GLYOL*, [D-Ala², MePhe⁴, gly-ol⁵]enkephalin; *DMPEA*, [D-Met², Pro⁵]enkephalinamide. (From Carroll et al. 1988)

A number of investigators have postulated the presence of μ-receptor subtypes in GPI (SCHULZ et al. 1981b; TAKEMORI and PORTOGHESE 1985; WARD et al. 1986). μ-Receptor heterogeneity in this tissue was first suggested by Schulz et al. (1981b), in order to explain their findings of incomplete cross-tolerance between μ-selective agonists. However, as has been discussed elsewhere (LESLIE 1987; IVARRSON and NEIL 1989), this lack of cross-tolerance does not constitute definitive proof of receptor hetero-geneity, but may reflect other factors, such as the use of agonists of differing efficacy. As discussed below, subsequent studies of the effects of irreversible receptor inactivation in GPI have provided further evidence of μ-receptor multiplicity, although the data are often inconsistent and must be interpreted carefully.

Two groups (TAKEMORI and PORTOGHESE 1985; WARD et al. 1986) have found that irreversible μ-receptor inactivation by β-FNA shifts the K_B values for naloxone antagonism of morphine and other alkaloid agonists by more than an order of magnitude, but not those for antagonism of DAGOL and related peptides. The increased K_B for naloxone antagonism of morphine in β-FNA-treated tissues presumably reflects interaction of the agonist at κ-receptors, which are less sensitive to naloxone and which are not inactivated by β-FNA (HUTCHINSON et al. 1975; HAYES and KELLY 1985). In contrast, the unaltered K_B for naloxone antagonism of DAGOL suggests that this peptide interacts with residual μ-receptors. Based on these findings, TAKEMORI and PORTOGHESE (1985) have proposed that GPI contains two populations of μ-receptors for which naloxone exhibits equal affinity, one (μ) which is sensitive to both alkaloid and peptide agonists and is inactivated by β-FNA, and another (μ') which is sensitive to peptides, but insensitive to alkaloid agonists and β-FNA.

Although WARD et al. (1986) have reported that increasing concen-trations of β-FNA do not produce further shifts in naloxone sensitivity, other groups, who have used either higher drug concentrations or longer inactivation times, have found significant increases in K_B values for naloxone antagonism of DAGOL (GINTZLER and HYDE 1983; CORBETT et al. 1985; HAYES et al. 1985). In their study, CORBETT et al. (1985) have concluded that the maximum concentrations of β-FNA which are tolerated by GPI do not completely inactivate all μ-receptors, and that differences in the sensitivities of DAGOL and morphine to naloxone antagonism in β-FNA-treated tissues reflect differences in the μ/κ selectivity ratios of these drugs. It should be noted, however, that this same study has found that, although β-FNA pretreatment of GPI produces a marked decrease in the functional activity of μ-agonists, it does not inhibit radioligand binding to μ-sites in GPI membranes as it does in brain homogenates. This finding suggests possible structural differences between μ-binding sites in GPI and brain.

These results are consistent with those of GINTZLER and PASTERNAK (1983), who reported differential effects of naloxonazine or oxymorphonazine pretreatment on [^{3}H]dihydromorphine binding to membranes of GPI and rat and guinea pig brain. Whereas these ligands selectively inactivated a significant proportion of μ-binding sites in brain, similarly treated GPI membranes were virtually unaffected. Based on these findings, the authors concluded that there is a significant population of naloxonazine-sensitive μ_1-sites in brain, while GPI contains a homogeneous population of naloxonazine-insensitive μ_2-sites.

2. κ-Receptors

Some benzomorphan drugs, such as ethylketocyclazocine (EKC), also produce an inhibition of electrically stimulated GPI twitch contraction which is antagonized by naloxone (Hutchinson et al. 1975). However, the K_B value for naloxone antagonism of EKC is almost an order of magnitude greater than for antagonism of morphine, indicating that these drugs interact with different opioid receptor types to produce the same biological effect (Table 1). Selective inactivation studies have provided further evidence that benzomorphans, arylacetamides, and certain peptides, such as dynorphin, interact with κ-receptors in GPI (Chavkin and Goldstein 1981b; Goldstein and James 1984; Miller et al. 1986; Sheehan et al., 1986a; Porreca et al. 1990). As with μ-agonists, there is significant receptor reserve for many κ-agonists in this tissue, such that IC_{50} is less than K_A (Miller et al. 1986; Porreca et al. 1990).

   The radioligand binding properties of κ-sites in GPI have recently been examined and compared to those of brain (Dissanayake et al. 1990). Whereas numerous studies have indicated that κ-binding sites in brain are heterogeneous (Rothman et al. 1990; and references therein), κ-sites in GPI longitudinal muscle-myenteric plexus appear to consist of a homogeneous population with pharmacological properties similar to that of κ_1-sites in brain. In contrast, a second population of binding sites, with pharmacological similarities to κ_2-sites in brain, has been identified in circular muscle.

3. δ-Receptors

There is limited evidence for functional δ-receptors on cholinergic neurons in GPI. Enkephalin and its derivatives do inhibit GPI longitudinal muscle contraction, but the K_B values for naloxone antagonism of their agonist actions are the same as for μ-agonists (Lord et al. 1977; Table 1). Receptor protection studies have further indicated an interaction of enkephalin-like peptides with μ-receptors in this tissue (Chavkin and Goldstein 1981b). Radioligand binding data suggest that GPI longitudinal muscle-myenteric plexus does contain binding sites with properties similar to those of δ-sites in brain (Leslie et al. 1980; Corbett et al. 1985), but the cellular localization and functional role of such sites is unknown. Autoradiographic and physiological studies are needed to further examine this issue.

II. Mouse Vas Deferens

The specific action of opioids in MVD is to inhibit electrically stimulated twitch via inhibition of excitatory neurotransmitter release. In this tissue opioids inhibit the release of the sympathetic neurotransmitter norepinephrine in contrast to the GPI, where parasympathetic cholinergic transmission is modulated by opioid receptor activation (HUGHES et al. 1975a; HENDERSON and HUGHES 1976). As with GPI, however, pharmacological analysis of opioid activity in MVD is complicated by the presence of multiple receptor types within the same tissue.

1. μ-Receptors

There is a high degree of correlation between the relative potencies of μ-agonists in MVD and GPI (HUGHES et al. 1975a; LORD et al. 1977; Fig. 5). However, the absolute potencies of μ-agonists are lower in MVD than in GPI, and the antagonist properties of partial agonists are more apparent (HUGHES et al. 1975a). Considerable strain differences have also been reported in the sensitivity of MVD preparations to the activity of μ-agonists. In particular, a limited μ-agonist response is detectable in MVD from the C57/BL strain (BERTI et al. 1978; WATERFIELD et al. 1978; MILLER et al. 1986). The differential sensitivity to the effects of μ-agonists and partial agonists appears to reflect differences in the degree of receptor

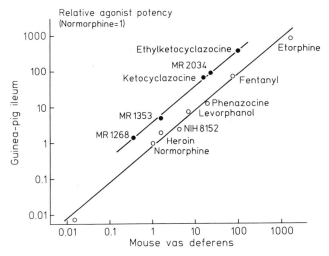

Fig. 5. Relative agonist activities of various μ-(*open circles*) and κ-(*closed circles*) agonists in the MVD and GPI (normorphine = 1). The values are plotted on a logarithmic scale. The two regression lines $y = 1.01x - 0.09$ (*open circles*) and $y = 1.0x + 0.61$ (*closed circles*) have been drawn. The correlation coefficients are $r = 0.993$ ($n = 8$) and $r = 0.999$ ($n = 5$), respectively. (From LORD et al. 1977)

reserve, rather than in the properties of the receptor (Miller et al. 1986; Porreca et al. 1990).

While there is much evidence to indicate that the μ-receptor population in MVD is similar to that of GPI (Hughes et al. 1975a; Lord et al. 1977; Miller et al. 1986), there have been some reports of subtle differences. Porreca et al. (1990), using the Furchgott method to calculate agonist K_A values, have reported a significant difference in the K_A of normorphine in GPI and MVD. Methadone also exhibits differential sensitivity to inactivation by β-CNA in these two preparations. Another group have observed similar differential effects of alkylating antagonists in MVD and GPI (Sayre et al. 1983a,b), and have reported significant differences in pA$_2$ values for naltrexone, but not naloxone, antagonism of morphine in these tissues (Takemori and Portoghese 1984). This latter finding contrasts with our own data, which indicate that the K_B values for a number of μ-antagonists, including naloxone and naltrexone, are consistently higher in MVD than GPI (Table 2). Such findings may reflect tissue differences in pharmacokinetic factors, such as drug penetration, rather than in μ-receptor properties.

2. κ-Receptors

As in the GPI, some benzomorphans, arylacetamides, and dynorphin-like peptides interact with κ-receptors to inhibit longitudinal muscle contractions of MVD. The actions of selective μ- and κ-agonists in MVD can be distinguished by selective inactivation paradigms (Goldstein and James 1984; Hayes et al. 1985; Takemori et al. 1986). Also, K_B values for naloxone antagonism of the actions of κ-agonists are an order of magnitude greater than for antagonism of μ-agonists (Lord et al. 1977; Miller et al. 1986; Table 1).

There is considerable evidence that the κ-receptor population of MVD is pharmacologically similar to that of GPI. A high correlation has been

Table 2. Antagonist potencies against normorphine in the guinea pig ileum and mouse vas deferens

Drug	K_B (nM)		K_B (MVD)
	GPI	MVD	K_B (GPI)
Naltrexone	0.38 ± 0.07	0.64 ± 0.02	1.7
MR2266	1.54 ± 0.09	1.90 ± 0.16	1.3
Naloxone	1.89 ± 0.15	3.66 ± 0.29	1.9
GPA1843	19.8 ± 3.9	29.1 ± 3.3	1.5
FR-13-J	37.2 ± 3.2	68.8 ± 7.1	1.8

Values represent the mean ± standard error of the mean of at least three independent observations. (Leslie 1977).

found between the relative potencies of κ-agonists in these two preparations (LORD et al. 1977; MILLER et al. 1986; Fig. 5). Although the absolute potencies of κ-agonists are lower in MVD than in GPI, this is postulated to result from differences in tissue receptor reserve (COX and CHAVKIN 1983). The reported similarities in agonist K_A values and antagonist K_B values support this view (LORD et al. 1977; MILLER et al. 1986; BIRCH et al. 1987; PORRECA et al. 1990; Table 1).

3. δ-Receptors

Unlike GPI, there appear to be functional δ-receptors in MVD. Enkephalin-like peptides are much more potent inhibitors of muscle contraction in MVD than in GPI (LORD et al. 1977), and have significantly lower K_A values in this tissue (PORRECA et al. 1990). The actions of enkephalin and its analogs in the two tissues can be further distinguished by the potency of naloxone as antagonist, with K_B values for naloxone antagonism of enkephalin-like peptides being more than an order of magnitude greater in MVD than in GPI (LORD et al. 1977; LESLIE et al. 1980; Table 1). Selective inactivation studies have further indicated that enkephalin analogs interact with a specific δ-receptor population in MVD (GOLDSTEIN and JAMES 1984; TAKEMORI et al. 1986).

In general, the relative potencies of δ-selective agonists for twitch inhibition in MVD correlate well with those for inhibition of radioligand binding to δ-sites in brain (LORD et al. 1977; LESLIE et al. 1980). The pharmacological profile of δ-binding sites in MVD membranes has also been reported to be similar to that of brain (LESLIE et al. 1980). Recent studies have suggested some possible differences in the pharmacology of these two δ-receptor populations, however. Several opioid peptides, including certain conformationally restricted or cyclic enkephalin analogs (SHIMOHIGASHI et al. 1987; BRYAN et al. 1989) and β-casomorphin analogs (BRANTL et al. 1982), are potent inhibitors of radioligand binding to δ-sites in brain, but are relatively inactive in MVD bioassay. Direct comparison of the potencies of conformationally restricted enkephalin analogs to inhibit radioligand binding in brain and MVD membranes suggests that these potency differences do reflect differences in the affinities of these drugs for δ-sites in the two tissues (VAUGHN et al. 1990).

III. Other Vasa Deferentia

1. Rat Vas Deferens

In contrast to other peptides and alkaloids, β-endorphin is a potent inhibitor of electrically evoked longitudinal muscle contractions of rat vas deferens (RVD) (LEMAIRE et al. 1978; SCHULZ et al. 1979; GARZON et al. 1985; SHOOK et al. 1988). This observation has led to the suggestion that RVD contains a novel population of ε-opioid receptors which have high affinity and selectivity for β-endorphin (Schulz et al. 1979; Garzon et al. 1985; Shook et al. 1988). The finding that the structure-activity relationships for β-endorphin and its analogs in RVD are distinct from those in GPI and MVD has provided further support for this hypothesis (Schulz et al. 1981a; Huidobro-Toro et al. 1982).

Subsequent studies have shown that RVD does contain a significant population of μ-receptors (Smith and Rance 1983; Miller et al. 1986; Sheehan et al. 1988). This tissue has a small μ-receptor reserve, however, such that only those agonists with high intrinsic activity can elicit a response, while other drugs, such as morphine, act as pure antagonists (Miller et al. 1986; Carroll et al. 1988). As with other tissue preparations, the efficiency of μ-receptor coupling in RVD is highly influenced by the concentration of calcium in the extracellular medium (Sheehan et al. 1988). A reduction in Ca^{2+} ion concentration from 2.5 to 1.25 mM produces a marked increase in the potency of μ full agonists in this preparation, and results in the expression of agonist activity for μ partial agonists such as morphine (Sheehan et al. 1988). The pharmacological properties of μ-receptors in RVD appear to be very similar to those of other tissues. A high correlation between K_B values for antagonism of DAGOL agonist activity in RVD and MVD has been reported (Miller et al. 1986; Fig. 6). K_B values for antagonism of DAGOL agonist activity in RVD are also highly correlated with K_I values for inhibition of [^{3}H]naloxone binding to rat brain membranes (Carroll et al. 1988; Fig. 7).

A small population of δ-receptors has also been identified in the vasa deferentia of Sprague-Dawley rats (Smith and Rance 1983; Nicolaou and Zioudrou 1985; Smith and Carter 1986). The coupling of these δ-receptors is also highly sensitive to manipulations of buffer ion concentrations, such that δ-agonist effects are most clearly demonstrable in reduced calcium buffers. Expression of δ-receptors in RVD is strain dependent, and is not detectable in vasa from PVG rats (Smith and Carter 1986; Sheehan et al. 1988).

With evidence for the presence of both μ- and δ-receptor populations in RVD, there has been considerable controversy as to whether β-endorphin produces its biological effects through interaction with these receptor types or with a specific ε-receptor. Garzon et al. (1985) have confirmed the presence of μ-receptors in RVD. However, their analysis of the combined effects of β-endorphin and μ-agonists in this preparation has suggested functional synergism following activation of two distinct receptors with a common effector, rather than interaction at the same receptor. Additional selective protection studies, in which pretreatment with β-endorphin has been shown to differentially protect against β-FNA-induced receptor inactivation, provides further support for this hypothesis.

In contrast to these data, other groups have failed to detect the existence of a unique ε-receptor in RVD (Smith and Rance 1983; Sheehan et al.

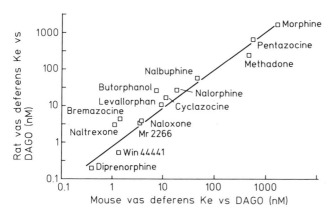

Fig. 6. Correlation between antagonist affinities (K_e) against DAGO in the MVD and RVD preparations. $r = 0.944$; *slope* $= 0.966$. DAGO, [D-Ala², MePhe⁴, gly-ol⁵]enkephalin. (From MILLER et al. 1986)

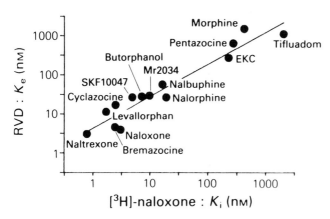

Fig. 7. Relationship between antagonist affinity (K_e) determined in the RVD and K_I values for inhibition of [³H]naloxone binding to rat whole brain homogenates for a range of opioid standards. Regression line by least squares analysis, $r = 0.96$; *slope* $= 0.82$. (From CARROLL et al. 1988) *EKC*, ethylketocyclazocine

1988). In particular, SHEEHAN et al. (1988) have shown that tissue responses to DAGOL and β-endorphin are blocked to the same extent by pretreatment with β-CNA. Furthermore, in a selective protection paradigm, pretreatment with DAGOL provides equivalent protection of the receptors activated by β-endorphin and DAGOL from inactivation by β-CNA. This group and others (GILLAN et al. 1981; KUNO et al. 1986) have reported small, but significant, differences in pA₂ values for naloxone antagonism of

DAGOL and β-endorphin in RVD. Furthermore, β-endorphin and PL017 exhibit differential sensitivity to antagonism by the μ-selective blocker CTOP (Shook et al. 1988). While these findings may indicate that β-endorphin and μ-agonists interact with different receptors, it has been suggested that enzymatic degradation of β-endorphin in RVD may disrupt equilibrium conditions and confound determination of accurate pA_2 values (Sheehan et al. 1988). It should be noted, however, that a cocktail of peptidase inhibitors, which increased met-enkephalin potency 200-fold in RVD (McKnight et al. 1983), had no effect on the potency of β-endorphin in this preparation (Sheehan et al. 1988). It is not presently known whether this reflects lack of degradation of β-endorphin in RVD or the use of inappropriate enzyme inhibitors.

2. Hamster Vas Deferens

There is good evidence that sympathetic transmission in the vas deferens of the Syrian Golden hamster is modulated by a homogeneous population of δ-receptors (McKnight et al. 1985; Sheehan et al. 1986b). Agonists which have high affinity for δ-receptors inhibit electrically stimulated longitudinal muscle contractions of HVD, while μ- and κ-agonists do not. K_B values for naloxone antagonism of agonist actions in this preparation are consistent with those for antagonism at δ-sites in MVD (Sheehan et al. 1986b; Table 1). Furthermore, the δ-selective antagonist ICI 174864 (Cotton et al. 1984) is a potent inhibitor of opioid agonist activity in HVD.

There is a high degree of enzymatic activity in HVD, such that the peptidase inhibitor cocktail which has been shown to be effective in other isolated tissue preparations, $30 \mu M$ bestatin, $0.3 \mu M$ thiorphan, $2 mM$ Leu-Leu, and $10 \mu M$ captopril, does not provide full protection of enkephalin and its analogs (McKnight et al. 1985). An increase in the thiorphan concentration of the inhibitor cocktail to $10 \mu M$ and the incorporation of an additional aminopeptidase inhibitor, amastatin ($10 \mu M$) greatly enhances the potency of met-enkephalin in HVD (McKnight et al. 1985). However, even when protected from enzymatic degradation, δ-agonists are considerably less potent in this tissue than in MVD. This potency difference appears to reflect a low receptor reserve in HVD as compared to MVD, rather than a difference in the properties of δ-receptors in the two tissues (Sheehan et al. 1986b).

3. Rabbit Vas Deferens

A number of studies have indicated that sympathetic transmission in LVD is modulated by a pure population of κ-receptors (Oka et al. 1980; Corbett et al. 1985; Hayes and Kelly 1985; Miller et al. 1986). Agonists with high affinity for κ-, but not μ- or δ-, receptors are potent inhibitors of electrically stimulated LVD twitch. The potencies of κ-agonists are approximately twofold higher in LVD than in MVD, and more than an order of magnitude lower than in GPI (MILLER et al. 1986). However, these potency differences appear to reflect differences in receptor reserve rather than in the properties of the receptor. Potencies for antagonism of EKC by naloxone, norBNI, and a number of other compounds are quite similar in these three tissue preparations (MILLER et al. 1986; BIRCH et al. 1987; Table 1).

Although the homogeneity of its receptor population makes LVD a valuable bioassay preparation, there are a number of technical difficulties associated with the use of this tissue. EKC, and other κ-agonists, are slow to equilibrate, with a single dose often taking as long as 30 or 40 min to achieve maximal effect (HAYES and KELLY 1985; VERLINDE and DE RANTER 1988). On washout, the twitch response also recovers slowly, necessitating the use of cumulative dosing schedules (OKA et al. 1980; VERLINDE and DE RANTER 1988). Significant changes in tissue sensitivity occur throughout the course of an experiment, making it difficult to relate the potency of a compound to that of a reference one in the same preparation (OKA et al. 1980; CORBETT et al. 1985; VERLINDE and DE RANTER 1988). Furthermore, significant interexperimental variability has been noted, with large differences between individual tissues in both agonist potency and maximal response (VERLINDE and DE RANTER 1988; HUNTER et al. 1990).

D. Conclusions

Over the last quarter of a century, organ system bioassays have provided an invaluable tool for studying the properties of opioid receptors and of the drugs which interact with them. In order to obtain the most accurate data, however, one must understand the methodological limitations of this technique. In particular, care must be taken to ensure that equilibrium conditions exist, since this is a fundamental assumption of the equations from which pharmacological constants are derived. It is also important to understand the theoretical framework which governs drug-receptor interaction and the measurement of tissue response. Thus, agonist potency and the manifestation of antagonist characteristics are a function, not only of a drug's affinity for the receptor, but also of its efficacy, which is a tissue-related parameter.

Since the pharmacological properties of opioid receptors in peripheral tissues are generally similar to those of brain, organ systems provide a good model of central nervous system function. However, subtle differences have been reported in some of the receptor characteristics of different tissues. While this may indicate receptor microheterogeneity, it may also result from a number of other factors which have been discussed above. Isolation of the genes encoding for opioid receptor proteins will be necessary to determine whether these pharmacological distinctions reflect structural differentiation.

References

Arunlakshana O, Schild HO (1959) Some quantitative uses of drug antagonists. Br J Pharmacol 14:48–58

Berti F, Bruno F, Omini C, Racagni G (1978) Genotype dependent response of morphine and methionine-enkephalin on the electrically induced contractions of the mouse vas deferens. Naunyn Schmiedebergs Arch Pharmacol 305: 5–8

Bill D, Hartley JE, Stephens RJ, Thompson AM (1983) The antinociceptive activity of meptazinol depends on both opiate and cholinergic mechanisms. Br J Pharmacol 79:191–199

Birch PJ, Hayes AG, Sheehan MJ, Tyers MB (1987) Norbinaltorphimine: antagonist profile at κ opioid receptors. Eur J Pharmacol 144:405–408

Black JW, Leff P (1983) Operational models of pharmacological agonism. Proc R Soc Lond [Biol] 220:141–162

Brantl V, Pfeiffer A, Herz A, Henschen A, Lottispeich F (1982) Antinociceptive properties of β-casomorphin analogs as compared to their affinities towards μ and δ opiate receptor sites in brain and periphery. Peptides 3:793

Broccardo M, Erspamer V, Falconieri Erspamer G, Improta G, Linari G, Melchiorri P, Montecucchi PC (1981) Pharmacological data on demorphins, a new class of potent opioid peptides from amphibian skin. Br J Pharmacol 73:625–631

Bryan WM, Callahan JF, Codd EE, Lemieuxc, Moore ML, Schiller PW, Walker RF, Huffman WF (1989) Cyclic enkephalin analogues containing α-amino-β-mercapto-β, β-pentamethylenepropionic acid at positions 2 or 5. J Med Chem 32:302–304

Budai D, Duckles SP (1989) Opioid-induced prejunctional inhibition of vasoconstriction in the rabbit ear artery: alpha-2 adrenoceptor activation and external calcium. J Pharmacol Exp Ther 251(2):497–501

Carroll JA, Shaw JS, Wickenden AD (1988) The physiological relevance of low agonist affinity binding at opioid μ-receptors. Br J Pharmacol 94:625–631

Chavkin C, Goldstein A (1981a) Specific receptor for the opioid peptide dynorphin: structure-activity relationships. Proc Natl Acad Sci USA 78:6543–6547

Chavkin C, Goldstein A (1981b) Demonstration of a specific dynorphin receptor in guinea pig ileum myenteric plexus. Nature 291:591–593

Chavkin C, Goldstein A (1984) Opioid receptor reserve in normal and morphine-tolerant guinea pig ileum myenteric plexus. Proc Natl Acad Sci USA 81: 7253–7257

Corbett AD, Paterson SJ, McKnight AT, Magan J, Kosterlitz HW (1982) Dynorphin (1–8) and dynorphin (1–9) are ligands for the κ-subtype of opiate receptor. Nature 299:79–81

Corbett AD, Kosterlitz HW, McKnight AT, Paterson SJ, Robson LE (1985) Pre-incubation of guinea-pig myenteric plexus with β-funaltrexamine: discrepancy between binding assays and bioassays. Br J Pharmacol 85:665–673

Cotton R, Giles MG, Miller L, Shaw JS, Timms D (1984) ICI174864: a highly selective antagonist for the opioid δ-receptor. Eur J Pharmacol 97:331–332

Cowie AL, Kosterlitz HW, Watt AJ (1968) Mode of action of morphine-like drugs on autonomic neuroeffectors. Nature 220:1040–1042

Cowie AL, Kosterlitz HW, Waterfield AA (1979) Factors influencing the release of acetylcholine from the myenteric plexus of the ileum of the guinea-pig and rabbit. Br J Pharmacol 64:565–580

Cox BM (1988) Peripheral actions mediated by opioid receptors. In: Pasternak GW (ed) The opiate receptors. Humana, Clifton, p 357

Cox BM, Chavkin C (1983) Comparison of dynorphin-selective kappa receptors in mouse vas deferens and guinea pig ileum. Mol Pharmacol 23:36–43

Cox BM, Padhya R (1977) Opiate binding and effect in ileum preparations from normal and morphine pretreated guinea-pigs. Br J Pharmacol 61:271–278

Cox BM, Weinstock M (1966) The effect of analgesic drugs on the release of acetyl-choline from electrically stimulated guinea pig ileum. Br J Pharmacol 27:81–92

Creese I, Snyder SH (1975) Receptor binding and pharmacological activity of opiates in the guinea-pig intestine. J Pharmacol Exp Ther 194:205–219

Dissanayake VUK, Hunter JC, Hill RG, Hughes J (1990) Characterization of κ-opioid receptors in the guinea-pig ileum. Eur J Pharmacol 182:73–82

Dixon DM, Traynor JR (1990) Evidence that the agonist action of dynorphin A (1–8) in the guinea-pig myenteric plexus may be mediated partly through conversion to [Leu⁵]enkephalin. Br J Pharmacol 101:674–678

Dougall IG, Leff P (1987) Pharmacological analysis of the calcium-dependence of μ-receptor agonism. Br J Pharmacol 92:723–731

Furchgott RF (1966) The use of β-haloalkylamines in the differentiation of receptors and in the determination of dissociation constants of receptor-agonist complexes. Adv Drug Res 3:21

Furchgott RF (1972) The classification of adrenoceptors (adrenergic receptors). An evaluation from the standpoint of receptor theory. In: Blaschko H, Muscholl E (eds) Catecholamines. Springer, Berlin Heidelberg New York, p 283 (Handbook of experimental pharmacology, vol 33)

Galli A (1985) Inhibition of cholinesterases by the opioid analgesic meptazinol. Biochem Pharmacol 34:1579–1581

Garzon J, Schulz R, Herz A (1985) Evidence for the ε-type of opioid receptor in the rat vas deferens. Mol Pharmacol 28:1–9

Gillan MGC, Kosterlitz HW, Magnan J (1981) Unexpected antagonism in the rat vas deferens by benzomorphans which are agonists in other pharmacological tests. Br J Pharmacol 72:13–15

Gintzler AR, Hyde D (1983) Unmasking myenteric delta receptors. Life Sci 33 [suppl 1]:323–325

Gintzler AR, Pasternak GW (1983) Multiple mu receptors: evidence for mu₂ sites in the guinea pig ileum. Neurosci Lett 39:51–56

Goldstein A, James IF (1984) Site-directed alkylation of multiple opioid receptors. Mol Pharmacol 25:343–348

Goldstein A, Tachibana S, Lowney LI, Hunkapiller M, Hood L (1979) Dynorphin-(1–13), an extraordinarily potent opioid peptide. Proc Natl Acad Sci USA 76:6666–6670

Goodall J, Hughes IE, Mackay D (1986) Quantification of the actions of agonists that simultaneously act on a particular type of receptor and have separate functional interactant properties. Br J Pharmacol 88:639–644

Gyang EA, Kosterlitz HW (1966) Agonist and antagonist actions of morphine-like drugs on the guinea-pig isolated ileum. Br J Pharmacol 27:514–527

Hayes AG, Kelly A (1985) Profile of activity of κ receptor agonists in the rabbit vas deferens. Eur J Pharmacol 110:317–322

Hayes AG, Sheehan MJ, Tyers MB (1985) Determination of the receptor selectivity of opioid agonists in the guinea-pig ileum and mouse vas deferens using β-FNA. Br J Pharmacol 86:899–904

Henderson G, Hughes J (1976) The effects of morphine on the release of noradrenaline from the mouse vas deferens. Br J Pharmacol 57:551–557

Hughes IE, Mackay D (1985) Quantification of the characteristics of antagonists exhibiting both competitive antagonism and functional interaction. Br J Pharmacol 85:271–275

Hughes J (1975) Isolation of an endogenous compound from the brain with pharmacological properties similar to morphine. Brain Res 88:195–306

Hughes J (1981) Peripheral opiate receptor mechanisms. Trends Pharmacol Sci 2: 21–24

Hughes J, Kosterlitz HW, Leslie FM (1975a) Effects of morphine on adrenergic transmission in the mouse vas deferens. Assessment of agonist and antagonist potencies of narcotic analgesics. Br J Pharmacol 53:371–381

Hughes J, Smith TW, Kosterlitz HW, Fothergill, LA, Morgan BA, Morris HR (1975b) Identification of two related pentapeptides from the brain with potent opiate agonist activity. Nature 258:577–579

Huidobro-Toro JP, Caturay EM, Ling N, Lee NM, Loh HH, Way EL (1982) Studies on the structual prerequisites for the activation of the β-endorphin receptor on the rat vas deferens. J Pharmacol Exp Ther 222:262–269

Hunter JC, Leighton GE, Meecham KG, Boyle S, Horwell DC, Rees DC, Hughes J (1990) CI-977, a novel and selective agonist for the κ-opioid receptor. Br J Pharmacol 101:183–189

Hurlbut DE, Evans CJ, Barchas JD, Leslie FM (1987) Pharmacological properties of a proenkephalin A-derived opioid peptide: BAM 18. Eur J Pharmacol 138:359–366

Hutchinson M, Kosterlitz HW, Leslie FM, Waterfield AA, Terenius L (1975) Assessment in the guinea-pig ileum and mouse vas deferens of benzomorphans which have a strong antinociceptive activity but do not substitute for morphine in the dependent monkey. Br J Pharmacol 55:541–546

Ivarsson M, Neil A (1989) Differences in efficacies between morphine and methadone demonstrated in the guinea pig ileum: a possible explanation for previous observations on incomplete opioid cross-tolerance. Pharmacol Toxicol 65:368–371

James IF, Fischli W, Goldstein A (1984) Opioid receptor selectivity of dynorphin gene products. J Pharmacol Exp Ther 228:88–93

Johnson SM, Fleming WW (1989) Mechanisms of cellular adaptive sensitivity changes: applications to opioid tolerance and dependence. Pharmacol Rev 41(4):435–488

Kenakin TP (1984) The classification of drugs and drug receptors in isolated tissues. Pharmacol Rev 36:165–183

Kosterlitz HW, Waterfield AA (1975a) An analysis of the phenomenon of acute tolerance to morphine in the guinea-pig isolated ileum. Br J Pharmacol 53:131–138

Kosterlitz HW, Waterfield AA (1975b) In vitro models in the study of structure-activity relationships of narcotic analgesics. Annu Rev Pharmacol 15:29–47

Kosterlitz HW, Watt AJ (1968) Kinetic parameters of narcotic agonists and antagonists, with particular reference to N-allylnoroxymorphone (naloxone). Br J Pharmacol 33:266–276

Kosterlitz HW, Leslie FM, Waterfield AA (1975) Rates of onset and offset of action of narcotic analgesics in isolated preparations. Eur J Pharmacol 32:10–16

Kuno Y, Aoki K, Kajiwara M, Ishii K, Oka T (1986) The relative potency of enkephalins and β-endorphin in guinea-pig ileum, mouse vas deferens and rat vas deferens after the administration of peptidase inhibitors. Jpn J Pharmacol 41:273–281

Lees GM, Kosterlitz HW, Waterfield AA (1972) Characteristics of morphine-sensitive release of neurotransmitter substances. In: Kosterlitz HW, Collier HOJ, Villareal JE (eds) Agonist and antagonist actions of narcotic analgesic drugs. Macmillan, London, pp 142–152

Leff P, Dougall IG (1989) Estimation of affinities and efficacies for κ-receptor agonists in the guinea-pig ileum. Br J Pharmacol 96:702–706

Lemaire S, Magnan J, Regoli D (1978) Rat vas deferens a specific bioassay for endogenous opioid peptides. Br J Pharmacol 64:327–329

Leslie FM (1977) Opiate receptor mechanisms: an in vitro analysis. PhD thesis, University of Aberdeen, Great Britain

Leslie FM (1987) Methods used for the study of opioid receptors. Pharmacol Rev 39(3):197–249

Leslie FM, Goldstein A (1982) Degradation of dynorphin (1–13) by membrane-bound rat brain enzymes. Neuropeptides 2:185–196

Leslie FM, Chavkin C, Cox BM (1980) Opioid binding properties of brain and peripheral tissues: evidence for heterogeneity in opioid ligand binding sites. J Pharmacol Exp Ther 214:395–402

Lord JAH, Waterfield AA, Hughes J, Kosterlitz HW (1977) Endogenous opioid peptides: multiple agonists and receptors. Nature 267:495–499

McKnight AT, Corbett AD, Kosterlitz HW (1983) Increase in potencies of opioid peptides after peptidase inhibition. Eur J Pharmacol 86:393–402

McKnight AT, Corbett AD, Marcoli M, Kosterlitz HW (1985) The opioid receptors in the hamster vas deferens are of the δ-type. Neuropharmacology 24: 1011–1017

Miller L, Rance MJ, Shaw JS, Traynor JR (1985) Conversion of dynorphin-(1–9) to [Leu^5]enkephalin by the mouse vas deferens in vitro. Eur J Pharmacol 116: 159–163

Miller L, Shaw JS, Whiting EM (1986) The contribution of intrinsic activity to the action of opioids in vitro. Br J Pharmacol 87:595–601

Nicolaou N, Zioudrou C (1985) The effects of calcium on the responses to opioid peptides and morphine in the rat vas deferens. Communication to the International Narcotics Research Conference Abstr Handbook p 160

Oka T, Negishi K, Suda M, Matsumiya T, Inazu T, Masaaki U (1980) Rabbit vas deferens: a specific bioassay for opioid κ-receptor agonists. Eur J Pharmacol 73:235–236

Opmeer FA, van Ree JM (1979) Competitive antagonism of morphine action in vitro by calcium. Eur J Pharmacol 53:395–397

Pasternak GW, Goodman R, Snyder SH (1975) An endogenous morphine-like factor in mammalian brain. Life Sci 16:1765–1769

Paton WDM (1957) The action of morphine and related substances on contraction and on acetylcholine output of coaxially stimulated guinea-pig ileum. Br J Pharmacol Chemother 12:119–127

Paton WDM, Zar MA (1968) The origin of acetylcholine released from guinea-pig intestine and longitudinal muscle fibres. J Physiol (Lond) 194:13–33

Porreca F, Burks TF (1983) Affinity of normorphine for its pharmacologic receptor in the naive and morphine-tolerant guinea-pig isolated ileum. J Pharmacol Exp Ther 225:688–693

Porreca F, LoPresti D, Ward SJ (1990) Opioid agonist affinity in the guinea-pig ileum and mouse vas deferens. Eur J Pharmacol 179:129–139

Portoghese PS, Sultana M, Takemori AE (1990) Design of peptidomimetic & opioid receptor antagonists using the message-address concept. J Med Chemistry 33: 1714–1720

Raffa RB, Vaught JL, Porreca F (1989) Can equal pA$_2$ values be compatible with receptor differences? Trends Pharmacol Sci 10:183–185

Rang HP (1964) Stimulant actions of volatile anaesthetics on smooth muscle. Br J Pharmacol 22:356–362

Rothman RB, Bykov V, de Costa BR, Jacobson AE, Rice KC, Brady L (1990) Interaction of endogneous opioid peptides and other drugs with four kappa opioid binding sites in guinea pig brain. Peptides 11:311–331

Sayre LM, Portoghese PS, Takemori AE (1983a) Difference between μ-receptors in the guinea pig ileum and the mouse vas deferens. Eur J Pharmacol 90:159–160

Sayre LM, Portoghese PS, Takemori AE (1983b) Alkylation of opioid receptor subtypes by α-chlornaltrexamine produces concurrent irreversible agonistic and irreversible antagonistic activities. J Med Chem 26:503–506

Schild HO (1957) Drug antagonism and pA$_x$. Pharmacol Rev 9:242–246

Schiller PW, DiMaio J (1982) Opiate receptor subclasses differ in their conformational requirements. Nature 297:74–76

Schulz R, Faase M, Wüster M, Herz A (1979) Selective receptors for beta-endorphin on the rat vas deferens. Life Sci 24:843–850

Schulz R, Wüster M, Herz A (1981a) Pharmacological characterisation of the epsilon opiate receptor. J Pharmacol Exp Ther 216:604–606

Schulz R, Wüster M, Rubini P, Herz A (1981b) Functional opiate receptors in the guinea-pig ileum: their differentiation by means of selective tolerance development. J Pharmacol Exp Ther 219:547–550

Sheehan MJ, Hayes AG, Tyers MB (1986a) Irreversible selective blockade of κ-opioid receptors in the guinea-pig ileum. Eur J Pharmacol 129:19–24

Sheehan MJ, Hayes AG, Tyers MB (1986b) Pharmacology of δ-opioid receptors in the hamster vas deferens. Eur J Pharmacol 130:57–64

Sheehan MJ, Hayes AG, Tyers MB (1988) Lack of evidence for ε-opioid receptors in the rat vas deferens. Eur J Pharmacol 154:237–245

Shimohigashi Y, Costa T, Pfeiffer A, Herz A, Kimura H, Stammer CH (1987) Δ^EPhe^4-enkephalin analogs. Delta receptors in rat brain are different from those in the mouse vas deferens. FEBS Lett 222:71–74

Shook JE, Kazmierski W, Wire WS, Lemcke PK, Hruby VJ, Burks TF (1988) Opioid receptor selectivity of β-endorphin in vitro and in vivo: mu, delta and epsilon receptors. J Pharmacol Exp Ther 246:1018–1025

Smith CFC (1984) Morphine, but not diacetyl morphine (heroin), possesses opiate antagonist activity in the mouse vas deferens. Neuropeptides 5:173–176

Smith CFC, Carter A (1986) Delta receptors in the rat vas deferens. Arch Int Pharmacodyn Ther 284:181–192

Smith CFC, Rance MJ (1983) Opiate receptors in the rat vas deferens. Life Sci 33 [Suppl 1]:327–330

Stephenson RP (1956) A modification of receptor theory. Br J Pharmacol 11: 379–393

Takemori AE, Portoghese PS (1984) Comparitive antagonism by naltrexone and naloxone of μ, κ, and δ agonists. Eur J Pharmacol 104:101–104

Takemori AE, Portoghese PS (1985) Receptors for opioid peptides in the guinea-pig ileum. J Pharmacol Exp Ther 235:389–235

Takemori AE, Ikeda M, Portoghese PS (1986) The μ, κ, and δ properties of various opioid agonists. Eur J Pharmacol 123:357–361

Terenius L, Wahlstrom A (1975) Search for an endogenous ligand for the opiate receptor. Acta Physiol Scand 94:74–81

Trendelenburg P (1917) Physiologische und pharmakologische Versuche über die Dünndarmperistaltik. Naunyn Schmeidebergs Arch Exp Pathol Pharmakol 81:55–129

Vaughn LK, Wire WS, Davis P, Shimohigashi Y, Toth G, Knapp RJ, Hruby VJ, Burks TF, Yamamura HI (1990) Differentiation between rat brain and mouse vas deferens δ opioid receptors. Eur J Pharmacol 177:99–101

Verlinde C, de Ranter C (1988) Assessment of the kappa-opioid activity of a series of 6, 7-benzomorphans in the rabbit vas deferens. Eur J Pharmacol 153:83–87

Walker JM, Moises HC, Coy DH, Baldrighi G, Akil H (1982) Nonopiate effects of dynorphin and des-tyr dynorphin. Science 218:1136–1138

Ward SJ, LoPresti D, James DW (1986) Activity of mu- and delta-selective opioid agonists in the guinea pig ileum preparation: differentiation into peptide and nonpeptide classes with β-funaltrexamine. J Pharmacol Exp Ther 238:625–631

Waterfield AA, Lord JAH, Hughes J, Kosterlitz HW (1978) Differences in the inhibitory effects of normorphine and opioid peptides on the responses of the vasa deferentia of two strains of mice. Eur J Pharmacol 47:249–250

CHAPTER 5
Anatomical Distribution of Opioid Receptors in Mammalians: An Overview

A. Mansour and S.J. Watson

A. Introduction

Of the peptide receptors examined, the opioid receptors are by far the most intensely studied and best characterized systems in the CNS. They consist of at least three receptor types, referred to as μ, δ, and κ, and have distinct anatomical distributions (Mansour et al. 1987, 1988; Sharif and Hughes 1988; Tempel and Zukin 1987), ligand selectivities (Goldstein and Naidir 1989; James and Goldstein 1984; Robson et al. 1983), and functions in the brain and periphery (Martin 1984; Wood 1982). With their first demonstration nearly 20 years ago (Pert and Snyder 1973; Simon et al. 1973; Terenius 1973), they heralded a new era in the neurosciences, paving the way for the eventual discovery of the opioid peptides and serving as model systems for peptidergic transmission. While the biochemical demonstration of opioid receptors took place in the 1970s, a wealth of pharmacological evidence in the preceding decades had suggested the existence of specific binding sites for the opiates (Beckett and Casey 1954; Portoghese 1965; Woods 1956). The characterization of opiate antagonists, such as naloxone and the stereoselective requirements of opiate agonists, clearly pointed to the existence of opioid receptors prior to the first receptor-binding assay.

Soon after their demonstration in tissue homogenates, the method of in vivo receptor autoradiography was developed to more accurately determine the anatomical localization of the opioid receptors in the brain and peripheral tissues (Atweh and Kuhar 1977a,b,c; Pert et al. 1976). Radiolabeled opiates of high specific activity were injected intravenously and animals were allowed to survive for 30–60 min, at which time tissues were either dissected and assayed for bound ligand or sectioned and mounted on microscope slides for receptor autoradiography. In vivo autoradiographic results confirmed earlier research with tissue homogenates and provided more precise anatomical resolution of the opioid-binding sites. This more physiological technique to label receptors was soon supplanted, however, by in vitro receptor autoradiographic methods which produced similar anatomical results (Herkenham and Pert 1982; Young and Kuhar 1979) but required significantly less radioactive ligand, allowed the analysis of serial tissue sections to simultaneously compare several receptors or other anatomical markers, and was not limited to ligands that crossed the blood-brain barrier.

This increased anatomical flexibility in conjunction with the development of highly selective ligands, such as DAGO (Tyr-D-Ala-Gly-MePhe-Gly-ol) (HANDA et al. 1981), DPDPE (D-Pen^2, D-Pen^5-enkephalin) (MOSBERG et al. 1983), and U69,593 (LAHTI et al. 1985), has allowed the specific labeling of μ-, δ-, and κ-opioid receptors respectively, in serial brain sections of numerous species including human, rat, and guinea pig (CROSS et al. 1987; MANSOUR et al. 1988; SHARIF and HUGHES 1988; TEMPEL and ZUKIN 1987). Despite these advances, a number of inherent complexities still remained. First and foremost is ligand specificity. While this was more of an issue prior to the development of selective ligands, such as DAGO and DPDPE, it continues to be a problem in labeling κ-receptors, where multiple subtypes have been proposed. A second complicating factor in describing the distribution of the opioid receptors is related to the inherent complexity of the nervous tissues. For example, as receptor-binding sites are localized on cell somatas and fibers, it is often difficult to determine whether the emulsion grains observed represent binding on specific cell bodies or on fibers from distant cells. Such anatomical complexities are further exacerbated by the marked species differences observed in the distributions of opioid receptors, the multiplicity of receptor subtypes, and the number of overlapping neuronal systems present in the nervous system.

Given these considerations, this chapter first provides an overview of the μ-, δ-, and κ-receptor distributions in the rat and monkey brain with an aim at identifying unifying principles concerning the anatomical distribution and function of the opioid receptors. This is followed by a discussion of the evidence pointing to the existence of multiple κ-receptor subtypes and their differential localization in the brain. The nigrostriatal and mesolimbic systems of the basal ganglia are next examined as model systems for studying opioid receptor-peptide interactions, and the chapter concludes with a discussion of how anatomical approaches in conjunction with receptor autoradiography might provide insights into the functions of the opioid receptors.

While other opioid receptor types (ε, λ) and subtypes (μ_1) have been proposed (CHANG et al. 1984; GOODMAN and PASTERNAK 1985; GREVEL et al. 1985; SCHULZ et al. 1981), there is no consensus as to the nature and distribution of these sites and, therefore, they will not be discussed. The following is a qualitative comparison of μ-, δ-, and κ-receptor distributions in the CNS. The relative receptor densities apply within a receptor distribution and species. For instance, a high level of κ-binding in the rat hypothalamus may be equivalent, in terms of receptor number, to a low or moderate level of μ-binding in the monkey cortex. To aid in this description, the binding conditions are such that the ligands occupy 75% of each receptor type in both monkey and rat. The μ- and δ-sites were labeled with [^{3}H]DAGO and [^{3}H]DPDPE, respectively, while the κ-sites were labeled with [^{3}H]bremzocine in the presence of a 300-fold excess of unlabled DAGO and DPDPE. Under these conditions [^{3}H]bremazocine should label all the known κ-receptor subtypes and in a later portion of the manuscript we make direct comparisons between the distribution of [^{3}H]bremazocine and [^{3}H]U69,593 (a κ-selective agonist) binding sites.

B. Anatomical Distributions

I. μ-Receptors

μ-Opioid receptors are widely distributed throughout the CNS with particularly dense binding observed in the basal ganglia, limbic structures, thalamic nuclei, and regions important for nociceptive and visceral regulation. As it is beyond the scope of this chapter to provide a comprehensive analysis of the species differences in the distributions of the opioid receptors, the more salient features have been emphasized in this overview in order to derive principles of anatomical organization. Schematic drawings demonstrating the distributions of the opioid peptides and receptors in the rat brain are provided (Fig. 1) to facilitate peptide-receptor comparisons.

Marked species variations are noted in the cerebral cortex, where regional as well as laminar differences in the distribution of opioid receptors are observed. In the rat, the frontal, parietal, and temporal corticies show dense μ-binding in layers I and IV, with only light to moderate densities in the remaining cortical layers (Fig. 2). Since the complexity of the monkey cortex precludes a detailed regional and cytoarchitectural analysis here, we present the distribution of μ-sites in several selected regions of monkey cortex in Table 1. As is evident from this table there is relatively little μ-binding in most neocortical areas, in sharp contrast with the rat. Palleocortical and cingulate cortex of the monkey, in contrast, demonstrate moderate to dense μ-receptor binding.

An area of dense μ-binding common to both rat and monkey is the amygdaloid nuclear complex. Species differences are observed in the central nucleus, where there is little or no μ-binding in the rat and moderate to dense binding in the monkey (Fig. 3). This observation is of particular interest since the central nucleus is an area of heavy opioid peptide innervation and may suggest a differential interaction between opioid peptides and receptor across these two species.

In the rat hippocampal formation, μ-binding is dense in the stratum lacunosum-moleculare, the pyramidal cell layer, and the molecular and granular cell layers of the ventral dentate gyrus. In the monkey, moderate to dense labeling is also observed in the pyramidal cell region and the stratum lacunosum-moleculare (Fig. 4). As can be seen from Fig. 4, the granular layer of the monkey dentate gyrus contains exclusively μ-binding sites,

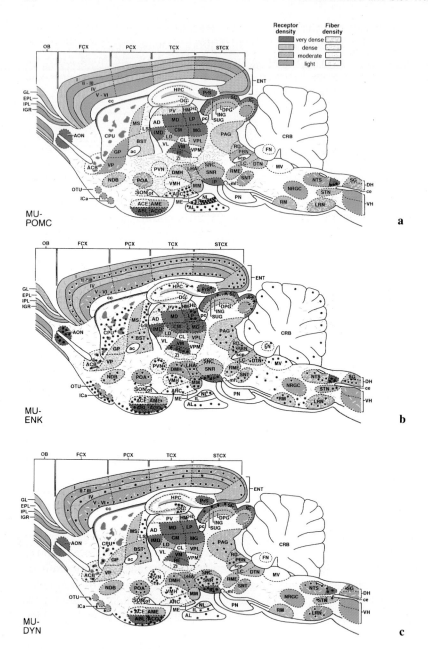

Fig. 1

Fig. 1a–i. Schematic representation of μ-, δ-, and κ-opioid receptors overlayed with cell and fiber distributions of the proopiomelanocortion (*POMC*), enkephalin (*ENK*), or dynorphin (*DYN*) peptides. There is a total of nine sagittal rat brain sections illustrating each peptide distribution in register with the three opioid receptors. μ-Sites were labeled with [^{3}H]DAGO, δ-sites with [^{3}H]DPDPE, and κ-sites with [^{3}H]bremazocine in the presence of μ- and δ-blockers (κ_1 and κ_2). The relative density of receptors has been encoded with use of four colors; *red*, very dense; *yellow*, dense; *green*, moderate; *blue*, light. Relative receptor densities are within a receptor type and do not represent absolute receptor capacity but are designed to transmit qualitatively the correspondence between the opioid peptides and receptors. Peptide cell bodies are represented by *small red dots*, while fibers are illustrated by *red lines*. Each map represents multiple parasagittal levels through the rat brain and was reconstructed using the atlas of PAXIONS and WATSON (1986). Peptide maps were adapted from KHACHATURIAN et al. (1985a).

ABL, basolateral amygdaloid nucleus; *ac*, anterior comissure; *ACB*, nucleus accumbens; *ACE*, central amygdaloid nucleus; *ACO*, cortical amygdaloid nucleus; *AD*, anteriodorsal thalamus; *AL*, anterior lobe, pituitary; *AME*, medial amygdaloid nucleus; *AON*, anterior olfactory nucleus; *ARC*, arcuate nucleus, hypothalamus; *BST*, bed nucleus stria terminalis; *cc*, corpus callosum; *ce*, central canal; *CL*, centrolateral thalamus; *CM*, centromedial thalamus; *CPU*, caudate-putamen; *CRB*, cerebellum; *DG*, dentate gyrus; *DH*, dorsal horn, spinal cord; *DMH*, dorsomedial hypothalamus; *DPG*, deep gray matter, superior colliculus; *DTN*, dorsal tegmental nucleus; *ENT*, entorhinal cortex; *EPL*, external plexiform layer, olfactory bulb; *FCX*, frontal cortex; *FN*, fastigial nucleus, cerebellum; *GL*, glomerular layer; *GP*, globus pallidus; *HL*, lateral habenula; *HM*, medial habenula; *HPC*, hippocampus; *IC*, inferior colliculus; *ICa*, Islands of Calleja; *IGR*, intermediate granular layer, olfactory bulb; *IL*, intermediate lobe, pituitary; *IMD*, intermediodorsal thalamus; *ING*, intermediate gray layer, superior colliculus; *IP*, interpeduncular nucleus; *IPL*, intermediate plexiform layer, olfactory bulb; *LC*, locus ceruleus; *LD*, laterodorsal thalamus; *LHA*, lateral hypothalamic area; *LP*, lateroposterior thalamus; *LRN*, lateral reticular nucleus; *LS*, lateral septum; *MD*, dorsomedial thalamus; *ME*, median eminence; *MG*, medial geniculate; *ML*, medial laminscus; *MM*, medial mammillary nucleus; *MS*, medial septum; *MV*, medial vestibular nucleus; *NDB*, nucleus diagonal band; *NL*, neural lobe, pituitary; *NRGC*, nucleus reticularis gigantocellularis; *NTS*, nucleus tractus solitarius; *ot*, optic tract; *OTU*, olfactory tubercle; *PAG*, periaquadual gray; *PBN*, parabrachial nucleus; *pc*, posterior commissure; *PCX*, parietal cortex; *PN*, pons; *POA*, preoptic area; *PrS*, presubiculum; *PV*, paraventricular thalamus; *PVN*, paraventricular hypothalamus; *RD*, dorsal raphe; *RE*, reuniens thalamus; *RM*, raphe magnus; *RME*, median raphe; *SC*, superior colliculus; *scp*, superior cerebellar preduncle; *SG*, substantia gelatinosa; *SNC*, substantia nigra, pars compacta; *SNR*, substantia nigra, pars reticulata; *SNT*, sensory nucleus trigeminal; *SON*, supraoptic nucleus; *STCX*, striate cortex; *STN*, spinal trigeminal nucleus; *SUG*, superficial gray layer, superior colliculus; *TCX*, temporal cortex; *VH*, ventral horn, spinal cord; *VL*, ventrolateral thalamus; *VM*, ventromedial thalamus; *VMH*, ventromedial hypothalamus; *VP*, ventral pallidus; *VPL*, ventroposteriolateral thalamus; *VPM*, ventroposteriormedial thalamus; *ZI*, zona incerta

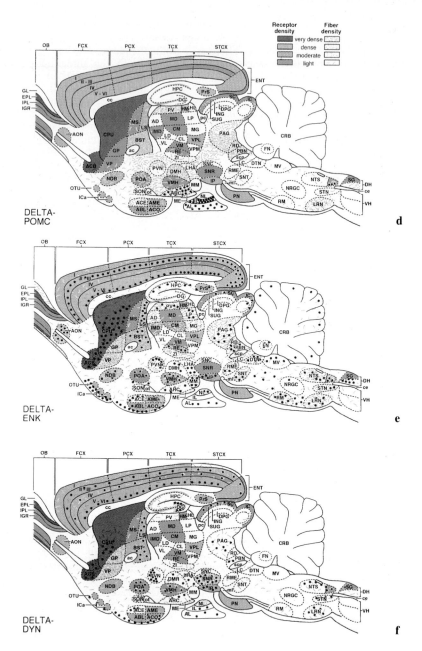

Fig. 1

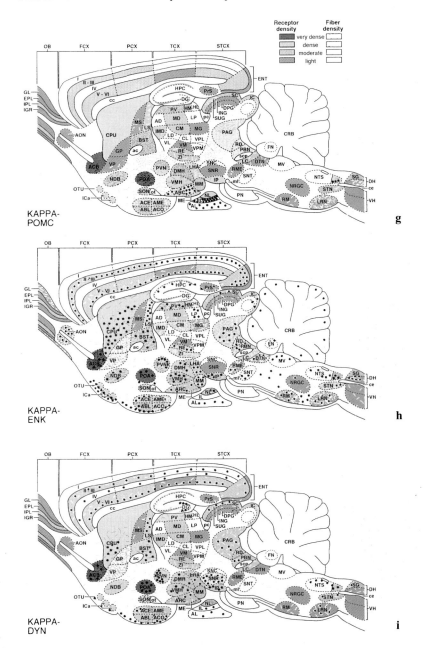

Fig. 1

86 A. MANSOUR and S.J. WATSON

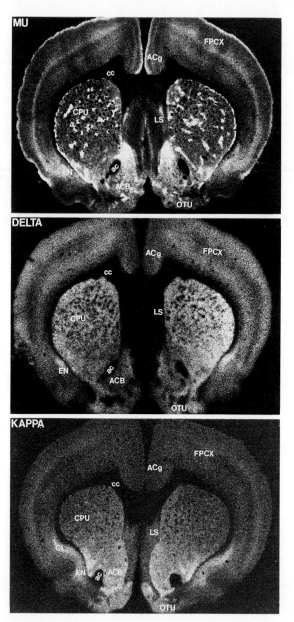

Fig. 2. Darkfield autoradiograms of μ-, δ-, and κ-binding in coronal rat brain sections. In the caudate-putamen (*CPU*) μ-sites form "patches", areas of high receptor density and the subcallosal streak, while δ- and κ-sites are diffusely localized in the *CPU*, being concentrated either laterally (δ) or medioventrally (κ). κ-Receptors are particularly prominent in the ventral striatum in the nucleus accumbens (*ACB*) and olfactory tubercle (*OTU*). Abbreviations not included in Fig. 1 are: *ACg*, anterior cingulate cortex; *CL*, claustrum; *EN*, endopiriform nucleus; *FPCX*, frontal-parietal cortex

Table 1. Relative density of opioid receptors in selected areas of monkey cerebral cortex

	μ	δ	κ
Frontal Cortex (FCBm)			
Layer I	+ +	+ + +	+ + +
II	+	+ + +	+ + +
III	+	+ +	+ + +
IV	+	+ +	+ +
V	+	+ +	+ +
VI	+	+ +	+ + +
Temporal cortex (Ta)			
Layer I	+ +	+ + +	+ +
II	+	+ + +	+ +
III	+	+ + +	+ +
IV	+	+ + +	+ +
V	+ +	+ + +	+ +
VI	+	+ + +	+ + +
Parietal cortex (PEm)			
Layer I	+	+ + +	+ +
II	+	+ + +	+ +
III	+	+ + +	+ +
IV	+	+ +	+ +
V	+	+ +	0
VI	+	+ +	+ + +
Occipital cortex (OB)			
Layer I	+	+ + + +	+ +
II	+	+ + + +	+ +
III	+	+ + + +	+ +
IV	+	+ + + +	+ +
V	+	+ + +	+ +
VI	+ +	+ + + +	+ + +

+ + + +, very dense; + + +, dense; + +, moderate; +, low; 0, nondetectable.

confirming the pharmacological and anatomical selectivity of the binding conditions.

In the caudate-putamen of the rat, μ-binding sites are densest in patches and in the subcallosal streak. The density of the μ-patches varies dramatically rostrocaudally, with the densest number of these patches found in the rostral portion of the caudate-putamen (Fig. 2). Similar regional variations are observed in the monkey, where μ-binding is densest in the medical aspects of the caudate and putamen and μ-patches demonstrate a rostrocaudal gradient. Only a light to moderate density of μ-binding is observed in the monkey and rat matrix portion of the caudate and putamen. The dense patches of μ-binding extend from the caudate-putamen of the rat to the nucleus accumbens (Fig. 2), an area of moderate and somewhat patchy μ-binding in the monkey.

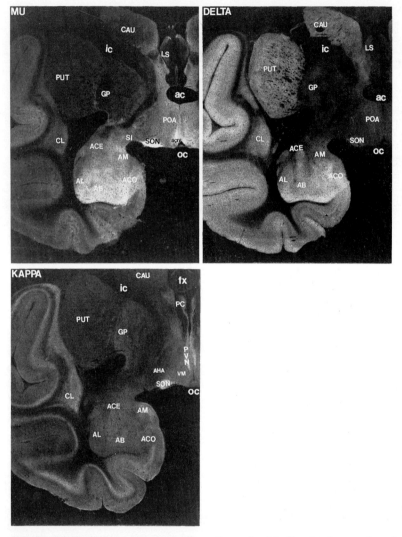

Fig. 3. Darkfield autoradiogram of μ-, δ-, and κ-binding in the monkey forebrain. Note the high levels of δ-binding in the caudate (*CAU*), putamen (*PUT*), amygdala, cortex, and claustrum (*CL*). In contrast, μ- and κ-binding sites are prominent in the hypothalamus, amygdala, and, in the case of κ-binding, the deep layers of cortex. Abbreviations not listed in Fig. 1 are *AB*, basal amygdala; *AHA*, anterior hypothalamic area; *AL*, lateral amygdala; *AM*, medial amygdala; *fx*, fornix; *ic*, internal capsule; *oc*, optic chiasm; *PC*, paracentral thalamus; *SCN*, suprachiasmatic nucleus; *SI*, substantia innominata; *VM*, ventromedial hypothalamus

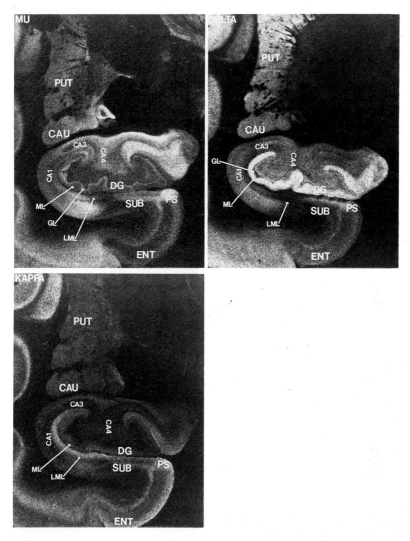

Fig. 4. μ-, δ-, and κ-darkfield autoradiograms of monkey hippocampus and dentate gyrus. Each receptor has a distinct laminar distribution, with μ-binding prominent in the granular layer (*GL*) of the dentate gyrus and the pyramidal cell layer (*CA1–CA4*) of the hippocampus. In contrast, note the lack of δ- and κ-binding in the granular layer of the dentate gyrus. δ- and κ-binding is prominent in the molecular layer (*ML*) of the dentate gyrus and the striatum lacunosum-moleculare (*LML*) of the hippocampus, respectively. Abbreviations include: *CA1–CA4*, fields 1–4 of Ammon's horn; *CAU*, caudate; *DG*, dentate gyrus; *ENT*, entorhinal cortex; *PS*, presubiculum; *PUT*, putamen; *SUB*, subiculum

In the diencephalon, marked species differences are observed in the hypothalamus. In the monkey, dense μ-binding is observed in most of the hypothalamic nuclei (Fig. 5), areas containing little or no μ-binding in the rat. μ-Binding is dense only in the medical mammillary nucleus of the rat, an area devoid of opioid receptor binding in the monkey. More dorsally, μ-receptors are densely distributed in the thalamus of both the monkey and the rat.

In the mesencephalon, the distribution of μ-sites is remarkably similar in the rat and monkey. μ-Binding sites are seen in the periaqueductal gray, superior and inferior colliculi, interpeduncular nucleus, substantia nigra, and raphe nuclei. In the superior and inferior colliculi, distinct regional patterns of receptor binding are observed in both species. In the rat superior colliculus, μ-binding is densest in the superficial gray layer with moderate amounts of binding in the intermediate and deep gray layers. A similar lamination pattern is observed in the superior colliculus of the monkey. The interpeduncular and raphe nuclei also appear to be similarly labeled in both species with very dense and moderate levels of binding sites, respectively.

The distribution of μ-sites in the rat and monkey substantia nigra do appear to differ, however. In the rat, dense μ-binding is restricted to the pars compacta, with light to moderate levels observed in the pars reticulata. In contrast, μ-sites in the monkey appear to be more homogeneously distributed in both divisions of the substantia nigra.

More caudally in the brainstem, dense levels of μ-binding sites are seen in the nucleus tractus solitarius and the spinal trigeminal and parabrachial nuclei of both the monkey and rat. Only low amounts of μ-binding are observed in the lateral reticular nucleus and no specific μ-binding is observed in the cerebellum.

II. δ-Receptors

Compared to the μ and κ sites, δ-opioid receptors are more restricted in their distribution and are densest in forebrain regions. Another and possibly related distinguishing feature of the δ-receptor distribution is that it is well conserved across mammalian species. For example, in both rat and monkey brain, δ-receptors are densest in the caudate, putamen, cerebral cortex, and amygdala, and are generally sparse to nonexistent in the thalamus and hypothalamus. While there are species differences that can easily be seen, the overall similarity of the δ-receptor distribution across these two mammalian species is remarkable.

Fairly diffuse and dense binding is observed in the cerebral cortex of the monkey and rat. In the rat, δ-binding is densest in layers II, III, V, and VI of the frontal, parietal, and temporal cortex, a pattern inverse to that observed with μ-binding in the rat (Fig. 2). It can be seen from Table 1 that, while δ-binding sites are distributed throughout monkey cerebral cortex, species differences can be observed in the striate cortex of the rat

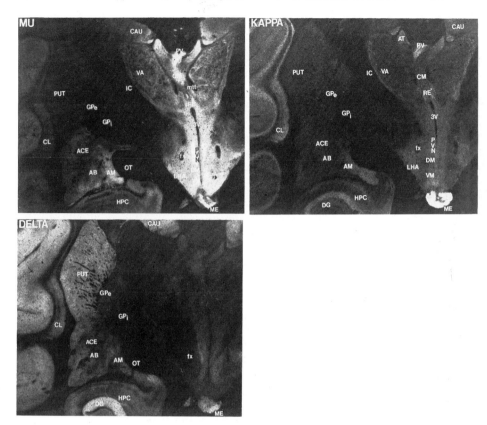

Fig. 5. Darkfield autoradiograms of μ-, δ-, and κ-binding in the monkey thalamus and hypothalamus. Note the prominent μ- and κ-binding and the comparatively poor δ-binding observed in the monkey hypothalamus. All three receptor types are localized in the median eminence (*ME*) and may modulate the release of hormones from the anterior lobe of the pituitary. Regions of dense δ-binding include caudate (*CAU*), putamen (*PUT*), amygdala, dentate gyrus (*DG*), and cortex. Abbreviations not listed in Fig. 1 include: *AB*, basal amygdala; *AM*, medial amygdala; *AT*, anterior thalamus; *CL*, claustrum; *DM*, dorsomedial hypothalamus; *fx*, fornix; *GPe*, globus pallidus, external division; *GPi*, globus pallidus, internal division; *ic*, internal capsule; *mtt*, mammillothalamic tract; *VA*, anterior ventral thalamus; *VM*, ventromedial hypothalamus; *3V*, third ventricle

and the occipital cortex of the monkey. Monkey occipital cortex shows uniformly dense δ-binding, while only layers V and VI of striate cortex of the rat are densely labeled with δ-sites.

Further species differences are observed in the dentate gyrus and amygdala. In the monkey, dense δ-binding is restricted to the stratum moleculare of the dentate gyrus (Fig. 4), with no binding in the granular cell layer, while in the rat only light labeling is observed in the molecular and granular layers of ventral dentate gyrus. δ-Binding is dense in the amygdala of both species (Fig. 3); however, in the monkey, the central nucleus is prominently labeled.

Within the basal ganglia, dense and rather diffuse binding is observed in the caudate and putamen of both monkey and rat. In the rat, δ-binding is more pronounced in the ventral-lateral portion of this region (Fig. 2), and in the monkey there tends to be more intense binding in the more lateral portions of the putamen (Fig. 3). In contrast to the very dense δ-binding observed in the rostral nucleus accumbens and olfactory tubercle of the rat, only moderate levels are seen in these areas of the monkey brain.

Compared to the telencephalon, diencephalic structures show considerably less δ-binding in both the monkey and rat. In the rat hypothalamus, only a low density of binding is observed in the ventromedial nucleus, with the remaining hypothalamic nuclei showing no apparent δ-binding. In the monkey, a low to moderate density of δ-binding sites is observed in several hypothalamic nuclei, including the preoptic area, supraoptic, and periventricular nuclei. Dense δ-binding is observed, however, in the median eminence of the monkey (Fig. 5), an area devoid of δ-receptors in the rat. As can be seen from Fig. 5, all three opioid receptors are present in the median eminence of the monkey, consistent with the localization of μ-, δ-, and κ-sites in the monkey neural lobe of the pituitary. In contrast, the rat neural lobe contains exclusively κ-sites, consistent with the relative abundance of κ-sites in the rat hypothalamus.

More caudally in the midbrain and brainstem, δ-binding is limited to a few neural structures in both monkey and rat. Areas of light δ-binding in the rat include the substantia nigra (pars reticulata), nucleus tractus solitarius, and the substantia gelatinosa of the spinal cord. The interpeduncular nucleus has relatively dense labeling, particularly in the central division, and moderate amounts of binding are seen in the pons. While clearly not as prominent, light δ-labeling is observed in the periaqueductal gray and interpeduncular nucleus of the monkey.

III. κ-Receptors

The distribution of κ-receptors demonstrates some of the most striking species differences observed among the opioid receptor types. In the rat, κ-sites comprise only approximately 10% of the total number of opioid receptor sites, while in most other species, such as guinea pig, monkey, and human, they represent at least a third of the total opioid receptor population. In all species examined so far, the κ-sites have been found to be widely distributed throughout the forebrain, midbrain, and brainstem.

In the telencephalon, marked species differences are observed in the cerebral cortex. In the rat, a diffuse, low to moderate density of binding sites is observed in layers II, III, V, and VI of the frontal and parietal cortices (Fig. 2), with light to undetectable amounts in the temporal cortex. The deep layers (V and VI) of the striate cortex, however, show moderate amounts of κ-labeling. In contrast to the rat, κ-binding is quite prominent throughout the monkey cerebral cortex. As can be seen from Table 1 and Fig. 3, it varies dramatically from the rat, with particularly dense labeling observed in the deep layers of the frontal, parietal, temporal, and occipital cortices.

Species differences are also observed in the hippocampus, where light labeling is observed in the CA1–CA4 regions of the rat and monkey. Of the hippocampal layers, only stratum lacunosum-moleculare shows light κ-binding in the rat, with no specific binding observed in the strata moleculare, oriens, or radiatum. The monkey stratum lacunosum-moleculare, on the other hand, shows fairly dense κ-labeling which can be easily distinguished from the μ- and δ-labeling in this region (Fig. 4). Moderate to light κ-binding is observed in the molecular layer of the monkey dentate gyrus, while light labeling is observed in the granular and molecular layers of the ventral dentate gyrus of the rat.

Other differences are observed in the basal ganglia, where in the rat κ-sites are densely and diffusely distributed in the ventromedial portion of the caudate-putamen, nucleus accumbens, and olfactory tubercle (Fig. 2). The monkey caudate and putamen, on the other hand, have only light to moderate κ-labeling with a somewhat patchy distribution in the caudate and putamen. Additionally, differences are observed in the globus pallidus, where the κ-binding appears to be much more prominent in the monkey (Fig. 3) as compared to the rat.

Hypothalamic regions that have dense κ-labeling in both rat and monkey include the medial preoptic area, median eminence, and the periventricular, ventromedial, and dorsomedial nuclei (Fig. 5). Moderate κ-labeling is observed in the supraoptic, arcuate, and medial mammillary nuclei of the rat. In contrast, very dense κ-labeling is observed in the supraoptic nucleus of the monkey (Fig. 3) and no specific binding is observed in the mammillary nucleus. Of the thalamic nuclei, κ-binding is concentrated in the medial nuclei of both the rat and monkey (Fig. 5).

In contrast to the marked species differences observed in the forebrain, the distribution of κ-sites appears to be similar in the rat and monkey in the midbrain and brainstem. In both species, a moderate density of κ-receptors is observed in the superior and inferior colliculi, periaqueductal gray, interpeduncular nucleus, raphe nuclei, parabrachial nucleus, and spinal trigeminal nucleus. Marked differences are observed, however, in the cerebellum, where there is dense κ-binding in the deep layers of monkey cerebellum and no detectable κ-binding in the rat. More subtle differences are also seen in the pars reticulata of the substantia nigra, which is prominently labeled in the monkey and only lightly labeled in the rat.

IV. Anatomical Conclusions

Several conclusions may be drawn by comparing the opioid receptor anatomy of the rat and monkey. First, the distribution of δ-sites appears well conserved between these two species, with dense binding found primarily in the cerebral cortex, caudate, putamen, and amygdala, with poor binding in most of midbrain and brainstem. This distribution, in conjunction with the low δ-binding observed in pigeons and reptiles, would suggest that this receptor may have fully developed later in evolution. Second, in both rat and monkey the greatest differences observed between the μ- and κ- distributions appear in the forebrain, with parallel distributions, to a large extent, in the midbrain and brainstem. Third, the distribution of the opioid receptor types appears to be well conserved across species within certain functional systems. The distribution of opioid receptors within the neural systems modulating pain and visceral functions are well conserved across species, while those underlying neuroendocrine regulation, for example, are not. And finally, the opioid receptors are heavily distributed in monoaminergic systems in both rat and monkey, suggesting an intimate relationship between opioids and monoamines.

It is tempting to speculate further about the function of the opioid receptor types given their anatomical distribution. Clearly the role of opiates as analgesics is supported by their localization in the dorsal horn of the spinal cord, periquaductal gray, and thalamus. Further, the moderate to dense distribution of μ- and κ-sites in the supraoptic and paraventricular nuclei of the monkey could provide the anatomical basis for the opposing effects of μ- and κ-agonists on fluid regulation. The diuretic effects of opiates may also be mediated at the level of the neural lobe, where in the monkey μ-, δ-, and κ-sites can be localized. It is not clear, however, whether all three receptor types are on hypothalamic terminals or pituicytes. The localization of opioid binding sites (particularly μ and κ) in several hypothalamic nuclei and in the median eminence is also consistent with the effects of opiates on other neuroendocrine systems including those modulating ACTH and prolactin secretion. Other functions in which opioid receptors may be involved include sensorimotor integration and the modulation of affect with high levels of binding observed in the basal ganglia and limbic systems.

C. Multiple κ-Receptor Subtypes

Despite their early pharmacological characterization (GILBERT and MARTIN 1976; MARTIN et al. 1976), the biochemical properties and anatomical distribution of κ-receptors in the nervous system remain as areas of controversy. While early in vitro studies were initially unsuccessful in demonstrating κ-receptor binding (e.g., HILLER and SIMON 1979), more recent experiments using enriched tissues, such as guinea pig brain, and improved binding conditions have been able to show specific binding (GILLAN and KOSTERLITZ 1982; JAMES et al. 1982; KOSTERLITZ et al. 1981), with some investigators suggesting multiple κ-receptor subtypes based on sensitivity to D-ala-D-leu-enkephalin (ATTALI et al. 1982; CASTASNAS et al. 1985) or dynorphin A

(1–9) (Morre et al. 1983). Physiological results (e.g., Iyengar et al. 1986) tended to support the suggestion of multiple κ-receptor subtypes, but these results failed to correspond to the multiple κ-sites suggested by either earlier group of investigators. It was not until the recent availability of selective radiolabeled κ-ligands that this issue was reexamined and some consensus emerged.

Several laboratories (Clark et al. 1989; Hunter et al. 1989; Nock et al. 1988a; Su 1985; Tiberi and Magnan 1990; Wood et al. 1989; Zukin et al. 1988) have demonstrated two populations of κ-receptors that can be differentiated based on their affinity for benzeneacetamides, such as U50,488, U69,593, and PD117302. κ-Sites sensitive to U69,593-like compounds have been referred to by some investigators as κ_1 and sites having a low affinity for these compounds have been referred to as κ_2. These conclusions are based on several lines of evidence. First, several laboratories have demonstrated that the total number of κ-receptors labeled using [^{3}H]bremazocine or [^{3}H]EKC in the presence of μ- and δ-receptor blockade is consistently higher than that observed with [^{3}H]U69,593 and the differences are especially great in the rat. Second, competition studies using either [^{3}H]EKC or [^{3}H]bremazocine (in the presence of μ- and δ-blockade) and unlabeled U50,488 demonstrate that U50,488 is either unable to completely displace all the κ-sites even at micromolar concentrations or produces in a curvilinear plot, suggesting two sites. Third, leftover or residual sites labeled with [^{3}H]bremazocine in the presence of unlabeled DAGO, DPDPE, and U69,593 designed to block μ-, δ-, and κ_1-sites demonstrate an opiate pharmacology; displaceable by κ-agonists and -antagonists, as well as naloxone and diprenorphine (Tiberi and Magnan 1990). And, fourth, there is anatomical evidence to suggest a differential distribution between U50,488-sensitive and -insensitive sites (Nock et al. 1988b; Zukin et al. 1988).

While there is apparent agreement concerning the κ_1-site and the existence of an additional benzeneacetamide-insensitive (κ_2-) site, the exact nature and distribution of the κ_2-site is a matter of controversy. For example, it is unclear whether the dynorphin peptides bind to the κ_2-sites. Some investigators (Zukin et al. 1988) find that DYN peptides can compete for the κ_2-sites, while others (e.g., Devlin and Shoemaker 1990) suggest that DYN peptides bind only κ_1-sites. There is also no agreement as to whether there is a single κ_2-site or multiple non-U69,593-sensitive κ-sites. Clark et al. (1989), for example, have presented data to suggest a second non-U69,593 sensitive site that is labeled with naloxone benzoylhydrazone. And, finally, perhaps most relevant to this chapter, the relative abundance of the U69,593-insensitive sites and their distributions in the nervous tissue vary markedly between laboratories. Some studies (Zukin et al. 1988) have suggested levels as high as 111 fmol/mg protein of κ_2-receptors in the rat brain when [^{3}H]ECK binding is performed at 4°C, while most studies report comparatively low levels of U69,593-sensitive and -insensitive κ-sites in the rat brain. In addition, some investigators have reported κ-sites in cerebellum and as patches in caudate-putamen of the rat (ZUKIN et al. 1988), while others fail to find this distribution (LYNCH et al. 1985; MANSOUR et al. 1987; MORRIS and HERZ 1986; SHARIF and HUGHES 1988).

Findings from our laboratory suggest that brain tissue from several animals contain a mixture of κ_1- and κ_2-sites and the ratio of κ_1/κ_2 varies with species. Pigeon brains, for example, contain predominantly κ_2-sites, while guinea pig and monkey brains are rich in κ_1-sites. Rat brains provide a third example and contain a low density of κ_1- and κ_2-sites. From the data presently available, the distribution of the κ-sites labeled with [^{3}H]U69,593 and [^{3}H]bremazocine in the presence of μ- and δ-blockade is not markedly different. Most regions of rat and guinea pig brain that contain κ_2 also demonstrate κ_1-sites as labeled by [^{3}H]U69,593. The differences that we have observed in the κ_1- and κ_2-distribution are those of relative density of sites within particular brain regions. Clear differences in the ratio of κ_1/κ_2-sites can be seen in the guinea pig, where, for example, κ_1 (labeled by [^{3}H]U69,593) and κ_2 ([^{3}H]bremazocine with μ- and δ-blockade) are seen in the dentate gyrus, but far fewer κ_1- than κ_2-sites are seen in the CA_2–CA_3 pyramidal cell layer of the hippocampus (Fig. 6). As can be seen from Fig. 6, κ_1-receptors are, in fact, so low in the CA_3 region of the hippocampus that they are not observeable with this film exposure. Similarly in the rat, comparable levels of κ_1- and κ_2-sites are seen in the superior colliculus, but the ratio of κ_1/κ_2-sites is low in the inferior colliculus. Regions of rat brain such as the mammillary nucleus and locus ceruleus that have been reported to contain κ_2-sites and no detectable [^{3}H]U69,593 binding need (NOCK et al. 1988b; ZUKIN et al. 1988) to be interpreted with caution, as low levels of κ_1-sites may be present and apparent differences reported

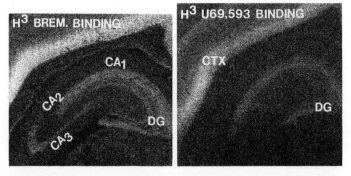

Fig. 6. Darkfield autoradiograms comparing the distribution of κ-sites (κ_1, κ_2) labeled with [^{3}H]bremazocine in the presence of a 300-fold excess of unlabeled DAGO and DPDPE (*left*), to κ_1-binding sites labeled with [^{3}H]U69,593 (*right*) in the guinea pig brain. Note that while there is a considerable overlap between the two distributions, some regions, such as the CA_2–CA_3 of hippocampus have proportionally fewer κ_1-sites and are not visible with this film exposure. Both κ_1- and κ_2-sites are observed in deep layers of guinea pig cortex and dentate gyrus (*DG*)

,may be due to low ratios of κ_1/κ_2-sites as opposed to differences in anatomical distribution. This is a particular problem in the rat where the total number of κ-receptors is quite low.

It is evident even from the brief review presented above that the pharmacological properties and anatomical distribution of the κ_2-receptor remains controversial. This is largely due to the fact that there is no clear means of labeling this site. As there is no specific κ_2-agonist or -antagonist, κ_2-sites have been visualized as the residual binding of [^{3}H]bremazocine or [^{3}H]EKC following μ-, δ-, or κ_1-blockade or by comparing [^{3}H]U69,593 binding to a mixed population of κ_1- and κ_2-sites. Both methods have their drawbacks, but it is clear that these issues will not be resolved without more selective κ_2-ligands and assay conditions.

D. Nigrostriatal and Mesolimbic Dopamine Systems as Models for Opioid Peptide and Receptor Interactions

As is evident from Fig. 1, it quickly becomes an overwhelming task to survey all the interactions between the multiple opioid receptor types and opioid peptides throughout the entire mammalian brain. A more heuristic and perhaps revealing approach, especially if the goal is to understand the possible function of these receptors, may be to examine the opioid receptors and peptides within specific neuroanatomical systems across species. Two systems that may be particularly informative are the nigrostriatonigral and mesolimbic dopamine systems of the basal ganglia. These neural systems are well defined anatomically, provide rich interactions between opioid peptides and receptors and, by comparing across species, one may derive principles of organization and function.

The following is a qualitative description of the opioid peptide and receptor distributions in the nigrostriatonigral and mesolimbic dopamine systems in the rat and monkey. Comparisons to the opioid receptors in the guinea pig are also provided to highlight certain anatomical features, but as there is little immunohistochemical information on opioid peptide distribution in the guinea pig, this species is not discussed extensively. As indicated earlier, relative receptor distributions are expressed within a species and receptor type. The binding conditions with [^{3}H]bremezocine are such that both κ_1 and κ_2 are labeled and will be described as a single population. While numerous investigators have contributed to this field, the peptide and receptor distributions are largely derived from studies performed in this laboratory (e.g., KHACHATURIAN et al. 1982, 1983a,b, 1984, 1985a,b; LEWIS et al. 1984, 1985a; MANSOUR et al. 1987, 1988). For a more complete description of the distinct opioid peptide distribution in the nervous system see Chap. 18.

Within the basal ganglia there are two separate yet interacting neural systems that have been differentiated both anatomically and functionally.

The dorsal system consisting of the caudate-putamen, globus pallidus, entopeduncular nucleus, and substantia nigra is thought to be involved primarily in motor control, while the ventral system consisting of the nucleus accumbens, olfactory tubercle, ventral pallidum, and ventral tegmental area is thought to be involved in reward and motivation. While these systems and their basic anatomy are common to all mammals, the interactions of the opioid peptides and receptors vary dramatically across species within these neural systems. Additional complex anatomical connections from other brain regions such as the thalamus, subthalamic nucleus, and cortex have been described for these systems (e.g., ALHEID and HEIMER 1988; GRAYBIEL 1990), but, because of space limitations, the discussion will focus on the neural structures outlined above.

All three opioid receptors and enkephalin and dynorphin peptides are prominent in the caudate and putamen. μ-Receptors and enkephalins form "patches," areas of dense binding or cell staining, in the caudate and putamen of the rat and monkey. A patch-matrix distinction has been described for other neurotransmitter systems and has been suggested to be a guiding principle in understanding basal ganglia anatomy (for reviews see GRAYBIEL 1990). The μ-receptor patches do not anatomically correspond to the enkephalin patches, however, and, in fact, appear to match the dynorphin peptide distribution better. The enkephalin patches in the rat are not as prominent as those observed in the monkey and are predominantly localized adjacent to the globus pallidus. Enkephalin patches in the monkey are more concentrated in the rostral caudate and putamen.

In contrast to the patch-matrix distinction of the μ-receptors and enkephalin peptides, δ- and κ-receptors are diffusely distributed, with δ-sites densest laterally and κ-sites densest in the medial-ventral caudate-putamen of the rat. κ-Receptors in the monkey, however, form patches in the caudate and putamen that extend throughout the rostral-caudal extent of these structures, with highest levels seen rostrally.

In addition to enkephalin cells and fibers, the caudate-putamen of the rat contains scattered dynorphin-positive cells and fibers. In the monkey, dynorphin cells are concentrated rostrally in the ventromedial caudate. No dynorphin cells are observed in the monkey putamen, but scattered fibers are present in the caudate and putamen. Some scattered POMC fibers are also observed in monkey putamen, in contrast to the rat caudate-putamen, where no fibers are observed.

The opioid receptors and peptides extend into the ventral striatum with moderate to dense μ-, δ-, and κ-binding seen in association with enkephalin and dynorphin cells and fibers and POMC fibers. μ-Receptor patches and δ-and κ-binding extend into the nucleus accumbens with the densest levels observed in the medial portion of the shell of the rat nucleus accumbens. The levels of κ-receptors in the nucleus accumbens of the rat, in fact, exceed those observed in the caudate-putamen. In contrast to the diffuse binding observed in the rat, patches of κ-receptor binding extend from the monkey caudate and putamen into the nucleus accumbens.

As seen with the opioid receptors, the opioid peptide distributions extend into the ventral striatum with enkephalin "patches" and a moderate number of dynorphin cells and fibers found in nucleus accumbens. A substantial number of POMC fibers are observed in the monkey nucleus accumbens as compared to the scattered POMC fibers seen in the medial portions of the rat nucleus accumbens and the occasional fiber seen in the olfactory tubercle. Species differences are also seen in the enkephalin distribution, with patches being particularly dense in the ventral nucleus accumbens of the monkey and extending into the olfactory tubercle, while in the rat enkephalin dense fibers and scattered cells are seen primarily medial to the anterior commissure, with the staining in the olfactory tubercle distinguished as a continuous band of cells extending laterally and dorsally to the rhinal fissure. The olfactory tubercle also contains scattered dynorphin cells and fibers with especially dense staining in the islands of Calleja.

More caudally in the pallidum, enkephalin projections from the striatum form a dense plexus of fibers in the rat and monkey referred to as "woolly fibers" and are a clear example of an enkephalinergic terminal field. These woolly fibers appear to synapse on large pallidal cells and extend in both the globus and ventral pallidum. Pronounced dynorphin fibers are also seen in the globus and ventral pallidum of the rat and monkey and have a woolly-like appearance. POMC fibers have not been observed in the pallidum of the rat or monkey.

In contrast to the dense enkephalin and dynorphin innervation, comparatively little μ-, δ-, and κ-binding is observed in the pallidum of the rat and monkey. The density of opioid receptors in the globus and ventral pallidum is indistinguishable in the rat, while considerably higher levels of κ-receptors are observed in the globus pallidus compared to the ventral pallidum of the guinea pig and monkey.

In the entopeduncular nucleus, a region receiving major projection from the globus pallidus, both dense levels of μ-receptors and moderate amounts of dynorphin staining are observed in the rat. No enkephalin or POMC fibers and only a light density of κ-sites are observed in this nucleus in the rat, suggesting a possible interaction of dynorphin peptides and μ-receptors. The region anatomically equivalent to the entopeduncular nucleus in the monkey (internal division of the globus pallidus) demonstrates dense dynorphin staining and a low density of μ- and κ-sites.

In the midbrain, dense enkephalin and dynorphin fiber staining is observed in the monkey substantia nigra, pars reticulata, particularly its medial aspect. This opioid peptide distribution corresponds well with the moderate μ-receptor binding prominent in the medial pars reticulata and pars compacta of the monkey. Moderate levels of κ-receptors are also seen in the monkey substantia nigra, but have a predominantly lateroventral distribution within the pars reticulata and pars compacta. Only a light density of δ-receptors is observed in the monkey substantia nigra, pars reticulata. No cellular opioid peptide staining has been observed in the monkey pars compacta, but scattered POMC fibers have been seen in the monkey and rat.

The distribution of opioid receptors in the substantia nigra varies markedly between species. In the rat, μ-receptors are predominantly in the substantia nigra, pars compacta, with moderate levels in pars reticulata, which also contains a low density or δ- and κ-sites. The case is reversed in the guinea pig where a high density of μ- and κ-sites is observed in the pars reticulata and only low levels of κ-binding are seen in pars compacta. In relation to the opioid receptor distributions in the rat, dense dynorphin fibers and a moderate number of dynorphin cells are seen in the pars reticulata, with some scattered POMC and enkephalin fibers observed in the pars compacta.

Low to moderate levels of μ-receptors and low amounts of δ- and κ-receptors as well as scattered enkephalin and dynorphin fibers have been seen in the ventral tegmental area of the rat and monkey. POMC fibers have also been reported to course through the ventral tegmental area.

I. Conclusions

Perhaps the most fundamental concept that has emerged from these studies comparing opioid peptide and receptor distributions is that there is no simple and consistent anatomical relationship between specific opioid receptors and peptides. Even within these well-delineated anatomical systems, enkephalin fibers are not consistently colocalized with δ-receptors nor are dynorphin projections consistently found with κ-receptors. These findings are not unique to the basal ganglia and can be observed in a number of neural areas as can be better appreciated in the overlayed peptide-receptor maps of Fig. 1. The advantage of using these neural systems for this analysis is that, aside from being more manageable, anatomically one can clearly identify peptidergic terminal fields in the globus pallidus, entopeduncular nucleus, and substantia nigra where opioid peptides are likely released and interact with the opioid receptors. These interactions are largely dependent on species and anatomical region.

While technical limitations, such as the inability of receptor autoradio-graphy to detect regions of low receptor density or immunohistochemical insensitivity to visualize finely scattered fibers may contribute to the results, they cannot be the entire explanation. The globus pallidus, for example, contains dense enkephalin and dynorphin fibers in both rat and monkey, yet the relative densities of opioid receptors varies across species with a pre-ponderance of κ-sites in the monkey and low levels of μ-, δ-, and κ-sites in the rat. Similarly in the substantia nigra, pars reticulata, dense enkephalin, and dynorphin fibers are found in relation to moderate levels of μ- and κ-sites in the monkey, while in the rat dense dynorphin fibers are codis-tributed with predominantly μ-sites.

These apparent inconsistencies between specific opioid peptides and receptors may reflect differences in posttranslational processing of the opioid peptides both across species and anatomical area. For example, in the processing of DYN (1–17) to DYN (1–8) there is a shift in the relative affinity of the resultant peptide from being κ-selective to having a good affinity for μ- and κ-sites (CORBETT et al. 1982). The conversion of DYN (1–17), in fact, is more complete in the rat substantia nigra, pars reticulata, than in the guinea pig (LEWIS et al. 1985b) and may be related to the predominance of μ-sites in the rat substantia nigra compared to the μ- and κ-sites seen in the guinea pig. Similarly, a number of the pro-enkephalin peptides, such as peptide E, BAM-12, and BAM-22, have affinities for both μ- and κ-receptors (QUIRION and WEISS 1983) and depending on the peptide form released can interact with μ-, δ-, or κ-sites. Differences, then, in peptide-receptor distributions may suggest differential posttranslational processing and are essential for understanding opioid receptor functioning and regulation.

E. Future Directions

A primary goal in studying the distribution of receptors in the nervous system is not simply to catalog the structures that contain a high or low density of binding sites. Rather, it is the first stage in understanding the possible function of these binding sites in the nervous system. Despite the fundamental anatomical importance of receptor autoradiographic studies, they ultimately cannot address the more basic issue of whether a receptor is functional and participates in neural transmission. These studies, for example, cannot easily differentiate nascent receptors traveling along axons from fully functional receptors that are inserted into synaptic membranes and coupled to second message systems. While understanding the precise codistribution of the opioid peptide and receptors has enhanced our appreciation of opioid circuits in the brain, this analysis needs to be coordinated with peptide and opiate antagonist microinjection studies to more clearly delineate whether these circuits are biologically significant. In addition, the more recent development of anatomical techniques to visualize second messengers, such as cAMP and phosphinositide (HWANG et al. 1990), when coupled with receptor autoradiographic and immunohisto-chemical methods will greatly aid our understanding of these receptors and their physiology.

Given the biochemical and physiological similarities of the opioid receptors and the monaminergic receptors, many of the recent molecular biological advances observed with these latter proteins will likely be applied to the opioid receptors. The application of in situ hybridization techniques to opioid receptors once they are cloned will aid not only in identifying and differentiating specific opioid receptor types and subtypes, but will be essential in understanding opioid circuitry and regulation. While receptor autoradiographic techniques label receptors both in cell bodies and fibers, in situ hybridization identifies the cell bodies capable of synthesizing these proteins. The combined use of both these methods provides not only a means of studying the regulation of the receptors within an anatomical context but also a clearer view of the biogenic origin and anatomical projections of these receptors. Such combined techniques have been successfully used in the study of dopaminergic receptors (Mansour et al. 1990) and will likely be applied to the opioid receptors once the nucleic acid sequences encoding these binding sites are identified.

Acknowledgements. We are grateful to Henry Khachaturian and Michael E. Lewis for the many years of productive and stimulating collaboration and friendship. We are also appreciative to Kamie Fulton for her secretarial help and the following grants for their financial support: NIDA (DA02265), T. Raphael, Gastrointestinal Hormone Research Core (P30 AM34933), NIMH Program Project (PO1MH422251).

References

Alheid GF, Heimer L (1988) New perspectives in basal forebrain organization of special relevance for neuropsychiatric disorders: the striatopallidal, amygdaloid, corticopetal components of substantia innominata. Neuroscience 27:1–39

Attali B, Gouarderes C, Mazarguil H, Audigier Y, Cros J (1982) Evidence for multiple "kappa" binding sites by use of opioid peptides in the guinea pig lumbo-sacral spinal cord. Neuropeptides 3:53–64

Atweh SF, Kuhar MJ (1977a) Autoradiographic localization of opiate receptors in rat brain. I. Spinal cord and lower medulla. Brain Res 124:53–67

Atweh SF, Kuhar MJ (1977b) Autoradiographic localization of opiate receptors in rat brain. II. The brain stem. Brain Res 129:1–12

Atweh SF, Kuhar MJ (1977c) Autoradiographic localization of opiate receptors in rat brain III. The telencephalon. Brain Res 134:393–405

Beckett AH, Casey AF (1954) Synthetic analgesics: stereochemical considerations. J Pharm Pharmacol 6:986–999

Castasnas E, Bourhim N, Giraud P, Boudouresque F, Cantan P, Oliver C (1985) Interaction of opiates with opioid binding sites in the bovine adrenal medulla. II. Interaction with kappa sites. J Neurochem 45:688–699

Chang KJ, Blanchard SG, Cuatrecasas P (1984) Benzomorphan sites are ligand recognition sites of putative epsilon receptors. Mol Pharmacol 26:484–488

Clark JA, Liu L, Price M, Hersh B, Edelson M, Pasternak GW (1989) Kappa opiate receptor multiplicity: evidence for two U50,488-sensitive K1 subtypes and a novel K3 subtype. J Pharmacol Exp Ther 251:461–468

Corbett AD, Paterson SJ, McKnight AT, Magnam J, Kosterlitz H (1982) Dynorphin (1–8) and dynorphin (1–9) are ligands for the kappa subtype of opiate receptor. Nature 299:79–81

Cross AJ, Hille C, Slater P (1987) Subtraction autoradiography of opiate receptor subtypes in human brain. Brain Res 418:343–348

Devlin T, Shoemaker WJ (1990) Characterization of kappa opioid binding using dynorphin A(1–13) and U69,593 in the rat brain. J Pharmacol Exp Ther 253:749–759

Gilbert PE, Martin WR (1976) The effects of morphine- and nalorphine-like drugs in the nondependent, morphine dependent and cyclazocine-dependent chronic spinal dog. J Pharmacol Exp Ther 198:66–82

Gillan MGC, Kosterlitz HW (1982) Spectrum of the mu, delta, and kappa binding sites in homogenates of rat brain. Br J Pharmacol 77:461–469

Goldstein A, Naidir A (1989) Multiple opioid receptors: ligand selectivity profiles and binding site signatures. Mol Pharmacol 36:265–272

Goodman RR, Pasternak GW (1985) Visualization of mul opiate receptors in rat brain by using a computerized autoradiographic subtraction technique. Proc Natl Acad Sci USA 82:6667–6671

Graybiel AM (1990) Neurotransmitters and neuromodulators in the basal ganglia. Trends Neurosci 13:244–254

Grevel J, Yu V, Sadee W (1985) Characterization of a labile naloxone binding site (lambda) in rat brain. J Neurochem 44:1647–1655

Handa BK, Lane AC, Lord JAH, Morgan BA, Rance MJ, Smith CFC (1981) Analogues of B-LPH 61–64 processing selective agonist activity at opiate receptors. Eur J Pharmacol 70:531–540

Herkenham M, Pert CB (1982) Light microscopic localization of brain opiate receptors: a general autoradiographic method which perserves tissue quality. J Neurosci 2:1129–1149

Hiller JM, Simon EJ (1979) [3H]Ethylketocyclazocine binding: lack of evidence for a separate kappa receptor in rats CNS. Eur J Pharmacol 60:389–390

Hunter JC, Birchmore B, Woodruff R, Hughes J (1989) Kappa opioid binding sites in the dog cerebral cortex and spinal cord. Neuroscience 31:735–743

Hwang PM, Bredt DS, Snyder SH (1990) Autoradiographic imaging of phosphoinositide turnover in the brain. Science 249:802–804

Iyengar S, Kim HS, Wood PL (1986) Effects of kappa agonists on neurochemical and neuroendocrine indices: evidence for kappa receptor subtypes. Life Sci 39:637–644

James IF, Goldstein A (1984) Site-directed alkylation of multiple opioid receptors. I. Binding selectivity. Mol Pharmacol 25:337–342

James IF, Chavkin C, Goldstein A (1982) Preparation of brain membranes containing a single type of opioid receptor highly selective for dynorphin. Proc Natl Acad Sci USA 79:7570–7574

Khachaturian H, Watson SJ, Lewis ME, Coy D, Goldstein A, Akil H (1982) Dynorphin immunocytochemistry in the rat central nervous system. Peptides 3:941–954

Khachaturian H, Lewis ME, Höllt V, Watson SJ (1983a) Telencephalic enkephalinergic systems in the rat brain. J Neurosci 3:844–855

Khachaturian H, Lewis ME, Watson SJ (1983b) Enkephalin systems in diencephalon and brainstem of the rat. J Comp Neurol 220:310–320

Khachaturian H, Lewis ME, Haber S, Akil H, Watson SJ (1984) Proopiomelanocortin peptide immunocytochemistry in rhesus monkey brain. Brain Res Bull 13:785–800

Khachaturian H, Lewis ME, Schafer MK-H, Watson SJ (1985a) Anatomy of the CNS opioid systems. Trends Neurosci 8:111–119

Khachaturian H, Lewis ME, Haber SN, Houghten RA, Akil H, Watson SJ (1985b) Prodynorphin peptide immunocytochemistry in rhesus monkey brain. Peptides 6:155–166

Kosterlitz HW, Paterson SJ, Robson LE (1981) Characterization of the kappa subtype of the opiate receptor in the guinea pig brain. Br J Pharmacol 73:939–949

Lahti RA, Mickelson MM, McCall JM, vonVoigtlander PF (1985) [3H]U69,593, a highly selective ligand for the opioid κ receptor. Eur J Pharmacol 109:281–284

Lewis ME, Khachaturian H, Akil H, Watson SJ (1984) Anatomical relationship between opioid peptides and receptors in rhesus monkey brain. Brain Res Bull 13:801–812

Lewis ME, Khachaturian H, Watson SJ (1985a) Combined autoradiographic-immunocytochemical analysis of opioid receptors and opioid peptide neuronal systems in brain. Peptides 6:37–47

Lewis ME, Lewis MS, Dores RM, Lewis JW, Khachaturian H, Watson SJ, Akil H
     (1985b) Characterization of multiple opioid receptors and peptides in rat and
     guinea pig substantia nigra. J Biophys 47:54a
Lynch WC, Watt J, Krall S, Paden CM (1985) Autoradiographic localization of
     kappa opiate receptors in CNS taste and feeding areas. Pharmacol Biochem
     Behav 22:699–705
Mansour A, Khachaturian H, Lewis ME, Akil H, Watson SJ (1987) Autoradiographic
     differentiation of mu, delta, and kappa opioid receptors in the rat forebrain and
     midbrain. J Neurosci 7:2445–2464
Mansour A, Khachaturian H, Lewis ME, Akil H, Watson SJ (1988) Anatomy of
     CNS opioid receptors. Trends Neurosci 11:308–314
Mansour A, Meador-Woodruff JH, Bunzow JR, Civelli O, Akil H, Watson SJ
     (1990) Localization of dopamine D2 receptor mRNA and D1 and D2 receptor
     binding in the rat brain and pituitary: an in situ hybridization-receptor
     autoradiographic analysis. J Neurosci 10:2587–2600
Martin WE (1984) Pharmacology of opioids. Pharmacol Rev 35:283–323
Martin WR, Eades CG, Thompson JA, Hupler RE, Gilbert PE (1976) The effects
     of morphine and nalophine-like drugs in the nondependent and morphine-
     dependent chronic spinal dog. J Pharmacol Exp Ther 197:517–532
Morre M, Bachy A, Gout B, Boigegrain R, Arnone M, Rocucci R (1983) Kappa
     binding sites in guinea pig brain membranes: evidence for a dynorphin resistant
     subtype. Life Sci 33:179–182
Morris BJ, Herz A (1986) Autoradiographic localization in rat brain of kappa opiate
     binding site labelled by [3H]bremazocine. Neuroscience 19:839–846
Mosberg HI, Hurst R, Hruby VJ, Gee K, Yamamura HI, Galligan JJ, Burks TF
     (1983) Bis-penicillamine enkephalin possess highly improved specificity toward
     opioid receptors. Proc Natl Acad Sci USA 80:5871–5874
Nock B, Rajpara A, O'Connor LH, Cicero TJ (1988a) [3H]U69,593 labels a subtype
     of kappa opiate receptor with characteristics different from that labeled by
     [3H]ethylketocyclazocine. Life Sci 42:2403–2412
Nock B, Rajpara A, O'Connor LH, Cicero TJ (1988b) Autoradiography of
     [3H]U69,593 binding sites in rat brain: evidence for kappa opioid receptor
     subtypes. Eur J Pharmacol 154:27–34
Paxinos G, Watson C (1986) The rat brain in sterotoxic coordinates. Academic, New
     York
Pert CB, Snyder SH (1973) Opiate receptor: demonstration in nervous tissue.
     Science 179:1011–1014
Pert CB, Kuhar MJ, Snyder SH (1976) Opiate receptor: autoradiographic localiza-
     tion in rat brain. Proc Natl Acad Sci USA 73:3729–3733
Portoghese PS (1965) A new concept in the mode of interaction of narcotic analgesics
     with receptors. J Med Chem 8:609–616
Quirion R, Weiss AS (1983) Peptide E and other proenkephalin-derived peptides are
     potent kappa opiate receptor agonists. Peptides 4:445–449
Robson LE, Paterson SJ, Kosterlitz HW (1983) Opiate receptors. In: Iversen SD,
     Iversen LL, Snyder SH (eds) Handbook of psychopharmacology, vol 14.
     Plenum, New York, pp 13–80
Schulz R, Wüster M, Herz A (1981) Pharmacological characterization of the epsilon
     opiate receptor. J Pharmacol Exp Ther 216:604–606
Sharif NA, Hughes J (1988) Discrete mapping of brain mu and delta opioid receptors
     using selective peptides: quantitative autoradiography, species differences and
     comparison with kappa receptors. Peptides 10:499–522
Simon EJ, Hiller JM, Edelman I (1973) Stereospecific binding of the potent narcotic
     analgesic 3H-etorphine to rat brain homogenate. Proc Natl Acad Sci USA
     70:1947–1949
Su T-S (1985) Further demonstration of kappa opioid binding sites in the brain:
     evidence for heterogeneity. J Pharmacol Exp Ther 232:144–148

Tempel A, Zukin RS (1987) Neuroanatomical patterns of the mu, delta, and kappa opioid receptors of rat brain as determined by quantitative in vitro auto-radiography. Proc Natl Acad Sci USA 84:4308–4312

Terenius L (1973) Characteristics of the "receptor" for narcotic analgesics in synaptic plasma membrane fractions from rat brain. Acta Pharmacol Toxicol (Copenh) 33:377–384

Tiberi M, Magnan J (1990) Demonstration of the heterogeneity of the kappa opioid receptors in guinea pig cerebellum using selective and nonselective drugs. Eur J Pharmacol 188:379–389

Wood MS, Rodriguez FD, Traynor JR (1989) Characterization of kappa opioid binding sites in rat and guinea pig spinal cord. Neuropharmacology 28: 1041–1046

Wood PL (1982) Multiple opiate receptors: support for unique mu, delta and kappa sites. Neuropharmacology 21:487–497

Woods LA (1956) The pharmacology of nalorphine (N-allylnormorphine). Pharmacol Rev 8:175–198

Young WS III, Kuhar MJ (1979) A new method for receptor autoradiography: [3H] opioid receptors in rat brain. Brain Res 179:255–270

Zukin RS, Eghabli M, Olive D, Unterwald EM, Tempel A (1988) Characterization and visualization of rat and guinea pig kappa opioid receptors: evidence for K1 and K2 opioid receptors. Proc Natl Acad Sci USA 85:4061–4065

CHAPTER 6

Opioid Receptor Regulation

R.S. Zukin, D.E. Pellegrini-Giampietro, C.M. Knapp, and A. Tempel

A. Introduction

The actions of opiates and opioid peptides upon nervous tissue are mediated by μ-, δ-, and κ-opioid receptors and (in the case of σ-opioids) the PCP site of the NMDA receptor (for a review see Chap. 1). The three opioid receptors exhibit different ligand selectivities, strikingly different neuroanatomical patterns, distinct physiological and behavioral profiles, and differing sensitivities to naloxone (or naltrexone) antagonism. In the central nervous system (CNS) these receptors are activated by three classes of structurally related peptides, β-endorphin, the enkephalins, and the dynorphin-related peptides, encoded by three different genes. The observation that opiate analgesics produce tolerance and dependence suggests that opioid systems can undergo plastic changes. This chapter focuses on studies of the regulation of μ- and δ-opioid receptors. A particular emphasis is placed upon examination of mechanisms by which chronic treatment of opioid drugs quantitatively regulates opioid receptors in adult, embryonic, and neonatal brain.

The μ-receptor is operationally defined as the receptor at which β-endorphin, morphine, and related opioids (normorphine, dihydromorphine, levorphanol) produce analgesia and other classical pharmacological effects. The δ-receptor is defined as the opioid receptor which predominates in the mouse vas deferens and exhibits highest affinity for the enkephalins. Receptor-binding assays have provided considerable evidence for the existence of multiple subtypes of both μ- and δ-opioid receptors. Most opioid peptides and opioid drugs interact with more than one of these receptor sites. Thus, the complex neuropharmacological actions of a given opioid would appear to reflect its interaction with varying potencies at a combination of these and other opioid receptor sites.

Insight into the functional consequences of opioid receptor activation comes from electrophysiological studies (see Chap. 30). Studies from the laboratories of MacDonald (WERZ and MacDONALD 1985; MacDONALD and WERZ 1986) and North (NORTH and WILLIAMS 1983; CHERUBINI and NORTH 1985; MIYAKE et al. 1989) have shown that in locus ceruleus and peripheral ganglion neurons μ- and δ-receptors can couple to voltage and/or Ca^{2+}-dependent K^+ channels through the local intermediary action of a

GTP-binding protein; activation of μ- and δ-receptors leads to opening of membrane potassium channels, causing a hyperpolarization of the cell membrane and closing of voltage-sensitive channels. Activation of all three opioid receptors ultimately decreases calcium entry, but by different mechanisms. If these receptors were located on presynaptic terminals, they would be expected to mediate inhibition of transmitter release (NORTH 1986).

Although to date no opioid receptor types have been cloned, a variety of studies indicate that opioid receptors are members of the large super-family of G protein-linked receptors. These receptors are coupled through various G proteins to any of a number of voltage-sensitive K^+ or Ca^{2+} channels. Coupling may involve diffusible components of the adenylyl cyclase or phosphoinositide second messenger systems or may be more direct. Members of this superfamily include rhodopsin, the α- and β-adrenergic, muscarinic acetylcholine (ACh), dopamine, 5-hydroxytryptamine $(5-HT_{1c})$, $5-HT_{2A}$, $5-HT_{2B}$, substance K, and substance P receptors. Each of the members of this receptor superfamily comprises a single subunit with significant sequence identity among the members. Predicted structural features include: (1) seven putative transmembrane-spanning domains; (2) a large extracellular N-terminal region which contains seven putative glycosylation sites, as well as the presumed transmitter binding site; (3) a very large fourth cytoplasmic loop of varying length, which is essential for binding of G protein; and (4) a large cytoplasmic C-terminal domain with consensus sequences for cAMP-dependent phosphorylation.

Studies in neuronal cell lines demonstrating opioid-induced inhibition of adenyl cyclase (SHARMA et al. 1975; KLEE and NIRENBERG 1976) and in brain and cell lines showing guanyl nucleotide modulation of opioid agonist binding (BLUME 1978) provided early evidence that μ- and δ-receptors are coupled to guanyl nucleotide binding proteins. More recent studies demonstrate that pertussis toxin blocks opioid-induced shortening of action potentials in dorsal root ganglion neurons, implicating linkage of some opioid receptors to G_i or G_o proteins (SHEN and CRAIN 1989). Cholera toxin selectivity blocks opioid-induced prolongation of the action potential in the same neurons (SHEN and CRAIN 1989). Intracellular injection of a cAMP-dependent protein kinase into dorsal-root ganglion neurons was shown to block opioid peptide-induced prolongation, but not shortening, of the action potential (CRAIN and SHEN 1990). These findings indicate that excitatory actions of opioids are mediated by opioid receptors coupled to channels via a cAMP-dependent system.

Opioid receptor regulation has received much attention as the result of efforts to elucidate mechanisms involved in the generation of opioid-induced tolerance and dependence. It would appear that these phenomena involve not only changes in opioid receptor numbers, but also changes in coupling of opioid receptors to G proteins or alterations in second messenger systems such as adenylyl cyclase (see Chap. 54 in part II this volume). Chronic, but not acute, administration of opioids has been reported to increase levels of $G_{i\alpha}$ and $G_{o\alpha}$, adenylate cyclase activity, cAMP-dependent protein kinase activity, and a number of morphine- and cAMP-regulated phosphoproteins (NESTLER and TALLMAN 1988; GUITART and NESTLER 1989; GUITART et al. 1990). Furthermore, acute or chronic morphine treatment decreases gene expression of the immediate early genes c-*fos* and c-*jun* in rat brain, whereas precipitation of withdrawal increases their expression two- to threefold (HAYWARD et al. 1990).

It should be noted that in some cells or tissues opioid receptor down-regulation may be sufficient to account for opioid-induced desensitization in vitro and tolerance in vivo (see below). Moreover, it is well established that opioid antagonist-induced supersensitivity is the result of opioid receptor upregulation. Long-term in vivo administration of the opioid antagonist naloxone (or naltrexone) to adult rats results in enhanced morphine-induced analgesia (TANG and COLLINS 1978; SCHULZ et al. 1979) and a coordinated increase in μ- and δ-receptors (ZUKIN et al. 1982; TEMPEL et al. 1984; see below). Brain regions in which maximal receptor increases occurred were cortical layers I and III, striatum, nucleus accumbens, periaqueductal gray, and ventral tegmental area (TEMPEL et al. 1984).

The study of opioid receptor regulation has taken on additional import-ance as the variety of opioid agents in clinical use has increased. The opioid antagonist naltrexone has recently been put into use clinically to treat heroin addicts and a variety of new opioid agonists have been developed as analgesics. Studies reviewed in this chapter demonstrate that chronic treat-ment of animals with either class of drugs can alter opioid receptor densities and properties and opioid peptide content in specific brain regions. Chronic treatment with opioid drugs can affect embryonic and neonatal animals differently than it does adults (see below).

Despite nearly 2 decades of research in the area of opioid receptor regulation, a number of questions are as yet unanswered. What is the molecular basis of opioid tolerance? Do antagonists regulate enkephalin and substance P at the transcriptional or posttranscriptional level? Do they regulate preproenkephalin (PPE) gene expression differentially throughout the brain? Is naltrexone-induced opioid receptor upregulation mediated by *fos* and *jun*? Does antagonist-induced receptor upregulation require forma-tion of synapses? How do chronic opiates affect peptides and receptors in the developing nervous system? The following sections review studies that have begun to provide some of the answers.

B. Regulation of Opioid Receptors in the Adult Brain by Chronically Administered Opioid Agonists and Antagonists

I. Chronic Administration of Opioid Agonists In Vivo

To date the question of whether opioid agonist-induced tolerance and dependence in vivo and desensitization in vitro are associated with altered receptor numbers remains unresolved. Most early studies failed to show a systematic change in receptor number following chronic administration of morphine to rats, guinea pigs, or mice (PERT et al. 1973; HITZEMANN et al. 1974; HÖLLT et al. 1975; KLEE et al. 1976). An exception was the study by DAVIS et al. (1979), who showed that the development of tolerance to morphine in rats is accompanied by a reduction in opioid receptor number. In this study receptor binding was carried out in the brainstem slice which was homogenized *after* ligand incubation. All early studies used non-selective radiolabeled opioids, such as [^{3}H]naloxone. In more recent studies in which the relatively specific μ-ligand [^{3}H]D-Ala^2, Me-Phe^4, Gly-ol^5-enkephalin (DAGO) was used, chronic administration of morphine modestly decreased μ-receptors in the guinea pig cerebral cortex (WERLING et al. 1989), but increased μ-receptors in several rat brain regions (BRADY et al. 1989). When [^{3}H]FK 33,824, another μ-selective ligand, was used, chronic morphine appeared to produce no change in rat spinal cord μ-receptors. More recent studies report that chronic morphine treatment of rats produces an upregulation of the low-affinity [^{3}H]D-Ala^2,D-Leu^5-enkephalin (DADLE) site in brain (ROTHMAN et al. 1986; DANKS et al. 1988; BRADY et al. 1989).

Opioid agonists other than morphine appear to induce receptor down-regulation in vivo. For example, chronic etorphine produces downregulation of μ- and δ-receptors in vivo (TAO et al. 1987). Opioid peptides administered to rats in vivo also induce opioid receptor downregulation. Long-term administration of D-Ala^2, D-Leu^5-enkephalin (DADLE; TAO et al. 1988) or methionine-enkephalin i.c.v. to rats (STEECE et al. 1986) decreases brain δ-receptors. Intrathecal administration of high concentrations of the μ-selective peptide [*N*-Me-Phe^3, D-Pro^4] morphiceptin leads to a reduction in the number of spinal cord, but not brain, μ-receptors (NISHINO et al. 1990). Only in the neonatal rat, however, has a correlation been demonstrated between *morphine*-induced receptor downregulation and the development of tolerance (TEMPEL et al. 1988; see below).

Although numerous studies have examined the effects of chronic μ- and δ-opioids on brain receptors, few have addressed the effects of chronic κ-agonist administration. Rats treated chronically with κ-opioids develop tolerance, as determined in behavioral paradigms measuring analgesia (BHARGAVA et al. 1989a). Chronic administration of bremazocine leads to a reduction in [^{3}H]bremazocine binding under conditions in which μ- and δ-binding has been suppressed (MORRIS and HERZ 1989). Moreover, chronic treatment of rats with U-50,488H (κ-opioid) leads to a decrease in [³H]ethylketocyclazocine binding to brain membranes (BHARGAVA et al. 1989b). Because ethylketocyclazocine is a nonselective μ-opioid and because [³H]bremazocine labels nonopioid sites in addition to μ-, δ-, and κ-receptors (ZUKIN et al. 1988), it is not clear whether the observed decreases are in κ-opioid receptors.

An important question is why chronic treatment with etorphine and opioid peptides, but not with morphine, produces opioid receptor downregulation in the adult animal. Several explanations are plausible. For example, it may be that morphine is a partial agonist. Alternatively, interaction of etorphine and enkephalin-like peptides with δ-receptors may be critical to long-term changes at the cellular level. Yet another possibility is that opioid peptides bind differently than do opioid narcotic agonists to the same receptor, thereby producing different effects.

II. Chronic Administration of Agonists to Cells Grown in Culture

Drug-induced downregulation of opioid receptors has been documented in several neurotumor cell lines. Cultured mouse neuroblastoma cells (N4TG-1) and neuroblastoma-glioma hybrid cells (NG108-15) express δ-, but not μ- or κ-, opioid receptors (CHANG and CUATRECASAS 1979). Early studies indicated that long-term exposure of NG108-15 cells to opiate drugs or opioid peptides leads to a time-dependent inhibition of adenylyl cyclase activity (SHARMA et al. 1975; LAMPERT et al. 1976). Continued exposure of the cells to agonist results in a return to normal cyclase activity; removal of agonist leads to an increase above normal levels, a phenomenon thought to be related to tolerance and dependence in animals. Cuatrecasas and coworkers used a rhodamine derivative of enkephalin to label opioid receptors in cell culture; visualization of the receptors by fluorescence microscopy provided evidence that they slowly form clusters, but do not appear to internalize (HAZUM et al. 1979). This finding is in contrast to findings for many other polypeptide hormone receptors which do appear to internalize; internalization in such cases is thought to be involved in agonist-induced receptor downregulation and desensitization.

More recently, several laboratories have shown that long-term exposure of neurotumor cell lines (CHANG et al. 1978, 1982; BLANCHARD et al. 1982; SIMANTOV et al. 1982; LAW et al. 1983; TAO et al. 1988) or aggregating fetal brain cells (LENOIR et al. 1983) to methionine-enkephalin or other opioid peptides results in a decrease in receptor density. Chronic exposure to alkaloid agonists, however, has no detectable effect (CHANG et al. 1981; LENOIR et al. 1983), except in the case of pituitary tumor cells, which show a 25% reduction of [³H]diprenorphine binding sites following a 5-h exposure to morphine (PUTTFARKEN and COX 1989). Studies of [³H]DADLE (D-Ala², D-Leu⁵-enkephalin) uptake by N4TG-1 cells (BLANCHARD et al. 1982) provide evidence that enkephalin is internalized by means of receptor-mediated endocytosis.

III. Chronic Administration of Opioid Antagonists

The first reports of antagonist-induced opioid supersensitivity and opiate receptor upregulation came from two laboratories. TANG and COLLINS (1978) found that long-term treatment with naloxone results in enhanced morphine-induced analgesia. Because naloxone is rapidly metabolized, it was necessary to prepare rats with indwelling venous cannulas. The same laboratory (LAHTI and COLLINS 1978) determined that the enhanced analgesia correlates with an increased number of [^{3}H]naloxone binding sites. Almost simultaneously, SCHULZ et al. (1979) reported that guinea pigs exposed to naloxone for 1–2 weeks by implantation with naloxone pellets show increased sensitivity to the inhibitory properties of opiates in the isolated ileum preparation. Chronic naloxone treatment also results in increased [^{3}H]etorphine binding in the ileum and brainstem of guinea pigs. It is important to point out that these studies were preliminary reports and, as such, did not control for (1) possible changes induced in endogenous opioid peptide levels that might give rise to apparent changes in receptor densities and (2) the effects of acute antagonist administration.

Later studies confirmed these findings and showed that chronic, but not acute, administration of the long-acting opioid antagonist naltrexone produces a dramatic (+95%) increase in brain opioid receptor density (ZUKIN et al. 1982; TEMPEL et al. 1985). In all experiments, brain tissue was incubated at 37°C for 30 min and washed by centrifugation before addition of radioligand in order to facilitate the removal of both endogenous ligands and naltrexone. Thus, it is unlikely that the receptor upregulation observed in response to chronic antagonist administration is due to an increased capacity of the same number of active receptors. In experiments designed to target specific opioid receptor types, it was shown that long-term treatment with naltrexone produces a coordinated upregulation of brain μ- and δ-receptors, but causes no significant change in the density or affinity of κ- and σ-receptors (TEMPEL et al. 1985; YOBURN et al. 1989). These findings indicate that the κ- and σ-receptor classes might be subject to independent control mechanisms.

Several neurochemical and functional correlates of opioid receptor upregulation have been found. First, the newly synthesized or unmasked receptors exhibit an enhanced sensitivity to guanyl nucleotide modulation (ZUKIN et al. 1982). Withdrawal from chronic naltrexone treatment results in a return to nearly control levels of receptor density and guanyl nucleotide sensitivity in a period of 6 days (TEMPEL et al. 1985). These results suggest that upregulation is accompanied by an increased coupling of the receptors to the inhibitory guanyl nucleotide binding protein G_i. Second, chronic in vivo administration of naloxone or naltrexone results in enhanced morphine-induced analgesia (TANG and COLLINS 1978; TEMPEL et al. 1985; YOBURN et al. 1985) and an enhanced effect of morphine on neurons of the locus ceruleus (BARDO et al. 1983). These findings suggest a functional significance for the naltrexone-induced opioid receptor upregulation.

The neuronanatomical pattern of brain opioid receptor upregulation in response to chronic naltrexone administration was elucidated by quantitative receptor autoradiography (TEMPEL et al. 1984). The radioligand used was [^{3}H]dihydromorphine, a relatively selective μ-opioid ligand. Table 1 summarizes the changes in μ-opioid receptor density throughout the brain following chronic naltrexone treatment. The largest increases occur in layer I of the neocortex, the nucleus accumbens, the amygdala, the ventral tegmental area, the ventromedial hypothalamus and the substantia nigra compacta. Moderate increases occur in layer III of the neocortex, the striatum, the lateral septum, the posterior thalamic nucleus, and the superior colliculus. No significant changes in density are found in areas surrounding the striatal patches, the medial septum, the ventral thalamic nuclei, the substantia nigra reticulata, or the locus ceruleus.

Brunello and coworkers (BRUNELLO et al. 1984) showed that chronic naltrexone administration results in a marked increase in the number of μ-

Table 1. Optical density measurements of opiate receptors in chronic naltrexone-treated and control rat brain. From TEMPEL et al. (1984)

Region	Control brain ($n = 2$)	Naltrexone-treated brain ($n = 2$)	% change
Neocortex			
Layer I	0.11 ± 0.04	0.22 ± 0.02	+100
Layer III	0.17 ± 0.03	0.27 ± 0.02	+59
Subcallosal streak	0.36 ± 0.06	0.31 ± 0.04	−14
Striatum			
Patches	0.38 ± 0.11	0.55 ± 0.02	+45
Other areas	0.22 ± 0.03	0.26 ± 0.04	+18
Nucleus accumbens	0.29 ± 0.06	0.55 ± 0.02	+90
Thalamus			
Post. thal. nucleus	0.33 ± 0.02	0.57 ± 0.03	+73
Dorsal thal. nucleus	0.46 ± 0.04	0.61 ± 0.02	+33
Ventral thal. nucleus	0.14 ± 0.01	0.13 ± 0.02	−7
Hippocampus			
Molecular layer	0.34 ± 0.03	0.51 ± 0.02	+50
Other areas	0.19 ± 0.03	0.23 ± 0.02	+21
Hypothalamus			
Ventromedial	0.12 ± 0.02	0.45 ± 0.02	+275
Central gray	0.20 ± 0.01	0.42 ± 0.04	+110
Substantia nigra			
Compacta	0.10 ± 0.02	0.30 ± 0.04	+200
Reticulata	0.21 ± 0.02	0.21 ± 0.03	–
Ventral tegmental area	0.12 ± 0.01	0.45 ± 0.02	+275
Locus ceruleus	0.24 ± 0.03	0.21 ± 0.0	−13

and δ-receptors in the striatum and brainstem of C$_{57}$BL/6J mice, but produces no change in methionine-enkephalin levels. The increase in receptor number is accompanied by an enhancement of morphine-induced locomotor activity. Chronic administration of opioid antagonists to neonatal rats or indirect exposure in utero also leads to alterations in opioid receptor development (see below). For example, Bardo et al. (1982) showed that rat pups treated chronically with naloxone exhibited significant increases in opiate receptors of the hypothalamus, striatum, and neocortex (Bardo et al. 1982). These antagonist-induced receptor increases are accompanied by the development of supersensitivity to morphine, as determined in analgesia paradigms, and are reversed following cessation of antagonist treatment.

A variety of studies in the adult CNS have documented that chronic administration of opioid drugs alters opioid peptide content in specific brain regions and that this regulation occurs at the level of gene expression (see also Chap. 24). Chronic administration of naltrexone to rats increases methionine enkephalin-like immunoreactivity in the striatum and nucleus accumbens (Tempel et al. 1984). Chronic naltrexone also increases substance P immunoreactivity in the striatum (Tempel et al. 1990) and decreases β-endorphin immunoreactivity in the hypothalamus, thalamus, and amygdala (Ragavan et al. 1983). To determine the mechanism by which opioids modify enkephalin and substance P levels, their effects on preproenkephalin (PPE) and preprotachykinin (PPT) mRNA levels were examined. Long-term blockade of opioid receptors by naltrexone leads to increases in both PPE and PPT mRNA in the striatum (Tempel et al. 1990). Chronic morphine treatment, on the other hand, decreases striatal PPE mRNA (Uhl et al. 1988). It is concluded that both chronic activation and blockade of opioid receptors influence PPE and PPT gene expression.

C. Regulation of Opioid Receptors by Other Drugs or Specific Brain Lesions

Other drug and lesion studies have provided further examples of opioid receptor upregulation in adult and neonatal animals. For example, Gardner et al. (1980) found that injection of the neurotoxin 6-hydroxydopamine into the lateral substantia nigra of the rat leads to an increase in δ-receptors in the striatum. Simantov and Amir (1983) reported that monosodium glutamate (MSG)-induced lesions of the arcuate nucleus of the hypothalamus led to an increase in μ-receptors in the midbrain of neonatal mice. Receptor upregulation correlates with an enhanced response to morphine and naltrexone in tests of the intact animal for thermal pain sensitivity. By contrast, MSG administration to neonatal rats produces a selective increase in receptor number in the thalamus, with no apparent change in μ-receptors or δ-receptors of other brain regions (Young et al. 1982).

Holaday and coworkers showed that repeated electroconvulsive shock treatment of rats produces significant increases in opioid receptor density in the olfactory bulb, nucleus accumbens, and caudate nucleus, as measured by binding of [^{3}H]DADLE (HOLADAY et al. 1982) or [^{3}H]diprenorphine (HOLADAY et al. 1986; HITZEMANN et al. 1987). Epileptic seizures may also lead to increases in opioid receptor density, as measured by positron emission tomography; maximal increases are in μ-receptors ipsilateral to the site of electrical focus (FROST et al. 1988). It has also been reported, however, that electroconvulsive shock causes downregulation of μ- and δ-receptors (NAKATA et al. 1985), possibly due to long-term occupation of receptors with endogenous opioids released during electroconvulsive shock. Chronic membrane depolarization produces upregulation of μ- and δ-opioid receptors in embryonic guinea pig brain cells (SIMANTOV and LEVY 1989). In contrast, treatment of cells with high concentrations of KCl or veratridine downregulates κ-receptors, indicating that neuronal activation can differentially regulate subpopulations of opioid receptors (BARG and SIMANTOV 1990).

D. Regulation of Opioid Receptor and Peptide Gene Expression in Embryonic and Neonatal Brain

Although opioid binding sites are detectable in rat brain prior to embryonic day E14, the pattern of distribution in the immature brain (CLENDENINN et al. 1976; COYLE and PERT 1976) differs from that in adult brain (YOUNG and KUHAR 1979; HERKENHAM and PERT 1981; TEMPEL et al. 1984) until 2 weeks after birth. Opioid receptors show a caudal to rostral sequence in their development (TSANG and NG 1980; TSANG et al. 1982). The different opioid receptor types are expressed at different times during brain development, although in each case the largest increases are observed between 3 and 15 days after birth (BARR et al. 1986; PETRILLO et al. 1987). μ-Opioid receptors are present in the mouse and rat brain at the time of birth (TAVANI et al. 1985; PETRILLO et al. 1987) and receptor density increases rapidly postnatally. By contrast, δ-receptors are not detectable until 7–10 days after birth (KENT et al. 1982; LESLIE et al. 1982; SPAIN et al. 1985; TAVANI et al. 1985; PETRILLO et al. 1987; TEMPEL et al. 1988), and by 15 days after birth they have reached 50% of adult levels (TAVANI et al. 1985). κ-Receptors are present at birth and their density reaches adult levels by 1 week after birth (LESLIE et al. 1982; BARR et al. 1985; LOUGHLIN et al. 1985; SPAIN et al. 1985). These diverse patterns of development suggest that different mechanisms may regulate expression of the various opioid receptor types.

Little is known about mechanisms regulating the initial expression of opioid receptors. However, receptor development may be influenced quantitatively by a variety of factors in the neuronal environment. Antenatal or perinatal exposure to opioid agonists or antagonists alters the apparent number of opioid receptors in the brain with concomitant changes in antinociceptive responses (Tsang and Ng 1980; Handelmann and Quirion 1983; Tempel et al. 1988). Similarly, stress, pain, and a variety of other drugs and toxins have been shown to alter receptor number (Torda 1978; Kirby et al. 1982; Watanabe et al. 1983; Moon 1984). However, the intracellular factors that regulate opioid receptor synthesis, insertion, and degradation are unknown.

I. Effects of Chronic Opioid Administration on Opioid Receptor Expression

1. Perinatal Treatment

It is well established that perinatal exposure to drugs may influence the ontogenesis of brain opioid systems. Chronic administration of opioid agonists to pregnant rats may alter the pattern and number of opioid receptors, as well as sensitivity to opioid drugs in offspring. Results from a variety of studies are complicated and contradictory, however, presumably due to differences in exposure time, dose and route of administration, and the age at which animals were tested. Exposure of rats to morphine in utero has been reported to decrease brain opioid receptors during the first week postnatal, relative to age-matched controls, (Kirby and Aronstam 1983; Tempel et al. 1988) but an increase at later ages (Iyengar and Rabii 1982; Tsang and Ng 1980; Tempel et al. 1988). Greatest changes are in μ-receptors (Tempel et al. 1988). Table 2 summarizes the time course of μ-receptor downregulation in offspring following chronic prenatal treatment with morphine. It should be noted that these studies controlled for protein content in morphine- and placebo-treated animals; thus it is unlikely

Table 2. Changes in brain μ-opioid receptor densities of infant rats following chronic prenatal treatment with morphine. Rat pups were put to death by decapitation on the day of parturition (day 0), and 5, 14, and 29 days postnatally. Values were generated by computer-assisted linear regression analysis. Receptor density values are reported as means ± SEM from a minimum of three independent experiments. The number of animals per group for each time point is indicated in parentheses

Postnatal day	[^{3}H]DAGO binding		% change
	Control (fmol/mg protein)	Morphine-treated (fmol/mg protein)	
0	(4) 77 ± 2.3	(4) 50 ± 3.5	−35%*
5	(4) 81 ± 4.3	(4) 59 ± 5.3	−27%
14	(3) 81 ± 4.1	(3) 83 ± 4.7	−
28	(4) 132 ± 12.5	(4) 128 ± 11.7	−

* Statistically significant difference (two-tailed t test, $p < 0.05$).

that the observed changes are due to differences in protein levels. Chronic treatment of neonatal rats with morphine does not produce changes in brain GABA receptors (TEMPEL et al. 1988). It is concluded that the observed change in opioid receptor number is a specific one.

2. Postnatal Treatment

Early studies of chronic morphine administration to neonates also provide conflicting results. In one study, morphine administration to neonates was reported to increase opioid receptor binding in the striatum and nucleus accumbens (HANDELMANN and QUIRION 1983), whereas in another study no such changes were detected (BARDO et al. 1982). More recent studies have used more selective radiolabeled opioids. Chronic administration of morphine to neonates decreases brain μ-receptors by 30%. In contrast, δ-and κ-receptors are unchanged. Further treatment with morphine fails to result in any significant change in receptors relative to saline-treated (control) animals. The degree of μ-opioid receptor downregulation decreases with age of the animal (Table 3). At postnatal day 14, there is no statistically significant difference in receptor density between brains of control and morphine-treated pups, as in adult rats. When rat pups are treated chronically with morphine beginning on postnatal day 14 and assayed on either postnatal day 22 or day 29, no significant differences in opioid receptor number, relative to that for saline-treated (control) animals, can be detected (TEMPEL et al. 1988). Thus, morphine-induced receptor downregulation is observed only during the first week of life.

In order to examine the neuroanatomical pattern of opioid receptor changes, receptor autoradiography at the level of the light microscope was carried out on frozen brain sections of chronic morphine-treated and control

Table 3. Changes in brain μ-opioid receptor densities of infant rats following chronic postnatal treatment with morphine. Neonatal rats were each given one daily s.c. injection of morphine or saline beginning on postnatal day 1. Rat pups were put to death by decapitation at the time indicated. Values were generated by computer-assisted linear regression analysis. Receptors density values are reported as means ± SEM from a minimum of three experiments. The number of animals per group for each time point is indicated in parentheses

Duration of treatment postparturition (days)	[^{3}H]DAGO binding		% change
	Control (fmol/mg protein)	Morphine-injected (fmol/mg protein)	
4	(6) 81 ± 3.8	(6) 57 ± 3.3	−30%*
8	(6) 74 ± 8.5	(6) 61 ± 11.5	−18%
21	(4) 156 ± 5.7	(4) 135 ± 10.4	−13%
28	(3) 132 ± 16.5	(3) 128 ± 8.4	0%

* Statistically significant difference (two-tailed t test, $p < 0.05$).

pups (TEMPEL, unpublished). Morphine treatment (4 days) decreases μ-opioid receptors in striatal patches and the nucleus accumbens. Longer treatment with morphine (8 days) does not significantly alter μ-receptors. It is concluded that the neonatal opioid receptor system is particularly responsive to chronic drug treatment for a transient period.

II. Effects of Chronic Opioid Administration on Opioid Peptide Expression

Studies of the effects of chronic morphine treatment on brain enkephalin levels have produced conflicting results. Chronic administration of morphine to mature rats has been reported to reduce brain enkephalin content (SHANI et al. 1979; BERGSTROM and TERENIUS 1983) or to have no effect (CHILDERS et al. 1977; FRATTA et al. 1977). β-Endorphin levels are markedly decreased (HÖLLT et al. 1978; PRZEWLOCKI et al. 1979). Chronic administration of morphine also decreased enkephalin content in monkey hippocampus (ELSWORTH et al. 1986). Chronic antagonist treatment also causes increases in methionine enkephalin and substance P content in the striatum (TEMPEL et al. 1990); these changes appear to arise at both the transcriptional and posttranscriptional levels (ROGINSKI et al., submitted).

In a preliminary study, TEMPEL and coworkers have examined the effects of chronic morphine treatment of neonatal rats on preproenkephalin (PPE) mRNA levels in the striatum (unpublished data). Four days of post-natal morphine treatment to 7-day-old rats produces a 24% *increase* in striatal PPE mRNA. In contrast, longer treatment (14 days) leads to a 30% *decrease* in striatal PPE mRNA, as observed for adults (UHL et al. 1988). Chronic treatment with opiate antagonists produces the opposite result. Four days of naltrexone treatment to neonates decreases striatal pre-proenkephalin mRNA by 33%, whereas 8 days of treatment increases PPE mRNA by 23%.

The effect of prolonged opioid use by pregnant women on opioid peptide levels in their newborns has received considerable attention. Babies born to morphine- and methadone-dependent mothers have elevated plasma β-endorphin levels for at least 40 days after birth and exhibit behavioral abnormalities (LESSER-KATZ 1982; BAUMAN and LEVINE 1986; DEREN 1986), but fail to exhibit either signs of withdrawal (GENAZZANI et al. 1986; PANERAI et al. 1983).

It is concluded that chronic opioid drugs affect the developing brain differently than they affect adult brain. Future research along these lines should provide further insights into mechanisms underlying opioid tolerance and addiction.

References

Bardo MT, Bhatnagar RK, Gebhardt GF (1982) Differential effects of chronic morphine and naloxone on opiate receptors, monoamines, and morphine-induced behaviors in preweanling rats. Dev Brain Res 4:139–147

Bardo MT, Bhatnagar RK, Gebhardt GF (1983) Chronic naltrexone increases opiate binding in brain and produces supersensitivity to morphine in the locus coeruleus of the rat. Brain Res 289:223–234

Barg J, Simantov R (1990) Depolarization regulates selectively the expression of different opioid receptors: a decreased number of kappa receptors in chronically activated guinea pig brain cell cultures. Neurosci Lett 111:222–227

Barr GA, Paredes W, Erickson KL, Zukin RS (1986) Kappa opioid receptor-mediated analgesia in the developing rat. Dev Brain Res 29:145–152

Bauman PS, Levine SA (1986) The development of children of drug addicts. Int J Addict 21:849–863

Bergstrom L, Terenius L (1983) Enkephalin levels decrease in rat striatum during morphine abstinence. Eur J Pharmacol 60:349–352

Bhargava HN, Ramarao P, Gulati A (1989a) Effects of morphine in rats treated chronically with U-50,488H, a kappa opioid receptor agonist. Eur J Pharmacol 162:257–264

Bhargava HN, Gulati A, Ramarao P (1989b) Effect of chronic administration of U-50,488H on tolerance to its pharmacological actions and on multiple opioid receptors in rat brain regions and spinal cord. J Pharmacol Exp Ther 251:21–26

Blanchard SG, Chang KJ, Cuatrecasas P (1982) Studies on the mechanism of enkephalin receptor down regulation. Life Sci 31:1311–1314

Blume AJ (1978) Interaction of ligands with the opiate receptors of brain membranes: regulation by ions and nucleotides. Proc Natl Acad Sci USA 75:1713–1717

Brady LS, Herkenham M, Long JB, Rothman RB (1989) Chronic morphine increases mu-opiate receptor binding in rat brain: a quantitative auto-radiographic study. Brain Res 477:382–386

Brunello N, Volterra A, DiGiulio AM, Cuomo V, Racagni G (1984) Modulation of opioid system in C57 mice after repeated treatment with morphine and naloxone: biochemical and behavioral correlates. Life Sci 34:1669

Chang KJ, Cuatrecasas P (1979) Multiple opiate receptors: enkephalins and morphine bind to receptors of different specificity. J Biol Chem 254:2610–2618

Chang KJ, Miller RJ, Cuatrecasas P (1978) Interaction of enkephalin with opiate receptors in intact cultured cells. Mol Pharmacol 14:961–970

Chang KJ, Hazum E, Killian A, Cuatrecasas P (1981) Interactions of ligands with morphine and enkephalin receptors are differentially affected by guanine nucleotide. Mol Pharmacol 20:1–7

Chang KJ, Eckel RW, Blanchard SG (1982) Opioid peptides induce reduction of enkephalin receptors in cultured neuroblastoma cells. Nature 296:446–448

Cherubini E, North RA (1985) Mu and κ opioids inhibit transmitter release by different mechanisms. Proc Natl Acad Sci USA 82:1860

Childers SR, Simantov R, Snyder SH (1977) Enkephalin: radioimmunoassay and radioreceptor assay in morphine dependent rats. Eur J Pharmacol 46:289–293

Clendeninn NJ, Petraitis M, Simon EJ (1976) Ontological development of opiate receptors in rodent brain. Brain Res 118:157–160

Coyle JT, Pert CB (1976) Ontogenetic development of [^{3}H]naloxone binding in rat brain. Neuropharmacology 15:555–560

Crain SM, Shen KF (1990) Opioids can evoke direct receptor-mediated excitatory effects on sensory neurons. Trends Pharmacol Sci 11:77–81

Danks JA, Tortella FC, Long JB, Bykov V, Jacobson KC, Rice JW, Holaday, Rothman RB (1988) Chronic administration of morphine and naltrexone upregulate [^{3}H] (D-Ala^2, D-Leu^5) enkephalin binding sites by different mechanisms. Neuropharmacology 27:965–974

Davis ME, Akera T, Brody TM (1979) Reduction of opiate binding to brainstem slices associated with the development of tolerance to morphine in rats. J Pharmacol Exp Ther 211:112–119

Deren S (1986) Children of substance abusers: a review of the literature. J Subst Abuse Treat 3:77–94

Elsworth JD, Redmond DE Jr, Roth RH (1986) Effect of morphine treatment and withdrawal on endogenous methionine- and leucine-enkephalin levels in primate brain. Biochem Pharmacol 35:3415–3417

Fratta W, Yang H-YT, Hong J, Costa E (1977) Stability of met-enkephalin content in brain structures of morphine-dependent or foot-shock stressed rats. Nature 268:452–453

Frost JJ, Mayberg HS, Fisher RS, Douglass KH, Dannals RF, Links JM, Wilson AA, Ravert HT, Rosenbaum AE, Snyder SH (1988) Mu-opiate receptors measured by positron emission tomography are increased in temporal lobe epilepsy. Ann Neurol 23:231–237

Gardner EL, Zukin RS, Makman MH (1980) Modulation of opiate receptor binding in striatum and amygdala by selective mesencephalic lesions. Brain Res 194:232–239

Genazzani AR, Petraglia F, Giudetti R, Volpe A, Facchinetti F (1986) Neonatal β-endorphin secretion in babies passively addicted to opiates. Excerpta Med Int Congr Ser 369:379–382

Guitart X, Nestler EJ (1989) Identification of morphine and cyclic AMP-regulated phosphoproteins (MARPPs) in the locus coeruleus and other regions of rat brain. Regulation by acute and chronic morphine. J Neurosci 9:4371–4387

Guitart X, Hayward MD, Nisenbaum LK, Beitner-Johnson DB, Haycock JW, Nestler EJ (1990) Identification of MARPP-58, a morphine- and cyclic AMP-regulated phosphoprotein of 58 kDa, as tyrosine hydroxylase: evidence for regulation of its expression by chronic morphine in the rat locus coeruleus. J Neurosci 10:2649–2659

Handelmann GE, Quirion R (1983) Neonatal exposure to morphine increases mu opiate binding in the adult forebrain. Eur J Pharmacol 94:357–358

Hayward MD, Duman RS, Nestler EJ (1990) Induction of the c-fos proto-oncogene during opiate withdrawal in the locus coeruleus and other regions of rat brain. Brain Res 525:256–266

Hazum E, Chang KJ, Cuatrecasas P (1979) Role of disulphide and sulphydryl groups in clustering of enkephalin receptors in neuroblastoma cells. Nature 282:626–628

Herkenham M, Pert CB (1981) Mosaic distribution of opiate receptors, parafascicular projections and acetylcholinesterase in rat striatum. Nature 291:415–418

Hitzemann RJ, Hitzemann BA, Loh HH (1974) Binding of ^{3}H-naloxone in the mouse brain: effect of ions and tolerance development. Life Sci 14:2393–2404

Hitzemann RJ, Hitzemann BA, Blatt S, Meyerhoff JL, Tortella FC, Kenner JR, Belenky GL, Holaday JW (1987) Repeated electroconvulsive shock: effect on sodium dependency and regional distribution of opioid-binding sites. Mol Pharmacol 31:562–566

Holaday JW, Hitzemann RJ, Curell J, Tortella FC, Belenky GL (1982) Repeated electroconvulsive shock or chronic morphine treatment increases the number of ^{3}H-D-Ala^2-D-Leu^5-enkephalin binding sites in rat brain membranes. Life Sci 31:2359–2362

Holaday JW, Tortella FC, Meyerhoff JL, Belenky GL, Hitzemann RJ (1986) Electroconvulsive shock activates endogenous opioids systems: behavioral and biochemical correlates. Ann NY Acad Sci 467:249–255

Höllt V, Dum J, Blasig J, Schubert P, Herz A (1975) Comparison of in vivo and in vitro parameters of opiate receptor binding in naive and tolerant/dependent rodents. Life Sci 16:1823–1828

Höllt V, Przewlocki R, Herz A (1978) β-Endorphin-like immunoreactivity in plasma, pituitaries and hypothalamus of rats following treatment with opiates. Life Sci 23:1057–1066

Iyengar S, Rabii J (1982) Effect of prenatal exposure to morphine on the postnatal development of opiate receptors. Fed Proc 41:1354–1357

Kent JL, Pert CB, Herkenham M (1982) Ontogeny of opiate receptors in rat forebrain: visualization by in vitro autoradiography. Dev Brain Res 2:487–504

Kirby ML, Aronstam RS (1983) Levorphanol-sensitive [^{3}H]naloxone binding in developing brainstem following prenatal morphine exposure. Neurosci Lett 35:191–195

Kirby ML, Gale TF, Mattio TG (1982) Effects of prenatal capsaicin treatment on fetal spontaneous activity, opiate receptor binding, and acid phosphatase in the spinal cord. Exp Neurol 76:298–308

Klee WA, Nirenberg M (1976) Mode of action of endogenous opiate peptides. Nature 248:609–612

Klee WA, Lampert A, Nirenberg M (1976) Dual regulation of adenylate cyclase by endogenous opiate peptides. In: Kosterlitz HW (ed) Opiates and endogenous opioid peptides. Elsevier/North-Holland, New York, pp 153–159

Lahti RA, Collins RJ (1978) Chronic naloxone results in prolonged increases in opiate binding sites in brain. Eur J Pharmacol 51:185–186

Lampert A, Nirenberg M, Klee WA (1976) Tolerance and dependence evoked by an endogenous opiate peptide. Proc Natl Acad Sci USA 73:3165–3167

Law PY, Hom DS, Loh HH (1983) Opiate receptor downregulation and desensitization in neuroblastoma × glioma NG108-15 hybrid cells are two separate cellular adaptation processes. Mol Pharmacol 24:413–424

Lenoir D, Barg J, Simantov R (1983) Down-regulation of opiate receptors in serum-free cultures of aggregating fetal brain cells. Life Sci 33[Suppl 1]:337–340

Leslie FM, Tso S, Hurlbut DE (1982) Differential appearance of opiate receptor subtypes in neonatal rat brain. Life Sci 31:1393–1396

Lesser-Katz M (1982) Some effects of maternal drug addiction on the neonate. Int J Addict 17:887–896

Loughlin SE, Massamiri T, Kornblum HI, Leslie FM (1985) Postnatal development of opioid systems in rat brain. Neuropeptides 5:469–472

McDonald RL, Werz MA (1986) Dynorphin A decreases voltage-dependent calcium conductance of mouse dorsal root ganglion neurones. J Physiol (Lond) 377:237–249

Miyake M, Christie MJ, North RA (1989) Single potassium channels opened by opioids in rat locus ceruleus neurons. Proc Natl Acad Sci USA 86:3419–3422

Moon SL (1984) Prenatal haloperidol alters striatal dopamine and opiate receptors. Brain Res 323:109–113

Morris BJ, Herz A (1989) Control of opiate receptor number in vivo: simultaneous kappa-receptor down-regulation and mu-receptor up-regulation following chronic agonists/antagonist treatment. Neuroscience 29:433–442

Nakata Y, Chang KJ, Mitchell CL, Hong JS (1985) Repeated electroconvulsive shock down regulates the opioid receptors in rat brain. Brain Res 346:160–163

Nestler EJ, Tallman JF (1988) Chronic morphine treatment increases cyclic AMP-dependent protein kinase activity in the rat locus coeruleus. Mol Pharmacol 33:127–132

Nishino K, Su YF, Wong CS, Watkins WD, Chang KJ (1990) Dissociation of mu opioid tolerance from receptor down-regulation in rat spinal cord. J Pharmacol Exp Ther 253:67–72

North RA (1986) Opioid receptor types and membrane ion channels. Trends Neurosci 9:114–117

North RA, Williams JT (1983) Opiate activation of potassium conductance inhibits calcium action potentials in rat locus coeruleus neurones. Br J Pharmacol 80: 225

Panerai AE, Martini A, di Giulio AM, Fraioli F, Vegni C, Pardi G, Marini A, Mantegazza P (1983) Plasma β-endorphin, β-lipotropin, and met-enkephalin concentrations during pregnancy in normal and drug-addicted women and their newborn. J Clin Endocrinol Metab 57:537–543

Pert CB, Pasternak GW, Snyder SH (1973) Opiate agonists and antagonists discriminated by receptor binding in brain. Science 182:1359–1361

Petrillo P, Tavani A, Verotta D, Robson LE, Kosterlitz HW (1987) Differential postnatal development of mu-, delta-, and kappa-opioid binding sites in rat brain. Brain Res 428:53–58

Przewlocki R, Höllt V, Duka T, Kleber G, Gramsch C, Haarmann I, Herz A (1979) Long-term morphine treatment decreases endorphin levels in rat brain and pituitary. Brain Res 174:357–361

Puttfarken PS, Cox BM (1989) Morphine-induced desensitization and down-regulation at mu-receptors in 7315C pituitary tumor cells. Life Sci 45:1937–1942

Ragavan VV, Wardlaw SL, Kreek MJ, Frantz AG (1983) Effect of chronic naltrexone and methadone administration on brain immunoreactive beta-endorphin in the rat. Neuroendocrinology 37:266–268

Rothman RB, Danks JA, Jacobson AE, Burke TR, Rice KC, Tortella F, Holaday JW (1986) Morphine tolerance increases mu-noncompetitive delta binding sites. Eur J Pharmacol 124:113–119

Schulz R, Wüster M, Herz A (1979) Supersensitivity to opioids following chronic blockade of endorphin activity by naloxone. Naunyn Schmiedebergs Arch Pharmacol 306:93–96

Shani J, Azov R, Weissman BA (1979) Enkephalin levels in rat brain after various regimens of morphine administration. Neurosci Lett 12:319–322

Sharma SK, Klee WA, Nirenberg M (1975) Dual regulation of adenylate cyclase accounts for narcotic dependence and tolerance. Proc Natl Acad Sci USA 72:3092–3096

Shen KF, Crain SM (1989) Dual opioid modulation of the action potential duration of mouse dorsal root ganglion neurons in culture. Brain Res 491:227–242

Simantov R, Amir S (1983) Regulation of opiate receptors in mouse brain: arcuate nuclear lesion induces receptor up-regulation and supersensitivity to opiates. Brain Res 262:168–171

Simantov R, Levy R (1989) Neuronal activation regulates the expression of opioid receptors: possible role of glial-derived factors and voltage-dependent ion channels. J Neurochem 52:305–309

Simantov R, Levy R, Baram D (1982) Down regulation of enkephalin (δ) receptors: demonstration in membrane bound and solubilized receptors. Biochem Biophys Acta 721:478–484

Spain JW, Roth BL, Coscia CJ (1985) Differential ontogeny of multiple opioid receptors (μ, δ, and κ). J Neurosci 5:584–588

Steece KA, DeLeon-Jones FA, Myerson LR, Lee JM, Fields JZ, Ritzman RF (1986) In vivo down-regulation of rat striatal opioid receptors by chronic enkephalin. Res Bull 17:255–257

Tang AH, Collins RJ (1978) Enhanced analgesic effects of morphine after chronic administration of naloxone in the rat. Eur J Pharmacol 47:473–474

Tao PL, Law PY, Loh HH (1987) Decrease in delta and mu opioid receptor binding capacity in rat brain after chronic etorphine treatment. J Pharmacol Exp Ther 240:809–816

Tao PL, Li R, Chang KL, Law PY, Loh HH (1988) Decrease in delta-receptor density in rat brain after chronic (D-Ala^2, D-Leu^5) enkephalin treatment. Brain Res 462:313–320

Tavani A, Robson L, Kosterlitz HW (1985) Differential postnatal development of mu, delta, and kappa opioid binding sites in mouse brain. Dev Brain Res 23:306–309

Tempel A, Gardner EL, Zukin RS (1984) Visualization of opiate receptor up-regulation by light microscopy autoradiography. Proc Natl Acad Sci USA 81:3893–3897

Tempel A, Gardner EL, Zukin RS (1985) Neurochemical and functional correlates of naltrexone-induced opiate receptor up-regulation. J Pharmacol Exp Ther 232:439–444

Tempel A, Habas JE, Paredes W, Barr GA (1988) Morphine-induced down-regulation of μ-opioid receptors in neonatal rat brain. Dev Brain Res 41:129–133

Tempel A, Kessler JA, Zukin RS (1990) Chronic naltrexone treatment increases expression of preproenekphalin and preprotachykinin mRNA in discrete brain regions. J Neurosci 10:741–747

Torda C (1978) Effects of recurrent postnatal pain-related stressful events on opiate receptor-endogenous ligand system. Psychoneuroendrocrinology 3:85–91

Tsang D, Ng SC (1980) Effect of antenatal exposure to opiates on the development of opiate receptors in rat brain. Brain Res 188:199–206

Tsang D, Ng SC, Ho KP (1982) Kappa opioid receptor-mediated analgesia in the developing rat. Brain Res 394:145–152

Uhl G, Ryan JP, Schwartz JP (1988) Morphine alters preproenkephalin gene expression. Brain Res 459:391–397

Watanabe Y, Shibuya T, Salafsky B, Hill HF (1983) Prenatal and postnatal exposure to diazepam: effects on opioid receptor binding in rat brain cortex. Eur J Pharmacol 96:141–144

Werling LL, McMahon PN, Cox BM (1989) Selective changes in mu opioid receptor properties induced by chronic morphine exposure. Proc Natl Acad Sci USA 86:6393–6397

Werz MA, McDonald RL (1985) Dynorphin and neoendorphin peptides decrease dorsal root ganglion enuron calcium-dependent action potential duration. J Pharmacol Exp Ther 234:49

Yoburn BC, Goodman RR, Cohen AH, Pasternak GW, Inturrisi CE (1985) Increased analgesic potency of morphine and increased brain opioid bindings sites in the rat following chronic naltrexone treatment. Life Sci 36:2325–2332

Yoburn BC, Sierra V, Lutfy K (1989) Chronic opioid antagonist treatment: assessment of receptor upregulation. Eur J Pharmacol 170:193–200

Young E, Olney J, Akil A (1982) Increase in delta, but not mu, receptors in MSG-treated rats. Life Sci 31:1343–1346

Young WS, Kuhar MJ (1979) A new method for receptor autoradiography: [3H]opioid receptors in rat brain. Brain Res 179:225–270

Zukin RS, Sugarman JR, Fitz-Syage ML, Gardner EL, Zukin SR, Gintzler AR (1982) Naltrexone-induced opiate receptor supersensitivity. Brain Res 245:285–292

Zukin RS, Eghbali M, Olive D, Unterwald E, Tempel A (1988) Characterization and visualization of rat and guinea-pig kappa opioid receptors: evidence for kappa1 and kappa2 receptors. Proc Natl Acad Sci USA 85:4061–4065

CHAPTER 7

Multiple Opioid Receptors and Presynaptic Modulation of Neurotransmitter Release in the Brain

A.H. MULDER and A.N.M. SCHOFFELMEER

A. Introduction

Many of the effects of opioids on animals and men, especially those on behaviour, motor activity and vegetative functions, are thought to involve modulation of neurotransmission processes in the brain. In this regard, effects of opiates and opioid peptides on noradrenergic, cholinergic, dopaminergic and serotonergic neuronal systems in particular have been studied extensively over the past 20–25 years. Many of these investigations have examined the changes brought about in (regional) brain neurotransmitter levels and/or turnover or in various behavioural activities thought to reflect primarily the activity of one or other of these neuronal systems after systemic, intracerebroventricular or local intracerebral administration of opioids. Other studies have measured changes in neurotransmitter release from certain brain areas in vivo after opioid drug administration, using the push-pull cannula, the cortical cup method or, more recently, the brain microdialysis technique (DI CHIARA and IMPERATO 1988; SPANAGEL et al. 1990a,b, see also Chap. 25).

However, although such in vivo studies undoubtedly yield important information with regard to the changes in activity of various neuronal systems brought about by opioids, they generally do not allow unambiguous conclusions to be drawn as to the primary cellular site(s) and mechanism(s) of action of these agents. After systemic or intracerebroventricular administration of an opioid drug its effects may be brought about either directly at the neuronal cell bodies and/or the nerve terminals or in an indirect manner, involving local neuronal circuits or polysynaptic neuronal feedback pathways, a possibility that cannot be disregarded even after local intracerebral injection of the drug. This has led several investigators to follow reductionistic approaches, exploring the functions and transduction mechanisms of opioid receptors in simplified in vitro systems, using brain slices, synaptosomes or cultured cells. For instance, in vitro methods have been used successfully in studies examining presynaptic inhibition of neurotransmitter release as one of the possible actions of opioid drugs, including the endogenous opioid peptides, in the brain (STARKE 1981; CHESSELET 1984; MULDER et al. 1984a; ILLES 1989).

The first evidence for presynaptic inhibition of neurotransmitter release by morphine and other opiates was obtained in studies using isolated peripheral tissue preparations. Thus, it was shown that the inhibitory effect of morphine and enkephalin on the electrically evoked contractions of the guinea pig ileum and the mouse vas deferens are due to an inhibition of the release of acetylcholine and noradrenaline, respectively (see references in LESLIE 1987; ILLES 1989). This chapter reviews studies on presynaptic modulation of neurotransmitter release in the brain and summarizes evidence indicating that, at least in certain cases, activation of different opioid receptor types may result in modulation of the release of different neurotransmitters. In most of these investigations neurotransmitter release was measured in vitro after selective labelling of the nerve terminals concerned by incubating brain slices with a low concentration of radiolabelled neurotransmitter or, in some cases, its precursor. Subsequent depolarization of the slices by electrical field stimulation or by increasing the K^+ concentration in the medium has been shown to result in a calcium-dependent and (at least in the case of electrical stimulation or a moderately increased K^+ concentration) tetrodotoxin-sensitive (exocytotic) release of neurotransmitter. Thus, depolarization-induced release of radiolabelled neurotransmitters in vitro appears to provide a legitimate model of action potential-induced neuronal transmitter release in vivo and has proven to be a convenient and reliable method for measuring release and its presynaptic modulation in small samples (a few milligrams) of brain tissue. Nevertheless, incubation of brain slices with the radiolabelled neurotransmitter or its precursor may result in an inhomogeneous labelling of different neurotransmitter pools (e.g., "storage pool" and "releasable pool") in the nerve terminals concerned. This may result in differences in release depending on the labelling conditions and also compared to the release of endogenous neurotransmitter, as has been shown for dopamine (DA) release from striatal slices (HERDON et al. 1985). However, in spite of quantitative differences in neurotransmitter release, presynaptic modulation of the release of, respectively, radiolabelled and endogenous neurotransmitter is not likely to be qualitatively different, as has been demonstrated for striatal DA release (HERDON et al. 1987), in agreement with the view that it is the stimulus-secretion-coupling process itself that is subject to modulation via activation of presynaptic receptors.

The majority of the studies reviewed here were published in the period 1984–1991; for studies published before that period the reader is referred to the reviews mentioned above. Most of these early studies did not adequately characterize the opioid receptors involved in the modulatory effects demonstrated, simply because sufficiently selective agonists and antagonists for opioid receptors were not available at the time. An extensive survey of the literature until 1988 with regard to the modulatory effects of opioids on neurotransmitter release in peripheral tissues and on hormone release can be found in the comprehensive review by ILLES (1989).

B. Modulation of Noradrenaline Release

In the 1970s various groups reported that the depolarization-induced release of [^{3}H]noradrenaline (NA) from rat brain cortex slices was depressed by morphine and other narcotic analgesics as well as by enkephalin and β-endorphin in a naloxone-reversible manner (see IWAMOTO and WAY 1979; ILLES 1989, and references therein). Later studies, utilizing opioid receptor-selective agonists and antagonists, demonstrated that depolarization-induced NA release from rat cortical slices is indeed inhibited by opioids only via activation of μ-receptors. Thus, HAGAN and HUGHES (1984) showed that the inhibitory effects of the highly μ-selective enkephalin analogue DAMGO and the δ/μ-agonist DADLE were antagonized by naloxone, but not by the δ-selective antagonist ICI 154129. Furthermore, whereas the electrically evoked release of [^{3}H]NA from rat cortical slices was strongly inhibited by DAMGO, it was not affected by the δ-selective agonist DPDPE, nor by the κ-selective agonist U50488 (WERLING et al. 1987; SCHOFFELMEER et al. 1988a; MULDER et al. 1989). Also other highly selective δ-agonists, DSTBULET and BUBU (DE VRIES et al. 1989) and κ-agonists, such as U69593 and PD117302 (MULDER et al. 1991a), did not affect cortical [^{3}H]NA release. Moreover, various conformationally restrained somatostatin analogues, such as CTOP and CTAP, that were previously found to be potent and highly selective μ-receptor antagonists in peripheral tissue preparations, were recently shown to display essentially the same potency and selectivity with regard to the μ-receptors mediating presynaptic inhibition of NA release in the rat brain (MULDER et al. 1991b). An ontogenetic study (DE VRIES et al. 1990) has demonstrated that these functional μ-receptors are already present during embryonic development.

The finding that μ-receptor agonists produce a strong inhibition of K$^+$-induced [^{3}H]NA release from rat cortical synaptosomes (MULDER et al. 1987) strongly supports the view that the μ-receptors involved truly are located on the noradrenergic varicosities, since in superfused synaptosomal preparations indirect effects are very unlikely (DE LANGEN et al. 1979a).

An interesting recent finding is the very high potency (IC$_{50}$ about 2 nM; compare to an IC$_{50}$ of about 0.1 μM for DAMGO) of the endogenous opioid peptide β-endorphin as an agonist at the presynaptic μ-receptors mediating inhibition of NA release (SCHOFFELMEER et al. 1991). β-Endorphin was also found to display a much higher degree of selectivity with regard to the functional opioid receptor types mediating inhibition of neurotransmitter release than with regard to the different opioid receptor recognition sites demonstrated in binding studies. It appeared to have a 200-fold higher affinity for the presynaptic μ-receptors than for the δ-receptors mediating inhibition of striatal acetylcholine (ACh) release and no significant affinity for the κ-receptors mediating inhibition of striatal DA release (SCHOFFELMEER et al. 1991; Fig. 1). Therefore, β-endorphin might be an important endogenous agonist for presynaptic μ-opioid receptors.

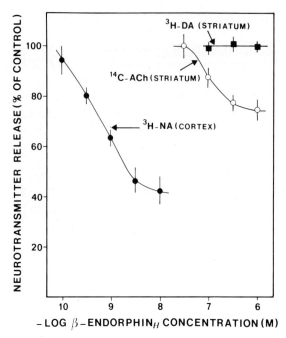

Fig. 1. Inhibitory effect of human β-endorphin$_{1-31}$ on the electrically evoked release of neurotransmitters from rat brain slices. After labelling with [^{3}H]NA (cortex) or with [^{3}H]DA and [^{14}C]choline (striatum), the slices were superfused with Krebs-Ringer-bicarbonate medium (gassed with 95% O_2/5% CO_2) at 37°C. During superfusion calcium-dependent neurotransmitter release was induced by exposing the slices to electrical field stimulation (striatal slices: 4-ms blockpulses, 1 pps, 24 mA; cortex slices: 4-ms blockpulses, 1 pps, 15 mA) for 10 min. Drugs were added 20 min before stimulation. Control release (in excess of spontaneous efflux) amounted to about 5% ([^{3}H]NA), 3% ([^{3}H]DA) and 9% ([^{14}C]ACh) of total tissue radioactivity, respectively. Data represent means ± SEM of 12 observations obtained in 3 separate experiments. (From Schoffelmeer et al. 1991)

Not only in the cortex, but also in other regions of the rat brain, i.e., hippocampus (Jackisch et al. 1986a; Werling et al. 1987), amygdala (Frankhuyzen et al. 1991), nucleus tractus solitarii (Arakawa et al. 1991), periaqueductal grey (Versteeg et al. 1991) and cerebellum (Werling et al. 1987), was the depolarization-induced release of [^{3}H]NA in vitro found to be inhibited by opioids only if they activate μ-receptors. A notable exception appears to be the mediobasal hypothalamus, a brain region of essential importance in the regulation of pituitary functions. The electrically evoked release of [^{3}H]NA from slices of this brain region was not inhibited by DAMGO, nor by the κ-agonist U50488 (Heijna et al. 1991). Thus, it seems that, in contrast to neurotransmitter release from noradrenergic neurons arising from the locus ceruleus and innervating most brain regions, release from some other noradrenergic neurons, e.g., those arising from the A1 and A2 nuclei in the brainstem and innervating the medial basal hypothalamus, is not subject to inhibition by opioids at the level of the nerve terminals.

Studies examining presynaptic modulation of NA release from brain slices of guinea pig or rabbit have revealed striking species differences. The electrically evoked release of [^{3}H]NA from slices of rabbit hippocampus or colliculus superior was shown to be inhibited by opioids only if they activate κ-receptors (JACKISCH et al. 1986a; WICHMANN and STARKE 1988). [^{3}H]NA release from slices of cortex, hippocampus or cerebellum of the guinea pig brain, known to contain κ-receptors as the predominant opioid receptor type, appeared to be inhibited by activation of either κ-, μ- or δ-receptors, although activation of δ-receptors was the least effective, at least in cortex and hippocampus (WERLING et al. 1987, 1989a). KINOUCHI et al. (1989) concluded that κ-receptors are the major type of receptors involved in inhibition of K$^+$-induced [^{3}H]NA release from guinea pig cortex slices, since activation of μ-receptors had little and that of δ-receptors no effect on release in their study.

The mechanisms involved in the inhibitory effect of opioid receptor activation on depolarization-induced NA release have been explored quite extensively. In our own laboratory we have compared the mechanisms by which activation of either μ-opioid or α$_2$-adrenoceptors results in inhibition of [^{3}H]NA release from rat cortical slices, utilizing different means for inducing transmitter release, viz. electrical field stimulation, K$^+$ depolarization, the alkaloid veratrine or the calcium ionophore A23187 (SCHOFFELMEER and MULDER 1983, 1984; MULDER and SCHOFFELMEER 1985; SCHOFFELMEER et al. 1986a,b, 1988b; MULDER et al. 1990). These studies indicated that, although activation of these presynaptic receptors results in the same effect, the primary transduction mechanisms involved are quite different. Thus, activation of presynaptic α$_2$-adrenoceptors, in contrast to that of μ-opioid receptors, appears to involve inhibition of an adenylate cyclase localized in the nerve terminals and activated during depolarization, whereas activation of presynaptic μ-receptors primarily results in an inhibition of voltage-dependent calcium channels. Furthermore, activation of both α$_2$-adrenoceptors and μ-opioid receptors appears to interfere with intracellular calcium stores in the noradrenergic nerve terminals and/or with the sensitivity of the stimulus-secretion coupling process to calcium. Other data from our laboratory (SCHOFFELMEER and MULDER 1983, 1984) support the view that activation of these presynaptic receptors is not directly linked to changes in the permeability of the nerve terminal membrane to K$^+$, Na$^+$ or Cl$^-$ ions. Therefore, it appears that the primary transduction mechanisms of μ-opioid receptors and α$_2$-adrenoceptors localized on noradrenergic nerve terminals are different from those localized on the cell bodies in the locus ceruleus, since electrophysiological studies have convincingly demonstrated that activation of the latter results in an increase in K$^+$ conductance and subsequently in hyperpolarization and a reduced firing rate of the nerve fibers (NORTH et al. 1987). Recent studies have also examined the possible involvement of G proteins in the presynaptic opioid receptor-mediated inhibition of NA release. Werling et al. (1989b) reported that previous intra-cerebroventricular injections of pertussis toxin attenuated the μ-receptor-mediated inhibition of (20 mM) K$^+$-induced [^{3}H]NA release from rat and guinea pig hippocampus slices, whereas the κ-receptor-mediated inhibition of release (only found in guinea pig brain, see above) remained unaffected, suggesting that, in contrast to the μ-receptors, the κ-receptors are not coupled to G proteins. On the other hand, Allgaier et al. (1989) showed that pretreatment of rabbit hippocampal slices with either pertussis toxin or N-ethylmaleimide strongly diminished the inhibitory effect of κ-receptor as well as α$_2$-adrenoceptor activation on electrically evoked [^{3}H]NA release.

Mutual interactions between different presynaptic receptors mediating inhibition of NA release and apparently localized on the same (noradrenergic) nerve terminals have been demonstrated in the case of μ-receptors and α$_2$-adrenoceptors in rat cortex slices (Schoffelmeer et al. 1986b) and κ-receptors, α$_2$-adrenoceptors and adenosine A$_1$ receptors in rabbit cortex slices (Limberger et al. 1986a, 1988a,b). Activation of one kind of pre-synaptic receptor was found to diminish or even obliterate the inhibition of NA release produced by subsequent activation of the other kind of receptor, a phenomenon that appeared not to be due to the reduction of release per se caused by the first drug. Allgaier et al. (1989) suggested that these interactions take place at the level of receptor-coupled transduction mechanisms, possibly through competition for a common pool of G proteins.

C. Modulation of Acetylcholine Release

Several studies before 1980 demonstrated that, after systemic or i.c.v. administration, morphine and related opiates as well as [Leu^5]- and [Met^5]enkephalin and some of their analogues depressed the release of endogenous ACh in vivo, measured in anesthetized cats or rats, using ventricular perfusion or "cortical cup" techniques (see Domino 1979; Jhamandas and Sutak 1980, and references therein). Occasional early studies on modulation of ACh release from brain tissue in vitro by opioids sometimes yielded apparently conflicting results, which upon further con-sideration may have been due to differences in methodology, e.g., nature and intensity of the stimulus used to induce ACh release, or to the use of tissue from different species or brain regions (for review and references see Illes 1989). In 1984 we reported that the release of [^{14}C]ACh and that of [^{3}H]DA induced by low-intensity (15 mM) K$^+$ depolarization from rat striatal slices was inhibited by activation of δ- and κ-opioid receptors, respectively (Mulder et al. 1984b). This initial finding, providing first evidence for differential modulation of neurotransmitter release via different opioid receptors, was corroborated by further studies in our laboratory. Thus, of several enkephalin- and dynorphin-related opioid peptides, some,

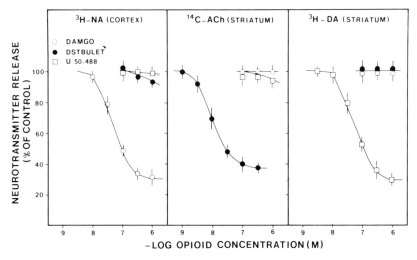

Fig. 2. Selective inhibitory effects of μ-, δ-, or κ-opioid receptor activation on the electrically evoked release of [³H]NA from rat cortex slices and of [³H]DA and [¹⁴C]ACh from rat striatal slices. For experimental details see legend to Fig. 1. Data represent means ± SEM of 12–16 observations obtained in 3–4 separate experiments

e.g., DPDPE, DSLET and DSTBULET, were potent inhibitors of the electrically evoked release of radiolabelled ACh from rat striatal slices, whereas others, e.g., DAMGO or dynorphin$_{1-13}$, were not effective, at least up to concentrations of 1 μM (Mulder et al. 1989; De Vries et al. 1989; see also Figs. 2 and 4). Further, various non-peptide κ-receptor agonists, which potently inhibited [³H]DA release, did not affect striatal [¹⁴C]ACh release (Mulder et al. 1991a). The inhibitory effects of DPDPE and other enkephalin analogues on ACh release were antagonized by the irreversible δ-selective ligand fentanyl-isothiocyanate and the competitive δ-antagonist naltrindole (Schoffelmeer et al. 1988a, 1992), but not by highly μ-selective somatostatin analogues, such as CTOP or CTAP (Mulder et al. 1991b; see also Fig. 3).

Inhibition of electrically evoked [³H]ACh release from slices of rat striatum as well as striatostriatal grafts by δ-, but not κ- or μ-, opioid agonists was also demonstrated by Wichmann and Starke (1990). Interestingly, it was recently reported that naloxone significantly enhanced the electrically evoked release of [³H]ACh from rat striatal slices when the nigrostriatal pathway had been destroyed with 6-hydroxydopamine or when D₂ DA receptors were blocked by sulpiride, indicating that under these experimental conditions striatal ACh release is partially inhibited by released endogenous enkephalins (Sándor et al. 1991).

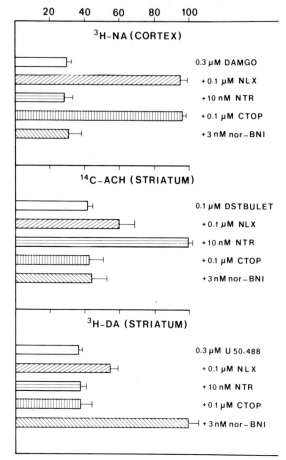

NEUTROTRANSMITTER RELEASE
(% OF CONTROL)

Fig. 3. Pharmacological characterization with selective antagonists of the opioid receptors mediating presynaptic inhibition of the release of [³H]NA from rat cortex slices and of [³H]DA and [¹⁴C]ACh from rat striatal slices. The opioid agonists DAMGO (μ), DSTBULET (δ) and U50488 (κ) were used at concentrations that cause near-maximal inhibition of release (see Fig. 2). The antagonists naloxone (*NLX*), naltrindol (*NTR*), CTOP and nor-binaltorphimine (*nor-BNI*) were added together with the agonists 20 min before electrical stimulation. For further experimental details, see legend to Fig. 1. Data represent means ± SEM of 12–16 observations obtained in 3–4 separate experiments

Striking regional differences have been demonstrated with regard to the modulation of ACh release from rat brain slices by opioids in studies using highly selective agonists and antagonists for the different opioid receptor types (HEIJNA et al. 1990; FRANKHUYZEN et al. 1991). In the frontal cortex the electrically evoked release of radiolabelled ACh in vitro was not affected by any of the opioids, indicating that not all cholinergic neurons are subject to presynaptic modulation by opioids. Furthermore, whereas ACh release from striatal slices was depressed only by activation of δ-receptors, release from nucleus accumbens and olfactory tubercle tissue was inhibited by both δ- and μ-agonists (HEIJNA et al. 1990) and that from hippocampus or amygdala slices by μ-agonists only (JACKISCH et al. 1986b; FRANKHUYZEN et al. 1991). Thus, it appears that the type(s) of opioid receptors involved in presynaptic inhibition of ACh release depend on the type and origin of the cholinergic neurons concerned.

Recently, ARENAS et al. (1990, 1991) reported that K^+- or glutamate-induced ACh release from rat striatal slices is inhibited by both δ- and μ-opioid agonists, contrary to the findings mentioned above. However, their conclusions are based on data that raise some doubts upon careful consideration. For instance, they found DADLE to be 10–20 times less potent than DPDPE in inhibiting ACh release (ARENAS et al. 1990), although the former peptide is known to be more potent at δ-receptors than the latter in the mouse vas deferens (MOSBERG et al. 1983) as well as the rat brain (MULDER et al. 1989). Moreover, in contrast to DADLE, dynorphin$_{1-13}$, was found to be ineffective, even at micromolar concentrations (ARENAS et al. 1990), in spite of the fact that this peptide, although being highly κ-selective, has been shown to be nearly as potent as DADLE as an agonist at μ-receptors, e.g., those involved in presynaptic modulation of NA release (MULDER et al. 1989). These anomalies are difficult to explain, but they might perhaps somehow be due to the chemoluminescent method used by these authors to measure ACh release (ARENAS et al. 1990, 1991), which involves the enzymatic production of H_2O_2, a highly reactive intermediate, to which the tissue is exposed.

Only few data are available on species differences with regard to the opioid receptor types involved in the modulation of ACh release in the brain. JACKISCH et al. (1986b) have shown that in the rabbit hippocampus ACh release is inhibited by opioids primarily through activation of κ-receptors, in contrast to the rat hippocampus, where μ-receptors are involved. In a comparative study LAPCHAK et al. (1989) examined the regulation of ACh release via opioid receptors using slices from hippocampus, striatum and cortex of guinea pig and rat brain. They measured the release of endogenous ACh during incubation of the slices in the presence of physostigmine. However, under these experimental conditions presynaptic muscarinic autoreceptors, mediating inhibition of ACh release, are likely to be maximally activated, which may diminish or even obliterate the inhibitory effects of opioid receptor activation on release, as has been shown for $α_2$-noradrenergic autoreceptors mediating inhibition of NA release (SCHOFFELMEER et al. 1986b; LIMBERGER et al. 1986a, 1988a,b). Furthermore, LAPCHAK et al. (1989) exposed the slices to a strong depolarizing stimulus, viz. 50 mM K^+, to induce ACh release, a condition known to be less favourable for presynaptic modulation to occur. Indeed, most of the inhibitory effects these authors demonstrated were small or were only found at relatively high (micromolar) drug concentrations. Surprisingly, they found no inhibitory effect at all of δ-agonists on rat striatal ACh release, in contrast to the findings consistently reported by others (see above). Lapchak et al. (1989) concluded that the types of opioid receptors involved in the regulation of ACh release in rat and guinea pig brain are different, primarily μ in the former and κ in the latter species, but we feel that this conclusion should be considered with some caution.

D. Modulation of Dopamine Release

Some occasional early studies suggested that morphine, enkephalin and β-endorphin inhibited the K^+-induced release of radiolabelled DA from rat striatal slices, presumably by activating μ-receptors, but others found no effect of these opioids (see Iwamoto and Way 1979; Illes 1989, and references therein). In fact, all subsequent investigations, using highly selective opioid-receptor agonists, indicate that activation of μ-receptors, in contrast to that of other opioid receptors, does not result in presynaptic modulation of DA release from rat or guinea pig brain tissue in vitro. As mentioned before, we reported that the K^+-induced release of [^{3}H]DA from rat striatal slices was inhibited by κ-agonists, but not affected by μ- or δ-agonists (Mulder et al. 1984b).

The conclusion that striatal DA release is subject to presynaptic inhibition by opioids only via activation of κ-receptors is strengthened by further studies, examining electrically evoked [^{3}H]DA release from rat striatal slices and using highly selective μ-, κ- and δ-agonists and antagonists (Schoffelmeer et al. 1988a, 1991; Mulder et al. 1989, 1991a,b; De Vries et al. 1989). In agreement with the κ-profile of the opioid receptors involved, drugs like bremazocine, U69593 and PD117302 selectively inhibited striatal DA release with EC_{50} values in the nanomolar range, whereas highly μ- or δ-selective agonists, such as DAMGO, DPDPE or DSTBULET, were ineffective up to concentrations of at least $1 \mu M$ (Figs. 2, 4). Furthermore, in contrast to the highly selective κ-antagonist nor-binaltorphimine, various cyclic somatostatin analogues, such as CTOP and CTAP, that are highly selective μ-opioid receptor antagonists as well as the δ-selective antagonist naltrindol, displayed very low affinity for these receptors (Fig. 3). Considering the action of endogenous opioid peptides on the κ-receptors mediating inhibition of striatal DA release, both $dynorphin_{1-13}$ and $dynorphin_{1-8}$ appeared to possess a high affinity, whereas the enkephalins and β-endorphin displayed a very low affinity, for these receptors (Mulder et al. 1989; Schoffelmeer et al. 1991). However, in contrast to $dynorphin_{1-13}$, $dynorphin_{1-8}$ also potently inhibited striatal ACh release in vitro and its affinity for the δ-receptors involved in this effect appeared to be similar to that for the κ-receptors mediating presynaptic inhibition of DA release (Mulder et al. 1989; Fig. 4). An ontogenetic study

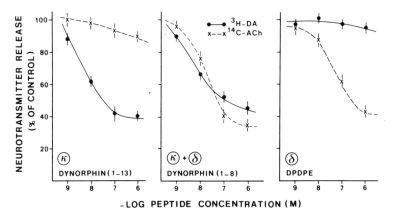

Fig. 4. Differential inhibition of the electrically evoked release of [^{3}H]DA and [^{14}C]ACh (measured simultaneously) from rat striatal slices by dynorphin$_{1-13}$ and DPDPE. Also note that dynorphin$_{1-8}$ activates both κ- and δ-opioid receptors with similar affinity. (From MULDER et al. 1989)

(DE VRIES et al. 1990) has demonstrated that these functional κ-receptors are already present during embryonic development.

Inhibitory effects of κ-, but not μ- or δ-, opioid receptor activation have also been reported by others, examining either (20 mM) K$^+$- or (100 μM) NMDA-stimulated [H^3]DA release from both rat and guinea pig striatal slices (WERLING et al. 1988, 1990). Recently, GAUCHY et al. (1991), using a subtle microsuperfusion technique to examine the (50 μM) acetylcholine-evoked release of [^{3}H]DA continuously synthesized from [^{3}H]tyrosine from striosome-enriched and matrix areas of cat caudate nucleus slices, also demonstrated strong DA release-inhibiting effects of dynorphin$_{1-13}$ and U50488. Previous studies by Glowinski's group have shown that μ-agonists do not affect the spontaneous or K$^+$-induced release of newly synthesized [^{3}H]DA from rat striatal slices (LUBETZKI et al. 1982; PETIT et al. 1986).

However, although studies from different laboratories agree on the inhibitory effect of κ-receptor activation on striatal DA release in vitro and the absence of μ-receptor-mediated presynaptic modulation, there is disagreement with regard to the involvement of δ-receptors. Thus, as mentioned above, MULDER et al. and WERLING et al. consistently found that δ-agonists did not affect or, if anything, slightly *inhibited* (at micromolar concentrations) the depolarization-induced release of [^{3}H]DA from rat striatal slices, prelabelled by incubation with [^{3}H]DA. In contrast, Glowinski and coworkers have reported that activation of δ-receptors *increased* the spontaneous release (LUBETZKI et al. 1982) as well as the K$^+$-induced release (PETIT et al. 1986) of radiolabelled DA continuously synthesized from [^{3}H]tyrosine from rat striatal slices. However, such a facilitatory effect of δ-receptor activation was not observed when using slices from rat nucleus accumbens (Petit et al. 1986). Particularly if the possibility of a stimulatory effect of the δ-agonists used (DSLET and DTLET) on DA synthesis is to be excluded, as the authors claim, the reasons for the differences between their findings and those of others using striatal slices previously labelled with [³H]DA remain enigmatic. The authors suggest an explanation involving different DA "pools" in the nerve terminal, a "main storage pool" and a "functional pool", which contains the newly synthesized DA and is used preferentially in the release process. According to Petit et al. (1986), it might be DA release from this latter pool that is specifically increased by δ-receptor activation. However, incubation of brain slices with [³H]DA will undoubtedly, in addition to the storage pool, also label the functional transmitter pool, from which release occurs anyhow (De Langen et al. 1979b) and, moreover, presynaptic modulatory effects on transmitter release are generally thought to be due to changes in the stimulus-secretion coupling process. Therefore, it is hard to understand why the increasing effect of δ-receptor activation on newly synthesized [³H]DA was not found by others examining release of previously accumulated [³H]DA, whereas the inhibitory effect of κ-opioid receptor activation (Gauchy et al. 1991; Mulder et al. 1984b, 1991a; Werling et al. 1988, 1990), and also the modulatory effects mediated by DA autoreceptors and muscarinic receptors, were found with both approaches (Chesselet 1984).

Using synaptosomal preparations from guinea pig striatum, evidence has been provided for the presynaptic localization of the κ-opioid receptors mediating inhibition of DA release (Werling et al. 1988). Recent regional studies have shown that these presynaptic κ-receptors are present not only in the caudate nucleus, but also in the frontal cortex, olfactory tubercle, nucleus accumbens (Heijna et al. 1990), mediobasal hypothalamus (Heijna et al. 1991) and amygdala (Frankhuyzen et al. 1991) of the rat brain, indicating that transmitter release from all dopaminergic neurons is subject to inhibition by opioids acting on κ-receptors. The importance of ensuring selective uptake of [³H]DA uptake into dopaminergic nerve terminals in these studies, by using, e.g., desipramine to prevent uptake into noradrenergic nerve endings, was demonstrated clearly by Heijna et al. (1990).

Recent in vivo brain microdialysis studies, examining the release of DA and its major metabolites, have shown that κ-receptor activation results in an inhibition of DA release, whereas activation of δ- or μ-receptors causes an enhanced release in the rat striatum and nucleus accumbens (Di Chiara and Imperato 1988; Spanagel et al. 1990a,b; Longoni et al. 1991). As mentioned before, these in vivo release studies do not allow unambiguous conclusions to be drawn with regard to the primary site of action of the opioid drugs that modulate DA release. Therefore, in view of the findings of in vitro studies the stimulatory effects of μ- and δ-agonists on DA release in striatum and/or nucleus accumbens shown in in vivo studies are likely to be a consequence of their inhibitory actions on neurons which tonically inhibit dopaminergic neurons at the level of the nerve terminals and/or the cell bodies.

E. Modulation of the Release of Other Neurotransmitters

Studies of the effects of opioids on the release of neurotransmitters other than acetylcholine, dopamine or noradrenaline are scarce and those concerning serotonin (5-HT), histamine, GABA and some neuropeptides will be summarized here together.

HAGAN and HUGHES (1984) reported that, in contrast to the electrically evoked release of [^{3}H]NA, that of [^{3}H]5-HT from rat cortical slices was not modulated by normorphine or DADLE. More recently, however, inhibitory effects of opioids have been demonstrated on [^{3}H]5-HT release from slices of another rat brain area, the hippocampus (PASSARELLI and COSTA 1989). In the latter study it was shown, by using DAMGO and DPDPE as selective agonists and CTAP and ICI174864 as selective antagonists, that 5-HT release induced by $20\,mM$ K^+ was inhibited by activation of both μ- and δ-receptors. However, DAMGO and DPDPE inhibited release with strikingly steep agonist concentration-effect curves, and naloxone appeared to antagonize the effect of DPDPE in a non-competitive fashion and also U50488 caused some inhibition of 5-HT release in the study by PASSARELLI and COSTA (1989), so that the nature of the opioid receptors involved remains somewhat uncertain. Data reported by WICHMANN et al. (1989) indicate that the electrically evoked release of [^{3}H]5-HT, like that of [^{3}H]NA, from rabbit superior colliculus slices is inhibited by activation of κ-, but not δ- or μ-, opioid receptors.

Recently, the first study on modulation by opioids of histamine release from brain slices was reported by GULAT-MARNAY et al. (1990). These authors demonstrated that the $K^+(30\,mM)$-induced release of [^{3}H]histamine, synthesized from [^{3}H]histidine during incubation of rat cortical slices, was inhibited by various κ-agonists, but not by DAMGO, DADLE or DPDPE. However, the inhibitory effects of the κ-agonists U50488, U69593, PD117302 and dynorphin A$_{1-13}$, although they were antagonized by nor-BNI, required concentrations more than 100-fold higher than those needed to inhibit DA release from rat striatal slices (MULDER et al. 1991a), suggesting that perhaps another κ-receptor subtype might be involved in the modulation of histamine release.

Regarding modulation by opioids of the release of amino acid neurotransmitters from brain tissue in vitro, only some studies examining GABA release have been reported. The inhibitory effects of opioids on GABA release demonstrated by STARR (1985) and BRADFORD et al. (1986) are very doubtful in view of the extremely high concentrations ($10–100\,\mu M$) needed for these effects. Furthermore, a careful study by LIMBERGER et al.

(1986b) failed to demonstrate modulation by opioids of electrically evoked [^{3}H]GABA release from rabbit caudate nucleus slices.

Finally, a few studies on the modulatory effects of opioids on neuro-peptide release from brain slices have been published. MYCEVICH et al. (1984a) reported that the K^+-induced release of vasoactive intestinal peptide (VIP), but not that of cholecystokinine (CCK), from cat frontal cortex slices was inhibited by morphine and DADLE, but whether only μ- or both μ- and δ-opioid receptors were involved in this effect remained somewhat uncertain. On the other hand, the release of CCK as well as that of substance P from cat hypothalamic slices was inhibited by morphine and DADLE, but not by U50488. Based on the sensitivity of the inhibitory effects to naloxone, it was concluded that inhibition of CCK release was mediated by μ-receptors only, whereas the inhibition of substance P release involved both μ- and δ-receptors (MICEVYCH et al. 1984b).

BUCKINGHAM and COOPER (1986) showed that the (basal) secretion of corticotropin-releasing factor (CRF) from rat hypothalami in vitro, deter-mined using a bioassay, was stimulated by activation of μ- and κ-, but not δ-, opioid receptors. However, these findings are difficult to reconcile with the more recent study by TSAGARAKIS et al. (1990), who measured CRF-41 using a radioimmunoassay and reported that activation of μ- and κ-, but not δ-, opioid receptors inhibited the K^+-induced release of this peptide from rat hypothalami in vitro, with no effect on basal CRF secretion. Interest-ingly, already in the nanomolar concentration range CRF itself appears to be able to stimulate the release of β-endorphin and dynorphin from rat hypothalamic slices, as shown by NIKOLARAKIS et al. (1987). These authors found that following an initial stimulation of opioid peptide release CRF caused a decline of release. Since naloxone by itself caused an increase in opioid peptide release and, in addition, prevented the decline of release upon prolonged exposure of the slices to CRF, the involvement of feedback inhibition via presynaptic opioid receptors was proposed. Indeed, in a subsequent study it was shown that selective blockade of δ-receptors in rat hypothalamus slices facilitated the release of β-endorphin and dynorphin as well as [Met^5]enkephalin, whereas blockade of μ-receptors enhanced the release of β-endorphin and dynorphin and blockade of κ-receptors caused an increase of dynorphin release only (NIKOLARAKIS et al. 1989).

F. Conclusions

Thus far, presynaptic modulation of the release of various neurotransmitters from brain tissue in vitro by opioids has been investigated most extensively in the rat. A smaller number of studies have used brain tissue from the guinea pig or, in some cases, other species, i.e., rabbit or cat. With this restriction in mind some general conclusions can be drawn tentatively from the studies reviewed in this chapter.

1. The depolarization-induced release of noradrenaline, acetylcholine and dopamine appears to be subject to (local) presynaptic modulation via opioid receptors in most, but not necessarily all, brain regions, as demonstrated in the rat and, to a lesser extent, the guinea pig. Whether or not neurotransmitter release is liable to presynaptic modulation by opioids may be related to the type of neuron, e.g., the nuclei from which they originate. In general, modulation of the release of other neurotransmitters, including neuropeptides, has been examined only in one particular brain region.

2. Virtually all studies published thus far, examining different neurotransmitters, species and brain regions, have demonstrated that activation of opioid receptors results in a (local) presynaptic *inhibition* of depolarization-induced neurotransmitter release.

3. Activation of different opioid receptor types may result in presynaptic inhibition of different neurotransmitters. In various rat brain regions (e.g., striatum, nucleus accumbens, amygdala) DA release is inhibited only through activation of κ-receptors, whereas ACh release is inhibited via δ- and/or μ-receptors. On the other hand, in rat hippocampus or amygdala both NA and ACh release are inhibited through activation of μ-receptors only. These conclusions are strengthened by the fact that, at least in our own laboratory, many of these studies were carried out using a double-label technique, i.e., labelling slices with both [^{3}H]DA (or [^{3}H]NA) and [^{14}C]ACh (via [^{14}C]choline), so that the effects of opioid drugs on the release of the two different neurotransmitters can be studied simultaneously. With regard to the guinea pig brain the situation is less clear, although the data available thus far suggest that in this species the κ-receptor is the only or main type involved in the inhibition of NA as well as DA and ACh release by opioids. However, further studies using this species as well as others (e.g., rabbit, cat) would be required to establish whether differential modulation of neurotransmitter release via different opioid receptor types in the brain is a frequent phenomenon or rather an exception.

4. Regarding the endogenous opioid peptide agonists for the presynaptic opioid receptors mediating inhibition of neurotransmitter release, [Leu^5]- and [Met^5]enkephalin appear to have a relatively high affinity and a fair selectivity for the δ-receptors, whereas dynorphin$_{1-13}$ and β-endorphin display both high affinity and selectivity for the κ-receptors and μ-receptors, respectively.

Finally, we would like to emphasize that the ultimate effects of opioids on neurotransmission processes in the brain of the living animal are the result of presynaptic and postsynaptic actions. For example, adenylate cyclase activity stimulated by activation of D_1 DA receptors in rat striatal slices appears to be profoundly reduced following activation of μ- or δ-, but not κ-opioid receptors (SCHOFFELMEER et al. 1988a). Therefore, even though μ- and δ-receptor agonists enhance DA release in vivo (DI CHIARA

and IMPERATO 1988; SPANAGEL et al. 1990a,b), their net effect on dopaminergic neurotransmission could well be inhibitory.

References

Allgaier C, Daschmann B, Sieverling J, Hertting G (1989) Presynaptic κ-opioid
    receptors on noradrenergic nerve terminals couple to G-proteins and interact
    with the α_2-adrenoceptors. J Neurochem 53:1629–1635
Arakawa K, de Jong W, Mulder AH, Versteeg DHG (1991) Electrically-stimulated
    release of [^{3}H]noradrenaline from nucleus tractus solitarii slices is modulated via
    μ-opioid receptors. Eur J Pharmacol 192:311–316
Arenas E, Alberch J, Arroyos RS, Marsal J (1990) Effect of opioids on acetylcholine
    release evoked by K$^+$ or glutamic acid from rat neostriatal slices. Brain Res
    523:51–56
Arenas E, Alberch J, Marsal J (1991) Dopaminergic system mediates only δ-opiate
    inhibition of endogenous acetylcholine release evoked by glutamate from rat
    striatal slices. Neuroscience 42:707–714
Bradford HF, Crowder JM, White EJ (1986) Inhibitory actions of opioid compunds
    on calcium fluxes and neurotransmitter release from mammalian cerebral
    cortical slices. Br J Pharmacol 88:87–93
Buckingham JC, Cooper TA (1986) Pharmacological characterization of opioid
    receptors influencing the secretion of corticotrophin releasing factor in the rat.
    Neuroendocrinology 44:36–40
Chesselet MF (1984) Presynaptic regulation of neurotransmitter release in the brain.
    Neuroscience 12:347–375
De Langen CDJ, Hogenboom F, Mulder AH (1979a) Presynaptic noradrenergic
    alpha-receptors and modulation of ^{3}H-noradrenaline release from rat brain
    synaptosomes. Eur J Pharmacol 60:79–89
De Langen CDJ, Stoof JC, Mulder AH (1979b) Studies on the nature of the
    releasable pool of dopamine in synaptosomes from rat corpus striatum:
    depolarization-induced release of ^{3}H-dopamine from superfused synaptosomes
    labeled under various conditions. Naunyn Schmiedebergs Arch Pharmacol
    308:41–49
De Vries TJ, Schoffelmeer ANM, Delay-Goyet P, Roques BP, Mulder AH (1989)
    Selective effects of [D-Ser^2(O-t-butyl), Leu^5]enkephalyl-Thr^6 and [D-Ser^2(O-t-
    butyl), Leu^5]enkephalyl-Thr^6(O-t-butyl), two new enkephalin analogues, on
    neurotransmitter release and adenylate cyclase in rat brain slices. Eur J
    Pharmacol 170:137–143
De Vries TJ, Hogenboom F, Mulder AH, Schoffelmeer ANM (1990) Ontogeny of
    μ-, δ-and κ-opioid receptors mediating inhibition of neurotransmitter release and
    adenylate cyclase activity in rat brain. Dev Brain Res 54:63–69
Di Chiara G, Imperato A (1988) Opposite effects of mu and kappa opiate agonists
    on dopamine release in the nucleus accumbens and in the dorsal caudate of
    freely moving rats. J Pharmacol Exp Ther 244:1067–1080
Domino EF (1979) Opiate interactions with cholinergic neurons. In: Loh HH, Ross
    DH (eds) Neurochemical mechanisms of opiates and endorphins. Raven, New
    York, pp 339–355
Frankhuyzen AL, Jansen FP, Schoffelmeer ANM, Mulder AH (1991) Mu-opioid
    receptor-mediated inhibition of the release of radiolabelled noradrenaline and
    acetylcholine from rat amygdala slices. Neurochem Int 19:543–548
Gauchy C, Desban M, Krebs MO, Glowinski H, Kemel ML (1991) Role of
    dynorphin-containing neurons in the presynaptic inhibitory control of the
    acetylcholine-evoked release of dopamine in the striosomes and the matrix of
    the cat caudate nucleus. Neuroscience 41:449–458

Gulat-Marnay C, Lafitte A, Arrang JM, Schwartz JC (1990) Modulation of histamine release in the rat brain by κ-opioid receptors. J Neurochem 55:47–53

Hagan RM, Hughes IE (1984) Opioid receptor sub-types involved in the control of transmitter release in cortex of the brain of the rat. Neuropharmacology 23: 491–495

Heijna MH, Padt M, Hogenboom F, Porthoghese PS, Mulder AH, Schoffelmeer ANM (1990) Opioid receptor-mediated inhibition of dopamine and acetylcholine release from rat brain slices: differences between nucleus accumbens, olfactory tubercle and frontal cortex in receptor types involved. Eur J Pharmacol 181:267–278

Heijna MH, Padt M, Hogenboom F, Schoffelmeer ANM, Mulder AH (1991) Opioid receptor-mediated inhibition of [³H]dopamine but not [³H]noradrenaline release from rat mediobasal hypothalamus slices. Neuroendocrinology 54:118–126

Herdon H, Strupisch J, Nahorski SR (1985) Differences between the release of radiolabelled and endogenous dopamine from superfused rat brain slices: effects of depolarizing stimuli, amphetamine and synthesis inhibition. Brain Res 348:309–319

Herdon H, Strupisch J, Nahorski SR (1987) Endogenous dopamine release from rat striatal slices and its regulation by D-2 autoreceptors: effects of uptake inhibitors and synthesis inhibition. Eur J Pharmcol 138:69–76

Illes P (1989) Modulation of transmitter and hormone release by multiple neuronal opioid receptors. Rev Physiol Biochem Pharmacol 112:139–233

Iwamoto ET, Way EL (1979) Opiate actions and catecholamines. In: Loh HH, Ross DH (eds) Neurochemical mechanisms of opiates and endorphins. Raven, New York, pp 357–407

Jackisch R, Geppert M, Illes P (1986a) Characterization of opioid receptors modulating noradrenaline release in the hippocampus of the rabbit. J Neurochem 46:1802–1810

Jackisch R, Geppert M, Brenner AS, Illes P (1986b) Presynaptic opioid receptors modulating acetylcholine release in the hippocampus of the rabbit. Naunyn Schmiedebergs Arch Pharmacol 332:156–162

Jhamandas K, Sutak M (1980) Action of enkephalin analogues and morphine on brain acetylcholine release: differential reversal by naloxone and an opiate pentapeptide. Br J Pharmacol 71:201–210

Kinouchi K, Maeda S, Saito K, Inoki R, Fukumitsu K, Yoshiya I (1989) Effects of pentazocine and other opioids on the potassium-evoked release of [³H]noradrenaline from guinea pig cortical slices. Eur J Pharmacol 164:63–68

Lapchak PA, Araujo DM, Collier B (1989) Regulation of endogenous acetylcholine release from mammalian brain slices by opiate receptors: hippocampus, striatum and cerebral cortex of guinea-pig and rat. Neuroscience 31:313–325

Leslie FM (1987) Methods used for the study of opioid receptors. Pharmacol Rev 39:197–249

Limberger N, Späth L, Hölting T, Starke K (1986a) Mutual interaction between presynaptic α₂-adrenoceptors and opioid κ-receptors at the noradrenergic axons of rabbit brain cortex. Naunyn Schmiedebergs Arch Pharmacol 334:166–171

Limberger N, Späth L, Starke K (1986b) A search for receptors modulating the release of γ-[³H]aminobutyric acid in rabbit caudate nucleus slices. J Neurochem 46:1109–1117

Limberger N, Singer EA, Starke K (1988a) Only activated but not non-activated presynaptic α₂-autoreceptors interfere with neighbouring presynaptic receptor mechanisms. Naunyn Schmiedebergs Arch Pharmacol 338:62–67

Limberger N, Späth L, Starke K (1988b) Presynaptic α₂-adrenoceptor, opioid κ-receptor and adenosine A₁-receptor interactions on noradrenaline release in rabbit brain cortex. Naunyn Schmiedebergs Arch Pharmacol 338:53–61

Longoni R, Spina L, Mulas A, Carboni E, Garau L, Melchiorri P, di Chiara G (1991) (D-Ala²)deltorphin II: D₁-dependent stereotypes and stimulation of dopamine release in the nucleus accumbens. J Neurosci 11:1565–1576

Lubetzki C, Chesselet MF, Glowinski J (1982) Modulation of dopamine release in rat striatal slices by delta opiate agonists. J Pharmacol Exp Ther 222:435–440

Micevych PE, Go VLW, Yaksh TL (1984a) Simultaneous measurement of the release of cholecystokinin- and vasoactive intestinal polypeptide-like immunoreactivity from cat frontal cortex in vitro: effect of morphine and D-Ala^2-D-Leu^5-enkephalin. Brain Res 291:55–62

Micevych PE, Yaksh TL, Go VLW (1984b) Studies on the opiate receptor-mediated inhibition of K$^+$-stimulated cholecystokinin and substance P release from cat hypothalamus in vitro. Brain Res 290:87–94

Mosberg HI, Hurst R, Hruby VJ, Gee K, Yamamura HI, Galligan JJ, Burks TF (1983) Bis-penicillamine enkephalins possess highly improved specificity toward δ opioid receptors. Proc Natl Acad Sci USA 80:5871–5874

Mulder AH, Schoffelmeer ANM (1985) Catecholamine and opioid receptors, presynaptic inhibition of CNS neurotransmitter release and adenylate cyclase. Adv Cyclic Nucleotide Protein Phosphorylation Res 19:273–286

Mulder AH, Frankhuyzen AL, Stoof JC, Wemer J, Schoffelmeer ANM (1984a) Catecholamine receptors, opiate receptors, and presynaptic modulation of neurotransmitter release in the brain. In: Usdin E, Carlsson A, Dahlstrom A, Engel J (eds) Catecholamines: neuropharmacology and central nervous system: theoretical aspects. Liss, New York, pp 47–58

Mulder AH, Wardeh G, Hogenboom F, Frankhuyzen AL (1984b) Kappa and delta-opioid receptor agonists differentially inhibit striatal dopamine and acetylcholine release. Nature 308:278–280

Mulder AH, Hogenboom F, Wardeh G, Schoffelmeer ANM (1987) Morphine and enkephalins potently inhibit ^{3}H-noradrenaline release from rat brain cortex synaptosomes: further evidence for a presynaptic localization of μ-opioid receptors. J Neurochem 48:1043–1047

Mulder AH, Wardeh G, Hogenboom F, Frankhuyzen AL (1989) Selectivity of various opioid peptides towards delta-, kappa- and mu-opioid receptors mediating presynaptic inhibition of neurotransmitter release in the brain. Neuropeptides 14:99–104

Mulder AH, Schoffelmeer ANM, Stoof JC (1990) On the role of adenylate cyclase in presynaptic modulation of neurotransmitter release mediated by monoamine and opioid receptors in the brain. Ann NY Acad Sci 604:237–249

Mulder AH, Burger DM, Wardeh G, Hogenboom F, Frankhuijzen AL (1991a) Pharmacological profile of various κ-agonists at κ-, μ- and δ-opioid receptors mediating presynaptic inhibition of neurotransmitter release in the rat brain. Br J Pharmacol 102:518–522

Mulder AH, Wardeh G, Hogenboom F, Kazmierski W, Hruby VJ, Schoffelmeer ANM (1991b) Cyclic somatostatin analogues as potent antagonists at μ-, but not δ- and κ-opioid receptors mediating inhibition of neurotransmitter release in the brain. Eur J Pharmacol 205:1–6

Nikolarakis KE, Almeida OFX, Herz A (1987) Feedback inhibition of opioid peptide release in the hypothalamus of the rat. Neuroscience 23:143–148

Nikolarakis KE, Almeida OFX, Yassouridis A, Herz A (1989) Presynaptic auto- and allelo-receptor regulation of hypothalamic opioid peptide release. Neuroscience 31:269–273

North RA, Williams JT, Surprenant A, Christie MJ (1987) Mu- and δ-receptors belong to a family of receptors that are coupled to potassium channels. Proc Natl Acad Sci USA 84:5487–5491

Passarelli F, Costa T (1989) Mu and delta opioid receptors inhibit serotonin release in rat hippocampus. J Pharmacol Exp Ther 248:299–305

Petit F, Hamon M, Fournie-Zaluski MC, Roques BP, Glowinski J (1986) Further evidence for a role of δ-opiate receptors in the presynaptic regulation of newly synthesized dopamine release. Eur J Pharmacol 126:1–9

Sándor NT, Kiss J, Sándor A, Lendvai B, Vizi ES (1991) Naloxone enhances the release of acetylcholine from cholinergic interneurons of the striatum if the dopaminergic input is impaired. Brain Res 552:343–345

Schoffelmeer ANM, Mulder AH (1983) Differential control of Ca^{2+}-dependent ^3H-noradrenaline release from rat brain slices through presynaptic opiate receptors and α-adrenoceptors. Eur J Pharmacol 87:449–458

Schoffelmeer ANM, Mulder AH (1984) Presynaptic opiate-receptor and $α_2$-adrenoceptor mediated inhibition of noradrenaline release in the rat brain: role of hyperpolarization? Eur J Pharmacol 105:129–135

Schoffelmeer ANM, Wieringa EA, Mulder AH (1986a) The role of adenylate cyclase in presynaptic $α_2$-adrenoceptor and μ-opioid receptor-mediated inhibition of ^3H-noradrenaline release from rat brain cortex slices. J Neurochem 46:1711–1717

Schoffelmeer ANM, Putters J, Mulder AH (1986b) Activation of presynaptic $α_2$-adrenoceptors attenuates the inhibitory effect of μ-opioid receptor agonists on noradrenaline release from brain slices. Naunyn Schmiedebergs Arch Pharmacol 333:377–380

Schoffelmeer ANM, Rice KC, van Gelderen JG, Hogenboom F, Heijna MH, Mulder AH (1988a) Mu, δ- and κ-opioid receptor-mediated inhibition of neurotransmitter release and adenylate cyclase activity in rat brain slices: studies with fentanylisothiocyanate. Eur J Pharmacol 154:169–178

Schoffelmeer ANM, Hogenboom F, Mulder AH (1988b) Sodium-dependent ^3H-noradrenaline release from rat neocortical slices in the absence of extracellular calcium: presynaptic modulation by μ-opioid receptor and adenylate cyclase activation. Naunyn Schmiedebergs Arch Pharmacol 338:548–552

Schoffelmeer ANM, Wardeh G, Hogenboom F, Mulder AH (1991) β-Endorphin: a highly selective endogenous opioid receptor agonist for presynaptic μ-opioid receptors. J Pharmacol Exp Ther 258:237–242

Schoffelmeer ANM, de Vries TJ, Hogenboom F, Hruby VJ, Portoghese PS, Mulder AH (1992) Opioid receptor antagonists discriminate between presynaptic μ- and δ-receptors and the adenylate cyclase coupled opioid receptor complex in the brain. J Pharmacol Exp Ther (in press)

Spanagel R, Herz A, Shippenberg TS (1990a) The effects of opioid peptides on dopamine release in the nucleus accumbens: an in vivo microdialysis study. J Neurochem 55:1734–1740

Spanagel R, Herz A, Shippenberg TS (1990b) Identification of the opioid receptor types mediating β-endorphin-induced alterations in dopamine release in the nucleus accumbens. Eur J Pharmacol 190:177–184

Starke K (1981) Presynaptic receptors. Annu Rev Pharmacol Toxicol 21:7–30

Starr MS (1985) Multiple opiate receptors may be involved in suppressing γ-aminobutyrate release in substantia nigra. Life Sci 37:2249–2255

Tsagarakis S, Rees LH, Besser M, Grossman A (1990) Opiate receptor subtype regulation of CRF-41 release from rat hypothalamus in vitro. Neuro-endocrinology 51:599–605

Versteeg DHG, Csikós T, Spierenburg H (1991) Stimulus-evoked release of tritiated monoamines from rat periaqueductal gray slices in vitro and its receptor-mediated modulation. Naunyn Schmiedebergs Arch Pharmacol 343:595–602

Werling LL, Brown SR, Cox BM (1987) Opioid receptor regulation of the release of norepinephrine in brain. Neuropharmacology 26:987–996

Werling LL, Frattali A, Portoghese PS, Takemori AE, Cox BM (1988) Kappa receptor regulation of dopamine release from striatum and cortex of rats and guinea pigs. J Pharmacol Exp Ther 246:282–286

Werling LL, McMahon PN, Portoghese PS, Takemori AE, Cox BM (1989a) Selective opioid antagonist effects on opioid-induced inhibition of release of norepinephrine in guinea pig cortex. Neuropharmacology 28:103–107

Werling LL, McMahon PN, Cox BM (1989b) Effects of pertussis toxin on opioid regulation of catecholamine release from rat and guinea pig brain slices. Naunyn Schmiedebergs Arch Pharmacol 339:509–513

Werling LL, Jacocks HM III, McMahon PN (1990) Regulation of [^{3}H]dopamine release from guinea pig striatum by NMDA receptor/channel activators and inhibitors. J Pharmacol Exp Ther 255:40–45

Wichmann T, Starke K (1988) Uptake, release and modulation of release of noradrenaline in rabbit superior colliculus. Neuroscience 26:621–634

Wichmann T, Starke K (1990) Modulation by muscarine and opioid receptors of acetylcholine release in slices from striato-striatal grafts in the rat. Brain Res 510:396–302

Wichmann T, Limberger N, Starke K (1989) Release and modulation of release of serotonin in rabbit superior colliculus. Neuroscience 32:141–151

CHAPTER 8

Opioid Receptor-G Protein Interactions: Acute and Chronic Effects of Opioids

B.M. Cox

A. Introduction

It has been accepted for several years that opioid action mediated through μ- and δ-type opioid receptors requires the interaction of the agonist-occupied receptor with a guanine nucleotide binding protein (G protein). Accumulating evidence suggests that a similar mechanism is an essential component of κ-type opioid receptor function. In this chapter, we will discuss the evidence supporting these conclusions and review similarities and differences between opioid receptor-G protein interactions and the functions of other G protein-linked receptor systems. The evidence that tolerance to opioid agonist actions and the development of dependence on opioid agonist after chronic exposure might also be related to modified interactions between receptor and G protein, and also to changes in the concentrations of individual forms of G proteins, will also be considered.

It was shown in early studies of radioligand binding to opioid receptors that ligand binding was inhibited by guanine nucleotides (BLUME 1978a,b; CHILDERS and SNYDER 1978). The major effect of guanine nucleotides was to increase the rate of dissociation of agonists, with essentially no effect on the dissociation rate of antagonists (CHILDERS and SNYDER 1980). The effects of guanine nucleotides were substantially enhanced when NaCl was present. GTP, GDP, and its nonhydrolysable analogue, guanyl-5'-yl imidophosphate (Gpp(NH)p), were approximately equiactive in reducing opioid agonist affinity for receptors in rat brain membranes, while other nucleotides (including ATP, ADP, AMP, CTP, UTP, and GMP) were much less active (BLUME 1978a,b). ITP reduced opioid binding, but to a lesser extent than GTP. GTP and sodium ions were also shown to be essential for opioid receptor-mediated inhibition of adenylyl cyclase in membranes from the neuroblastoma X glioma hybrid cell NG 108-15 (BLUME et al. 1979).

These results suggested that opioid receptors were similar to other types of receptor where agonist-binding affinity was known to be reduced by guanine nucleotide in the presence of NaCl. Such receptors included the angiotensin II receptor in adrenal glomerulosa cells (GLOSSMAN et al. 1974) and β-adrenoceptors (MAGUIRE et al. 1976; LEFKOWITZ et al. 1976). By the mid-1970s it was recognized that hormone activation of adenylyl cyclase, for example by epinephrine or glucagon, was dependent on the presence of

GTP. Early models proposed to account for the stimulatory actions of hormones of adenylyl cyclase suggested that GTP bound to a regulatory component of the adenylyl cyclase enzyme complex. Hormones or neuro-transmitter activators of the enzyme appeared to facilitate the stimulatory effects of GTP (RODBELL et al. 1974). The mechanisms by which hormones or transmitters inhibited adenylyl cyclase were not initially clear. Subsequently, RODBELL (1980) suggested that there might be more than one GTP-binding regulatory protein capable of regulating the catalytic activity of adenylyl cyclase, and he proposed the terms N_s and N_i to describe the stimulatory and inhibitory forms of the GTP-binding regulatory proteins. Since it was apparent that the regulatory proteins do not bind all nucleotides indiscriminately but are preferentially regulated by guanine nucleotides, the descriptors N_s and N_i have been replaced by G_s and G_i. Subsequently, other guanine nucleotide binding proteins (G proteins) have been discovered; their functional roles are not limited to regulation of adenylyl cyclase. Many other receptor-effector transduction systems, including enzymes and receptor-controlled ion channels, are known to be regulated by G proteins apparently acting in a manner similar to the role exerted by G_s and G_i in the regulation of adenylyl cyclase. Opiate receptors are but one of many sets of receptors for various hormones, transmitters, and growth factors that regulate the activities of a subset of the numerous forms of G protein that have now been identified. The regulatory effects of opioids on adenylyl cyclase are discussed in detail in Chap. 9; the effects of opioids on G protein regulated ion channels are discussed in Chap. 30.

    G proteins exist as heterotrimers composed of α-, β-, and γ-subunits in which GDP is associated with the α-subunit under basal conditions. Receptor-mediated activation of G proteins results in a reduction in the affinity of the α-subunit for GDP leading to GDP dissociation. In the presence of an excess of GTP (a situation presumed to prevail in the intra-cellular milieu of intact cells), GTP moves to occupy the α-subunit site previously occupied with GDP. The association of GTP with the α-subunit results in dissociation of the agonist receptor-complex and the components of the G protein heterotrimer. The α-subunit with bound GTP is now free to interact with components of the effector system (e.g., adenylyl cyclase). This interaction causes hydrolysis of the bound GTP to GDP, with release of phosphate. The GDP-bound α-subunit dissociates from the effector system and reassociates with the β- and γ-subunits, again becoming competent to interact with agonist-activated receptors. (For a review of the development of the model of G protein function proposed here, see BIRNBAUMER 1990.)

    This model requires that agonist activation of an effector system via G protein transduction is associated with activation of the intrinsic GTPase activity of the G protein α-subunit. Agonist-induced stimulation of GTPase activity therefore provided evidence of receptor-mediated G protein activation. Analysis of the roles of G proteins as transducers of the effects of receptor activation has also been facilitated by the identification of treatments selectively activating or inhibiting G protein function. Cholera toxin (CT) persistently activates the G protein, G_s, resulting in a persistent and sustained activation of adenylyl cyclase in G_s-containing systems (G.L. JOHNSON et al. 1978). G_s can also be activated by forskolin. Pertussis toxin (PT) inhibits G_i and some other G proteins by ADP-ribosylation of the α-subunit (KATADA and UI 1982). Studies of the effects of CT and PT pretreatments on the receptor binding and agonist actions of opioids have provided evidence confirming the transducer roles of certain G proteins in opioid action.

B. Effects of Guanine Nucleotides on Ligand Binding to Opioid Receptors

I. Opioid μ- and δ-Receptors Are Functionally Linked to Guanine Nucleotide Binding Proteins

1. Guanine Nucleotides Lower Agonist Affinity at μ- and δ-Receptors

Binding of agonists to either μ- or δ-types of opioid receptor is substantially reduced in the presence of GTP, GDP, or their nonhydrolyzable analogues. Early studies demonstrating the ability of GTP to reduce agonist binding to opioid-binding sites in rat or guinea pig brain used the radiolabeled agonist [³H]dihydromorphine (DHM) (BLUME 1978a,b; CHILDERS and SNYDER 1978, 1980; ZUKIN and GINTZLER 1980). This ligand has reasonably good selectivity for the μ-type of opioid receptor, suggesting that GTP regulates agonist affinity at this type of opioid receptor. Later studies with the more selective μ-agonist [³H]Tyr-D-Ala-Gly-MePhe-Gly-ol (DAMGO) confirmed that μ-receptor binding was regulated by GTP (WERLING et al. 1984; ZAZAC and ROQUES 1985). The sensitivity of δ-receptors in NG 108-15 cells to GTP was established by BLUME (1978b) using [³H]-labeled enkephalins and etorphine. Subsequently, δ-binding sites in guinea pig brain and in rat brain were also shown to be regulated by guanine nucleotides (WERLING et al. 1984; ZAZAC and ROQUES 1985).

Additional studies suggest that the guanine nucleotides do not interact directly with μ- or δ-receptors, but bind to guanine nucleotide binding proteins (G proteins) associated with the receptors. Opioid effects mediated by δ-receptors in NG 108-15 cells (BURNS et al. 1983; KUROSE et al. 1983) and in guinea pig cerebral cortex (WERLING et al. 1989a), or mediated by μ-receptors in guinea pig ileum (TUCKER 1984), in 7315c cells (AUB et al. 1986), in rat locus ceruleus (AGHAJANIAN and WANG 1986), and in guinea pig cortex (Werling et al. 1989a) are prevented if the tissues are previously treated with pertussis toxin (PT). PT prevents receptor-mediated activation of the G protein G_i and G_o by ADP-ribosylating a Cys residue close to the carboxyl-terminus of the α-subunit of these G proteins (Sullivan et al. 1987). Thus, it is probable that PT-sensitive G proteins such as G_i and G_o mediate some or all of the actions of activated μ- and δ-receptors. In NG 108-15 cell membranes, DADLE-stimulated GTPase activity is specifically inhibited by an antiserum selective for two forms of G_i (G_{i-1} and G_{i-2}), but not by antisera specific for G_{i-3} or G_o (McKenzie and Milligan 1990). Since there is no detectable G_{i-1} mRNA or protein in NG 108-15 cell membranes, the major G protein mediating the effects of δ-receptor activation in NG 108-15 cells is probably G_{i-2}.

2. Guanine Nucleotides Increase Agonist Dissociation Rates

At both μ- and δ-receptors the primary effect of guanine nucleotides was to increase the rates of dissociation of agonists from the receptors (Blume 1978a,b; Childers and Snyder 1980). The dissociation of radiolabeled agonists from μ- or δ-receptors in neural membrane homogenates may be either monophasic or multiphasic, apparently depending in part on the specific radioligand used (Blume 1978b). Other factors influencing opioid agonist dissociation rates include the ionic and nucleotide composition of the medium, membrane pretreatments (Blume 1978a; Childers and Snyder 1980; Spain and Coscia 1987), and the type of membrane preparation. Agonist binding to receptors in the synaptosomal P_2 fraction of a brain membrane homogenate (sedimenting at $20\,000\,g$ in $0.32\,M$ sucrose) is inhibited by GTP, while binding to receptors in the microsomal fraction of the homogenate (P_3, sedimenting at $100\,000\,g$ or higher) is insensitive to guanine nucleotides (Roth et al. 1981; Ott et al. 1989). Binding sites in the P_3 fraction may reflect the presence of opioid receptors being transported from the Golgi apparatus for insertion in the plasma membrane or of receptors that have been internalized from the plasma membrane. However, proteins in the P_3 fraction prepared from intact NG 108-15 cells are readily labeled by treatment of the intact cells with hydrophilic protein modifying reagents, and the δ-receptors in the P_3 fraction are as sensitive as those in the P_2 fraction to treatment of the intact cells by a receptor-selective alkylating agent or PT (Ott et al. 1989). These results suggest that the P_3 fraction contains a significant amount of plasma membrane. The concentration of G protein in the P_3 fraction of NG 108-15 cells is only about 30%–50% of the concentration in the P_2 fraction. It is probable that the extent of δ-receptor-G protein interaction is determined in part by the concentration of G protein in the membrane, even though there may be a molar excess of G protein in both fractions.

The effect of GTP or its nonhydrolysable analogues (e.g., Gpp(NH)p; guanosine 5'-O-(3-thio)triphosphate, GTPγS) is to increase the rate of dissociation of agonist from a substantial fraction of the binding sites in the membrane preparation. This action is greatly facilitated in the presence of Na^+. In contrast, divalent ions such as Mn^{2+} or Mg^{2+} tend to reduce agonist dissociation rates in the absence or presence of guanine nucleotides (BLUME 1978a,b; CHILDERS and SNYDER 1980; CHANG et al. 1983; ZAZAC and ROQUES 1985). There are some quantitative differences between the effects of nucleotides on μ- and δ-receptors, but these may reflect differences in the specific properties of the selective labeled ligands used to measure binding affinity rather than differences in the mechanism of regulation of binding site affinity between the receptor types. In general, the regulation of agonist binding at the two types of receptors by ions and nucleotides shows qualitative similarities, suggesting that similar processes are involved at each receptor type.

Detailed measurements of the effects of guanine nucleotides on agonist association and dissociation rates at δ-receptors have utilized NG 108-15 cell membranes (BLUME 1978b; LAW et al. 1985a). This membrane preparation carries a homogeneous population of δ-receptors; low affinity opioid binding in these membranes therefore reflects the presence of low agonist-affinity states of the δ-receptor, and not binding of incompletely selective labeled ligands to other forms of opioid receptor for which they have low affinity. The monophasic dissociation rate of [^{3}H]DADLE in the presence of $10\,mM$ Mg^{2+} ($t_{0.5}$ approx., 180 min) was shifted to a biphasic dissociation in the presence of $100\,mM$ Na^+ ($t_{0.5}$, 5 min and 130 min) or in the presence of Na^+ and $5\,\mu M$ Gpp(NH)p ($t_{0.5}$, 6 min and 110 min; calculated from data in LAW et al. 1985). These dissociation rates were not influenced by the level of receptor occupancy. In contrast, association rates for agonists in NG 108-15 cell membranes were reduced as the level of receptor occupancy by agonist was increased. At both high and low levels of occupancy, association rates were increased by guanine nucleotides in the presence of $100\,mM$ Na^+ (LAW et al. 1985), but this increase was not sufficient to offset the accelerated dissociation in the presence of Na^+ and guanine nucleotides.

3. Guanine Nucleotide Effects on Equilibrium Binding of Opioids

The effects of ion and nucleotide treatments on association and dissociation rates are reflected in measurements of equilibrium dissociation constants for agonists. When radiolabeled agonists are used, Na^+ and guanine nucleotides reduce specific binding at equilibrium of radiolabeled agonists to levels not very much higher than the nonspecific binding of the ligand (WERLING et al. 1984). Thus, radiolabeled agonist binding does not usually provide quantitatively reliable estimates of the affinities of low agonist-affinity states of the receptor. However, the equilibrium binding of opioid antagonists is not substantially affected by guanine nucleotides or ions (CHILDERS and SNYDER 1980; LAW et al. 1985a; WERLING et al. 1988b). It is therefore possible to estimate the low affinities of agonists for opioid receptors in the presence of Na$^+$ and guanine nucleotides by determining their potencies in competing against labeled antagonist binding.

a) δ-Receptors

In studies of opioid receptors, this method of characterizing the multiple agonist-affinity states generated by coincubation of membranes with ions and nucleotides was first employed in studies of δ-binding sites in NG 108-15 cell membranes. Cell membrane suspensions were incubated in Tris-HCl buffer using [^{3}H]diprenorphine ([^{3}H]DIP) as the radiolabeled ligand and DADLE as the competing agonist (LAW et al. 1985). Nonlinear regression analysis of the competition curves was used to determine if the experimental data was best fit by a one-site model of binding or two- or three-site models. In the absence of Na$^+$ and guanine nucleotides a single-site model provided the best fit, with an estimated K_D for DADLE of 1.9 nM. In the presence of Na$^+$ (100 mM) and the nonhydrolysable GTP analogue, Gpp(NH)p (10 μM), a two-site model was required to fit the experimental data, with a $K_{D\ high}$ of 3.9 nM, and a $K_{D\ low}$ of 250 nM. Approximately 60% of the sites remained in the higher affinity state. Qualitatively similar results were obtained when the competition of the partially δ-selective agonist [D-Ser^2]-enkephalyl-D-Thr (DSLET) against [^{3}H]DIP binding to δ-receptors in the presence and absence of GTP or its nonhydrolyzable analogue, GTPγS, was analyzed in the same way (WERLING et al. 1988b). The GDP analogue, GDPβS, was also shown to significantly reduce agonist affinity, although a single low agonist-affinity state was the predominant form in the presence of this nucleotide. In this study, δ-receptors in NG 108-15 cell membranes and in guinea pig cerebral cortex membranes showed similar sensitivity to the nucleotides. These results indicate that δ-receptors in mammalian neural tissue behave similarly to those in the NG 108-15 neuroblastoma × glioma hybrid cell line in their interactions with guanine nucleotides. It appears that δ-receptors can exist in at least two states with differing affinities for agonists. This conclusion, based on studies using equilibrium binding techniques, is consistent with the multiple rates of agonist dissociation from δ-binding sites in bovine hippocampus membranes (SPAIN and COSCIA 1987). Finally, the existence of multiple affinity states of the δ-receptor is not an artifact arising from disruption of the cell membrane. Multiple affinity states for δ-receptor agonists were observed in NG 108-15 cells (COSTA et al. 1985), suggesting that endogenous guanine nucleotides normally regulate agonist affinity in intact cells.

b) μ-Receptors

Interpretation of guanine nucleotide effects on agonist binding affinities at μ-receptors has been impeded by the few cell or membrane preparations in which the only form of opioid receptor present is of the μ type. When both μ- and δ-receptors are present, as in almost all mammalian neural membrane preparations, low-affinity binding of μ-selective agonists in the presence of guanine nucleotides and Na^+ might reflect either the binding of the agonist to a low-affinity state of the μ-receptor or binding of the μ-selective agonist at δ-receptors with low affinity. The discovery that a rat pituitary tumor cell type, 7315c, carries a homogeneous population of μ-receptors (FREY and KEBABIAN 1984; PUTTFARCKEN et al. 1986) made it possible to examine the effects of guanine nucleotides in a pure population of μ-receptors. Guanine nucleotides reduced agonist binding affinity at μ-receptors in 7315c cells and exposed at least two affinity states of the receptor (WERLING et al. 1988). Similar results were obtained in guinea pig cortical membranes under conditions in which labeled ligand binding to δ- and κ-receptors was blocked by co-incubation with the selective competing ligands ICI 174864 (5 μM; δ) and U50488H (1 μM; κ). Thus, μ-receptors, like δ-receptors, exist in multiple agonist-affinity states, the relative proportions of each form being influenced by the presence or absence of guanine nucleotides.

c) Multiple Agonist Affinity States at μ- and δ-Receptors

The effects of guanine nucleotides on opioid agonist binding can be considered in the framework of a complex equilibrium among free agonist and agonist bound free receptors or to receptors associated with G proteins (Fig. 1). The existence of multiple agonist affinity states supports this model. However, the determination of which affinity states corresponds to which G protein-complexed or free form of the ligand-receptor complex is still a matter of conjecture. Affinity states associated with binding to free receptor, and to receptor-G protein complexes in the absence and presence of GDP and GTP, are assumed to exist, at least transiently, following agonist activation. It is also possible that the receptor from which G protein and GTP has recently dissociated (i.e., L.R' in Fig. 1) is initially in a conformation with a different affinity for agonist from that displayed by free receptor (L.R). Indications of the agonist dissociation constants associated with differing complexed forms of the receptor are provided by membrane treatments that are likely to shift the equilibria in the direction of specific free or complexed forms of bound ligand (Table 1). The table reports apparent dissociation constants (K_{app}) for DSLET at δ-receptors in NG 108-15 cell membranes and guinea pig cerebral cortex membranes, and for DAMGO at μ-receptors in 7315c cell membranes and in guinea pig cortex membranes. The reported K_{app} values are presumed to approximate to macroscopic dissociation constants describing subsets of the equilibria in Fig. 1, determined by the treatments to which the membranes have been exposed.

The binding affinity of agonists at μ- and δ-binding sites is significantly reduced by PT treatment of the cells or membranes (COSTA et al. 1983; WERLING et al. 1988b, 1989b). Agonist affinity is also reduced by other membrane treatments affecting G protein function. *N*-Ethylmaleimide (NEM), an agent that inactivates G proteins (Asano and Ogasawara 1986), reduces or abolishes opioid agonist binding (Larsen et al. 1981; Childers 1984). However, unlike PT, NEM may also modify opioid receptor function by direct interaction with the receptor itself (Larsen et al. 1981; Ueda et al. 1990a). Further evidence of the association of opioid receptors with G proteins is provided by the demonstration that binding of the nonselective opioid agonists [^{3}H]DADLE and [^{3}H]etorphine is reduced by treatment of rat brain membranes with 5′-*p*-fluorosulfonylbenzoyl guanosine (Wong et al. 1990), an agent that covalently modifies the GTP-binding site of G proteins. Agonist affinity at δ-receptors in NG 108-15 cell membranes is significantly reduced by an antiserum selective for G_{i-1} and G_{i-2}, but is not influenced by antisera selective for G_{i-3} and G_o (McKenzie and Milligan 1990). Since each of these agents functionally inactivates G_i and/or G_o, it is probable that measurements of agonist affinity after PT or other treatments characterize the equilibrium between free agonist and agonist bound to receptors functionally uncoupled from G proteins (equilibrium 2 in Fig. 1). This affinity is significantly lower than that observed in washed membranes that have not been exposed to PT or other G protein inactivators (see Table 1). After PT treatment, the dissociation constants for DAMGO binding to μ-receptors in 7315c cells and in guinea pig cortex membranes are very similar. Relatively low affinity for agonists has also been noted in preparations of solubilized and partially purified δ-receptors from NG 108-15 cells, where the receptor-G protein complex appears to have been dissociated during the purification procedure (Scheideler and Zukin 1990).

Since receptors functionally uncoupled from G protein have a low agonist affinity, the factors leading to the presence of high-affinity states for agonist in untreated neural membranes must be determined. Ueda et al. (1988) have shown that opioid agonist potency in competing against [^{3}H]naloxone binding to solubilized rat brain opioid receptors is increased about 50-fold by co-incubation of the receptors with purified G_i or G_o. Addition of GTPγS to the receptor-G protein complex again reduced the agonist potency. This suggests that high-affinity agonist binding in untreated membranes reflects binding of agonist to receptor-G protein complexes with no associated guanine nucleotide (equilibrium 4, Fig. 1), and not to free receptors (equilibrium 2). It is possible that a fraction of the opioid receptors are closely associated with G protein even in the absence of agonist, since Costa et al. (1990) have shown that, in NG 108-15 cell membranes with δ-receptors, the basal low K_m GTPase activity typical of G protein in the absence of agonist is actually reduced significantly when some (but not all) antagonists at δ-receptors are added. However, Frances et al. (1990) have reported that μ-receptors solubilized from rabbit cerebellum membranes by digitonin in the absence of added agonist are not associated with G protein. [In contrast, Frances et al. (1990) found that κ-receptors solubilized from guinea pig cerebellum membranes sedimented more slowly in

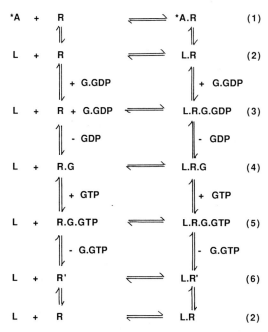

Fig. 1. Assumed equilibria in agonist competition against labeled antagonist binding to opioid receptors coupled to G proteins. Transitions among the various agonist affinity states are regulated by the binding of guanine nucleotides by the G protein. *A indicates labeled antagonist; L, agonist; R, receptor; G, guanyl nucleotide binding protein; R' represents a hypothetical conformation of the receptor formed after the dissociation of G.GTP. The affinity of R' for L may differ from that of R; R' is presumed to revert to R

the presence of Gpp(NH)p than in its absence, suggesting that Gpp(NH)p was able to dissociated a preexisting complex of κ-receptor and G protein.] Clearly, further study is required to determine the extent of "precoupling" of the various forms of opioid receptors in normal mammalian neurons.

Two affinity states for agonist are usually discriminable when washed neural membranes are incubated with labeled antagonist and a wide range of concentrations of unlabeled agonist (WERLING et al. 1988b; Table 1). Quantitatively, the high and low apparent dissociation constants for DSLET at δ-receptors in NG 108-15 membranes were similar to the dissociation constants observed in guinea pig cortical membranes. The high and low apparent dissociation constants for DAMGO at μ-receptors in 7315c and guinea pig cortex membranes were also comparable. The presence of two similar sets of agonist-affinity states in each membrane preparation is more likely to be explained by the presence of two or more interconverting forms of a single receptor type in each membrane preparation than to the presence of fortuitously similar ratios of two unrelated binding components. The lower affinity state(s) may reflect agonist binding to the GDP-bound

Table 1. Agonist dissociation constants at μ- and δ-receptors; effects of guanine nucleotides

Membrane treatments	Bound forms of ligand receptor complex assumed present	DSLET, K_{app} δ-sites		DAMGO, K_{app} μ-sites	
		NG 108-15 membranes	Guinea pig cortex	7315c membranes	Guinea pig cortex
PT pretreated	L.R	100	n.d.	90	90*
No treatment	[L.R.G / L.R. / L.R.G.GDP]	3 (77%) 400	5 (68%) 400	7 (64%) 500	11 (61%)*, 60 (64%) 200*, 800
GDPβS	L.R.G.GDPβS	20	40	300	50
GTPγS	[L.R / L.R.G.GTPγS / L.R']	20 (48%) 5000	20 (55%) 3000	40 (41%) 4000	100 (54%) 5000

Apparent macroscopic dissociation constants for DSLET binding to δ-receptors in NG 108-15 cell membranes or guinea pig cortex membranes and for DAMGO binding to μ-receptors in 7315 c cell membranes or guinea pig cortex membranes. K_{app} values were calculated by analysis of agonist competition curves against labeled antagonist binding, using the nonlinear curve-fitting program LIGAND, and have been rounded to one significant figure. Figures in parenthesis indicate the percentage of binding sites in the higher affinity state when more than one binding site was present. Reported values are from WERLING et al. (1988b), except for values indicated by asterisk (*) which are from WERLING et al. (1989b). In the latter study the membranes were washed more extensively before assay, resulting in an increase in apparent affinities for DAMGO. This may indicate that extensive washing is required to remove guanine nucleotides from the binding sites. The forms of the ligand-receptor-G protein complex assumed present under each condition are based on the hypothetical set of equilibria in Fig. 1. n.d., not determined.

form of the receptor-G protein complex (L.R.G.GDP), binding to free receptor (L.R), or possibly to receptor-G protein to which GTP is bound (L.R.G.GTP) or has recently been bound (L.R'; see Fig. 1). It is very probable that several of these presumed low-affinity forms are actually present in the membrane preparations.

When GDP or its nonhydrolyzable analogue GDPβS is added in excess, binding is assumed to be shifted toward equilibrium 3 in Fig. 1, with the predominant bound form of agonist being L.R.G.GDPβS. At both δ- and μ-receptors this complexed form appears to exhibit lower affinities than the L.R.G. form (Table 1). Treatment with the nonhydrolyzable GTP analogue GTPγS consistently results in the appearance of two affinity states, one of which is substantially lower than any detected in the absence of GTP. It is reasonable to assume that the two affinity states observed after GTP treatment reflect equilibria 5, 6, and 1 (Fig. 1; Table 1), although it is not yet possible to assign specific complexed forms to the two discriminable K_{app} values observed under these conditions.

d) Estimation of Agonist Affinity by Measurement of Opioid Effects

The functional significance of receptor conformations with low affinity for agonists is still a matter for conjecture. In intact cells, unoccupied opioid receptors appear to reside predominantly in a form associated with G protein and GDP. This is a state of relatively low affinity for agonists. It is also clear that the presence of GTP is required for the induction of opioid-receptor mediated effects (BLUME et al. 1979), supporting the view that formation of the L.R.G.GTP complex is essential for opioid action. This receptor complex also has a low affinity for agonists. Thus, agonist action may require binding to low-affinity receptor complexes. Attempts to measure agonist affinity in functional assays using the partial receptor occlusion method developed by FURCHGOTT (1978) have been made. PORRECA and BURKS (1983) and CHAVKIN and GOLDSTEIN (1984) have reported a K_A for normorphine of about $1.5\,\mu M$ in the isolated guinea pig ileum myenteric plexus preparation. Using a similar approach in slices of rat locus ceruleus, WILLIAMS and NORTH (1984) have reported a K_A for normorphine of approximately $12\,\mu M$. In each case, these estimated K_A values are at least an order of magnitude higher than the concentrations of normorphine required to give 50% of maximal inhibition in each system. These low estimates of agonist apparent affinity based on functional assays support the conclusion that low-affinity forms of the receptor generated by association with G protein and guanine nucleotides are critical components of opioid action.

However, the partial receptor occlusion method does not provide a true reflection of agonist affinity for receptors that must form a ternary complex to induce an agonist affect. The estimated affinity is influenced by the relative concentrations of the interacting species and their rates of association and dissociation. For G protein linked receptors, the concentration of

G protein may become a critical factor in determining the apparent affinity of the agonist when intracellular concentrations of GTP are high (MACKAY 1990). It is difficult to determine to what extent the formation of a ternary complex has biased the estimation of opioid agonist affinity in the studies noted above. It has been argued that in some systems the affinities of partial agonists at G protein-coupled receptors can be estimated by the partial receptor occlusion method with reasonable reliability (LEFF et al. 1990). Since morphine and normorphine appear to be partial agonists (relative to etorphine or opioid peptides) in both the isolated guinea pig ileum and the locus ceruleus preparations (CHAVKIN and GOLDSTEIN 1984; WILLIAMS and NORTH 1984), the estimates of normorphine K_A may provide some indication of its true affinity. Generally, measurements of opioid action appear to support the view that the low-affinity form of the receptor are important in the mediation of opioid effect.

4. Sodium Regulates Agonist Affinity at μ- and δ-Receptors

The earliest studies on ligand binding to opioid receptors demonstrated that sodium was more potent than other monovalent and divalent ions in reducing the affinity of agonists for opioid receptors (SIMON et al. 1973; PERT and SNYDER 1974; PATERSON et al. 1986). Sodium is essential for opioid inhibition of adenylate cyclase activity (BLUME et al. 1979). At both μ- and δ-receptors in guinea pig cortical membranes, the concentration of Na^+ giving half maximal inhibition of agonist binding is in the range $10-30\,mM$ (WERLING et al. 1986). It seems likely that if Na^+ exerts any physiologically significant role in the regulation of opioid agonist affinity at μ- and δ-receptors, then the regulatory site must be at an intracellular location since an extracellular site with this sensitivity to Na^+ would be permanently activated by the high extracellular concentration of this ion. In contrast, resting intracellular concentration of Na^+ may be close to or just below the concentration range at which this ion regulates opioid agonist affinity. Further evidence that the Na^+ regulatory site is intracellular has been provided by consideration of the effects of the sodium selective ionophore monensin on agonist binding to intact NG 108-15 cells and 7315c cells (PUTTFARCKEN et al. 1986). In the presence of extracellular Na^+, monensin reduced agonist binding at δ-receptors in intact NG 108-15 cells and at μ-receptors in intact 7315c cells. Monensin had no effect on agonist binding in the absence of extracellular Na^+, or in homogenized membrane preparations from the same cells in the presence of Na^+, indicating that monensin probably reduced agonist binding in intact cells by allowing the intracellular concentration of Na^+ to rise toward the level in the extracellular medium.

The molecular mechanism by which sodium acts to regulate opioid binding is not yet determined, although indirect evidence suggests an interaction of the ion with opioid receptors themselves rather than with G protein associated with the receptors. WÜSTER et al. (1984) showed that PT treatment of NG 108-15 cells, inactivating G_i and abolishing opioid inhibition of adenylate cyclase, did not reduce the ability of Na^+ to inhibit [^{3}H]DADLE binding. Some association between receptor and G protein apparently remained after PT treatment, however, since the ability of GDPβS (in the presence of Na^+) to inhibit agonist binding was potentiated by PT treatment. Since GDP affinity for G protein is reduced by agonists, this suggests that Na^+ impairs the ability of agonist-occupied receptors to dissociate GDP from G protein.

A number of studies suggest similarities in the properties of $α_2$-adrenergic receptors and opioid receptors; agonist binding at both sets of receptors is regulated by Na^+ and by guanine nucleotides and agonist activation of both sets of receptors inhibits adenylate cyclase. The Na^+ site at $α_2$-adrenoceptors also appears to be located at an intracellular site. The amino acid sequence of $α_2$-adrenoceptors is known. Recent studies by HORSTMAN et al. (1990) using site-directed mutagenesis have shown that Na^+ ions interact specifically with Asp-79 in the $α_2$-adrenergic receptor sequence to reduce agonist affinity. This Asp residue is known to be located at the intracellular end of the second transmembrane region of the $α_2$-receptor protein. It is possible that the functional similarities between $α_2$-adrenergic receptors and opioid receptors extend to regions of sequence homology, supporting the proposal emerging from functional studies suggesting that Na^+ regulates opioid agonist binding at an intracellular site on the receptor protein itself. This site may have a significant role in the interaction of the receptor with G protein subunits.

5. Stimulation of GTPase Activity by Activation of μ- and δ-Receptors

It has become accepted after the pioneering studies of CASSEL and SELINGER (1976) that receptor-mediated activation of G proteins is associated with activation of a GTPase activity of the G protein. The cleavage of the GTP bound to the α-subunit of the G protein to GDP, with release of phosphate, inactivates the G protein and thus inactivates the effector system. The α-, β-, and γ-subunits of the G protein are now free to reassociate, making the heterotrimer available for interaction again with agonist-occupied receptors (for review, see BIRNBAUMER 1990). Since the G protein can pass through several cycles of activation and GTP hydrolysis within the life span of each agonist-receptor complex, the G protein transduction system provides an amplification mechanism.

The demonstration by KOSKI and KLEE (1981) that opiates acting at δ-receptors can stimulate a low K_m GTPase in membranes from NG 108-15 cells indicated that GTPase stimulation is a critical feature of opioid receptor-effector coupling. Naloxone was shown to inhibit the opioid stimulation of GTPase with a K_i of about 20 nM, consistent with its affinity for δ-receptors. These observations have subsequently been confirmed and extended by VACHON et al. (1986). In the NG 108-15 cell membranes, δ-agonists were able to increase the GTPase activity by two- or three-fold above basal values. In brain membrane preparations, the lower concentration of opioid receptors and the presence of a high basal level of GTPase activity makes it much more difficult to measure opioid stimulation of the enzyme quantitatively. Nevertheless, BARCHFIELD and MEDZIHRADSKY (1984) reported that levorphanol (in concentrations from $10\,nM$ to $10\,\mu M$) increased the low K_m GTPase activity of rat striatum membranes by about 20%–30% above basal levels in a naloxone-reversible manner. The selective μ-agonist sufentanil and the partially δ-receptor selective agonist DSLET both stimulated the enzyme by a similar amount; κ-agonists also stimulated GTPase activity but to a lesser extent than the μ- and δ-agonists (CLARK and MEDZIHRADSKY 1987). Prior treatment of the membranes with the μ-selective alkylating antagonist β-FNA inhibited the stimulation by levorphanol, but not by DSLET. In contrast, the δ-selective alkylating agent Superfit inhibited the response to DSLET more than the response to sufentanil, suggesting that both δ- and μ-receptors can activate GTPase in brain membranes.

II. Evidence for κ-Receptor Interactions with G Proteins

Guanine nucleotides and their nonohydrolyzable analogues generally have less effect on agonist affinity at κ-receptors than at μ- and δ-type opioid receptors (WERLING et al. 1984; MACK et al. 1985). Interpretation of these early studies is complicated by the probability that more than one form of κ-receptor is present in mammalian neural membranes (SIMON and GIOANNINI, this volume). Recently, evidence has accumulated suggesting that κ-receptor activation results in inhibition of the G protein-regulated enzyme adenylyl cyclase in guinea pig cerebellum (KONKOY and CHILDERS 1989) and in rat spinal cord-dorsal root ganglion cultures (ATTALI et al. 1989a). CLARK et al. (1986) have suggested that κ-agonists stimulated a low-K_m GTPase in rat brain membranes. However, the high concentrations of κ-agonists needed in this study (ethylketocyclazocine EC_{50}, $3.5\,\mu M$; U50488H, $12\,\mu M$) makes it uncertain that the effect was mediated through κ-receptors.

In contrast, UEDA et al. (1987) have reported that U50488H ($1-100\,nM$) inhibited the low-K_m GTPase activity in guinea pig cerebellar membranes. In the same preparation, the μ-selective agonist DAMGO ($10\,nM$ to $1\,\mu M$) stimulated the low-K_m GTPase. The inhibitory effect of U50488H was prevented by coincubation with the benzomorphan opiate antagonist Mr2266 ($10\,nM$) but not by naloxone ($1\,\mu M$). The ability of Gpp(NH)p to induce the release of $[\alpha\text{-}^{32}P]GDP$ from guinea pig cerebellar membranes reconstituted with G_{i-1} or G_{i-2} prelabeled with $[\alpha\text{-}^{32}P]GDP$ (but not with prelabeled G_o) was also reduced by U50488H (UEDA et al. 1990b). The high potency of U50488H suggests that these effects were mediated through κ-receptors. MISAWA et al. (1990) have now reported that $100\,nM$ U50488H inhibits GTP-stimulated phospholipase C activity, reducing the GTP-induced formation of IP_3 in guinea pig cerebellum membranes. This appears to be a unique example of receptor-mediated inhibition of low-K_m GTPase and phospholipase C activities. The importance of this action in mediating κ-opioid effects is unclear; it has not been shown that inhibition of phospholipase C is required for κ-agonist action in most systems in which κ effects have been demonstrated.

1. Effects of Guanine Nucleotides on Agonist Binding at κ₁-Sites

The ligand used for κ-receptor characterization in the early studies was usually ethylketocyclazocine. This ligand is one of the prototypic κ-opioids, and has significant affinity for each of the forms of κ-binding site that have been discriminated to date. Studies with arylacetamide compounds such as U50488H which are selective for a subset (now characterized as κ₁ sites; ZUKIN et al. 1988) of the binding sites labeled by ethylketocyclazocine and related benzomorphans suggest that ethylketocyclazocine may not be a full agonist at κ₁-sites. In guinea pig cerebellum membranes which appear to have κ-binding sites (ROBSON et al. 1984), the inhibition of [^{3}H]DIP binding by the arylacetamide U50488H was markedly reduced by the nonhydrolyzable GTP analogue Gpp(NH)p in the presence of Na$^+$ (FRANCES et al. 1985).

When labeled κ-selective arylacetamides became available, it was shown that their dissociation rate from κ₁-receptors was significantly accelerated by Gpp(NH)p (SMITH et al. 1989), in much the same way as it had previously been shown that agonist dissociation rates at μ- and δ-receptors were significantly increased by guanine nucleotides. GAIRIN et al. (1989) have examined the effects of Gpp(NH)p on the binding affinity at guinea pig cerebellum κ₁-receptors of a series of analogues of dynorphin A, a very potent and selective κ-agonist. The Gpp(NH)p-induced shift in peptide IC_{50} in competing against [^{3}H]DIP binding in the cerebellar membranes was compared with the agonist or antagonist potency of the same series of peptides at κ-receptors in isolated rabbit vas deferens. For four peptides with κ-agonist activity in the rabbit vas deferens preparation the Gpp(NH)p-induced shift in IC_{50} was about 60-fold, and was not lower than 22-fold for any tested peptide. For the five peptides that behaved as antagonists in the bioassay, the Gpp(NH)p-induced shift in IC_{50} was about 8-fold, and did not exceed 15-fold for any antagonist peptide. It appears that at κ-receptors, as at μ- and δ-receptors, agonist affinity is more sensitive to guanine nucleotides than antagonist affinity. Direct evidence for an association of κ-receptors with a Gpp(NH)p binding protein in solubilized extracts of guinea pig cerebellum membranes has been presented (FRANCES et al. 1990).

2. Effects of Guanine Nucleotides on Binding at κ₂-Sites

The properties and distribution of the benzomorphan-binding sites described as κ₂ by ZUKIN et al. (1988) and TIBERI and MAGNAN (1990) have not been fully characterized. NOCK et al. (1990) have reported that this binding site, measured by [³H]EKC binding in rat brain homogenates in the presence of blocking concentrations of selective μ-, δ-, and κ₁-ligands, is the major binding site for [³H]EKC in rat brain with a site density greater than those of the μ-, δ-, and κ₁-sites. They suggest that this site is similar to the putative ε-binding site with high affinity for β-endorphin described by SCHULZ et al. (1980) in rat vas deferens and CHANG et al. (1984) in rat brain. A site with apparently similar properties has also been reported in bovine adrenal medulla (CASTANAS et al. 1985). The functional consequences, if any, of occupying these sites in brain are unknown. Thus, the agonist or antagonist activities of ligands occupying κ₂-sites are unknown. TIBERI and MAGNAN (1990) have reported that at least two affinity states for the κ₂-binding site can be discriminated, suggesting that this site, like μ- and δ-receptors, might be linked to G proteins regulating agonist affinity. However, it is also possible that these two affinity states reflect the existence of two (or more) independent sites with similar but nonidentical ligand affinities (ROTHMAN et al. 1990). The affinity of [³H]bremazocine for κ₂-sites measured under conditions of μ-, δ-, and κ₁-blockade was unaffected by the addition of 100 μM Gpp(NH)p (TIBERI and MAGNAN 1990). This might indicate either that these sites are not coupled to G proteins in the same way as other G protein-linked receptors, that bremazocine has relatively pure antagonist properties at these sites, or that bremazocine binds with comparable affinity to coupled and uncoupled forms of these sites. NOCK et al. (1990) have demonstrated that the K_i for several benzomorphans at the κ₂ site was reduced by the inclusion of high concentrations of NaCl in the assay medium, while the K_i for β-endorphin was increased from about 20 nM in the absence of NaCl to greater than 1 μM in its presence. These results might also indicate that the benzomorphans are antagonists while β-endorphin behaves as an agonist at the κ₂-sites. However, until a functional assay for κ₂-mediated effects is developed, it will remain uncertain if these sites are receptors that require an association with a G protein for receptor-effector transduction. It is also uncertain if the effects of activation of the proposed κ₃-subtype of κ-receptor are mediated though G protein transducers (CLARK et al. 1989).

III. Stimulatory Effects of Opioids: Possible Interactions of Opioid Receptors with G_s

The studies discussed above indicate that many effects of opioids are mediated by the interaction of agonist-occupied receptors with the PT-sensitive G proteins G_i and G_o. Recent evidence suggests that under some circumstances opioid receptors can interact with other G proteins. MAKMAN et al. (1988) have reported that in primary cultures of fetal mouse spinal cord-dorsal root ganglia, the basal activity of adenylyl cyclase (i.e., in the absence of forskolin or other added stimulants) was increased by 2 μM levorphanol. Naloxone (2 μM) also stimulated adenylyl cyclase activity, and antagonism of the stimulatory effect of levorphanol by naloxone was not demonstrated. When the enzyme was activated by forskolin, the anticipated inhibitory effect of levorphanol was observed, and this inhibitory effect was naloxone reversible. Chronic treatment of the cultures with morphine resulted in an enhancement of the stimulatory effects of levorphanol and a reduction of its inhibitory effects on adenylyl cyclase. Crain and his colleagues have attempted to correlate the stimulation of adenylyl cyclase with an increase in the duration of calcium-dependent action potentials in dorsal root ganglion neurons in the cultures. Low concentrations $(1-10\,nM)$ of opioids with μ-, δ-, and κ-receptor selectivity are all reported to increase action potential duration in about two-thirds of neurons tested, while high concentrations (around $1\,\mu M$) of the same agonist reduced action potential duration (SHEN and CRAIN 1989). PT treatment of the cultures enhanced the stimulatory effects and reduced or abolished the inhibitory effects of the opioids. A role for cAMP in the stimulatory effects of opioids is suggested by the observations that the opioid-induced prolongation of the action potential was blocked by an inhibitor of cAMP-dependent protein kinase (CHEN et al. 1988), by treatment with CT, or with the A-subunit of CT, which is known to activate G_s and therefore might prevent further activation by opioids (SHEN and CRAIN 1990a). These results suggest that in this preparation low concentrations of opioids are activating G_s, resulting in an increase in adenylyl cyclase activity, an activation of cAMP-dependent protein kinase to modify ion channel function, and extending action potential duration. (This proposed action is discussed further in Chap. 30).

It should be noted, however, that MAKMAN et al. (1988) reported an increased in adenylyl cyclase activity only after treatment with a high concentration of levorphanol $(2\,\mu M)$. SHEN and CRAIN (1989) found that in this concentration range for opioids the primary effect was a reduction in action potential duration. The very low concentrations of opioids reported by SHEN and CRAIN to increase action potential duration have not yet been demonstrated to increase adenylate cyclase activity. The report that the B-subunit of CT inhibited the stimulatory effect of low concentrations of opioids (SHEN and CRAIN 1990b) also casts some doubt about the role for G_s in the stimulatory effects of opioids. The B-subunit of the toxin is presumed to participate in the penetration of the cells by the toxin by binding to ganglioside GM1 on the cell surface and allowing the A-subunit to penetrate and interact with G_s. SHEN and CRAIN (1990b) suggest that the B-subunit of CT in some way interferes with opioid activation of Gs through a GM1-dependent mechanism since they also report that an antiserum against GM1 also blocked the action potential prolongation induced by dynorphin A.

There are other reports suggesting that low concentrations of opioids may exert stimulatory effects in different assay systems. GINTZLER and XU (1991) report that low concentrations $(1-5\,nM)$ of μ-, δ-, and κ-selective agonists enhance electrically stimulated release of [Met[5]]enkephalin from superfused guinea pig myenteric plexus preparations, and that this effect is blocked by CT treatment. Higher concentrations of the same opioids ($100\,nM$–$1\,\mu M$) inhibited release of the peptide. The inhibitory action was unaffected by CT but inhibited by prior PT treatment. As in the studies of CRAIN and coworkers, these results suggest that in some tissues activated opioid receptors can modify the function of G_s. It remains unclear if this is a direct opioid receptor interaction with G_s, or occurs as a result of cross-regulation among the many G proteins present.

C. Cellular Consequences of Sustained Exposure to Opiate Drugs

I. Characteristics of Opioid Tolerance and Dependence

Sustained or repeated exposure to opiate drugs or opioid peptides results in the development of tolerance to the action of agonist at opioid receptors. The effectiveness of the agonist is reduced, and a larger dose (or concentration) of agonist is required to induce the same intensity of opioid effect. In opiate-drug treated animals, removal of opiates after a period of sustained exposure usually results in the expression of a characteristic set of behaviors known as a withdrawal syndrome. These symptoms are often the opposite of the acute effects of opiate drugs in the same animal. Some in vitro opioid bioassay preparations demonstrate a similar type of effect. Removal of a tolerance-inducing opiate drug treatment results in hyper-activity of the system suppressed by opiate drug. This phenomenon is known as dependence. The features of opioid tolerance and dependence have been reviewed in more detail elsewhere (JOHNSON and FLEMING 1989; Cox 1990).

A significant feature of opioid tolerance is that the opioid agonist concentration-response curve, measured in vivo in assays of antinociceptive effect (BLÄSIG et al. 1979) or in vitro in isolated autonomically innervated smooth muscle preparations (S.M. JOHNSON et al. 1978; Cox 1978), is shifted to the right, and with higher intensities of opioid pretreatments shows a reduction in the maximum attainable response with agonist. Tolerance to opiate drug action has been shown to occur in isolated cells in culture. The induction of tolerance to opioid-induced inhibition of adenylyl cyclase following treatment with morphine was first demonstrated in the neuroblastoma X glioma hybrid cell line NG108-15 (SHARMA et al. 1975, 1977) and subsequently confirmed in several other cell types. In these in vitro systems, the maximum attainable response to opioids is often reduced with little rightward shift of the concentration-response curve (Fig. 2). These results suggest that tolerance is associated with a transient inactivation of functional opioid receptors. In systems where there is an excess of functional receptors, the concentration curve is initially shifted to the right by the tolerance-inducing treatment until the receptor reserve is abolished,

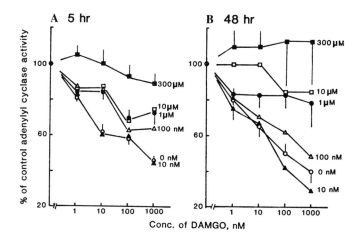

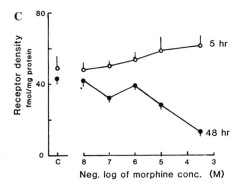

Fig. 2A–C. Inhibition of forskolin-stimulated adenylyl cyclase activity by DAMGO (**A,B**), and opioid receptor densities (**C**) measured by [³H]DIP binding in membranes from untreated (control) and morphine-treated 7315c pituitary tumor cells. Tolerance to the inhibitory effect of DAMGO was observed after 5h of morphine treatment, at a time when there was no change in the number of opioid binding sites. Tolerance in this system was manifested as a reduction in the maximum inhibition of adenylyl cyclase activity with little change in the IC_{50} for DAMGO. After 48h of morphine treatment, a significant reduction in opioid receptor density was also apparent, but the tolerance to the inhibitory effect of DAMGO on adenylyl cyclase activity was not much greater than after 5h of treatment. (From PUTTFARCKEN and COX 1989). Primary cultures of 7315c pituitary cells were treated with morphine at the concentration indicated *on the right side* of **A** and **B**, and on the *x*-axis of the graph in **C**, for 5h (**A,C**) or 48h (**B,C**), then rinsed in drug-free medium, homogenized, and washed membrane suspensions prepared. **A** and **B** show the inhibition of forskolin-stimulated adenylyl cyclase by the μ-receptor selective agonist DAMGO, expressed as a percentage of the control adenylyl cyclase activities in cultures maintained for the same periods in morphine-free medium. Control levels of forskolin-stimulated adenylyl cyclase activity were not significantly changed by the morphine treatments. **C** shows the density of [³H]DIP-binding sites (B_{max}, fmol/mg membrane protein) in the same washed membranes suspensions, after 5h and 48h of culture in medium containing the indicated concentrations of morphine; **C** binding site densities in control cells incubated in morphine-free medium for 5 or 48h

at which point further treatment reduces the maximum response. Similar effects are observed following treatment of guinea pig myenteric plexus longitudinal muscle preparations with irreversible opioid receptor antagonists (CHAVKIN and GOLDSTEIN 1984). Under experimental situations where there is initially no excess of functional receptors, the only observed effect of the tolerance-inducing treatment is a reduction in the maximum attainable response to agonist (Fig. 2). This effect might be a consequence of a reduction in the number of functional receptors, either as a result of a reduction in total receptor number, or as a result of the effective uncoupling of opioid receptors from their effector systems following their activation by agonists.

II. Changes in the Number of Opioid Receptors Following Sustained Exposure to High Concentrations of Opiate Drugs

1. In Vitro Studies Employing Tissue Culture

The development of methods for the direct measurement of the binding of radiolabeled ligands to their receptors made it possible to determine if changes occurred in the binding of agonists after chronic opioid treatments. The clearest evidence for an agonist-induced reduction in opioid receptor number comes from studies of cell lines and primary cultures exposed to high concentrations of opioids for periods of hours or days. CHANG et al. (1982) reported that incubation of NG 108-15 cells with DADLE, $100\,nM$, resulted in a 70% reduction in binding of a labeled agonist. LAW et al. (1982, 1983) demonstrated that etorphine, an agonist with higher affinity at δ-receptors than morphine, was more effective than morphine at inducing tolerance in the δ-receptor-carrying NG 108-15 cells. After 5 or more h of etorphine ($10\,nM$) treatment, a significant reduction in the number of [^{3}H]DIP-binding sites in these cells was observed. Control studies made it unlikely that this reduction was due to the presence of residual etorphine in the membranes of the pretreated cells. It is important to note that no change in the number of binding sites was observed after incubation with etorphine for 1 or 2 h, even though at this time the ability of etorphine to inhibit adenylyl cyclase was already significantly impaired. Thus, it is unlikely that the reduction in receptor number is the critical event on the loss of opioid responsiveness in these cells. The reduction in receptor number after 24 h of treatment with etorphine was specific for δ-receptors in the NG 108-15 cells; there was no change in the densities of muscarinic, α_2-adrenoceptors, or PGE_2 receptors at a time when the δ-receptor density was reduced by 60%–70% (LAW et al. 1983). The opiate-induced reduction δ-receptor number in NG 108-15 cells has since been confirmed by other groups (MOSES and SNELL 1984; MALOTEAUX et al. 1989).

More recently it has been shown that chronic exposure to morphine can reduce the density of μ-type opioid receptors in primary cultures of rat pituitary 7315c tumor cells (PUTTFARCKEN et al. 1988; PUTTFARCKEN and COX 1989; Fig. 2). A downregulation of μ-receptors in aggregating cultures of fetal rat brain cells (LENOIR et al. 1984) and in primary culture of fetal rat brain cells (MALOTEAUX et al. 1990) has also been reported after sustained exposure to the potent opiate agonists etorphine, DADLE, alfentanil, or sufentanil. The reduction in μ-receptor number induced by alfentanil was prevented by co-incubation with naloxone (MALOTEAUX et al. 1990), suggesting that activation of the receptors is necessary for downregulation to be observed. DINGLEDINE et al. (1983) found a reduction in the number of δ-receptors, but not μ-receptors, in rat hippocampal slices following superfusion of the slice preparations for 4 h with DADLE ($1 \mu M$). Thus, it now seems well established that downregulation of opioid receptors can be induced in vitro in neural cell lines, in primary cultures of tumor tissue or fetal brain cells, and in intact adult rat neurons in brain slices maintained under superfusion.

2. Effects of Chronic Opioid Treatment in Brain

a) Agonist-Induced Downregulation; μ- and δ-Binding Sites

Early studies using brain tissue from adult rats or other species failed to find significant changes in either the binding affinity or the number of opioid-binding sites following morphine treatments that induced significant tolerance to the analgesic actions of morphine (KLEE and STREATY 1974; DUM et al. 1979). However, subsequent studies, usually using more intense chronic opiate drug treatments with agonists with higher efficacy than morphine, have demonstrated that changes in the numbers of specific types of opioid receptor can be induced by sustained exposure to opioid drugs. It appears that relatively high concentrations of opiate agonist are necessary, and down-regulation is more readily observed after treatment with highly efficacious agonists than with partial agonists.

STEECE et al. (1986) used intracerebroventicular applications of [Met^5]enkephalin in rat for 5 days to achieve high local concentrations of the opioid peptide. At 24 h after the last injection, saturation analysis of binding in striatum with the selective δ-receptor agonist [^{3}H]DSLET indicated that the number of δ-receptors in this brain region had declined by about 30%. Intracerebroventricular injections of DADLE on an increasing dose regimen for 5 days in rats has also been shown to cause a reduction of about 30% in the number of [^{3}H]DIP-binding sites in rat cortex, striatum, and midbrain (TAO et al. 1988). The reduction in total [^{3}H]DIP-specific binding was attributable to a reduction of 70% or more in δ-sites, with little change in μ-site density. However, the interpretation of these results is complicated by the use of labeled agonists, since there is accumulating evidence to suggest that agonist affinity is reduced to the extent that some sites may not be detectable by labeled agonists after chronic opioid treatments (see Sect. C.III).

   Chronic opioid treatment may also induce changes in the numbers of
μ-opioid receptors in brain regions. TEMPEL et al. (1988) reported that
implantation of a morphine pellet into pregnant rats at gestational day
16 resulted in a 35% reduction in the number of μ-receptors in brain
homogenates prepared from the pups on neonatal day 0. A similar reduction
in μ-receptors was also observed when neonatal rats were given daily
subcutaneous injections of morphine injections for 4 days from postnatal
day 1. The reduction in receptors was accompanied by a tolerance to the
analgesic effects of morphine. If the morphine injections were continued
for 28 days in the neonatal rats, there was no difference in the number of
μ-receptors in treated and saline-injected control animals. These results
might indicate an agonist-induced downregulation of the μ-receptors, but
could also reflect a delay in neuronal development caused by the morphine
treatments. There was no evidence that the change in receptor density was
unique to the μ-receptors through which morphine acts.
   More recent studies have indicated that chronic treatment with morphine can induce a significant downregulation of μ-receptors in brain and
spinal cord of adult rodents. Subcutaneous infusions of morphine (1.7 mg/h
per kg body wt.) for 6 days from indwelling osmotic minipumps in guinea pigs
induced a reduction in the high-affinity μ-sites measured by labeled agonist
by about 45%, and a reduction in the total of high- and low-affinity forms of
the μ-receptor measured with labeled antagonist by about 20%–25%
(WERLING et al. 1989b). There was no change in the affinities or numbers of
δ- and κ-receptors. Thus, the morphine treatment induced both a change in
the relative proportions of the high- and low-affinity forms, and also a small
net reduction in the total number of μ-receptors without affecting other
opioid receptor types. A selective downregulation of μ-receptors of about
20%–30% (with no change in δ-receptor density) in cortex, striatum, midbrain, and spinal cord has also been reported after 5 days of intraventricular
injections of the selective μ-agonist [N-MePhe^3, D-Pro^4]morphiceptin
(PL017) (TAO et al. 1990; NISHINO et al. 1990). Collectively, these results
indicate that it is possible to induce a downregulation of μ-receptors by
sustained treatment with high doses of μ-agonists. However, in vivo, the
extent of μ-receptor downregulation is modest. It is unlikely that the degree
of functional tolerance observed after these μ-agonist treatments could
be completely explained on the basis of the small reported reduction in
receptor density.

b) Agonist-Induced Upregulation; μ-Binding Sites

An upregulation of a subset of μ-binding sites has been reported after
induction of morphine tolerance by the subcutaneous implantation of
morphine pellets (ROTHMAN et al. 1986; BRADY et al. 1989). Autoradiographic analysis indicated that the increased density of μ-binding was
limited to discrete brain regions; hypothalamus, basolateral and medial

nuclei of amygdala, and striatum. No significant increases were observed in cortex, hippocampus, or thalamus (BRADY et al. 1989). An upregulation of μ-binding has also been reported after heroin pellet implantation (BOLGER et al. 1988). It is not clear if the failure to observe any increase in μ-binding in the studies discussed above by WERLING et al. (1989b), TAO et al. (1990), and NISHINO et al. (1990) resulted from the analysis of different brain regions from those studied by the Rothman group, or from differing treatment protocols. The studies that have reported a μ-binding site down-regulation have used repeated injections or minipump infusions of morphine (or more efficacious agonists) to induce tolerance. Downregulation does not appear to be observed reliably after morphine pellet implantation (BOLGER et al. 1988). The maintenance of a steady rate of morphine release throughout the period after pellet administration is not certain. Again, the importance of sustained high concentrations of agonist in the induction of μ-binding site downregulation in vivo is emphasized.

c) Antagonist-Induced Upregulation of Opioid Binding Sites

Chronic treatment with opiate antagonists has been shown to increase the number of opioid receptors in brain (LAHTI and COLLINS 1978; ZUKIN et al. 1982; TEMPEL et al. 1986; MORRIS and HERZ 1989). These studies have used μ-selective labeled opioid ligands to demonstrate an increase in receptor-density following chronic treatment with naloxone or naltrexone, two opiate antagonists with a moderate selectivity for μ-receptors. There is therefore strong evidence of upregulation of μ-binding sites. It is assumed that the increase in receptor density occurs as a result of adaptive responses to the reduced level of μ-receptor activation in vivo during chronic naloxone or naltrexone treatment. The extent of upregulation of δ- and κ-binding sites following μ-selective antagonist treatment was not carefully assessed in these studies. GIORDANO et al. (1991) have confirmed that μ-opioid binding sites are upregulated 5 days or more after implantation of the rats with naltrexone pellets. In the same study they also report an upregulation of κ_2-binding sites for [^{3}H]EKC (described by GIORDANO et al. as putative ε-sites; see Sect. B.II.2) with a time course similar to that observed for μ-sites. In contrast, the density of δ- and κ_1-sites increased more slowly, with no significant change in the number of sites being apparent until 25 days of naltrexone treatment.

3. Effects of Chronic Treatment with κ-Agonists

The effects on opioid receptor populations of chronic treatments with κ-selective agonists are uncertain. MORRIS and HERZ (1989) found that infusion of bremazocine (at about 4 mg/kg per day for 7 days from an implanted reservoir) resulted in a substantial reduction in high-affinity sites for the κ-agonist [^{3}H]bremazocine (in the presence of receptor-blocking concentrations of μ- and δ-ligands), and an increase in the number of sites with low affinity for agonists. Because of the difficulty of quantifying the number of low-affinity sites, it is uncertain if the bremazocine treatment reduced total receptor number, or simply shifted a fraction of the receptors from a high-affinity to a low-affinity state for κ-agonists. Agonist-induced shifts in μ-binding site affinity states have also been reported after chronic treatments with μ-agonists (see Sect. C.III). Bremazocine is an antagonist at μ-receptors. As expected, the number of μ-receptors was substantially increased after chronic bremazocine treatment. Nalorphine, an antagonist at μ-receptors but a partial agonist at κ-receptors, increased μ-binding sites but did not alter κ-binding site density (MORRIS and HERZ 1989).

4. Mechanisms Implicated in Changes in Receptor Site Density

Collectively, these results suggest that the concentrations of μ-, δ-, and κ-receptors in the central nervous system can be regulated by sustained exposure to ligands. Agonist treatment may result in a reduction in receptor number, while antagonist treatment increases receptor number. Agonists must be present for significant periods and in high concentration to induce downregulation. It also appears that agonists capable of inducing down-regulation have reasonably high efficacy; partial agonists at μ- and κ-receptors produce neither up- or downregulation of μ- or κ-sites (MORRIS and HERZ 1989; MORRIS and MILLAN 1990). Recently, COSTA and HERZ (1989; COSTA et al. 1990) have proposed that competitive opioid antagonists at δ-receptors in NG 108-15 cells can be discriminated into two classes; those that inhibit the δ-receptor-coupled G protein GTPase and are there-fore described as possessing negative intrinsic activity, and those that do not affect GTPase activity. MORRIS and MILLAN (1990) suggest that antagonists lacking negative intrinsic activity, such as MR2266, are unable to induce opioid receptor upregulation, suggesting that the receptor-G protein inter-action is one of the factors determining the density of opioid receptors in the plasma membrane.

   The mechanisms by which opioid agonist and antagonists can decrease or increase opioid receptor number are not yet fully understood. In NG 108-15 cells, opioid δ-receptor agonists can induce receptor clustering (HAZUM et al. 1979) and internalization (CHANG et al. 1982; LAW et al. 1984). These results suggest that opioid receptors are removed from the plasma membrane by an endocytotic mechanism. In other systems, intern-alized plasma membrane proteins have been shown to be associated with a clathrin-enriched membrane fraction. BENNETT et al. (1985) have reported that clathrin-containing membrane vesicles from bovine brain homogenates contain opioid binding sites. It is therefore probable that the number of receptors in the plasma membrane is determined in part by the rate at which they are first sequestered and then internalized by endocytosis. It is possible that this rate is modified during sustained exposure to agonists or antag-onists, although direct evidence to support this statement is lacking. After internalization, receptors are probably destroyed by lysozomal enzymes (Law et al. 1984) or recycled to the plasma membrane after dissociation of bound ligand. The possibility that chronic agonist or antagonist treatments might also change the rates of receptor synthesis and/or insertion into plasma membranes has not yet been evaluated experimentally.

III. Chronic Opioid Treatment Uncouples Opioid Receptors from Their Associated G Proteins

1. Receptor Desensitization; μ- and δ-Receptors

Treatments inducing tolerance to opioid action cause a loss of opioid responsiveness before a significant reduction in receptor number can be demonstrated (Law et al. 1982; Puttfarcken et al. 1988). Receptor down-regulation is unlikely to be the primary cause of the loss of opioid effect. The term "receptor desensitization" has come to be used to describe the generation by agonists of nonfunctional receptor forms, where the total number of receptors measured by labeled antagonist binding is unchanged. Desensitization of opioid inhibition of adenylyl cyclase activity in NG 108-15 neuroblastoma X glioma hybrid cells and in 7315c pituitary tumor cells has been studied extensively. Desensitization is manifested as a time-dependent progressive reduction in the maximum inhibition of adenylyl cyclase activity as the duration and intensity of the tolerance-inducing treatment is increased. In some studies, the agonist concentration-response curve is shifted to the right; in others, there is little or no change in the concentration of agonist giving 50% of maximum effect despite a large reduction in maximum effect (Law et al. 1982; Puttfarcken et al. 1988; Puttfarcken and Cox 1989). In NG 108-15 cells, the opioid-induced desensitization after short exposures to etorphine was homologous; the inhibitory effects of muscarinic and α_2-adrenergic agonists were not modified at a time when there was significant attenuation of the opioid response (Law et al. 1983). Chronic treatment with cholinergic agonists has been reported to induce a desensitization of carbachol-mediated inhibition of adenylyl cyclase without significantly reducing opioid inhibition of the enzyme (Green and Clark 1982). Desensitization of opioid-activated GTPase activity has also been observed in NG 108-15 cells (Vachon et al. 1987). Loss of GTPase stimulation occurred rapidly; after 1 h of treatment with DADLE, the GTPase stimulatory response was reduced by 65% while the maximum inhibition of adenylyl cyclase activity was only 20%. It is probable that this apparent discrepancy is desensitization rates reflects the large amplification factor provided by the catalytic regulation of adenylyl cyclase activity by activated G proteins; a small number of activated G protein α-subunits are able to regulate the activity of a significantly larger number of adenylyl cyclase molecules.

Desensitization following activation by κ-agonists has been much less extensively studied, although it is well known that chronic treatment of animals in vivo results in tolerance to κ-receptor-mediated effects (e.g., WERLING et al. 1988a). ATTALI et al. (1989b) have reported that treatment of rat dorsal root ganglia-spinal cord cocultures (DRG-SC cultures) results in a reduced ability of κ-agonists to inhibit adenylyl cyclase. Unlike the homologous desensitization reported in NG 108-15 cells, the desensitization to κ-agonists in spinal cord cultures was heterologous; the responses to muscarinic and α_2-adrenergic agonists were also reduced after chronic exposure to the κ-agonist U50488H. The form of κ-receptor mediating this effect in the rat DRG-SC cultures is uncertain in view of the high concentration of U50488H required to inhibit the enzyme in this tissue. The absence of suitable cell preparations in which the effects of long-term drug treatments on defined κ_1-responses has precluded the study of desensitization at κ_1-receptors.

2. Mechanisms Implicated in Receptor Desensitization

WÜSTER et al. (1983) suggested that desensitization might result from an uncoupling of receptors from associated G proteins. If the form of the opioid receptor with high affinity for agonists is the form in which receptor is coupled to G protein in the absence of guanine nucleotides (see Sect. II above), then uncoupling of the receptor as a result of agonist treatment should be associated with a decrease in the fraction of opioid binding sites in washed membrane homogenates with high affinity for agonists. LAW et al. (1983) demonstrated that etorphine-induced desensitization was accompanied by a significant reduction in the affinity of the δ-receptors in NG 108-15 cells for the agonist DADLE although naloxone affinity was unchanged. Similar observations have been made with respect to μ-receptors. PUTTFARCKEN et al. (1988) reported that exposure of 7315c pituitary tumor cells to high concentrations of morphine for 5 h resulted in the binding sites for the μ-agonist DAMGO being shifted to a low-affinity state (DAMGO K_D, approx. 400 nM, relative to a DAMGO K_D of about 10 nM for the high-affinity form in membranes from untreated cells). In membranes from cerebral cortex of guinea pigs given a subcutaneous infusion of a high concentration of morphine for 7 days there is also evidence that morphine tolerance is associated with an increase in the fraction of μ-binding sites in a form with low affinity for agonists. In washed membranes from control guinea pigs, approximately 50% of the site displayed high affinity for DAMGO; after chronic morphine treatment only about 30% of the sites were in a form with high agonist affinity (WERLING et al. 1989b). Functional uncoupling of receptors from G protein is also induced by PT treatments that render tissues insensitive to the agonist effects of opioids (see Sect. II). The similarities between the effects of PT treatments and opioid tolerance were first noted by WÜSTER and COSTA (1984), and confirmed by

PUTTFARCKEN et al. (1988) and WERLING et al. (1989b). The similarities between the functional consequence of PT treatment and chronic opiate treatments support the view that one of the primary events in opioid tolerance is uncoupling of receptors from G proteins.

Opioid tolerance is induced by agonists but not by antagonists, yet competitive antagonists prevent activation of the receptor-associated G proteins apparently by functionally uncoupling receptor occupation from G protein activation. However, the effects of antagonists can be immediately overcome by high concentrations of agonist, while the inactivated receptors induced following agonist treatment cannot be reactivated by exposure to higher agonist concentrations. Thus, the nonfunctional form of receptor associated with antagonist must differ from that induced following activation of G proteins by agonist-occupied receptors. After dissociation of the antagonist, the receptors rapidly return to a form that can effectively transduce agonist action. In contrast, the agonist-occupied form of the receptor appears to remain inactivated for a significant time. There is no evidence indicating that this inactivation is caused by tight binding of agonist; agonist affinity is reduced in the desensitized state. An agonist-induced change in receptor structure or conformation seems a more probable explanation.

In other receptor systems, there is evidence that desensitization results from phosphorylation of receptors, either by cAMP-dependent protein kinases or by a kinase that specifically recognizes and phosphorylates agonist-occupied receptors (BENOVIC et al. 1986; HUGANIR and GREENGARD 1990). HARADA et al. (1989, 1990) have shown that c-AMP-dependent protein kinase treatment prevents μ-receptor-mediated activation of the GTPase activity of G_i in rat striatal membranes or after reconstitution in lipid vesicles, suggesting that phosphorylation of μ-receptors results in functional inactivation. The relevance of the cAMP-dependent kinase mechanism to opioid tolerance is not clear since most studies have reported that opioids inhibit adenylyl cyclase (see Chap. 8). However, in some systems, an opioid-induced increase in adenylyl cyclase activity has been reported and this effect appears to be enhanced after chronic opioid treatment (MAKMAN et al. 1988; see this chapter, Section C.V). It is also possible that cAMP-dependent mechanisms are involved in heterologous desensitization processes. It remains to be determined if other kinases, including a kinase with selectivity for agonist-occupied receptors, participate in agonist-induced opioid receptor desensitization.

The significance of the functional uncoupling of receptors from G proteins for the receptor downregulation that occurs at later times during tolerance is uncertain. As noted above (Sect. B), a functional uncoupling leading to opioid insensitivity can be induced by PT treatment (KUROSE et al. 1983). WERLING et al. (1988b) found a reduction of μ- and δ-binding sites in 7315c cells and NG 108-15 cells, respectively, after incubation of intact cells with PT for 36 h. A much shorter PT treatment (3 h) of NG

108-15 cells that abolished opioid agonist action but which did not alter receptor number also did not alter the rate of DADLE-induced reduction in receptor density (LAW et al. 1985), indicating that δ-binding site downregulation does not require activation of the receptors by the agonist. Thus receptor-G protein uncoupling, which appears to precede downregulation (LAW et al. 1983; PUTTFARCKEN et al. 1988), might be a triggering event leading to receptor clustering, sequestration, and internalization.

IV. Sustained Opioid Exposure Induces Changes in the Cellular Concentrations of Some G Proteins

1. Neuroblastoma × Glioma (NG 108-15) Hybrid Cells

Changes induced by chronic opioid treatments are not limited to the receptors mediating their effects. Studies have now suggested that opioid treatments may in some systems alter the amounts of G protein subunits present in neural membranes. Changes in the concentrations of G protein subunits might be expected to significantly affect the function of the opioid effector transduction system. In view of the well-documented occurrence of receptor desensitization and downregulation in NG 108-15 cells, changes in G protein concentrations in these cells might be expected during tolerance development. However, treatment of NG 108-15 cells with DADLE or morphine for up to 72 h did not alter the concentrations of $G_{o\alpha}$ and $G_{i-2\alpha}$, measured immunologically (LANG and COSTA 1989). Thus desensitization and receptor downregulation are not necessarily accompanied by changes in the levels of G protein subunits.

2. Guinea Pig Ileum Myenteric Plexus

Despite the lack of changes in NG 108-15 cells, LANG and SCHULZ (1989) report that treatment of guinea pigs with the potent μ-selective agonist fentanyl (5 μg/h for 6 days; a dose inducing significant tolerance to μ-receptor-mediated inhibition of electrically stimulated contractions of the ileum myenteric plexus-longitudinal muscle preparation) resulted in a significant increase in $G_{i\alpha}$ and $G_{o\alpha}$ subunit concentrations, and a reduction in $G_{s\alpha}$ subunits, in neural soma fractions from homogenates of the myenteric plexus-longitudinal muscle preparation. The most marked change, however, was an apparent increases of more than 150% in the concentration of G_β subunits. The significance of these changes in G protein subunit concentrations is not certain. However, it is possible that the higher concentration of β-subunits reduces the concentration of activated free α-subunits, thus reducing the activity of effector systems regulated by G proteins. It should be noted that in the guinea pig ileum preparation chronic opioid treatment does not appear to induce an homologous desensitization, but causes generalized changes in the responsiveness of the tissue to transmitters, reducing sensitivity to inhibitory agents while facilitating responses to stimulatory agents (FLEMING and JOHNSON 1989).

3. Central Nervous System

Opioid-induced reductions in the concentrations of G protein subunits have been reported in tissue of the mammalian central nervous system. ATTALI and VOGEL (1989) found that chronic treatment of rat dorsal root ganglion-spinal cord preparations with the κ-agonist U50488H for 4 days reduced the level of $G_{i-1\alpha}$ by about 30%. No changes were found in the concentrations of $G_{o\alpha}$, $G_{s\alpha}$, or G_β subunits. In aggregating cultures of fetal rat hindbrain, exposure to the κ-agonist U50488H also reduced $G_{i\alpha}$ (VOGEL et al. 1990). In the same system, the μ-agonist DAMGO was reported to reduce both $G_{i\alpha}$ and $G_{o\alpha}$ levels, while chronic treatment with the δ-agonist DPDPE increased the levels of the same G protein subunits. These results cannot be generalized to other brain regions; in aggregating cultures of forebrain, DAMGO treatment increased $G_{i\alpha}$ and $G_{o\alpha}$ levels by as much as 60% or more (VOGEL et al. 1990). Treatment of rats by implantation of morphine pellets each day for 5 days is reported to increase levels of $G_{i\alpha}$ and $G_{o\alpha}$ in the locus ceruleus and amygdala and to reduce their levels in the nucleus accumbens, while leaving the levels of these G protein subunits unchanged in other brain regions including the frontal cortex, hippocampus, thalamus, periaqueductal gray region, ventral tegmental area, substantia nigra, dorsal raphe, and cerebellum (NESTLER et al. 1989; TERWILLIGER et al. 1991).

4. Agonist Regulation of G Protein Levels

The studies discussed above indicate that is not possible to predict from the types of receptors in each region whether G protein levels will be increased, decreased, or unaltered by tolerance-inducing opioid treatments (see also Chap. 54 in part II, this volume). It is likely that any observed changes in concentrations of G protein subunits are not the invariable result of sustained agonist-occupation of specific types of receptor, but reflect adaptive responses to continued opioid agonist treatment that vary among neural cell types and among neural pathways. TERWILLIGER et al. (1991) have suggested that brain regions that show heterologous desensitization after chronic opioid treatment (e.g., DRG-SC and the guinea pig myenteric plexus) may show decreases in levels of $G_{i\alpha}$ subunits resulting in reduced effectiveness of all inhibitory receptor systems depending on coupling through G_i or G_o. In contrast, regions showing homologous desensitization will exhibit a different pattern of adaptive responses in which impairment of receptor-G protein coupling (receptor desensitization) as a result of a change in receptor properties is one contributing factor. This may lead to an upregulation of $G_{i\alpha}$ and $G_{o\alpha}$, thus permitting and even enhancing the continued effectiveness of transmitters such as norepinephrine and acetylcholine acting at other non-desensitized receptors to inhibit effector systems through these G proteins. This interesting hypothesis obviously requires further study.

In other systems, it has been shown that prolonged activation of receptors regulating adenylyl cyclase activity can change the levels of specific G proteins (MILLIGAN and GREEN 1991). Sustained activation of adenylate cyclase by forskolin or by the β-adrenoceptor agonist isoproterenol in S49 mouse lymphoma cells resulted in transient increases in the rates of synthesis of the mRNAs for $G_{\alpha i-2}$ and $G_{\alpha s}$, but at later times the half-life of $G_{\alpha s}$ protein was reduced. As a consequence, 24 h after the initiation of forskolin treatment $G_{\alpha i-2}$ protein levels were increased about threefold, and there was a modest (27%) decrease in the levels of $G_{\alpha s}$ protein (HADCOCK et al. 1990). In contrast to the effects of activators of adenylyl cyclase, stimulation of adenosine A_1 receptors causing inhibition of adenylyl cyclase in rat adipocytes resulted in an increase in the level of $G_{\alpha s}$ and a decrease in the level of $G_{\alpha i-2}$ proteins at 6 days after initiation of treatment (LONGABAUGH et al. 1989). It has been shown that the levels of G_β subunits do not change after prolonged activation of adenylyl cyclase with forskolin (HADCOCK et al. 1989) or isoproterenol (WANG et al. 1989). In general, the levels of the α-subunits of G proteins appear to be more susceptible than the levels of their β- or γ-subunits to regulation by chronic agonist exposure, although changes in the levels of β-subunits in guinea pig myenteric plexus after chronic morphine treatment were reported by LANG and SCHULZ (1989).

The levels of α-subunits of G proteins controlling the activity of adenylyl cyclase appear to be regulated in part by the products of adenylyl cyclase activity. Prolonged activation or inhibition of this enzyme can result in changes in G protein α-subunit mRNA synthesis rates, in mRNA stability, and in the turnover rates of the α-subunits. Cyclic AMP-dependent protein kinase may play a significant role in these regulatory mechanisms (HADCOCK et al. 1990). Changes in the relative balance of the α-subunits of the various G protein species, and in the ratios of α-subunits to βγ-subunits, will also significantly alter receptor regulation of G protein coupled effector systems (GRIFFIN et al. 1985). Evidence discussed above indicates that altered levels of G protein subunits may contribute to tolerance to opioids in some neural systems.

V. Effector System Function May Be Enhanced After Sustained Opiate Drug Treatment

The opioid withdrawal syndrome is characterized by a rebound increase in the activity or response to external stimulation in many systems that are sensitive to inhibition by opiate drugs (Cox 1990). An enhanced activity of effector systems in opioid-sensitive neurons occurs in some but not all opioid-sensitive neurons as part of the adaptive response to the sustained activation of opioid receptors. Increased activity in effector systems that are normally inhibited by opioids may play a significant role both in opioid tolerance (since a greater fractional reduction in effector activity may be needed to reduce the response to the same level as in noninduced cells) and in the expression of opioid withdrawal symptoms (since removal of the inhibitory opioid will result in an increase above basal levels in the activity of the opioid-sensitive effector system).

1. Guinea Pig Ileum Myenteric Plexus

Among in vitro preparations, one of the best-documented withdrawal responses is the contraction of the longitudinal and circular muscles of the guinea pig ileum from animals chronically treated with opiate drugs when exposed to opiate antagonists such as naloxone (SCHULZ and HERZ 1976; JOHNSON et al. 1989). The magnitude of the contraction is related to the intensity of the tolerance-inducing treatment, and requires the integrity of the cholinergic myenteric neurons innervating the muscle fibers although other transmitters may also be involved. The naloxone-induced contraction appears to be neurogenic in origin, since it is prevented by treatment of the tissue with tetrodotoxin. Naloxone also induces a dramatic increase in the rate of firing of myenteric neurons from morphine-treated guinea pigs, or of myenteric neurons in ileum preparations exposed to morphine, $1 \mu M$, for 24 h in vitro (NORTH and KARRAS 1978). Ileum preparations from morphine-treated guinea pigs show tolerance to inhibition of neurogenically induced contractions by opioids, and are supersensitive to treatments inducing contractions by releasing neurotransmitters from the myenteric plexus neurons (S.M. JOHNSON et al. 1978). The basis for these general changes in neuronal sensitivity is not known. It has been suggested that a small reduction in the neuronal membrane potential, perhaps resulting from reduced electrogenic pumping by Na^+/K^+-ATPase, might account for the sensitivity changes and the enhanced responses to excitatory neurotransmitters released by naloxone (JOHNSON and FLEMING 1989), but this proposal requires experimental confirmation.

2. Neuroblastoma × Glioma (NG 108-15) Hybrid Cells

It has been known since the first studies of the effects of chronic opioid exposure in NG 108-15 cells that in addition to changes in opioid receptor function an increase in the basal activity of the enzyme, adenylyl cyclase, also occurred (SHARMA et al. 1975, 1977; LAW et al. 1983). The increased activity of the enzyme is demonstrated by addition of naloxone to cultures treated with morphine or DADLE for periods of 12 h or with etorphine for 3 h (SHARMA et al. 1975; GRIFFIN et al. 1985; MUSACCHIO and GREENSPAN 1986). The mechanism by which this increase in enzyme activity is induced and maintained is not yet clear. The enhanced basal activity after opioid treatment is lower than the maximum levels of enzyme activity that can be induced by receptor stimulation by PGE_1, or by direct activation of G_s with non-hydrolysable guanine nucleotides or fluoride (SHARMA et al. 1977), or by forskolin (GRIFFIN et al. 1985). GRIFFIN et al. (1985) noted that PT treatment of NG 108-15 cells induced a similar increase in basal activity of adenylyl cyclase, and suggested that the effects of chronic opioid treatment and of PT treatment might both result from the removal of a tonic inhibitory effect of G_i on the basal activity of the enzyme. Changes in the activity of adenylyl cyclase in NG 108-15 cells are not induced only by sustained exposure to opioid agonists. The α_2-adrenoceptor agonist, clonidine, inhibits adenylyl cyclase activity in NG 108-15 cells; chronic treatment with this drug results in tolerance to the inhibitory effects of clonidine, and enzyme activity is increased above baseline values when the α_2-adrenoceptor antagonist idazoxan is applied to clonidine-treated cells (LEE et al. 1988). Since α_2-receptor-induced inhibition of adenylyl cyclase in NG 108-15 cells is mediated by G_i, it is probable that the increase in cAMP levels seen after opioid or clonidine treatment is a general response to sustained activation of G_i and not a specific effect of opioids. Recent studies have suggested that the increased cAMP levels in cells after chronic exposure to inhibitors is also due in part to a reduction in the degradation rate for cAMP in the treated cells (THOMAS et al. 1990). This action may contribute significantly to apparent increases in enzyme activity in studies where cAMP production has been measured in intact cells (e.g., SHARMA et al. 1975, 1977; MUSACCHIO and GREENSPAN 1986; LEE et al. 1988). It is less likely to be a factor where increased adenylyl cyclase activity following chronic opioid treatment has been demonstrated in NG 108-15 membrane homogenates (GRIFFIN et al. 1985), since THOMAS et al. (1990) found no change in phosphodiesterase activity in homogenates of NG 108-15 cells treated with inhibitors of adenylyl cyclase.

3. Dorsal Root Ganglion-Spinal Cord Cultures

Chronic morphine treatment is reported to increase levels of adenylyl cyclase activity in primary cultures of fetal mouse dorsal root ganglion-spinal cord (DRG-SC) cultures (MAKMAN et al. 1988). CRAIN and his colleagues have suggested that this action may be relevant to their observation that opioids can either prolong action potential duration (a stimulatory effect) by a mechanisms that can be inhibited by CT, or reduce action potential duration (an inhibitory effect) by a PT-sensitive mechanism (SHEN and CRAIN 1989; see Sect. B.III). In control DRG-SC cultures, 49% of cells were shown to respond to a high concentration of DADLE with a shortening of the action potential duration, while 34% showed a prolongation of action potential duration. After treatment of the cultures for 4 days or more with opioids, inhibitory effects were now observed in only 5% of tested cells while the stimulatory effects were recorded in 77% of tested cells (CRAIN et al. 1988). The reasons for the reduction in the inhibitory effect of opioids in the DRG-SC cultures after agonist treatment are not known.

4. Locus Ceruleus

The locus ceruleus (LC) receives inputs from a limited number of brain structures, but sends axons to most brain regions, including the cortex, hippocampus, cerebellum, and spinal cord (ASTON-JONES et al. 1986). The LC of the rat has been implicated as a significant site in the generation of opioid withdrawal responses in this species. Administration of naloxone to the LC of opioid-dependent animals induces a significant increase in the firing rates of the noradrenergic neurons (AGHAJANIAN 1978). The mechanisms responsible for the increase in firing rate in withdrawal are complex; several factors appear to be involved. Part of the increase in firing probably occurs as a result of antagonism by naloxone of residual opioid in the LC from the dependence-inducing treatment. When the LC region from morphine-dependent rats is removed and studied in vitro in a superfusion system, tolerance to the membrane hyperpolarization induced by μ-opioid agonists is observed, but there is no increase in firing rates above the baseline rates observed in LC neurons from control rats when naloxone is administered without prior or concurrent administration of opioid (CHRISTIE et al. 1987). It is quite likely that the failure to observe enhanced firing in vitro in LC neurons during withdrawal also results in part from the disconnection of the LC neurons from afferent inputs, especially those from the nucleus paragigantocellularis of the ventral medulla, which probably play a significant role in the expression of the opioid withdrawal syndrome (RASMUSSEN and AGHAJANIAN 1989; TUNG et al. 1990). Nevertheless, some neurochemical changes in LC have now been associated with the development of opioid tolerance and dependence.

The activities of adenylyl cyclase and cAMP-dependent protein kinase were increased in the microdissected LC region of rats after chronic morphine treatment (DUMAN et al. 1988; NESTLER and TALLMAN 1988). Increased levels of the G proteins G_i and G_o were also observed (NESTLER et al. 1989; see Sect. C.IV.3). These effects appeared to be specific to the LC; no changes in enzyme activity were observed in other selected brain regions. Several proteins in the LC have been reported to show increased levels of phosphorylation after chronic morphine treatment (GUITART and NESTLER 1989). One of these probable substrates for the enhanced cAMP-dependent protein kinase activity during chronic morphine treatment showed an apparent molecular weight of 58 kDa. Enhanced phosphorylation of a 58-kDa protein has also been reported in the synaptosomal (crude P_2) fraction of mouse brain homogenates after chronic morphine treatment (NAGAMATSU et al. 1989). The 58-kDa protein in rat LC has now been identified by GUITART et al. (1990) as tyrosine hydroxylase. Enhanced phosphorylation of the protein probably reflects an increase in the amounts of the protein present in LC, and not a change in the ratio of phosphorylated to nonphosphorylated forms. The significance of an increase in tyrosine hydroxylase levels in LC is not clear in view of the failure of CHRISTIE et al.

(1987) to detect changes in the activity of LC neurons in vitro during withdrawal, and the apparent absence (in in vitro studies) of increases in the K^+- or veratridine-stimulated release of norepinephrine from the forebrain terminal fields of the LC noradrenergic neurons of morphine-tolerant guinea pigs in the presence or absence of naloxone (Cox and WERLING 1988). It is noteworthy that BEITNER-JOHNSON and NESTLER (1991) have also found an increase in the levels of tyrosine hydroxylase in the ventral tegmental area of morphine-treated rats, but found no changes in the levels of the enzyme protein in the terminals of the VTA neurons in the nucleus accumbens. Activity of tyrosine hydroxylase in nucleus accumbens may actually have been reduced after morphine treatment since the ratio of phosphorylated (activated) to nonphosphorylated forms was reduced in the morphine-treated animals.

The enhanced adenylyl cyclase, cAMP-dependent protein kinase activities, and the increased levels of G_i and G_o return to levels not significantly different from the levels observed in untreated animals within about 6 h of precipitation of withdrawal by naloxone administration to the morphine-treated rats (RASMUSSEN et al. 1990). This time course is consistent with the initial rapid decay of behavioral withdrawal symptoms, and in the decline to baseline levels of the firing rates of the LC neurons following precipitation of withdrawal. However, some withdrawal symptoms were still apparent up to 72 h after the onset of withdrawal, despite the rapid return to baseline levels of the biochemical correlates of chronic morphine treatment. Thus other factors contributing to the prolonged withdrawal symptoms remain to be defined.

5. Summary

Collectively, these results suggest that opioid withdrawal may be associated with an increase in adenylyl cyclase activity in some but not all opioid-sensitive neurons. The processes contributing to the enhanced enzyme activity are not yet clearly resolved, although there is accumulating evidence to suggest that changes in the levels of expression of specific G protein α-subunits or in their rates of degradation may result in a shift in the relative balance of stimulatory and inhibitory α-subunits. Alterations in the ratio of α- to βγ-subunits, may also play a significant role in the expression of withdrawal responses. The activities of neurons showing an increase in adenylyl cyclase activity in opioid-dependent animals are probably modified as a result of alterations in the state of phosphorylation of a few critical .regulatory enzymes or ion channels subject to control by cAMP-dependent protein kinase. Alterations in effector function are probably not limited to those dependent on increased activity of adenylyl cyclase. In some peripheral neurons, small changes in resting membrane potential may affect the sensitivity of the neurons to inhibitory and excitatory regulatory agents.

Table 2. Summary of changes in opioid receptor and G protein functions after chronic exposure to opioids

Event	Functional consequences	Mechanisms
A. Changes specific to opioid receptor mediated functions		
Receptor desensitization (homologous desensitization) (see Sect. C.III)	Rapidly occurring reduction in response to opioid agonist; no change in number of binding sites (measured with labeled antagonists)	Uncertain (possibly phosphorylation of agonist-activated receptors)
Receptor downregulation (homolous downregulation) (see Sect. C.II)	More slowly developing reduction in the number of opioid receptors; reduced opioid response	Uncertain (presumed to involve an increased rate of receptor sequestration, internalization, and degradation)
B. Changes affecting neuronal sensitivity to many regulatory agents		
Heterologous desensitization, downregulation, and supersensitivity (see Sect. C.III)	Altered responses to nonopioid agonists; desensitization or supersensitivity; opioid tolerance, possible involvement in opioid withdrawal effects	Many (possibly including nonspecific receptor phosphorylation, and increases in nonopioid receptor density and coupling efficiency)
Changes in levels of G protein subunits (see Sect. C.IV)	Altered receptor-effector coupling efficiency resulting in modified responses to activation of heterologous receptors coupled to G proteins through increased or reduced availability of G protein α-subunits; reduced sensitivity to opioids, possible involvement in opioid withdrawal effects	Changes in G protein subunit mRNA synthesis rates and steady state levels, and in G protein degradation rates; altered ratios of α- to $\beta\gamma$-subunits
Increased function of effector systems (see Sect. C.V)	Altered neuronal sensitivity to excitatory and inhibitory agents; tolerance to opioid effects, possible involvement in opioid withdrawal effects	Many, including changes in G protein subunit concentrations and in other regulatory controls on neuronal function

VI. Summary: G Proteins and Opioid Tolerance and Dependence

Alterations in the function of G proteins subject to regulation by opioid receptors probably play a significant role in opioid tolerance and dependence, although other functions not subject to regulation by G proteins also play a role. A summary of the changes induced by chronic opioid treatments in the functions of opioid receptors and G proteins is presented in Table 2. At the cellular level, functional uncoupling of opioid receptors appears to be an important factor contributing significantly to the reduced sensitivity to opioid agonists. Receptor uncoupling (desensitization) precedes a reduction in the number of opioid receptors available in the plasma membrane to interact with agonist (downregulation), and may be one of the factors increasing the rate of receptor sequestration, internalization, and degradation. Opioid-induced changes in the rates of synthesis and/or degradation of specific G protein subunits may be important not only in opioid tolerance, but also in the enhanced responsiveness of some effector systems after chronic opioid treatments that contribute to the opioid withdrawal syndrome. Changes in the function of other effector systems probably also contribute to the overall withdrawal syndrome. This chapter has concentrated only on the cellular changes associated with chronic opioid treatments. In vivo, behavioral factors play an important role in opioid tolerance and dependence.

References

Aghajanian GK (1978) Tolerance of locus coeruleus neurons to morphine and suppression of withdrawal response by clonidine. Nature 276:186–188

Aghajanian GK, Wang Y-Y (1986) Pertussis toxin blocks the outward currents evoked by opiate and α_2-agonists in locus coeruleus neurons. Brain Res 371: 390–394

Asano T, Ogasawara N (1986) Uncoupling of γ-aminobutyric acid B receptors from GTP-binding proteins by N-ethylmaleimide: effect of N-ethylmaleimide on purified GTP-binding proteins. Mol Pharmacol 29:244–249

Aston-Jones G, Ennis M, Pieribone VA, Nickel WT, Shipley MT (1986) The brain locus coeruleus: restricted afferent control of a broad efferent network. Science 234:734–737

Attali B, Vogel Z (1989) Long-term opiate exposure leads to reduction of the α_{i-1} subunit of GTP-binding proteins. J Neurochem 53:1636–1639

Attali B, Saya D, Nah S-Y, Vogel Z (1989a) κ-Opiate agonists inhibit Ca^{2+} influx in rat spinal cord-dorsal root ganglion cocultures: involvement of a GTP-binding protein. J Biol Chem 264:347–353

Attali B, Saya D, Vogel Z (1989b) κ-Opiate agonists inhibit adenylate cyclase and produce heterologous desensitization in rat spinal cord. J Neurochem 52: 360–369

Aub DL, Frey EA, Sekura RD, Cote TE (1986) Coupling of the thyrotropin-releasing hormone receptor to phospholipase C by a GTP-binding protein distinct from the inhibitory or stimulatory GTP binding proteins. J Biol Chem 261:9333–9340

Barchfield CC, Medzihradsky F (1984) Receptor-mediated stimulation of brain GTPase by opiates in normal and dependent rats. Biochim Biophys Acta 121: 641–648

Beitner-Johnson D, Nestler EJ (1991) Morphine and cocaine exert common chronic actions on tyrosine hydroxylase in dopaminergic brain reward regions. J Neurochem 57:344–347

Bennett DB, Spain JW, Lakowski MB, Roth BL, Coscia CJ (1985) Stereospecific opiate binding sites occur in coated vesicles. J Neurosci 5:3010–3015

Benovic JL, Strasse RH, Caron MG, Lefkowitz RJ (1986) β-Adrenergic receptor kinase: identification of a novel protein kinase that phosphorylates the agonist-occupied form of the receptor. Proc Natl Acad Sci USA 83:2797–2801

Birnbaumer L (1990) Transduction of receptor signal into modulation of effector activity by G proteins: the first 20 years or so. FASEB J 4:3068–3078

Bläsig J, Meyer G, Höllt V, Hengstenburg J, Dum J, Herz A (1979) Non-competitive nature of the antagonistic mechanism responsible for tolerance development to opiate-induced analgesia. Neuropharmacol 18:473–481

Blume AJ (1978a) Interactions of ligands with opiate receptors of brain membranes; regulation by ions and nucleotides. Proc Natl Acad Sci USA 75:1713–1717

Blume AJ (1978b) Opiate binding to membrane preparations of neuroblastoma X glioma hybrid cells NG 108-15: effects of ions and nucleotides. Life Sci 22: 1843–1852

Blume AJ, Lichtshtein D, Boone G (1979) Coupling of opiate receptors to adenylate cyclase: requirement for Na^+ and GTP. Proc Natl Acad Sci USA 76:5626–5630

Bolger GT, Sklonick P, Rice KC, Weisman BA (1988) Differential regulation of μ-opiate receptors in heroin- and morphine-dependent rats. FEBS Lett 234: 22–26

Brady LS, Herkenham M, Long JB, Rothman RB (1989) Chronic morphine increases μ-opiate receptor binding in rat brain: a quantitative autoradiographic study. Brain Res 477:382–386

Burns DL, Hewlett EL, Moss J, Vaughan M (1983) Pertussis toxin inhibits enkephalin stimulation of GTPase of NG 108-15 cells. J Biol Chem 258:1435–1438

Cassel D, Selinger Z (1976) Catecholamine-stimulated GTPase activity in turkey erythrocyte membranes. Biochim Biophys Acta 252:538–551

Castanas E, Bourhim N, Giraud P, Boudouresque F, Cantau P, Oliver C (1985) Interaction of opiates with opioid binding sites in the bovine adrenal medulla: interaction with κ sites. J Neurochem 45:688–699

Chang K-J, Eckel RW, Blanchard SG (1982) Opioid peptides induce reduction of enkephalin receptors in cultures neuroblastoma cells. Nature 296:446–448

Chang K-J, Blanchard SG, Cuatrecasas P (1983) Unmasking of magnesium-dependent high-affinity binding sites for [D-Ala^2, D-Leu^5] enkephalin after pretreatment of brain membranes with guanine nucleotides. Proc Natl Acad Sci USA 80:940–944

Chang K-J, Blanchard SG, Cuatrecasas P (1984) Benzomorphan sites are ligand recognition sites of putative ε-receptors. Mol Pharmacol 26:484–488

Chavkin C, Goldstein A (1984) Opioid receptor reserve in normal and morphine-tolerant guinea pig ileum myenteric plexus. Proc Natl Acad Sci USA 81: 7253–7257

Chen G-C, Chalazonitis A, Shen K-F, Crain SM (1988) Inhibitor of cyclic AMP-dependent protein kinase blocks opioid-induced prolongation of the action potential of mouse sensory ganglion neurons in dissociated cell cultures. Brain Res 462:372–377

Childers SR (1984) Interaction of opiate receptor binding sites and guanine nucleotide regulatory sites: selective protection from N-ethylmaleimide. J Pharmacol Exp Ther 230:684–691

Childers SR, Snyder SH (1978) Guanine nucleotides differentiate agonist and antagonist interactions with opiate receptors. Life Sci 23:759–762

Childers SR, Snyder SH (1980) Differential regulation by guanine nucleotides of opiate agonist and antagonist receptor interactions. J Neurochem 34:583–593

Christie MJ, Williams JT, North RA (1987) Cellular mechanisms of opioid tolerance; studies in single brain neurons. Mol Pharmacol 32:632–638

Clark JA, Lui L, Price M, Hersh B, Edelson M, Pasternak GW (1989) Kappa opiate receptor multiplicity: evidence for two U50488-sensitive κ_1 subtypes and a novel κ_3 subtype. J Pharmacol Exp Ther 251:461–468

Clark MJ, Medzihradsky F (1987) Coupling of multiple opioid receptors to GTPase following selective receptor alkylation in brain membranes. Neuropharmacology 26:1763–1770

Clark MJ, Levenson SD, Medzihradsky F (1986) Evidence for coupling of the κ opioid receptor to brain GTPase. Life Sci 39:1721–1727

Costa T, Herz A (1989) Antagonists with negative intrinsic activity at delta opioid receptors coupled to GTP-binding proteins. Proc Natl Acad Sci USA 86:7321–7325

Costa T, Aktories K, Schultz G, Wüster M (1983) Pertussis toxin decreases opiate receptor binding and adenylate inhibition in a neuroblastoma X glioma hybrid cell line. Life Sci 33 [Suppl 1]:219–222

Costa T, Wüster M, Gramsch C, Herz A (1985) Multiple states of opioid receptor may modulate adenylate cyclase in intact neuroblastoma X glioma hybrid cells. Mol Pharmacol 28:146–154

Costa T, Lang G, Gless C, Herz A (1990) Spontaneous association between opioid receptors and GTP-binding regulatory proteins in native membranes: specific regulation by antagonists and sodium. Mol Pharmacol 37:383–394

Cox BM (1978) Multiple mechanisms in opiate tolerance. In: van Ree J, Terenius L (eds) Characteristics and functions of opioids. Elsevier/North-Holland, Amsterdam, pp 13–23

Cox BM (1990) Drug tolerance and physical dependence. In: Pratt WB, Taylor P (eds) Principles of drug action: the basis of pharmacology. Churchill Livingstone, New York, pp 639–690

Cox BM, Werling LL (1988) Regulation of norepinephrine release by opioids: role of noradrenergic pathways in opiate withdrawal. In: Illes P, Farsang C (eds) Regulatory roles of opioid peptides. VCH, Weinheim, pp 259–267

Dingledine R, Valentino RJ, Bostock E, King ME, Chang K-J (1983) Down-regulation of δ but not μ opioid receptors in the hippocampal slice associated with loss of physiological response. Life Sci 33 [Suppl 1]:333–336

Dum J, Meyer J, Höllt V, Herz A (1979) In vivo opiate binding unchanged in tolerant/dependent mice. Eur J Pharmacol 58:453–460

Duman RS, Tallman JF, Nestler EJ (1988) Acute and chronic opiate-regulation of adenylate cyclase in brain: specific effects in locus coeruleus. J Pharmacol Exp Ther 246:1033–1039

Frances B, Moisand C, Meunier J-C (1985) Na$^+$ ions and Gpp (NH) p selectively inhibit agonist interactions at κ opioid receptor sites in rabbit and guinea-pig cerebellum membranes. Eur J Pharmacol 117:223–232

Frances B, Puget A, Moisand C, Meunier J-C (1990) Apparent precoupling of κ- but not μ-opioid receptors with a G protein in the absence of agonist. Eur J Pharmacol 189:1–9

Frey E, Kebabian J (1984) A μ-opiate receptor in 7315c tumor tissue mediates inhibition of immunoreactive prolactin release and adenylate cyclase activity. Endocrinology 115:1797–1804

Furchgott RF (1978) Pharmacological characterization of receptors: its relation to radioligand binding studies. Fed Proc 37:115–120

Gairin JE, Botanch C, Cros J, Meunier J-C (1989) Binding of dynorphin A and related peptides to κ- and μ-opioid receptors: sensitivity to Na$^+$ and Gpp (NH)p. Eur J Pharmacol 172:381–384

Gintzler AR, Xu H (1991) Different G proteins mediate the opioid inhibition or enhancement of evoked [5-methionine] enkephalin release. Proc Natl Acad Sci USA 88:4741–4745

Giordano AL, Nock B, Cicero TJ (1991) Antagonist-induced up-regulation of the putative epsilon opioid receptor in rat brain: comparison with kappa, mu and delta opioid receptors. J Pharmacol Exp Ther 255:536–540

Glossman H, Baukal AJ, Catt KJ (1974) Properties of angiotensin II receptors in bovine and rat adrenal cortex. J Biol Chem 249:825–834

Green DA, Clark RB (1982) Specific mucarinic-cholinergic desensitization in the neuroblastoma-glioma hybrid NG108-15. J Neurochem 39:1125–1131

Griffin MT, Law P-Y, Loh HH (1985) Involvement of both inhibitory and stimulatory guanine nucleotide binding proteins in the expression of chronic opiate regulation of adenylate cyclase activity in NG108-15 cells. J Neurochem 45: 1585–1589

Guitart X, Nestler EJ (1989) Identification of morphine- and cyclic AMP-regulated phosphoproteins (MARPPs) in the locus coeruleus and other regions of rat brain: regulation by acute and chronic morphine. J Neurosci 9:4371–4387

Guitart X, Hayward M, Nisenbaum LK, Beitner-Johnson DB, Haycock JW, Nestler EJ (1990) Identification of MARPP-58, a morphine- and cyclic AMP-regulated phosphoprotein of 58 KDa, as tyrosine hydroxylase: evidence for regulation of its expression by chronic morphine in rat locus coeruleus. J Neurosci 10: 2649–2659

Hadcock JR, Ros M, Malbon CC (1989) Agonist regulation of β-adrenergic receptor mRNA: analysis in S49 mouse lymphoma mutants. J Biol Chem 264: 13956–13961

Hadcock JR, Ros M, Watkins DC, Malbon CC (1990) Cross-regulation between G-protein-mediated pathways: stimulation of adenylyl cyclase increases expression of the inhibitory G-protein, $G_{i\alpha2}$. J Biol Chem 265:14784–14790

Harada H, Ueda H, Wada Y, Katada T, Ui M, Satoh M (1989) Phosphorylation of μ-opioid receptors – a putative mechanism of selective uncoupling of receptor-G_i interaction, measured with low K_m GTPase and nucleotide-sensitive agonist binding. Neurosci Lett 100:221–226

Harada H, Ueda H, Katada T, Ui M, Satoh M (1990) Phosphorylated μ-opioid receptor purified from rat brains lacks functional coupling with G_i1, a GTP-binding protein in reconstituted lipid vesicles. Neurosci Lett 113:47–49

Hazum E, Chang K-J, Cuatrecasas P (1979) Opiate (enkephalin) receptors of neuroblastoma cells: occurrence in clusters on the cell surface. Science 206:1077–1079

Horstman DA, Brandon S, Wilson AL, Guyer CA, Cragoe EJ Jr, Limbird LE (1990) An aspartate conserved among G-protein receptors confers allosteric regulation of α_2 adrenergic receptors by sodium. J Biol Chem 265:21590–21595

Huganir RL, Greengard P (1990) Regulation of neurotransmitter receptor desensitization by protein phosphorylation. Neuron 5:555–567

Johnson GL, Kaslow HR, Bourne HR (1978) Genetic evidence that cholera toxin substrates are regulatory components of adenylyl cyclase. J Biol Chem 253: 7120–7123

Johnson SM, Costa M, Humphreys CMS (1989) Opioid dependence in myenteric neurons innervating the circular muscle of guinea-pig ilcum. Naunyn-Schmiedeberg's Arch Pharmacol 339:166–172

Johnson SM, Fleming WW (1989) Mechanisms of cellular adaptive sensitivity changes: applications to opioid tolerance and dependence. Pharmacol Rev 41: 435–488

Johnson SM, Westfall DP, Howard SA, Fleming WW (1978) Sensitivities of the isolated ileal longitudinal smooth muscle-myenteric plexus and hypogastric nerve-vas deferens of the guinea pig after chronic morphine pellet implantation. J Pharmacol Exp Ther 204:54–66

Katada T, Ui M (1982) Direct modification of the membrane adenylate cyclase system by islet-activating protein due to ADP-ribosylation of a membrane protein. Proc Natl Acad Sci USA 79:3129–3133

Klee WA, Streaty RA (1974) Narcotic receptor sites in morphine-dependent rats. Nature 248:61–63

Konkoy CS, Childers SR (1989) Dynorphin-selective inhibition of adenylyl cyclase in guinea pig cerebellum membranes. J Pharmacol Exp Ther 36:627–633

Koski G, Klee WA (1981) Opiates inhibit adenylate cyclase by stimulating GTP hydrolysis. Proc Natl Acad Sci USA 78:4185–4189

Kurose H, Katada T, Ui M (1983) Specific uncoupling by islet activating protein, pertussis toxin, of negative signal transduction via α-adrenergic, cholinergic, and opiate receptors in neuroblastoma × glioma hybrid cells. J Biol Chem 258: 4870–4875

Lahti R, Collins R (1978) Chronic naloxone results in prolonged increases in opiate binding sites in rat brain. Eur J Pharmacol 51:185–186

Lang J, Costa T (1989) Chronic exposure of NG 108-15 cells to opiate agonists does not alter the amount of the guanine nucleotide-binding proteins G_i and G_o. J Neurochem 53:1500–1506

Lang J, Schulz R (1989) Chronic opiate receptor activation in vivo alters the level of G-protein subunits in guinea-pig myenteric plexus. Neuroscience 32:503–510

Larsen NE, Mulliken-Kilpatrick D, Blume AJ (1981) Two different modifications of the neuroblastoma × glioma hybrid opiate receptors induced by N-ethylmaleimide. Mol Pharmacol 20:255–262

Law P-Y, Hom DS, Loh HH (1982) Loss of opiate receptor activity in neuroblastoma × glioma NG108-15 hybrid cells after chronic opiate treatment: a multistep process. Mol Pharmacol 22:1–4

Law P-Y, Hom DS, Loh HH (1983) Opiate receptor down-regulation and desensitization in neuroblastoma × glioma NG108-15 hybrid cells are two separate cellular adaptation processes. Mol Pharmacol 24:413–424

Law P-Y, Hom DS, Loh HH (1984) Down-regulation of opioid receptor in neuroblastoma × glioma NG108-15 hybrid cells: chloroquine promotes accumulation of tritiated enkephalin in the lysosomes. J Biol Chem 259:4096–4104

Law P-Y, Hom DS, Loh HH (1985a) Multiple affinity states of opiate receptor in neuroblastoma × glioma NG108-15 hybrid cells. J Biol Chem 260:3561–3569

Law P-Y, Louie AK, Loh HH (1985b) Effect of pertussis toxin treatment on the down-regulation of opiate receptors in neuroblastoma × glioma NG108-15 hybrid cells. J Biol Chem 260:14818–23

Lee S, Rosenberg CR, Musacchio JM (1988) Cross-dependence to opioid and α_2-adrenergic receptor agonists in NG1208-15 cells. FASEB J 2:52–55

Leff P, Harper D, Dainty IA, Dougall IG (1990) Pharmacological estimation of agonist affinity; detection of errors that may be caused by the operation of receptor isomerization or ternary complex mechanism. Br J Pharmacol 101: 55–60

Lefkowitz RJ, Mullikan D, Caron MG (1976) Regulation of β-adrenergic receptors by guanyl-5′-yl imidophosphate and other purine nucleotides. J Biol Chem 254:44686–44692

Lenoir D, Barg J, Simantov R (1984) Characterization and downregulation of opiate receptors in aggregating fetal rat brain cells. Brain Res 304:295–290

Longabaugh JP, Didbury J, Spiegal A, Stiles GL (1989) Modification of rat adipocyte A_1 adenosine receptor-adenylate cyclase system during chronic exposure to an A_1 adenosine receptor agonist: alterations in the quantity of $G_{s\alpha}$ and $G_{i\alpha}$ are not associated with changes in their mRNAS. Mol Pharmacol 36:681–688

Mack KJ, Lee MF, Weyhenmeyer JA (1985) Effects of guanyl nucleotides and ions on kappa opioid binding. Brain Res Bull 14:301–306

Mackay D (1990) Agonist potency and apparent affinity: interpretation using classical and steady-state ternary-complex models. Trends Pharmacol Sci 11: 17–22

Maguire ME, van Arsdale PM, Gilman AG (1976) An agonist-specific effect of guanine nucleotides on binding to the beta adrenergic receptor. Mol Pharmacol 12:335–339

Makman MH, Dvorkin B, Crain SM (1988) Modulation of adenylate cyclase activity of mouse spinal cord-ganglion explants by opioids, serotonin and pertussis toxin. Brain Res 445:303–313

Maloteaux JM, Octave JN, Laterre EC, Laduron PM (1989) Downregulation of ^{3}H-lofentanil binding to opiate receptors in different cultured neuronal cells. Naunyn Schmiedebergs Arch Pharmacol 339:192–199

McKenzie FR, Milligan G (1990) δ-Opioid receptor mediated inhibition of adenylate cyclase is transduced specifically by the guanine nucleotide binding protein G_{i2}. Biochem J 267:391–398

Milligan G, Green A (1991) Agonist control of G-protein levels. Trends Pharmacol Sci 12:207–209

Misawa H, Ueda H, Satoh M (1990) κ-Opioid agonist inhibits phospholipase C, possibly via an inhibition of G-protein activity. Neurosci Lett 112:324–327

Morris BJ, Herz A (1989) In vivo regulation of opioid receptors: simultaneous down-regulation of kappa sites and up-regulation of mu sites following chronic agonist/antagonist treatment. Neuroscience 29:433–442

Morris BJ, Millan MJ (1990) Inability of an opioid antagonist lacking negative intrinsic activity to induce opioid receptor up-regulation in vivo. Br J Pharmacol 102:883–886

Moses MA, Snell CR (1984) The regulation of δ-opiate receptor density on 108cc15 neuroblastoma X glioma hybrid cells. Br J Pharmacol 81:169–174

Musacchio JM, Greenspan DL (1986) The adenylate cyclase rebound response to naloxone in the NG 108-15 cells: effects of etorphine and other opiates. Neuropharmacology 25:833–837

Nagamatsu K, Suzuki K, Teshima R, Ikebuchi H, Terao T (1989) Morphine enhances the phosphorylation of a 58 kDa protein in mouse brain membranes. Biochem J 257:165–171

Nestler EJ, Tallman JF (1988) Chronic morphine treatment increases cyclic AMP-dependent protein kinase activity in the rat locus coeruleus. Mol Pharmacol 33:127–132

Nestler EJ, Erdos JJ, Terwilliger R, Duman RS, Tallman JF (1989) Regulation of G proteins by chronic morphine in the rat locus coeruleus. Brain Res 476:230–239

Nishino K, Su YF, Wong C-S, Watkins WD, Chang K-J (1990) Dissociation of μ-opioid tolerance from receptor downregulation in rat spinal cord. J Pharmacol Exp Ther 253:67–72

Nock B, Giodano AL, Cicero TJ, O'Connor LH (1990) Affinity of drugs and peptides for U-69593-sensitive and -insensitive kappa opiate binding sites: the U-69593-insensitive site appears to be the beta-endorphin-specific epsilon receptor. J Pharmacol 254:412–419

North RA, Karras PJ (1978) Opiate tolerance and dependence induced in vitro in single myenteric neurons. Nature 272:73–75

Ott S, Costa T, Herz A (1989) Opioid receptors of neuroblastoma cells are in tow domains of the plasma membrane that differ in content of G protein. J Neurochem 52:619–626

Paterson SJ, Robson LE, Kosterlitz HW (1986) Control by cations of opioid binding in guinea pig brain membranes. Proc Natl Acad Sci USA 83:6216–6220

Pert CB, Snyder SH (1974) Opiate receptor binding of agonists and antagonists affected differentially by sodium. Mol Pharmacol 10:868–879

Porreca F, Burks TF (1983) Affinity of normorphine for its pharmacologic receptor in the naive and morphine-tolerant guinea pig isolated ileum. J Pharmacol Exp Ther 225:688–693

Puttfarcken PS, Cox BM (1989) Morphine-induced desensitization and down-regulation at mu-receptors in 7315c pituitary tumor cells. Life Sci 45:1937–1942

Puttfarcken P, Werling LL, Brown SR, Cote TE, Cox BM (1986) Sodium regulation of agonist binding at opioid receptors. I. Effects of sodium replacement on binding to μ- and δ-type opioid receptors in 7315c and NG 108-15 cells and cell membranes. Mol Pharmacol 30:81–89

Puttfarcken PS, Werling LL, Cox BM (1988) Effects of chronic morphine exposure on opioid inhibition of adenylyl cyclase in 7315c cell membranes: a useful model for the study of tolerance at μ opioid receptors. Mol Pharmacol 33:520–527

Rasmussen K, Aghajanian GK (1989) Withdrawal-induced activation of locus coeruleus neurons in opiate-dependent rats: attentuation by lesions of the nucleus paragigantocellularis. Brain Res 505:346–350

Rasmussen K, Beitner-Johnson DB, Krystal JH, Aghajanian GK, Nestler EJ (1990) Opiate withdrawal and the rat locus coeruleus: behavioral, electrophsiological and biochemical correlates. J Neurosci 10:2308–2317

Robson LE, Foote RW, Maurer R, Kosterlitz HW (1984) Opioid binding sites of the κ-type in guinea pig cerebellum. Neuroscience 12:621–627

Rodbell M (1980) The role of hormone receptors and GTP-regulatory proteins in membrane transduction. Nature 284:17–22

Rodbell M, Lin MC, Salomon Y (1974) Evidence for interdependent action of glucagon and nucleotides of the hepatic adenylate cyclase system. J Biol Chem 249:59–65

Roth RL, Laskowski MB, Coscia CJ (1981) Evidence for distinct subcellular sites of opiate receptors: demonstration of opiate receptors in smooth microsomal fractions isolated from rat brain. J Biol Chem 256:10117–10123

Rothman RB, Danks JA, Jacobson AE, Burke TR Jr, Rice KC, Tortella FC, Holaday JW (1986) Morphine tolerance increases μ-non-competitive δ binding sites. Eur J Pharmacol 124:113–119

Pothman RB, Bykov V, de Costa BR, Jacobson AE, Rice KC, Brady LS (1990) Interaction of endogenous opioid peptides and other drugs with four kappa opioid binding sites in guinea pig brain. Peptides 11:311–331

Scheideler MA, Zukin RS (1990) Reconstitution of solubilized delta-opiate receptor binding sites in lipid vesicles. J Biol Chem 265:15176–15182

Schulz R, Herz A (1976) Aspects of opiate dependence in the myenteric plexus of the guinea pig. Life Sci 19:1117–1128

Schulz R, Wüster M, Herz A (1980) Pharmacological characterization of the epsilon sopiate receptor. J Pharmacol Exp Ther 216:604–606

Sharma SK, Klee WA, Nirenberg M (1975) Dual regulation of adenylate cycclase accounts for narcotic dependence and tolerance. Proc Natl Acad Sci USA 72:3092–3096

Sharma SK, Klee WA, Nirenberg M (1977) Opiate-dependent modulation of adenylate cyclase. Proc Natl Acad Sci USA 74:3365–3369

Shen K-F, Crain SM (1989) Dual opioid modulation of the action potential duration of mouse dorsal root ganglion neurons in culture. Brain Res 491:227–242

Shen K-F, Crain SM (1990a) Cholera toxin-A subunit blocks opioid excitatory effects on sensory neuron action potentials indicating mediation by G_s-linked opioid receptors. Brain Res 525:225–231

Shen K-F, Crain SM (1990b) Cholera toxin-B subunit blocks opioid excitatory effects on sensory neuron action potentials indicating that GM1 ganglioside may regulate G_s-linked opioid receptor functions. Brain Res 531:1–7

Simon EJ, Hiller JM, Edelman I (1973) Stereospecific binding of the potent narcotic analgesic [^{3}H]etorphine to rat brain homogenate. Proc Natl Acad Si USA 70:1947–1949

Smith JAM, Hunter JC, Hill RG, Hughes J (1989) A kinetic analysis of κ-opioid agonist binding using the selective radioligand [^{3}H]U69593. J Neurochem 53: 27–36

Spain JW, Coscia CJ (1987) Multiple interconvertible affinity states for the δ opioid agonist receptor complex. J Biol Chem 262:8948–8951

Steece KA, DeLeon-Jones FA, Meyerson LR, Lee JM, Fields JZ, Ritzman RF (1986) In vivo down-regulation of rat striatal opioid receptors by chronic enkephalin. Brain Res Bull 17:255–257

Sullivan KA, Miller RT, Masters SB, Beidermann B, Heidman W, Bourne HR (1987) Identification of receptor contact site involved in receptor-G protein coupling. Nature 330:758–762

Tao P-L, Chang L-R, Law PY, Loh HH (1988) Decrease in δ-receptor density in rat brain after chronic [D-Ala^2, D-Leu^5]enkephalin treatment. Brain Res 462: 313–320

Tao P-L, Lee H-Y, Chang L-R, Loh HH (1990) Decrease in μ-opioid receptor binding capacity in rat brain after chronic PL017 treatment. Brain Res 526: 270–275

Tempel A, Crain SM, Peterson ER, Simon EJ, Zukin RS (1986) Antagonist-induced opiate receptor upregulation in cultures of fetal mouse spinal cord-ganglion explants. Dev Brain Res 25:287–291

Tempel A, Habas JE, Paredes W, Barr GA (1988) Morphine-induced down-regulation of μ-opioid receptors in neonatal rat brain. Dev Brain Res 41: 129–133

Terwilliger R, Beitner-Johnson D, Sevarino KA, Crain SM, Nestler EJ (1991) A general model for adaptations in G proteins and the cyclic AMP system in mediating the chronic actions of morphine and cocaine on neuronal function. Brain Res 548:100–110

Thomas JM, Vagelos R, Hoffman BB (1990) Decreased cyclic AMP degradation in NG 108-15 neuroblastoma X glioma hybrid cells and S49 lymphoma cells chronically treated with drugs that inhibit adenylate cyclase. J Neurochem 54: 402–410

Tiberi M, Magnan J (1990) Quantitative analysis of multiple κ-opioid receptors by selective and non-selective ligand binding in guinea pig spinal cord: resolution of high and low affinity states of the κ$_2$ receptors by a computerized model-fitting technique. Mol Pharmacol 37:694–703

Tucker JF (1984) Effects of pertussis toxin on normorphine dependence and on acute inhibitory effects of normorphine and clonidine in guinea pig isolated ileum. Br J Pharmacol 83:326–328

Tung C-S, Grenhoff J, Svennson TH (1990) Morphine withdrawal responses of rat locus coeruleus neurons are blocked by an excitatory amino acid antagonist. Acta Physiol Scand 138:581–582

Ueda H, Misawa H, Fukushima N, Takagi H (1987) The specific opioid κ-agonist U50488H inhibits low K_m GTPase. Eur J Pharmacol 138:129–132

Ueda H, Harada H, Nozaki M, Katada T, Ui M, Satoh M, Takagi H (1988) Reconstitution of rat brain μ opioid receptors with purified guanine nucleotide-binding regulatory proteins. G$_i$ and G$_o$. Proc Natl Acad Sci USA 85:7013–7017

Ueda H, Misawa H, Katada T, Ui M, Takagi H, Satoh M (1990a) Functional reconstitution of purified G$_i$ and G$_o$ with μ-opioid receptors in guinea pig striatal membranes pretreated with micromolar concentrations of N-ethylmaleimide. J Neurochem 54:841–848

Ueda H, Uno S, Harada J, Kobayashi I, Katada T, Ui M, Satoh M (1990b) Evidence for receptor-mediated inhibition of intrinsic activity of GTP-binding protein, G_i1 and G_i2, but not G_o in reconstitution experiments FEBS Lett 266:178–182

Vachon L, Costa T, Herz A (1986) Differential sensitivity of basal and opioid-stimulated low K_m GTPase to guanine nucleotide analogs. J Neurochem 47: 1361–1369

Vachon L, Costa T, Herz A (1987) GTPase and adenylate cyclase desensitize at different rates in NG 108-15 cells. Mol Pharmacol 31:159–168

Vogel Z, Barg J, Attali B, Simantov R (1990) Differential effect of μ, δ, and κ ligands on G protein α subunits in cultured brain cells. J Neurosci Res 27:106–111

Wang H-Y, Berrios M, Malbon CC (1989) Localization of β-adrenergic receptors in A431 cells in situ: effect of chronic exposure to agonist. Biochem J 263:533–538

Werling LL, Brown SR, Cox BM (1984) The sensitivity of opioid receptor types to regulation by sodium and GTP. Neuropeptides 5:137–140

Werling LL, Brown SR, Puttfarcken P, Cox BM (1986) Sodium regulation of agonist binding at opioid receptors. II. Effects of sodium replacement on opioid binding in guinea pig cortical membranes. Mol Pharmacol 30:90–95

Werling LL, McMahon PN, Cox BM (1988a) Selective tolerance at mu and kappa opioid receptors modulating norepinephrine release in guinea pig cortex. J Pharmacol Exp Ther 247:1103–1106

Werling LL, Puttfarcken PS, Cox BM (1988b) Multiple agonist-affinity states of opioid receptors: regulation of binding by guanyl nucleotides in guinea pig cortical, NG 108-15, and 7315c cell membranes. Mol Pharmacol 33:423–431

Werling LL, McMahon PN, Cox BM (1989a) Effects of pertussis toxin on opioid regulation of catecholamine release from rat and guinea pig brain slices. Naunyn Schmiedebergs Arch Pharmacol 339:509–513

Werling LL, McMahon PN, Cox BM (1989b) Selective changes in μ opioid receptor properties induced by chronic morphine exposure. Proc Natl Acad Sci USA 86:6393–6397

Williams JT, North RA (1984) Opiate-receptor interactions on single locus coeruleus neurones. Mol Pharmacol 26:489–497

Wong YH, Demohou-Mason CD, Hanley MR, Barnard EA (1990) Agonist-selective protection of the opioid receptor-coupled G proteins from inactivation by 5'-p-fluorosulphonylbenzoyl guanosine. J Neurochem 54:39–45

Wüster M, Costa T (1984) The opioid-induced desensitization (tolerance) in neuroblastoma X glioma NG 108-15 hybrid cells: results from receptor uncoupling. NIDA Res Monogr 54:136–145

Wüster M, Costa T, Gramsch C (1983) Uncoupling of receptors is essential for opiate-induced desensitization (tolerance) in neuroblastoma X glioma hybrid cells NG 108-15. Life Sci 33 [Suppl 1]:341–344

Wüster M, Costa T, Aktories K, Jacobs KH (1984) Sodium regulation of opioid agonist binding is potentiated by pertussis toxin. Biochem Biophys Res Commun 123:1107–1115

Zazac J-M, Roques B (1985) Differences in binding properties of μ and δ opioid receptor subtypes from rat brain: kinetic analysis and effects of ions and nucleotides. J Neurochem 44:1605–1614

Zukin RS, Gintzler AR (1980) Guanyl nucleotide interactions with opiate receptors in guinea pig brain and ileum. Brain Res 186:486–491

Zukin RS, Sugarman JR, Fitz-Syage ML, Gardner EL, Zukin SR, Gintzler AR (1982) Naltrexone-induced opiate-receptor supersensitivity. Brain Res 25:287–291

Zukin RS, Eghbali M, Olive D, Unterwald EM, Tempel A (1988) Characterization and visualization of rat and guinea pig brain κ opioid receptors: evidence for $κ_1$ and $κ_2$ opioid receptors. Proc Natl Acad Sci USA 85:4061–4065

CHAPTER 9
Opioid Receptor-Coupled Second Messenger Systems

S.R. CHILDERS

A. Introduction

Most neurotransmitter and hormone receptors can be grouped into a series of receptor "superfamilies." Receptors in each of these groups share a number of common properties, including general protein subunit structure, primary sequence homologies, and general gene structure and regulation. Receptors within each of these groups also share common effector systems and, in many cases, the effector systems themselves actually define the individual receptor superfamilies. Most neurotransmitters belong to two major receptor groups: the oligomeric receptor-ion channel complexes, and the G-protein-linked receptors. For neurotransmitters like GABA (acting at $GABA_A$ receptors) and acetylcholine (acting at nicotinic sites), receptors are large multisubunit structures which complex together to form ion channels integrated with the receptor-binding sites. For dopamine, norepinephrine, acetylcholine (acting at muscarinic receptors), and many neuropeptides, receptors are coupled to specific G proteins which activate a series of effector systems, several of which are associated with diffusible second messenger systems.

All known opioid receptors are coupled to G proteins, with the possible exception of the OBCAM molecule purified by Loh and colleagues (SCHOFIELD et al. 1989), whose exact relationship to G-protein-coupled opioid receptors is not yet clear. G-protein-coupled opioid receptors should exhibit many of the same properties which have already been characterized for other neurotransmitter receptors in this class. In addition to the structural features which such receptors should possess, they should also be coupled to one or more of a defined set of effector systems. At this time, the effector systems associated with G proteins include:

1. Stimulation of adenylyl cyclase (e.g., β-adrenergic receptors)
2. Inhibition of adenylyl cyclase (e.g., α_2-adrenergic receptors)
3. Stimulation of phosphoinositol turnover (e.g., muscarinic M_1-receptors)
4. Direct G protein coupling to potassium channels (e.g., muscarinic M_2-receptors)
5. Direct G protein coupling to close calcium channels (e.g., k-opioid receptors)

Table 1. Effector systems coupled through G proteins to opioid receptors

Effector	G protein	Receptor type	Tissue	Reference
Inhibit adenylyl cyclase	Gi/o	μ	SK-N-SH cells	Yu and Sadee 1986
		δ	NG 108–15 cells	Sharma et al. 1975a
		κ	Guinea pig cerebellum	Konkoy and Childers 1989
Stmulate adenylyl cyclase	Gs?	Unknown	Spinal cord explants	Makman et al. 1988
Increase potassium conductance	Gi/o	μ, δ	Locus ceruleus	North et al. 1987
Decrease calcium conductance	Gi/o	κ	Spinal cord cultures	Gross et al. 1990
	Go	δ	NG 108–15 cells	Hescheler et al. 1987
Stimulate phosphoinositol turnover (?)	Gp?	κ	Rat hippocampus	Periyasamy and Hoss 1990

Entries in the table represent typical examples and are not meant to describe all known occurrences of these actions of opioid receptors.

6. Direct G protein coupling to open calcium channels (e.g., β-adrenergic receptors)

With varying degrees of success, opioid receptors have been associated with most of the above effector systems (Table 1). The only known exception at this time is the β-adrenergic-like action of opening calcium channels directly through G protein coupling. The best-known opioid effector system is opioid-inhibited adenylyl cyclase, and this review will concentrate mostly on this activity. However, it will also briefly review opioid effects on phosphoinositol turnover and on stimulation of adenylyl cyclase where significant effects have been obtained. The GTP-dependent effects of opioids on calcium and potassium channel function represent other significant actions of opioids, but these effects will be reviewed in another chapter. Also, direct actions of opioids on G protein function will be discussed in Chap. 8.

Several earlier reviews have also discussed the relationship between opioids and cyclic nucleotides (Wolleman 1981; Childers 1988b; Marckel and Childers 1989). For a more complete description of receptors and G protein structure and functions, a number of general reviews on G protein structure and function are recommended (Rodbell 1980; Schramm and Selinger 1984; Gilman 1984; Bourne 1988; Neer and Clapham 1988; Birnbaumer et al. 1990).

B. G Protein Coupling to Receptors

I. General G Protein Structure and Function

The detailed evidence which demonstrates that opioid receptors are coupled to G proteins is provided elsewhere in this book (Chap. 7). However, a brief

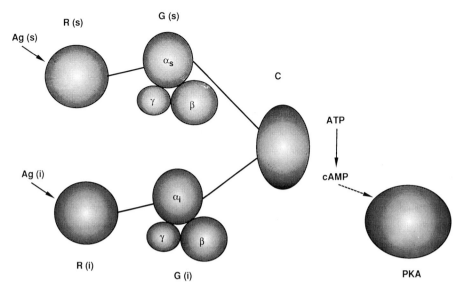

Fig. 1. Interactions between stimulatory receptors (*Rs*) and inhibitory receptors (*Ri*), G proteins, adenylyl cyclase, and protein phosphorylation. Agonist binding (*Ags* and *Agi*) to the high-affinity states of their respective receptors increases binding of GTP to the α-subunits of either G_s or G_i. The presence of GTP causes dissociation of the G protein subunits, which produces low-affinity states for agonist binding at the receptors, and either stimulation or inhibiton of the adenylyl cyclase catalytic unit (*C*). The final output of the system will be modulation of cyclic AMP-dependent protein kinase (*PKA*), thus increasing or decreasing phosphorylation of specific proteins

summary of G protein structure and function, together with their association with opioid receptors, is presented below.

The prototypical effector system mediated by G-protein-linked receptors is adenylyl cyclase. Receptor-mediated stimulation or inhibition of adenylyl cyclase requires the presence of guanine nucleotides, specifically GTP. Nonhydrolyzable GTP analogs (such as Gpp(NH)p and GTPγS) do not support agonist-induced inhibition of adenylyl cyclase in brain. In addition to supporting receptor-mediated adenylyl cyclase activity, GTP (and its nonhydrolyzable analogs) also directly affect receptor function by increasing agonist dissociation rates and thus decreasing agonist affinity. This effect of guanine nucleotides is apparent only with the binding of agonists, since GTP does not affect antagonist binding. Therefore, the receptor exists in two different affinity states for agonists depending on the presence of guanine nucleotides, while antagonists bind with a single high affinity to both states (KENT et al. 1980). These effects are unifying actions that occur with all G-protein-coupled receptors.

Figure 1 shows the general scheme for interactions of receptors with G proteins to regulate the activity of adenylyl cyclase. This model has become the basis for understanding interactions between receptors and other effector systems as well. The basis of this model is the ternary complex (De Lean et al. 1980): the interaction between three different membrane proteins (the receptor, the G protein, and the effector protein) to provide the complete receptor-effector system. Unlike the oligomeric receptor ion channel complex, where subunits complex together to form an integrated ion channel effector, this complex is transient, and is partially controlled by diffusion of these proteins through the lipid bilayer of the plasma membrane. The nature of the effector is provided by the identity of the G protein. The stimulatory guanine nucleotide regulatory protein G_s mediates receptor-stimulated adenylyl cyclase, while the inhibitory guanine nucleotide regulatory protein G_i mediates receptor inhibition of activity. Both proteins are heterotrimers of subunit composition α, β, and γ. Although α_s and α_i are different proteins, they exhibit considerable similarities. Both subunits bind and hydrolyze GTP (Cassel and Selinger 1976; Sunyer et al. 1984; Milligan and Klee 1985) and have considerable parallels in primary structure (Manning and Gilman 1983). The α-subunits contain several highly conserved regions which contain the GTP-binding site (Itoh et al. 1986), while other regions, containing much of the variability between subtypes, may be responsible for selectivity of coupling with effector systems or with receptors. The molecular mechanism of G protein activation and inhibition of adenylyl cyclase has been the subject of much investigation, leading to several different models. However, details of these models are beyond the scope of this review, and are covered in more detail elsewhere (Gilman 1984; Neer and Clapham 1988; Birnbaumer et al. 1990; Cerione et al. 1984, 1986b; Katada et al. 1986).

Other GTP-binding proteins exhibit striking parallels to α_s and α_i. One is the α-subunit of G_o (Sternweis and Robishaw 1984; Neer et al. 1984), whose amino acid sequence is highly homologous with both α_i and α_s (Tsai et al. 1987). While the function of G_o is not yet clear, muscarinic (Florio and Sternweis 1985) and α_2-adrenergic receptors (Cerione et al. 1986a) have been reconstituted with α_o. G_o may couple opioid receptors and a G-protein-linked Ca^{2+} channel in NG108-15 cells (Hescheler et al. 1987). Multiple gene products exist for both α_s and α_i, as well as β-subunits (Amatruda et al. 1988); recent evidence suggests that different receptor types are coupled to different subtypes of α-subunits (Kobilka et al. 1988) and β-subunits (Cerione et al. 1987). Thus, the identification of the precise G protein subtype coupled to different receptors is important in characterizing the receptor-second messenger system. Indeed, recent studies suggest that δ-opioid receptors may be coupled to G_{i1} in NG108-15 cells (McKenzie and Milligan 1990) while κ-receptors in the guinea pig cerebellum are coupled to G_{i1} and G_{i2} but not G_o (Ueda et al. 1990b).

Cholera toxin and pertussis toxin (islet-activating protein) interact with specific α-subunits, by catalyzing ADP ribosylation of the proteins. Paradoxically, the functional consequences of toxin reactions with both G_s

and G_i proteins lead to the same result: an increase in adenylyl cyclase activity and an increase in intracellular cyclic AMP. Cholera toxin-mediated ribosylation blocks the α_s-GTPase responsible for inactivation of adenylyl cyclase (CASSEL and SELINGER 1976; NORTHUP et al. 1983), thus irreversibly stimulating the enzyme. On the other hand, pertussis toxin inactivates the inhibitory function of the α_i-subunit, thus stimulating adenylyl cyclase by removing the inhibitory component of the cycle (KATADA and UI 1982).

The identification of several homologous gene products among a class of GTP-binding proteins implies that several second messenger systems are coupled to receptors via G proteins. One example is transducin in the retinal rod outer segment, where the second messenger system is cyclic GMP phosphodiesterase. In mast cells, pertussis toxin blocked receptor-mediated stimulation of phospholipase A_2 and arachidonic acid release (NAKAMURA and UI 1985). In other cells, receptor-mediated changes in phosphoinositide turnover (NISHIZUKA 1984) have been associated with G-protein-coupling mechanisms. The precise G proteins responsible for mediating phosphoinositol turnover have not yet been identified, but for the time being are named G_p. However, in most systems, G-protein-mediated phosphoinositol turnover is not sensitive to pertussis toxin (BIRNBAUMER et al. 1990).

Receptor-coupled ion channels are other G-protein-linked systems. Well-known examples include the muscarinic receptor coupled via G proteins to K^+ channels in the heart (BREIWEISER and SZABO 1985; PFAFFINGER et al. 1985; CODINA et al. 1987) and β-adrenergic receptors coupled to Ca^{2+} channels in the heart (YATANI et al. 1987; MATTERA et al. 1989). In these systems, receptor function is mediated by direct coupling of receptors to ion channels through the relevant G proteins, without the intervention of diffusible second messenger systems (BIRNBAUMER et al. 1990).

II. Opioid Receptors Are Coupled to G Proteins

Two pieces of evidence indicate that opioid receptors are directly coupled to G proteins. First, guanine nucleotides regulate opioid receptor binding by decreasing binding of agonists (BLUME 1978a,b; CHILDERS and SNYDER 1979, 1980). When guanine nucleotide effects on binding are studied in the presence of sodium (which is also required for agonist inhibition of adenylyl cyclase), guanine nucleotides have no effect on opioid antagonist binding (CHILDERS and SNYDER 1980). These effects of guanine nucleotides have been observed for μ- (CHILDERS and SNYDER 1980), δ- (BLUME 1987a; CHANG et al. 1981; PFEIFFER et al. 1982; ZAJAC and ROQUES 1985), and κ- (MACK et al. 1985; FRANCIS et al. 1985) receptors. μ_1-receptors, the receptor type described by Pasternak and colleagues to be the common high-affinity binding sites for a number of opioids (WOLOZIN and PASTERNAK 1981), are also regulated by guanine nucleotides (CHILDERS and PASTERNAK 1982; CLARK et al. 1988). Two recent studies reported guanine nucleotide inhibition of σ-receptor binding (Itzhak 1989; Beart et al. 1989), but this finding is controversial at the present time, and σ-receptors are not normally considered as true opioid receptor types. The guanine nucleotide regulation of opioid receptor binding is typical of other members of the G-protein-linked receptor superfamily, including effects on binding kinetics, guanine nucleotide specificity, and additivity with sodium.

The second indication that opioid receptors are coupled to G proteins is the finding that opioid agonists stimulate GTPase activity in cells and membranes which contain opioid receptors (Koski and Klee 1981). Again, this activity has been associated with μ- (Yu and Sadee 1986), δ- (Koski and Klee 1981), and κ- (Clark and Medeihradsky 1987; Clark et al. 1986) receptor types and is typical of G-protein-coupled receptors. The final test of G protein coupling to opioid receptors is the purification of the separate components of this signal transduction system and their functional reconstitution. Several reports (Ueda et al. 1990a,b) have indicated that such reconstitution experiments have been successful with purified opioid receptors and G proteins. Details of all of these G-protein-associated functions are discussed in Chap. 7.

Coupling of opioid receptors to G proteins may have some properties which are different from other G-protein-coupled receptors. One case in point is the recent finding of "negative intrinsic activity" in NG108-15 cells (Costa and Herz 1989; Costa et al. 1990). These studies showed that some classes of δ-receptor antagonists behaved differently from normal competitive antagonists. Instead of producing no change in GTPase activity in NG108-15 cells, these antagonists inhibited GTPase in the same preparations where opioid agonists stimulated GTPase. These data suggest that some antagonists may have negative intrinsic activity when binding to G proteins. It will be interesting to see whether this phenomenon is peculiar to the δ-receptor system or whether it will become a novel mechanism for a variety of different receptors.

C. Opioid-Inhibited Adenylyl Cyclase

Experiments which characterize the opioid-regulated GTPase activities and guanine nucleotide regulation of opioid receptor binding have provided a great deal of information about the interactions between opioid receptors and G proteins. Unfortunately, they provide no information about the effector systems to which these receptor-G-protein complexes are coupled. Of all of the effector systems which have been implicated with opioid receptors (see Table 1), the best studied is opioid inhibition of adenylyl cyclase in transformed cell lines and in brain membranes.

I. Acute Effects of Opioid Agonists on Adenylyl Cyclase in Transformed Cell Lines

The discovery of opioid receptors on transformed cell types has been a tremendous boost to the analysis of opioid receptor-coupled effector systems. These cells are derived from neural tissue, represent relatively homogeneous cell populations and, unlike neurons from nontransformed tissue, undergo regular cell division. NG108-15 cells, which contain high levels of opioid receptor binding sites (HAMPRECHT 1977), have been an excellent model system to study mechanisms of receptor coupling to adenylyl cyclase (TRABER et al. 1975; SHARMA et al. 1957a, 1977). The pharmacological characteristics of these opioid sites correspond to δ-receptors (CHANG et al. 1981). Other transformed cell types, including N4TG1, N1E-115, and N18TG2 cells, also contain δ-receptors and δ-inhibited adenylyl cyclase (GILBERT and RICHELSON 1983). In all of these cell lines, opioid inhibition of adenylyl cyclase occurred not only for PGE_1-stimulated activity but also for basal, adenosine-stimulated and cholera toxin-stimulated adenylyl cyclase (PROPST and HAMPRECHT 1981). Like other inhibitory receptor systems, opioid inhibition of adenylyl cyclase required both sodium and GTP (BLUME et al. 1979). Also, incubation of NG108-15 cells with pertussis toxin abolished opioid inhibition of adenylyl cyclase (HSIA et al. 1984), suggesting that G_i (or G_o) proteins were required for inhibitory activity.

Because of their homogeneous cell populations, clonal cell lines were useful to study the relationship between receptor occupancy and efficacy of opioid inhibition of adenylyl cyclase. In one study (FANTOZZI et al. 1981), this relationship was explored by blocking receptor binding sites with the irreversible antagonist β-chlornaltrexamine (β-CNA). Blockade of 95% of opioid receptor binding sites did not alter the inhibition of adenylyl cyclase by opioid agonists, suggesting the presence of a large population of spare receptors in the NG108-15 cells. In detailed receptor binding studies by LAW et al. (1985b), sodium and GTP produced three distinct agonist binding states of opioid receptors in NG108-15 cells whose agonist association rates were functions of receptor occupancy. Other studies (COSTA et al. 1985; OTT et al. 1989) demonstrated several agonist affinity states in NG108-15 cell membranes, and showed that the sites coupled to adenylyl cyclase did not correspond to the high-affinity δ-sites identified in binding studies. These studies point to the complicated relationship which must occur between receptor-binding sites and second messenger systems, even in a simplified cell system like NG108-15 cells.

Other transformed cell types contain different opioid receptor types. YU et al. (1986, 1990) located a human neuroblastoma cell line, SH-SY5Y, with both μ- and δ-receptor binding sites. FREY and KEBABIAN (1984) identified μ-receptors in the pituitary tumor 7315c. In both cell types, opioid agonists inhibited adenylyl cyclase, with morphine and other μ-agonists being more potent than enkephalin and other δ-analogs. These results suggested that μ-receptors as well as δ-receptors were negatively coupled to adenylyl cyclase in transformed cells.

II. Acute Effects of Opioid Agonists on Adenylyl Cyclase in Brain

Although much of the early progress in understanding this second messenger system came from transformed cell lines such as NG108-15 cells, the first reports of opioid-inhibited adenylyl cyclase were from brain membranes (CHOU et al. 1971; COLLIER and ROY 1974). The study from Collier's laboratory can be considered as the breakthrough report in this field, since it was the first to demonstrate that a second messenger system effect was mediated by true opioid receptor actions. These experiments showed that morphine inhibited PGE_1-stimulated adenylyl cyclase from rat striatal membranes, and that this action of the opioid agonist was blocked by naloxone. Although this finding made an immediate impact, at the time it was considered relatively controversial because other early studies in brain membranes provided contradictory evidence. While some groups were able to reproduce the finding (MINNEMAN and IVERSEN 1976; HAVEMANN and KUSCHINSKY 1978; TSANG et al. 1978), other groups found no effects of opioid agonists on brain adenylyl cyclase activity (WILKENING et al. 1976; TELL et al. 1975; VAN INVEGEN et al. 1975). This controversy was probably due to at least two reasons. First, opioid-inhibited adenylyl cyclase in brain membranes represented an extremely low signal due to the heterogeneous nature of brain and the well-known finding that coupling between receptors and second messenger systems is disrupted by cell lysis and homogenization. Second, the requirement for guanine nucleotides in receptor-mediated adenylyl cyclase activities was not yet clear. More reproducible results were obtained with the realization that GTP was required for receptor-adenylyl cyclase coupling. LAW et al. (1981) and COOPER et al. (1982) showed that opioid-inhibited activity in brain was GTP dependent. Although some disagreement on sodium dependence of opioid inhibition was reported, careful removal of sodium from all components of the assay revealed that opioid-inhibited adenylyl cyclase was sodium dependent in brain (KONKOY and CHILDERS 1989). The pharmacological properties of opioid-inhibited adenylyl cyclase in brain were similar to a δ-receptor response, since opioid peptides were more potent than opioid alkaloids. However, this activity remained difficult to quantitate since the actual level of inhibition by opioid agonists was small, averaging around 20%.

Recognizing that opioid effects on adenylyl cyclase activity were small even under ideal conditions, other studies focused on techniques which selectively altered the function of G proteins. In one such technique, brain membranes were preincubated at pH 4.5 before assay at physiological pH (CHILDERS and JACKSON 1984). Low pH pretreatment increased guanine nucleotide regulation of agonist binding but had no effect on agonist binding in the absence of guanine nucleotides (LAMBERT and CHILDERS 1984). These results suggested that low pH pretreatment of brain membranes altered the interaction of G proteins with receptors. Other experiments (CHILDERS et al. 1983; CHILDERS and LARIVIERE 1984) showed that low pH pretreatment blocked G_s-stimulated adenylyl cyclase with no effect on basal enzyme activity. As G_s-stimulated activity was decreased by low pH pretreatment, opioid-inhibited activity was increased. These results suggested that there was an inverse correlation between G_s-stimulated and G_i-inhibited adenylyl cyclase in brain membranes (RASENICK and CHILDERS 1989), and that significant opioid receptor-inhibited activity in brain membranes was masked when a large amount of G_s-stimulated activity was present. Low pH treatment also showed that the two actions of GTP on the opioid receptor system (regulation of agonist binding and support of agonist-inhibited adenylyl cyclase) were independent from each other (CHILDERS and LARIVIERE 1984).

The mechanism of the low pH pretreatment has now been explored in brain membranes (RASENICK and CHILDERS 1989). Stimulation of adenylyl cyclase in brain membranes requires exchange of guanine nucleotides from the α-subunit of G_i to the α-subunit of G_s (HATTA et al. 1986). In low pH pretreated brain membranes, this exchange does not occur, thus eliminating the ability of G_s to stimulate adenylyl cyclase. Interestingly, binding of guanine nucleotides to G_i is unaffected by low pH pretreatment, so that receptor inhibition of activity has not been attenuated. The mechanism by which low pH pretreatment eliminated the ability of GTP to exchange between G_i and G_s is not known, but it is known that the effects of low pH pretreatment are reversed by addition of phospholipids to membranes (CHILDERS and LARIVIERE 1984), indicating that the principal effect may be due to alterations of membrane structure.

The properties of opioid-inhibited adenylyl cyclase in brain have now been examined in low pH pretreated membranes (CHILDERS 1988a). Like all other receptor-inhibited activities, this reaction required guanine nucleotides and sodium. Opioid inhibition of adenylyl cyclase was noncompetitive, decreasing V_{max} of the enzyme without affecting K_m of the enzyme for ATP. Regional distribution showed that opioid inhibition occurred primarily in striatum, frontal cortex, and amygdala, with small inhibition in other regions. This distribution was similar, but not identical, to that of classical δ-receptor binding sites. The pharmacological profile of opioid-inhibited adenylyl cyclase in striatum did not follow any known receptor binding site. For example, the agonist profile resembled δ-receptors, with enkephalin and enkephalin analogs more potent than μ-agonists, but other opioid peptides such as β-endorphin and dynorphin were equipotent to enkephalin. These data suggested that multiple opioid receptors might be coupled to adenylyl cyclase in brain. Detailed studies in rat thalamus (S. CHILDERS, manuscript submitted) have revealed the presence of μ-inhibited activity, since inhibition by DAGO was highest in that region, and since inhibition by DAGO and DPDPE were partially additive. Also, the μ-antagonist naloxone was more potent in blocking DAGO inhibition than DPDPE inhibition.

μ-Inhibited adenylyl cyclase has also been identified in the rabbit cerebellum (POLASTRON et al. 1990b), in primary cultures of rat striatal neurons (VAN VLIET et al. 1990), and in the rat periaqueductal gray (FEDYNSHYN and LEE 1989). In rat locus ceruleus, BEITNER et al. (1989) reported that morphine produced a small inhibition of adenylyl cyclase activity which remained after washing.

The evidence that κ-receptors are also coupled to adenylyl cyclase may be somewhat controversial. One recent study (POLASTRON et al. 1990a) identified μ-inhibited adenylyl cyclase in rabbit cerebellum, but failed to identify any effect of κ-agonists on adenylyl cyclase in the guinea pig cerebellum, a tissue which contains 85% κ-receptor binding sites. Other studies in frog brain (MAKIMURA and MURAKOSHI 1989) also failed to identify any κ effects on adenylyl cyclase. However, another report demonstrated κ-inhibited adenylyl cyclase in membranes from rat spinal cord neurons (ATTALI et al. 1989a). In other studies using guinea pig cerebellar membranes (KONKOY and CHILDERS 1989), various dynorphin analogs were potent in inhibiting adenylyl cyclase, while μ- and δ-agonists had no effect. The κ nature of the dynorphin effect was confirmed by the finding that selective κ-agonists like U-50488H were also potent in inhibiting adenylyl cyclase, and by the finding that the selective κ-antagonist nor-binaltorphimine was 20 times more potent than naloxone in blocking the agonist inhibition. Further experiments (C. KONKOY and S. CHILDERS, manuscript in preparation) showed that the κ-inhibited activity in this tissue was highly localized to cerebellar granule cells, similar to adenosine A_1- and $GABA_B$-inhibited adenylyl cyclase (WOJCIK et al. 1985).

III. Chronic Effects of Opioid Agonists

The effects of chronic opioid agonist treatment on opioid-inhibited adenylyl cyclase represents one of the best-known models for a biochemical analogy to opioid tolerance. As discussed below, the response of opioid receptor coupled adenylyl cyclase to chronic agonist treatment varies between different tissues. However, a common finding is that the adenylyl cyclase system acts to compensate for the acute effect of opioid agonist inhibition by increasing basal adenylyl cyclase activity. In many systems, opioid-inhibited adenylyl cyclase continues to function under these conditions; however, the effect of opioid inhibition is blunted because of the general increase in adenylyl cyclase activity. This phenomenon is summarized in Fig. 2, which compares hypothetical opioid agonist inhibition in control and chronic agonist-treated systems. The increase in basal activity shifts the agonist dose-response curve upwards. Thus, although opioid inhibition is still observed in the treated system, the effect of the agonist is diminished; in the example in Fig. 2, the maximum inhibition produced in the treated system only brings adenylyl cyclase activity back to the original control basal activity. This is not the classical rightward shift in dose response curves

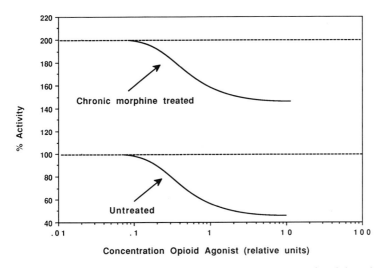

Fig. 2. Effect of chronic opioid agonist treatment on adenylyl cyclase activity to produce "upwards" shift in agonist dose-response curves (hypothetical data derived from studies in NG108-15 cells [SHARMA et al. 1975b] and brain membranes [DUMAN et al. 1988; L. FLEMING and S. CHILDERS, submitted]). Opioid agonists inhibit activity in both control and treated systems. However, in the agonist-treated system, basal activity has been increased; therefore, the maximum effect of opioid inhibition reaches the same level as basal activity without agonist in the untreated system

which is observed in many desensitization studies, but still represents an attenuation of the cell response to opioids. As discussed below, this effect is observed for adenylyl cyclase in NG108-15 cells treated with morphine and in brain membranes from rats treated with morphine. Moreover, the same response occurs with opiate-inhibited protein phosphorylation (see Sect. D.IV below).

When NG108-15 cells were treated chronically with morphine, a biphasic response of adenylyl cyclase was observed. Initially, basal activity was decreased by acute opioid agonist treatment due to direct inhibition of the enzyme by agonist occupation of opioid receptors. After 12 h of exposure to morphine, cells showed a gradual increase of adenylyl cyclase activity to normal (nontreated) levels. When morphine was removed from chronically treated NG108-15 cells, or when naloxone was added, a rebound effect occurred, in which a large (but transient) increase in adenylyl cyclase was observed (SHARMA et al. 1975b, 1977). These effects on basal adenylyl cyclase have been used as a model system for tolerance and dependence, where the slow increase from inhibited levels of adenylyl cyclase activity represents the development of tolerance and the rebound actions of naloxone represent withdrawal (SHARMA et al. 1975b). However, chronic morphine treatment of NG108-15 cells did not produce significant downregulation of opioid receptors nor did it decrease opioid-inhibited adenylyl cyclase, although it did attenuate the stimulatory response of adenylyl cyclase to fluoride and Gpp(NH)p. It is important to note that chronic treatment of NG108-15 cells with muscarinic or α-adrenergic agonists (both of which inhibit adenylyl cyclase in these cells) produced the same response as that seen by chronic exposure of cells to morphine (GILBERT and RICHELSON 1983) except that downregulation of receptors occurred. Therefore, the gradual increase in adenylyl cyclase during chronic treatment with inhibitory agonists was a general homeostatic principle of these cells. Later experiments (GREENSPAN and MUSSACHIO 1984) demonstrated that the rebound effect of naloxone could only be observed if agnoist-treated cells were effectively washed before treatment with naloxone.

Since NG108-15 cells contain δ-, not μ-, receptors, chronic morphine treatment may not be the most appropriate test for desensitization of opioid receptor-coupled adenylyl cyclase. Other experiments have used different agonists in chronic treatment studies. LAW et al. (1982) showed that chronic treatment of NG108-15 cells with the nonselective opioid agonist etorphine produced significant downregulation (i.e., decreased B_{max}) of opioid receptor binding sites. Also, desensitization of adenylyl cyclase to opioid agonists (determined by loss of opioid-inhibited adenylyl cyclase) occurred in etorphine-treated cells. These two effects were later shown to be two separate processes (LAW et al. 1983a,b), with desensitization occurring first, followed by receptor downregulation. These processes were homologous responses to etorphine, since there was no change in muscarinic, α_2-adrenergic, and PGE_1 receptor binding and little change in their regulation of adenylyl cyclase. Desensitization to opioids also occurred in isolated NG108-15 cell membranes treated with etorphine (LOUIE et al. 1986). Other studies (COSTA et al. 1988; VACHON et al. 1986) showed that opioid-stimulated GTPase and opioid-inhibited adenylyl cyclase desensitized at different rates after exposure of NG108-15 cells to chronic agonist treatment. In 7315c tumor cells, which express a homogeneous μ-opioid receptor population, a similar downregulation and desensitization of μ-receptors and μ-inhibited adenylyl cyclase occurred (PUTTFARCKEN and COX 1989; PUTTFARCKEN et al. 1988).

Studies on opioid-inhibited adenylyl cyclase have also been conducted in brain membranes isolated from animals chronically treated with opioid agonists. Some studies (e.g., CHILDERS et al. 1986) have revealed no effect of chronic morphine treatment on opioid-inhibited adenylyl cyclase. However, in guinea pig, chronic morphine treatment eliminated guanine nucleotide regulation of binding to μ-receptors in brain membranes (WERLING et al. 1989a). TAO et al. (1987) showed that chronic treatment of rats with etorphine decreased both μ- and δ-opioid receptors in brain, while treatment with DADLE decreased δ-receptor binding (TAO et al. 1988). These effects occurred with a concomitant small increase in IC_{50} value of DADLE in inhibiting adenylyl cyclase. DUMAN et al. (1988) showed that chronic morphine treatment increased basal, GTP-, and forskolin-stimulated adenylyl cyclase specifically in locus ceruleus; however, the extent of DADLE-inhibited adenylyl cyclase was unchanged after chronic morphine treatment. These results agree with the general model shown in Fig. 2, where adenylyl cyclase activity has increased after chronic morphine treatment to compensate for acute opioid-inhibited adenylyl cyclase.

IV. Biological Roles for Opioid-Inhibited Adenylyl Cyclase

One of the final physiological endpoints for opioids is modulation of neuro-transmitter release (PATON 1957; COX and WEINSTOCK 1966; PASSARELLI and COSTA 1989), and a considerable effort has examined the relationship between opioid-inhibited adenylyl cyclase and opioid-inhibited neuro-transmitter release. Some studies (JOHNSON 1990) have shown that opioid effects on neurotransmitter release are not mediated through cyclic AMP. Other studies have revealed a more complex relationship. MULDER et al. (1984, 1990) found that μ-receptors inhibited norepinephrine release in brain slices. Since the inhibitory effects of the α_2-agonists but not morphine were blocked by 8-bromo-cyclic AMP, these results suggested that the μ-opioid effect, unlike α_2-adrenoceptor-inhibited NE release, was not mediated by inhibition of adenylyl cyclase (SCHOFFELMEER et al. 1986). In striatal slices, μ- and δ-, but not κ-, receptors, inhibited adenylyl cyclase which was stimulated by release of endogenous dopamine (HEIJNA et al. 1989). Other results (SCHOFFELMEER et al. 1988) demonstrated that μ- and δ-inhibited adenylyl cyclase in striatal slices shared a common site, since the antagonism of DAGO inhibition by naloxone (but not the DAGO inhibition itself) was blocked by the irreversible δ-antagonist FIT. These data provide functional support for the μ-/δ- complex model of ROTHMAN et al. (1988). Interestingly, the effects of μ- and δ-agonists, but not κ-agonists, on inhibition of norepinephrine release from brain slices were blocked by pertussis toxin (WERLING et al. 1989b), suggesting that κ-receptors may modulate neurotransmitter release by a different mechanism than μ- and δ-receptors.

Are any of the effects of opioids on ion channels mediated through adenylyl cyclase? Most of the electrophysiological evidence would suggest that cyclic AMP does not play a direct role in these opioid-mediated processes (DUGGAN and NORTH 1983; CHERUBINI and NORTH 1985; NORTH et al. 1987; TATSUMI et al. 1990; GROSS et al. 1990), and that opioid receptors couple to ion channels through direct G protein coupling. However, one possible exception to this general finding may be the spinal cord. Crain and colleagues (CHEN et al. 1988) showed that opioid effects on Ca^{2+} conductance in spinal cord explant cultures may be mediated by cyclic AMP-dependent protein kinase. ATTALI et al. (1989b) demonstrated that κ-agonists inhibited both adenylyl cyclase activity and Ca^{2+} influx in spinal cord-dorsal root ganglion cells. The finding that κ-agonists inhibited forskolin-stimulated Ca^{2+} influx suggested that at least a portion of these κ-actions may be mediated through inhibition of adenylyl cyclase.

Other studies have focused on long-term regulatory roles for opioid-inhibited adenylyl cyclase. One area of interest is the role of opioid-inhibited adenylyl cyclase in modulating neuropeptide synthesis. Several neuropeptide genes, including pro-enkephalin, contain cyclic AMP-responsive promoter elements (CRE). The function of these promoters is to increase mRNA synthesis when stimulated by cyclic AMP-dependent protein kinase (QUACH et al. 1984; COMB et al. 1986, 1988). It is conceivable that opioid-inhibited adenylyl cyclase may act as a negative feedback mechanism to attenuate cyclic AMP-stimulated pro-enkephalin mRNA synthesis. This model would suggest that opioid agonists decrease pro-enkephalin mRNA levels. Interestingly, in vivo administration of opioid agonists inhibited pro-enkephalin mRNA levels in striatum (UHL et al. 1988). Moreover, chronic treatment of rats with the opioid antagonist naltrexone, which increased opioid receptor binding sites and produced supersensitivity to morphine analgesia (TEMPEL et al. 1982, 1985; ZUKIN et al. 1982), stimulated pro-enkephalin mRNA levels (TEMPEL et al. 1990). Experiments in our laboratory (D. MARCKEL and S. CHILDERS, submitted for publication) tested this hypothesis directly in primary neuronal culture. This system was chosen because it contains measurable amounts of both opioid-inhibited adenylyl cyclase and pro-enkephalin mRNA. In these cells, both forskolin and dibutyryl cyclic AMP stimulated pro-enkephalin mRNA levels. Forskolin-stimulated pro-enkephalin mRNA was inhibited by opioid agonists. This opioid effect was blocked by pertussis toxin and by naloxone, indicating that it was mediated through a G-protein-coupled opioid receptor response. However, opioid agonists had no effect on stimulation of proenkephalin mRNA by dibutyryl cyclic AMP, which bypassed the normal receptor-adenylyl cyclase coupling step. Therefore, this action of opioids was probably mediated through receptor inhibition of adenylyl cyclase. These results suggest that opioid-inhibited adenylyl cyclase might play a role in the long-term regulation of neuropeptide levels through control of mRNA synthesis. A model for this function of opioid-inhibited adenylyl cyclase is shown in Fig. 3. In this model, agents which increase cyclic AMP levels increase pro-enkephalin mRNA synthesis by activation of the cyclic AMP responsive element (CRE) on the pro-enkephalin gene. An inhibitory agonist (either an exogenous opiate or an opioid peptide) binding to an opioid receptor would inhibit adenylyl cyclase, thus decreasing intracellular cyclic AMP levels and decreasing pro-enkephalin mRNA synthesis. For presynaptic opioid receptors, this system would represent a negative feedback loop, in which high concentrations of enkephalin released into the synaptic cleft would eventually attenuate its own synthesis by inhibition of adenylyl cyclase. This model also predicts that other receptors that inhibit adenylyl cyclase would also play the same role if present on an enkephalinergic neuron. The recent finding that D_2 dopamine receptors (which also inhibit adenylyl cyclase)

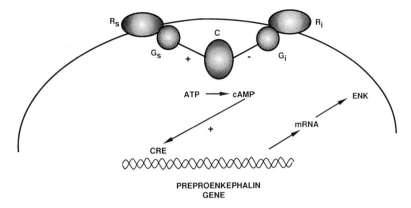

Fig. 3. Regulation of pro-enkephalin mRNA synthesis by opioid-inhibited adenylyl cyclase. Release of enkephalin (or exogenous opiates) bind to presynaptic receptors and inhibit adenylyl cyclase. Decreased intracellular cyclic AMP levels attenuate pro-enkephalin mRNA synthesis through inhibition at the cyclic AMP-responsive element (*CRE*)

are highly localized in striatal neurons that contain pro-enkephalin mRNA (LE MOINE et al. 1990) suggest that this relationship may be important in regulating neuropeptide levels.

D. Other Second Messenger Systems

I. Stimulation of Adenylyl Cyclase

Some evidence has accumulated for the existence of opioid-stimulated adenylyl cyclase. At least one early study (PURI et al. 1975) reported that morphine stimulated adenylyl cyclase in brain membranes. Indirect evidence was provided by Crain and colleagues (CHEN et al. 1988), who demonstrated that opioid agonists both stimulated and inhibited neuronal firing in spinal cord DRG cells. Since both of these electrophysiological effects appeared to be mediated through cyclic AMP, these studies suggested the existence of both opioid-stimulated and -inhibited adenylyl cyclase in these cells. MAKMAN et al. (1988) confirmed this suggestion by directly showing both types of opioid activities in these cells. However, the opioid stimulation of adenylyl cyclase was not fully characterized. Experiments in our laboratory (D. MARCKEL and S. CHILDERS, submitted for publication) have also shown opioid-stimulated adenylyl cyclase in C-6 gliomas cells. This activity was small in magnitude, however, and its significance is not yet clear.

II. Cyclic GMP

Opiate-induced increase of cyclic GMP levels in cells and brain slices was demonstrated soon after the discovery of opiate-inhibited adenylyl cyclase. There was a brief flurry of interest in coupling of opioid receptors to cyclic GMP metabolism, but this field has not advanced as far as the adenylyl cyclase field.

MINNEMAN and IVERSEN (1976) found that enkephalin increased intracellular cyclic GMP levels in rat striatal slices and that this stimulation was blocked by naloxone. This study, however, has not been followed by any detailed pharmacological studies. In 1977, Gullis showed an opiate-induced increase in cyclic GMP levels in NG108-15 cells. This finding later proved to be unreliable and was withdrawn (GULLIS 1977). Nevertheless, later studies showed opiate stimulatory effects on cyclic GMP levels in N4TG1 cells (GWYNN and COSTA 1982) and in various peripheral tissues in the C57BL mouse (MURAKI et al. 1984). Since guanylate cyclase is largely soluble, the molecular properties of receptor-coupled guanylate cyclase are less well characterized than those of adenylate cyclase, and direct coupling between receptors and guanylate cyclase has been difficult to establish. Therefore, experiments are conducted with whole cells, using radio-immunoassays to determine levels of cyclic GMP. The studies in N4TG1 cells used cyclic GMP phosphodiesterase inhibitors, thus eliminating the possibility that opiates increased cyclic GMP levels by inhibition of cyclic GMP phosphodiesterase. In N4TG1 cells, stimulation of cyclic GMP levels appeared to be mediated by a δ-receptor (GWYNN and COSTA 1982). Thus, occupation of δ-receptors in N4TG1 cells may simultaneously increase cyclic GMP levels while decreasing levels of cyclic AMP.

III. Phosphatidylinositol Turnover and Effects on Membrane Lipids

Receptor-mediated stimulation of phosphatidylinositol turnover is another second messenger system linked to several neurotransmitters. In this system, release of inositol-bisphosphate through a receptor-G-protein-linked phosphatidylinositol phosphodiesterase causes release of calcium from intracellular stores. Since changes in calcium flux have been associated with opioid receptor function, and since all opioid receptor types are coupled to G proteins (even in tissues where inhibition of adenylyl cyclase is very low), one potential opioid-coupled second messenger system is phosphatidylinositol turnover. However, in both NG108-15 and SK-N-SH cells, where phosphatidylinositol turnover systems were stimulated by bradykinin and acetylcholine, respectively, opioid agonists had no effect on phosphatidylinositol turnover (YU and SADEE 1986). In cultured bovine adrenal chromaffin cells, opioid agonists failed to produce any effect on either basal or stimulated total inositol accumulation (BUNN et al. 1988). More recent data (PERIYASAMY and HOSS 1990) have suggested that κ-agonists stimulate phosphoinositol turnover in rat hippocampal slices. However, these effects occurred at high concentrations of agonists (even higher than those required for opioid-inhibited adenylyl cyclase in brain membranes), and pharmacological experiments have not yet confirmed the κ-opioid selectivity of this response.

In phosphoinositol turnover reactions, receptor agonists presumably stimulate phospholipase C activity to begin the cascade which leads to phosphoinositol turnover. In an interesting variation upon this theme, recent studies (MISAWA et al. 1990) have shown that GTP stimulated phospholipase C activity in the guinea pig cerebellum. Moreover, a κ-agonist inhibited GTP-stimulated, but not basal, phospholipase C activity. If this effect is confirmed, it may suggest a novel second messenger system which would have an action opposite from the normal receptor-stimulated phosphoinositol turnover system. Unfortunately, blockade of this presumed κ-response with an antagonist was not reported, so that the opioid specificity of this response is not yet clear.

An important concept in second messenger research is communication between different second messenger systems. For example, stimulation of protein kinase C is known to phosphorylate and inactivate G_i (JAKOBS et al. 1985; KATADA et al. 1985). Similar results have been obtained in NG108-15 cells (LOUIE et al. 1990) and in brain membranes (S. CHILDERS, unpublished data), where treatment with phorbol esters to stimulate protein kinase C attenuated opioid-inhibited adenylyl cyclase. Cyclic AMP-dependent protein phosphorylation can also play a role in regulating opioid receptor function. In rat striatal membranes (HARADA et al. 1990), cyclic AMP-dependent protein kinase abolished the ability of G_i to reconstitute opioid-stimulated GTPase after pertussis toxin treatment.

Other studies have demonstrated the role of lipids and protein glycosylation in opiate receptor function. For example, incorporation of cerebroside sulfate increased the ability of enkephalin analogs to inhibit PGE-stimulated adenylate cyclase in N18TG2 cells, with no effect on receptor number or affinity (LAW et al. 1983b). Incubation of NG108-15 cells with tunicamycin, a protein glycosylation inhibitor, decreased receptor binding without affecting etorphine-inhibited adenylate cyclase (LAW et al. 1985a).

Other experiments demonstrated effects of opiates on membrane lipid composition. For example, in neuroblastoma cells, opiate agonists inhibited ganglioside synthesis (DAWSON et al. 1980). In these systems, 24-h incubation of cells with enkephalin analogs did not alter phospholipid content, but decreased total ganglioside content in a naloxone-reversible manner. Moreover, the opiate-induced decrease in gangliosides was reversed by addition of cyclic AMP, suggesting that these effects of opiates may be mediated through inhibition of adenylate cyclase, presumably through inhibition of cyclic AMP-induced phosphorylation of glycosyltransferases. However, these effects may be limited to certain cell lines, since other cell lines that contain δ-opiate receptors and opiate-inhibited adenylate cyclase did not possess this action on gangliosides (GILBERT and RICHELSON 1983).

IV. Opioid-Dependent Protein Phosphorylation

It is generally agreed that the immediate target of cyclic AMP actions in cells is cyclic AMP-dependent protein phosphorylation. Protein phosphorylation is a common reaction in brain membranes, with more than 70 protein substrates for phosphorylation reactions (NESTLER et al. 1984). Several reports have identified opioid-induced changes in protein phosphorylation in brain membranes. EHRLICH et al. (1978) showed that enkephalin inhibited phosphorylation of two brain membrane proteins of molecular weight 47 kDa and 10–20 kDa. WILLIAMS and CLOUET (1982) showed a biphasic response of brain membrane protein phosphorylation following acute administration of opioid agonists. Nestler's group (NESTLER and TALLMAN 1988; GUITART and NESTLER 1989) showed that chronic morphine administration increased cyclic AMP-dependent protein kinase activity in rat locus ceruleus but not in other regions. Interestingly, as discussed earlier, the same group demonstrated that chronic morphine increased adenylyl cyclase in the same region (DUMAN et al. 1988). It is interesting to speculate that all of these effects are related mechanisms which compensate for the acute inhibition of cyclic AMP by opioids. The finding that levels of G proteins are also regulated by chronic morphine treatment (NESTLER et al. 1989) provides evidence that the entire signal transduction machinery may be affected by opiate tolerance.

Experiments by our laboratory (L. FLEMING and S. CHILDERS, submitted) have identified phosphoproteins inhibited by opioid-inhibited adenylyl cyclase in rat striatal membranes. Membranes were preincubated with App(NH)p as a substrate for adenylyl cyclase. The cyclic AMP formed by this reaction stimulated protein phosphorylation through cyclic AMP-dependent protein kinase, and opioid-inhibited adenylyl cyclase produced a small but significant decrease in forskolin-stimulated phosphorylation. At least two bands (M_r 85 and 63 kDa) were identified in this fashion on SDS PAGE gels. Two-dimensional gel electrophoresis suggested that these bands were probably synapsin I and II. These proteins, therefore, are among candidates for the final targets of the biochemical actions of opioid-inhibited adenylyl cyclase. In further experiments, where rats were chronically treated for 2 days with morphine pellets, the phosphorylation of both of these proteins were significantly increased in membranes from thalamus, a region particularly high in μ-receptors. It is interesting to speculate that increase in phosphorylation of these proteins may be an early event occurring in the development of morphine tolerance. Moreover, the role of synapsin in regulation of neurotransmitter release provides a biological rationale for these effects. In the squid giant axon, stimulation of synapsin phosphorylation increased neurotransmitter release (LLINAS et al. 1985). Inhibition of neurotransmitter release is a commonly observed physiological endpoint for the actions of opioid agonists (PATON 1957; Cox and WEINSTOCK 1966; CHERUBINI and NORTH 1985; MUDGE et al. 1979; PASSARELLI and COSTA 1989). It is possible that acute inhibition of synapsin phosphorylation by opioid agonists through opioid-inhibited adenylyl cyclase may play a role in the inhibition of neurotransmitter release by opioids. Conversely, stimulation of synapsin phosphorylation in morphine-treated brains may overcome the opioid inhibition and increase neurotransmitter release, thus counteracting the effects of opioids.

Since other G-protein-linked receptors are phosphorylated in the presence of agonist (LEFKOWITZ et al. 1990), opioid receptors may be similarly phosphorylated. Although (as of this date) opioid receptors have not yet been cloned, several preliminary studies have been completed on purified preparations of receptors. In mouse brain membranes, opioid agonists stimulated phosphorylation of a 58-kDa band (NAGAMATSU et al. 1989). Although this band has not yet been fully characterized, its size was consistent with opioid receptors. In other studies (HARADA et al. 1989, 1990), μ-receptors purified from rat brain membranes were phosphorylated in vitro with cyclic AMP-dependent protein kinase. When these purified receptors were reconstituted with purified G_{i1} into phosphatidylcholine vesicles, the opioid-stimulated GTPase which resulted from reconstitution was markedly reduced by phosphorylation. These data suggest that opioid receptors are regulated by phosphorylation like other G-protein-coupled receptors (LEFKOWITZ et al. 1990).

E. Conclusions

Data concerning the nature of the coupling of opioid receptors to their respective effector systems has provided significant information not only about the acute actions of opioids but also about mechanisms involved in tolerance and dependence. The latter problems are particularly relevant in the study of the opioid receptor-coupled second messenger system, since most investigators would agree that opioid receptor downregulation is not the rate-limiting step in the development of tolerance. The techniques for studying these systems in detail at the molecular level have just recently become available, and it will be interesting to see where they lead us. For the time being, it is useful to divide opioid receptor-coupled effector systems into two categories: short-term effectors, like K^+ and Ca^{2+} channels where opioid effects may be mediated through direct coupling of receptors with G-protein-linked ion channels, and longer-term effectors which involve diffusible second messenger systems. It is conceivable that although these different effector systems may be quite different in terms of the detail of their operation, the mechanism by which they are regulated during the development of opioid tolerance and dependence may be quite similar.

References

Amatruda TT, Gautam N, Fong HKW, Northup JK, Simon MI (1988) The 35- and 36-kDa β subunits of GTP-binding regulatory proteins are products of separate genes. J Biol Chem 263:5008–5011

Attali B, Saya D, Vogel Z (1989a) Kappa-opiate agonists inhibit adenylate cyclase and produce heterologous desensitization in rat spinal cord. J Neurochem 52:360–369

Attali B, Saya D, Nah SY, Vogel Z (1989b) Kappa opiate agonists inhibit Ca^{2+} influx in rat spinal cord-dorsal root ganglion cocultures. Involvement of a GTP-binding protein. J Biol Chem 264:347–353

Beart PM, O'Shea RD, Manallack DT (1989) Regulation of sigma-receptors: high- and low-affinity agonist states, GTP shifts and up-regulation by rimcazole and 1,3-di(2-tolyl)guanidine. J Neurochem 53:779–788

Beitner DB, Duman RS, Nestler EJ (1989) A novel action of morphine in the rat locus coeruleus: persistent decrease in adenylate cyclase. Mol Pharmacol 35:559–564

Birnbaumer L, Abramowitz J, Brown AM (1990) Receptor-effector coupling by G-proteins. Biochim Biophys Acta 1031:163–224

Blume AJ (1978a) Interactions of ligands with opiate receptors of brain membranes: regulation by ions and nucleotides. Proc Natl Acad Sci USA 75:1713–1717

Blume AJ (1978b) Opiate binding to membrane preparations of neuroblastoma-glioma hybrid cells NG108-15: effects of ions and nucleotides. Life Sci 22: 1843–1852

Blume AJ, Lichtshtein L, Boone G (1979) Coupling of opiate receptors to adenylate cyclase: requirement for sodium and GTP. Proc Natl Acad Sci USA 76:5626–5630

Bourne H (1988) Cold Spring Harbor Symp Quant Biol 53:203–208

Breiweiser GE, Szabo G (1985) Uncoupling of cardiac muscarinic and β-adrenergic receptors from ion channels by a guanine nucleotide analogue. Nature 316: 538–540

Bunn SJ, Marley PD, Livett BG (1988) Effects of opioid compounds on basal and muscarinic induced accumulation of inositol phosphates in cultured bovine chromaffin cells. Biochem Pharmacol 37:395–399

Cassel D, Selinger Z (1976) Catecholamine-stimulated GTPase activity in turkey erythrocyte membranes. Biochim Biophys Acta 452:538–551

Cerione RA, Codina J, Benovic JL, Lefkowitz RJ, Birnbaumer L, Caron MG (1984) The mammalian beta-adrenergic receptor: reconstitution of functional interactions between pure receptor and pure stimulatory guanine nucleotide binding protein of the adenylate cyclase system. Biochemistry 23:4519–4525

Cerione RA, Regan JW, Nakata H, Codina J, Benovic JL, Geirschik P, Somers RL, Spiegel AM, Birnbaumer L, Lefkowitz RJ, Caron MG (1986a) Functional reconstitution of alpha(2)-adrenergic receptors with guanine nucleotide regulatory proteins in phospholipid vesicles. J Biol Chem 261:3901–3909

Cerione RA, Staniszewski C, Gierschik P, Codina J, Somers R, Birnbaumer L, Spiegel AM, Caron MG, Lefkowitz RJ (1986b) Mechanism of guanine nucleotide regulatory protein-mediated inhibition of adenylate cyclase: studies with isolated subunits of transducin in a reconstituted system. J Biol Chem 261:9514–9520

Cerione RA, Gierschik P, Staniszewski C, Benovic JL, Codina J, Somers R, Birnbaumer L, Spiegel AM, Lefkowitz RJ, Caron MG (1987) Functional differences in the $β_γ$ complexes of transducin and the inhibitory guanine nucleotide regulatory protein. Biochemistry 26:1485–1491

Chang KJ, Hazum E, Killian A, Cuatrecasas P (1981) Interactions of ligands with morphine and enkephalin receptors are differentially affected by guanine nucleotides. Mol Pharmacol 20:1–7

Chen GG, Chalazonitis A, Shen KF, Crain SM (1988) Inhibitor of cyclic AMP-dependent protein kinase blocks opioid-induced prolongation of the action potential of mouse sensory ganglion neurons in dissociated cell cultures. Brain Res 462:372–377

Cherubini E, North RA (1985) μ and κ opioids inhibit transmitter release by different mechanisms. Proc Natl Acad Sci USA 82:1860–1863

Childers SR (1988a) Opiate-inhibited adenylate cyclase in rat brain membranes depleted of G_s-stimulated adenylate cyclase. J Neurochem 50:543–553

Childers SR (1988b) Opioid receptor-coupled second messenger systems. In: Pasternak GW (ed) The opiate receptors. Humana, Clifton, pp 231–270

Childers SR, Jackson JL (1984) pH Selectivity of N-ethylmaleimide reactions with opiate receptor complexes in rat brain membranes. J Neurochem 43:1163–1170

Childers SR, LaRiviere G (1984) Modification of guanine nucleotide regulatory components in brain membranes: II. Relationship of guanosine-5'triphosphate effects on opiate receptor binding and coupling receptors with adenylate cyclase. J Neurosci 4:2764–2771

Childers SR, Pasternak GW (1982) Naloxazone a novel opiate antagonist: irreversible blockade of rat brain opiate receptors in vitro. Cell Mol Neurobiol 2:93–103

Childers SR, Snyder SH (1979) Guanine nucleotides differentiate agonist and antagonist interactions with opiate receptors. Life Sci 23:759–762

Childers SR, Snyder SH (1980) Differential regulation by guanine nucleotide of opiate agonist and antagonist receptor interactions. J Neurochem 34:583–593

Childers SR, Lambert SM, LaRiviere G (1983) Selective alterations in guanine nucleotide regulation of opiate receptor binding and coupling with adenylate cyclase. Life Sci 33 (Suppl I): 215–218

Childers SR, Nijssen P, Nadeau P, Buckhannan P, Li P-V, Harris J (1986) Opiate-inhibited adenylate cyclase in mammalian brain membranes. Natl Inst Drug Abuse Res Monogr Ser 71:65–80

Chou WS, Ho AKS, Loh HH (1971) Effect of acute and chronic morphine and norepinephrine on brain adenylate cyclase activity. Proc West Pharmacol Soc 14:42–46

Clark MJ, Medzihradsky F (1987) Coupling of multiple opioid receptors to GTPase following selective receptor alkylation in brain membranes. Neuropharmacology 26:1763–1770

Clark MJ, Levenson SD, Medzihradsky F (1986) Evidence for coupling of the κ opioid receptor to brain GTPase. Life Sci 39:1721–1727

Clark JA, Houghten R, Pasternak GW (1988) Opiate binding in calf thalamic membranes: a selective mu_1 binding assay. Mol Pharmacol 34:308–317

Codina J, Yatani A, Grenet D, Brown AM, Birnbaumer L (1987) The α subunit of the GTP binding protein G_K opens atrial potassium channels. Science 236: 442–445

Collier HOJ, Roy AC (1974) Morphine-like drugs inhibit the stimulation by E prostaglandins of cyclic AMP formation by rat brain homogenates. Nature 248:24–27

Comb M, Birnberg NC, Seasholtz A, Herbert E, Goodman HM (1986) A cyclic AMP- and phorbol ester-inducible DNA element. Nature 323:353–356

Comb M, Mermod N, Hyman SE, Pearlberg J, Ross ME, Goodman HM (1988) Proteins bound at adjacent DNA elements act synergistically to regulate human proenkephalin cAMP inducible transcription. EMBO J 7:3793–3805

Cooper DMF, Londos C, Gill DL, Rodbell M (1982) Opiate receptor-mediated inhibition of adenylate cyclase in rat striatal plasma membranes. J Neurochem 38:1164–1167

Costa T, Herz A (1989) Antagonists with negative intrinsic activity at delta opioid receptors coupled to GTP-binding proteins. Proc Natl Acad Sci USA 86: 7321–7325

Costa T, Wuster M, Gramsch C, Herz A (1985) Multiple states of opioid receptors may modulate adenylate cyclase in intact neuroblastoma × glioma hybrid cells. Mol Pharmacol 28:146–154

Costa T, Klinz FJ, Vachon L, Herz A (1988) Opioid receptors are coupled tightly to G proteins but loosely to adenylate cyclase in NG108-15 cell membranes. Mol Pharmacol 34:744–754

Costa T, Lang J, Gless C, Herz A (1990) Spontaneous association between opioid receptors and GTP-binding regulatory proteins in native membranes: specific regulation by antagonists and sodium ions. Mol Pharmacol 37:383–394

Cox BM, Weinstock M (1966) The effects of analgesic drugs on the release of acetylcholine from electrically stimulated guinea-pig ileum. Br J Pharmacol 27:81–92

Dawson G, McLawhon R, Miller RJ (1980) Inhibition of sialoglycosphingolipid (ganglioside) biosynthesis in mouse clonal lines N4TG1 and NG108-15 by beta endorphin, enkephalins, and opiates. J Biol Chem 255:129–137

De Lean A, Stadel JM, Lefkowitz RJ (1980) A ternary complex model explains the agonist-specific binding proterties of the adenylate cyclase-coupled beta-adrenergic receptor. J Biol Chem 255:1108–1111

Duggan AW, North RA (1983) Electrophysiology of opioids. Pharmacol Rev 35:219–281

Duman RS, Tallman JF, Nestler EJ (1988) Acute and chronic opiate-regulation of adenylate cyclase in brain: specific effects in locus coeruleus. J Pharmacol Exp Ther 246:1033–1039

Ehrlich YH, Bonnet KA, Davis LG, Brunngraber EG (1978) Decreased phosphorylation of specific proteins in neostriatal membranes from rats after long-term narcotics exposure. Life Sci 23:137–146

Fantozzi R, Mullikin-Kirkpatrick D, Blume AJ (1981) Irreversible inactivation of the opiate receptors in neuroblastoma × glioma hybrid NG108-15 cells by chlornaltrexamine. Mol Pharmacology 20:8–15

Fedynyshyn JP, Lee NM (1989) Mu type opioid receptors in rat periaqueductal gray-enriched P2 membrane are coupled to G-protein-mediated inhibition of adenylyl cyclase. Brain Res 476:102–109

Florio VA, Sternweis PC (1985) Reconstitution of resolved muscarinic cholinergic receptors with purified GTP-binding proteins. J Biol Chem 260:3477–3483

Francis B, Moisand C, Meunier JC (1985) Na^+ and Gpp(NH)p selectively inhibit agonist interactions at μ- and κ-opioid receptor sites in rabbit and guinea-pig cerebellum membranes. Eur J Pharmacol 117:223–232

Frey A, Kebabian JW (1984) μ-Opiate receptor in 7315c tumor tissue mediates inhibition of immunoreactive prolactin release and adenylate cyclase activity. Endocrinology 115:1797–1804

Gilbert JA, Richelson E (1983) Function of delta opioid receptors in cultured cells. Mol Cell Biochem 55:83–91

Gilman AG (1984) G proteins and dual control of adenylate cyclase. Cell 36: 577–579

Greenspan DL, Mussachio JM (1984) The effect of tolerance on opiate dependence as measured by the adenylate cyclase rebound response in the NG108-15 model system. Neuropeptides 5:41–44

Gross RA, Moises HC, Uhler MD, Macdonald RL (1990) Dynorphin A and cAMP-dependent protein kinase independently regulate neuronal calcium currents. Proc Natl Acad Sci USA 87:7025–7029

Guitart X, Nestler EJ (1989) Identification of morphine- and cyclic AMP-regulated phosphoproteins (MARPPs) in the locus coeruleus and other regions of rat brain: regulation by acute and chronic morphine. J Neurosci 9:4371–4387

Gullis RJ (1977) Statement. Nature 265:764

Gwynn CJ, Costa E (1982) Opioids regulate cyclic GMP formation in cloned neuroblastoma cells. Proc Natl Acad Sci USA 79:690–694

Hamprecht B (1977) Sturctural, electrophysiological, biochemical, and pharmacological properties of neuroblastoma × glioma cell hybrids in cell culture. Int Rev Cytol 49:99–170

Harada H, Ueda H, Wada Y, Katada T, Ui M, Satoh M (1989) Phosphorylation of mu-opioid receptors – a putative mechanism of selective uncoupling of receptor – Gi interaction, measured with low-Km GTPase and nucleotide-sensitive agonist binding. Neurosci Lett 100:221–226

Harada H, Ueda H, Katada T, U M, Satoh M (1990) Phosphorylated mu-opioid receptor purified from rat brains lacks functional coupling with Gi1, a GTP-binding protein in reconstituted lipid vesicles. Neurosci Lett 113:47–49

Hatta S, Marcus MM, Rasenick MM (1986) Exchange of guanine nucleotide between GTP-binding proteins that regulate neuronal adenylate cyclase. Proc Natl Acad Sci USA 83:5439–5443

Havemann U, Kuschinsky K (1978) Interactions of opiates and prostaglandin E with regard to cyclic AMP in striatal tissue of rats in vitro. Arch Pharmacol 302: 103–106

Heijna MH, Hogenboom F, Portoghese PS, Mulder AH, Schoffelmeer AN (1989) Mu- and delta-opioid receptor-mediated inhibition of adenylate cyclase activity stimulated by released endogenous dopamine in rat neostriatal slices; demonstration of potent delta-agonist activity of bremazocine. J Pharmacol Exp Ther 249:864–868

Hescheler J, Rosenthal W, Trautwein W, Schultz G (1987) The GTP-binding protein, G_o, regulates neuronal calcium channels. Nature 325:445–447

Hsia JA, Moss J, Hewlett EL, Vaughan M (1984) ADP-ribosylation of adenylate cyclase by pertussis toxin: effects on inhibitory agonist binding. J Biol Chem 259:1086–1090

Itoh H, Kozasa T, Nagata S, Nakamura S, Katada T, Ui M, Iwai S, Ohtsuka E, Kawasaki H, Suzuki K, Kaziro Y (1986) Molecular cloning and sequence determination of cDNAs for the subunits of the guanine nucleotide-binding proteins G_s, G_i, and G_o from rat brain. Proc Natl Acad Sci USA 83:3776–3780

Itzhak Y (1989) Multiple affinity binding states of the sigma receptor: effect of GTP-binding protein-modifying agents. Mol Pharmacol 36:512–517

Jakobs KH, Bauer S, Watanabe Y (1985) Modulation of adenylate cyclase of human platelets by phorbol ester. Impairment of the hormone-sensitive inhibitory pathway. Eur J Biochem 151:425–340

Johnson SM (1990) Opioid inhibition of cholinergic transmission in the guinea-pig ileum is independent of intracellular cyclic AMP. Eur J Pharmacol 180:331–338

Katada T, Ui M (1982) Direct modification of the membrane adenylate cyclase system by islet-activating protein due to ADP-ribosylation of a membrane protein. Proc Natl Acad Sci USA 79:3129–3133

Katada T, Gilman AG, Watanabe Y, Bauer S, Jakobs KH (1985) Protein kinase C phosphorylates the inhibitory guanine-nucleotide-binding regulatory component and apparently suppresses its function in hormonal inhibition of adenylate cyclase. Eur J Biochem 151:431–437

Katada T, Oinuma M, Ui M (1986) Mechanisms for inhibition of the catalytic activity of adenylate cyclase by the guanine nucleotide-binding proteins serving as the substrate of islet-activating protein, pertussis toxin. J Biol Chem 261:5215–5221

Kent RS, De Lean A, Lefkowitz RJ (1980) A quantitative analysis of beta-adrenergic receptor interactions: resolution of high and low affinity states of the receptor by computer modeling of ligand binding data. Mol Pharmacol 17:14–23

Kobilka BK, Kobilka TS, Daniel K, Regan JW, Caron MG, Lefkowitz RJ (1988) Chimeric α_2-β_2-adrenergic receptors: delineation of domains involved in effector coupling and ligand binding specificity. Science 240:1310–1316

Konkoy CS, Childers SR (1989) Dynorphin-selective inhibition of adenylyl cyclase in guinea pig cerebellum membranes. Mol Pharmacol 36:627–633

Koski G, Klee WA (1981) Opiates inhibit adenylate cyclase by stimulating GTP hydrolysis. Proc Natl Acad Sci USA 78:4185–4189

Lambert SM, Childers SR (1984) Modification of guanine nucleotide regulatory components in brain membranes: I. Changes in guanosine-5'-triphosphate regulation of opiate receptor binding sites. J Neurosci 4:2755–2763

Law PY, Wu J, Koehler JE, Loh HH (1981) Demonstration and characterization of opiate inhibition of the striatal adenylate cyclase. J Neurochem 36:1834–1846

Law PY, Hom DS, Loh HH (1982) Loss of opiate receptor activity in neuroblastoma × glioma NG108-15 hybrid cells after chronic opiate treatment: a multi-step process. Mol Pharmacol 22:1–4

Law PY, Hom DS, Loh HH (1983a) Opiate receptor down-regulation and desensitization in neuroblastoma × glioma NG108-15 hybrid cells are two separate cellular adaptation processes. Mol Pharm 24:413–424

Law PY, Griffin MT, Koehler JE, Loh HH (1983b) Attenuation of enkephalin activity in neuroblastoma × glioma NG108-15 hybrid cells by phospholipases. J Neurochem 40:267–275

Law PY, Ungar HG, Hom DS, Loh HH (1985a) Effects of cycloheximide and tunicamycin on opiate receptor activities in neuroblastoma × glioma NG108-15 hybrid cells. Biochem Pharmacol 34:9–17

Law PY, Hom DS, Loh HH (1985b) Multiple affinity states of opiate receptors in neuroblastoma × glioma NG108-15 hybrid cells: opiate agonist association rate is a function of receptor occupancy. J Biol Chem 260:3561–3569

Lefkowitz RJ, Hausdorff WP, Caron MG (1990) Role of phosphorylation in desensitization of the beta-adrenoceptor. Trends Pharmacol Sci 11:190–194

Le Moine C, Normand E, Guitteny AF, Fouque B, Teoule R, Bloch B (1990) Dopamine receptor gene expression by enkephalin neurons in rat forebrain. Proc Natl Acad Sci USA 87:230–234

Llinas R, McGuinness TL, Leonard CS, Sugimori M, Greengard P (1985) Intraterminal injection of synapsin I or calcium/calmodulin-dependent protein kinase II alters neurotransmitter release at the squid giant synapse. Proc Natl Acad Sci USA 82:3035–3039

Louie AK, Law PY, Loh HH (1986) Cell-free desensitization of opioid inhibition of adenylate cyclase in neuroblastoma × glioma NG108-15 hybrid cell membranes. J Neurochem 47:733–737

Louie AK, Bass ES, Zhan J. Law PY, Loh HH (1990) Attenuation of opioid receptor activity by phorbol esters in neuroblastoma × glioma NG108-15 hybrid cells. J Pharmacol Exp Ther 253:401–407

Mack KJ, Lee MF, Wehenmeyer JA (1985) Effects of guanine nucleotides and ions on kappa opioid binding. Brain Res Bull 14:301–306

Makimura M, Murakoshi Y (1989) Kappa-opioid agonists do not inhibit adenylate cyclase. J Pharmacobiodyn 12:125–131

Makman MH, Dvorkin B, Crain SM (1988) Modulation of adenylate cyclase activity of mouse spinal cord-ganglion explants by opioids, serotonin and pertussis toxin. Brain Res 445:303–313

Manning DR, Gilman AG (1983) The regulatory components of adenylate cyclase and transducin: a family of structurally homologous guanine nucleotide binding proteins. J Biol Chem 258:7059–7063

Marckel DR, Childers SR (1989) Opioid receptor second messenger systems. In: Watson RR (ed) Biochemistry and physiology of substance abuse. CRC Press, Boca Raton, pp 155–180

Mattera R, Graziano MP, Yatani A, Zhou Z, Graf R, Codina J, Birnbaumer L, Gilman AG, Brown AM (1989) Splice variants of the alpha subunit of the G protein G_s activate both adenylyl cyclase and calcium channels. Science 243:804–807

McKenzie FR, Milligan G (1990) Delta-opioid-receptor-mediated inhibition of adenylate cyclase is transduced specifically by the guanine-nucleotide-binding protein G_{i2}. Biochem J 267:391–398

Milligan G, Klee WA (1985) The inhibitory guanine nucleotide-binding protein (N$_i$) purified from bovine brain is a high affinity GTPase. J Biol Chem 260:2057–2063

Minneman KP, Iversen LL (1976) Enkephalin and opiate narcotics increase cyclic GMP accumulation in slices of rat neostriatum. Nature 261:313–314

Misawa H, Ueda H, Satoh M (1990) Kappa-opioid agonist inhibits phospholipase C, possibly via an inhibition of G-protein activity. Neurosci Lett 112:324–327

Mudge AW, Leeman SE, Fischbach GD (1979) Enkephalin inhibits release of substance P from sensory neurons and decreases action potential duration. Proc Natl Acad Sci USA 76:526–530

Mulder AH, Wardeh G, Hogenboom F, Frankhuyzen AL (1984) κ- and ∂-opioid receptor agonists differentially inhibit striatal dopamine and acetylcholine release. Nature 308:278–280

Mulder AH, Schoffelmeer AN, Stoof JC (1990) On the role of adenylate cyclase in presynaptic modulation of neurotransmitter release mediated by monoamine and opioid receptors in the brain. Ann NY Acad Sci 60:237–249

Muraki T, Usamaki H, Kato R (1984) Effect of morphine on the tissue cyclic AMP and cyclic GMP content in two strains of mice. J Pharm Pharmacol 36:490–492

Nagamatsu K, Suzuki K, Teshima R, Ikebuchi H, Terao T (1989) Morphine enhances the phosphorylation of a 58 kDa protein in mouse brain membranes. Biochem J 257:165–171

Nakamura T, Ui M (1985) Simultaneous inhibitions of inositol-phospholipid breakdown, arachidonic acid release and histamine secretion in mast cells by islet activating protein, pertussis toxin: a possible involvement of the toxin-specific substrate in the calcium-moblizing receptor-mediated biosignalling system. J Biol Chem 260:3584–3593

Neer EJ, Clapham DE (1988) Roles of G-protein subunits in transmemebrane signalling. Nature 133:129–133

Neer EJ, Lok JM, Wolf LG (1984) Purification and properties of the inhibitory guanine nucleotide regulatory unit of brain adenylate cyclase. J Biol Chem 259:14222–14229

Nestler EJ, Tallman JF (1988) Chronic morphine treatment increases cyclic AMP-dependent protein kinase activity in the rat locus coeruleus. Mol Pharmacol 33:127–132

Nestler EJ, Walaas SI, Greengard P (1984) Neuronal phosphoproteins: physiological and clinical implications. Science 225:1357–1364

Nestler EJ, Erdos JJ, Terwilliger R, Duman RS, Tallman JF (1989) Regulation of G proteins by chronic morphine in the rat locus coeruleus. Brain Res 476:230–239

Nishizuka Y (1984) Turnover of inositol phospholipids and signal transduction. Science 225:1365–1370

North RA, Williams JT, Surprenant A, Christie MJ (1987) μ and ∂ receptors belong to a family of receptors that are coupled to potassium channels. Proc Natl Acad Sci USA 84:5487–5491

Northup JK, Smigel MD, Sternweis PC, Gilman, AG (1983) The subunits of the stimulatory regulatory component of adenylate cyclase: resolution of the activated 45,000-dalton (alpha) subunit. J Biol Chem 258:11369–11376

Ott S, Costa T, Herz A (1989) Opioid receptors of neuroblastoma cells are in two domains of the plasma membrane that differ in content of G proteins. J Neurochem 52:619–626

Passarelli F, Costa T (1989) Mu and delta opioid receptors inhibit serotonin release in rat hippocampus. J Pharmacol Exp Ther 248:299–305

Paton WDM (1957) The action of morphine and related substances on contraction and on acetylcholine output of coaxially stimulated guinea-pig ileum. Br J Pharmacol 12:119–127

Periyasamy S, Hoss W (1990) Kappa opioid receptors stimulate phosphoinositide turnover in rat brain. Life Sci 47:219–225

Pfaffinger PJ, Martin JM, Hunter D, Nathanson NM, Hille B (1985) GTP-binding proteins couple cardiac muscarinic receptors to a potassium channel. Nature 317:536–538

Pfeiffer A, Sadee W, Herz A (1982) Differential regulation of mu-, delta-, and kappa-opiate receptor subtypes by guanine nucleotides and metal ions. J Neurosci 2:912–917

Polastron J, Boyer MJ, Quertermont Y, Thouvenot JP, Meunier JC, Jauzac P (1990a) Mu-opioid receptors and not kappa-opioid receptors are coupled to the adenylate cyclase in the cerebellum. J Neurochem 54:562–570

Polastron J, Boyer MJ, Thouvenot JP, Meunier JC, Jauzac P (1990b) Coupling of mu-opioid receptors with adenylate cyclase in naive and morphine tolerant rabbits. Prog Clin Biol Res 328:25–28

Propst F, Hamprecht B (1981) Opioids, noradrenaline and GTP analogs inhibit cholera toxin activated adenylate cyclase in neuroblastoma × glioma hybrid cells. J Neurochem 36:580–588

Puri SK, Cochin J, Volicer L (1975) Effect of morphine sulfate on adenylate cyclase and phosphodiesterase activities in rat corpus striatum. Life Sci 16:759–768

Puttfarcken PS, Cox BM (1989) Morphine-induced desensitization and down-regulation at mu-receptors in 7315C pituitary tumor cells. Life Sci 45:1937–1942

Puttfarcken PS, Werling LL, Cox BM (1988) Effects of chronic morphine exposure on opioid inhibition of adenylyl cyclase in 7315c cell membranes: a useful model for the study of tolerance at μ opioid receptors. Mol Pharmacol 33:520–527

Quach TT, Tang F, Kageyama H, Mocchetti I, Guidotti A, Meek JL, Costa E, Schwartz JP (1984) Enkephalin biosynthesis in adrenal medulla. Modulation of proenkephalin mRNA content of cultured chromaffin cells by 8-bromo-adenosine 3′,5′-monophosphate. Mol Pharmacol 26:255–260

Rasenick MM, Childers SR (1989) Modification of G_s-stimulated adenylate cyclase in brain membranes by low pH treatment: correlation with altered guanine nucleotide exchange. J Neurochem 53:219–225

Rodbell M (1980) The role of hormone receptors and GTP-regulatory proteins in membrane transduction. Nature 284:17–21

Rothman RB, Long JB, Bykov V, Jacobson AE, Rice KC, Holaday JW (1988) β-FNA binds irreversibly to the opiate receptor complex: in vivo and in vitro evidence. J Pharmacol Exp Ther 247:405–416

Schoffelmeer ANM, Wierenga EA, Mulder AH (1986) Role of adenylate cyclase in presynaptic a_2-adrenoceptor- and μ-opioid receptor-mediated inhibition of [^{3}H]-noradrenaline release from rat brain cortex slices. J Neurochem 46:1711–1717

Schoffelmeer AN, Rice KC, Heijna MH, Hogenboom F, Mulder AH (1988) Fentanyl isothiocyanate reveals the existence of physically associated mu- and delta-opioid receptors mediating inhibition of adenylate cyclase in rat neostriatum. Eur J Pharmacol 149:179–182

Schofield PR, McFarland KC, Hayflick JS, Wilcox JN, Cho TM, Roy S, Lee NM, Loh HH, Seeburg PH (1989) Molecular characterization of a new immunoglobulin superfamily protein with potential roles in opioid binding and cell contact. EMBO J 8:489–495

Schramm M, Selinger Z (1984) Message transmission: receptor-controlled adenylate cyclase system. Science 225:1350–1356

Sharma SK, Niremberg M, Klee W (1975a) Morphine receptors as regulators of adenylate cyclase activity. Proc Natl Acad Sci USA 72:590–594

Sharma SK, Klee WA, Niremberg M (1975b) Dual regulation of adenylate cyclase accounts for narcotic dependence and tolerance. Proc Natl Acad Sci USA 72:3092–3096

Sharma SK, Klee WA, Niremberg M (1977) Opiate dependent modulation of adenylate cyclase activity. Proc Natl Acad Sci USA 74:3365–3369

Sternweis PC, Robishaw JD (1984) Isolation of two proteins with high affinity for guanine nucleotides from membranes of bovine brain. J Biol Chem 259: 13806–13813

Sunyer T, Codina J, Birnbaumer L (1984) GTP hydrolysis by pure N_i, the inhibitory regulatory component of adenylyl cyclases. J Biol Chem 259:15447–15451

Tao P, Law P, Loh HH (1987) Decrease in delta and mu opioid receptor binding capacity in rat brain after chronic etorphine treatment. J Pharm Exp Ther 240:809–816

Tao PL, Chang LR, Law PY, Loh HH (1988) Decrease in delta-opioid receptor density in rat brain after chronic [D-Ala^2,D-Leu^5]enkephalin treatment. Brain Res 462:313–320

Tatsumi H, Costa M, Schimerlik M, North RA (1990) Potassium conductance increased by noradrenaline, opioids, somatostatin, and G-proteins: whole-cell recording from guinea pig submucous neurons. J Neurosci 10:1675–1682

Tell GP, Pasternak GW, Cuatrecasas P (1975) Brain and caudate nucleus adenylate cyclase: effects of dopamine, GTP, E prostaglandins and morphine. FEBS Lett 51:242–245

Tempel A, Zukin RS, Gardner EL (1982) Supersensitivity of brain opiate receptor subtypes after chronic naltrexone treatment. Life Sci 31:1401–1404

Tempel A, Gardner EL, Zukin RS (1985) Neurochemical and functional correlates of nal-trexone-induced opiate receptor up-regulation. J Pharmacol Exp Ther 232:439–444

Tempel A, Kessler JA, Zukin RS (1990) Chronic naltrexone treatment increases expression of preproenkephalin and preprotachykinin mRNA in discrete brain regions. J Neurosci 10:741–747

Traber F, Gullis R, Hamprecht B (1975) Influence of opiates on levels of adenosine 3',5'-monophosphate in neuroblastoma × glioma hybrid cells. Life Sci 16: 1863–1868

Tsai S, Adamik R, Kanaho Y, Halpern JL, Moss J (1987) Immunological and biochemical differentiation of guanyl nucleotide binding proteins: interaction of $G_{o\alpha}$ with rhodopsin, anti-$G_{o\alpha}$ polyclonal antibodies, and a monoclonal antibody against transducin a subunit and $G_{i\alpha}$. Biochemistry 26:4728–4733

Tsang D, Tan AT, Henry JL, Lal S (1978) Effect of opioid peptides on noradrenaline-stimulated cyclic AMP formation in homogenates of rat cerebral cortex and hypothalamus. Brain Res 152:521–527

Ueda H, Uno S, Harada J, Kobayashi I, Katada T, Ui M, Satoh M (1990a) Evidence for receptor-mediated inhibition of intrinsic activity of GTP-binding protein, G_{i1} and G_{i2}, but not G_0 in reconstitution experiments. FEBS Lett 266:178–182

Ueda H, Misawa H, Katada T, Ui M, Takagi H, Satoh M (1990b) Functional reconstruction of purified Gi and Go with mu-opioid receptors in guinea pig striatal membranes pretreated with micromolar concentrations of N-ethylmaleimide. J Neurochem 54:841–848

Uhl GR, Ryan JP, Schwartz JP (1988) Morphine alters preproenkephalin gene expression. Mol Brain Res 391–397

Vachon L, Costa T, Herz A (1986) GTPase and adenylate cyclase desensitize at different rates in NG108-15 cells. Mol Pharmacol 31:159–168

Van Inwegen RG, Strada SJ, Robison GA (1975) Effects of prostaglandins and morphine on brain adenylate cyclase. Life Sci 16:1875–1876

Van Vliet BJ, Mulder AH, Schoffelmeer AN (1990) Mu-opioid receptors mediate the inhibitory effect of opioids on dopamine-sensitive adenylate cyclase in primary cultures of rat neostriatal neurons. J Neurochem 55:1274–1280

Werling LL, McMahon PN, Cox BM (1989a) Selective changes in mu opioid receptor properties induced by chronic morphine exposure. Proc Natl Acad Sci USA 86:6393–6397

Werling LL, McMahon PN, Cox BM (1989b) Effects of pertussis toxin on opioid regulation of catecholamine release from rat and guinea pig brain slices. Naunyn Schmiedebergs Arch Pharmacol 339:509–513

Wilkening D, Mishra RK, Makman MH (1976) Effects of morphine on dopamine-stimulated adenylate cyclase and on cyclic GMP formation in primate brain amygdaloid nucleus. Life Sci 19:1129–1138

Williams N, Clouet DH (1982) The effect of acute opioid administration on the phosphorylation of rat striatal synaptic membrane proteins. J Pharmacol Exp Ther 220:278–286

Wojcik WJ, Cavalla D, Neff NH (1985) Co-localized adenosine A1 and gamma-aminobutyric acid B (GABA$_B$) receptors of cerebellum may share a common adenylate cyclase catalytic unit. J Pharmacol Exp Ther 232:62–66

Wolleman M (1981) Endogenous opioids and cyclic AMP. Prog Neurobiol 16: 145–154

Wolozin BL, Pasternak GW (1981) Classification of multiple morphine and enkephalin binding sites in the central nervous system. Proc Natl Acad Sci USA 78:6181–6185

Yatani A, Codina J, Imoto Y, Reeves JP, Birnbaumer L, Brown AM (1987) A G protein directly regulates mammalian cardiac calcium channels. Science 238:1288–1292

Yu VC, Saddee W (1986) Phosphatidylinositol turnover in neuroblastoma cells: regulation by bradykinin, acetylcholine, but not μ- and ∂-opioid receptors. Neurosci Lett 71:219–223

Yu VC, Richards ML, Sadee W (1986) A human neuroblastoma cell line expresses mu and delta opioid receptor sites. J Biol Chem 261:1065–1070

Yu VC, Eiger S, Duan DS, Lameh J, Sadee W (1990) Regulation of cyclic AMP by the mu-opioid receptor in human neuroblastoma SH-SY5Y cells. J Neurochem 55:1390–1396

Zajac J-M, Roques BP (1985) Differences in binding properties of mu and delta opioid receptor subtypes from rat brain, kinetic analysis and effects of ions and guanine nucleotides. J Neurochem 44:1605–1614

Zukin RS, Sugarman JR, Fitz-Syage ML, Gardner EL, Zukin SR, Gintzler AR (1982) Naltrexone-induced opiate receptor supersensitivity. Brain Res 245: 285–292

Allosteric Coupling Among Opioid Receptors: Evidence for an Opioid Receptor Complex

R.B. ROTHMAN, J.W. HOLADAY, and F. PORRECA

A. Introduction

The existence of several distinct and physically separable types of opioid receptor, termed μ, δ, and κ, is well supported by biochemical (SIMONDS et al. 1985; CHO et al. 1986; GIOANNINI et al. 1985; SIMON et al. 1987; SZÜCS et al. 1987), ligand binding, bioassay, and autoradiographic data (ROBSON et al. 1983). Although the multiplicity of opioid receptors provides a basis for explaining the diverse and complex pharmacology of the opioids, several investigators reported observations in the late 1970s and 1980s which are difficult to explain solely on the basis of distinct opioid receptors. Instead, these observations have led to the postulated existence of an opioid receptor complex, composed of μ-, δ-, and perhaps κ-binding sites (VAUGHT et al. 1982; D'AMATO and HOLADAY 1984; LEE and SMITH 1980b; BALS-KUBIK et al. 1990).

Figure 1 provides an overview of this hypothesis. The opioid receptor complex is thought to be composed of distinct but physically interacting μ-, δ-, and κ-binding sites. The hatched arrows indicate the ability to physically interact, not interconvert. The subscript "cx" indicates a binding site associated with the receptor complex. In addition, the existence of distinct μ-, δ-, and κ-sites not associated with the complex are hypothesized, as indicated by the "ncx" subscript.

This chapter will (a) review past and current data which speak of the existence of an opioid receptor complex, and (b) provide an historical perspective on the development of the concept of an opioid receptor complex.

B. Evidence for a μ-δ-Opioid Receptor Complex

I. Ligand-Binding Data

1. Evidence that μ-Ligands Noncompetitively Inhibit δ-Receptor Binding

The first in vitro binding data which provided evidence for a μ-δ-opioid receptor complex was the observation that morphine noncompetitively inhibited [^{3}H]leu^5-enkephalin ([^{3}H]LE) binding, shown as a Scatchard plot

218   R.B. ROTHMAN et al.

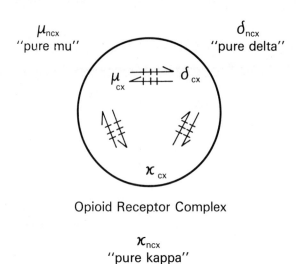

μ_{ncx} "pure mu" δ_{ncx} "pure delta"

Opioid Receptor Complex

κ_{ncx}
"pure kappa"

Fig. 1. Schematic model of the opioid receptors. The subscript *ncx* refers to binding sites which are not part of the opioid receptor complex. The subscript *cx* refers to binding sites which are part of the opioid receptor complex. *Arrows* do not indicate interconversion, but the ability to influence

in Fig. 2 (ROTHMAN and WESTFALL 1980; ROTHMAN and WESTFALL 1982a). These data demonstrated that morphine decreased the B_{max}, and increased the K_d, of [³H]LE-binding sites. The data were analyzed according to two models. Model 1 ("the two-site competitive model") postulated that [³H]LE labeled two binding sites (μ and δ) and that morphine was a weak competitive inhibitor at the δ-binding site, and a potent competitive inhibitor at the μ-binding site. Model 2 (the "one-site allosteric" model) postulated that [³H]LE labeled a single class of δ-binding sites, and that morphine potently decreased the B_{max} by binding to a physically adjacent μ-binding site (noncompetitive inhibition), and less potently increased the apparent K_d by binding directly to the δ-binding site (competitive mechanism). Computer-assisted analysis of the data demonstrated that model 2 fitted the data better than model 1.

In 1981 BOWEN et al. (1981) reported that the metabolically stable enkephalin analog [³H][D-ala²,D-leu⁵]enkephalin ([³H]DADL) labeled two anatomically and biochemically distinct binding sites in the rat striatum. Whereas the binding of [³H]DADL to the site present in the striatal matrix (type II site) was not affected by manipulations of the in vitro assay conditions, [³H]DADL binding to the site present in the striatal patches was increased by the addition of 100 mM NaCl, 3 mM MnCl₂ and 2 µM GTP, and decreased by the inclusion of MnCl₂ only. Since [³H]dihydromorphine binding to striatal patches was decreased by the addition of 100 mM NaCl, 3 mM MnCl₂, and 2 µM GTP, and increased by the inclusion of MnCl₂ only,

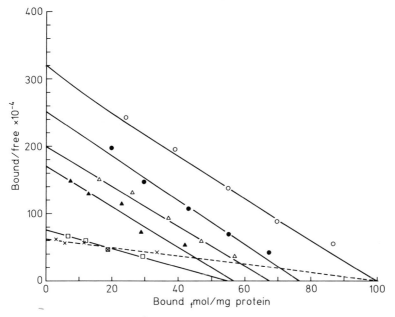

Fig. 2. Scatchard plot of [³H]leucine enkaphalin binding in the absence (*open circles*) or presence of 10 n*M* morphine (*closed circles*), 50 n*M* morphine (*open triangles*), 100 n*M* morphine (*closed triangles*), 500 n*M* morphine (*open squares*), or 5 n*M* ME (*X*). (Illustration taken from ROTHMAN and WESTFALL 1982a)

these investigators suggested that the opioid receptor present in the striatal patches interconverted between µ- and δ-forms.

Since an assumption of the one-site allosteric model described above is that [³H]LE labels a single class of binding sites, the observations of BOWEN et al. (1981) prompted a reformulation of model 2 into the "two-site allosteric model" (model 3). This model postulates that µ-ligands are competitive inhibitors at one [³H]DADL site, and noncompetitive inhibitors at a second [³H]DADL site. The subtle differences between the two-site competitive model on the one hand, and either the one-site or two-site allosteric models on the other hand, necessitated the development of a novel method of experimental design and data analysis, called "binding surface analysis," which would be sensitive enough to distinguish among these models (ROTHMAN 1983, 1986; ROTHMAN et al. 1983). Variations of the binding surface analysis technique have subsequently been adopted by laboratories which specialize in the quantitative analysis of ligand-binding data (NEVE et al. 1986; MCGONIGLE et al. 1986; ROVATI et al. 1990).

Binding surface analysis of [³H]DADL binding to rat brain membranes demonstrated that the two-site allosteric model (model 3) fits the data better than the two-site competitive model (model 1) (ROTHMAN et al. 1985b). [³H]DADL was shown to label two binding sites distinguished by the inhibitory mechanism of the μ-ligands: (1) a higher affinity binding site (localized in the striatal matrix) at which μ-ligands are weak, competitive inhibitors, i.e., the δ-binding site labeled by $[^3H][D\text{-}Pen^2,D\text{-}Pen^5]$enkephalin (DPDPE), and (2) a lower affinity binding site (localized in the striatal patches) at which μ-ligands are potent, noncompetitive inhibitors (ROTHMAN et al. 1984a, 1985b). These $[^3H]$DADL binding sites were initially named the μ-competitive and μ-noncompetitive binding sites, respectively. By common agreement, they are now called the δ_{ncx}- and δ_{cx}-binding sites, for the δ-binding site not associated with ("ncx"), and the δ-binding site in ("cx") the opioid receptor complex. Since the anatomical distribution of the lower affinity $[^3H]$DADL-binding site was apparently identical to that of μ-binding sites, ROTHMAN et al. (1985b) proposed that the lower-affinity $[^3H]$DADL-binding site was the δ-binding site of the opioid receptor complex, and that the noncompetitive inhibition produced by μ-ligands is mediated through the μ-binding site of the receptor complex. In that the observations of noncompetitive interactions are incompatible with the "interconversion" model, it is likely that the condition-dependent labeling of the striatal patches by $[^3H]$DADL reflects condition-dependent altera-tions in the affinity of $[^3H]$DADL for its lower-affinity binding site.

A limitation of the study discussed above (ROTHMAN et al. 1985b) was its reliance on computer analysis of the binding data. Therefore, in subsequent studies, the site-directed irreversible ligands 2-(4-ethoxybenzyl)-1-diethylaminoethyl-5-isothiocyanatobenzimidazole · HCl (BIT) and N-phenyl-N-[1-(2-(4-isothiocyanato)phenethyl)-4-piperidinyl]propanamide · HCl (FIT), developed by Rice and associates (RICE et al. 1983), were used to selectively deplete membranes of the δ_{cx}- and δ_{ncx}-binding sites, respec-tively. Several studies have since demonstrated that, using $[^3H]$DADL as the ligand, BIT- and FIT-pretreated membranes permit selective measurement of the δ_{ncx}- and δ_{cx}-binding sites, respectively (DANKS et al. 1988; ROTHMAN et al. 1984a,c, 1985b, 1988b). Thus, using FIT-pretreated membranes, it was possible to demonstrate directly that morphine noncompetitively inhibited $[^3H]$LE binding at the δ_{cx}-binding site, confirming previous reports (Fig. 3) (ROTHMAN et al. 1984b). Table 1 provides a brief summary of the nomencla-ture of these different binding sites.

2. Evidence that δ-Ligands Noncompetitively Inhibit μ-Receptor Binding

Given that μ-ligands noncompetitively inhibit $[^3H]$DADL binding to the δ_{cx}-site, one would predict that δ-ligands should noncompetitively inhibit the binding of $[^3H]$μ-ligands to the μ-site of the receptor complex. This has proven to be more difficult to demonstrate convincingly. Using $[^3H]$etorphine to label μ-binding sites, Rothman and Westfall presented evidence that LE and met⁵-enkephalin (ME) decreased the B_{max} (noncompetitive interaction) and increased the K_d (competitive interaction) of $[^3H]$etorphine-binding sites (ROTHMAN and WESTFALL 1982b). Although evidence was presented in

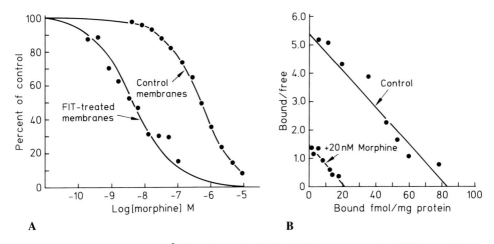

Fig. 3. A Displacement of [³H]leucine enkephalin binding to control or FIT-treated membranes. Notice the increased potency in FIT-treated membranes, in which [³H]leucine enkephalin is labeling the δ_{cx}-binding site. **B** Scatchard plot of [³H]leucine enkephalin binding to FIT-treated membranes in the absence or presence of 20 nM morphine. These data demonstrate that morphine is a noncompetitive inhibitor of [³H]leucine enkephalin binding to the δ_{cx}-binding site. (Illustration taken from ROTHMAN et al. 1984b)

Table 1. Selected characteristics of opioid binding sites

	μ_{ncx}	μ_{cx}	δ_{cx}	δ_{ncx}
Labeled by [³H]cycloFOXY[a]	No	Yes	No	No
Labeled by [³H]DADL[b]	No	No	Yes	Yes
Labeled by [³H]DAMGO[c]	Yes	Yes	No	No
B_{max} increased by chronic morphine[d]	No	Yes	Yes	No
B_{max} increased by chronic naltrexone[d]	Yes	Yes	Yes	Yes
Sensitive to β-FNA[e]	No	Yes	Yes	No
Commonly accepted nomenclature	μ	μ	μ	δ

A partial tabulation of the properties of opioid receptor subtypes is provided. The table is taken from ROTHMAN et al. (1989). Citations are as follows: [a] ROTHMAN et al. (1987b); [b] ROTHMAN et al. (1985b); [c] ROTHMAN et al. (1987a); [d] DANKS et al. (1988); [e] ROTHMAN et al. (1988b).

that study that [³H]etorphine selectively labeled μ-binding sites, it is now known that under some conditions [³H]etorphine can also label δ- and κ-binding sites, suggesting the obvious need for additional experiments.

In view of data indicating that [³H]naloxone selectively labels the μ-receptor when the assay is conducted at 0°C in the presence of 100 mM NaCl (PERT and SNYDER 1974; CREESE and SNYDER 1975), subsequent experiments examined the interaction of LE with [³H]naloxone-binding sites under these conditions. In the first study, saturation binding studies with [³H]naloxone conducted in the absence and presence of different concentrations of LE demonstrated that LE decreased the B_{max} and increased the K_d in a dose-dependent manner (ROTHMAN and WESTFALL 1983b). Computer-assisted analysis of the data demonstrated that the one-site allosteric model (model 2) fitted the data better than the two-site competitive model (model 1).

A subsequent study of the interaction of LE with [^{3}H]naloxone binding, which used binding surface analysis, demonstrated that the two-site allosteric model (model 3) fitted the data better than the two-site competitive model (model 1) (ROTHMAN et al. 1985a). According to the two-site allosteric model, [^{3}H]naloxone labels two binding sites distinguished by the inhibitory mechanism of LE: (1) a µ-site at which LE is a potent noncompetitive inhibitor and (2) a second site, at which LE is a weak competitive inhibitor, identified subsequently as a κ_2-binding site (ROTHMAN and MCLEAN 1988). The µ-binding site labeled by [^{3}H]naloxone has been identified as the µ-binding site of the opioid receptor complex (μ_{cx}) based upon: (1) the noncompetitive interaction of LE; (2) the concurrent upregulation of it and the δ_{cx}-binding site by chronic morphine, which does not upregulate either κ- or δ_{ncx}-binding sites (ROTHMAN et al. 1987b, 1989; DANKS et al. 1988); and (3) the concurrent sensitivity of this site and the δ_{cx}-binding site to the irreversible µ-antagonist β-FNA (ROTHMAN et al. 1985a, 1988b).

An intrinsic weakness of the above data is that [^{3}H]naloxone labels two binding sites, necessitating the use of computer analysis to demonstrate that LE noncompetitively inhibits [^{3}H]naloxone binding to the μ_{cx}-binding site. Unfortunately, a site-directed irreversible ligand is not available to deplete membranes of the κ_2-binding site labeled by [^{3}H]naloxone, which would permit the selective labeling of the μ_{cx}-binding site, and a direct demonstration of noncompetitive interactions.

Identifying noncompetitive interactions using µ-agonist ligands such as [^{3}H][D-ala^2-MePhe^4,gly-ol^5]enkephalin ([^{3}H]DAMGO) have not been successful (R.B. ROTHMAN, unpublished data). Possible reasons for this include: (1) the noncompetitive interactions might be detected only with antagonist ligands, or only with certain µ-agonist ligands; (2) the probable existence of µ-binding sites not associated with the receptor complex (μ_{ncx}) in addition to the μ_{cx}-site (ROTHMAN et al. 1978a); and (3) the possibility that the interactions between the µ- and δ-binding sites of the complex are not bidirectional.

The probable existence of μ_{ncx}-binding sites was suggested by differences in the B_{max} values of the δ_{cx}- and µ-binding sites (ROTHMAN et al. 1985b), and the partial sensitivity of µ-binding sites to pretreatment with β-FNA (ROTHMAN et al. 1987a). Since [^{3}H]DAMGO binds to an apparent single class of binding site, this ligand must have similar K_d values at μ_{cx}-and μ_{ncx}-binding sites. Therefore, the ability to demonstrate noncompetitive interactions might depend in part on the relative ratio of μ_{cx}- to μ_{ncx}-binding sites. This hypothesis is supported by the report that the δ-selective peptide [D-Ser^2(O-$tert$-butyl), Leu^5]enkephanyl-Thr^6 (DSTBULET) noncompetitively inhibits [^{3}H]DAMGO binding to striatal membranes, an area of the rat brain the authors suggest is enriched with the opioid receptor complex (SCHOFFELMEER et al. 1990).

In summary, the data reviewed in this section support the hypothesis of an opioid receptor complex, composed of distinct but interacting μ- and δ-binding sites, as well as μ-, δ- and κ-binding sites not associated with the receptor complex. Although binding data directly demonstrating the existence of a κ-binding site associated with the receptor complex has not been observed, this does not rule out its existence. In other words, absence of evidence is not evidence of absence.

II. δ-Agonist–μ-Agonist Interactions

1. Early Studies: Analgesia Model

The term "agonist-agonist interactions" in this hypothesis refers to the ability of subeffective doses of δ-agonists to modulate morphine-induced antinociception. In 1979 Vaught and Takemori reported that subeffective doses of LE potentiated morphine antinociception (VAUGHT and TAKEMORI 1979). Lee et al. (1980a) subsequently reported that subeffective doses of met^5-enkephalin (ME) attenuated morphine antinociception (LEE et al. 1980), and Rothman and Westfall reported that morphine was an apparent noncompetitive inhibitor of [^{3}H]LE binding (ROTHMAN and WESTFALL 1980; ROTHMAN and WESTFALL 1982a). To explain these data it was suggested that morphine produces antinociception via an interaction at the μ-site of the receptor complex, and that LE potentiates, and ME attenuates, morphine antinociception via interactions at the δ-site of the receptor complex (ROTHMAN 1981).

Several predictions of the model were formulated (ROTHMAN 1981). Among these were: (1) coadministration of subeffective doses of ME should reverse the LE-induced potentiation of morphine antinociception and (2) coadministration of subeffective doses of LE should reverse the ME-induced attenuation of morphine antinociception. These predictions were experimentally verified in a collaborative study with Dr. Jeffry L. Vaught (VAUGHT et al. 1982). The observations reported in that study (Fig. 4) suggested two possible hypotheses: (1) the opposing effects of the pentapeptides are mediated via the same δ-receptor; (2) the opposing effects reflect selective interactions of LE and ME with different δ-receptors, located, perhaps, on different neuronal elements. A direct prediction of hypothesis two is that binding studies should detect LE- and ME-specific δ-binding sites, whereas hypothesis 1 predicts that binding studies with [^{3}H]LE and [^{3}H]ME should demonstrate that each labels the same population of binding sites, albeit with different properties, reflecting, perhaps, a different mode of interaction with the δ-binding site of the opioid receptor complex. Moreover, in that

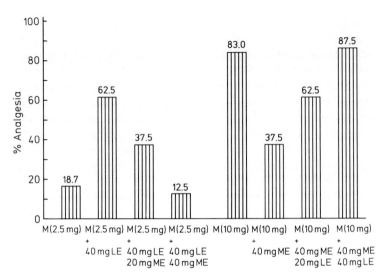

Fig. 4. Effects of simultaneous i.c.v. administration of varying doses of ME on a fixed potentiating dose of LE, and vice versa. (Illustration taken from Vaught et al. 1982)

subeffective doses of DADL, [D-Ser^2,Leu^5,Thr^6] enkephalin (DSLET), and DPDPE (Barrett and Vaught 1982; Heyman et al. 1989a) have been shown to potentiate, and subeffective doses of [D-Ala^2,Met^5]enkephalinamide (DAMA) (Vaught et al. 1982) have been shown to attenuate morphine antinociception, DADL, DSLET, and DPDPE would be expected to inter-act selectively with the LE-specific δ-binding site, whereas DAMA would be expected to interact selectively with the ME-specific δ-binding site.

Direct binding studies demonstrated that [^{3}H]LE and [^{3}H]ME label the same population of binding sites, and that the number of [^{3}H]ME binding sites was twice that of the [^{3}H]LE binding sites (Rothman and Westfall 1983a). Although the relationship between the different B_{max} values and the opposing effects of subeffective doses of ME and LE on morphine antinociception remains to be clarified, the lack of evidence for LE-specific and ME-specific δ-binding sites make a compelling case that the opposing effects of the pentapeptides are mediated via interactions at the same recep-tor. More recent data obtained by Porreca and associates (see below) considerably strengthens this hypothesis.

2. More Recent Studies: Analgesia Model

The work of Porreca and associates has considerably extended the early work of Vaught and associates. Of major importance is the finding that the selective δ-antagonist, N,N-diallyl-Tyr-Aib-Aib-Phe-Leu-OH (ICI174,864) (Cotton et al. 1984), which by itself does not affect morphine antinocicep-tion, blocks the potentiating action of subeffective doses of DPDPE or LE, and also blocks the attenuating action of subeffective doses of DAMA or ME (HEYMAN et al. 1989b). Given the high degree of selectivity of DPDPE (MOSBERG et al. 1983) and ICI174864 for δ-receptors, these data strongly suggest that modulation of morphine antinociception is mediated by a δ-receptor, although the data do not permit a conclusion as to whether it is the δ_{cx}- or δ_{ncx}-binding site.

Additionally, it was demonstrated that δ-agonists such as DPDPE and ME modulated not only the potency of μ-agonists such as morphine, but the efficacy as well (JIANG et al. 1990b). Thus in cases of severe nociceptive stimuli, or in situations of reduced maximal effect due to chronic exposure to the agonist (tolerance), the efficacy of μ-agonists could be enhanced. Importantly, the modulation of potency and efficacy could be achieved selectively, without enhancing the rate of development of antinociceptive tolerance to morphine (JIANG et al. 1990a). The modulatory effects were demonstrated to be mediated within the CNS, in that peripheral injection of LE could produce modulation of intracerebroventricular (i.c.v.) morphine antinociception, which was antagonized by i.c.v. ICI174,864 (JIANG et al. 1990c). This study also demonstrated that the interaction between LE and morphine was synergistic, rather than additive, a finding which supported the concept of an opioid receptor complex (JIANG et al. 1990c).

Experiments utilizing receptor-selective irreversible antagonists have clarified the issue of which δ-site mediates modulation of morphine antinociception (HEYMAN et al. 1989b). Pretreatment with the μ-opioid antagonists β-FNA and naloxonazine did not alter the direct analgesic actions of DPDPE or DAMA (HEYMAN et al. 1987). However, pretreatment with β-FNA prevented the modulation of morphine antinociception by both DPDPE and DAMA, while pretreatment with the long-acting μ_1-antagonist naloxonazine (PASTERNAK et al. 1980) failed to affect modulation of morphine antinociception by either DPDPE or DAMA. Thus, in light of the finding that i.c.v. administration of β-FNA selectively alkylates the δ_{cx}-binding site defined on the basis of in vitro binding studies (ROTHMAN et al. 1988b), these data demonstrate that the β-FNA-sensitive δ-receptor-modulating morphine antinociception can be identified as the δ_{cx}-binding site.

The simplest interpretation of the finding that naloxonazine attenuates morphine antinociception without altering its modulation by DPDPE or DAMA is that naloxonazine blocks the μ_{ncx}-binding site (see Sect. 2.12). However, this is apparently incompatible with the notion that the μ_1-binding site as most recently defined in vitro (CLARK et al. 1988) is similar to the δ_{cx}-binding site, as it is defined in vitro. Although it is possible that naloxonazine alters the opioid receptor complex so as to increase the ED_{50} for morphine antinociception and not alter the modulatory effects of DPDPE and DAMA, additional experiments are needed to clarify these issues.

The development of the irreversible δ-receptor ligand [D-Ala^2,Leu^5,Cys^6]enkephalin (DALCE) by BOWEN et al. (1987) provided an additional tool with which to explore the mechanism of δ-receptor-mediated modulation of morphine antinociception. As reported by JIANG et al. (1990d), administration of DALCE produced a transient antinociception, which was antagonized by ICI174864. DALCE pretreatment up to 24 h before testing, a time at which no remaining antinociception could be detected, blocked the i.c.v. antinociceptive effects of DPDPE and DALCE, but not that of morphine, suggesting long-lasting DALCE antagonism at the δ_{ncx}-receptor. Constituent this notion, recent studies demonstrated that pretreatment of membranes with DALCE decreases the B_{max} of the δ_{ncx} not the δ_{cx}, binding site (ROTHMAN et al., in prep.). Pretreatment of mice with DALCE did not alter the ability of subeffective doses of i.c.v. DPDPE or ME to potentiate or attenuate morphine antinociception. Subeffective doses of i.c.v. DALCE did not modulate morphine antinociception.

More recent studies (Q. JIANG et al. unpublished observations) have shown that, while DALCE fails to antagonize the modulatory actions of δ-agonists, a novel irreversible δ-antagonist, naltrindole-5'-isothiocyanate (5'-NTII), does (PORTOGHESE et al. 1990). Unlike DALCE, 5'-NTII does not produce any detectable antinociception, and does not block either direct μ- or DPDPE-mediated antinociception. In addition, recent studies with the DALCE analog [D-Ala^2,Leu^5,Ser^6]enkephalin (DALES) (MATTIA et al. 1990) have shown that this peptide does not modulate morphine anti-nociception, but does produce antinociception which is antagonized by both DALCE and ICI174864. These, and the data reviewed above, suggest that the δ-receptor which mediates modulation of morphine antinociception can be characterized as being sensitive to β-FNA and 5'-NTII, and insensitive to DALCE and naloxonazine. Studies of direct antinociception mediated via opioid δ receptors have been carried out using DALCE and 5'NTII as selective antagonists. On this basis, the receptors have been classified as either sensitive to the effects of DALCE and termed the δ_1 receptor or sensitive to the effects of 5'NTII and termed the δ_2 receptor (JIANG et al. 1991; MATTIA et al. 1991; MATTIA et al. 1992). Given the sensitivity of the μ-modulatory actions of opioid δ agonists to 5'NTII, it would appear reasonable to conclude that the δ receptor in the complex (δ_{cx}) would be analogous to the δ_2 receptor (MATTIA et al. 1992).

Ligand-binding data demonstrate that β-FNA selectively alkylates the μ-δ-opioid receptor complex, altering the conformation of the δ_{cx}-, but not the δ_{ncx}-site (ROTHMAN et al. 1988b). Moreover, pretreatment of membranes with DALCE irreversibly inhibits [^{3}H]DADL binding to the δ_{ncx}-site to a much greater extent than to the δ_{cx}-site (R.B. ROTHMAN et al. unpublished data). Thus the δ_{cx}-binding site, as characterized in vitro, is sensitive to β-FNA, but not to DALCE.

The in vitro and in vivo data reviewed above, and summarized in Table 2, provide a compelling case that (1) the site which mediates modulation of morphine antinociception is a δ-receptor; (2) that this site is sensitive to β-FNA and 5'-NTII, and is synonymous with the δ_{cx}-binding site defined on the basis of in vitro binding studies; (3) the site mediating the direct

Table 2. Tentative classification of opioid receptor responses based on i.c.v. administration and the mouse tail flick test

Agent	Opioid receptor complex		
	δ_{ncx} [9]	δ_{cx} [b]	μ_{cx}
A. Irreversible agents			
DALCE	Reversible agonist and irreversible antagonist	No known agonist effect	No known agonist effect
β-FNA	No known effect	Irreversible antagonist	Irreversible antagonist
5'-NTII	No known effect	Irreversible antagonist	No known effect
BIT	No known effect	Depletes the binding site	Depletes the binding site
FIT	Depletes the binding site	Alters the conformation of the binding site	Depletes the binding site
B. Reversible agents			
DPDPE	Agonist	Agonist, direct agonist	No known effect
DSLET[c] Deltorphin II	No known agonist effects	Agonist and direct agonist	No known effect
Oxymorphindole LE	No known agonist effect	Agonist	No known effect
DALES	Agonist	No known agonist effect	No known effect
ME	No effect	Inverse agonist	No known effect
DAMA4[d]	No effect	Inverse agonist	No known effect
ICI174864[d]	Antagonist	Antagonist at δ_{cx}	No known effect

Summarized above are the pharmacological actions of various agents at the μ_{cx}-, δ_{cx}-, and δ_{ncx}-binding sites.

[a] An agonist action at the δ_{ncx}-receptor is defined as antinociception blocked by pretreatment with DALCE but not by pretreatment with 5'-NTII.

[b] The terms agonist, antagonist, and inverse agonist at the δ_{cx}-site refer to agents which, at subantinociceptive doses, potentiate morphine antinociception, have no effect on morphine antinociception, or antagonize morphine antinociception, respectively. The term "direct agonist" refers to an agent which is thought to produce its direct antinociception via the δ_{cx}-binding site. The antinociception produced by these agents is insensitive to pretreatment with DALCE, but is antagonized by pretreatment with 5'-NTII.

[c] The direct antinociceptive effects of these agents are not blocked by DALCE, but are blocked by 5'-NTII (JIANG et al. 1992). In addition, a component of DSLET-induced antinociception occurs via the μ-receptor

[d] It is possible that a component of DAMA-induced antinociception occurs via the δ_{cx}-receptor, but this point has not yet been studied.

analgesic actions of DPDPE is sensitive to DALCE, is insensitive to β-FNA, naloxonazine, and 5'-NTII, and is synonymous with the δ_{ncx}-binding site; and (4) the data are most simply explained by the hypothesis of a μ-δ-opioid receptor complex. Similar data have also obtained in a model of urinary bladder motility, demonstrating that the pattern of δ-agonist–μ-agonist opioid responses reviewed above is not limited to the antinociceptive effects of morphine (SHELDON et al. 1989).

As illustrated in Table 2, the in vivo data suggest that DPDPE acts as an agonist at the δ_{cx}-binding site. However, in vitro binding studies demonstrate that it is highly selective for the δ_{ncx}-binding site, and binds weakly to the δ_{cx}-binding site (ROTHMAN et al. 1988a). Moreover, δ-receptor-mediated modulation of morphine-induced antinociception can always be demonstrated at doses lower than those needed to produce direct antinociception. Thus the in vivo and in vitro data are apparently incompatible. However, other data demonstrate that pretreatment of membranes with FIT alters the conformation of the δ_{cx}-binding site (ROTHMAN et al. 1985c), which results in a high-affinity interaction of DPDPE with that site (R.B. ROTHMAN et al. 1991). For example, pretreatment of membranes with (+)-trans-SUPERFIT, which is a more potent analog of FIT (KIM et al. 1989), decreased the IC_{50} of DPDPE for the δ_{cx}-binding site from $1523 \pm 59\,nM$ in lysed-P2 membranes to $49.6 \pm 8.0\,nM$, and increased the IC_{50} of naloxone from $30.5 \pm 2.1\,nM$ to $40.2 \pm 5.3\,nM$ (R.B. ROTHMAN et al. 1991). The finding that DPDPE does interact with high affinity at the δ_{cx}-binding site is consistent with the in vivo observations mentioned above. Alternatively, it is possible that even weak binding of DPDPE at the δ_{cx}-site is adequate to produce modulation of morphine-induced antinociception. Such a view is consistent with the finding that Leu-enkephalin and Het-enkephalin can produce modulatory effects on morphine antinociception without eliciting direct antinociception (JIANG et al. 1990c; HORAN et al. 1992).

III. μ-Antagonist–δ-Antagonist Interactions

As pointed out in a recent review article (HOLADAY et al. 1990), in order to demonstrate interactions among opioid receptor types, it is necessary to evaluate responses following combinations of agonist and antagonist ligands. Using this approach, HOLADAY and associates obtained data in three different experimental systems which is most simply explained by a μ-δ-opioid receptor complex (Table 3).

In the endotoxic shock model, D'AMATO and HOLADAY (1984) demonstrated that whereas the μ-selective antagonists β-FNA, naloxazone [and later naloxonazine (HAHN and PASTERNAK 1982; LING et al. 1986)] and dynorphin(1–13) failed to reverse endotoxic hypotension, high doses of naloxone or the δ-selective antagonists ICI154129 and ICI174864 were effective, indicating that endogenous opioids contribute to endotoxic hypotension by acting at δ-receptors. However, pretreatment of rats with β-FNA, naloxazone, or dynorphin(1–13) attenuated the ability of the δ-antagonists to reverse endotoxic hypotension presumably produced by endogenous δ-receptor ligands.

A similar pattern was demonstrated by TORTELLA et al. (1985) in a model of flurothyl-induced seizures in the rat. In this model, activation of both μ- and δ-receptors elevated the seizure threshold. For example, the anticonvulsant effects of etorphine were completely blocked by the μ-antagonist β-FNA, but not by the δ-antagonist ICI154129. Conversely, the anticonvulsant effects of DADL were partially antagonized by β-FNA, but completely antagonized by ICI154129. However, pretreatment of rats with β-FNA attenuated the ability of ICI154129 to antagonize DADL. Thus, as observed in the endotoxic shock model, pretreatment with a μ-antagonist attenuated the ability of a δ-antagonist to block δ-agonist effects. Similar results were also observed where the pharmacological endpoint was striatal cAMP levels (HOLADAY et al. 1986), an important observation in view of the binding data demonstrating enrichment of the opioid receptor complex in the striatum (reviewed above).

The occurrence of this same pattern of responses across three separate models of opioid responses is most simply explained by a μ-δ-opioid receptor complex. Occupation of either the μ_{cx}- or the δ_{cx}-site by the corresponding selective agonist produces a response which is antagonized by the appropriate selective antagonist. Administration of a μ-antagonist such as β-FNA produces a conformational change in the δ_{cx}-site, which does not affect the binding of an agonist, but decreases the affinity of an antagonist for the δ_{cx}-site. In vitro binding studies described in the next section support this hypothesis.

IV. Linkage Studies

The in vivo evidence for a μ-δ-opioid receptor complex reviewed in the previous sections is somewhat paradoxical. In the antinociception model, the receptor complex is detected by the ability of subeffective doses of enkephalin-related peptides to modulate morphine antinociception. In the models developed by Holaday and associates (D'AMATO and HOLADAY 1984; TORTELLA et al. 1985; HOLADAY et al. 1986), the receptor complex is detected by a μ-antagonist attenuating the ability of a δ-antagonist to

Table 3. Experimental systems demonstrating antagonist-antagonist interactions

System	μ-Antagonist	δ-Antagonist
Endotoxic shock	β-FNA naloxazone dynorphin(1–13)	High-dose naloxone ICI174864 ICI154129
Seizures	β-FNA dynorphin(1–13)	ICI154129 high-dose naloxone
Striatal cAMP	β-FNA dynorphin(1–13)	ICI174864 high-dose naloxone

reverse the effects of a δ-agonist. Thus the former model detects δ-agonist-μ-agonist interactions, while the latter detects μ-antagonist-δ-antagonist interactions. Although the symmetry of this formulation is appealing, the question arises of whether the μ-δ-receptor complex defined on the basis of in vitro ligand binding studies is the same entity as the μ-δ-receptor complexes postulated to mediate the interactive effects reviewed in previous sections.

To address this issue, ROTHMAN et al. (1988b) formulated and experimentally tested the following prediction: (1) if the μ-δ-receptor complex defined on the basis of ligand binding studies is the same as that defined by μ-antagonist-δ-antagonist interactions in vivo, then i.c.v. administration of β-FNA to rats, at the same dose used in the in vivo studies, should alter the conformation of the δ_{cx}-binding site such that the K_d of [^{3}H]DADL (an agonist) is not altered, but the IC_{50} of the antagonist for displacement of [^{3}H]DADL from the δ_{cx}-binding site is increased. To test this prediction, 20 nmol β-FNA was administered i.c.v. and brain membranes were prepared 18–24 h later. The results demonstrated that β-FNA selectively altered the δ_{cx}-, but not the δ_{ncx}-binding site. Although the K_d of [^{3}H]DADL for the δ_{cx}-site was not altered, pretreatment of rats with β-FNA increased the IC_{50} value for naloxone and naltrexone to displace [^{3}H]DADL from the δ_{cx}-site by a factor of two. Similar data were obtained when membranes were pretreated with β-FNA in vitro. In other words, these in vitro data complemented in vivo findings that the μ-antagonist β-FNA attenuated the actions of high concentrations of naloxone and naltrexone at the δ_{cx}-binding site.

The selective effect of β-FNA on the δ_{cx}-binding site suggested a way to test the linkage between the receptor complex defined on the basis of in vitro binding studies with that defined by the antinociception model: administration of β-FNA should prevent the modulatory effects of δ-ligands, which are mediated via the δ_{cx}-site, but not their direct antinociceptive effects, which are mediated via the δ_{ncx}-site. As described in Sect. B.II, this prediction was experimentally confirmed (HEYMAN et al. 1989b).

C. Evidence for a κ-Binding Site Associated with the μ-δ-Opioid Receptor Complex

The consistent observation (Table 3) that compounds described as κ-agonists, i.e., β-FNA and dynorphin(1–13), are μ-antagonists and additionally attenuate the action of δ-antagonists, supports the hypothesis that the μ-δ-opioid receptor complex also has an associated κ-binding site (HOLADAY et al. 1986, 1990).

The work of SHELDON et al. (1987) provides additional support for this concept. Their study demonstrated that subeffective doses of the κ-agonists, U50,488H, ethylketocyclazocine, and tifluadom attenuated the ability of morphine and normorphine, but not several other μ-agonists, to inhibit the micturition reflex. Moreover, i.c.v. administration of subeffective doses of DPDPE potentiated the effects of morphine and normorphine on the micturition reflex, but not the effects of other μ-agonists (SHELDON et al. 1989). Additionally, HEYMAN et al. (1989a) demonstrated that i.c.v. administration of DPDPE potentiated morphine and normorphine antinociception, but not antinociception produced by several other μ-agonists. Further, PORRECA and TORTELLA have demonstrated that the κ-agonist U50,488H selectively antagonizes morphine in the rat flurothyl seizure model (PORRECA and TORTELLA 1987). These observations in three different model systems demonstrating selective modulation of morphine- and normorphine-induced effects suggests that the inhibitory effects of κ-agonists are mediated via the μ-δ-opioid receptor complex.

Some ligand binding studies provide support for a κ-binding site associated with the μ-binding sites (DEMOLIOU-MASON and BARNARD 1986a,b). However, this μ-κ-receptor complex has not been shown to be synonymous with the μ-δ-opioid receptor complex. Although the data reviewed above are most simply explained by an interaction of κ-agonists with a κ-binding site associated with the μ-δ-opioid receptor complex, they can also be explained by an interaction of the κ-agonists with the μ_{cx}-binding site.

I. In Vitro, Electrophysiological, Anatomical, and Biochemical Evidence for a μ-δ-Opioid Receptor Complex

Until recently, the data supporting the hypothesis of a μ-δ-opioid receptor complex were obtained from in vitro ligand binding studies and experiments measuring opioid responses in whole animals. The work by SCHOFFELMEER et al. (1988) provided data from an in vitro slice preparation. These investigators demonstrated that dopamine D1 receptor-stimulated-cAMP efflux from striatal slices was inhibited by DAMGO or DPDPE, and that these effects were blocked by either low-dose naloxone or pretreatment of the slices with FIT, respectively. Although FIT did not alter the effect of DAMGO, it blocked the ability of naloxone to reverse the effect of DAMGO. The authors suggested that these data provided evidence for a functional μ-δ-opioid receptor complex, and complement the cAMP data of HOLADAY et al. (1986). Consistent with these observations are the findings reviewed earlier that pretreatment of membranes with (+)-*trans*-SUPERFIT increases the IC_{50} of naloxone at the δ_{cx}-binding site (ROTHMAN et al. 1990).

Electrophysiological studies demonstrated that both μ- and δ-receptors are coupled to potassium channels (NORTH et al. 1987). Consistent with their colocalization in a μ-δ-opioid receptor complex, both ZIEGLGÄNSBERGER (personal communication to J.W. HOLADAY) and SHEN and CRAIN (1989) found μ- and δ-receptors coexisting on the same neurons. However, no interaction studies have been reported in electrophysiological model systems.

Anatomical studies demonstrating a differential distribution of μ- and δ-receptors in the brain are compatible with the model of the opioid receptors presented in Fig. 1 (Goodman et al. 1980; McLean et al. 1986), since these studies are optimized to label the δ_{ncx}-binding site. On the other hand, experiments optimized to label the δ_{cx}-site demonstrate colocalization with μ-binding sites (Rothman et al. 1985b).

Schoffelmeer et al. (1990) recently reported biochemical evidence for a μ-δ-opioid receptor complex in rat caudate. In this study, both DAMGO and δ-selective ligand, DSTBULET, displaced [^{125}I]β-endorphin binding in a monophasic manner, consistent with the labeling of a single class of binding sites. DSTBULET noncompetitively inhibited [^{3}H]DAMGO binding. Cross-linking experiments determined that the apparent molecular weight of the [^{125}I]β-endorphin binding site was about 80 kDa, about twice that of separately isolated μ- or δ-binding sites. These data collectively demonstrate the biochemical identification of a μ-δ-opioid receptor complex. It would be of interest to perform a "linkage" study, and determine if the μ-δ-opioid receptor complex as biochemically defined is synonymous with the receptor complex defined on the basis of the ligand binding and whole animal studies reviewed in earlier sections of this chapter.

D. Conclusions

The in vivo data reviewed in this chapter clearly illustrate that examining the effects of combinations of selective opioid agonists and antagonists on opioid pharmacological responses reveals different patterns of response than observed in single agent studies. In particular, independently conducted studies using six different model systems generate data compatible with the hypothesis of a μ-δ-opioid receptor complex. Several hypotheses must be considered when attempting to explain these repeating patterns of pharmacological responses observed in whole animal studies, the results obtained with slice preparations (Schoffelmeer et al. 1988), the in vitro binding data demonstrating allosteric interaction between μ- and δ-binding sites, and recently reported biochemical demonstration of a μ-δ-opioid receptor complex (Schoffelmeer et al. 1990).

1. Combinations of ligands may alter the uptake or metabolism of other ligands.
2. Interpretation of experiments conducted in vivo and with brain slices are complicated by the existence of neuronal networks.
3. Combinations of ligands may result in alterations in coupling to second messenger systems.
4. There exists a μ-δ-opioid receptor complex.

The fact that interactions among opioid receptor types have been demonstrated using many structurally diverse compounds suggests that altered metabolism or uptake are unlikely hypotheses. Moreover, the effects of β-FNA and dynorphin(1–13) are seen at a time when these agents have no effect on their own. Although the neuronal network hypothesis cannot be entirely ruled out, in view of the absence of data demonstrating LE- and ME-specific binding sites, and in view of the general concordance of biochemical, ligand binding and pharmacological experiments, it is difficult to conceive of how the neuronal network hypothesis can explain the data.

Although the existence of a μ-δ-opioid receptor complex is not conclusively proven, this hypothesis provides the simplest explanation of the data. The third hypothesis that combinations of ligands may result in alterations in coupling to second messenger systems provides a possible mechanism for how occupation of the μ-δ-receptor complex by different ligands might result in altered responses, as has been proposed for antinociception (VAUGHT et al. 1982).

The recognition of the existence of a μ-δ-opioid receptor complex as well as μ-, δ-, and κ-binding sites not associated with the receptor complex (Fig. 1) presents new opportunities for drug development, since it is likely that the μ-, δ-, and perhaps κ-binding sites associated with the opioid receptor complex will have a different ligand-selectivity pattern than the opioid binding sites not associated with the receptor complex. Although it is certainly premature to speculate on this point, it is possible that a greater understanding of the structure and function of the μ-δ-opioid receptor complex in relation to the spectrum of opioid-induced pharmacological responses will lead to the development of nonaddicting analgesics and new treatments for substance abuse.

References

Bals-Kubik R, Shippenberg TS, Herz A (1990) Involvement of central mu and delta opioid receptors in mediating the reinforcing effects of beta-endorphin in the rat. Eur J Pharmacol 175:63–69

Barrett RW, Vaught JL (1982) The effects of receptor selective opioid peptides on morphine-induced analgesia. Eur J Pharmacol 80:427–430

Bowen WD, Gentlemen S, Herkenham M, Pert CB (1981) Interconverting mu and delta forms of the opiate receptors in rat striatal patches. Proc Natl Acad Sci USA 78:4818–4822

Bowen WD, Hellewell SB, Kelemen M, Huey R, Stewart D (1987) Affinity labeling of delta-opiate receptors using [D-Ala^2,Leu^5,Cys^6]enkephalin. Covalent attachment via thiol-disulfide exchange. J Biol Chem 262:13434–13439

Cho TM, Hasegaua J, Ge BL, Loh HH (1886) Purification to homogeneity of a mu-type of opioid receptor from rat brain. Proc Natl Acad Sci USA 83: 4138–4142

Clark JA, Houghten R, Pasternak GW (1988) Opiate binding in calf thalamic membranes: a selective μ_1 binding assay. Mol Pharmacol 34:308–317

Cotton R, Giles MG, Miller L, Shaw JS, Tims D (1984) ICI174,864: a highly selective anatgonist for the opioid delta-receptor. Eur J Pharmacol 97:331–332

Creese I, Snyder SH (1975) Receptor binding and pharmacological activity of opiates in the guinea-pig intestine. J Pharmacol Exp Ther 194:205–219

D'Amato R, Holaday JW (1984) Multiple opiate receptors in endotoxic shock: evidence for delta involvement and mu-delta interactions in vivo. Proc Natl Acad Sci USA 81:2898–2901

Danks JD, Tortella FC, Long JB, Bykov V, Jacobson AE, Rice KC, Holaday JW, Rothman RB (1988) Chronic administration of morphine and naltrexone up-regulate ^{3}H-[D-ala^2,D-leu^5]enkephalin binding sites by different mechanisms. Nauropharmacology 27:965–974

Demoliou-Mason CD, Barnard EA (1986a) Distinct subtypes of the opioid receptor with allosteric interactions in brain membranes. J Neurochem 46:1118–1128

Demoliou-Mason CD, Barnard EA (1986b) Characterization of opioid receptor subtypes in solution. J Neurochem 46:1129–1136

Gioannini TL, Howard AD, Hiller JM, Simon EJ (1985) Purification of an active opioid binding protein from bovine striatum. J Biol Chem 260:15117–15121

Goodman RR, Synder SH, Kuhar MJ, Young WS III (1980) Differentiation of delta and mu receptor localizations by light microscopic autoradiography. Proc Natl Acad Sci USA 77:6239–6243

Hahn EF, Pasternak GW (1982) Naloxonazine, a potent, long-lasting inhibitor of opiate binding sites. Life Sci 31:1385–1388

Heyman JS, Mulvaney SA, Mosberg HI, Porreca F (1987) Opioid delta-receptor involvement in supraspinal and spinal antinociception in mice. Brain Res 420:100–108

Heyman JS, Vaught JL, Mosberg HI, Haaseth RC, Porreca F (1989a) Modulation of mu-mediated antinociception by delta agonists in the mouse: selective potentiation of morphine and normorphine by [D-Pen^2,D-Pen^5]enkephalin. Eur J Pharmacol 165:1–10

Heyman JS, Jiang Q, Rothman RB, Mosberg HI, Porreca F (1989b) Modulation of mu-mediated antinociception by delta agonists: characterization with antagonists. Eur J Pharmacol 169:43–52

Holaday JW, Tortella FC, Maneckjee R, Long JB (1986) In vivo interaction among opiate receptor agonists and antagonists. In: Brown RM, Clouet DH, Friedman DP (eds) Opiate receptor subtypes and brain function. Natl Inst Drug Abuse Res Monogr Ser 71:173–188

Holaday JW, Porreca F, Rothman RB (1990) Functional coupling among opioid receptor types: implications for anesthesiology. In: Estafanous FG (ed) Opioids in anesthesia II. Butterworth-Heineman, Boston, pp 50–60

Horan P, Tallarida RJ, Haaseth R, Matsunaga T, Hruby VJ, Porreca, F (1992) Antinociceptive interactions of opioid delta receptor agonists with morphine in mice: supra- and subadditivity. Life Sciences 50

Jiang Q, Mosberg HI, Porreca F (1990a) Selective modulation of morphine antinociceptive potency, but not development of tolerance, by delta agonists in the mouse. J Pharmacol Exp Ther 186:137–141

Jiang Q, Mosberg HI, Porreca F (1990b) Modulation of the potency and efficacy of mu-mediated antinociception by delta agonists in the mouse. J Pharmacol Exp Ther 254:683–689

Jiang Q, Tallarida RJ, Porreca F (1990c) Modulation of morphine antinociception by peripherally-administered [Leu^5]enkephalin: demonstration of a synergistic interaction. Eur J Pharmacol 179:463–468

Jiang Q, Bowen WD, Mosberg HI, Rothman RB, Porreca F (1990d) Opioid agonist and antagonist antinociceptive properties of [D-Ala^2,Leu^5,Cys^6]enkephalin: selective actions at the delta(noncomplexed) site. J Pharmacol Exp Ther 255: 636–641

Jiang Q, Takemori AE, Sultana M, Portoghese PS, Bowen WD, Mosberg HI, Porreca F (1991) Differential antagonism of opioid delta antinociception by [D-Ala^2,Leu^5,Cyc^6]enkephalin (DALCE) and Naltrindole 5'isothiocyanate (5'-NTII): Evidence for δ receptor subtypes. J Pharmacol Exp Ther 257:1069–1075

Kim C-H, Rothman RB, Jacobson AE, Mattson MV, Bykov V, Streaty RA, Klee WA, George C, Long JB, Rice KC (1989) Probes for narcotic receptor mediated phenomena. 15. (3S,4S)-(+)-*trans*-3-methylfentanyl isothiocyanate, a potent site-directed acylating agent for the delta opioid receptors in vitro. J Med Chem 32:1392–1398

Lee NM, Smith AP (1980) A protein-lipid model of the opiate receptor. Life Sci 26:1459–1464

Lee NM, Leybn L, Chang J-K, Loh HH (1980) Opiate and peptide interaction: effect of enkephalins on morphine analgesia. Eur J Pharmacol 68:181–185

Ling GS, Simantov R, Clark JA, Pasternak GW (1986) Naloxonazine actions in vivo. Eur J Pharmacol 129:33–38

Mattia A, Vanderah T, Mosberg HI, Bowen WD, Porreca F (1991) Pharmacological characterization of [D-Ala^2,Leu^5,Ser^6]enkephalin (DALES): antinociceptive actions at the delta(non-complexed) receptor. Eur J Pharmacol 192:371–376

Mattia A, Vanderah T, Mosberg HI, Porreca F (1991) Lack of antinociceptive cross-tolerance between [D-Pen^2,D-Pen^5]enkephalin and [D-Ala^2]deltorphin II in mice: Evidence for delta receptor subtypes. J Pharmacol Exp Ther 258:583–587

Mattia A, Farmer SC, Takemori AE, Sultana M, Portoghese PS, Mosberg HI, Bowen WD, Porreca F (1992) Spinal opioid delta antinociception in the mouse: mediation by a single subtype of opioid delta receptor. J Pharmacol Exp Ther 260:518–525

McGonigle P, Neve KA, Molinoff PB (1986) A quantitative method of analyzing the interaction of slightly selective radioligands with multiple receptor subtypes. Mol Pharmacol 30:329–337

McLean S, Rothman RB, Herkenham M (1986) Autoradiographic localization of mu and delta opiate receptors in the forebrain of the rat. Brain Res 378:49–60

Mosberg HI, Hurst R, Hruby VJ, Gee K, Yamamura HI, Galligan JJ, Burkes TF (1983) Bis-penicillamine enkephalins possess highly improved specificity toward delta opioid receptors. Proc Natl Acad Sci USA 80:5871–5874

Neve KA, McGonigle P, Molinoff PB (1986) Quantitative analysis of the selectivity of radioligands for subtypes of beta adrenergic receptors. J Pharmacol Exp Ther 238:46–53

North RA, Williams JT, Surprenant A, Christie MJ (1987) MU and delta receptors belong to a family of receptors that are coupled to potassium channels. Proc Natl Acad Sci USA 84:5487–5491

Pasternak GW, Childers SR, Snyder SH (1980) Naloxazone, a long-acting opiate antagonist: effects on analgesia in intact animals and on opiate receptor binding in vitrol. J Pharmacol Exp Ther 214:455–462

Pert CB, Snyder SH (1974) Opiate receptor binding of agonists and antagonists affected differentially by sodium. Mol Pharmacol 10:868–879

Porreca F, Tortella FC (1987) Differential antagonism of mu agonists by U50,488H in the rat. Life Sci 41:2511–2516

Portoghese PS, Sultana M, Takemori AE (1990) Naltrindole 5'-isothiocyanate: a nonequilibrium, highly selective delta opioid receptor antagonist [letter]. J Med Chem 33:1547–1548

Rice KC, Jacobson AE, Burke TR Jr, Bajwa BS, Streaty RA, Klee WA (1983) Irreversible ligands with high selectivity toward mu or delta opiate receptors. Science 220:314–316

Robson LE, Paterson SJ, Kosterlitz HW (1983) Opiate receptors. Handb Psychopharmacol 17:13–80

Rothman RB (1981) Evidence for an opioid receptor complex. PhD Thesis, University of Virginia, Charlottesville, Virginia

Rothman RB (1983) Analysis of binding surfaces: a methodology appropriate for the investigation of complex receptor mechanisms and multiple neurotransmitter receptors. Neuropeptides 4:41–44

Rothman RB (1986) Binding surface analysis: an intuitive yet quantitative method for the design and analysis of ligand binding studies. Alcohol Drug Res 6: 309–325

Rothman RB, McLean S (1988) An examination of the opiate receptor subtypes labeled by [^{3}H]cycloFOXY: an opiate antagonist suitable for positron emission tomography. Biol Psychol 23:435–458

Rothman RB, Westfall TC (1980) Noncompetitive inhibition by morphine of the binding of ^{3}H-leucine enkephalin to crude membranes prepared from rat brain. Fed Proc 39:385–385

Rothman RB, Westfall TC (1982a) Morphine allosterically modulates the binding of ^{3}H-leucine enkephalin to a particulate fraction of rat brain. Mol Pharmacol 21:538–547

Rothman RB, Westfall TC (1982b) Allosteric coupling between morphine and enkephalin receptors in vitro. Mol Pharmacol 21:548–557

Rothman RB, Westfall TC (1983a) Further evidence for an opioid receptor complex. J Neurobiol 14:341–351

Rothman RB, Westfall TC (1983b) Interaction of leucine enkephalin with ^{3}H-naloxone binding in rat brain: evidence for an opioid receptor complex. Neurochem Res 8:913–931

Rothman RB, Barrett RW, Vaught JL (1983) Multidimensional analysis of ligand binding data: application to opioid receptors. Neuropeptides 3:367–377

Rothman RB, Bowen WD, Bykov V, Schumacher UK, Pert CB, Jacobson AE, Burke TR Jr, Rice KC (1984a) Preparation of rat brain membranes greatly enriched with either type-I-delta or type-II-delta opiate binding sites using site directed alkylating agents. Neuropeptides 4:201–215

Rothman RB, Pert CB, Jacobson AE, Burke TR Jr, Rice KC (1984b) Morphine noncompetitively inhibits the binding of [^{3}H]leucine enkephalin to a preparation of rat brain membranes lacking type-II delta receptors. Neuropeptides 4: 257–260

Rothman RB, Danks JA, Pert CB (1984c) Ionic conditions differentially affect ^{3}H-DADL binding to type-I and type-II opiate delta receptors in vitro. Neuropeptides 4:261–268

Rothman RB, Danks JA, Jacobson AE, Burke TR Jr, Rice KC (1985a) Leucine enkephalin noncompetitively inhibits the binding of [^{3}H]naloxone to the opiate mu recognition site: evidence for delta – >mu binding site interactions in vitro. Neuropeptides 6:351–363

Rothman RB, Bowen WD, Herkenham M, Jacobson AE, Rice KC, Pert CB (1985b) A quantitative study of [^{3}H]D-Ala^2-D-Leu^5-enkephalin binding to rat brain membranes. Evidence that oxymorphone is a noncompetitive inhibitor of the lower affinity delta-binding site. Mol Pharmacol 27:399–409

Rothman RB, Danks JA, Herkenham M, Jacobson AE, Burke TR Jr, Rice KC (1985c) Evidence that the delta-selective alkylating agent, FIT, alters the mu-noncompetitive opiate delta binding site. Neuropeptides 6:227–237

Rothman RB, Jacobson AE, Rice KC, Herkenham M (1987a) Autoradiographic evidence for two classes of mu opioid binding sites in rat brain using [^{125}I]FK33824. Peptides 8:1015–1021

Rothman RB, McLean S, Sykov V, Lessor RA, Jacobson AE, Rice KC, Holaday JW (1987b) Chronic morphine up-regulates a mu-opiate binding site labeled by ^{3}H-cycloFOXY: a novel opiate antagonist suitable for positron emission tomography. Eur J Pharmacol 142:73–81

Rothman RB, Bykov V, Ofri D, Rice KC (1988a) LY164929: a highly selective ligand for the lower affinity [^{3}H]D-ala^2-D-leu^5-enkephalin binding site. Neuropeptides 11:13–16

Rothman RB, Mahboubi A, Bykov V, Kim C-H, Jacobson AE, Rice KC (1991) Probing the opioid receptor complex with (+)-trans-SUPERFIT I. Evidence that [D-Pen^2,D-Pen^5]enkephalin interacts with high affinity at the δ_{cx} binding site. Peptides 12:359–364

Rothman RB, Long JB, Bykov V, Jacobson AE, Rice KC, Holaday JW (1988b) Beta-FNA binds irreversibly to the opiate receptor complex: in vivo and in vitro evidence. J Pharmacol Exp Ther 247:405–416

Rothman RB, Bykov V, Long JB, Brady LS, Jacobson AE, Rice KC, Holaday JW (1989) Chronic administration of morphine and naltrexone up-regulate opioid binding sites labeled by ^{3}H-[D-ala^2-MePhe^4,Gly-ol^5]enkephalin: evidence for two mu binding sites. Eur J Pharmacol 160:71–82

Rovati GE, Rodbard D, Munson PJ (1990) DESIGN: computerized optimization of experimental design for estimating K_d and B_{max} in ligand binding experiments: II. Simultaneous analysis of homologous and heterologous competition curves and analysis blocking and of "multiligand" dose-response surfaces. Anal Biochem 184:173–183

Schoffelmeer AN, Rice KC, Heijna MH, Hogenboom F, Mulder AH (1988) Fentanyl isothiocyanate reveals the existence of physically associated mu- and delta-opioid receptors mediating inhibition of adenylate cyclase in rat neostriatum. Eur J Pharmacol 149:179–182

Schoffelmeer AN, Yao YH, Gioannini TL, Hiller JM, Ofri D, Roques BP, Simon EJ (1990) Cross-linking of human [^{125}I]beta-endorphin to opioid receptors in rat striatal membranes: biochemical evidence for the existence of a mu/delta opioid receptor complex. J Pharmacol Exp Ther 253:419–426

Sheldon RG, Nunan L, Porreca F (1987) Mu antagonist properties of kappa agonists in a model of rat urinary bladder motility in vivo. J Pharmacol Exp Ther 243:234–240

Sheldon RJ, Nunan L, Porreca F (1989) Differential modulation by [D-Pen^2,D-Pen^5]enkephalin and dynorphin A-(1-17) of the inhibitory bladder motility effects of selected mu agonists in vivo. J Pharmacol Exp Ther 249:462–469

Shen K-F, Crain SM (1989) Dual modulation of the action potential duration of mouse dorsal root ganglion neurons in culture. Brain Res 491:227–242

Simon J, Benyhe S, Hepp J, Khan A, Borsodi A, Szücs M, Medzihradszky K, Wollemann M (1987) Purification of a kappa-opioid receptor subtype from frog brain. Neuropeptides 10:19–28

Simonds WF, Burke TR Jr, Rice KC, Jacobson AE, Klee WA (1985) Purification of the opiate receptor of NG108-15 neuroblastoma-glioma hybrid cells. Proc Natl Acad Sci USA 82:4974–4978

Szücs M, Borsodi A, Bogdány A, Gaäl J, Batke J, Töth G (1987) Detailed analysis of heterogeneity of [^{3}H]naloxone binding sites in rat brain synaptosomes. Neurochem Res 12:581–587

Tortella FC, Robles L, Holaday JW (1985) The anticonvulsant effects of DADL are primarily mediated by activation of delta opioid receptors: interaction between delta and mu-receptor antagonists. Life Sci 37:497–503

Vaught JL, Takemori AE (1979) Differential effects of leucine and methionine enkephalin on morphine-induced analgesia, acute tolerance and dependence. J Pharmacol Exp Ther 208:86–90

Vaught JL, Rothman RB, Westfall TC (1982) Mu and delta receptors: their role in analgesia and in the differential effects of opioid peptides on analgesia Life Sci 30:1443–1455

Section B: Chemistry of Opioids with Alkaloid Structure

CHAPTER 11

Chemistry of Nonpeptide Opioids

S. ARCHER

A. Introduction

During the past three decades interest in nonpeptide opioids has been rekindled in part by the introduction of a clinically acceptable analgesic of the mixed agoinst-antagonist type with reduced addiction liability (ARCHER et al. 1962), which was followed by the seminal papers by Martin (MARTIN 1967; MARTIN et al. 1976) on multiple opioid receptors. The next several years were marked by the development of more analgesics of the mixed agonist-antagonist class, pure narcotic antagonists devoid of agonist action, and the discovery of higher potent opioids in the oripavine, fentanyl, and meperidine series. On a parallel front the past few decades were marked by the introduction of a methadone maintenance program for narcotic addicts (DOLE and NYSWANDER 1965); and the realization that heroin abusers are particularly susceptible to AIDS has stimulated research on new modalities for treating opiate addicts.

Because of space limitations this chapter has focused on the chemistry of nonpeptide opioids, which have been of interest to biologists working in opioid research. Omitted from the discussion are such clinical standbys as dihydromorphinone, propoxyphene, and opioids which are used as anti-diarrheals. Portoghese and Takemori discuss in Chap. 12 certain antagonists which are not covered here. Several recent monographs (LENDICER 1982; CASY and PARFITT 1986; LENZ et al. 1987) have appeared in which the chemistry of nonpeptide opioids is discussed in greater detail.

B. Biosynthesis of Morphine, Codeine, and Thebaine

Opium is the dried juice of the unripe seed capsules of the poppy, Papaver somniferum. It contains about 10% morphine (1), 0.5% codeine (2), and 0.2% thebaine (3). In addition to these epoxymorphinans several benzylisoquinolines such as papaverine (13) and noscapine are present in opium. All these alkaloids are derived from a common biosynthetic inter-mediate, nor-reticuline (11), as shown in Schemes 1 and 2 (TORSELL, 1983).

Tyrosine (4) is oxidatively deaminated to p-hydroxyphenylpyruvic acid (5), which in turn is converted to 3,4-dihydroxyphenylpyruvic acid (6). By a separate pathway tyrosine is hydroxylated to furnish L-DOPA (7), which

Scheme 1

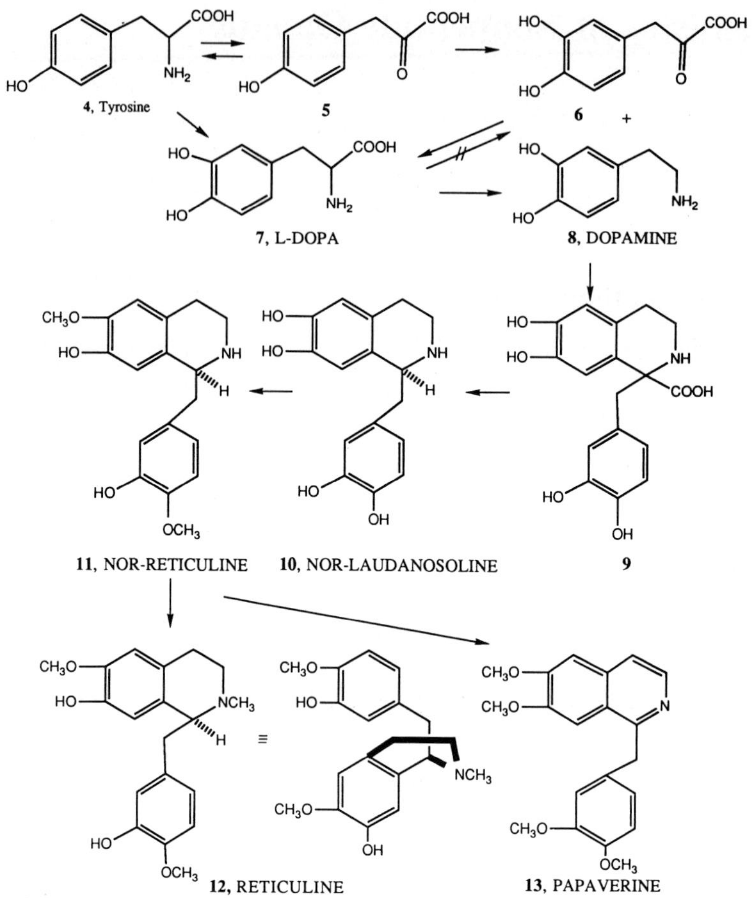

on decarboxylation gives dopamine (8). 3,4-Dihydroxyphenylpyruvic acid is also reductively aminated to L-DOPA but the reverse process is very slow. Coupling of structures 6 and 8 gives the amino acid (9), which is decarboxylated to nor-laudanosoline (10), methylation of which furnishes nor-reticuline (11). The latter is methylated to give S-reticuline (12), the precursor of the epoxymorphinan alkaloids as shown in Scheme 2. In a parallel pathway nor-reticuline is methylated and aromatized to afford the benzylisoquinoline, papaverine (13).

The biosynthetic conversion of S-reticuline to the epoxymorphinan alkaloids is shown in Scheme 2.

S-Reticuline (12) is oxidized to the diketone (14), which undergoes o-p coupling to give the ketone (15). Reduction furnishes salutaridine (16), a minor alkaloid which is found in various species of Papaver. Compound 16 is transformed to thebaine (3) via a ring closure, reduction, and dehydration. Hydrolysis of structure 3 gives neopinone, reduction of which followed

Scheme 2

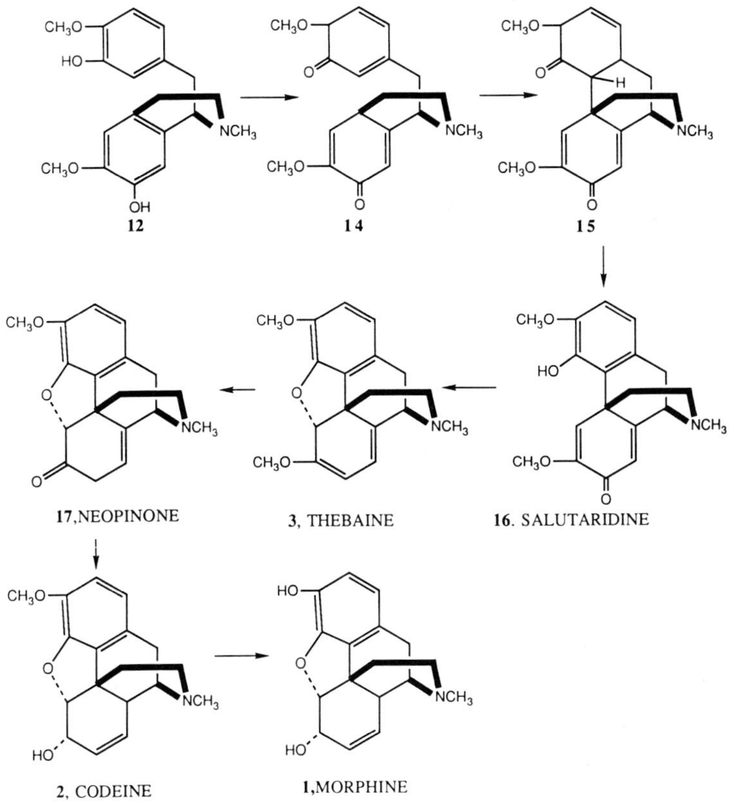

17,NEOPINONE   3, THEBAINE   16. SALUTARIDINE

2, CODEINE   1,MORPHINE

by isomerization affords codeine (2). Finally, enzymatic demethylation gives morphine. Since morphine is derived from S-reticuline it too must have the S configuration.

The presence of morphine in mammalian tissues has been established unequivocally and is the subject of Chap. 12. Until very recently the only evidence that this alkaloid was biosynthesized in mammals by the same pathway established in plants rested on the observations of Spector and his colleagues, who showed that administration of (+)salutaridine, (−)thebaine, and (−)codeine resulted in a marked increase in morphine levels in rat tissues (DONNERER et al. 1986). The recent careful demonstration of the conversion of (R)-[$N^{14}CH_3$]reticuline to salutaridine (16) by a cytochrome P-450 enzyme from pig liver by AMANN and ZENK (1991) confirmed and strengthened the earlier observations of Weitz, Faull, and Goldstein (WEITZ et al. 1987), who found that [^{3}H]reticuline was converted to salutaridine by rat liver. The experiments strongly support the view that mammalian tissues can biosynthesize opium alkaloids using the same pathways found in the poppy.

C. Morphine and Its Companions

Ever since the total synthesis of morphine was reported by Gates (GATES and TSCHUDI 1956) and Ginsburg (ELAD and GINSBURG 1954), many ingenious partial and total syntheses have been reported in an attempt to achieve a practical synthesis of this important alkaloid (TOTH et al. 1988; EVANS and MITCH 1982; SCHULTZ et al. 1985; SCHWARTZ et al. 1975; SZANTAY et al. 1982; WELL et al. 1985).

In an attempt to apply his eminently successful approach to the synthesis of morphinans, Grewe (GREWE and FRIEDRICHSON 1967) prepared the 1-benzylhexahydroisoquinoline (18), which underwent cyclization. Unfortunately, the predominant isomer was structure 19, obtained in 37% yield, instead of the desired structure 20, which was formed in only 3% yield.

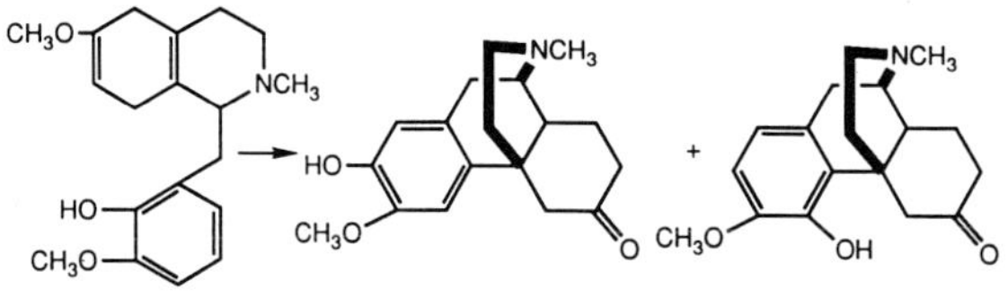

18 19 (37%) 20 (3%)

Beyerman (BEYERMAN et al. 1976) modified the Grewe approach by the simple but ingenious expedient of adding another hydroxyl group to structure 18 in such a way as to make the substitution on the benzyl group symmetrical (Scheme 3).

1-(3,5-Dihydroxy-4-methoxybenzyl-6-methoxy-tetrahydroisoquinoline (21) was subjected to a Birch reduction to give the previously reported 1-(3,5-dihydroxy-4-methoxybenzyl)hexahydroisoquinoline (22) (DEGRAW et

Scheme 3

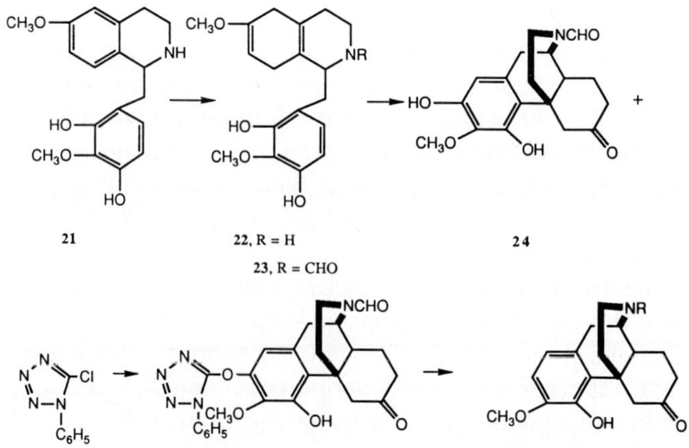

21 22, R = H 23, R = CHO 24

25 26 27, R = CHO 28, R = CH3

al. 1974). Treatment with ethyl formate gave the *N*-formyl derivative (23), which underwent a Grewe cyclization to the morphinan 24. The 2-hydroxyl group, having served its purpose, was removed by treating structure 24 with 5-chloro-1-phenyltetrazole (25), to give the ether 26, which on catalytic hydrogenation furnished racemic *N*-formyl nordihydrothebainone (27), whose spectral data (MS, IR, NMR) were identical with that of a sample prepared from (−)-dihydrothebainone (20). Since the latter has been converted to (−)codeine and (−)morphine (GATES and SHEPPARD 1962; WELLER and RAPOPORT 1976), this sequence almost constitutes a formal total synthesis of these alkaloids. (Strictly speaking, structure 26 must be resolved before this partial synthesis can qualify as a true formal total synthesis).

A complete total synthesis of both (+) and (−)morphine, as well as (+) and (−)codeine, was accomplished successfully in high overall yield by K.C. Rice and his group (RICE 1985) as shown in Scheme 4.

Scheme 4

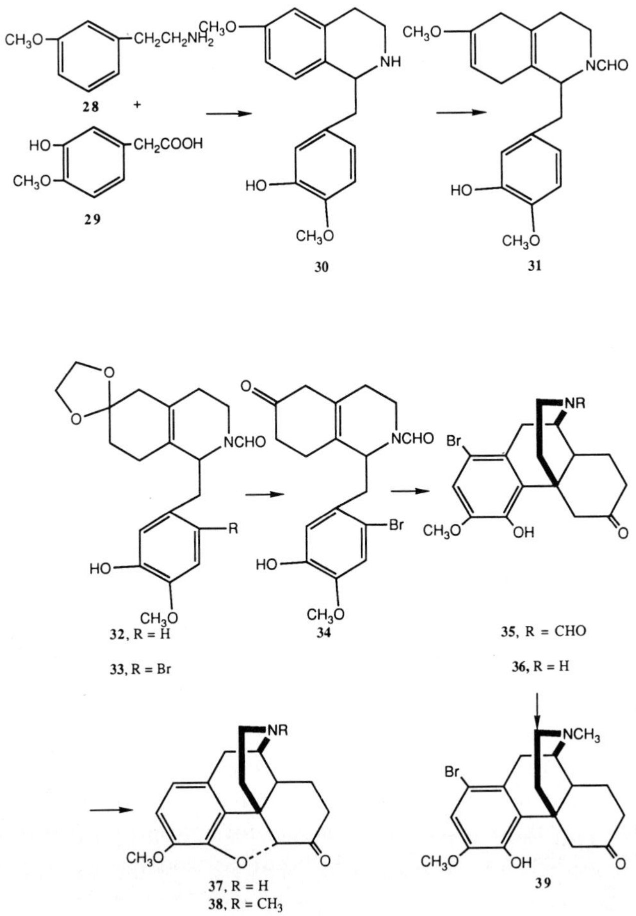

Condensation of the amine (28) with homoisovanillic acid (29) gave an amide which, on cyclization and subsequent catalytic hydrogenation, afforded the tetrahydroisoquinoline (30). Formylation followed by a Birch reduction furnished the enol ether (31), which was converted to the ketal (32). Bromination with *N*-bromosuccinimide gave the bromophenol (33), which was then hydrolyzed to the ketone (34). Treatment with trifluoromethanesulfonic acid resulted in the formation of the morphinan (35), which was readily transformed to the secondary amine (36). Treatment of the latter with bromine, followed by base, resulted in the formation of an epoxymorphinan which was reductively debrominated to structure 37 and then methylated to form (±)dihydrocodeinone (38). Catalytic debromination followed by methylation gave (±)dihydrothebainone [(±)-39]. Resolution of structure 30 gave both the "unnatural" (+) and "natural" (−) isomers which were carried through the same sequence to give (+) and (−)-39. A method was developed to racemize structure 30 efficiently so that the unwanted isomer could be recycled through the resolution step. (−)Dihydrothebainone (39) was converted to codeine and thebaine in high yield (WELLER and RAPOPORT 1976) as shown in Scheme 5.

Scheme 5

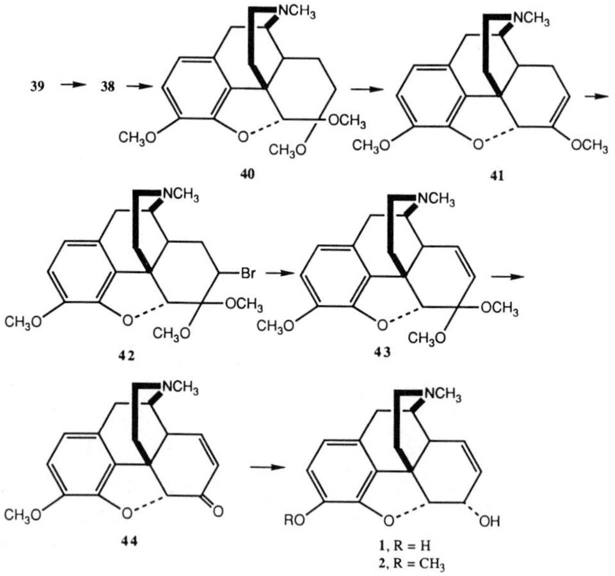

(−)Dihydrothebainone (39) was converted to structure 38, which in turn was treated with trimethyl orthoformate to yield the ketal (40). Acid-catalyzed elimination of methanol gave Δ^6-dihydrothebainone (41), which was treated with methyl hypobromite to furnish structure 42. Treatment with potassium *t*-butoxide resulted in the formation of codeinone dimethyl ketal (43), which was easily hydrolyzed to codeinone (44). Reduction with sodium borohydride gave natural codeine (2). The overall yield from dihydrothebainone was 71%. RICE (1977) converted codeine to morphine (1) in very high yield. The overall yield of (±)dihydrothebainone (39) from *m*-methoxyphenylethyl amine was 37%. Recently Noyori (NOYORI and TAKAYA 1990) reported that his group was able to prepare the Rice inter-mediate (30) by an enantioselective reduction using BINAP catalysts (45a, 45b). This procedure eliminates the necessity for resolution and subsequent racemization of the unwanted isomer.

45a, R-BINAP   45b, S-BINAP

D. Transformation Products of Thebaine

Oxidation of thebaine (3) with hydrogen peroxide gave an intermediate, which readily hydrolyzed to 14β-hydroxycodeinone (46), which, on *O*-demethylation, was transformed to oxymorphone (47) (WEISS 1955). Reduction followed by acetylation furnished a diacetate (48), which, on *N*-demethylation, afforded the norbase (49). Alkylation with allyl bromide afforded naloxone (50) (LEWENSTEIN and FISHMAN 1966). Similarly, treat-ment of structure 49 with cyclopropylmethyl bromide afforded naltrexone (51) (BLUMBERG et al. 1967). Acylation of structure 49 with cyclobutyl-carbonyl chloride, followed by reduction with lithium aluminum hydride, gave nalbuphine (53) (PACHTER and MATOSSIAN 1968) as shown in Scheme 6.

Naloxone (50) is a pure narcotic antagonist devoid of any dysphoric effects (JASINSKI et al. 1967). Naltrexone (51) is a more potent antagonist than naloxone and does not produce dysphoric effects in man (GRITZ et al. 1976). Nalbuphine (53) is a mixed agonist-antagonist which produces less dysphoric effects than pentazocine (JAFFE and MARTIN 1990).

It has been suggested that agonist-antagonist behavior was regulated by different low-energy equatorial N-substituent conformers and in the 14β-hydroxy series the C_{14} hydroxyl, the protonated nitrogen, and the anionic site on the receptor form a ternary complex which was predicted to be stable over a small range of N-substituent conformations. The role of the 14β-hydroxyl group in reducing agonist effects in compounds such as naloxone or naltrexone was to select only one of the many low-energy conformers among the several possible. On the basis of this analysis, it was predicted that a 14β-substituent such as an ethoxyl group would restore agonist activity (LOEW and BERKOWITZ 1978).

Scheme 6

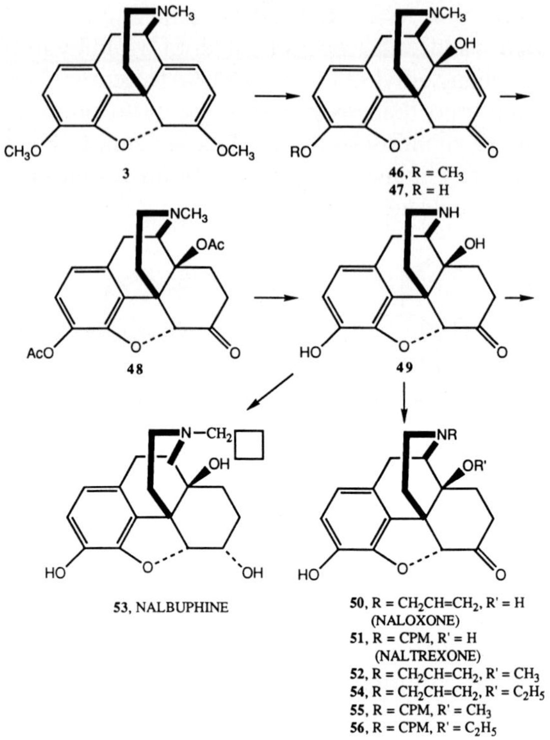
NCH3
CH3O
O
OCH3
3
OH
RO
46, R = CH3
47, R = H
OAc
AcO
48
NH
HO
49
N—CH2
53, NALBUPHINE
NR
OR'
50, R = CH2CH=CH2, R' = H
(NALOXONE)
51, R = CPM, R' = H
(NALTREXONE)
52, R = CH2CH=CH2, R' = CH3
54, R = CH2CH=CH2, R' = C2H5
55, R = CPM, R' = CH3
56, R = CPM, R' = C2H5

KOBYLECKL et al. (1982) tested this hypothesis by preparing four 14β-alkoxy analogs of naloxone and naltrexone. Alkylation of 14β-hydroxydihydrocodeinone with methyl and ethyl sulfates gave the corresponding 14β-alkoxy ethers, which were N-demethylated with vinyl chloroformate. The resulting nor-bases were then alkylated with either allyl or cyclopropylmethyl bromide and O-demethylated to give the naloxone analogs (52, 54) and the naltrexone analogs (55, 56). All four derivatives turned out to be pure antagonists.

Treatment of thebaine or *N*-cyclopropylnorthebaine with thiocyanogen gave the 14β-thiocyanato compounds (57, 58), which were converted to 14β-mercaptomorphine (59) and 14β-mercapto-*N*-cyclopropyl normorphine (60) by reduction with lithium aluminum hydride. The 14β-bromo and 14β-chloro derivatives were prepared by treating thebaine or *N*-cyclopropylnorthebaine with *N*-bromosuccinimide or *N*-chlorosuccinimide, procedures which gave structures 61, 62, 63, and 64, respectively. Demethylation with boron tribromide resulted in the formation of the corresponding morphinones 65, 66, 67, and 68 (OSEI-GYIMAH and ARCHER 1980; OSEI-GYIMAH et al. 1981). The transformations are shown in Scheme 7.

The introduction of the 14β-nitro group was first carried out by ALLEN and KIRBY (1970), who used the potentially hazardous reagent

Scheme 7

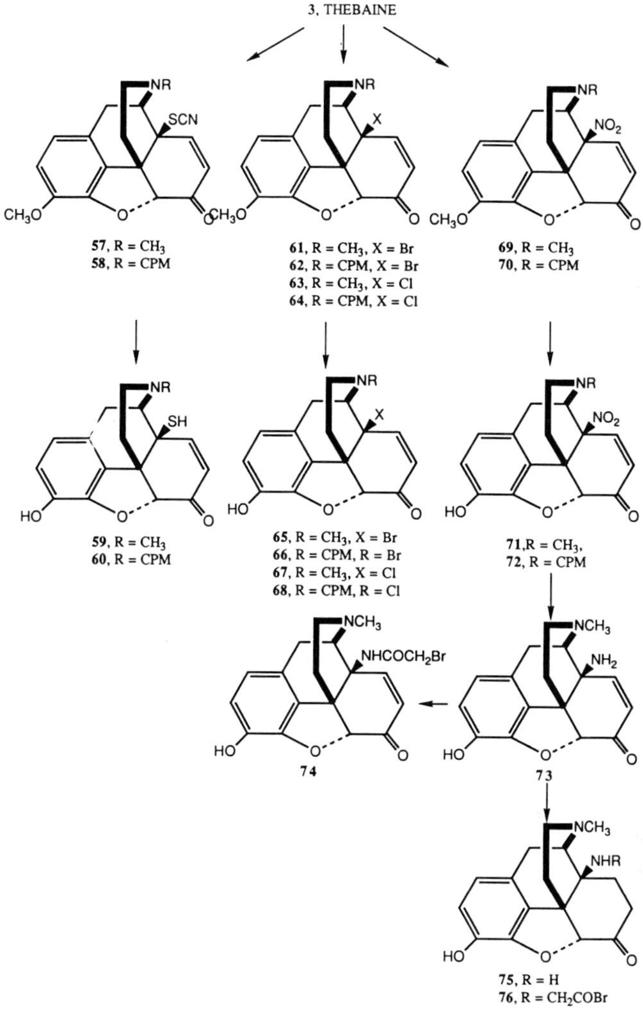

3, THEBAINE

57, R = CH$_3$
58, R = CPM

61, R = CH$_3$, X = Br
62, R = CPM, X = Br
63, R = CH$_3$, X = Cl
64, R = CPM, X = Cl

69, R = CH$_3$
70, R = CPM

59, R = CH$_3$
60, R = CPM

65, R = CH$_3$, X = Br
66, R = CPM, R = Br
67, R = CH$_3$, X = Cl
68, R = CPM, R = Cl

71, R = CH$_3$,
72, R = CPM

74

73

75, R = H
76, R = CH$_2$COBr

tetranitromethane. ARCHER and OSEI-GYIMAH (1979) used the readily available dinitrogen tetroxide obtained (69) accompanied by 8-nitrothebaine, which resulted from 1,2-addition of N_2O_4 followed by elimination of the elements of nitrous acid. O-Demethylation afforded structure 71. The sequence was repeated in the N-cyclopropylmethyl series whereby the 14β-nitro compound 72 was obtained, via the intermediate compound 70. Both the N-cyclopropyl-14β-halomorphinones 66 and 68 were pure antagonists. On the other hand, the 14β-mercapto analog 60 was about as active as naloxone as an antagonist but more potent than morphine as an agonist (OSEI-GYIMAH and ARCHER 1980).

Other 14β-substituted morphine derivatives were prepared from thebaine (OSEI-GYIMAH and ARCHER 1980; OSEI-GYIMAH et al. 1981) as shown in Scheme 7. It should be noted in passing that *N*-cyclopropylmethyl-14β-nitronormorphinone (72) was about three to four orders of magnitude more potent as an agonist than the corresponding *N*-methyl compound (71), in the guinea pig ileum preparation (OSEI-GYIMAH et al. 1981).

Reduction of structure 71 followed by O-demethylation gave the 14β-aminomorphinone (73) which, on bromoacetylation, gave 14β-bromoacetamidomorphine (74), a ligand which under proper conditions binds irreversibly to the μ-receptor (BIDLACK et al. 1989). Reduction of structure 73 furnished structure 75, which was converted to structure 76 by bromoacetylation (ARCHER et al. 1983). The latter is another ligand which binds selectively and irreversibly to the μ-receptor (BIDLACK et al. 1990).

A superior procedure for preparing 14-aminocodeinone (82) was reported by KIRBY and MCLEAN (1985) as shown in Scheme 8.

Scheme 8

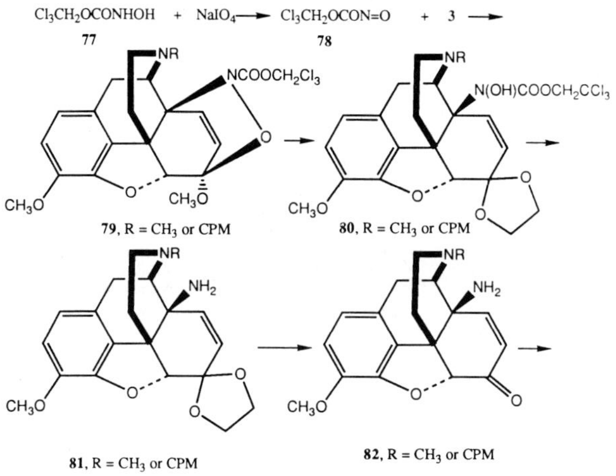
Cl3CH2OCONHOH + NaIO4 → Cl3CH2OCON=O + 3 →
77
78
NR
NCOOCH2Cl3
O
CH3O
CH3O
79, R = CH3 or CPM
N(OH)COOCH2CCl3
80, R = CH3 or CPM
NH2
81, R = CH3 or CPM
82, R = CH3 or CPM

Condensation of trichloroethyl chloroformate with hydroxylamine gave the carbamate (77), which was oxidized to the nitroso compound (78) with sodium periodate. Condensation with thebaine (3) afforded the adduct (79), which on treatment with ethylene glycol in the presence of acid was converted to the ketal (80), which on reduction yielded the ketal (81) and, after hydrolysis, 14β-aminocodeinone (82).

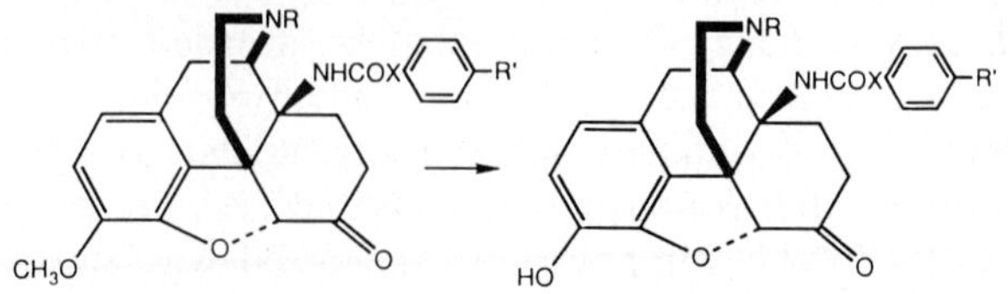
NR
NHCOX
R'
CH3O
HO
O

83, R = CH_3, X = CH=CH or CH_2-CH_2, R' = OCH_3 or Br
84, R = CPM, X = CH=CH or CH-CH_2, R' = OCH_3 or Br

85, R = CH_3, X = CH=CH or CH_2-CH_2, R' = OCH_3, or Br
86, R = CPM, X = CH=CH, or CH_2-CH_2, R' = OCH_3 or Br

The availability of structure 82 permitted Lewis and his colleagues (Lewis et al. 1988; Rance et al. 1981) to prepare a short series of 14β-cinnamoylamido and dihydrocinnamoylamido morphinone and codeinones (83, 84, 85, and 86).

The most striking feature of this series is that the *N*-CPM dihydro-morphinones have shown very long lasting antagonist effects in monkeys (Aceto et al. 1989).

E. Morphinans

The first practical synthesis of the morphinan ring system was reported by Grewe and Mondon (1948), who exploited the insightful biogenetic speculations of Robinson (Robinson and Sugasawa 1931), who pointed out the structural similarities between the benzylisoquinoline and morphine families of alkaloids. The original synthesis was superseded by the one developed by Schnider and Hellerbach (1950) and is shown in Scheme 9.

Scheme 9

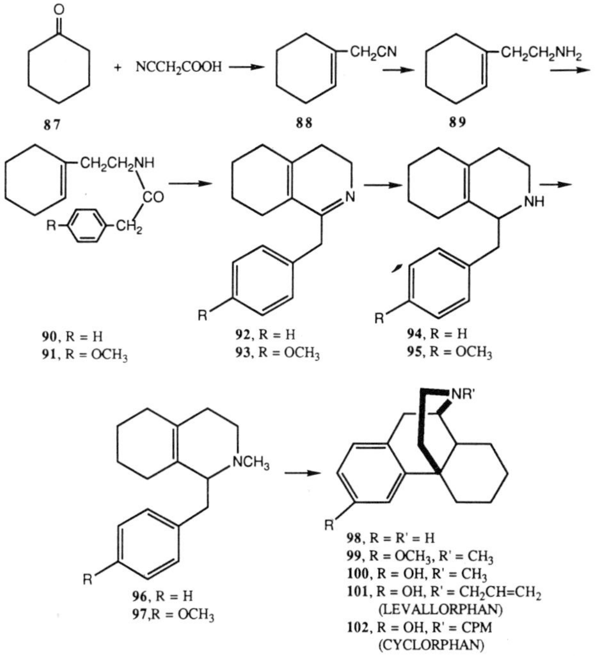

Cyclohexanone (87) was condensed with cyanoacetic acid to give the nitrile (88), which, on reduction with either lithium aluminum hydride or Raney cobalt, gave cyclohexenylethylamine (89). Condensation with phenylacetic acid or *p*-methoxyphenylacetic acid furnished the amides (90, 91), respectively, which were then caused to undergo cyclization with the aid of phosphorus oxychloride to afford the 1-benzylhexahydro-benzylisoquinolines

(92, 93). Catalytic reduction gave structures 94 and 95. Heating with formic acid or catalytic reduction in the presence of formaldehyde gave the *N*-methylamines 96 and 97, which were smoothly transformed to the (±)-morphinans 98 and 99.

Resolution of structures 94 or 95 with the aid of tartaric acid gave the (+) and (−) optical isomers. Demethylation of (−)99 gave (−)100 (levorphanol). The (+)-isomer is devoid of analgesic activity. However, (+)99 is a widely used antitussive agent (dextromethorphan). Resolution in this series is best carried out prior to cyclization. Heating structure 94 or 95 in the presence of a specially prepared palladium-zinc-iron catalyst resulted in complete racemization (HOLLANDER 1958). In this way, it is possible to recycle the unwanted optical isomer.

Replacement of the *N*-methyl group in structure 100 with an allyl group furnished levallorphan (101), a mixed agonist-antagonist (LEIMGRUBER et al. 1973). Cyclorphan (102), prepared by GATES and MONTZKA (1964), is more potent than levallorphan as an agonist and an antagonist.

Other morphinans of interest are the 14β-hydroxy compounds synthesized by Monkovic and his colleagues (MONKOVIC et al. 1973, 1975) as shown in Scheme 10.

Scheme 10

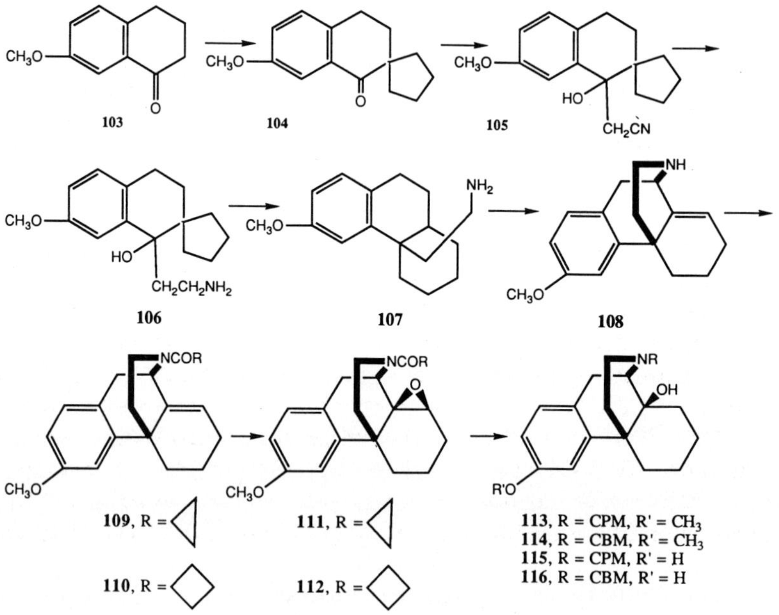

Alkylation of 7-methoxy-1-tetralone (103) with 1,4-dibromobutane gave the spiroketone (104), which was cyanomethylated to give the tertiary alcohol (105). This was reduced with lithium aluminum hydride, without prior isolation to the amino alcohol (106). Acid-catalyzed rearrangement furnished the unsaturated amine (107), which, on treatment with bromine followed by sodium bicarbonate, afforded structure 108. Acylation of this amine with cyclopropylcarbonyl chloride or cyclobutylcarbonyl chloride afforded the amides 109 and 110, respectively. Epoxidation gave predominantly the β-epoxides 111 and 112 which, on reduction with lithium aluminum hydride, were transformed to the desired 14β-hydroxy derivatives 113 and 114. These were resolved with tartaric acid, and demethylation of the optically active compounds gave structures 115 and 116. The former was a potent antagonist with moderate activity in the mouse writhing test whereas the latter, structure 116, was a potent agonist and antagonist and is used clinically (butorphanol).

A far more efficient way of preparing either optical isomer in the morphinan series was reported by Noyori (KITAMURA et al. 1988; NOYORI

Scheme 11

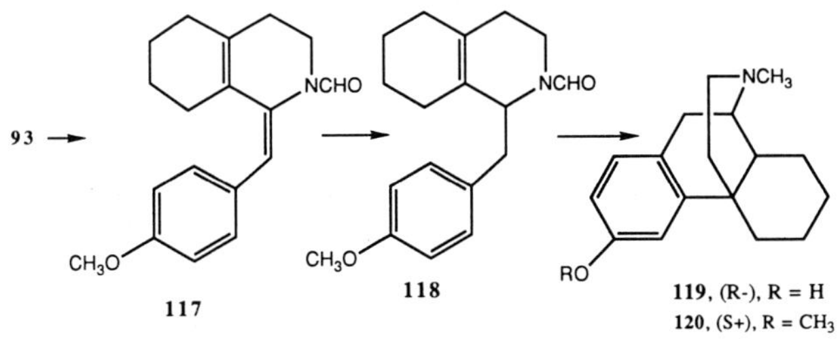

and TAKAYA 1990) as shown in Scheme 11. Conversion of structure 93 to the formamide (117) was readily accomplished. Reduction in the presence of R-BINAP (45a) gave the R (−)-isomer (118) in high enantiomeric excess. Cyclization followed by O-demethylation gave (R-)levallorphan (119). Using S-BINAP (45b) the same chemical conversions led to dextromethorphan (S+) (120).

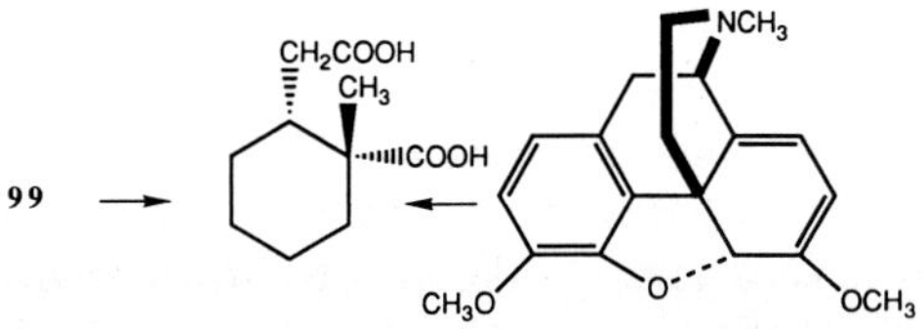

The absolute configuration of levorphan (99) was shown to be the same as that of thebaine by conversion of structure 99 to the diacid (121), which was identical with the same product derived from thebaine (3) (CORRODI et al. 1958). Since thebaine and its companion alkaloids have been configurationally related to (+)glyceraldehyde (STORK 1952; RAPOPORT and LAVIGNE 1953), the absolute configurations of the morphinans, benzomorphans (see below), and morphines are opposite of that of the amino acids. An interesting asymmetrical synthesis of dextromethorphan, using a chiral auxiliary, was reported by Meyers (MEYERS and BAILEY 1986) as shown in Scheme 12.

Scheme 12

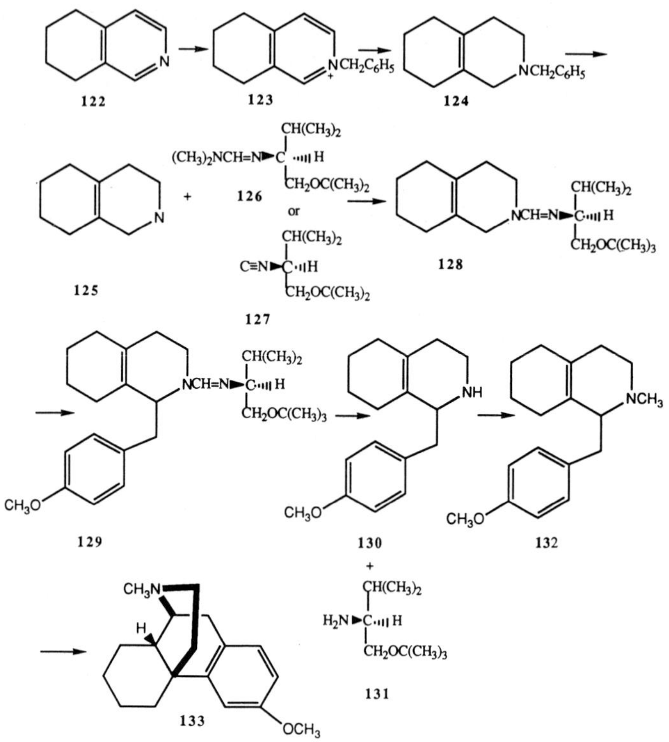

The tetrahydroisoquinoline (122), prepared by reduction of isoquinoline, was benzylated and the resulting quaternary salt (123) was reduced with sodium borohydride to the N-benzyloctahydroisoquinoline (124). Catalytic debenzylation gave structure 125. The chiral auxiliaries 126 and 127 prepared from L-valine were coupled with structure 125 to form the adduct 128. The anion of structure 128 prepared with the aid of n-butyllithium was alkylated with p-methoxybenzyl chloride to give structure 129, which was treated with hydrazine to furnish structure 130 and the t-butyl ether of valinol (131), which was recycled to give structures 126 and 127. The benzyloctahydroisoquinoline (130) was obtained in >98% enantiomeric excess. The usual N-methylation afforded structure 132, which, after a Grewe-type cyclization followed by demethylation, gave dextromethorphan (133), which is devoid of analgesic activity, but is a useful antitussive agent. In order to prepare the pharmacologically active isomer, using this procedure, it is necessary to employ the chiral auxiliary obtained from the unnatural isomer of valine.

F. Diene Adducts Derived from Thebaine

Bentley and his group (BENTLEY 1971; BENTLEY and HARDY 1963) carried out an extensive investigation of the chemistry and pharmacology (BLANE et al. 1967) of a group of compounds derived from the Diels-Alder adducts of thebaine and dienophiles. The synthesis of the pharmacologically more interesting compounds is shown in Scheme 13.

Scheme 13

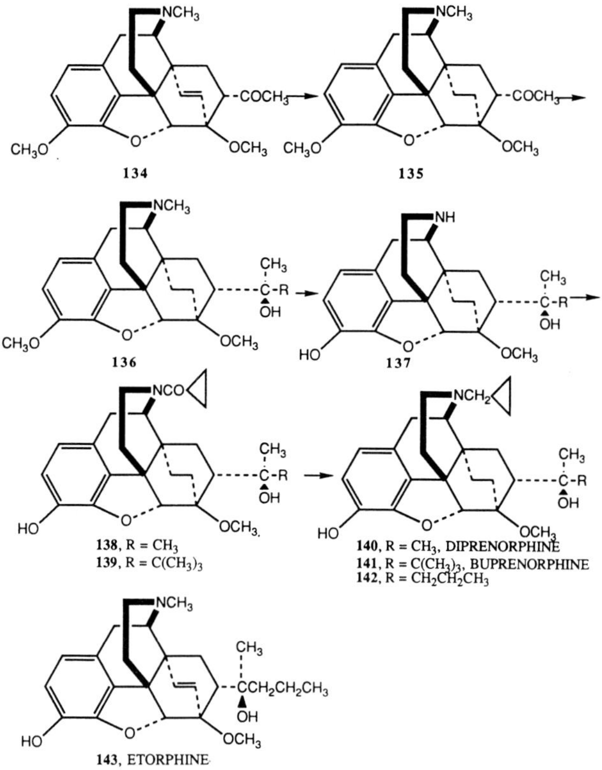

Thebaine (3) was allowed to react with methyl vinyl ketone to furnish the adduct 134. The etheno bridge was catalytically reduced to the ethano-bridged analog 135. This was treated with an organolithium reagent such as methyllithium or *t*-butyllithium to give the tertiary carbinol 136 (R = CH₃ or C(CH₃)₃). This was successfully O- and N-demethylated to the phenolic secondary base 137 which, in turn, was acylated with cyclopropanecarbonyl chloride. The resulting amides (138, 139), on reduction with lithium aluminum hydride gave diprenorphine (140), a powerful antagonist with little agonist activity. When similar transformations were carried out on structure 139 buprenorphine (141), a mixed agonist-antagonist with low abuse potential (JASINSKI et al. 1978), was formed. Treatment of structure 134 with propylmagnesium bromide, followed by O-demethylation, gave etorphine (143), an extremely potent μ-agonist. The etheno analog (142) is also a potent agonist.

Rapoport and Sheldrich (RAPOPORT and SHELDRICH 1963) found that, when thebaine was allowed to react with dimethyl acetylenedicarboxylate, the expected adduct (144) was obtained in high yield accompanied by structure 146. When ethyl propiolate was used as the dienophile, the adduct (145) was obtained in only 6% yield.

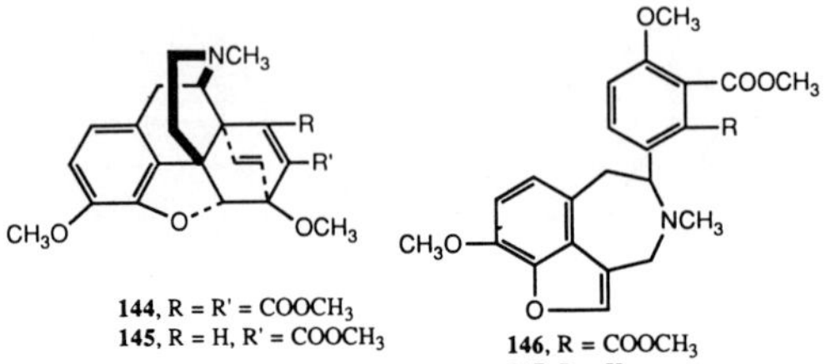

144, R = R' = COOCH₃
145, R = H, R' = COOCH₃
146, R = COOCH₃
147, R = H

Hayakawa (HAYAKAWA et al. 1981) and Singh (SINGH et al. 1982) re-investigated the reaction of thebaine and acetylene dienophiles and found that the reactions were more complex than originally thought (Scheme 14). For example, when methyl propiolate (148) was allowed to react with thebaine in refluxing tetrahydrofuran, the enol ether (150) was the major product accompanied by the thermolysis product (147). Mild hydrolysis of structure 150 gave the ketone (152), whose structure was secured by single crystal X-ray analysis (SINGH et al. 1982). When the reaction of thebaine with structure 148 was carried out in methanol, the ketal (153) was the major product accompanied by the enol ether (150). Treatment of structure 153 with acid resulted in the formation of structure 150. Thus carrying out the reaction in methanol traps a putative intermediate which, in the absence of methanol, cyclizes to structure 150. This type of ring opening

Scheme 14

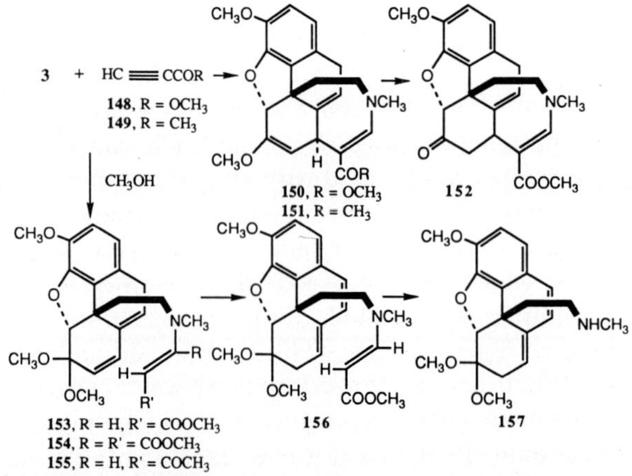

148, R = OCH₃
149, R = CH₃

150, R = OCH₃
151, R = CH₃

152

153, R = H, R' = COOCH₃
154, R = R' = COOCH₃
155, R = H, R' = COCH₃

156

157

of the piperidine ring in thebaine was also successfully carried out with 1-butyne-3-one to give structures 151 and 155 and with dimethyl acetylene-dicarboxylate to give structure 154. Treatment of structure 153 with strong base resulted in isomerization of the diene system, resulting in the formation of the fully conjugated compound 156, which was hydrolyzed to structure 157.

Catalytic reduction of the ketone (152) resulted in the formation of the dihydro compound (158). When a methanolic solution of structure 158 was allowed to stand in air for a few days, another substance was obtained whose structure was shown to be structure 161 by means of single crystal X-ray analysis (SINGH et al. 1986). Compound 161 is the result of an oxidative rearrangement as shown in Scheme 15. On standing in air, structure 158 is

Scheme 15

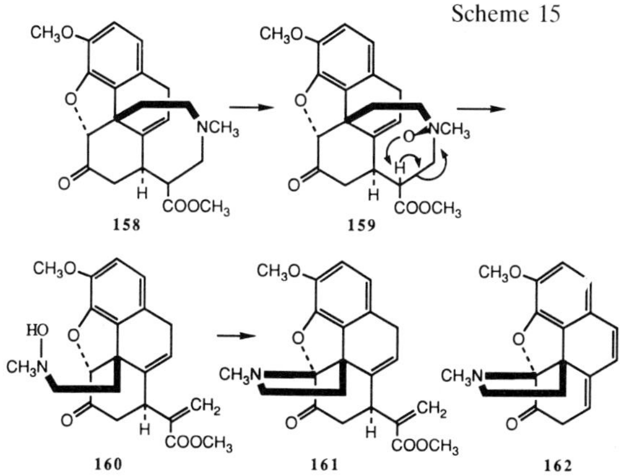

converted to the N-oxide (159), which then undergoes a rearrangement to structure 161 via the intermediacy of the hydroxylamine (160). Theuns (THEUNS et al. 1984) reported that an N-oxide of thebaine underwent a similar rearrangement to give structure 162.

G. 6,7-Benzomorphans

The first synthesis of a 6,7-benzomorphan was reported by Barltrop (1947) as shown in Scheme 16. Although this method has been superseded, it has been used to introduce a hydroxyl group at C-11 (MAY and KUGITA 1961; MAY et al. 1961).

In Barltrop's synthesis the methyltetralone (163) was alkylated and the basic ketone (165) was brominated to give the bromoketone (167). Warming yielded the quaternary salt (169), which, on heating, lost methyl bromide to yield the 6,7-benzomorphan (171), which, on reduction, yielded structure 173.

May (MAY and KUGITA 1961; MAY et al. 1961) used the methoxytetralone (164) as their starting material, which furnished the quaternary salt (170)

Scheme 16

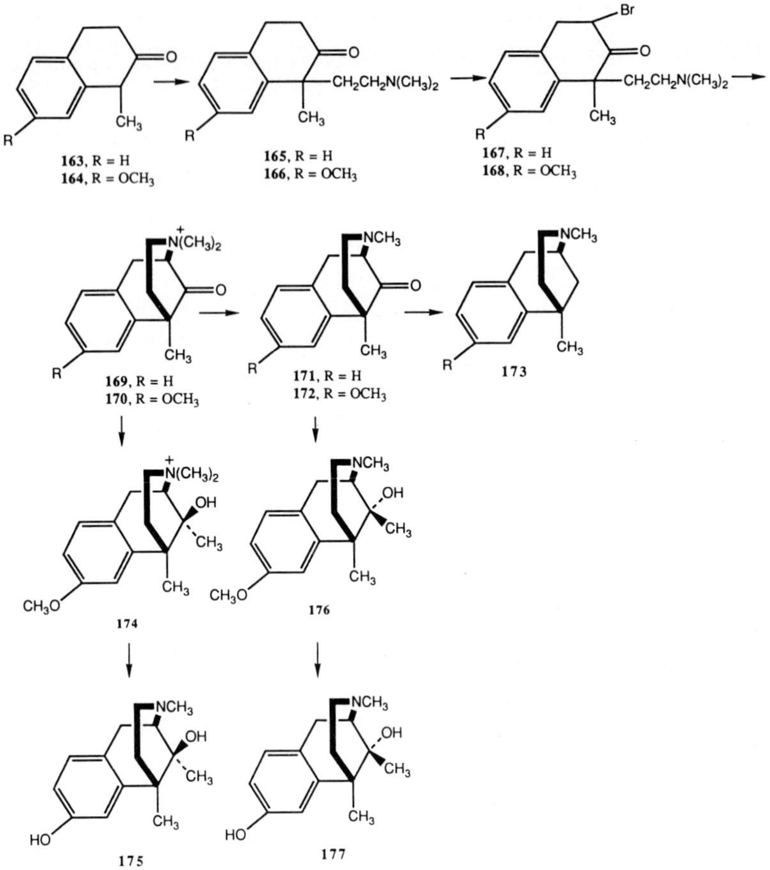

via the intermediates 166 and 168. When structure 170 was treated with methylmagnesium bromide the adduct (174) was formed by equatorial attack at the carbonyl group. Pyrolysis, followed by O-demethylation, afforded structure 175, in which the hydroxyl group was in the 11β-position. When the conversion of 170 to 172 preceded the treatment with methylmagnesium bromide, the isomeric 11α-hydroxy compound 176 was formed which, on O-demethylation, was converted to structure 177.

A preparation involving a Grewe-type cyclization was used by MAY and FRY (1957) to prepare 6,7-benzomorphans. This synthesis was modified by ALBERTSON and WETTERAU (1970) in that 1-benzyl-3,4-dimethylpyridinium chloride (179) was used instead of the corresponding methyl quaternary (178) as shown in Scheme 17.

The quaternary salt (179) was treated with p-methoxybenzylmagnesium chloride and the resulting dihydropyridine was catalytically reduced to the dihydropyridine (181). Cyclization to the 6,7-benzomorphan (182) required the usual acidic conditions. Debenzylation to the nor-base (183) was accom-

Scheme 17

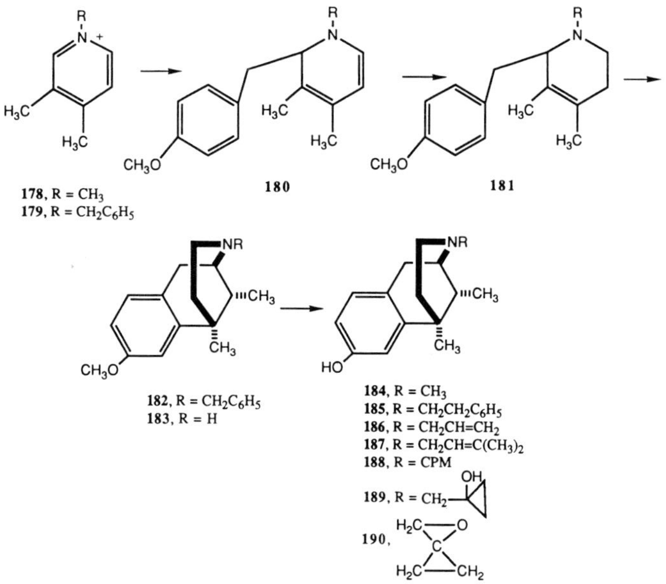

178, R = CH₃
179, R = CH₂C₆H₅

180   **181**

182, R = CH₂C₆H₅
183, R = H

184, R = CH₃
185, R = CH₂CH₂C₆H₅
186, R = CH₂CH=CH₂
187, R = CH₂CH=C(CH₃)₂
188, R = CPM

189, R = CH₂—

190,

plished by catalytic hydrogenation. Alkylation with a variety of alkyl halides followed by O-demethylation yielded a group of pharmacologically interesting compounds. Among them were metazocine (184) (MAY and AGER 1959), phenazocine (185) (AGER and MAY 1960), SKF-10047 (186) (GORDON et al. 1961), pentazocine (187) (ARCHER et al. 1962), cyclazocine (188) (ARCHER et al. 1964), and bremazocine (189) (RAHTZ et al. 1977), prepared by condensing structure 183 with the spirooxypentane (190). Single crystal X-ray analysis of L-cyclazocine hydrobromide showed that it had the same absolute configuration as natural morphine (KARLE et al. 1969).

A chiral synthesis of 6,7-benzomorphans was reported by Noyori (NOYORI and TAKAYA 1990) as shown in Scheme 18.

Tiglic acid (191) was converted to the amine (192), which was acylated with p-methoxyphenylacetic acid to yield the amide (193). Cyclization furnished structure 194, which was converted to the N-formyl compound (195). Hydrogenation in the presence of either R-BINAP or S-BINAP gave either R or S (196) in high enantiomeric excess. A Grewe cyclization furnished the optically active R or S 6,7-benzomorphan (197), which could be converted to R or S N-alkylbenzomorphans by alkylation with the appropriate alkyl halides.

Brossi and his coworkers (ZIERING et al. 1970) prepared the keto compound (198) by direct oxidation of metazocine O-methyl ether. MICHNE and ALBERTSON (1972) oxidized the corresponding nor-base to the ketone (199), which was then converted to a number of N-substituted compounds, the most interesting from a pharmacological standpoint being ketocyclazocine (200) and the homologous 6-ethyl analog (201) known as ethylketocyclazocine or

Scheme 18

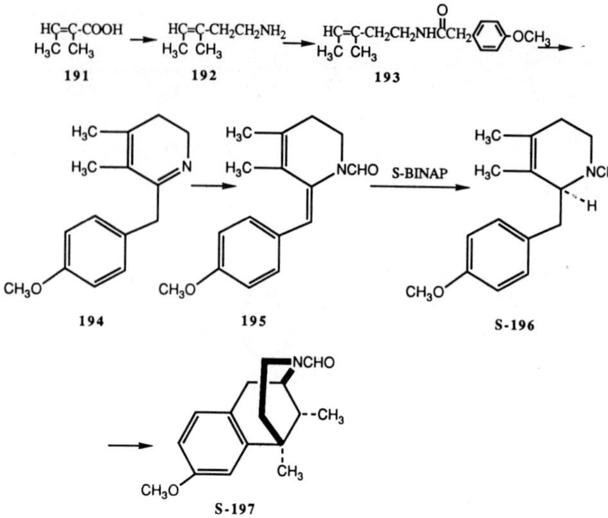

191 → **192** → **193** →

194 → **195** —S-BINAP→ **S-196**

→ **S-197**

EKC. The κ/μ-ratio of the K_i values for EKC was approximately 2.0 whereas that for cyclazocine was 0.75 (MAGNAN et al. 1982). This difference was due to the decrease in the K_i for μ-binding in the case of EKC rather than an increase in the K_i for κ-binding.

198   **199**   **200**, R = CH_3
                              201, R = C_2H_5

202, R = H   **207**, R =   (S)

203, R =

204, R =

205, R =   **208**, R =   (R)

206, R =

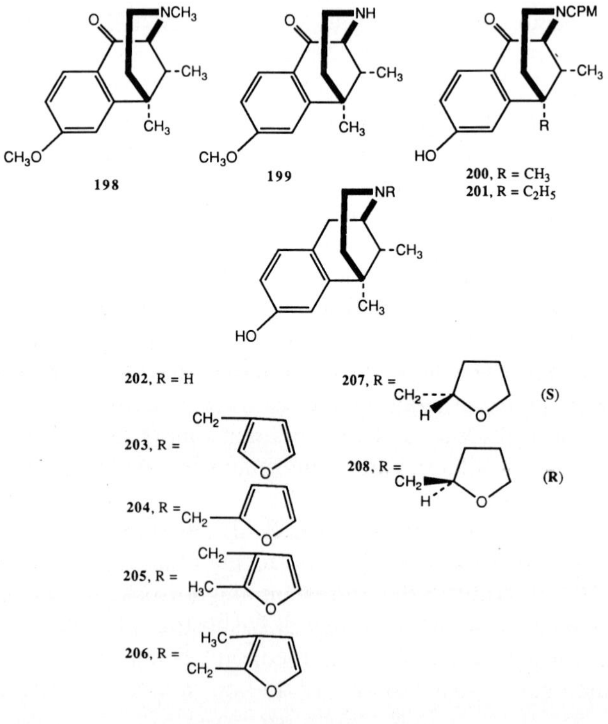

Another series of 6,7-benzomorphans of biological interest was prepared by Merz and his collaborators (MERZ et al. 1973, 1975). A few examples are shown below:

In the furylmethyl series wherein the side chains are achiral, structure 203 proved to be a pure antagonist, whereas structure 206 was a pure agonist. Compounds 204 and 205 were mixed agonist-antagonists (MERZ et al. 1973).

The 1975 paper dealt with the tetrahydrofurylmethyl side chains, which introduced a new chiral carbon atom in the N-substituent. The nor-base 202 had the same absolute configuration as morphine. The S-isomer (207) (M_r 2034) is pharmacologically active whereas the stereoisomeric R isomer (208) is inactive.

Structure 207 is active at the μ-and κ-receptor but is inactive as a δ-ligand (MAGNAN et al. 1982). It is also inactive at the ω-(phencyclidine) receptor. When administered to man it produced naloxone-reversible dysphoric effects (PFEIFFER et al. 1986). It was suggested by Martin (MARTIN 1967; MARTIN et al. 1976) that the dysphoric effects of the mixed agonists-antagonists such as SKF-10047 were mediated via the ω-receptor. The ivestigation of Herz and his coworkers (PFEIFFER et al. 1986) strongly suggests that the unpleasant effects of these compounds are mediated through κ-receptors.

A series of 6,7-benzomorphans modeled after Bentley's oripavines (BENTLEY 1971) was reported by Michne (MICHNE 1976, 1978; MICHNE et al. 1977, 1979), which were prepared according to the equations shown in Scheme 19.

The dihydropyridine (180) condensed with ethyl acrylate to give the Diels-Alder adduct (209), which cyclized in the presence of hydrogen fluoride to give structure 210. Hydrolysis of this ester followed by treatment with methyllithium gave the ketone (211). When the latter was heated with formic acid two reactions occurred. One was a retro-Mannich reaction which gave structure 212, which was transformed to structure 214. The other was a retro-Michael reaction which gave structure 213. This secondary amine cyclized spontaneously to furnish the ion 215, which was reduced to structure 216. In order to avoid the latter pathway the ester (210) was acylated to give structure 217. This compound could only undergo a retro-Mannich reaction. Treatment with formic acid afforded structure 218. Replacement of the N-benzyl group by a methyl group followed by O-demethylation furnished a series of alkanones which were obtained by simply varying the size of R in structure 217. One of the more interesting compounds was structure 219, which is inactive in the rat-tail flick assay, active in the writhing and bradykinin assays, and as active as naloxone as an antagonist (MICHNE et al. 1979). In this respect it resembles buprenorphine (141).

Scheme 19

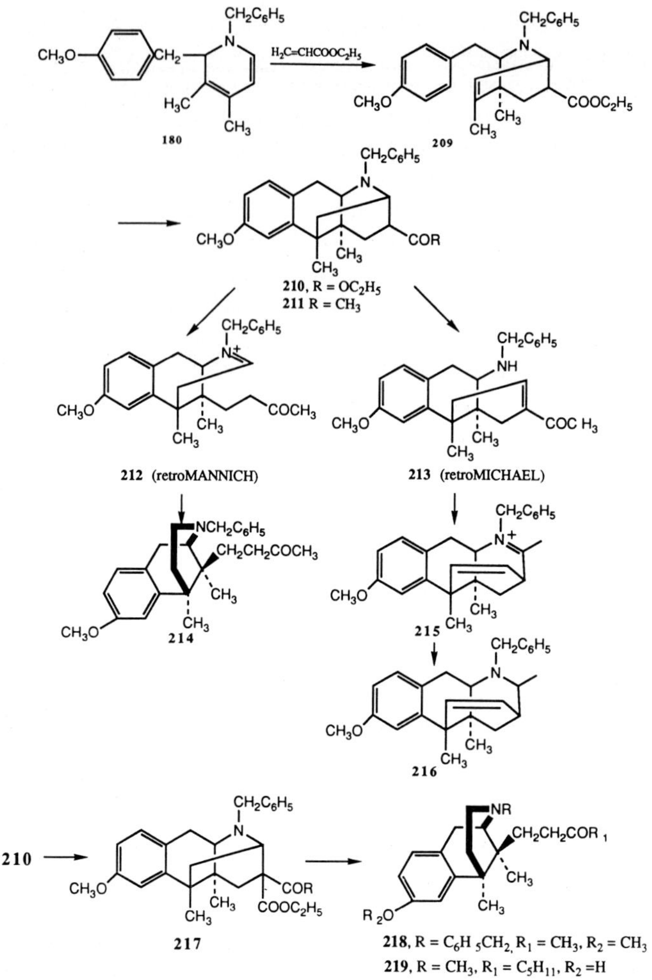

H. Piperidine-Based Opioids

Meperidine (225) was the first totally synthetic opioid introduced into clinical practice and is the simplest cyclic opioid. The original synthesis (EISLEB 1941) is shown in Scheme 20.

Scheme 20

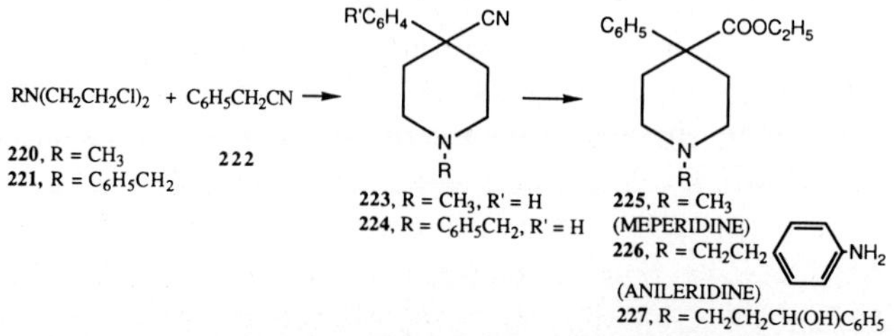

Alkylation of phenylacetonitrile (222) with bis(2-chloroethyl)methyl amine (nitrogen mustard) (220) gave the nitrile (223), which, on ethanolysis, was transformed to meperidine (225). Owing to the vesicant nature of structure 220, other less toxic alkylating agents were investigated. The N-benzyl derivative (221) proved to be less hazardous. Alkylation of structure 222 gave the nitrile 224, which after ethanolysis, debenzylation, and methylation afforded meperidine (BERGEL and MORRISON 1948). Condensation of m-methoxyphenylacetonitrile with structure 220 gave a nitrile, which, after treatment with ethylmagnesium bromide, followed by O-demethylation, was converted to ketobemidone (228), which is slightly more potent than meperidine (ARIDON and MORRISON 1950).

228, (KETOBEMIDONE)   229, R = R' = CH₃   231, R = CH₃
                       230, R = CH₂CH₂CH(OH) C₆H₅   232, R = CH₂CH₂CH(OH)C₆H₅
                       R' = CH₃

Major increases in potency were achieved by replacing the N-methyl group with phenylalkyl substituents. For example, anileridine (226) (WEIJLARD et al. 1956) is about three times as potent as meperidine but the secondary alcohol (227) is 150 times as potent (JANSSEN and EDDY 1960).

The most active piperidine-based opioid is structure 230 (CARABATEAS and GRUMBACH 1962). It is about 3200 times as active as meperidine. It is an analog of the "reversed ester" α-prodine (229), which itself is about five times as active as meperidine (ZIERING and LEE 1947).

Generally speaking, replacement of N-methyl groups in piperidine analgesics by allyl or cyclopropylmethyl groups does not convert agonists to either pure antagonists or mixed agonist-antagonists. ZIMMERMAN et al. (1975) reported that the N-methyl compound (231) was a moderately active pure antagonist and both the (+) and (−)-isomers of structure 232 were as active as naloxone as opioid antagonists.

Fentanyl (234) is a potent analgesic (JANSSEN et al. 1963). Introduction of a methyl group cis to the nitrogen atom results in a marked increase in potency. Thus (−)cis (237) is about 120 times as potent as fentanyl (VAN BEVER et al. 1974, 1976). Sufentanil (234) (VAN DAELE et al. 1976) is over 2000 times as potent as morphine. The synthesis of these compounds is shown in Scheme 21.

N-Phenethyl-4-piperidone was converted to a Schiff's base with aniline and the product was reduced to structure 233, which was acylated with propionic anhydride to give structure 234. The amide (237) was prepared similarly from the 3-methyl-N-phenethyl-4-piperidone (235). In this case,

Scheme 21

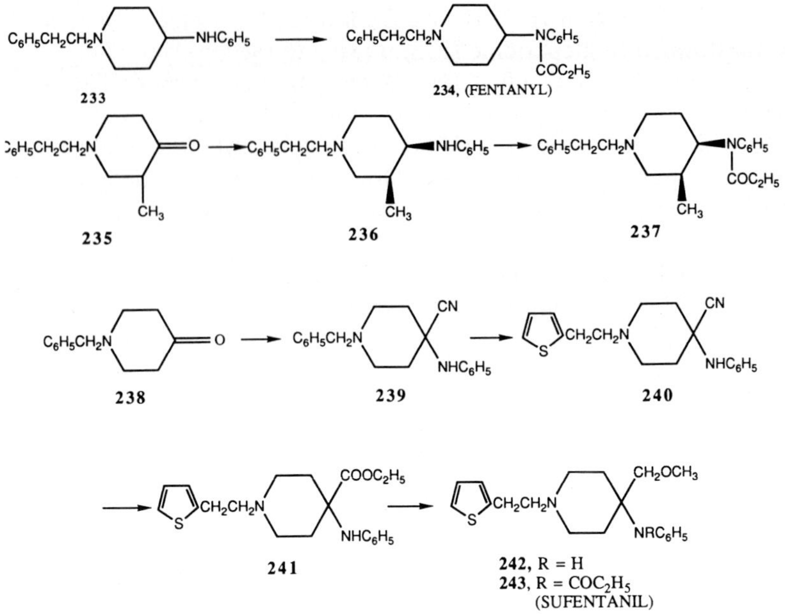

the *cis*-isomer (236) was resolved and acylated to give structure 237, the
(−)-isomer of which was the active analgesic.

Sufentanil (243) was prepared by a multistep synthesis starting from *N*-
benzyl-4-piperidone (238). This ketone was converted to the anilinonitrile
(239), which, after catalytic debenzylation and alkylation with 2-(2-thienyl)-
ethyl bromide, gave structure 240. This nitrile was converted to the corresponding ester (241), which was reduced with lithium aluminum hydride
and the resulting alcohol was methylated to give structure 242. Acylation
with propionic anhydride gave sufentanil (243).

Rice and his colleagues described two irreversible ligands which bind
selectively to δ-receptors in NG-108-15 neuroblastoma-glioma hybrid cells.
These are FIT (244) (KLEE et al. 1982) and SUPERFIT (251) (BURKE et al.
1984, 1986; SIMONDS et al. 1985), which were tritium-labeled as shown in
Scheme 22. These authors preferred using [^{3}H]-SUPERFIT (250) rather
than structure 244, because less nonspecific binding was encountered when
the former was used to label receptors.

Cis-3-methyl-4-anilinopiperidine (246) was alkylated with 2-(4-
nitrophenyl)-ethyl bromide to give structure 247, which is an analog of
structure 237. Resolution of structure 247 furnished the (+)-isomer, which
was acylated with propionic anhydride, reduced, and brominated to afford
structure 248. Reductive debromination with tritium followed by treatment with thiophosgene gave structure 250 (specific activity, 13 Ci/mmol).
Nonradiolabeled SUPERFIT (251) was prepared from structure 249 and
thiophosgene. It is interesting that the SUPERFIT analog without the

Scheme 22

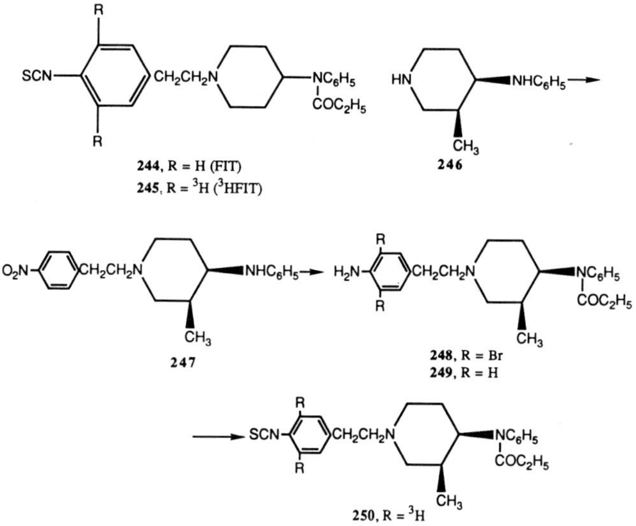

244, R = H (FIT)
245, R = ³H (³HFIT)

246

247

248, R = Br
249, R = H

250, R = ³H
251, R = H

isothiocyanate group (237) is a highly selective μ-ligand whereas structure 251 binds covalently to δ-receptors. BIT (253), an isothiocyanate derived from etonitazene, a potent μ-agonist (252), binds covalently to μ-receptors (RICE et al. 1983).

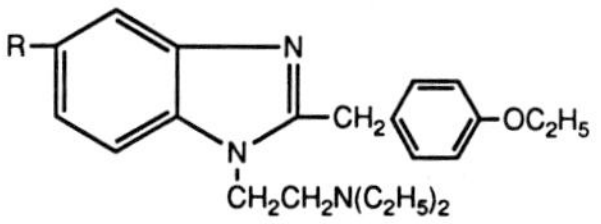

252, R = NO₂ (ETONITAZENE)
253, R = SNC (BIT)

I. Ethylene Diamines

SZMUSZKOVICZ and VAN VOIGHTLANDER (1982) described a series of amides which were κ-selective opioid ligands. The most potent was U-50488 (257) (VAN VOIGHTLANDER et al. 1983), whose synthesis is shown in Scheme 23.

Scheme 23

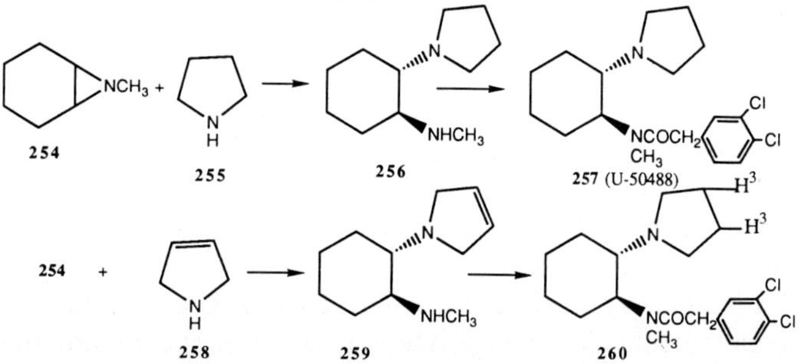

254

255

256

257 (U-50488)

254

258

259

260

The ethylene imine (254) was treated with pyrrolidine (255) to give the trans diamine (256), which was acylated with 3,4-dichlorophenylacetic acid to afford U50488 (257). Rice et al. (THURKAUF et al. 1989) prepared the tritium-labeled analog (260), by substituting the pyrrolline (258) for structure 255. The resulting base (259) was reduced in the presence of tritium gas. Condensation with 3,4-dichlorophenylacetic acid gave structure 260 (specific activity, 21 Ci/mmol).

The discovery of a nonpeptide κ-selective opioid ligand led to the synthesis and biological evaluation of other such ligands. For example, KAPLAN (1984) reported the synthesis of U-69,593 (273) as shown in Scheme 24 (LAHTI et al. 1985).

Scheme 24

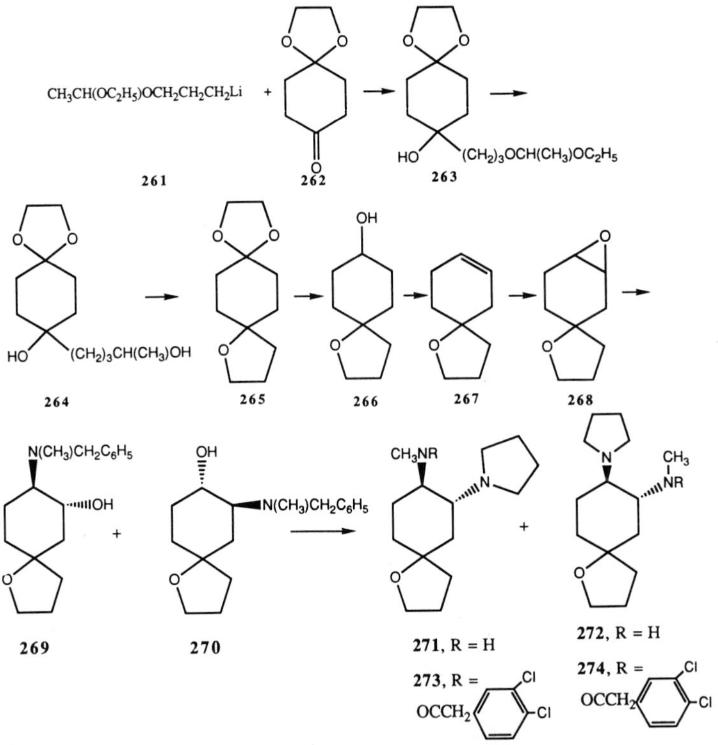

The acetal (261) prepared from the corresponding bromide was allowed to react with the cyclohexanone ketal (262) to furnish the alcohol (263), which was hydrolyzed to the diol (264). Cyclization of structure 264 to structure 265 followed by hydrolysis and reduction gave the alcohol 266. Dehydration to the cyclohexene 267 was followed by epoxidation to the oxide 268. Treatment with N-methylbenzyl amine gave a mixture of the amino alcohols 269 and 270. The alcohols were tosylated and the resulting esters were treated with pyrrolidine. The mixture was separated chromatographically and the pure diamines were catalytically debenzylated to give the secondary amines 271 and 272. Acylation with 3,4-dichlorophenylacetic acid gave U-69593 (273) and the isomeric structure 274.

CLARK et al. (1988) found that the optimum analgesic and μ/κ-ratios occurred in a series of diamines which were acylated by 4-benzo[b]thiophenacyl, 4-benzo[b]furanacyl, and 4-chlorophenoxyacetyl groups related to U-50488. HALFPENNY et al. (1989) reported that structure 276, prepared by acylation of the diamine 275 had high in vitro κ-opioid receptor affinity and was equal to morphine as an analgesic after administration to rats.

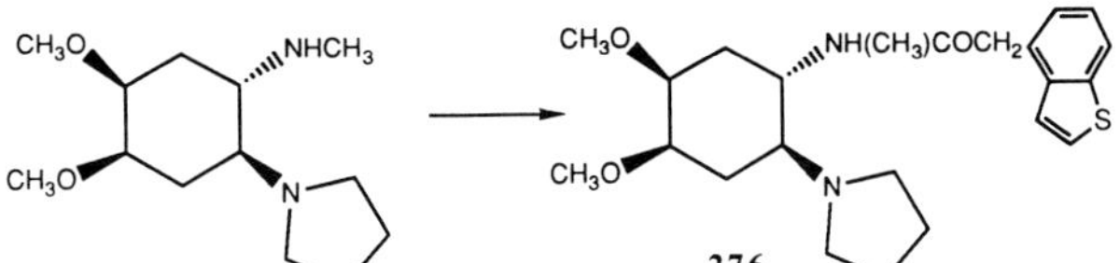

275   276

DeCOSTA et al. (1989) prepared the (−)- and (+)-isomers of U-50488, as well as the (−)- and (+)-isomers of the diasteromeric cisisomer of U-50488 as shown in Scheme 25. The (−)-isomer of U-50488 (288) showed the

Scheme 25

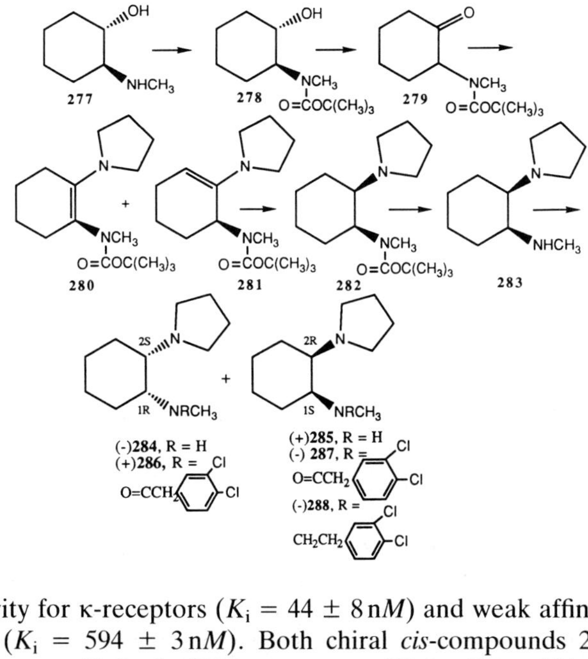

highest activity for κ-receptors ($K_i = 44 \pm 8\,nM$) and weak affinity for PPP-ω-receptors ($K_i = 594 \pm 3\,nM$). Both chiral cis-compounds 286 and 287 showed moderate affinity for PPP ω-receptors (K_i for 286 = 221 ± 36 nM; K_i for 287 = 81 ± 13 nM) but negligible affinity for κ-receptors.

Trans-2-methylaminocyclohexanol (277) was converted to the T-butylcarbamate (278), which was oxidized to the cyclohexanone (279). Condensation with pyrrolidine gave a mixture of enamines (280, 281), which, on reduction, give predominantly the cis-isomer (282), which, on treatment with hydrogen fluoride, afforded structure 283, which was resolved into its optocal antipodes 284 and 285. These bases were converted to the corresponding 3,4-dichlorophenylacetamides (+) (286) and (−) (287), respectively.

Reduction of structure 287 with lithium aluminum hydride gave structure 288, which showed high affinity for the PPP-ω-receptor (K_i = 1.3 ± 3 nM) and very little affinity for the PCP-ω- or κ-receptors (DeCosta et al. 1990a).

Another series of κ-selective agonists was reported by Costello (COSTELLO et al. 1988) and is represented by the general structures 289, 290, and 291. The more potent were structures 289 and 290, which showed IC_{50} values vs. bremazocine of 6.3 nM and 6.9 nM, respectively.

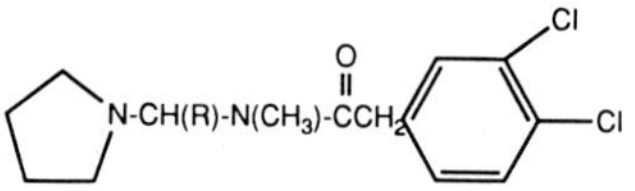

289, R = CH(CH$_3$)$_2$ (ICI 197,067)
290, R = C$_6$H$_5$ (ICI 199,441)

291, R = 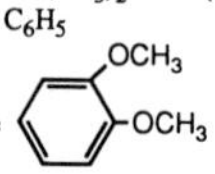 (ICI 204,871)

DeCosta (DeCOSTA et al. (1990b) prepared a series of isothiocyanates in the U-50488 series. Compound 292 bound specifically and irreversibly to κ-receptors.

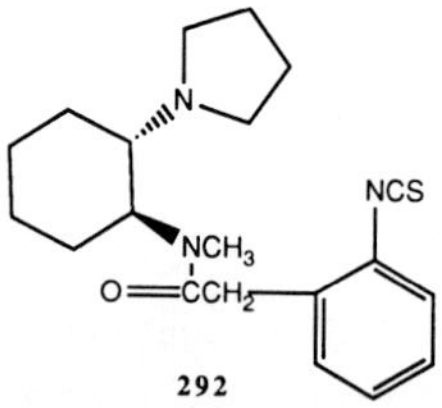

292

Interest in κ-selective agonists was reinforced by the belief that such compounds which demonstrated activity in in vivo functional assays for analgesics may be clinically active without addiction liability. However, it should be kept in mind that Herz (PFEIFFER et al. 1986) showed that a κ-agonist [(Mr 2034, (207)] without ω-activity produced psychotomimetic effects in man, an observation which strongly suggests that the dysphoric and psychotomimetic effects produced by clinically active analgesics such as cyclazocine and SKF 10047 may be mediated through κ-receptors.

Scheme 26

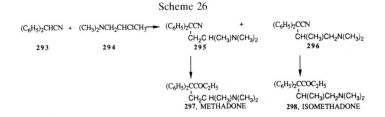

J. Acyclic Opioids

Methadone (297) and its companion isomethadone (298) were first prepared by EISLEB (1945) as shown in Scheme 26.

Diphenylacetonitrile (293) was converted to its anion, which was treated with dimethylaminoisopropyl chloride (294). The resulting mixture of nitriles 295 and 296 was separated and each was allowed to react with ethylmagnesium bromide to give methadone (297) and isomethadone (298). Both are active analgesics by the parenteral and oral routes although methadone is the isomer used clinically.

Racemic methadone has been resolved and the analgesic activity was shown to reside in the (−)-isomer (THORP et al. 1947). However, reduction of the inactive (+)-methadone gave 2-(−)-methadol (299), which on acetylation gave 2-acetyl(−)-methadol (300), which is a potent long-lasting analgesic in man (EDDY et al. 1952) (Scheme 27).

Scheme 27

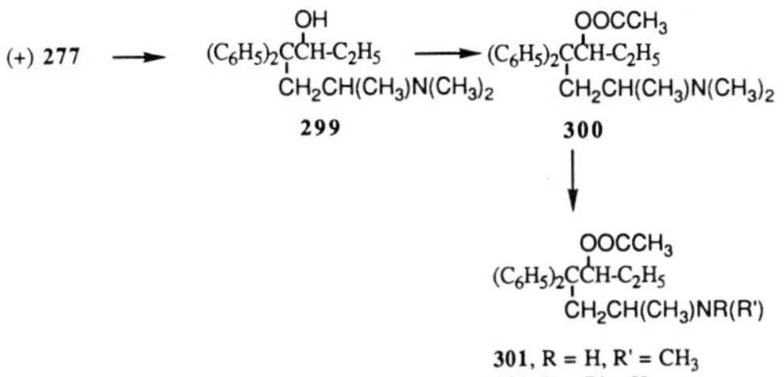

$$(+)\ 277 \longrightarrow \underset{\underset{299}{\overset{}{\text{CH}_2\text{CH(CH}_3)\text{N(CH}_3)_2}}}{(\text{C}_6\text{H}_5)_2\overset{\overset{\text{OH}}{|}}{\text{C}}\text{CH-C}_2\text{H}_5} \longrightarrow \underset{\underset{300}{\overset{}{\text{CH}_2\text{CH(CH}_3)\text{N(CH}_3)_2}}}{(\text{C}_6\text{H}_5)_2\overset{\overset{\text{OOCCH}_3}{|}}{\text{C}}\text{CH-C}_2\text{H}_5}$$

$$\underset{\underset{\begin{matrix}301,\ R = H,\ R' = CH_3\\302,\ R = R' = H\end{matrix}}{\overset{}{\text{CH}_2\text{CH(CH}_3)\text{NR(R')}}}}{(\text{C}_6\text{H}_5)_2\overset{\overset{\text{OOCCH}_3}{|}}{\text{C}}\text{CH-C}_2\text{H}_5}$$

The pioneering studies of DOLE and NYSWANDER (1965) led to the use of methadone maintenance as a modality in heroin abuse. A major disadvantage of this treatment procedure is the necessity for daily administration of the drug. L-α-Acetylmethadol (300) (LAAM) is an orally effective long-acting congener of methadone. Heroin addicts have been maintained at doses of 100 mg LAAM given thrice weekly. BILLINGS et al. (1973, 1974) found that LAAM is metabolized in man to nor-LAAM (301) and bis-nor-LAAM (302), both of which are active as analgesics (BOOHER and POHLAND 1975). It is possible that the long duration of activity of LAAM may be due to its metabolic conversion of structure 300 to the metabolites (301, 302), both of which have to be synthesized.

K. Concluding Remarks

With the exception of the ethylene diamines, which are κ-selective ligands, the agonists discussed in this chapter are for the most part μ-selective. Despite the enormous variation in chemical structures, which range from acyclic opioids such as methadone to polycyclic types represented by etorphine, the pharmacology of these compounds is remarkably similar.

Many years ago in his introduction to Bentley's monograph *The Chemistry of the Morphine Alkaloids* (BENTLEY 1954), Sir Robert Robinson referred to morphine as "this veritable Proteus among molecules" because of its tendency to undergo complex transformations when exposed to a variety of reagents. He could well have included thebaine and codeine and some of their simple derivatives as protean molecules. For example, it has been reported that codeine is photostable but recently we have found that *N*-carbomethoxynorcodeinone (303), when irradiated at 366 nm in the presence of methanol, rearranges via the intermediate (304) to furnish structure 305, which on reduction affords structure 307. If the photolysis is carried out in the presence of water instead of methanol, structure 306 is formed, as shown in Scheme 28 (SCHULTZ et al. 1991).

Scheme 28

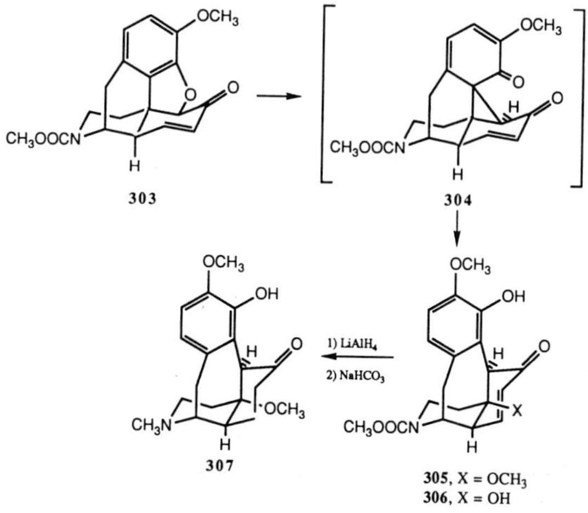

When 5β-methylcodeinone (308) was photolysed, compound 310 was produced, presumably via the dienone (309), as shown in Scheme 29.

Scheme 29

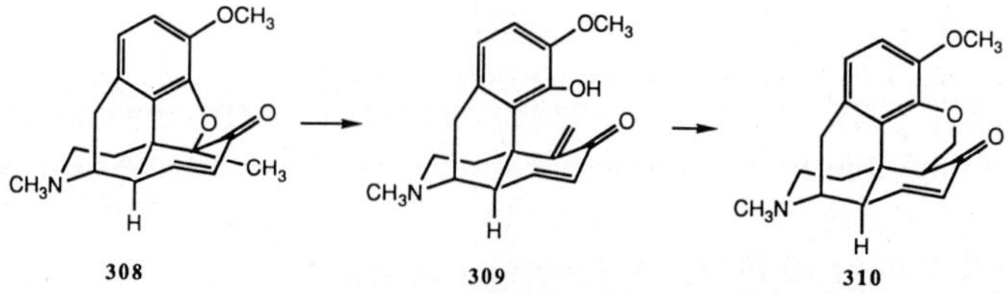

If codeinone can be considered to be a tetrahydrofuran, then structure 310 is its tetrahydropyran homolog. This is a new ring system whose chemistry and pharmacology is under investigation.

References

Aceto MD, Bowman ER, May EL, Harris LS, Woods JH, Smith CB, Medzihradsky F, Jacobson AE (1989) Very long-acting narcotic antagonists: the 14β-p-substituted cinnamoylaminomorphinones and their partial mu agonist codeinone relatives. Arzneimittelforschung 39:570–575

Ager JH, May EL (1960) Structures related to morphine: XIII. 2-Alkyl-2'-hydroxy-5,9-dimethyl-6,7-benzomorphans and a more direct synthesis of the 2-phenethyl compound. J Org Chem 25:984–986

Albertson NF, Wetterau WF (1970) The synthesis of pentazocine. J Med Chem 13:302–303

Allen RM, Kirby GW (1970) Iodination of thebaine: a new route to 9-substituted indolinocodeinone derivatives. Chem Commun 1346

Amann T, Zenk MH (1991) Formation of the morphine precursor salutaridine is catalyzed by a cytochrome P-450 enzyme in mammalian liver. Tetrahedron Lett 32:3675–3678

Archer S, Osei-Gyimah P (1979) Reaction of thebaine with dinitrogen tetroxide. J Heterocycl Chem 16:389

Archer S, Albertson NF, Harris LS, Pierson AK, Bird JG, Keats AS, Telford J, Papadopoulos CH (1962) Narcotic antagonists as analgesics. Science 137:541–543

Archer S, Albertson NF, Harris LS, Pierson AK, Bird JG (1964) Pentazocine. Strong analgesics and analgesic antagonists in the benzomorphan series. J Med Chem 7:123–127

Archer S, Seyed-Mozaffari A, Osei-Gyimah P, Bidlack JM, Abood LG (1983) 14β-(2-Bromoacetamido)morphine and 14β-(2-Bromoacetamido)-morphinone. J Med Chem 26:1775–1777

Aridon AWD, Morrison AL (1950) Synthetic analgesics: VI. The synthesis of ketobemidone. J Chem Soc:1469–1471

Barltrop JA (1947) Synthesis in the morphine series: 1. Derivatives of bicyclo[3:3:1]-2-azanonane. J Chem Soc:399–401

Bentley KW (1954) The chemistry of the morphine alkaloids. Oxford University Press, London

Bentley KW (1971) The morphine alkaloids. In: Manske RF (ed) The alkaloids, vol 13. Academic, New York, pp 75–120

Bentley KW, Hardy DG (1963) New potent analgesics in the morphine series. Proc Chem Soc London, p 220

Bergel F, Morrison AL (1948) Synthetic analgesics. Quart Revs (Lond) 2:349–382

Beyerman HC, Lie TS, Maat T, Bosman HH, Buurman E, Bijsterveld EJM, Sinnige HJM (1976) A convenient synthesis of codeine and morphine. Rec Trav Chim Pay Bas 95:24–25

Bidlack JM, Frey DK, Seyed-Mozaffari A, Archer S (1989) 14β-(Bromoacetamido)morphine irreversibly labels μ opioid receptors in rat brain membranes. Biochemistry 28:4333–4339

Bidlack JM, Frey DK, Kaplan RA, Seyed-Mozaffari A, Archer S (1990) Affinity labeling of μ opioid receptors by sulfhydryl alkylating derivatives of morphine and morphinone. Mol Pharmacol 37:50–59

Billings RE, Booher R, Smits S, Pohland A, McMahon RE (1973) Metabolism of acetylmethadol. A sensitive assay for noracetylmethadol and the identification of a new active metabolite. J Med Chem 16:305–306

Billings RE, McMahon RE, Blake DA (1974) I-Acetylmethadol (LAM) treatment of opiate dependence. Plasma and urine levels of two pharmacologically active metabolites. Life Sci 14:1437–1446

Blane GF, Boura ALA, Fitzgerald AE, Lister RE (1967) Actions of etorphine hydrochloride (M99): a potent morphine-like agent. Br J Pharmacol Chem 30:11–22

Blumberg H, Pachter IJ, Metossian Z (1967) 14β-Hydroxydihydromorphinones. US Patent 3 332 950, 25 July; Chem Abstr (1967) 67:P100301a

Booher RN, Pohland A (1975) Synthesis of a new metabolite of acetylmethadol. J Med Chem 18:266–268

Burke JR Jr, Bajwa BS, Jacobson AE, Rice KC, Streaty RA, Klee WR (1984) Probes for narcotic receptor mediated phenomena: 7. Synthesis and pharmacological properties of irreversible ligands specific for μ and δ opiate receptors. J Med Chem 27:1570–1574

Burke TR Jr, Jacobson AE, Rice KC, Silverton JV, Simonds WF, Streaty RA, Klee W (1986) Probes for narcotic receptor mediated phenomena. 12. cis-(+)-3-methylfentanyl isothiocyanate, a potent site-directed acylating agent for δ opioid receptors. Synthesis, absolute configuration and receptor enantioselectivity. J Med Chem 29:1087–1093

Carabateas PM, Grumbach L (1962) Strong analgesics. Some 1-substituted 4-phenyl-4-propioxypiperidines. J Med Chem 5:913–919

Casy AF, Parfitt RT (1986) Opioid analgesics. Plenum, New York

Clark CR, Halfpenny PR, Hill RG, Horwell DC, Hughes J, Jarvis JC, Rees DC, Hofield DS (1988) Highly selective κ opioid analgesics. Synthesis and structure-activity relationships of novel N-[(1-aminocyclohexyl)aryl]acetamide and N-[aminocyclohexy)aryloxy]-acetamido derivatives. J Med Chem 31:831–836

Corrodi H, Hellerbach J, Zuest A, Hardegger E, Schnider O (1958) Hydroxymorphinans: XII. Configuration of morphinan. Helv Chim Acta 42:212–217

Costello GF, Main BG, Barlow JJ, Carroll JA, Shaw JS (1988) A novel series of potent and selective agonists at the opioid κ-receptor. Eur J Pharmacol 151: 475–478

deCosta BR, Bowen WD, Hellewell SB, George C, Rothman RB, Reid AA, Walker JM, Jacobson AE, Rice KC (1989) Alterations in the stereochemistry of the κ-selective opioid agonist U50,488 result in high-affinity σ ligands. J Med Chem 32:1996–2002

deCosta BR, Rice KC, Bowen WD, Thurkauf A, Rothman RB, Band L, Jacobson AE, Radesca L, Conteras PC, Gray NM, Daly I, Iyengar S, Finn DT, Vazirini S, Walker JM (1990a) Synthesis and evaluation of N-substituted cis-N-methyl-2-(1-pyrrolidinyl)cyclohexylamines as high affinity σ receptor ligands. Identification of a new class of highly potent and selective σ receptor probes. J Med Chem 32:3100–3108

deCosta BR, Rothman RB, Bykov RB, Bykov V, Band L, Pert A, Jacobson AE, Rice KC (1990b) Probes for narcotic receptor mediated phenomena: 17. Synthesis and evaluation of a series of trans-3,4-dichloro-N-methyl-N-[2-(1-pyrrolidinyl)cyclohexyl]benzamide (U50,488) related isothiocyanate derivatives as opioid receptor affinity ligands. J Med Chem 33:1171–1176

DeGraw JI, Christiansen JC, Brown VH, Cory MJ (1974) Grewe codeine method. Attempts to achieve a practical synthesis. J Heterocycl Chem 11:363–367

Dole VP, Nyswander M (1965) A medical treatment for diacetylmorphine (heroin) addiction: a clinical trial with methadone hydrochloride. JAMA 193:640–650

Donnerer J, Oka K, Brossi A, Rice KC, Spector S (1986) Presence and formation of codeine and morphine in the rat. Proc Natl Acad Sci USA 83:4566–4567

Eddy NB, May EL, Mosettig E (1952) Chemistry and pharmacology of the methadols and acetylmethadols. J Org Chem 17:321–326

Eisleb O (1941) New syntheses using sodamide. Chem Ber 74:1433–1450

Eisleb O (1945) Office of the Publication Board, Department of Commerce Report No. PB-981, 9611

Elad D, Ginsburg D (1954) Synthesis in the morphine series: VI. The synthesis of morphine. J Chem Soc:3052–3056

Evans DA, Mitch CH (1982) Studies directed toward the total synthesis of morphine alkaloids. Tetrahedron Lett 23:285–289

Gates M, Montzka TA (1964) Some potent morphine antagonists possessing high analgesic activity. J Med Chem 7:127–131

Gates M, Sheppard MS (1962) The closure of the oxide bridge in the morphine series. J Am Chem Soc 84:4125–4130

Gates M, Tschudi G (1956) The synthesis of morphine. J Am Chem Soc 78:1380–1393

Gordon M, Lafferty JJ, Tedeschi DA, Eddy NB, May EL (1961) A new potent analgesic antagonist. Nature 92:1089

Gritz ER, Shiffman SM, Jarvik ME, Schlesinger J, Charu V, Astra VC (1976) Naltrexone: physiological and psychological effects of single doses. Clin Pharmacol Ther 19:773–776

Grewe R, Friedrichson W (1967) Cyclization of octahydroisoquinoline derivatives by morphinan ring closure. Synthesis of dihydrothebainone. Chem Ber 100:1550–1558

Grewe R, Mondon A (1948) Synthesis in the phenanthrene Series: VI. Synthesis of morphinan. Chem Ber 81:279–286

Halfpenny PR, Hill RG, Horwell DC, Hughes J, Hunter DC, Johnson S, Rees DC (1989) Highly selective κ opioid analgesics: 2. Synthesis and structure-activity relationships of novel N-[(2-aminocyclohexyl)aryl]acetamide derivatives. J Med Chem 32:1620–1626

Hayakawa K, Motohiro S, Fujii I, Kanematsu K (1981) Novel addition reaction of thebaine with acetylenic dienophiles: construction of a new morphine skeleton. J Am Chem Soc 103:4605–4606

Hollander CWD (1958) Racemization. US Patent 2819272, 7 Jan; Chem Abstr (1958) 52:9223i

Hollander CWD (1959) Racemization catalysts. US Patent 2915479, 1 Dec; Chem Abstr (1960) 54:12165d

Jaffe JH, Martin WR (1990) Opioid analgesics and antagonists. In: Gilman AG, Rall TW, Nies AS, Taylor P (eds) Goodman and Gilman's the pharmacological basis of therapeutics, 8th edn. Pergamon, New York, p 512

Janssen PAJ, Eddy NB (1960) Compounds related to pethidine: IV. New general chemical methods of increasing the analgesic activity of pethidine. J Med Chem 2:31–45

Janssen PAJ, Niemegeers CJE, Dony JGH (1963) The inhibitory effect of fentanyl and other morphine-like analgesics on the warm water induced tail withdrawal reflex in the rat. Arzneimittelforschung 13:502–507

Jasinski DR, Martin WR, Haerzten CA (1967) The human pharmacology and abuse potential of N-allylnoroxymorphone (Naloxone). J Pharmacol Exp Ther 157:420–426

Jasinski DR, Pevnick JS, Griffith JD (1978) Human pharmacology and abuse potential of the analgesic buprenorphine. A potential agent for treating narcotic addiction. Arch Gen Psychiatry 35:501–516

Kaplan LJ (1984) Analgesic 1-oxa-, aza- and thia-spirocyclic compounds. US Patent 4438130; Chem Abstr (1984) 101:54192w

Karle IL, Gilardi RD, Fratini AV, Karle J (1969) Crystal structures of DL-cyclazocine and L-cyclazocine, and the absolute configuration of L-cyclazocine HBr·H₂O. Acta Crystallogr Sect B 25:1469–1479

Kirby GW, McLean D (1985) An efficient synthesis of 14β-aminocodeinone from thebaine. J Chem Soc Perkin Trans 1:1443–1445

Kitamura M, Hsiao Y, Noyori R, Takaya H (1988) General asymmetric synthesis of benzomorphans and morphinans via enantioselective hydrogenation. Tetrahedron Lett 28:4829–4832

Klee WA, Simonds WF, Sweat FW, Burke TR Jr, Jacobson AE, Rice KC (1982) Identification of a M_r 58000 glycoprotein subunit of the opiate receptor. FEBS Lett 150:125–128

Kobylecki RJ, Guest IG, Lewis JW, Kirby GW (1978a) Morphine derivatives. Ger Offen 2 812 580, 5 Oct; Chem Abstr (1979) 90:87709t
Kobylecki RJ, Guest IG, Lewis JW, Kirby GW (1978b) Morphine derivatives. Ger Offen 2 812 581; Chem Abstr (1979) 90:39099r.
Kobylecki RJ, Carling RW, Lord JAH, Smith CFC, Lane AC (1982) Common anionic receptor site hypothesis: its relevance to the antagonist action of naloxone. J Med Chem 25:116–120
Lahti RA, Mickelson MM, McCall JM, Von Voightlander PF (1985) [^{3}H] U-69593 a highly selective Ligand for the opioid κ receptor. Eur J Pharmacol 109:281–284
Lednicer D (1982) Medicinal chemistry of central analgesics. In: Lednicer D (ed) Central analgesics. Wiley, New York, p 137
Leimgruber W, Mohacsi E, Baruth H, Randall LO (1973) Levallorphan and related compounds. In: Braude MC, Harris LS, May EL, Smith JP, Villareal JE (eds) Narcotic antagonists. Raven, New York, pp 45–50
Lenz GR, Evans SM, Walters DE, Hopfinger AJ (1987) Opiates. Academic, Orlando
Lewenstein MJ, Fishman J (1966) 14-Hydroxymorphine and codeine carboxymethyl oximes. US Patent 3 320 262, 16 May; Chem Abstr (1967) 67:90989g
Lewis J, Smith C, McCarthy P, Walter D, Kobylecki R, Myers M, Haynes A, Lewis C, Waltham K (1988) New 14-aminomorphinones and codeinones. problems of drug dependence. Natl Inst Drug Abuse Res Monogr Ser 90:136–143
Loew GH, Berkowitz DS (1978) Quantum chemical studies of N-substituent variation in the oxymorphone series of opiate narcotics. J Med Chem 21: 101–106
Magnan J, Paterson SJ, Tavani A, Kosterlitz HW (1982) The binding spectrum of narcotic analgesic drugs with different agonist and antagonist properties. Naunyn Schmiedebergs Arch Pharmacol 319:197–205
Martin WR (1967) Opioid antagonists. Pharmacol Rev 19:463–521
Martin WR, Eades CG, Thompson JA, Huppler RE, Gilbert PE (1976) The effects of morphine- and nalorphine-like drugs in the nondependent and morphine-dependent chronic spinal dog. J Pharmacol Exp Ther 197:517–532
May EL, Ager JH (1959) Structures related to morphine: XI. Analogs and a diastereoisomer of 2'-hydroxy-2,5,9-trimethyl-6,7-benzomorphan. J Org Chem 24:1432–1435
May EL, Fry EM (1957) Structures related to morphine: VIII. Further synthesis in the benzomorphan series. J Org Chem 22:1366–1369
May EL, Kugita H (1961) Structures related to morphine: XV. Stereochemical control of methyl-metallo additions to 9-oxobenzo-morphans. J Org Chem 26:158–163
May EL, Kugita H, Ager JH (1961) Structures related to morphine: XVII. Further stereochemical studies with 9-oxobenzomorphans. J Org Chem 26:1621–1624
McMurry JE, Farina V, Scott WJ, Davidson AH, Summers DR, Shenyi A (1984) A new approach to morphinans: total synthesis of O-methylpallidinine. J Org Chem 49:3803–3812
Merz H, Langbein A, Stockhaus K, Walther G, Wick H (1973) Structure activity relationships in narcotic antagonists with N-furylmethyl substituents. In: Braude MC, Harris LS, May EL, Smith JP, Villareal JE (eds) Narcotic antagonists. Raven, New York, pp 91–108
Merz H, Stockhaus K, Wick H (1975) Stereoisomeric 5,9-dimethyl-2'-hydroxy-2-tetrahydrofuryl-6,7-benzomorphans. Strong analgesics with non-morphine-like action profiles. J Med Chem 18:996–1000
Meyers AI, Bailey TR (1986) An asymmetric synthesis of (+) morphinans in high enantiomeric purity. J Org Chem 51:872–876
Michne WF (1976) A 2,6-Methano-3-benzazocine related to the Thebaine Diels-Alder adduct derivatives. J Org Chem 41:894–896

Michne WF (1978) 2,6-methano-3-benzazocine-11-propanols. Lack of antagonism between optical antipodes and observation of potent narcotic antagonism by two N-methyl derivatives. J Org Chem 21:1322-1324

Michne WF, Albertson NF (1972) Analgesic 1-oxidized-2,6-methano-3-benzazocines. J Med Chem 15:1278–1281

Michne WF, Salsbury RL, Michalec SJ (1977) Synthesis and narcotic agonist-antagonist evaluation of some 2,6-methano-3-benzazocine-11-propanols. Analogues of the ring C bridged oripavine-7-methanols. J Med Chem 20: 682–686

Michne WF, Lewis TR, Michalec SJ, Pierson AK, Rosenberg FJ (1979) (2,6-Methano-3-benzazocin-11β-yl)alkanones: 1. Alkylalkanones: a new series of N-methyl derivatives with novel opiate activity profiles. J Med Chem 22:1158–1163

Monkovic I, Conway TT, Wong H, Perron YG, Pachter IJ, Belleau B (1973) Total synthesis and pharmacological activities of N-substituted 3,14-dihydroxymorphinans I. J Am Chem Soc 95:7910–7912

Monkovic I, Wong H, Pircio AW, Perron YG, Pachter IJ, Belleau B (1975) Oxilorphan and butorphanol. Potent narcotic antagonists and non-addicting analgesics in the 3,14-dihydroxymorphinan series V. Can J Chem 53:3094–3102

Moos WH, Gless RD, Rapoport H (1983) Codeine analogs. Synthesis of 4a-aryldecahydroisoquinolines containing nitrogen ring functionality and of octahydro-1H-indeno[1,2,3-ef]isoquinolines. A total synthesis of codeine. J Org Chem 48:227–238

Niemegeers CJE, Schellekens KHF, Van Bever WFM, Janssen PAJ (1976) Sufentanil, a very potent and extremely safe intravenous morphine-like compound in mice, rats and dogs. Arzneimittelforschung 26:1551–1556

Noyori R, Takaya H (1990) BINAP: an efficient chiral element for asymmetric catalysis. Acc Chem Res 23:345–350

Osei-Gyimah P, Archer S (1980) Synthesis and analgesic activity of some 14β-substituted analogues of morphine. J Med Chem 23:162–166

Osei-Gyimah P, Archer S, Gillan MGC, Kosterlitz HW (1981) Some 14β-substituted analogues of N-(cyclopropylmethy)normorphine. J Med Chem 24:212–214

Pachter IJ, Matossian Z (1968) 14-Hydroxydihydromorphinone. British Patent 1 119 270, 10 July; Chem Abstr (1968) 69:87282q.

Pfeiffer A, Brante V, Herz A, Emreich HM (1986) Psychotomimesis mediated by κ opiate receptors. Science 233:774–776

Rahtz D, Paschelke G, Shroeder E (1977) New N-2-hydroxyalkyl-6,7-benzomorphan derivatives. Synthesis and preliminary pharmacology. Eur J Chim Ther 12: 271–278

Rance MJ, Kobylecki RJ, Lane AC, Holgate MJ, Barnard EA (1981) In: Advances in endogenous and exogenous opioids. Proceedings of the international narcotics research conference, Kyoto, Japan, p 408

Rapoport H, Lavigne JB (1953) Stereochemical studies in the morphine series. The relative configurations at carbons thirteen and fourteen. J Am Chem Soc 75:5320–5324.

Rapoport H, Sheldrich PS (1963) Diels-Alder reaction with thebaine: thermal rearrangement of some adducts from acetylenic dienophiles. J Am Chem Soc 85:1636–1642

Rice KC (1977) A rapid high-yield conversion of codeine to morphine. J Med Chem 20:164–165

Rice KC (1985) The development of a practical total synthesis of natural and unnatural codeine, morphine and thebaine, In: Phillipson JD, Roberts MF, Zenk MH (eds) The chemistry and biology of isoquinoline alkaloids. Springer, Berlin Heidelberg New York, pp 191–203

Rice K, Jacobson AE, Burke TR Jr, Bajwa BS, Streaty RA, Klee WA (1983) Irreversible ligands with high selectivity toward δ or μ opiate receptors. Science 220:314–316

Robinson R, Sugasawa S (1931) Synthetical experiments in the morphine group I. J Chem Soc:3163–3172

Schnider O, Hellerbach J (1950) Synthesis of morphinans II. Helv Chim Acta 33:1437–1448

Schultz AG, Lucci RD, Napier JJ, Kinoshita H, Ravichandran R, Shannon P, Yee YK (1985) Studies directed at a synthesis of the morphine alkaloids. A photochemical approach. J Org Chem 50:217–231

Schultz AG, Green NJ, Archer S, Tham FS (1991) Photochemistry of codeinone derivatives. Development of potential photoaffinity labelling techniques for opiate receptors. J Am Chem Soc 113:6280–6281

Schwartz MA, Mami IS (1975) A biogenetically patterned synthesis of morphine alkaloids. J Am Chem Soc 97:1238–1240

Simonds WF, Burke TR Jr, Rice KC, Jacobson AE, Klee W (1985) Purification of the opiate receptor of NG-108-15 neuroblastoma-glioma hybrid cells. Proc Natl Acad Sci USA 82:4974–4978

Singh A, Archer S, Hoogsteen K. Hirshfield J (1982) Thebaine and acetylenic dienophiles. J Org Chem 47:752–754

Singh A, Kulling RK, Seyed-Mozaffari A, Archer S (1986) Methyl-9,14-didehydro-4,5-epoxy-3-methoxy-17-methyl-2-methylene-6-oxothebinan-β-acetate. J Org Chem 51:3378–3380.

Stork G (1952) Stereochemistry and reaction mechanisms of the morphine alkaloids. In: Manske RHF, Holmes HL (eds) The alkaloids, vol 2. Academic, New York, p 171

Szantay C, Barbzai-Beke M, Pechy P, Blasko G, Dornyhei G (1982) Studies aimed at the synthesis of morphine: 3. Synthesis of (±)-salutaridine via phenolic oxidative coupling of (±)-reticuline. J Org Chem 47:594–596

Szmuszkovicz J, Von Voightlander PF (1982) Benzeneacetamide amines. Structurally novel non-mu opioids. J Med Chem 25:1125–1126

Theuns HG, Janssen RHAM, Biessels HWA, Menichini F, Salemin KCA (1984) A new rearrangement product of thebaine isolated from *Papaver bracteatum* Lindl. Structural assignment of thebaine N-oxides. J Chem Soc Perkin Trans I: 1701–1706

Thorp RH, Walton E, Ofner P (1947) Optical isomers of amidone, with a note on isoamidone. Nature 160:605–606

Thurkauf A, deCosta B, Rice KC (1989) Synthesis of tritium labelled (−)-U 50 488. A selective kappa opioid agonist. J Labelled Compds Radiopharmaceut 27: 577–582

Toth JE, Fuchs PL (1987) Total synthesis of (dl)-morphine. J Org Chem 52:473–475

Toth JE, Hamann PR, Fuchs PL (1988) Studies culminating in the total synthesis of (*dl*)-morphine. J Org Chem 53:4694–4708

Van Bever WFM, Niemegeers CJE, Janssen PAJ (1974) Synthetic analgesics. Synthesis and pharmacology of the diastereoisomers of N-[methyl-1-(2-phenyl)-4-piperidyl]-N-phenylpropanamide and N-[3-methyl-1-(1-methyl-2-phenethyl]-4-piperidyl-N-phenylpropanamide. J Med Chem 17:1047–1054

Van Bever WFM, Niemegeers CFE, Schellekens KHF, Janssen PAJ (1976) N-4-Substituted 1-(2-arylethyl)-4-piperidinyl-N-phenylpropanamides, a novel series of extremely potent analgesics with unusually high safety margin. Arzneimittelforschung 26:1548–1551

Van Daele GHP, DeBruyn MLF, Boev JM, Sanczuk S, Agten JTM, Janssen PAJ (1976) Synthetic analgesics: N-(1-[2-arylethyl]-4-substituted 4-piperidinyl)-N-arylalkanamides. Arzneimittelforschung 26:1521–1531

Von Voightlander PF, Lahti Ra, Ludens JH (1983) U-50488. A selective and structurally novel non-mu (Kappa) opioid agonist. J Pharmacol Exp Ther 224: 7–12

Weijlard J, Orohovats PD, Sullivan AP Jr, Purdue G, Heath FK, Pfister KIII (1956) A new synthetic analgesic. J Am Chem Soc 78:2342–2343

Weiss U (1955) Derivatives of morphine: I. 14-hydroxydihydromorphinone. J Am Chem Soc 77:5891–5892

Weitz CJ, Faull KF, Goldstein A (1987) Synthesis of the skeleton of the morphine molecule by mammalian liver. Nature 330:674–677

Weller DD, Rapoport H (1976) A practical synthesis of codeine from dihydrothebainone, J Med Chem 19:1171–1175; Barber RB, Rapoport H, (1976) Conversion of thebaine to codeine. J Med Chem 19:1175–1180

Weller DD, Stirchak EP, Weller DL (1983) Synthesis of 3-methyl-5,6-dihydro-3H-benzofuro[3,2-e]isoquinolin-7(7aH)-ones. J Org Chem 48:4597–4605.

Ziering A, Lee J (1947) Piperidine derivatives: V. 1,3-Dialkyl-4-aryl-4-accyloxypiperidines. J Org Chem 12:911–914

Ziering A, Malatestinic N, Williams T, Brossi A (1970) 3'-Methyl, 8-methyl, and 8-phenyl derivatives of 5,9-dimethyl-6,7-benzomorphans. J Med Chem 13:9–13

Zimmerman DM, Nickander R, Horng JS, Wong DT (1975) New structural concepts for narcotic antagonists defined in a 4-phenylpiperidine series. Nature 275:332–334

CHAPTER 12
Selective Nonpeptide Opioid Antagonists

P.S. PORTOGHESE

A. Introduction

Opioid antagonists have been indispensable as tools in opioid research (ZIMMERMAN and LEANDER 1990). In fact, the chief criterion for the classification of an agonist effect as opioid receptor-mediated is the ability of naloxone (SAWYNOK et al. 1979) or naltrexone (GOLD et al. 1982) to reversibly antagonize this effect in a competitive fashion. The usefulness of these ligands for this purpose stems from the fact that they are universal opioid antagonists; that is, they are capable of antagonizing the agonist effects mediated by multiple opioid receptor types.

Since it is now firmly established that there are a minimum of three opioid receptor types (HERZ 1987), it has become increasingly evident that selective opioid antagonists are valuable pharmacological tools to identify receptor types involved in the interaction with opioid agonists (ZIMMERMAN and LEANDER 1990). One of the major advantages of selective opioid antagonists over selective agonists is their utility in probing the interaction of endogenous opioid peptides with opioid receptor types. Also, they can be used to evaluate the selectivity of new opioid agonists. Established, selective opioid agonists complement antagonists in their utility as pharmacological tools. However, since it is sometimes not easy to distinguish between μ-, δ-, and κ-opioid receptor-mediated effects if the pharmacological endpoints are identical (e.g., antinociception or inhibition of smooth muscle preparation by agonists), selective antagonists clearly have wider utility as tools than selective agonists.

A general aspect of selective antagonists that deserves mention is that their utility as pharmacological tools depends upon the linkage of in vitro with in vivo activity. This can be accomplished more easily with nonpeptide ligands because they can generally penetrate the blood-brain barrier and therefore can be administered peripherally in vivo. Also, they are less subject to metabolism than peptides. On the other hand, peptides may offer the opportunity to study effects mediated by peripheral opioid receptors if they possess limited access to the CNS.

In addition to their uses as pharmacological tools, selective opioid antagonists with nonpeptide structures have potential clinical applications in the treatment of a variety of disorders where endogenous opioids play a modulatory role. These include food intake, shock, constipation, immune function, behavior, CNS injury, and alcoholism (OLSON et al. 1989).

This chapter focuses on nonpeptide, selective antagonists that interact noncovalently with opioid recognition sites. The number that qualify as pharmacologic tools is miniscule compared to the hundreds of compounds that have been synthesized. This disparity reflects the apparently rigorous structural requirements for selective opioid antagonist activity.

B. Receptor Selectivity

It is important to make a distinction between "selectivity" and "specificity," as these terms are sometimes erroneously used interchangeably. A selective ligand has a greater pharmacological effect or higher affinity associated with the target receptor than it has for other receptors, whereas "specificity" pertains to an effect or affinity that involves a single receptor to the exclusion of all others (PORTOGHESE 1970). Clearly, few, if any, opioid ligands appear to be specific.

The selectivity of an opioid antagonist in part emanates from its *relative* binding affinity for multiple sites. For example, the highly selective δ-antagonist (allyl)$_2$Tyr-Aib-Aib-Phe-Leu-OH (ICI174864) (COTTON et al. 1984) has about the same affinity for δ-sites as the μ-selective antagonist naltrexone. Here the difference in binding selectivity of ICI174864 arises from very low binding affinity for non-δ-sites. On the other hand, the nonpeptide antagonist naltrindole (PORTOGHESE et al. 1988a) derives its δ-selectivity primarily through an affinity for δ-sites that is orders of magnitude greater than that of ICI174864 or naltrexone (PORTOGHESE et al. 1990).

This illustrates that there are basically two different modes of enhancing selectivity through molecular modification. This can occur when there is (1) little change in affinity for the target site coupled with a very large decrease in affinity for sites other than the target site (e.g., ICI174864) or (2) greatly enhanced affinity for the target site, with reduced or no affinity changes for other sites.

Ligands that fall into the first category cannot be employed as models to study the topography of the target site because their selectivity is derived from unfavorable interactions with other sites. On the other hand, those ligands that fit into the second category are better suited for modeling the target site, as it is more likely that the high selectivity in this case reflects specific interactions that enhance molecular recognition.

Finally, it should be borne in mind that there are no "gold standards" for selective antagonists. Until homogeneous opioid receptor types and subtypes have been characterized unequivocally with respect to binding and function, the closed circle of reasoning concerning selectivity permits only tentative conclusions to be drawn on the true selectivity of opioid ligands.

C. μ-Selective Opioid Antagonists

Although naloxone and naltrexone are employed as universal opioid antagonists, they are in fact μ-selective. In smooth muscle preparations, pA_2 analysis indicates that they have five to ten times greater antagonist potency at μ-over κ-receptors and 13–33 over δ-receptors (TAKEMORI and PORTOGHESE 1984). Binding data parallel these results (TAKEMORI et al. 1988; PATERSON et al. 1984). The fact that the unnatural enantiomer (+)-naloxone is inactive as an opioid antagonist and has virtually no affinity for opioid sites underscores the critical stereochemical requirements of opioid recognition sites, particularly when the ligands possess little or no conformational freedom (IIJIMA et al. 1978).

In conjunction with pA_2 analysis (SCHILD 1957), naloxone has been used to identify different opioid receptor types in vivo (SMITS and TAKEMORI 1970; TALLARIDA et al. 1979). Indeed, prior to the advent of the variety of the selective opioid receptor antagonists presently available, in vivo pA_2 analysis was one of the principal methods of differentiating the effects mediated by different receptor types.

A compound that has been reported to have greater μ-selectivity in vitro than naltrexone is cyprodime (SCHMIDHAMMER et al. 1989), a naltrexone-related opioid antagonist. Cyprodime possesses four to five times greater κ/μ K_e ratios in smooth muscle preparations when compared to naloxone and naltrexone. Its potency is lower by over one order of magnitude relative to these antagonists, and its binding affinity also is lower. Thus, cyprodime is less selective by virtue of its substantially reduced binding to δ- and κ-receptors. Cyprodime is pharmacologically active after peripheral administration in mice, but requires doses that are 10–100 times greater than that of naltrexone for an equivalent antagonist effect.

Naloxonazine (PASTERNAK and HAHN 1980) is a long-lasting (>24 h) μ-opioid receptor antagonist in vivo when administered in relatively high doses (LING et al. 1986). Based upon radioligand binding studies at μ- and δ-sites, it has been proposed that it selectively interacts with a putative μ-receptor subtype, μ-1 (JOHNSON and PASTERNAK 1984). A tenfold higher affinity for μ- over putative μ-1-sites has been reported, but the relevance of this binding site to pharmacologic antagonism in vivo requires clarification.

Because of its long duration of action in vivo and apparent resistance to removal from brain membranes by washing, naloxonazine originally was thought to be involved in covalent binding to opioid receptors (JOHNSON and PASTERNAK 1984). However, further characterization of the binding revealed that the interaction is noncovalent (CRUCIANI et al. 1987). More recently, it was reported that naltrexonazine is transformed in brain membranes to the fatty acylhydrazone of the opiate (GARZON-ABURBEH et al. 1989). The proposed steps involved in this transformation (Fig. 1) are a receptor-based sulfydryl-catalyzed hydrolysis of the azine to the opiate hydrazone, followed by nucleophilic attack by the hydrazone moiety upon an ester carbonyl

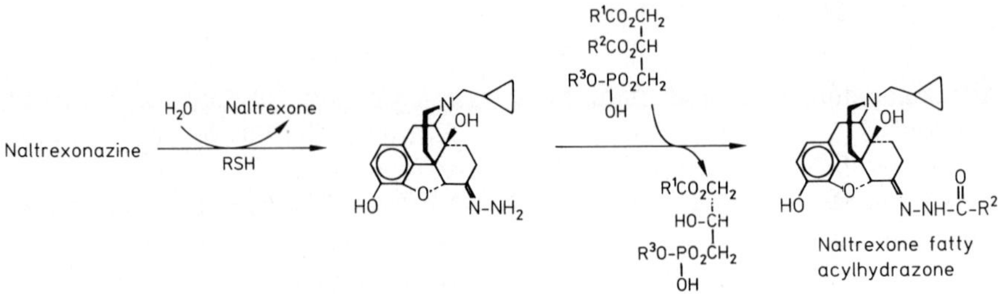

Fig. 1. Proposed pathway for the transformation of naltrexonazine to the fatty acylhydrazone derivative of naltrexone

group of a proximal phosphatide. The fatty acylhydrazone product is not easily removed from the membranes because of the lipophilic fatty acyl group. The observation that synthetic fatty acylhydrazone opiates also were difficult to remove by washing provided additional support for this mechanism. Thus, the apparent resistance of naltrexonazine to removal from brain membranes by washing may be due to accumulation of the fatty acylhydrazone of naltrexone rather than to intact naltrexonazine. Also, this may account for its long duration of action in vivo.

D. δ-Selective Opioid Antagonists

Until relatively recently, only analogues of enkephalin were reported to possess δ-selective antagonist activity and binding. The most widely employed of these ligands, ICI174864 (COTTON et al. 1984), has served as a useful tool for studying δ-opioid effects in vitro and in vivo. However, its peptidic nature and the relatively low affinity for δ-sites has prompted the search for potent, nonpeptide, δ-selective antagonists.

The rationale for the design of such compounds was based on the message-address model of SCHWYZER (1977), which was employed to analyze structure-activity relationships of ACTH and related peptide hormones. Accordingly, peptide hormones are termed "sychnologic" if their information content is organized so that the "message" and "address" domains are proximal to one another in the peptide chain. The message component is required for triggering signal transduction at the receptor site; the address confers additional binding affinity and is not essential to the transduction process.

It was pointed out by CHAVKIN and GOLDSTEIN (1981) that the endogenous opioid peptides conform to the message-address model in that they contain a constant tetrapeptide sequence, Tyr-Gly-Gly-Phe, that can be viewed as the message, and a variable sequence that may serve as an address to confer selectivity for a receptor type.

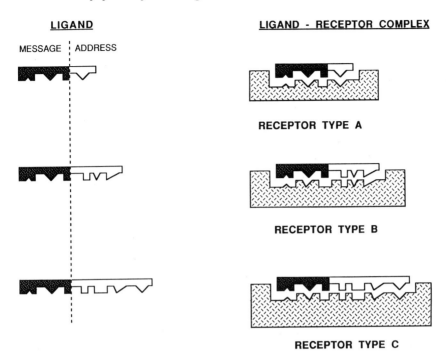

Fig. 2. Message address model for the selectivity of flexible peptide hormones. Note that all three message components are identical while the addresses are different from one another

A modified interpretation of the message-address model (PORTOGHESE et al. 1988b; PORTOGHESE 1989), as applied to opioid peptides, is that the Tyr[1] residue comprises the message component, and the sequence starting with Phe[4] constitutes the address; in this context, Gly[2]-Gly[3] serves as a spacer to connect the message and address elements. This modified view is consistent with the well-known structure-activity relationships of nonpeptide opioid ligands (e.g., morphine) that contain only one aromatic ring, which presumably mimics the Tyr[1] residue.

Figure 2 illustrates the concept with respect to a family of receptor types, depicting the receptor sites of each receptor type as having two subsites. There are (1) a message subsite which is similar or invariant for all of the receptor types and (2) an address subsite that is unique for each receptor type.

This model was evaluated by the attachment of the address segments of leucine-enkephalin and dynorphin to oxymorphone, which contains a nonpeptide message component (LIPKOWSKI et al. 1986) (Fig. 3). The binding data revealed that a typically μ-selective ligand such as oxymorphone can be transformed to a δ-selective ligand simply by attachment of the

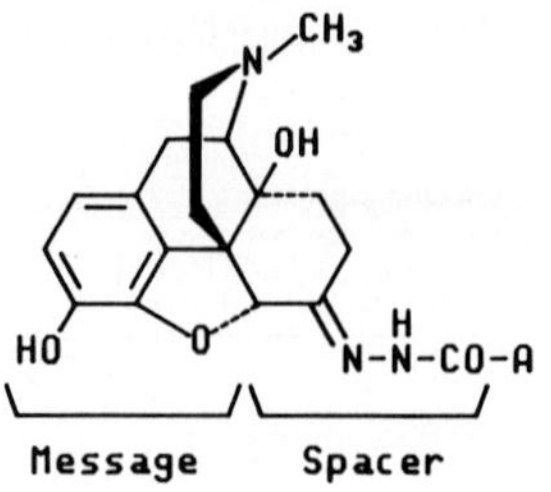

A (address)	Selectivity
Phe-Leu-OH	delta
Phe-Leu-Arg-Arg-Ile-OMe	kappa

Fig. 3. An opiate structure (message) with an attached address peptide (*A*) which modulates opioid receptor selectivity

"δ-address" (Phe-Leu) of leucine-enkephalin through a spacer to the C-6 position of the opiate. Similarly, a κ-selective ligand was obtained by attachment of a segment of the "κ-address" (Phe-Leu-Arg-Arg-Ile-OMe) that is common to the endogenous κ-selective agonist, dynorphin A.

These studies suggested the feasibility of developing nonpeptide, δ-selective opioid antagonists by the attachment of a nonpeptide moiety to an opiate structure in order to mimic a key recognition element in the address. Although the message-address concept was originally proposed for endogenous agonists, it may serve as a useful model for the design of selective antagonists if they also interact with the message and address subsites of the receptor site.

The information content of the address is encoded by the amino acid sequence and its conformational constraints. The latter, which can be considered to be a hidden part of the address, determines the facility with which the address adapts conformationally to an address subsite. The conformational mobility of the opioid peptides may contribute to cross-recognition of opioid receptor types. Presumably, this can take place by conformational adaption of the flexible peptide to the address subsite during the binding process. This may explain the relatively low binding selectivities of the endogenous opioid peptides (HRUBY and GEHRIG 1989).

A strategy for the design of nonpeptide, δ-selective antagonists was to employ a naltrexone-derived structure for the message component and a key element of the leucine-enkephalin δ-address (PORTOGHESE et al. 1988c, 1990). This element, which was hypothesized to be the benzene moiety of Phe^4, was fused to the morphinan structure of naltrexone through a rigid pyrrole spacer. The relationship of the functional components of the nonpeptide antagonist to leucine-enkephalin is illustrated in Fig. 4.

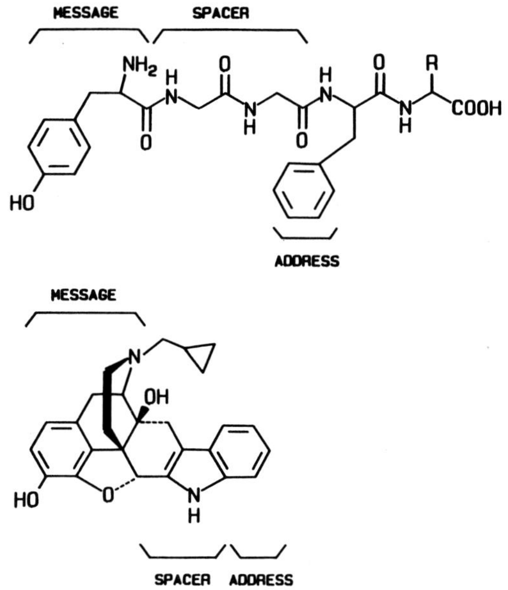

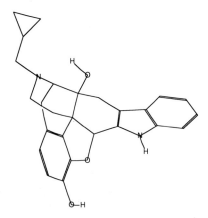

Fig. 4. Comparison of the functional components of enkephalin (*upper*) with those of the δ-selective opioid antagonist naltrindole (*lower*)

Fig. 5. The three-dimensional structure of naltrindole (*NTI*)

The pyrrole spacer confers conformational rigidity to the benzene moiety (δ-address mimic), as it was hoped that this would confer greater δ-selectivity by precluding conformational adaption of the molecule in binding to non-δ-sites on other opioid receptor types.

The geometry of this rigid ligand, known as naltrindole (NTI), is shown in Fig. 5. While alternative naltrexone-derived ligands that contain a

Table 1. Opioid receptor binding of δ-opioid antagonists

Antagonist	χ	K_i (nM)			K_i ratio	
		δ	μ	κ	μ/δ	κ/δ
NTI	NH	0.031	3.8	332	127	11066
NTB	O	0.013	188	1524	1446	11723
ICI174864	–	35	>1000	>1000	>29	>29
Naltrexone	–	36	0.8	20	0.02	0.6

benzene moiety fixed in a different conformation are possible, NTI was synthesized because it was accessible from naltrexone in a single synthetic step. Since the receptor-bound conformation of Phe[4] in enkephalin was not known, an expeditious synthetic route was best suited to explore this design.

Naltrindole (NTI) and related ligands were the first reported nonpeptide δ-opioid receptor antagonists. The in vitro δ-antagonist potency is about 500 times greater than the enkephalin analogue, ICI174864, and 240-fold greater than its precursor, naltrexone. In terms of binding, NTI has over a 1000-fold greater affinity for δ-sites than do ICI174864 and naltrexone (Table 1).

The high antagonist and binding selectivities of NTI are related to its greatly increased affinity for δ-sites and its reduced affinity for other receptor types (PORTOGHESE et al. 1990). This suggests that the benzene moiety of the indole system confers selectivity by binding to a part of the δ-address subsite while hindering binding to other opioid receptor types.

It is noteworthy that NTB, which contains an isosteric furan spacer to hold the benzene moiety in the same orientation as NTI, is also δ-selective, but with lower in vitro antagonist potency (PORTOGHESE et al. 1991). This benzofuran compound, NTB, possesses greater binding affinity at δ-sites than NTI and it also has greater binding selectivity. A possible explanation for the lack of correlation between the in vitro antagonist potency and binding may be related to the presence of δ-receptor subtypes.

Evidence for the existence of δ-receptor subtypes in vivo was obtained from studies in mice (SOFUOGLU et al. 1991). The antinociceptive ED_{50} of the δ-agonist, [D-Ser[2],Leu[5],Thr[6]]enkephalin (DSLET), was shifted fourfold by either NTB or NTI. However, the ED_{50} shift of another δ-agonist, [D-Pen[2],D-Pen[5]]enkephalin (DPDPE), was marginal, with NTI exhibiting

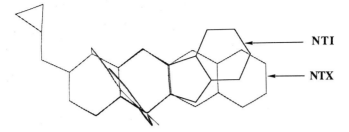

Fig. 6. Superposition of NTI with NTX. Note the different positions of the benzene moiety of the indole (*NTI*) and quinoxaline (*NTX*) systems

slightly greater antagonist potency than NTB. No antagonism of μ- or κ-selective agonists by NTB or NTI was observed. This suggested that DSLET and DPDPE were mediating their antinociceptive effect through different δ-receptor subtypes. The fact that there was no cross-tolerance between DSLET and DPDPE was consistent with this conclusion.

Analogues that contain quinoline (NTQ) or quinoxaline (NTX) ring systems replacing the indole of NTI are less potent δ-antagonists and have lower affinity for δ-sites than NTI or NTB (PORTOGHESE et al. 1991). This may be due to the geometry of the spacer, since they are six-membered rather than five-membered rings in NTQ and NTX. As is illustrated from the superimposed structures (Fig. 6), this orients the benzene moiety differently, reducing the affinity for δ-sites with a concomitant increase at non-δ-sites.

Molecular dynamics simulations were consistent with the idea that Phe[4] of enkephalin serves an address function (PORTOGHESE et al. 1991). The simulations of leucine enkephalin were carried out with the tyramine moiety of Tyr[1] immobilized in the same conformation as in the opiate structure, with the remainder of the peptide unrestrained (Fig. 7). This approach was taken in an effort to mimic a zipper-type mechanism (BURGEN et al. 1975) for binding of the peptide to the δ-site. The zipper model was employed because it offered a more reasonable alternative to the binding of flexible peptides than a lock and key model. Thus, leucine-enkephalin is envisaged to undergo nucleation of Tyr[1] at the message subsite followed by binding of the Phe[4] residue with a δ-address subsite. Presumably, mutual conformational changes of the recognition site also occur during this process and it is this perturbation of the receptor system that triggers signal transduction.

The results of these simulations showed that the conformational space occupied by the phenyl group of Phe[4] was restricted to the region of the indolic benzene moiety of NTI (Fig. 7). The bent leucine-enkephalin backbone is consistent with conformational studies of δ-selective enkephalin-related peptides by NMR and energy calculations (BELLENEY et al. 1989; ISHIDA et al. 1988; KAWAI et al. 1989; RENUGOPALAKRISHNAN et al. 1990;

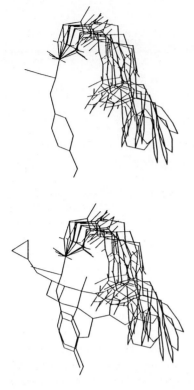

Fig. 7. Molecular dynamics simulation of enkephalin (*upper*) over a 5-ps period divided into 0.5-ps intervals. The message component (Tyr[1]) has been fixed in the same conformation as NTI, which is superposed upon it (*lower*)

SCHILLER 1984; YONEDA et al. 1988). This conformation of enkephalin would permit binding of Phe[4] to a δ-address subsite in the locus of the indolic benzene moiety. However, it is unlikely that the Phe[4] phenyl group would conformationally adapt to an orientation identical with that of the indolic benzene moiety because complete superposition of both rings was not observed during the simulation. It is possible that the conformation of the indolic benzene moiety in NTI may stabilize the δ-receptor in the antagonist state.

E. κ-Selective Opioid Antagonists

Prior to 1982 there were no reports of truly κ-selective opioid antagonists. The first κ-selective opioid antagonist, TENA, was developed from the bivalent ligand approach to design selective ligands (EREZ et al. 1982). TENA is a potent antagonist (PORTOGHESE and TAKEMORI 1985), with a $K_e \sim 0.2\,\mathrm{n}M$ for the antagonism of the κ-agonist, U50488H (SZMUSZKOVICZ and

VON VOIGTLANDER 1982), in the guinea pig ileum preparation (GPI) and it did not antagonize the δ-agonist, [D-Ala^2,D-Leu^5]enkephalin (FOURNIE-ZALUSKI et al. 1981), in the mouse was deferens (MVD). By way of comparison, the two compounds M_r2266 (JACOB and RAMABADRAN 1977) and WIN44441 (MICHNE et al. 1978), reputed to possess κ-antagonist activity, have been reported to be nonselective (PORTOGHESE and TAKEMORI 1985).

The term "bivalent ligands" is defined as a molecule that contains two recognition units linked through a spacer (EREZ et al. 1982; PORTOGHESE 1987). Bivalent ligands can be classified into those that contain either two pharmacophores or a single pharmacophore connected to a non-pharmacophore recognition unit (PORTOGHESE 1989).

The expectation of enhanced potency and selectivity for a receptor type was based on a model that involved the occupation of two neighboring recognition sites by a single bivalent ligand. Each of the sites may be located on separate but identical receptors or on a single receptor. When two neighboring sites are occupied by a bivalent ligand, its affinity should be considerably greater than that of the sum of the individual recognition units. In theory, it should be equal to the product of the binding constants of the individual recognition units.

The design of TENA was originally based on the idea that a spacer could modulate selectivity for a receptor type (EREZ et al. 1982). Such modulation was later demonstrated from in vitro structure-activity-relationship studies of a related series of bivalent ligands with succinyl oligoglycyl spacers. The antagonist bivalent ligand with the shortest spacer conferred significantly enhanced κ-antagonist potency (PORTOGHESE et al. 1986). These studies led to the investigation of bivalent ligands whose pharmacophores are linked through a short spacer, pyrrole, in order to rigidify the molecule and hence immobilize the pharmacophores with respect to one another.

The parent member of this series, norbinaltorphimine (norBNI), possessed unprecedented in vitro κ-opioid antagonist potency and selectivity (PORTOGHESE et al. 1987). Selectivity K_e ratios (μ/κ and δ/κ) in smooth muscle preparations were reported to be in the range of 30–50; another group subsequently determined the selectivity ratios to be considerably higher (250–400) (BIRCH et al. 1987). The high κ-antagonist selectivity is paralleled by its high binding selectivity, with K_i ratios >150 (TAKEMORI et al. 1988).

Animal studies have revealed that norBNI is a κ-selective antagonist with respect to antinociception (TAKEMORI et al. 1988). The selectivity and potency of norBNI in antagonizing opioid agonists in mice using the writhing assay is lower when compared to the in vitro data. This may reflect the nature of the assay, as it was reported (ENDOH et al. 1990) that the tail-pinch assay afforded considerably longer duration of action and higher selectivity ratios. Numerous in vitro and in vivo studies which utilized norBNI as a tool have been reported.

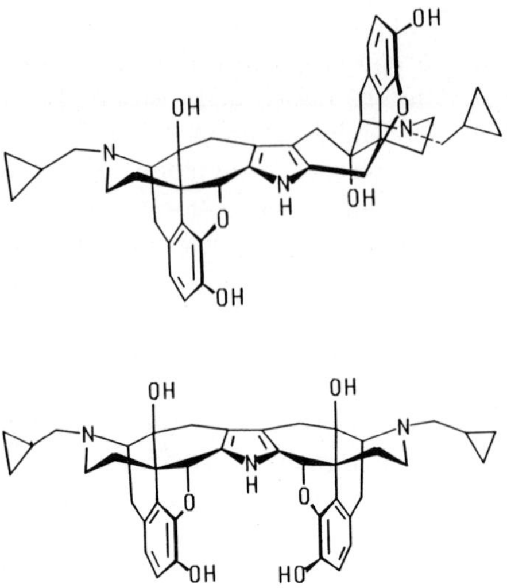

Fig. 8. Conformational representation of norBNI (*upper*) and meso-norBNI (*lower*). Note that the basic nitrogen in the second half of each of the molecules is in nearly the same position relative to the pharmacophore

Structure-activity relationship studies revealed that the two pharmacophores of norBNI are not required for high κ-antagonist potency and selectivity (PORTOGHESE et al. 1988d). In fact, when one of the naltrexone-derived pharmacophores was replaced with its inactive enantiomer, the resulting meso-isomer possessed five times greater κ-antagonist potency than norBNI and was nearly as selective (PORTOGHESE et al. 1988e). These results indicated that the two neighboring sites which interact with norBNI are actually subsites of a single recognition site on the κ-receptor system. The major subsite recognizes the opioid antagonist pharmacophore, and the second subsite is unique for the κ-receptor. A possible clue for the functional significance of this second subsite is the nearly identical positions of the basic nitrogens in the right halves of norBNI and its meso-isomer when these molecules are viewed as three-dimensional structures (Fig. 8). It has been suggested that this nitrogen may confer κ-selectivity by mimicking the Arg[7] basic group of the endogenous κ-selective opioid peptide dynorphin (PORTOGHESE et al. 1988e).

In other words, this model represents another example of the message-address concept that was described earlier in the design of the δ-antagonist, naltrindole. In this case the second half of norBNI contains a rigidly held basic nitrogen which may mimic a key element of the κ-address domain of dynorphin.

References

Belleney J, Gacel G, Fournie-Zaluski MC, Maigret B, Roques BP (1989) δ opioid receptor selectivity induced by conformational constraints in linear enkephalin-related peptides: ^{1}H 400-MHz NMR study and theoretical calculations. Biochemistry 28:7392–7400

Birch PJ, Hayes AG, Sheehan MJ, Tyers MB (1987) Norbinaltorphimine: antagonist profile at κ opioid receptors. Eur J Pharmacol 144:405–408

Burgen ASV, Roberts GCK, Feeny J (1975) Binding of flexible ligands to macromolecules. Nature 253:753–755

Chavkin C, Goldstein A (1981) Specific receptor for the opioid peptide dynorphin. Proc Natl Acad Sci USA 78:6543–6547

Cotton R, Giles MG, Miller L, Shaw JS, Timms D (1984) A highly selective antagonist for the delta receptor. Eur J Pharmacol 97:331–332

Cruciani RA, Lutz RA, Munson PJ, Rodbard D (1987) Naloxonazine effects on the interaction of enkephalin analogs with mu-1, mu-2, and delta opioid binding sites in rat brain membranes. J Pharmacol Exp Ther 242:15–20

Endoh T, Koike H, Matsura H, Nagase H (1990) Nor-binaltorphimine (nor-BNI); a potent and selective kappa opioid receptor antagonist with ultralong-lasting activity in vivo. In: van Ree JM, Mulder AH, Wiegant VM, van Wimersma Greidanus TB (eds) New leads in opioid research. Excerpta Medica, Amsterdam, pp 82–83

Erez M, Takemori AE, Portoghese PS (1982) Narcotic antagonistic potency of bivalent ligands which contain β-naltrexamine. Evidence for bridging between proximal recognition sites. J Med Chem 25:847–849

Fournie-Zaluski M-C, Gacel G, Maigret B, Premilat S, Roques BP (1981) Structural requirements for specific recognition of μ or δ opiate receptors. Mol Pharmacol 20:484–491

Garzon-Aburbeh A, Lipkowski AW, Larson DL, Portoghese PS (1989) Transfer of fatty acyl groups from membrane phospatides to opiate ligands. Neurochem Int 15:207–214

Gold MS, Dackis CA, Pottash ALC, Sternbach HH, Annetto WJ, Martin D, Dakis MP (1982) Naltrexone, opiate addiction, and endorphins. Med Res Rev 2: 211–246

Herz A (1987) The multiplicity of opioid receptors and their functional significance. In: Mutschler E, Winterfeldt E (eds) Trends in medicinal chemistry. VCH, Weinheim, pp 337–350

Hruby VJ, Gehrig CA (1989) Recent developments in the design of receptor specific opioid peptides. Med Res Rev 9:343–401

Iijima I, Minamikawa J, Jacobson AE, Brossi A, Rice K, Klee WA (1978) Studies in the (+)-morphinan series: 5. Synthesis and biological properties of (+)-naloxone. J Med Chem 21:398–400

Ishida T, Yoneda S, Doi M, Inoue M, Kitamura K (1988) Molecular-dynamics simulations of [Met[5]]- and [D-Ala[2],Met[5]]-enkephalins. Biochem J 255:621–628

Jacob JJC, Ramabadran K (1977) Opioid antagonists, endogenous ligands and antinociception. Eur J Pharmacol 46:393–394

Johnson N, Pasternak GW (1984) Binding of [^{3}H]naloxonazine to rat brain membranes. Mol Pharmacol 26:477–483

Kawai H, Kikuchi T, Okamoto Y (1989) A prediction of tertiary structures of peptide by the Monte Carlo simulated annealing method. Protein Eng 3:85–94

Ling GSF, Simantov R, Clark JA, Pasternak GW (1986) Naloxonazine actions in vivo. Eur J Pharmacol 129:33–38

Lipkowski AW, Tam SW, Portoghese PS (1986) Peptides as receptor selectivity modulators of opiate pharmacophores. J Med Chem 29:1222–1225

Michne WF, Lewis TR, Michalec SJ, Pierson AK, Gillan MGC, Paterson SJ, Robson LE, Kosterlitz HW (1978) Novel developments of Nmethylbenzomorphan narcotic antagonists. In: Van Ree JM, Terenius L (eds) Characteristics and functions of opioids. Elsevier, Amsterdam, pp 197–206

Olson GA, Olson RD, Kastin AJ (1989) Endogenous opiates: 1987. Peptides 10: 205–236

Pasternak GW, Hahn EF (1980) Long-acting opiate agonists and antagonists: 14-Hydroxydihydromorphinone hydrazones. J Med Chem 23:674–676

Paterson SJ, Robson LE, Kosterlitz HW (1984) Opioid receptors. In: Udenfriend S, Meienhofer J (eds) The peptides, vol 6. Academic, New York, pp 147–187

Portoghese PS (1970) Relationship between stereostructure and pharmacological activities. Annu Rev Pharmacol 10:51–76

Portoghese PS (1987) Bivalent ligands in the development of selective opioid receptor antagonists. In: Mutschler E, Winterfeldt E (eds) Trends in medicinal chemistry. VCH, Weinheim, pp 327–336

Portoghese PS (1989) Bivalent ligands and the message-address concept in the design of selective opioid antagonists. Trends Pharmacol Sci 10:230–235

Portoghese PS, Takemori AE (1985) TENA, a selective kappa opioid receptor antagonist. Life Sci 36:801–805

Portoghese PS, Larson DL, Sayre LM, Yim CB, Ronsisvalle G, Tam SW, Takemori AE (1986) Opioid agonist and antagonist bivalent ligands. The relationship between spacer length and selectivity at multiple opioid receptors. J Med Chem 29:1855–1861

Portoghese PS, Lipkowski AW, Takemori AE (1987) Binaltorphimine and norbinaltorphimine, potent and selective κ-opioid receptor antagonists. Life Sci 40:1287–1292

Portoghese PS, Sultana M, Takemori AE (1988a) Naltrindole, a highly selective and potent non-peptide δ-opioid receptor antagonist. Eur J Pharmacol 146:185–186

Portoghese PS, Sultana M, Nagase H, Takemori AE (1988b) The message-address concept in the design of highly potent and selective opioid receptor antagonists. In: Melchiorre C, Gianella M (eds) Recent advances in receptor chemistry. Elsevier, Amsterdam, pp 307–317

Portoghese PS, Sultana M, Takemori AE (1988c) Application of the message-address concept in the design of highly potent and selective non-peptide δ-opioid receptor antagonists. J Med Chem 31:281–282

Portoghese PS, Nagase H, Lipkowski AW, Larson DL, Takemori AE (1988d) Binaltorphimine-related bivalent ligands and their κ opioid receptor antagonist selectivity. J Med Chem 31:836–841

Portoghese PS, Nagase H, Takemori AE (1988e) Only one pharmacophore is required for the κ opioid antagonist selectivity of norbinaltorphimine. J Med Chem 31:1344–1347

Portoghese PS, Sultana M, Takemori AE (1990) Design of peptidomimetic δ opioid receptor antagonists using the message-address concept. J Med Chem 33: 1714–1720

Portoghese PS, Nagase H, MaloneyHuss KE, Lin C-E, Takemori AE (1991) Investigation of the spacer and address components in δ opioid antagonists related to naltrindole. J Med Chem 34:1715–1720

Renugopalakrishnan V, Rapaka RS, Bhargava HN (1990) Conformational features of opioid peptides: ligand-receptor interactions. In: Szekely J, Ramabadran K (eds) Biochemistry and applied physiology. CRC Press, Boca Raton, pp 53–114 (Opioid peptides, vol 4)

Sawynok J, Pinsky C, LaBella FS (1979) Minireview on the specificity of naloxone as an opiate antagonist. Life Sci 25:1621–1632

Schild HO (1957) Drug antagonism and pAx. Pharmacol Rev 9:242–246

Schiller P (1984) Conformational analysis of enkephalin and conformation-activity relationships. In: Udenfriend S, Meienhofer J (eds) The peptides, vol 6. Academic, New York, pp 219–268

Schmidhammer H, Burkhard WP, Eggstein-Aeppli L, Smith CFC (1989) Synthesis and biological evaluation of 14-alkoxymorphinans: 2. (−)-N-(cyclopropylmethyl)-4,14-dimethoxymorphinan-6-one, a selective μ opioid receptor antagonist. J Med Chem 32:418–421

Schwyzer R (1977) ACTH: a short introductory review. Ann NY Acad Sci 297:3–26

Smits SE, Takemori AE (1970) Quantitative studies on the antagonism by naloxone of some narcotic-antagonist analgesics. Br J Pharmacol 39:627–638

Sofuoglu M, Portoghese PS, Takemori AE (1991) Differential antagonism of delta opioid agonists by naltrindole (NTI) and its benzofuran analog (NTB) in mice: evidence for delta opioid receptor subtypes. J Pharmacol Exp Ther (in press)

Szmuszkovicz J, von Voigtlander PF (1982) Benzeneacetamide amines: structurally novel non-mu opioids. J Med Chem 25:1125–1126

Takemori AE, Portoghese PS (1984) Comparative antagonism by naltrexone and naloxone of μ, κ, and δ agonists. Eur J Pharmacol 154:101–104

Takemori AE, Ho BY, Naeseth JS, Portoghese PS (1988) Nor-binaltorphimine, a highly selective kappa-opioid antagonist in analgesic and receptor binding assays. J Pharmacol Exp Ther 246:255–258

Tallarida RJ, Cowan A, Adler MW (1979) pA_2 and receptor differentiation: a statistical analysis of competitive antagonism. Life Sci 25:637–654

Yoneda S, Kitamura K, Doi M, Inoue M, Ishida T (1988) Importance for folded monomer and extended antiparallel dimer structures as enkephalin active conformation. FEBS Lett 239:271–275

Zimmerman DM, Leander JD (1990) Selective opioid receptor agonists and antagonists: research tools and potential therapeutic agents. J Med Chem 33:895–902

CHAPTER 13

Presence of Endogenous Opiate Alkaloids in Mammalian Tissues

S. SPECTOR and J. DONNERER

A. Introduction

The finding that mammalian tissues contain the opiate alkaloid morphine endogenously arose as a fallout of having developed morphine antibodies (SPECTOR and PARKER 1970). Initially these antibodies were used to monitor exogenously administered opiates and to study their disposition in body fluids (GINTZLER et al. 1976a). The advantages that these antibodies served in the detection of opiate alkaloids were their sensitivity and specificity (SPECTOR 1971). It became feasible to speculate and ask whether morphine, an opiate alkaloid synthesized in a very complex and stereospecific pathway in the poppy plant *Papaver somniferum* (see Fig. 1), or a closely related compound, also existed as an endogenous compound in mammalian body fluids and tissues.

With the discovery of the family of endogenous opioid peptides (enkephalins: HUGHES et al. 1975; β-endorphin: Cox et al. 1976; dynorphins: GOLDSTEIN et al. 1979) and the pharmacological characterization of a multiplicity of opiate receptors (μ, δ, κ: MARTIN et al. 1976), the relative selectivities of several endogenous peptides in their interaction with the different opioid receptors made them candidates for endogenous ligands of the postulated receptor types. Although β-endorphin can bind to the μ-site with a relatively high affinity, the prototypic agonist for the μ-receptor is the alkaloid morphine (KOSTERLITZ 1985). This recognition further stimulated and justified the search for an endogenous morphine in mammalian tissue.

B. Technical Principles Used in the Isolation of Alkaloid Compounds from Animal Tissue

Several morphine antibodies developed from immunogens, in which a protein was conjugated to morphine at either C_3 or C_6 or at the N-atom, recognizing different epitopes of the morphine molecule but displaying no interaction with opioid peptides, were used in various stages of the isolation and purification process over the years. The early strategy was to use these antibodies as surrogate receptors to which only an unknown substance very similar to morphine in a tissue extract would bind (GINTZLER et al. 1976b).

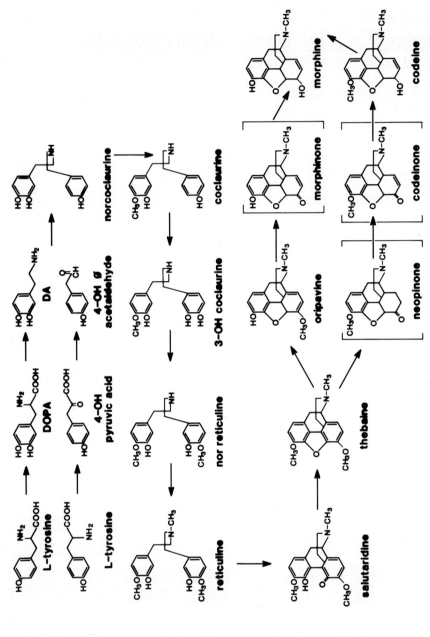

Fig. 1. Proposed biosynthetic pathway of morphine alkaloids starting from tyrosine building blocks in *Papaver somniferum* plants

Since there are a limited number of ways that a small molecule can present itself to a protein, whether it be a receptor, an enzyme, or an antibody, there may be some homology, i.e., receptors and antibodies see at least part of the same three-dimensional structure of the molecule. To detect this binding the principle of the radioimmunoassay (RIA) was employed. Thereby nonpeptide compounds capable of competing with labeled morphine for a limited amount of available binding sites of the antibody were found in animal tissue extracts and, since no definite purification and identification had yet been performed, was referred to as morphine-like compounds (MLC: GINTZLER et al. 1976b, 1978; KILLIAN et al. 1981).

These MLC extracts from beef brain or human urine were also shown to interact with opiate receptors (BLUME et al. 1977). Using the receptors found in the neuroblastoma and glioma hybrid cell line NG 108-215, shown by KLEE and NIRENBERG (1974) to exhibit the appropriate stereospecificity and selectivity for opiate agonist and opiate antagonist binding, it was found that MLC competes in a dose-dependent manner with the binding of [^{3}H]Leu-enkephalin, [^{3}H]etorphine, and [^{3}H]naloxone to the opiate receptor present on these cells (BLUME et al. 1977).

In a further attempt to characterize MLC, various high-performance liquid chromatography (HPLC) purification steps were added to the organic solvent extraction procedures and to the gel chromatography to purify the compound to homogeneity, always monitoring the MLCs with RIA. Finally the endogenous nonpeptide opioid was identified at the molecular level as morphine in an extract from toad skin using gas chromatography and mass spectrometry (OKA et al. 1985). Toad skin was chosen at that time for the isolation of morphine from an animal tissue because it had the greatest concentration of MLC among several tissues from various species analyzed. These studies also made clear that the quantitative determination of the morphine activity by RIA following two different HPLC-purification steps (reversed-phase and ion-exchange HPLC) gave the same results as mass spectrometry.

C. Identification of Endogenous Opiate Alkaloids in Mammalian Tissue

Using the methodology described above, two research groups simultaneously identified the opiate alkaloid morphine as an endogenous compound in several mammalian tissues: Spector's group demonstrated the presence of morphine in rat and rabbit skin as well as in beef brain and adrenals (OKA et al. 1985), whereas GOLDSTEIN et al. (1985), employing a powerful array of purification techniques and using a different set of morphine antibodies, reported the presence of morphine and several closely related compounds in beef hypothalamus and adrenal. At that time it became evident that there were other compounds, very closely related to morphine, also present in mammalian tissue that reacted with the morphine antibodies but eluted on HPLC at distinct positions. The first of these compounds identified was codeine in rat brain, liver, kidney, and intestine (Donnerer et al. 1986). Goldstein's group confirmed the presence of codeine in their extracts from bovine brain (Weitz et al. 1986). The identification of codeine as a natural endogenous alkaloid in mammalian tissue gave for the first time definite support to the existence of an endogenous biosynthetic pathway for morphine, because codeine is considered the immediate precursor of morphine in the poppy plant (Fig. 1).

The levels of morphine and codeine in mammalian tissues were not as high as in the toad skin and they were lower than the levels of opioid peptides in mammalian brain and adrenals (Kosterlitz 1987). However, the fact that at the μ-opiate receptor they could locally reach levels high enough for effective interaction cannot be excluded. Furthermore, more extensive biochemical studies revealed that only a small fraction of morphine in animal tissue exists in a free form and that the major fraction is present in a conjugated form from which the free alkaloids can be released either by acid hydrolysis or by the action of an arylsulfatase or a glucuronidase (Cardinale et al. 1987; Donnerer et al. 1987). Interestingly morphine-6-glucuronide and morphine-6-sulfate conjugate themselves have been recognized as very potent analgesics (Brown et al. 1985; Paul et al. 1989). Morphine, codeine, and their conjugates have also been identified as endogenous components of human cerebrospinal fluid (Cardinale et al. 1987).

Interestingly 6-acetylmorphine, which is known as a metabolite of the synthetic opiate alkaloid heroin (3,6-diacetylmorphine), has also been identified in bovine brain (Weitz et al. 1988). 6-Acetylmorphine has so far not been described as a metabolite of morphine or codeine, but only methodological limitations could have prevented its detection. Its known addictive and analgesic properties add new significance to a possible physiological role of endogenous morphinans.

The identification of the opiate thebaine, an intermediate of morphine biosynthesis in Papaver somniferum, as an endogenous compound in ovine brain (Kodaira et al. 1989), provided another link in the chain of precursor molecules for morphine in animal tissue that are similar to those in the plant (Fig. 1). Thereby it has to be considered that precursors, such as codeine or thebaine, can exert an additional function apart from just being precursors for morphine. Thebaine can stimulate the CNS and cause convulsions (Tortella et al. 1984).

D. Biosynthesis of Mammalian Morphine

One of the issues raised by Hazum et al. (1981), who found immunoreactive morphine in human and cow milk, was that morphine could be derived from dietary sources. Therefore, before one can definitively affirm that the opiate alkaloid is endogenously present and not derived from an exogenous source, one must demonstrate its synthesis in mammalian tissues.

In Papaver somniferum, morphine is synthesized from tyrosine by way of several intermediates (Fig. 1). This biosynthesis has been extensively investigated (BATTERSBY et al. 1965; BARTON et al. 1965; STADLER et al. 1987). (+)-Salutaridine, (−)-thebaine, and (−)-codeine are the direct precursors of (−)-morphine (BROCHMANN-HANSSEN 1984). It has recently been found that norcoclaurine and coclaurine are the precursors of reticuline and thebaine (STADLER et al. 1987), though tetrahydropapaveroline (norlaudanosoline) had been for a long time assumed to be the precursor of thebaine (BATTERSBY et al. 1964).

The possible role of tetrahydropapaveroline as a precursor in the biosynthesis of morphine is unclear. Tetrahydropapaveroline, which is formed by the condensation between dopamine and an aldehyde derived from a second dopamine molecule, has been identified in the brain of rats given L-3,4-dihydroxyphenylalanine (TURNER et al. 1974) as well as in the urine of Parkinsonian patients who had been given L-dopa (SANDLER et al. 1973), and much speculation has been made about the possible consequences of the formation of this compound in mammalian brain. However, it has not been detected in normal mammalian tissue nor has it been shown to be a precursor for reticuline in mammalian tissue.

In the investigation of the putative pathway for a mammalian biosynthesis of morphine it was taken as a prerequisite that this pathway might be identical to that in poppy plants and indeed the findings so far support this assumption. Using established precursor compounds for morphine such as codeine, thebaine, salutaridine, reticuline, or norcoclaurine, the potential mechanisms for converting these precursors in mammals in vivo and in vitro were investigated. Thus, conversion of codeine to morphine involves demethylation of the methoxy group at C3 only and a rather good rate for such conversion was demonstrated in laboratory animals (GINTZLER et al. 1976a; DONNERER et al. 1986) and in man (FINDLAY et al. 1978). DONNERER et al. (1986) also described an increase in the concentrations of codeine and morphine in brain, intestine, liver, kidney, and blood following intravenous injection of salutaridine and thebaine in the rat. Thus the first evidence for a conversion of several precursors to morphine in mammals was provided. The preparation of unambiguously pure samples of the precursors (+)-salutaridine and (−)-thebaine (DUMONT et al. 1986) made it possible to rule out any contamination or resolve questioning about the endogenous origin of the opiates formed from them. Finally the transformation of thebaine to oripavine, codeine, and morphine by rat liver, kidney, and brain microsomes in the presence of an NADPH-generating system provided direct evidence for the enzymatic formation of morphine in mammalian tissues (KODAIRA and SPECTOR 1988; Fig. 2). It was thereby demonstrated that morphine biosynthesis from thebaine in mammalian tissues can occur by the same two routes as demonstrated for Papaver somniferum (BROCHMANN-HANSSEN

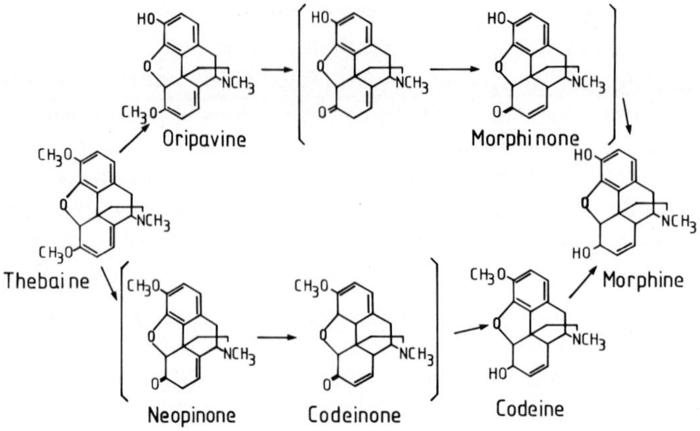

Fig. 2. Two alternative pathways have been described for the transformation of thebaine to morphine in Papaver somniferum as well as in rat liver microsomes

1984): (1) thebaine–neopinone–codeinone–codeine–morphine; and (2) thebaine–oripavine–3-O-demethylated neopinone–morphinone–morphine (Fig. 2). Either pathway requires the 3- and 6-O-demethylation of thebaine, and their respective different cofactor requirements (NADH for the 6-O-demethylations and NADPH for the 3-O-demethylations) indicated that different enzymes may be involved in the transformation (KODAIRA and SPECTOR 1988).

The oxidative intramolecular coupling of reticuline to form salutaridine is the critical step that generates the chiral four-ring arrangement defined as the morphinan structure (BARTON et al. 1965; Fig. 3). Using radioactive-labeled reticuline, WEITZ et al. (1987) have demonstrated that this compound can be converted to salutaridine by rat liver in vivo and in vitro (Fig. 3). Although neither reticuline nor salutaridine has yet been identified in animal tissue, the unusual features of this intramolecular coupling reaction suggest that it is catalyzed by a specific enzyme in mammalian liver. Since the conversion of reticuline to salutaridine could not be detected in brain and adrenal, but the presence of morphine and codeine has been confirmed there, it is suggested that one or more steps in mammalian biosynthesis of morphine take place only in the liver (WEITZ et al. 1987).

As demonstrated for the poppy plant, norcoclaurine, derived from an enzymatic and stereospecific condensation of dopamine with (4-hydroxyphenyl) acetaldehyde, is the first isoquinoline in the biosynthesis of the critical intermediate, reticuline (STADLER et al. 1987; Fig. 1). The O-methylation of norcoclaurine, catalyzed by mammalian catechol-O-methyltransferase, has been examined by CREVELING et al. (1990) and found to be stereoselective, only the 6-O-methylester being derived from the (−)-enantiomer, an obligatory pathway for the biosynthesis of (−)-reticuline.

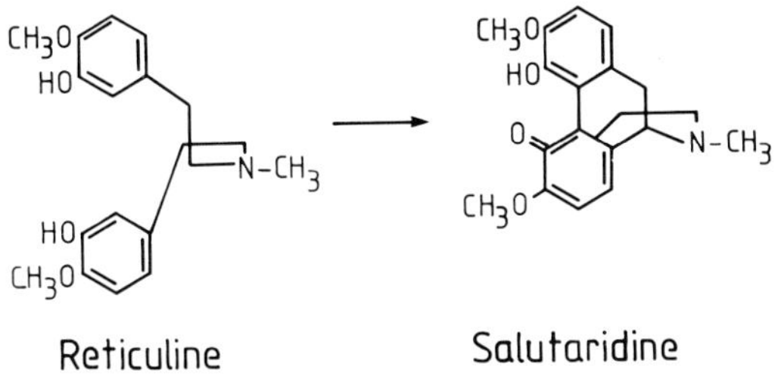

Reticuline   Salutaridine

Fig. 3. Oxidative cyclization of reticuline to yield salutaridine, the first compound with the morphine skeleton in the biosynthetic pathway of morphine alkaloids in the opium poppy, has also been demonstrated for rat liver

Taken together, all the studies performed to date suggest that the mammalian liver has the potential to perform several critical enzymic conversion steps of the morphine precursors and that the putative pathway for the mammalian biosynthesis of morphine may be identical to the pathway in poppy plants.

E. Regulation of Endogenous Morphine and Search for a Physiological Role

In two excellent commentaries, KOSTERLITZ (1985, 1987) has presented several critical thoughts regarding a true physiological role of endogenous morphine, as well as its relationship to the opioid peptides and their functions. With more and more data accumulating on the endogenous regulation of the opiate alkaloid levels under different situations, more evidence is provided for them being a flexible biosystem and not just an issue of pure chemical-analytical interest. Since the proper methods for fast and reliable determination of endogenous opiate alkaloid levels have already been established, the interest can now shift and focus upon the biological regulation of these compounds.

In rats with adjuvant-induced arthritis the spinal cord content of morphine was found increased four times and there was also a significant increase in urinary excretion of morphine (DONNERER et al. 1987). This elevation of morphine content and turnover during painful arthritis could reflect a functional, endogenous analgesic, adaptation process. It was also found that the endogenous content of the opiate alkaloids morphine and codeine became elevated in various brain regions of the rat during food deprivation (LEE and SPECTOR 1991) and this has been seen as an endogenous adaptation of the rate of metabolism.

Some of the precursors, such as codeine or thebaine, can also have a physiological function of their own (see above) and undergo alterations during pathophysiological situations (HABERMAN et al. 1988; RUMEYSA et al.

1990). However, there are still a number of open questions and several studies should be performed before we can fully understand the physiological role of the endogenous opiate alkaloids.

References

Barton DHR, Kirby GW, Steglich W, Thomas GM, Battersby AR, Dobson TA, Ramuz H (1965) Investigations on the biosynthesis of morphine alkaloids. J Chem Soc: 2423–2428

Battersby AR, Binks R, Francis RJ, McCaldin DJ, Ramuz H (1964) Alkaloid biosynthesis: IV. 1-Benzylisoquinolines as precursors of thebaine, codeine, and morphine. J Chem Soc: 3600–3610

Battersby AR, Foulkes DM, Binks R (1965) Alkaloid biosynthesis: VIII. Use of optically active precursors for investigations on the biosynthesis of morphine alkaloids. J Chem Soc: 3323–3332

Blume AJ, Shorr J, Finberg JPM, Spector S (1977) Binding of the endogenous non-peptide morphine-like compound to opiate receptors. Proc Natl Acad Sci USA 74:4927–4931

Brochmann-Hanssen E (1984) A second pathway for the terminal steps in the biosynthesis of morphine. Planta Med 4:343–345

Brown CE, Roerig SC, Burger VT, Cody RB, Fujimoto JM (1985) Analgesic potencies of morphine 3- and 6-sulfates after intracerebroventricular administration in mice: relationship to structural characteristics defined by mass spectrometry and nuclear mahnetic resonance. J Pharm Sci 74:821–824

Cardinale GJ, Donnerer J, Finck AD, Kantrowitz JD, Oka K, Spector S (1987) Morphine and codeine are endogenous components of human cerebrospinal fluid. Life Sci 40:301–306.

Cox BA, Goldstein A, Li CH (1976) Opiate activity of a peptide, β-lipotropin (61–91) derived from β-lipotropin. Proc Natl Acad Sci USA 73:1821–1823

Creveling CR, Bell ME, Sekine Y, Tadic D, Brossi A (1990) The biosynthesis of mammalian morphine: the role of enzymatic O-methylation of (R)- and (S)-enantiomers of norcoclaurine, and 3-demethylnorreticuline in the formation of (S)-reticuline. Soc Neurosci Abstr 16 1:802

Donnerer J, Oka K, Brossi A, Rice KC, Spector S (1986) Presence and formation of codeine and morphine in the rat. Proc Natl Acad Sci USA 83:4566–4567

Donnerer J, Cardinale G, Coffey J, Lisek CA, Jardine I, Spector S (1987) Chemical characterization and regulation of endogenous morphine and codeine in the rat. J Pharmacol Exp Ther 242:583–587

Dumont R, Newmann AH, Rice KC, Brossi A, Toome V, Wegrzynski B (1986) Precursors of the mammalian synthesis of morphine: (+)-salutaridine and (−)-N-13CH3-thebaine from (−)-northebaine. FEBS Lett 206:125–129

Findlay JWA, Jones EC, Butz RF, Welch RM (1978) Plasma codeine and morphine concentrations after therapeutic oral doses of codeine-containing analgesics. Clin Pharmacol Ther 24:60–68

Gintzler AR, Mohacsi E, Spector S (1976a) Radioimmunoassay for the simultaneous determination of morphine and codeine. Eur J Pharmacol 38:149–156

Gintzler AR, Levy A, Spector S (1976b) Antobodies as a means of isolating and characterizing biologically active substances: presence of a non-peptide, morphine-like compound in the central nervous system. Proc Natl Acad Sci USA 73:2432–2436

Gintzler AR, Gershon MD, Spector S (1978) A nonpeptide morphine-like compound: immunocytochemical localization in the mouse brain. Science 199:447–448

Goldstein A, Tachibana S, Lowney LI, Hunkapiller M (1979) Dynorphin (1–13) an extraordinary potent opioid peptide. Proc Natl Acad Sci USA 76:6666–6670

Goldstein A, Barrett RW, James IF, Lowney LI, Weitz CJ, Knipmeyer LL, Rapoport H (1985) Morphine and other opiates from beef brain and adrenal. Proc Natl Acad Sci USA 82:5203–5207

Haberman F, Lavicky J, Marcum E, Spector S (1988) Elevation of endogenous levels of codeine and morphine following the administration of tumor necrosis factor and lipopolysaccharide. FASEB J 2:A1260

Hazum E, Sabatka JJ, Chang KJ, Brent DA, Findlay JWA, Cuatrecasas P (1981) Morphine in cow and human milk: could dietary morphine constitute a ligand for specific morphine(μ) receptors? Science 213:1010–1012

Hughes J, Smith TW, Kosterlitz HW, Fothergrill JA, Morgan BA, Morris HR (1975) Identification of two related pentapeptides from the brain with potent opiate agonist activity. Nature 258:577–579

Killian AK, Schuster CR, House JT, Shell S, Connors VA, Warner BH (1981) A non-peptide morphine-like compound from brain. Life Sci 28:811–817

Klee WA, Nirenberg M (1974) A neuroblastoma x glioma hybrid cell with morphine receptors. Proc Natl Acad Sci USA 71:3474–3477

Kodaira H, Spector S (1988) Transformation of thebaine to oripavine, codeine, and morphine by rat liver, kidney, and brain microsomes. Proc Natl Acad Sci USA 85:1267–1271

Kodaira H, Lisek CA, Jardine I, Arimura A, Spector S (1989) Identification of the convulsant opiate thebaine in mammalian brain. Proc Natl Acad Sci USA 86:716–719

Kosterlitz HW (1985) Has morphine a physiological function in the animal kingdom? Nature 317:671–672

Kosterlitz HW (1987) Biosynthesis of morphine in the animal kingdom. Nature 330:606

Lee CS, Spector S (1991) Changes of endogenous morphine and codeine contents in the fasting rat. J Pharmacol Exp Ther 257:647–650

Martin WR, Eades CG, Thompson JA, Huppler RE, Gilbert PE (1976) The effects of morphine and nalorphine drugs in the nondependent and morphine dependent chronic spinal dog. J Pharmacol Exp Ther 197:517–532

Oka K, Kantrowitz JD, Spector S (1985) Isolation of morphine from toad skin. Proc Natl Acad Sci USA 82:1852–1854

Paul D, Standifer KM, Inturrisi CE, Pasternak GW (1989) Pharmacological characterization of morphine-6-glucuronide, a very potent morphine metabolite. J Pharmacol Exp Ther 251:477–483

Rumeysa S, Suna D, Dilek ED, Bilge S, Eymire O (1990) Endogenous thebaine: cause of epileptic convulsions? In: Van Ree (ed) New leads in opioid research. ICS 914, pp 349–350

Sandler M, Carter SB, Hunter KR, Stern GM (1973) Tetrahydroisoquinoline alkaloids: in vivo metabolites of L-dopa in man. Nature 241:439–443

Spector S (1971) Quantitative determination of morphine in serum by radioimmunoassay. J Pharmacol Exp Ther 178:253–258

Spector S, Perker C (1970) Morphine: radioimmunoassay. Science 168:1347–1348

Stadler R, Kutchan TM, Loeffler S, Nagakura N, Cassels B, Zenk MH (1987) Revision of the early steps of reticuline biosynthesis. Tetrahedron Lett 28:1251–1254

Tortella FC, Cowan A, Adler MW (1984) Studies on the Excetatory and inhibitory influence of intracerebroventricularily injection of opioids on seizure thresholds in rats. Neuropharmacology 23:749–754

Turner AJ, Baker KM, Algeri S, Frigerio A, Garattini S (1974) Tetrahydropapaveroline: formation in vivo and in vitro in rat brain. Life Sci 14:2247–2257

Weitz CJ, Lowney LI, Faull KF, Feistner G, Goldstein A (1986) Morphine and codeine from mammalian brain. Proc Natl Acad Sci USA 83:9784–9788
Weitz CJ, Faull KF, Goldstein A (1987) Synthesis of the skeleton of the morphine molecule by mammalian liver. Nature 330:674–677
Weitz CJ, Lowney LI, Faull KF, Jeisner G, Goldstein A (1988) 6-Acetylmorphine: a natural product present in mammalian brain. Proc Natl Acad Sci USA 85: 5335–5338

Section C: Opioid Peptides

CHAPTER 14

Regulation of Opioid Peptide Gene Expression

V. HÖLLT

A. Introduction

Mammalian opioid peptides are encoded by three different genes (Fig. 1):

1. The proopiomelanocortin (POMC) gene is transcribed into an mRNA which is translated into a protein of 267 amino acids. Posttranslational processing of this precursor molecule generates several biologically active peptides, such as β-endorphin, ACTH, and various peptides with melanocyte-stimulating activity (α-MSH, β-MSH, γ-MSH).
2. The proenkephalin (PENK) gene encodes the PENK precursor, a protein of 267 amino acids. This protein contains four copies of methionine-enkephalin (met-ENK) and one copy each of leucine-enkephalin (leu-ENK), the heptapeptide met-ENK-arg^6-phe^7, and the octapeptide met-ENK-arg^6-gly^7-(or ser^7)-leu^8. The PENK precursor can also be processed into larger ENK-containing peptides, such as peptide E, peptide F, BAM-18P, methorphamide, and amidorphin.
3. The prodynorphin (PDYN) gene gives rise to a protein of 254 amino acids and is a precursor of leu-ENK and of several opioid peptides containing leu-ENK at the N-terminus, such as dynorphin A (DYN), DYN B, and α- and β-neoendorphin.

The tissue-specific processing of the three precursor proteins and the characteristics of the generated opioid peptides will be reviewed in Chaps. 17 and 18.

In the present chapter an attempt has been made to summarize findings concerning the structures and regulation of the three opioid peptide genes. This review will provide an overview of the regulation of all three opioid peptide genes in several tissues. The regulation of the POMC gene in the pituitary and of that of the PENK gene in the adrenal medulla will be described in more detail in Chaps. 15 and 26.

B. Structure and Regulatory Elements of the Opioid Peptide Genes

I. Proopiomelanocortin

The structure of the human POMC gene has been completely sequenced (TAKAHASHI et al. 1983). It is 7665 base pairs (bp) long and comprises the following: exon 1 (86 bp), exon 2 (152 bp), exon 3 (833 bp); intron A (3708 bp), intron B (2886 bp) (Fig. 1). A similar structural organization has also been found for the bovine (NAKANISHI et al. 1981), mouse (NOTAKE et al. 1983a; UHLER et al. 1983), and rat (DROUIN et al. 1985) genes.

The size of the POMC mRNA in the pituitary is about 1200 nucleotides. An mRNA species with a longer poly (A) tail has been detected in the hypothalamus (JEANNOTTE et al. 1987a). In some peripheral tissues shorter POMC transcripts have been found, which are derived from aberrant transcription initiations next to the 5'-end of exon 3 and, thus, do not contain any exon 1 or exon 2 sequences (JINGAMI et al. 1984; JEANNOTTE et al. 1987a). In the intermediate pituitary of the rat, a different splicing occurs between exon 1 and exon 2, giving rise to two POMC mRNAs which differ in 30 nucleotides within the 5'-untranslated portion of the POMC mRNA (OATES and HERBERT 1984). In addition, larger, 5'-extended POMC transcripts have been observed in human tumors. These mRNA species result from a variable mode of transcription induced by promoters located at upstream start sites of transcription between −400 and −100 (DEBOLD et al. 1988c; DE KEYZER et al. 1989; CHANG et al. 1989).

Transfection of fusion genes revealed a DNA element located 53–59 bp upstream of the capping site which exerts a suppressive effect on POMC gene transcription (MISHINA et al. 1982; NOTAKE et al. 1983b). Recently, negative elements have also been localized further upstream of the human POMC promoter region between nt −676 and nt −414 (KRAUS and HÖLLT 1990, 1992). Transfection of a human POMC thymidine kinase fusion gene into mouse fibroblast revealed that the sequences responsible for the negative regulation by glucocorticoids are located within a DNA segment that extends 670 bp upstream from the cap site (ISRAEL and COHEN 1985). Further deletion analysis revealed that no more than 417 bp of the 5'-flanking region of the human POMC gene are required for transcriptional repression by glucocorticoids (NAKAI et al. 1991). The mechanisms whereby glucocorticoids inhibit transcription of the POMC gene have been analyzed in more detail for the rat POMC gene. Gene transfer studies indicated that sequences responsible for negative regulation of transcription by glucocorticoids reside within 706 nucleotides upstream of the capping site (CHARRON and DROUIN 1986). Similarly, expression of a rat POMC fusion gene in transgenic mice revealed that no more than 769 base pairs of the rat POMC promoter sequences are required for glucocorticoid inhibition of the POMC gene in the anterior pituitary (TREMBLAY et al. 1988). A

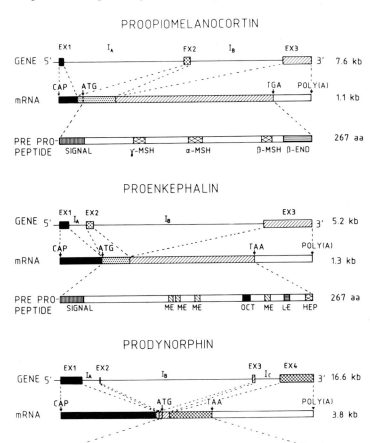

Fig. 1. Structural organization of the genes, mRNAs, and propeptides of the three opioid peptide systems. *CAP*, transcription initiation site; *ATG*, start of translation; *TAA/TGA*, end of translation; *Poly (A)*, polyadenylation site; *Ex*, exon; *I*, intron; *MSH*, melanocyte-stimulating hormone; B-*END*, β-endorphin; *M-E*, met-enkephalin; *L-E*, leu-enkephalin; *OCT*, octapeptide (met-enkephalin-arg[6]-gly[7]-leu[8]); *HEP*, heptapeptide (met-enkephalin-arg[6]-phe[7]); *α-NE*, α-neoendorphin; *DYN*, dynorphin

negative glucocorticoid recognition element (nGRE) that binds to purified glucocorticoid receptors in vitro has been identified at position −63 of the rat POMC gene (DROUIN et al. 1989). This nGRE differs significantly from the known glucocorticoid responsive element (GRE) consensus sequence. The nGRE was also shown to contain a binding site for a nuclear protein of the COUP (chicken *o*valbumin *u*pstream *p*romoter) family of transcription factors. Since the binding sites for COUP and the glucocorticoid receptor overlap, glucocorticoid-dependent repression of POMC transcription has been suggested to result from mutually exclusive binding of these two nuclear transcription factors (DROUIN et al. 1989). The region between −71 and −51 was also shown to be important in negative regulation of the rat POMC gene (RIEGEL et al. 1991). These authors also found that the region from −480 to −320 contribute to the negative regulation by glucocorticoids.

Sequences conferring tissue specificity have been localized 480–34 bp upstream of the capping site of the rat POMC gene (JEANNOTTE et al. 1987b). Moreover, the tissue specificity of the rat promoter was also shown in transgenic mice in which a chimeric rat POMC *neo* gene was introduced into the germ line. In these mice, high levels of the fusion transcripts were detected in the intermediate and the anterior pituitary. They were not detected in any other tissue except for very low levels in the testes (TREMBLAY et al. 1988). Recent experiments revealed that tissue-specific expression of the human POMC gene resides on an element between −414 and −223 (KRAUS and HÖLLT 1992).

A fragment of the rat POMC gene containing DNA sequences 794–38 nucleotides upstream of the capping site confers both elevated basal activity and inducibility by corticotropin-releasing hormone (CRH) or by forskolin when a POMC *tk* CAT fusion gene was transiently expressed in AtT-20 cells. DNA sequences extending from 478 to 320 bp upstream of the capping site were identified which confer elevated basal activity and a moderate inducibility by CRH. Another fragment extending from 320 to 133 nucleotides upstream of the start of transcription was shown to be required for the strong inducibility (ROBERTS et al. 1987). Since this DNA fragment does not have significant homology with the cAMP-responsive elements of other cAMP-regulated genes, it appears that there are other elements which are responsible for mediating the cAMP responsiveness of the rat POMC gene. In addition the rat POMC gene can be induced by fos oncoprotein, as recently shown in transactivation experiments (BOUTILLIER et al. 1991). The precise element of the POMC gene with which Fos interacts, is not known. The POMC gene appears to depend on the interaction of several transcription factors, since multiple regulatory elements have been defined in the rat and human POMC gene (THERRIEN and DROUIN 1992; KRAUS and HÖLLT 1992).

II. Proenkephalin

The structures of the human and rat PENK genes have been eludicated (NODA et al. 1982; ROSEN et al. 1984). The human gene contains four exons separated by two large and one short intron. The gene is about 5200 bp long and consists of exon 1 (70 bp), intron A (87 bp), exon 2 (56 bp), intron B (469 bp), exon 3 (141 bp), intron C (about 3400 bp), and exon 4 (980 bp). In contrast, the rat gene contains three exons only (Fig. 1): The portion of PENK mRNA that is contained between exon 1 and exon 2 in the human gene is located in a single exon (exon 1) in the rat gene. All of the species investigated appear to have only a single PENK gene.

The size of the PENK mRNA in the brain and the adrenal medulla is about 1400 nucleotides (JINGAMI et al. 1984; PITTIUS et al. 1985). A second slightly larger mRNA species which results from alternate splicing and contains the 87 nucleotides of intron A has been detected as a minor component in bovine hypothalamus (NODA et al. 1982). A larger form of PENK mRNA was also found in haploid rat sperm cells. This larger transcript contains an additional 5'-flanking sequence which is derived from alternate splicing of the PENK gene within intron A (YOSHIKAWA et al. 1989a). There is also some evidence for a shorter PENK mRNA species which occurs together with the 1400-nucleotide species in the human caudate and in pheochromocytoma tissues (MONSTEIN and GEIJER 1988). Whether these different mRNA species result from alternative splicing or from aberrant transcription of the gene has not been investigated.

The sequence requirement for transcription of the human PENK gene was analyzed by transfection of a vector containing 946 bp of the 5'-flanking regions and 63 bp of the 5'-noncoding region fused to SV 40 sequences in COS monkey cells (TERAO et al. 1983). Deletion up to 172 bp upstream of the capping site exerted no effect on the efficient transcription of the fusion product. However, deletion up to 145, 111, 81, and 67 bp upstream of the capping site resulted in a gradual decrease in the transcriptional efficiency, indicating that these sequences contain functional enhancer and/or promoter sites.

These sequences also confer cAMP and phorbol ester inducibility. Transfection of a human PENK CAT fusion plasmid into monkey CV1 cells revealed that DNA sequences required for regulation by both cAMP and phorbol esters map to the same 37-bp region located 107–71 bp 5' to the mRNA cap site of the PENK gene and exert properties of transcriptional enhancers (COMB et al. 1986) (Fig. 2). Further studies provided evidence that that two DNA elements (ENKCRE-1 and ENKCRE-2) are located within this enhancer region which are responsible for the transcriptional response to CAMP and phorbol ester (Fig. 2). The proximal promoter element, ENKCRE-2, is essential for both basal and regulated enhancer function. The distal promoter element, ENKCRE-1, has no inherent capacity to activate transcription, but snyergistically augments cAMP and phorbol ester inducible transcription in the presence of ENKCRE-2 (COMB et al. 1988; HYMAN et al. 1988). Several transcription factors bind to the enhancer regions in vitro: a transcription factor, termed ENKFT-1, binds to the DNA region encompassing ENKCRE-1. AP-1 and AP-4 bind to overlapping sites spanning ENKCRE-2. *Fos* and *Jun* polypeptides have been shown to bind directly to ENKCRE-2 (AP-1 site) in a cooperative manner (SONNENBERG et al. 1989). Moreover, a synergistic transactivation of the human PENK enhancer-promoter was found by cotransfection of plasmids expressing c-*fos* and c-*jun* in F9 teratocarcinoma cells (SONNENBERG et al.

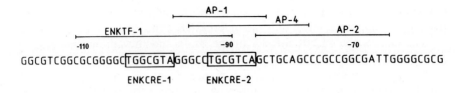

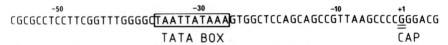

Fig. 2. Promoter and enhancer elements within the 5′-flanking region of the human proenkephalin gene. *ENKCRE*, cAMP-responsive elements; *AP-1, AP-2, AP-4*, and *ENKFT-1* are binding sites for transcription factors; *TATA*, TATA box. (Modified according to Comb et al. 1986)

1989). Recently, further upstream of the ENKCRE sequences, a novel regulatory element, was identified which binds the transcription factor NF-KB and a brain-specific transcription factor BETA (Korner et al. 1989; Rattner et al. 1989). NF-KB appears to play a role in lymphocyte specific expression of the gene. In fact, T-helper cells have been shown to increase PENK mRNA synthesis (Zurawski et al. 1986). A fourth transcription factor (AP-2) binds to a site immediately downstream of ENKCRE-2 (Comb et al. 1988). This AP-2 DNA-binding element acts synergistically with the enhancer elements to confer maximal response to cAMP and phorbol esters (Hyman et al. 1989). JunD, a component of the AP-1 transcription factor complex has recently been shown to activate transcription of the PENK gene in a fashion that is completely dependant upon the cAMP-dependent protein kinase, protein kinase A (Kobierski et al. 1991). JunD has been shown to bind to ENKCRE-2. Since multiple factors can bind to the 5′ control region, it is likely that the PENK gene is controlled by a combinatorial interaction of several transcription factors which may be constitutive or inducible.

III. Prodynorphin

The structural organization of the human PDYN gene has been clarified (Horikawa et al. 1983). The gene contains four exons separated by three introns (Fig. 1): exon 1 (1.4 kb), intron A (1.2 kb), exon 2 (60 bp), intron B (9.9 kb), exon 3 (145 bp), intron C (1.7 kb), and exon 4 (2.2 kb). As compared to the other opioid peptide genes, exons 1 and 4, which contain nontranslated sequences, are very large. It is possible that the 5′-terminal region of this gene contains an additional intron (Horikawa et al. 1983). A similar structural organization has recently been reported for the rat PDYN gene (Douglass et al. 1989). Exon 1 and exon 2 encode the majority of the

5'-untranslated sequence of the mRNA while exons 3 and 4 contain the translated regions. As revealed by Southern and Northern blotting experiments, only a single gene appears to exist in man, pigs, and rats. The size of the mRNA in porcine brain is about 3200 nucleotides (JINGAMI et al. 1984). The PDYN mRNA possesses a very long nontranslated 3'-terminal end of about 1500 nucleotides. The size of the rat PDYN mRNA in brain is smaller (about 2400 nucleotides (CIVELLI et al. 1985)). mRNA species which are about 100 nucleotides smaller have been found in the adrenal cortex (DAY et al. 1990) and in Sertoli cells of rats (GARRETT et al. 1989). The different mRNA species derive from an alternate splicing of the gene which result in the deletion of exon 2 (GARRETT et al. 1989).

Triple tandem-repeated sequences at the 5'-flanking region of the PDYN genes were suggested to be involved in the regulation of the expression of the PDYN gene (HORIKAWA et al. 1983). In transfection studies, 5'-flanking regions of the rat PDYN gene were joined with a CAT reporter gene and introduced into 2RC Leydig cells (McMURRAY et al. 1989). The fusion genes were positively regulated by cAMP analogs in these cells. The cAMP-responsive DNA sequence has been localized to a 210-bp fragment comprising 122 bp 5'-flanking sequences, and 88 bp of exon 1 of the rat PDYN gene. This sequence contains a DNA fragment which is 80% homologous to the cAMP consensus sequence located downstream to the cap site. Recently, a functional AP-1 element has been localized within the rat PDYN gene promoter region (NARANJO et al. 1991). This DNA element is constituted by the non-canonical TGACAACA sequence which was shown to be a target of Fos/Jun transactivation (NARANJO et al. 1991).

C. Gene Regulation

I. Proopiomelanocortin

The proopiomelanocortin (POMC) gene is predominantly expressed in the pituitary. In addition, cells expressing POMC have also been found in the brain, particularly in the arcuate nucleus of the hypothalamus, and in a variety of peripheral tissues, such as the gonads and lymphocytes, and in several pituitary and nonpituitary tumors.

1. Adenohypophysis

In the anterior pituitary, POMC gene expression is under the negative feedback control of adrenal steroids. Thus, adrenalectomy results in a marked increase in the POMC mRNA levels (NAKANISHI et al. 1979; BIRNBERG et al. 1983). Time course studies revealed that there was a rapid and sustained increase in the levels of POMC primary transcript followed by a slower rise in the accumulation of cytoplasmic mRNA levels (AUTELITANO et al. 1989). An increased transcription rate per cell and an increased number of POMC-synthesizing cells was observed in the anterior pituitaries of the adrenalectomized rats by in situ hybridization experiments (FREMEAU et al. 1986), although individual corticotrophes show marked differences in POMC gene expression (HATFIELD et al. 1989).

Injection of dexamethasone into adrenalectomized rats causes a rapid fall in POMC transcription (GAGNER and DROUIN 1985) and of the level of the POMC primary transcript (AUTELITANO et al. 1989) followed by a more protracted decline in POMC mRNA levels (BIRNBERG et al. 1983). In addition, glucocorticoids inhibit POMC gene expression in primary cultures of anterior pituitaries and in mouse AtT-20 tumor cells (NAKAMURA et al. 1978; ROBERTS et al. 1979; GAGNER and DROUIN 1985; EBERWINE et al. 1987; THIELE and EIPPER 1990). This inhibition appears to be mediated by a direct interaction of the glucocorticoid receptor with a negative regulatory DNA-binding element within the upstream promoter region of the POMC gene (DROUIN et al. 1989).

In contrast, POMC gene expression in the anterior pituitary is under positive control by CRH. A single injection of CRH caused a rapid increase in the POMC primary transcript in the anterior pituitaries of rats (AUTELITANO et al. 1990). Chronic administration of exogenous CRH for 3–7 days results in marked increases in the levels of the POMC primary transcript and of the cytoplasmic mRNA in the anterior pituitaries of rats (BRUHN et al. 1984; HÖLLT and HAARMANN 1984; AUTELITANO et al. 1990).

An increase in POMC mRNA levels in the anterior pituitary is also seen after various stress treatments, such as chronic foot-shock (HÖLLT et al. 1986; SHIOMI et al. 1986), hypoglycemic shock induced by insulin (TOZAWA et al. 1988), restraint stress, and swim stress (HARBUZ and LIGHTMAN 1989). It is very likely that these treatments exert their action on POMC gene expression by releasing hypothalamic CRH. This suggestion is supported by the finding that mRNA levels coding for CRH in the paraventricular nucleus of the rat are increased after various stress treatments (HARBUZ and LIGHTMAN 1989).

Repeated administration of morphine has also been shown to increase POMC mRNA levels in the anterior pituitary of rats (HÖLLT and HAARMANN 1985). It is reasonable to assume that CRH mediates this effect, since morphine has been shown to release CRH from rat hypothalamic slices (BUCKINGHAM 1982). High doses of morphine, however, appear to be required, since smaller doses did not alter POMC mRNA in the anterior pituitary (LIGHTMAN and YOUNG 1988). In addition, naloxone-precipitated withdrawal in morphine-tolerant rats increased POMC mRNA levels, indicating that withdrawal stress activates POMC gene expression in the anterior pituitary (LIGHTMAN and YOUNG 1988).

Moreover, administration of interleukin-1α and 1β stimulates POMC gene expression in the anterior pituitary of rats (SUDA et al. 1990). This effect appears to be predominantly mediated via the release of CRH, since interleukin in-1α and 1β did not consistently alter POMC gene expression in cultured rat anterior pituitary cells (SUDA et al. 1988b).

Chronic treatment of rats with ethanol in a vapor chamber decreased levels of POMC mRNA in the adenohypophysis (DAVE et al. 1986). However, other experiments in which ethanol was chronically administered by liquid diet revealed an increase in the biosynthesis of POMC in the anterior pituitary (SEIZINGER et al. 1984a). The different findings might be related to the different modes of ethanol administration. In addition, there appears to exist marked genetic differences concerning this effect. Thus, administration of ethanol resulted in a threefold higher increase in the POMC mRNA level in the adenohypophysis of "long sleep" mice than of "short sleep mice" (WAND 1990).

In primary cultures of rat anterior pituitary cells and in AtT-20 mouse tumor cells, CRH has been shown to increase POMC mRNA levels (LOEFFLER et al. 1985; AFFOLTER and REISINE 1985; VON DREDEN et al. 1988; KNIGHT et al. 1987; THIELE and EIPPER 1990) as a result of increased gene transcription (GAGNER and DROUIN 1985; EBERWINE et al. 1987). The effect of CRH appears to be predominantly mediated via cAMP followed by activation of protein kinase A. Thus, insertion of a protein kinase A inhibitor in AtT-20/D16-16 tumor cells blocked the ability of CRH and 8-bromo-cAMP to increase POMC mRNA levels (REISINE et al. 1986). Moreover, in primary cultures of rat anterior pituitary cells, 8-bromo-cAMP, forskolin, cholera toxin, and drugs which elevate cellular cAMP levels by inhibiting phosphodiesterases (e.g., Ro 20–1724) increase POMC mRNA levels (LOEFFLER et al. 1986a; AFFOLTER and REISINE 1985; SIMARD et al. 1986; DAVE et al. 1987; STALLA et al. 1989a; SUDA et al. 1988a). In addition, imidazole derivatives, such as ketoconazole or isoconazole, which inhibit adenylate cyclase, block the CRH- or forskolin-induced increase in POMC mRNA levels in rat anterior pituitary cultures (STALLA et al. 1988, 1989a). CRH also enhances POMC gene expression in cultured human corticotrophic tumor cells (STALLA et al. 1989b). The inducing effect of CRH on POMC mRNA levels in cultured anterior lobe cells and in mouse AtT-20/D-16v cells was partially inhibited by inhibitors of voltage-dependent Ca^{2+} channel blockers, such as verapamil and nifedipine (LOEFFLER et al. 1986a; VON DREDEN et al. 1988). This indicates that CRH exerts its effect on POMC gene expression partially via entry of Ca^{2+} ions. It is possible that this effect of CRH is also mediated by cAMP, since cAMP analogues can elevate intracellular Ca^{2+} levels (LUINI et al. 1985).

Although arginine vasopressin (AVP) releases POMC peptides from anterior pituitary cells and potentiates the secretory effect of CRH in vitro, it does not exert a major effect on POMC biosynthesis (VON DREDEN and HÖLLT 1988; STALLA et al. 1989b; SUDA et al. 1989; LEVIN et al. 1989). On the contrary, AVP decreased the levels of POMC primary transcript when applied to anterior pituitary cultures (LEVIN et al. 1989). Moreover, AVP does not potentiate the stimulation of POMC gene expression by CRH. The mechanism whereby AVP exerts its secretory effect on corticotrophic cells appears to be the activation of phospholipase C, which causes an increase in intracellular diacylglycerol and phosphatidyl-inositol-phosphates. Bombesin has been shown to activate phospholipase C in and to release POMC peptides from mouse AtT-20/D-16v cells (Höllt and Sincini 1988; Kessler et al. 1989). However it failed to increase POMC mRNA levels in these cells. Phorbol esters, such as phorbol 12-myristate 13-acetate (TPA), which activate protein kinase C, have been shown to increase POMC mRNA levels in AtT-20/D16-16 tumor cells (Affolter and Reisine 1985; Vyas et al. 1990) The inducing effect of TPA was depressed in AtT-20 cells with downregulated protein kinase C activity (Vyas et al. 1990). On the other hand, TPA had no effect on POMC mRNA levels in primary cultures of rat anterior pituitary cells or in AtT-20/D16-v cells (another mouse tumor cell line) (Suda et al. 1989). This suggests that the protein kinase C-dependent signal transduction system predominantly contributes to the release, but less to the biosynthesis, of POMC peptides.

2. Intermediate Pituitary

Proopiomelanocortin gene expression in the intermediate pituitary is, in general, differently regulated from that in the anterior pituitary. Thus, adrenalectomy alters POMC mRNA levels in this lobe only slightly (Schachter et al. 1982). Although the melanotrophic cells of the intermediate pituitary do not contain glucocorticoid receptors, glucocorticoid receptors are expressed after denervation in vivo or after prolonged culture in vitro (Antakly et al. 1985). Interestingly, glucocorticoids cause an elevation of POMC mRNA levels in the intermediate pituitary of rats after denervation of the pituitary by hypothalamic lesions (Seger et al. 1988). These findings indicate that the structure of the POMC gene does not necessarily predict the direction in which POMC gene expression is altered. In primary cultures of rat intermediate pituitaries, however, glucocorticoids only slightly inhibit POMC transcription (Eberwine and Roberts 1984) or have no effect (Jeannotte et al. 1987b).

Corticotropin-regulating hormone increases POMC gene expression also in the intermediate pituitary by a mechanism which involves the activation of adenylate cyclase. Thus, CRH, 8-bromo-cAMP, forskolin, cholera toxin, and the phosphodiesterase inhibitor Ro 20–1724 increased POMC mRNA levels in intermediate lobe cultures (Loeffler et al. 1985, 1986a, 1988). The effect of forskolin was partially blocked by Ca^{2+} channel antagonists (Loeffler et al. 1986a). This indicates that Ca^{2+} entry possibly triggered by cAMP is also involved in the induction of POMC gene expression in the melanotrophic cells of the intermediate lobe. In cultured porcine intermediate lobe cells, calmodulin antagonists and phorbol esters decrease POMC mRNA levels. This indicates that activation of Ca^{2+}/calmodulin- and protein kinase C-dependent signal pathways can modulate POMC gene expression in these cells (LOEFFLER et al. 1989). Surprisingly, long-term administration of CRH to rats in vivo decreases POMC mRNA levels (HÖLLT and HAARMANN 1984; LUNDBLAD and ROBERTS 1988). Various stress treatments, such as insulin shock or chronic foot-shock for up to 7 days, increase POMC mRNA levels in the anterior, but not in the intermediate pituitary (HÖLLT et al. 1986; TOZAWA et al. 1988). Prolonged foot-shock stress (administered for 2 weeks), however, causes an increase of POMC mRNA levels also in the intermediate lobe (SHIOMI et al. 1986).

The release of POMC-derived peptides from the intermediate pituitary is tonically inhibited by DA via D_2 receptors. Blockade of these receptors by haloperidol causes an increase in the levels of POMC mRNA (HÖLLT et al. 1982; CHEN et al. 1983) and of POMC gene transcription (PRITCHETT and ROBERTS 1987) in the intermediate lobe of the rats. On the contrary, chronic injections of the DA agonist bromocriptine decreased POMC mRNA levels in the intermediate pituitary (CHEN et al. 1983; LEVY and LIGHTMAN 1988). A combined morphometric analysis by light and electron microscopy, as well as by in situ hybridization, revealed differences in the biosynthetic activity of individual melanotrophic cells. Haloperidol treatment increased the number of dark melanotrophic cells and the amount of POMC in each cell (CHRONWALL et al. 1988). DA and bromocryptine also inhibited POMC gene expression in explanted rat intermediate lobes (COTE et al. 1986) or intermediate lobe cells (LOEFFLER et al. 1988) in vitro. The inhibitory effect of the DAergic compounds was abolished by pretreatment with pertussis toxin. Conversely, compounds that activate the cAMP pathway counteracted the DAergic inhibition of POMC biosynthesis (LOEFFLER et al. 1986c, 1988). These findings suggest that the inhibitory guanyl nucleotide binding protein G_i, and possibly the adenylate cyclase, mediate DAergic inhibition of POMC biosynthesis.

In addition to DA, GABA has also been shown to inhibit the release of POMC-derived peptides from the intermediate pituitary (TOMIKO et al. 1983). When endogenous GABA levels in the hypothalamus and pituitary of rats were elevated by GABA-transaminase inhibitors, a decrease in the levels of POMC mRNA was found (LOEFFLER et al. 1986b). In addition, GABA also caused a reduction of POMC mRNA levels, when applied to primary cultures of intermediate lobe cells (LOEFFLER et al. 1986b).

Chronic administration of morphine decreased POMC mRNA levels in the intermediate pituitary lobe (HÖLLT and HAARMANN 1985). Similarly, a decrease of POMC biosynthesis in this lobe was also seen after chronic ethanol treatment (SEIZINGER et al. 1984b; DAVE et al. 1986). This effect, however, may result from the dehydrating action of ethanol. Thus, salt loading has also been shown to decrease POMC mRNA levels in the intermediate lobe of mice (ELKABES and LOH 1988). In contrast, ethanol administered by a controlled drinking schedule (liquid diet) increased POMC biosynthesis in the intermediate lobe of rats (SEIZINGER et al. 1984a).

3. Hypothalamus

In the hypothalamus POMC is synthesized by cells localized in the periarcuate region (GEE et al. 1983).

Proopiomelanocortin mRNA levels in the hypothalamus were initially reported to be unchanged after adrenalectomy (BIRNBERG et al. 1983). However, a recent paper reported that POMC mRNA levels in the hypothalamus increase after adrenalectomy and that glucocortiocoids reverse this response (BEAULIEU et al. 1988). Such findings indicate that glucocorticoid regulation of POMC gene expression is similar in the anterior pituitary and hypothalamus.

Also gonadal steroids influence hypothalamic POMC mRNA levels. Thus, estrogen treatment decreased hypothalamic POMC mRNA levels in ovarectomized rats (WILCOX and ROBERTS 1985). Moreover, castration resulted in decreased POMC mRNA levels in the arcuate nucleus of rats, an effect that can be reversed by testosterone (CHOWEN-BREED et al. 1989a,b). Other studies, however, showed that castration of male rats resulted in an increase in POMC mRNA levels in the medial basal hypothalamus (MBH) and that testosterone replacement reverses this effect, indicating that androgens have an inhibitory effect on POMC gene expression in the MBH (BLUM et al. 1989). The reason for this discrepant result is not known. Evidence for an involvement of POMC-derived peptides in the control of gonadotropin-releasing hormone (GnRH) came from studies showing that a marked increase in the levels of hypothalamic POMC mRNA occurs contemporaneously with the onset of puberty (WIEMANN et al. 1989). Thus, the increase in POMC mRNA during the onset of puberty may be important for pulsatile GnRH secretion.

Chronic administration of morphine has been reported to decrease POMC mRNA levels in the rat hypothalamus (MOCCHETTI et al. 1989). In our hands, however, POMC mRNA levels in the hypothalamus were unchanged following chronic administration of morphine according to various schedules (HÖLLT et al. 1989b). Exposure to ethanol for 3 weeks resulted in an increased accumulation of POMC mRNA in the hypothalamus of rats (ANGELOGIANNI and GIANOULAKIS 1990).

4. Peripheral Tissues

Apart from the anterior pituitary, POMC mRNA has been localized in many peripheral tissues, such as adrenal medulla, thyroid gland, duodenum, colon, stomach, liver, kidney, spleen, mononuclear cells, gonads, and placenta.

Analysis of the mRNA of bovine (JINGAMI et al. 1984), rat (DEBOLD et al. 1988a), and human (DEBOLD et al. 1988b) tissues revealed that the major mRNA species in these tissues is 200–300 bases smaller than the species found in pituitary and hypothalamus. The truncated POMC mRNA lacked exon 1 and exon 2 and few nucleotides of the 5' end of exon 3 (DEBOLD et al. 1988a). These smaller POMC mRNA forms which lack the signal sequence appear to be much less efficiently translated, since the ratio of POMC-like mRNA to POMC-derived peptide concentrations is 1000 times higher in these nonpituitary tissues than in the pituitary. Moreover, very few, if any, POMC-derived peptides are released from human peripheral mononuclear cells expressing the smaller POMC mRNA species (McLoughlin et al. 1990). This finding largely excludes the possibility that the low content in the peripheral tissues is due to an extensive release of the peptides.

The localization and regulation of the small POMC mRNA has been extensively studied in gonadal tissues. In the rat testis POMC mRNA was initially reported to be localized in Leydig cells (Pintar et al. 1984; Gizang-Ginsberg and Wolgemuth 1985). In addition POMC mRNA was shown to be present in testicular germ cells (Kilpatrick et al. 1987; Gizang-Ginsberg and Wolgemuth 1985). Recent studies, however, revealed that administration of ethane dimethane sulfonate (EDS), a drug which selectively destroys Leydig cells, did not alter POMC-mRNA levels in the testis of rats (Li et al. 1989). Moreover, other authors were unable to detect POMC transcripts in cultured Leydig cells (Garrett and Douglass 1989). These data suggest that the predominant site of rat POMC gene expression is in testicular interstitial and germ cells rather than Leydig cells.

Small POMC transcripts were also found in the ovary and the placenta (Chen et al. 1986). Gonadotropins and androgens markedly increase the ovarian levels of POMC mRNA (Chen et al. 1986; Melner et al. 1986; Chen and Madigan 1987). Moreover, higher levels of ovarian POMC mRNA have been found in pregnant than in nonpregnant rats (Chen and Madigan 1987; Jin et al. 1988).

5. Tumors

Proopiomelanocortin mRNA has been detected in many nonpituitary tumors, such as thymic carcinoid tumors (de Keyzer et al. 1985), pheochromocytomas (DeBold et al. 1988c), and small cell lung cancer (Chang et al. 1989). The size of the POMC transcripts in these tumors is frequently larger than the 1400-nucleotide species found in normal human pituitaries. These longer mRNA forms can result from a variable mode of transcription induced by promoters located at upstream sites of transcription (DeBold et al. 1988c; de Keyzer et al. 1989; Chang et al. 1989). However, another study, in which a variety of human tumors was analyzed, indicated that most POMC transcripts in tumors originated from the conventional promoter. The size heterogeneity observed was due to longer poly (A) tails (Clark et al. 1989). In addition, some tumors espressed a short POMC mRNA (800 nucleotides) which may lack the first two exons.

Expression of POMC gene in a human small cell lung cancer cell line was not suppressible by glucocorticoids although significant glucocorticoid receptor binding could be measured (CLARK et al. 1990), indicating that nonsuppression of the POMC gene by glucocorticoids lies distal to steroid binding in the nucleus of these cells.

II. Proenkephalin

1. Striatum

Very high levels of proenkephalin (PENK) mRNA have been found in the striatum, where more than half of the neurons express the gene. The majority of these cells are projection neurons which innervate the globus pallidus (GRAYBIEL 1986). PENK gene expression in these neurons is under negative control of DA. Thus, chronic treatment of rats with haloperidol increases the levels of PENK mRNA in the striatum (TANG et al. 1983; BLANC et al. 1985; SIVAM et al. 1986a,b; ANGULO et al. 1987; ROMANO et al. 1987; MORRIS et al. 1988d; LE MOINE et al. 1990). The increase in PENK mRNA was associated with an increase in D2-DA receptor mRNA (LE MOINE et al. 1990). On the other hand, a marked ipsilateral increase in the levels of PENK mRNA was observed after 6-hydroxy-DA lesion of the substantia nigra and/or the ventral tegmental area of rats (TANG et al. 1983; NORMAND et al. 1988; VERNIER et al. 1988; MORRIS et al. 1989).

There appears to be a different regulation of the PENK mRNA via D1 and D2 receptors. However, there is some discrepancy in the reports: Whereas MOCCHETTI et al. (1987) reported that chronic treatment of rats with the selective D1 antagonist SCH 23390 increases PENK mRNA levels in the striatum, a clear decrease in the striatal PENK mRNA was found by others (MORRIS et al. 1988d). A recent study (POLLACK and WOOTEN 1992) suggests that the inhibition of PENK biosynthesis by DA is mediated via an interaction with D_2DA receptors.

Dopamine also causes a slight decrease in PENK mRNA levels in primary cultures of rat striatal cells (KOWALSKI et al. 1989), indicating that DA directly inhibits PENK gene expression. cAMP analogues and phorbol esters increase PENK mRNA levels in these cells, suggesting that protein kinase A and protein kinase C dependent pathways are involved in the induction of striatal gene expression.

An increase in PENK mRNA levels in the striatum was also observed after chronic treatment of rats with reserpine, indicating that reserpine increases enkephalin synthesis by eliminating the DAergic inhibition (MOCCHETTI et al. 1985).

In contrast to the DAergic drugs, administration of serotonergic drugs and/or lesioning of the raphe muclei with 5,7-dihydroxytryptamine failed to alter striatal PENK mRNA content (MOCCHETTI et al. 1984; MORRIS et al. 1988b).

Specific alterations in striatal levels of PENK mRNA have been found after administration of drugs influencing GABAergic transmission. Chronic treatment of rats with the GABA transaminase inhibitor amino oxyacetic acid (AOAA) causes an increase in PENK mRNA levels in the striatum (SIVAM and HONG 1986). On the other hand, our group observed a decrease in the level of PENK mRNA in rats chronically treated with the GABA transaminase inhibitors (REIMER and HÖLLT 1990a). Biphasic changes in striatal levels of PENK mRNA (an initial decrease followed by an increase) were observed after a combined administration of the GABA agonist muscimol and diazepam into mice (LLORENS-CORTES et al. 1990).

An increase in striatal PENK mRNA levels has also been found after chronic treatment of rats with lithium (SIVAM et al. 1988). Similarly, electroacupuncture of rats has been shown to markedly increase the levels of PENK mRNA in the striatum (ZHENG et al. 1988). On the other hand, chronic electroconvulsive shock did not alter PENK mRNA levels in the striatum, although this treatment increased PENK mRNA levels in the amygdala (LEVIEL et al. 1990).

Discrepant results have been reported with regard to the effect of opiates on striatal PENK mRNA levels. Chronic treatment with morphine was reported to cause a slight decrease in the levels of adult and neonatal rats (UHL et al. 1988; TEMPEL 1990). In contrast, no significant effect of chronic morphine treatment on striatal PENK mRNA levels could be found by our group (HÖLLT et al. 1989b). Inactivation of μ-opiate receptors by local injection of the irreversible μ-antagonist β-funaltrexamine into the striatum did not change the levels of PENK mRNA in this structure. In contrast, local administration of the nonselective irreversible antagonist β-chlornaltrexamine caused a marked increase in PENK mRNA levels at the site of injection (MORRIE et al. 1988c). This indicates that activation of non-μ, possibly δ- and/or κ-opioid receptors tonically suppresses striatal PENK gene expression. Moreover, a chronic blockade of σ-opiate receptors by treatment of rats with BMY 14802 for 2 weeks increased the level of PENK mRNA in the striatum, indicating that σ-opiate receptor activity suppresses PENK gene expression in striatal neurons (ANGULO et al. 1990).

2. Hypothalamus

Cells expressing the PENK gene are concentrated in the ventromedial hypothalamus.

Treatment of ovariectomized rats with estrogens markedly increases PENK mRNA levels in the ventromedial nucleus. Time-course studies revealed that estrogen stimulates PENK mRNA levels in the ventromedial hypothalamus very rapidly (within 1 h). Following estrogen removal, the PENK mRNA levels decline rapidly (ROMANO et al. 1989), indicating that estrogen might stimulate PENK mRNA by affecting the rates of both mRNA appearance and degradation. In addition, progesterone treatment attenuated the decline of the PENK mRNA after estrogen removal, suggesting that the ENKergic system in the ventromedial hypothalamus is regulated by both estrogen and progesterone during the estrous cycle.

Chronic morphine treatment has been reported to decrease PENK mRNA levels in the hypothalamus of rats (UHL et al. 1988). Other groups failed to find any effect of morphine and/or NAL treatment (LIGHTMAN and YOUNG 1987a; HÖLLT et al. 1989a). However, NAL-precipitated withdrawal in morphine-tolerant rats resulted in a dramatic increase in PENK mRNA levels in cells of the paraventricular nucleus (LIGHTMAN and YOUNG 1987a). These data suggest that the activation of hypothalamic PENK-producing neurons are important in the neuroendocrine response to stress. Moreover, stress due to administration of hypertonic saline stress resulted in an increase of prooxytocin and PENK mRNAs in the magnocellular nuclei of the hypothalamus (LIGHTMAN and YOUNG 1987b). On the other hand, hypothalamic PENK mRNA levels were unaffected by restraint, swim, and cold stress (HARBUZ and LIGHTMAN 1989), whereas daily applications of electroconvulsive shock increased PENK mRNA levels in the hypothalamus of rats (YOSHIKAWA et al. 1985). It is tempting to speculate that an enhancement of PENK biosynthesis in areas belonging to the limbic system might contribute to the antidepressive action of electroconvusive shock treatment in human.

3. Hippocampus and Cortex

Proenkephalin mRNA has also been found in the hippocampus of rats (PITTIUS et al. 1985; NARANJO et al. 1986a; WHITE et al. 1987; MORRIS et al. 1988a; MONETA and HÖLLT 1990). Within the hippocampus, cells producing PENK-derived peptides have been localized to the granule cell layer of the dentate gyrus and to various interneurons within the hippocampal formation (GALL et al. 1981). Moreover, using in situ hybridization techniques, PENK mRNA has been located in the granule cells of the dentate gyrus after electrical stimulation (MORRIS et al. 1988a). Repetitive stimulation of the amygdala (kindling) of rats, which resulted in a progressive development of generalized seizures, causes a marked increase in hippocampal levels of PENK mRNA (NARANJO et al. 1986a). These data suggest that the PENK system might participate in the development of kindling phenomena. A similar increase in hippocampal PENK mRNA levels was found in rats with recurrent limbic seizures induced by contralateral lesions of the dentate gyrus hilus (GALL et al. 1981). Moreover, direct electrical stimulation of the dentate gyrus granule cells markedly increases the levels of PENK mRNA at the site of stimulation (MORRIS et al. 1988a). In addition, repetitive electrical stimulation of the perforant pathway results in an increase in PENK mRNA levels in the ipsilateral dentate gyrus, indicating that PENK gene expression in granule cells can be induced transynaptically (MONETA and HÖLLT 1990).

Electrical stimulation of the amygdala also increases PENK mRNA levels in the entorhinal cortex, frontal cortex, nucleus accumbens, and the amygdala itself (NARANJO et al. 1986a). Similarly, repeated electroconvulsive shock increases levels of PENK mRNA in the hippocampus and the entorhinal cortex of rats (XIE et al. 1989). The degree of increase was highest in the entorhinal cortex, which contains ENKergic neurons projecting to the dentate gyrus granule cells as part of the tractus perforans. It thus appears that several ENKergic neurons within the entorhinal-hippocampal formation are sensitive to seizure activity. The finding that PENK mRNA is also induced in other brain areas such as the frontal cortex implies that electrically induced recurrent seizures activate multisynaptic excitatory chains in several brain regions.

4. Spinal Cord and Lower Brainstem

Inflammatory stimuli have been found to be associated with an increase in the level of PENK mRNA in the spinal cord of rats (IADAROLA et al. 1986, 1988b), although the effects were much smaller than those seen for PDYN mRNA. In arthritic rats suffering from chronic inflammation or chronic pain, no major change in the level of PENK mRNA in the whole spinal cord has been found (WEIHE et al. 1989). Increased levels of PENK mRNA were also found in the spinal cord after spinal injury or after dissection (PRZEWLOCKI et al. 1988). In situ hybridization experiments, however, indicated substantial, but localized alterations in the PENK gene expression in the spinal cord and lower brainstem after manipulation of primary afferent input. Thus, in situ hybridization experiments revealed that the PENK gene is expressed in many neurons of lamina I and lamina II of the nucleus caudalis of the trigeminal nuclear complex (HARLAN et al. 1987; NISHIMORI et al. 1988). Levels of PENK mRNA were decreased in nucleus caudalis and spinal cord dorsal horn neurons following lesions of the primary afferents (NISHIMORI et al. 1988). Moreover, electrical stimulation of the trigememinus nerve elicited a rapid and dramatic induction of PENK mRNA in lamina I and lamina II neurons (NISHIMORI ct al. 1989). Taken together, the electrical stimulation, deafferentiation, and inflammation experiments suggest a function-related plasticity in expression of PENK in these neurons following changes in primary afferent stimulation. Primary afferent stimulation can also enhance the expression of c-*fos* in subsets of lamina I and II neurons; this precedes and expression of PENK and PDYN (HUNT et al. 1987; DRAISCI and IADAROLA 1989). The 5′-flanking region of the PENK gene contains a recognition sequence for the *Fos/Jun* heterodimeric complex (AP1) (COMB et al. 1986; CURRAN et al. 1988). This supports the hypothesis that the modulatory effects of primary afferent stimulation on PENK (and/or PDYN) gene expression in the spinal cord and nucleus caudalis are mediated via the transcription factor *Fos*.

5. Pituitary

In addition to nervous tissues, PENK mRNA has been reported in the pineal gland (ALOYO et al. 1990) and in the pituitary (PITTIUS et al. 1985; SCHÄFER et al. 1990). In situ hybridization techniques have shown that within the rat pituitary PENK mRNA is localized in the anterior and in the neural lobe of the pituitary, but not in the intermediate pituitary (SCHÄFER et al. 1990). The localization of PENK mRNA in the neural lobe suggests that pituicytes (a special class of astroglial cells) synthesize ENKs. In fact, PENK mRNA has recently been demonstrated in astrocyte cultures of neonatal rat brain (VILIJN et al. 1988; SCHWARTZ and SIMANTOV 1988).

6. Adrenal Medulla

In situ hybridization of sections derived from bovine adrenal medullae revealed that PENK mRNA was localized selectively in cells at the outer margin of the medulla, a region rich in epinephrine-containing cells (WAN et al. 1989a; BLOCH et al. 1985). Incubation of primary cultures of chromaffin cells from bovine adrenal medulla with 8-bromo-cAMP, forskolin, or cholera toxin resulted in an increase in PENK mRNA content (QUACH et al. 1984; EIDEN et al. 1984a; KLEY et al. 1987a).

Membrane depolarization induced by nicotine, high K^+, or veratridine causes a marked increase in PENK mRNA levels in cultured bovine chromaffin cells (EIDEN et al. 1984a; KLEY et al. 1986; NARANJO et al. 1986b). The effect is inhibited by drugs which block voltage-dependent Ca^{2+} channels (e.g., verapamil, nifedipine, D_{600}) or by reduced Ca^{2+} ion concentration in the medium (SIEGEL et al. 1985; KLEY et al. 1986; NARANJO et al. 1986b; WASCHEK and EIDEN 1988; WASCHEK et al. 1987). These findings indicate that the influx of extracellular Ca^{2+} through voltage-dependent Ca^{2+} channels is a prerequisite for the induction of PENK gene expression. Ba^{2+} ions stimulate PENK mRNA and ENK release from chromaffin cells (KLEY et al. 1986; WASCHEK et al. 1987). In low Ca^{2+} medium the effect of Ba^{2+} on PENK gene expression is blocked, but it still causes a release of ENKs, indicating that Ba^{2+} can substitute for extracellular Ca^{2+} in mediating peptide secretion. Ca^{2+} might act at two different targets to activate secretion versus biosynthesis.

Initially, glucocorticoids were reported to increase PENK mRNA levels in chromaffin cells. In addition, they were shown to exert a marked permissive action on the stimulation of PENK gene expression by depolarizing agents (NARANJO et al. 1986b). However, a recent study failed to find any glucocorticoid-induced changes in PENK mRNA levels in bovine chromaffin cells although the steroids markedly induced the mRNA coding for phenyl ethanolamine N-methyl transferase (PNMT) in these cells (WAN and LIVETT 1989).

Since the majority of drugs which affect PENK mRNA levels release PENK peptides, it is possible that release per se might be the stimulus for increased PENK synthesis. This possibility, however, appears to be unlikely, since the nicotine-induced increase in PENK mRNA can be blocked by nicotine antagonists, such as hexamethonium or tubocurare, even if added 1–3 h after the addition of nicotine (FARIN et al. 1990b).

Histamine, bradykinin, or angiotensin-induced activation of phospholipase C, which gives rise to the second messengers diacylglycerol and inositol-3-phosphate, causes an increase in the levels of PENK mRNA in chromaffin cells (KLEY et al. 1987b; BOMMER et al. 1987; WAN et al. 1989b; FARIN et al. 1900). Activation of protein kinase C appears to be an important trigger for the induction of PENK gene expression, since tumor-promoting phorbol esters increase PENK mRNA levels (KLEY 1988). Although the activation of protein kinase C by phorbol esters can enhance PENK mRNA levels, phorbol esters inhibit the stimulatory effect of depolarizing agents on PENK biosynthesis (KLEY 1988; PRUSS and STAUDERMAN 1988). Phorbol esters appear to inhibit PENK gene expression by inactivating voltage-dependent Ca^{2+} channels, indicating that sustained elevation of intracellular Ca^{2+} is necessary to increase ENK synthesis in chromaffin cells. Although muscarine activates phospholipase C (NOBLE et al. 1986), it does not activate PENK gene expression. However, following coincubation of muscarine with the Ca^{2+} ionophore A 23187, at concentrations which do not increase PENK mRNA levels, a clear increase in the expression of the PENK was observed (FARIN et al. 1990a). Nuclear runoff experiments indicated that the increase of PENK mRNA by histamine is mediated by an increased rate of transcription. Measurements of PENK mRNA half-life indicated that histamine does not alter the stability of the mRNA coding for PENK (FARIN et al. 1990b).

Depletion of catecholamine stores by reserpine causes a decrease in the levels of PENK mRNA (EIDEN et al. 1984b). Since reserpine has been reported to block the release of ENKs from chromaffin cells, it has been proposed that the intracellular accumulation of these peptides may activate a negative feedback system, whereby PENK biosynthesis is turned off (MOCCHETTI et al. 1985; NARANJO et al. 1988).

In rat adrenal medulla, regulation of PENK mRNA appears to be different from that in primary cultures of bovine adrenal chromaffin cells. Thus, denervation, by sectioning of the splanchnic nerve, markedly increases the level of PENK mRNA in the adrenal gland of rats (KILPATRICK et al. 1984), indicating that splanchnic innervation exerts a tonic inhibitory influence on PENK gene expression. Such an innervation-dependent suppression is supported by experiments in which rat adrenal medullae were explanted. In such an organ culture system, levels of PENK mRNA rise 74-fold after 4 days (LAGAMMA et al. 1985; INTURRISI et al. 1988b). Depolarization with either elevated K^+ or veratridine inhibited this increase. Inhibition of Ca^{2+} influx by verapamil or D_{600} prevented the effect of the depolarizing agents (LAGAMMA et al. 1988). Calmodulin inhibitors had no effect, whereas trifluperazine, a drug which also inhibits protein kinase C, partially antagonized the effect of K^+ depolarization. These data suggest that the inhibitory effect of membrane depolarization on adrenal PENK gene expression occurs through Ca^{2+} and possibly through protein kinase C. An inhibitory effect of membrane depolarization on PENK gene transcription could be demonstrated using runoff assays (La Gamma et al. 1989).

Derivatives of cAMP also inhibit the increase of PENK mRNA during culture (LaGamma et al. 1988). In contrast, glucocorticoids have been shown to markedly increase PENK mRNA levels in adrenal medullary explants from control and hypophysectomized rats (LaGamma and Adler 1987; Inturrisi et al. 1988a).

Denervated or explanted adrenal medullae from neonatal rats do not show any increase in ENK content, indicating that there is an ontogenetic development of the factors regulating PENK gene expression induced by membrane depolarization (LaGamma et al. 1988). These in vitro results contrast those obtained in rats in which increased splanchnic nerve activity, generated by insulin, caused a dramatic increase in the levels of adrenal medullary mRNA (Kanamatsu et al. 1986; Fischer-Colbrie et al. 1988). The effect of insulin was blocked by combined treatment of rats with chlorisondamine and atropine, or by bilateral transsection of the splanchnic nerves, indicating that insulin exerts its effect on PENK gene expression via splanchnic nerve activation.

Recently, we found that treatment of rats with morphine markedly increase the levels of PENK mRNA in the adrenal medulla (Höllt et al. 1989b). Moreover, morphine can also exert its effect after intracerebroventricular administration, indicating that morphine activates PENK gene expression by increasing splanchnic nerve activity (Reimer and Höllt 1990b). An explanation of the increase in PENK mRNA following denervation might be that the denervation causes an induction of PENK gene expression by stimulating the release of acetylcholine from splanchnic nerve endings, rather than by the unmasking of a tonic inhibition of an intact nerve.

In experiments with primary cultures of rat adrenal medullary cells, we found that depolarizing stimuli and 8-bromo-cAMP increase PENK mRNA levels, indicating that rat chromaffin cells respond similarly to bovine cells. Moreover, depolarizing stimuli and 8-bromo-cAMP have been shown to increase PENK mRNA in cultured fetal rat brain cells (Simantov and Höllt 1990). Although glucocorticoids modulate PENK gene expression in bovine chromaffin cells (Naranjo et al. 1986b) and in rat adrenal medullary explants (Keshet et al. 1989; Inturrisi et al. 1988a), no specific alteration in PENK mRNA has been found in rats after hypophysectomy and/or glucocorticoid treatment (Stachowiak et al. 1988; Fischer-Colbrie et al. 1988).

7. Heart

High concentrations of PENK mRNA have been found in the rat heart ventricle. Although the levels of PENK mRNA are higher than in the brain, the content of PENK-derived peptides is only 3% of that in brain (Howells et al. 1986). In primary cardiac muscle cell cultures, PENK mRNA was induced by 8-bromo-cAMP and 3-isobutyl-1-methylxanthine (IBMX), whereas the phorbol ester TPA only elicited a transient increase of PENK gene expression (SPRINGHORN and CLAYCOMB 1989).

8. Gonads

Regulation of PENK gene expression has been studied in male and female gonads. A PENK mRNA species of 1450 nucleotides in size was found in the uterus, oviduct and ovary and in testis, vas deferens, epididymidis, seminal vesicles and prostate of rats and hamsters (KILPATRICK et al. 1985; KILPATRICK and MILLETTE 1986; KILPATRICK and ROSENTHAL 1986). Such data indicate that PENK-derived peptides are synthesized at multiple sites within the male and female reproductive tracts and may locally regulate reproductive function. In the rat testis, an additional mRNA species of 1700–1900 nucleotides was observed. This species contains a distinct 5'-nontranslated mRNA sequence derived by alternate splicing within intron A of the rat gene (YOSHIKAWA et al. 1989a). PENK mRNA was present in mouse spermatocytes and in spermatids, but not in extracts of mature sperm, suggesting that developing germ cells may be a major site of PENK synthesis in the testis and that PENK-derived peptides may function as germ cell-associated autocrine and/or paracrine hormones (KILPATRICK and ROSENTHAL 1986; KILPATRICK and MILLETTE 1986). In rats, PENK mRNA levels were markedly changed during the estrous cycle in both the ovary and uterus. The highest concentrations occurred at estrus in the rat ovary, and at metestrus and diestrus in the rat uterus (JIN et al. 1988). In the uterus of rhesus monkeys, PENK mRNA is expressed primarily in the endometrium of the uterus. PENK gene expression in the endometrium is induced by 17 β-estradiol, an action antagonized by progesterone (Low et al. 1989).

The regulation of PENK gene expression has recently been studied in cultured rat testicular peritubular cells. PENK mRNA was found to be increased by forskolin and by the phorbol ester TPA. Both drugs synergistically increase PENK mRNA in these cells. Moreover, glucocorticoids potentiated the effect of forskolin, but not that of TPA. These findings indicate that regulation of PENK gene expression in the testicular peritubular cells is similar to that in the chromaffin cells, and that PENK gene expression can be induced by activation of protein kinase C and by a cAMP-dependent pathway. Furthermore, they indicate that glucocorticoids exert a permissive effect (YOSHIKAWA et al. 1989b).

9. Immune System

Activation of mouse T-helper cells in vitro by concanavalin A results in a dramatic induction of PENK mRNA (ZURAWSKI et al. 1986). In activated mouse T-helper cells, as much as 0.4% of the total mRNA coded for PENK, allowing for the cloning of mouse PENK mRNA. Interestingly, the predicted amino acid sequence of mouse PENK contains a different sequence for the octapeptide (see above). PENK mRNA was also found in normal rat B cells. The expression of PENK mRNA in these cells was markedly enhanced by LPS or *Salmonella typhimurium* in vitro (Rosen et al. 1989).

10. Cell Lines

Proenkephalin mRNA has been detected in various cell lines. Low levels of PENK mRNA have been found in PC12 cells, a cell line derived from a rat pheochromocytoma (Byrd et al. 1987). Although PENK mRNA levels in PC12 cells can be increased by treatment with sodium butyrate, they are still too low to make PC12 cells a useful tool for studying PENK gene expression. A greater abundance of PENK mRNA was found in cultured C6 rat glioma cells. In this cell line activation of β-adrenergic receptors by norepinephrine increased cAMP levels and stimulated PENK mRNA. Glucocorticoids have no effect, but potentiate the inducing effect of norepinephrine on PENK gene expression (Yoshikawa and Sabol 1986). In addition, PENK mRNA is also present in mouse neuroblastoma-rat glioma hybrid cells (NG108CC15). Treatment of the cells with opiates (etorphine, D-ala$_2$-D-met$_5$-ENK) increased PENK mRNA levels by an effect not involving adenylate cyclase (Schwartz 1988). PENK mRNA has also been found in several human neuroblastoma cell lines (SK-N-MC; SH-SY5Y; Folkesson et al. 1988). In addition, PENK mRNA has been found in human leukocytes from patients with chronic lymphoblastic leukemia (Monstein et al. 1986). In human neuroblastoma SK-N-MC cells, dibutyryl-cAMP and β-receptor agonists increased PENK mRNA (Folkesson et al. 1989). Glucocorticoids had no effect per se, but inhibited the effect of norepinephrine, in contrast to earlier results obtained with rat C6 glioma cells (Yoshikawa and Sabol 1986).

III. Prodynorphin

Regulation of PDYN gene expression has been studied in hypothalamus, striatum, hippocampus and spinal cord, pituitary, adrenal gland, and gonadal tract.

1. Hypothalamus

In the rat hypothalamus, PDYN mRNA has been localized in the magnocellular divisions of supraoptic and paraventricular nuclei (Sherman et al. 1986; Morris et al. 1986). With chronic osmotic challenge, PDYN mRNA levels in the suproptic and paraventricular nuclei are increased, in parallel with those for provasopressin (Sherman et al. 1986). These findings indicate a coordinate regulation of mRNA expression for coexisting peptide systems. A coordinate increase in the levels of PDYN and of provasopressin mRNA in the hypothalamus has also been found in rats treated with nicotine (HÖLLT and HORN 1989; V. HÖLLT and HORN 1992). The regulation of these mRNAs can also differ, however, since repeated electroconvulsive shock concomitantly activates PDYN and provasopressin gene expression in the supraoptic, but not in the paraventricular, hypothalamic nuclei (SCHÄFER et al. 1989).

2. Striatum

The striatum contains many GABAergic neurons projecting to the substantia nigra and the external segment of the pallidum which express PDYN (GRAYBIEL 1986). PDYN mRNA in the striatum, the nucleus accumbens, and the olfactory tubercle has been demonstrated by in situ hybridization (YOUNG et al. 1986; MORRIS et al. 1986, 1989).

Destruction of the substantia nigra with 6-hydroxy-DA resulted in a slight decrease (YOUNG et al. 1986) or had no effect on PDYN mRNA levels in the striatum (MORRIS et al. 1989), indicating that the mesostriatal DA system does not exert a major influence on PDYN synthesis in this brain region. Similarly, chronic treatment with the DA antagonist haloperidol did not change the PDYN levels in the striatum (MORRIS et al. 1989). On the other hand, chronic treatment with the DA agonist apomorphine has been shown to increase the levels of PDYN mRNA in the striatum (LI et al. 1988). Recent results of our group showed that, after lesion of the medial forebrain bundle, the PDYN mRNA levels in the nucleus accumbens – an area which contains a high proportion of D_1 receptors – were decreased (S. REIMER et al. 1992). These findings suggest that there appears to exist a slight tonic enhancement of PDYN synthesis in the basal ganglia via D_1 receptors.

The raphe-striatal serotonergic pathway tonically enhances PDYN gene expression in striatal target cells, since destruction of the dorsal raphe nucleus by microinjection of 5,7-dihydroxytryptamine caused significant reductions in PDYN mRNA levels in the medial nucleus accumbens and the caudomedial striatum – regions which contain a particularly dense serotonergic innervation (MORRIS et al. 1988b).

Enhancement of GABAergic transmission by chronic administration of GABA transaminase inhibitors (AOAA; EOS; γ-vinyl-GABA) causes a decrease in striatal levels of PDYN (REIMER and HÖLLT 1990a). This might reflect a type of autoinhibition, since the dynorphinergic neurons in the striatum contain GABA as neurotransmitter.

In addition, irreversible inactivation of striatal opioid receptors by local administration of β-chlornaltrexamine caused an increase in PDYN mRNA levels at the site of injection (MORRIS et al. 1988c), indicating that endogenous opioids tonically inhibit striatal PDYN biosynthesis. This effect, however, appears to be mediated via δ- and κ-receptors rather than μ-opioid receptors, since local injection of the irreversible antagonist β-funaltrexamine and administration of the μ-agonist morphine or the antagonist NAL have no effect on the striatal levels of PDYN (Morris et al. 1988c; V. Höllt, unpublished).

Prodynorphin biosynthesis in the striatum was also slightly increased after electrical kindling of the deep prepyriform cortex, indicating that the striatum participates in the neuronal circuits activated by cortical kindling (Lee et al. 1989).

3. Hippocampus

Within the hippocampus, DYN peptides are synthesized in the granule cells of the dentate gyrus and transported within the mossy fiber pathways which innervate the pyramidal cells (McGinty et al. 1983; Morris et al. 1986). Following brief trains of high-frequency electrical stimulation to the dentate gyrus of rats, the levels of PDYN mRNA were markedly decreased on the stimulated, but not the unstimulated side (Morris et al. 1988a). Similarly, chronic electrical stimulation of the dentate gyrus, which resulted in stage 4 kindling seizures in rats, caused a marked decrease in PDYN mRNA levels in the granule cells of the dentate gyrus. This decrease was seen in the stimulated and unstimulated hemispheres (Morris et al. 1987). The contralateral decrease in PDYN mRNA levels might be due to the activation of commissural projections. A bilateral decrease in PDYN levels can also be induced by unilateral electrical stimulation of the perforant pathway, which results in stage 3 kindling seizures in rats (Moneta and Höllt 1990), indicating that PDYN gene expression in the hippocampus can be altered transsynaptically. The perforant path stimulation-induced decrease in PDYN mRNA levels could be blocked by a glutamate antagonist indicating that endogenous glutamate at perforans synapses may regulate biosynthesis of PDYN in dentate granule cells (Yie et al. 1991). PDYN mRNA levels in the hippocampus are also decreased during the development of deep prepyriform cortex kindling (Lee et al. 1989) and after repeated electroconvulsive shocks (Xie et al. 1989). The altered PDYN mRNA levels in the hippocampus return to normal 1–6 weeks following cessation of stimulation (Lee et al. 1989; Moneta and Höllt 1990). However, a further single stimulus was still effective in producing kindling seizures. These findings indicate that opioid peptides may play a role in the development, but not maintenance, of kindling. There is electrophysiological evidence for an inhibitory action of PDYN peptides on hippocampal pyramidal cells (Henricksen et al. 1982). A decrease in PDYN biosynthesis might, therefore, contribute to the hyperexcitability found in the kindling state. Thus, in contrast to the PENK gene, the PDYN gene is negatively regulated by neuronal activity.

In aged rats an increase in hippocampal levels of PDYN mRNA was observed (Lacaze-Masmonteil et al. 1987). An age-related loss of perforant path afferents which inhibit dynorphin biosynthesis in the granule cells might be responsible for this effect.

4. Spinal Cord

In the spinal cord, a prominent role for PDYN-derived peptides has been suggested by the observation that PDYN mRNA in the cord is markedly enhanced by acute or chronic inflammatory processes (IADAROLA et al. 1986, 1988a,b; HÖLLT et al. 1987; WEIHE et al. 1989). In polyarthritic rats a pronounced elevation in PDYN mRNA was found in the lumbosacral spinal cord (HÖLLT et al. 1987; WEIHE et al. 1989). In rats with unilateral inflammation, a pronounced increase in PDYN mRNA was observed only in those spinal cord segments that received sensory inputs from the affected limb (IADAROLA et al. 1988a,b). These changes were rapid in onset, being significantly elevated as early as 4h after the injection of the inflammatory agent into the paw (DRAISCI and IADAROLA 1989). PDYN mRNA levels peaked after about 3 days, returning to normal after about 2 weeks (IADAROLA et al. 1988a). In situ hybridization revealed that the increase in the PDYN mRNA occurs in the superficial dorsal-horn laminae I and II, and in the deep dorsal-horn laminae V and VI (RUDA et al. 1988). In addition to inflammation, traumatic injury and cord transection also increased PDYN mRNA levels in the spinal cord (PRZEWLOCKI et al. 1988). This marked increase in PDYN biosynthesis suggests a highly specific role for PDYN-derived peptides in the modulation of pain associated with inflammation and tissue injury. It was shown recently that an increased PDYN gene expression provoked by noxious thermal stimulation or inflammation is preceded by an early induction of c-*fos* in the same neurones (NARANJO et al. 1991; NOGUCHI et al. 1991). In addition, an AP-1 like element has been localized within the promoter region of the rat PDYN gene and shown to be a target of Fos/Jun oncoproteins (NARANJO et al. 1991). These findings suggest that fos/Inn oncoproteins may function as third messengers in the signal transduction mechanisms in response to painful stimuli.

5. Pituitary

Prodynorphin mRNA has been localized in the anterior pituitary of rats (CIVELLI et al. 1985; SCHÄFER et al. 1990) and pigs (PITTIUS et al. 1987). It is still unclear which cell type produces PDYN, although the parallel release of luteinizing hormone together with PDYN peptides in response to GnRH suggests that both peptides are produced by gonadotrophic cells. PDYN mRNA in the rat anterior pituitary is decreased by estrogens and increased by anti-estrogens (SPAMPINATO et al. 1990). In the rat, in situ hybridization experiments revealed that PDYN mRNA is also produced in melanotrophic cells of the intermediate pituitary (SCHÄFER et al. 1990). In the pig, however, no PDYN mRNA could be demonstrated in the neurointermediate lobe when Northern blot analysis was employed (PITTIUS et al. 1987).

6. Peripheral Tissues

Northern blot and solution analysis revealed the presence of PDYN mRNA in the porcine heart ventricle, gut, and lung; these tissues contain low, but significant, levels of PDYN-derived peptides (PITTIUS et al. 1987). However, the mRNA species found in the gut and lung are smaller than those found in the brain and heart ventricle and appear to derive from a different gene which possesses a high homology to the PDYN gene (PITTIUS et al. 1987). In the rat adrenal gland, a unique PDYN mRNA species, which is about 350 bases shorter than the PDYN transcripts in the hypothalamus (2100 vs. 2400 nucleotides), has been found (CIVELLI et al. 1985). The observed size difference of the PDYN mRNA in the adrenal may be due to alternate splicing, resulting in the deletion of exon 2 of the PDYN gene (DAY et al. 1990). In situ hybridization studies localized PDYN mRNA in the zona fasciculata and zona reticularis of the adrenal cortex (DAY et al. 1990). PDYN mRNA has been shown to be influenced by pituitary-dependent factors, since there is a dramatic loss of PDYN mRNA in the zona fasciculata following hypophysectomy in rats (DAY et al. 1990).

In the gonads, PDYN mRNA has been found in the testes of rats, rabbits, and guinea pigs, and in the rat ovary and uterus (CIVELLI et al. 1985; DOUGLASS et al. 1987). Within the rat testis, PDYN peptides have been found in Leydig cells. Moreover, PDYN mRNA is found in the R2C Leydig tumor cell line (McMURRAY et al. 1989) and in cultured Sertoli cells. The testicular PDYN mRNA species is about 100 bases smaller than that found in the hypothalamus. This may be due to alternate splicing leading to the loss of exon 2 of the PDYN gene. In R2C rat Leydig cells the PDYN gene is positively regulated by cAMP analogs, whereas phorbol esters exert a slight negative regulation on PDYN mRNA levels. The presence of mRNA together with PDYN-derived peptides in the reproductive tract suggests that these peptides exert paracrine and/or autocrine effects.

D. Summary

The three opioid peptide genes (see also Fig. 1) are strikingly similar in their general organization. They all contain a main exon which codes for the vast majority of the protein sequences. The signal peptide and the translational initiation site are coded by another exon. This exon has an almost identical site in all three genes. These similarities in structural organization suggest that the three opioid peptide genes may have evolved from a common ancestor.

All three genes are positively regulated by cAMP, although only the *PENK* gene possesses an identified cAMP-responsive element within the 5'-flanking region. Moreover, all three genes are expressed in tissues (pituitary, adrenal gland, hypothalamus) which are known to play an important role in the response of the organism to stressful conditions.

References

Affolter HU, Reisine T (1985) Corticotropin releasing factor increases proopiomelanocortin messenger RNA in mouse anterior pituitary tumor cells. J Biol Chem 260:15477–15481

Aloyo VJ, Lewis ME, Walker RF (1990) Opioid peptide mRNAs in the rat pineal gland. In: Quirion R, Jhamandas K, Giounalakis C (eds) The international narcotics research conference (IRNC) '89. Liss, New York, pp 235–238

Angelogianni P, Gianoulakis C (1990) Ethanol regulation of proopiomelanocortin biosynthesis in the rat hypothalamus. In: Van Ree J, Molder AH, Wiegant VM, van Wimersma Greidanus TB (eds) New leads in opioid research. Elsevier, Amsterdam, pp 117–118

Angulo JA, Christoph GR, Manning RW, Burkhart BA, Davis LG (1987) Reduction of dopamine receptor activity differentially alters striatal neuropeptide mRNA levels. Adv Exp Med Biol 221:385–391

Angulo JA, Cadet JL, McEwen BS (1990) Sigma receptor blockade by BMY 14802 affects enkephalinergic and tachykinin cells differentially in the striatum of the rat. Eur J Pharmacol 175:225–228

Antakly T, Sasaki A, Liotta AS, Palkovits M, Krieger DT (1985) Induced expression of the glucocorticoid receptor in the rat intermediate pituitary lobe. Science 229:277–279

Autelitano DJ, Blum M, Roberts JL (1989) Changes in rat pituitary nuclear and cytoplasmic pro-opiomelanocortin RNAs associated with adrenalectomy and glucocorticoid replacement. Mol Cell Endocrinol 66:171–180

Autelitano DJ, Blum M, Lopingco M, Allen RG, Roberts JL (1990) Corticotropin-releasing factor differentially regulates anterior and intermediate pituitary lobe proopiomelanocortin gene transcription, nuclear precursor RNA and mature mRNA in vivo. Neuroendocrinology 51:123–130

Beaulieu S, Gagne B, Barden N (1988) Glucocorticoid regulation of proopiomelanocortin messenger ribonucleic acid content of rat hypothalamus. Mol Endocrinol 2:727–731

Birnberg NC, Lissitzky JC, Hinman M, Herbert E (1983) Glucocorticoids regulate proopiomelanocortin gene expression in vivo at the levels of transcription and secretion. Proc Natl Acad Sci USA 80:6982–6986

Blanc D, Cupo A, Castanas E, Bourhim N, Giraud P, Bannon MJ, Eiden LE (1985) Influence of acute, subchronic and chronic treatment with neuroleptic (haloperidol) on enkephalins and their precursors in the striatum of rat brain. Neuropeptides 5:567–570

Bloch B, Le-Guellec D, de-Keyzer Y (1985) Detection of the messenger RNAs coding for the opioid peptide precursors in pituitary and adrenal by "in situ" hybridization: study in several mammal species. Neurosci Lett 53:141–148

Blum M, Roberts JL, Wardlaw SL (1989) Androgen regulation of proopio-melanocortin gene expression and peptide content in the basal hypothalamus. Endocrinology 124:2283–2288

Bommer M, Liebisch D, Kley N, Herz A, Noble E (1987) Histamine affects release and biosynthesis of opioid peptides primarily via H1-receptors in bovine chromaffin cells. J Neurochem 49:1688–1696

Boutillier AL, Sassone-Corsi P, Loeffler JP (1991) The protooncogene c-fos is induced by corticotropin-releasing factor and stimulates proopiomelanocortin gene transcription in pituitary cells. Mol Endocrinol 5:1301–1310

Bruhn TO, Sutton RE, Rivier CL, Vale WW (1984) Corticotropin-releasing factor regulates proopiomelanocortin messenger ribonucleic acid levels in vivo. Neuroendocrinology 39:170–175

Buckingham JC (1982) Secretion of corticotrophin and its hypothalamic releasing factor in response to morphine and opioid peptides. Neuroendocrinology 35:111–116

Byrd JC, Naranjo JR, Lindberg I (1987) Proenkephalin gene expression in the PC12 pheochromocytoma cell line: stimulation by sodium butyrate. Endocrinology 121:1299–1305

Chang AC, Israel A, Gazdar A, Cohen SN (1989) Initiation of pro-opiomelanocortin mRNA from a normally quiescent promoter in a human small cell lung cancer cell line. Gene 84:115–126

Charron J, Drouin J (1986) Glucocorticoid inhibition of transcription from episomal proopiomelanocortin gene promoter. Proc Natl Acad Sci USA 83:8903–8907

Chen CL, Madigan MB (1987) Regulation of testicular proopiomelanocortin gene expression. Endocrinology 121:590–596

Chen CL, Dionne FT, Roberts JL (1983) Regulation of the pro-opiomelanocortin mRNA levels in rat pituitary by dopaminergic compounds. Proc Natl Acad Sci USA 80:2211–2215

Chen CL, Chang CC, Krieger DT, Bardin CW (1986) Expression and regulation of proopiomelanocortin-like gene in the ovary and placenta: comparison with the testis. Endocrinology 118:2382–2389

Chowen-Breed J, Fraser HM, Vician L, Damassa DA, Clifton DK, Steiner RA (1989a) Testosterone regulation of proopiomelanocortin messenger ribonucleic acid in the arcuate nucleus of the male rat. Endocrinology 124:1697–1702

Chowen-Breed JA, Clifton DK, Steiner RA (1989b) Regional specificity of testosterone regulation of proopiomelanocortin gene expression in the arcuate nucleus of the male rat brain. Endocrinology 124:2875–2881

Chronwall BM, Hook GR, Millington WR (1988) Dopaminergic regulation of the biosynthetic activity of individual melanotropes in the rat pituitary intermediate lobe: a morphometric analysis by light and electron microscopy and in situ hybridization. Endocrinology 123:1992–2002

Civelli O, Douglass J, Goldstein A, Herbert E (1985) Sequence and expression of the rat prodynorphin gene. Proc Natl Acad Sci USA 82:4291–4295

Clark AJ, Lavender PM, Besser GM, Rees LH (1989) Pro-opiomelanocortin mRNA size heterogeneity in ACTH-dependent Cushing's syndrome. J Mol Endocrinol 2:3–9

Clark AJ, Stewart MF, Lavender PM, Farrell W, Crosby SR, Rees LH, White A (1990) Defective glucocorticoid regulation of proopiomelanocortin gene expression and peptide secretion in a small cell lung cancer cell line. J Clin Endocrinol Metab 70:485–490

Comb M, Liston D, Martin M, Rosen H, Herbert E (1985) Expression of the human proenkephalin gene in mouse pituitary cells: accurate and efficient mRNA production and proteolytic processing. EMBO J 4:3115–3122

Comb M, Birnberg NC, Seasholtz A, Herbert E, Goodman HM (1986) A cyclic AMP- and phorbol ester-inducible DNA element. Nature 323:353–356

Comb M, Mermod N, Hyman SE, Pearlberg J, Ross ME, Goodman HM (1988) Proteins bound at adjacent DNA elements act synergistically to regulate human proenkephalin cAMP inducible transcription. EMBO J 7:3793–3805

Cote TE, Felder R, Kebabian JW, Sekura RD, Reisine T, Affolter HU (1986) D-2 dopamine receptor-mediated inhibition of pro-opiomelanocortin synthesis in rat intermediate lobe. Abolition by pertussis toxin or activators of adenylate cyclase. J Biol Chem 261:4555–4561

Curran T, Rauscher FJ, Cohen DR, Franza BR Jr (1988) Beyond the second messenger: oncogenes and transcription factors. Cold Spring Harb Symp Quant Biol 53(2):769–777

Dave JR, Eiden LE, Karanian JW, Eskay RL (1986) Ethanol exposure decreases pituitary corticotropin-releasing factor binding, adenylate cyclase activity, proopiomelanocortin biosynthesis, and plasma beta-endorphin levels in the rat. Endocrinology 118:280–286

Dave JR, Eiden LE, Lozovsky D, Waschek JA, Eskay RL (1987) Calcium-independent and calcium-dependent mechanisms regulate corticotropin-releasing factor-stimulated proopiomelanocortin peptide secretion and messenger ribonucleic acid production. Endocrinology 120:305–310

Day R, Schäfer MK-H, Watson SJ, Akil H (1990) Effects of hypophysectomy on dynorphin mRNA and peptide content in the rat adrenal gland. In: Quirion R, Jhamandas K, Giounalakis C (eds) The international narcotics conference (IRNC) '89. Liss, New York, pp 207–210

De Keyzer Y, Bertagna X, Lenne F, Girard F, Luton JP, Kahn A (1985) Altered proopiomelanocortin gene expression in adrenocorticotropin-producing nonpituitary tumors. Comparative studies with corticotropic adenomas and normal pituitaries. J Clin Invest 76:1892–1898

De Keyzer Y, Bertagna X, Luton JP, Kahn A (1989) Variable modes of proopiomelanocortin gene transcription in human tumors. Mol Endocrinol 3:215–223

DeBold CR, Nicholson WE, Orth DN (1988a) Immunoreactive proopiomelanocortin (POMC) peptides and POMC-like messenger ribonucleic acid are present in many rat nonpituitary tissues. Endocrinology 122:2648–2657

DeBold CR, Menefee JK, Nicholson WE, Orth DN (1988b) Proopiomelanocortin gene is expressed in many normal human tissues and in tumors not associated with ectopic adrenocorticotropin syndrome. Mol Endocrinol 2:862–870

DeBold CR, Mufson EE, Menefee JK, Orth DN (1988c) Proopiomelanocortin gene expression in a pheochromocytoma using upstream transcription initiation sites. Biochem Biophys Res Commun 155:895–900

Douglass J, Cox B, Quinn B, Civelli O, Herbert E (1987) Expression of the prodynorphin gene in male and female mammalian reproductive tissues. Endocrinology 120:707–713

Douglass J, McMurray CT, Garrett JE, Adelman JP, Calavetta L (1989) Characterization of the rat prodynorphin gene. Mol Endocrinol 3:2070–2078

Draisci G, Iadarola MJ (1989) Temporal analysis of increases in c-*fos*, preprodynorphin and preproenkephalin mRNAs in rat spinal cord. Brain Res Mol Brain Res 6:31–37

Drouin J, Chamberland M, Charron J, Jeannotte L, Nemer M (1985) Structure of the rat pro-opiomelanocortin (POMC) gene. FEBS Lett 193:54–58

Drouin J, Trifiro MA, Plante RK, Nemer M, Erikson P, Wrange Y (1989) Glucocorticoid receptor binding to a specific DNA sequence is required for hormone-dependent repression of pro-opiomelanocortin gene transcription. Mol Cell Biol 9:5305–5314

Eberwine JH, Roberts JL (1984) Glucocorticoid regulation of pro-opiomelanocortin gene transcription in the rat pituitary. J Biol Chem 259:2166–2170

Eberwine JH, Jonassen JA, Evinger MJ, Roberts JL (1987) Complex transcriptional regulation by glucocorticoids and corticotropin-releasing hormone of pro-opiomelanocortin gene expression in rat pituitary cultures. DNA 6:483–492

Eiden LE, Giraud P, Dave JR, Hotchkiss AJ, Affolter HU (1984a) Nicotinic receptor stimulation activates enkephalin release and biosynthesis in adrenal chromaffin cells. Nature 312:661–663

Eiden LE, Giraud P, Affolter HU, Herbert E, Hotchkiss AJ (1984b) Alternative modes of enkephalin biosynthesis regulation by reserpine and cyclic AMP in cultured chromaffin cells. Proc Natl Acad Sci USA 81:3949–3953

Elkabes S, Loh YP (1988) Effect of salt loading on proopiomelanocortin (POMC) messenger ribonucleic acid levels, POMC biosynthesis, and secretion of POMC products in the mouse pituitary gland. Endocrinology 123:1754–1760

Farin C-J, Höllt V, Kley N (1990a) Proenkephalin gene expression in cultured chromaffin cells is regulated at the transcriptional level. In: Quirion R, Jhamandas K, Giounalakis C (eds) The international narcotics research conference (IRNC) '89. Liss, New York, pp 239–242

Farin CJ, Kley N, Höllt V (1990b) Mechanisms involved in the transcriptional activation of proenkephalin gene expression in bovine chromaffin cells. J Biol Chem 265:19116–19121

Fischer-Colbrie R, Iacangelo A, Eiden LE (1988) Neural and humoral factors separately regulate neuropeptide Y, enkephalin, and chromogranin A and B mRNA levels in rat adrenal medulla. Proc Natl Acad Sci USA 85:3240–3244

Folkesson R, Monstein HJ, Geijer T, Pahlman S, Nilsson K, Terenius L (1988) Expression of the proenkephalin gene in human neuroblastoma cell lines. Brain Res 427:147–154

Folkesson R, Monstein HJ, Geijer T, Terenius L (1989) Modulation of proenkephalin A gene expression by cyclic AMP. Brain Res Mol Brain Res 5:211–217

Fremeau RT Jr, Lundblad JR, Pritchett DB, Wilcox JN, Roberts JL (1986) Regulation of pro-opiomelanocortin gene transcription in individual cell nuclei. Science 234:1265–1269

Gagner JP, Drouin J (1985) Opposite regulation of pro-opiomelanocortin gene transcription by glucocorticoids and CRH. Mol Cell Endocrinol 40:25–32

Gall C, Brecha N, Karten HJ, Chang KJ (1981) Localization of enkephalin-like immunoreactivity to identified axonal and neuronal populations of the rat hippocampus. J Comp Neurol 198:335–350

Garrett JE, Douglass JO (1989) Human chorionic gonadotropin regulates expression of the proenkephalin gene in adult rat Leydig cells. Mol Endocrinol 3:2093–2100

Garrett JE, Collard MW, Douglass JO (1989) Translational control of germ cell-expressed mRNA imposed by alternative splicing: opioid peptide gene expression in rat testis. Mol Cell Biol 9:4381–4389

Gee CE, Chen CL, Roberts JL, Thompson R, Watson SJ (1983) Identification of proopiomelanocortin neurones in rat hypothalamus by in situ cDNA-mRNA hybridization. Nature 306:374–376

Giraud P, Kowalski C, Barthel F, Becquet D, Renard M, Grino M, Boudouresque S, Loeffler JP (1991) Striatol proenkephalin turnover and gene transcription are regulated by cyclic AMP and protein kinase C-related pathways. Neuroscience 43:67–79

Gizang-Ginsberg E, Wolgemuth DJ (1985) Localization of mRNAs in mouse testes by in situ hybridization: distribution of alpha-tubulin and developmental stage specificity of pro-opiomelanocortin transcripts. Dev Biol 111:293–305

Graybiel AM (1986) Neuropeptides in the basal ganglia. Res Publ Assoc Res Nerv Ment Dis 64:135–161

Harbuz MS, Lightman SL (1989) Responses of hypothalamic and pituitary mRNA to physical and psychological stress in the rat. J Endocrinol 122:705–711

Harlan RE, Shivers BD, Romano GJ, Howells RD, Pfaff DW (1987) Localization of preproenkephalin in the rat brain and spinal cord by in situ hybridization. J Comp Neurol 258:159–184

Hatfield JM, Daikh DI, Adelman JP, Douglass J, Bond CT, Allen RG (1989) In situ hybridization detection of marked differences in pre-proopiomelanocortin messenger ribonucleic acid content of individual corticotropes and melanotropes. Endocrinology 124:1359–1364

Henricksen SJ, Chouvet G, Bloom FE (1982) In vivo cellular responses to electrophoretically applied dynorphin in the rat hippocampus. Life Sci 31:1785–1788

Höllt V, Haarmann I (1984) Corticotropin-releasing factor differentially regulates proopiomelanocortin messenger ribonucleic acid levels in anterior as compared to intermediate pituitary lobes of rats. Biochem Biophys Res Commun 124:407–415

Höllt V, Haarmann I (1985) differential alterations by chronic treatment with morphine of pro-opiomelanocortin mRNA levels in anterior as compared to intermediate pituitary lobes of rats. Neuropeptides 5:481–484

Höllt V, Horn G (1989) Nicotine and opioid peptides. In: Nordberg A, Fuxe K, Holmstedt B, Sundwall A (eds) Nicotinic receptors in the CNS: their role in synaptic transmission. Prog Brain Res 79:187–193

Höllt V, Horn G (1992) Effect of nicotine on mRNA levels encoding opioid peptides, vasopressin and α_3 nicotinic receptor submit in the rat. Clin Investig 70:224–231

Höllt V, Sincini E (1988) Bombesin and structurally related peptides increase inositol-1-phosphate production in a corticotrophic cell line of the pituitary (AtT-20). Acta Endocrinol (Copenh) 117 [Suppl 287]:206–206

Höllt V, Haarmann I, Seizinger BR, Herz A (1982) Chronic haloperidol treatment increases the level of in vitro translatable messenger ribonucleic acid coding for the beta-endorphin/adrenocorticotropin precursor proopiomelanocortin in the pars intermedia of the rat pituitary. Endocrinology 110:1885–1891

Höllt V, Przewlocki R, Haarmann I, Almeida OF, Kley N, Millan MJ, Herz A (1986) Stress-induced alterations in the levels of messenger RNA coding for proopiomelanocortin and prolactin in rat pituitary. Neuroendocrinology 43:277–282

Höllt V, Haarmann I, Millan MJ, Herz A (1987) Prodynorphin gene expression is enhanced in the spinal cord of chronic arthritic rats. Neurosci Lett 73:90–94

Höllt V, Haarmann I, Reimer S (1989a) Opioid peptide gene expression in rats after chronic morphine treatment. Adv Biosci 75:711–714

Höllt V, Haarmann I, Reimer S (1989b) Opioid gene expression in rats after chronic morphine treatment. Adv Biosci 75:711–714

Horikawa S, Takai T, Toyosato M, Takahashi H, Noda M, Kakidani H, Kubo T, Hirose T, Inayama S, Hayashida H, Miyata T, Numa S (1983) Isolation and structural organization of the human preproenkephalin B gene. Nature 306:611–614

Howells RD, Kilpatrick DL, Bailey LC, Noe M, Udenfriend S (1986) Proenkephalin mRNA in rat heart. Proc Natl Acad Sci USA 83:1960–1963

Hunt SP, Pini A, Evan G (1987) Induction of c-fos-like protein in spinal cord neurons following sensory stimulation. Nature 328:632–634

Hyman SE, Comb M, Lin YS, Pearlberg J, Green MR, Goodman HM (1988) A common trans-acting factor is involved in transcriptional regulation of neurotransmitter genes by cyclic AMP. Mol Cell Biol 8:4225–4233

Hyman SE, Comb M, Pearlberg J, Goodman HM (1989) An AP-2 element acts synergistically with the cyclic AMP- and phorbol ester-inducible enhancer of the human proenkephalin gene. Mol Cell Biol 9:321–324

Iadarola MJ, Douglass J, Civelli O, Naranjo JR (1986) Increased spinal cord dynorphin mRNA during peripheral inflammation. Natl Inst Drug Abuse Res Monogr Ser 75:406–409

Iadarola MJ, Brady LS, Draisci G, Dubner R (1988a) Enhancement of dynorphin gene expression in spinal cord following experimental inflammation: stimulus specificity, behavioral parameters and opioid receptor binding. Pain 35:313–326

Iadarola MJ, Douglass J, Civelli O, Naranjo JR (1988b) Differential activation of spinal cord dynorphin and enkephalin neurons during hyperalgesia: evidence using cDNA hybridization. Brain Res 455:205–212

Inturrisi CE, Branch AD, Robertson HD, Howells RD, Franklin SO, Shapiro JR, Calvano SE, Yoburn BC (1988a) Glucocorticoid regulation of enkephalins in cultured rat adrenal medulla. Mol Endocrinol 2:633–640

Inturrisi CE, LaGamma EF, Franklin SO, Huang T, Nip TJ, Yoburn BC (1988b) Characterization of enkephalins in rat adrenal medullary explants. Brain Res 448:230–236

Israel A, Cohen SN (1985) Hormonally mediated negative regulation of human pro-opiomelanocortin gene expression after transfection into mouse L cells. Mol Cell Biol 5:2443–2453

Jeannotte L, Burbach JPH, Drouin J (1987a) Unusual proopiomelanocortin ribonucleic acids in extrapituitary tissues: intronless transcripts in testes and long poly (A) tails in the hypothalamus. Mol Endocrinol 1:749–757

Jeannotte L, Trifiro MA, Plante RK, Chamberland M, Drouin J (1987b) Tissue-specific activity of the pro-opiomelanocortin gene promoter. Mol Cell Biol 7:4058–4064

Jin DF, Muffly KE, Okulicz WC, Kilpatrick DL (1988) Estrous cycle- and pregnancy-related differences in expression of the proenkephalin and pro-opiomelanocortin genes in the ovary and uterus. Endocrinology 122:1466–1471

Jingami H, Nakanishi S, Imura H, Numa S (1984) Tissue distribution of messenger RNAs coding for opioid peptide precursors and related RNA. Eur J Biochem 142:441–447

Kanamatsu T, Unsworth CD, Diliberto EJ Jr, Viveros OH, Hong JS (1986) Reflex splanchnic nerve stimulation increases levels of proenkephalin A mRNA and proenkephalin A-related peptides in the rat adrenal medulla. Proc Natl Acad Sci USA 83:9245–9249

Keshet E, Polakiewicz RD, Itin A, Ornoy A, Rosen H (1989) Proenkephalin A is expressed in mesodermal lineages during organogenesis. EMBO J 8:2917–2923

Kessler U, Sincini E, Stalla GK, Höllt V (1989) Bombesin stimulates release of β-endorphin in corticotrophic pituitary cells in vitro. Acta Endocrinol (Copenh) 120 [Suppl 1]:206–206

Kilpatrick DL, Millette CF (1986) Expression of proenkephalin messenger RNA by mouse spermatogenic cells. Proc Natl Acad Sci USA 83:5015–5018

Kilpatrick DL, Rosenthal JL (1986) The proenkephalin gene is widely expressed within the male and female reproductive systems of the rat and hamster. Endocrinology 119:370–374

Kilpatrick DL, Howells RD, Fleminger G, Udenfriend S (1984) Denervation of rat adrenal glands markedly increases preproenkephalin mRNA. Proc Natl Acad Sci USA 81:7221–7223

Kilpatrick DL, Howells RD, Noe M, Bailey LC, Udenfriend S (1985) Expression of preproenkephalin-like mRNA and its peptide products in mammalian testis and ovary. Proc Natl Acad Sci USA 82:7467–7469

Kilpatrick DL, Borland K, Jin DF (1987) Differential expression of opioid peptide genes by testicular germ cells and somatic cells. Proc Natl Acad Sci USA 84:5695–5699

Kley N (1988) Multiple regulation of proenkephalin gene expression by protein kinase C. J Biol Chem 263:2003–2008

Kley N, Loeffler JP, Pittius CW, Höllt V (1986) Proenkephalin A gene expression in bovine adrenal chromaffin cells is regulated by changes in electrical activity. EMBO J 5:967–970

Kley N, Loeffler JP, Pittius CW, Höllt V (1987a) Involvement of ion channels in the induction of proenkephalin A gene expression by nicotine and cAMP in bovine chromaffin cells. J Biol Chem 262:4083–4089

Kley N, Loeffler JP, Höllt V (1987b) Ca^{2+}-dependent histaminergic regulation of proenkephalin mRNA levels in cultured adrenal chromaffin cells. Neuroendocrinology 46:89–92

Knight RM, Farah JM, Bishop JF, O'Donohue TL (1987) CRF and cAMP regulation of POMC gene expression in corticotrophic tumor cells. Peptides 8:927–934

Kobierski LA, Chu H-M, Comb MJ (1991) cAMP-dependent regulation of proenkephalin by JunD and JunB: Positive and negative effects of AP-1 proteins. Proc Natl Acad Sci 88:10222–10226

Korner M, Rattner A, Manxion F, Sen T, Citri Y (1989) A brain-specific transcription activator. Neuron 3:563–572

Kowalski C, Giraud P, Boudouresque F, Lissitzky JC, Cupo A, Renard M, Saura RM, Oliver C (1989) Enkephalins expression in striatal cell cultures. Adv Biosci 75:225–228

Kraus J, Höllt V (1990) A negative regulatory element in the upstream promoter region of the human proopiomelanocortin gene. In: Van Ree J, Mulder AJ, Wiegant VM, van Wimersma Greidanus TB (eds) New leads in opioid research. Elsevier, Amsterdam, pp 115–117

Kraus J, Buchfelder M, Höllt V (1992) Regulatory elements of the human proopiomelanocortin gene promoter. DNA Cell Biol (in press)

Lacaze-Masmonteil T, de-Keyzer Y, Luton JP, Kahn A, Bertagna X (1987) Characterization of proopiomelanocortin transcripts in human nonpituitary tissues. Proc Natl Acad Sci USA 84:7261–7265

LaGamma EF, Adler JE (1987) Glucocorticoids regulate adrenal opiate peptides. Mol Brain Res 2:125–130

LaGamma EF, White JD, Adler JE, Krause JE, McKelvy JF, Black IB (1985) Depolarization regulates adrenal preproenkephalin mRNA. Proc Natl Acad Sci USA 82:8252–8255

LaGamma EF, White JD, McKelvy JF, Black IB (1988) Second messenger mechanisms governing opiate peptide transmitter regulation in the rat adrenal medulla. Brain Res 441:292–298

LaGamma EF, Goldstein NK, Snyder Jr SB, Weisinger G (1989) Prerproenkephalin DNA-binding proteins in the rat: 5'-flanking region. Mol Brain Res 5:131–140

Le Moine C, Normand E, Guitteny AF, Fouque B, Teoule R, Bloch B (1990) Dopamine receptor gene expression by enkephalin neurons in rat forebrain. Proc Natl Acad Sci USA 87:230–234

Lee PHK, Zhao D, Xie CW, McGinty JF, Mitchell CL, Hong JS (1989) Changes of proenkephalin and prodynorphin mRNAs and related peptides in rat brain during the development of deep prepyriform cortex kindling. Mol Brain Res 6:263–273

Leviel V, Fayada C, Guibert B, Chaminade M, Machek G, Mallet J, Biguet NF (1990) Short- and long-term alterations of gene expression in limbic structures by repeated electroconvulsive-induced seizures. J Neurochem 54:899–904

Levin N, Blum M, Roberts JL (1989) Modulation of basal and corticotropin-releasing factor-stimulated proopiomelanocortin gene expression by vasopressin in rat anterior pituitary. Endocrinology 125:2957–2966

Levy A, Lightman SL (1988) Quantitative in-situ hybridization histochemistry in the rat pituitary gland: effect of bromocriptine on prolactin and pro-opiomelanocortin gene expression. J Endocrinol 118:205–210

Li H, Risbridger GP, Funder JW, Clements JA (1989) Effect of ethane dimethane sulphonate on proopiomelanocortin (POMC) mRNA and POMC-derived peptides in the rat testis. Mol Cell Endocrinol 65:203–207

Li SJ, Sivam SP, McGinty JF, Jiang HK, Douglass J, Calavetta L, Hong JS (1988) Regulation of the metabolism of striatal dynorphin by the dopaminergic system. J Pharmacol Exp Ther 246:403–408

Lightman SL, Young WS (1987a) Changes in hypothalamic preproenkephalin A mRNA following stress and opiate withdrawal. Nature 328:643–645

Lightman SL, Young WS (1987b) Vasopressin, oxytocin, dynorphin, enkephalin and corticotrophin-releasing factor mRNA stimulation in the rat. J Physiol (Lond) 394:23–39

Lightman SL, Young WS (1988) Corticotrophin-releasing factor, vasopressin and pro-opiomelanocortin mRNA responses to stress and opiates in the rat. J Physiol (Lond) 403:511–523

Llorens-Cortes C, Giros B, Quach T, Schwartz J-C (1990) Adaptive changes in two indices of enkephalin neuron activity in mouse striatum following gabaergic stimulation. In: Quirion R, Jhanmandas K, Gianoulakis C (eds) The international narcotics research conference (INRC) '89. Liss, New York, pp 203–206

Loeffler JP, Kley N, Pittius CW, Höllt V (1985) Corticotropin-releasing factor and forskolin increase proopiomelanocortin messenger RNA levels in rat anterior and intermediate cells in vitro. Neurosci Lett 62:383–387

Loeffler JP, Kley N, Pittius CW, Höllt V (1986a) Calcium ion and cyclic adenosine 3',5'-monophosphate regulate proopiomelanocortin messenger ribonucleic acid levels in rat intermediate and anterior pituitary lobes. Endocrinology 119:2840–2847

Loeffler JP, Demeneix BA, Pittius CW, Kley N, Haegele KD, Höllt V (1986b) GABA differentially regulates the gene expression of proopiomelanocortin in rat intermediate and anterior pituitary. Peptides 7:253–258

Loeffler JP, Kley N, Pittius CW, Höllt V (1986c) Regulation of proopiomelanocortin (POMC) mRNA levels in primary pituitary cultures. Natl Inst Drug Abuse Res Monogr Ser 75:397–400

Loeffler JP, Demeneix BA, Kley NA, Höllt V (1988) Dopamine inhibition of proopiomelanocortin gene expression in the intermediate lobe of the pituitary. Interactions with corticotropin-releasing factor and the beta-adrenergic receptors and the adenylate cyclase system. Neuroendocrinology 47:95–101

Loeffler JP, Kley N, Louis JC, Demeneix BA (1989) Ca^{2+} regulates hormone secretion and proopiomelanocortin gene expression in melanotrope cells via the calmodulin and the protein kinase C pathways. J Neurochem 52:1279–1283

Low KG, Nielsen CP, West NB, Douglass J, Brenner RM, Maslar IA, Melner MH (1989) Proenkephalin gene expression in the primate uterus: regulation by estradiol in the endometrium. Mol Endocrinol 3:852–857

Luini A, Lewis D, Guild S, Corda D, Axelrod J (1985) Hormone secretagogues increase cytosolic calcium by increasing cAMP in corticotropin-secreting cells. Proc Natl Acad Sci USA 82:8034–8038

Lundblad JR, Roberts JL (1988) Regulation of proopiomelanocortin gene expression in pituitary. Endocr Rev 9:135–158

McGinty JF, Henriksen SJ, Goldstein A, Terenius L, Bloom FE (1983) Dynorphin is contained within hippocampal mossy fibers: immunochemical alterations after kainic acid administration and colchicine-induced neurotoxicity. Proc Natl Acad Sci USA 80:589–593

McLoughlin L, Buzzetti R, Lavender PM, Clark A, Rees LH (1990) Pro-opiomelanocortin derived peptides in cells of the human immune system. In: Van Ree J, Mulder AH, Wiegant VM, van Wimersma Greidanus TB (eds) New leads in opioid research. Elsevier, Amsterdam, pp 373–374

McMurray CT, Devi L, Calavetta L, Douglass JO (1989) Regulated expression of the prodynorphin gene in the R2C Leydig tumor cell line. Endocrinology 124:49–59

Melner MH, Young SL, Czerwiec FS, Lyn D, Puett D, Roberts JL, Koos RD (1986) The regulation of granulosa cell proopiomelanocortin messenger ribonucleic acid by androgens and gonadotropins. Endocrinology 119:2082–2088

Mishina M, Kurosaki T, Yamamoto T, Notake M, Masu M, Numa S (1982) DNA sequences required for transcription in vivo of the human corticotropin-beta-lipotropin precursor gene. EMBO J 1:1533–1538

Mocchetti A, Ritter A, Costa E (1989) Down-regulation of proopiomelanocortin synthesis and beta-endorphin utilization in hypothalamus of morphine-tolerant rats. J Mol Neurosci 1:33–38

Mocchetti I, Giorgi O, Schwartz JP, Costa E (1984) A reduction of the tone of 5-hydroxytryptamine neurons decreases utilization rates of striatal and hypothalamic enkephalins. Eur J Pharmacol 106:427–430

Mocchetti I, Guidotti A, Schwartz JP, Costa E (1985) Reserpine changes the dynamic state of enkephalin stores in rat striatum and adrenal medulla by different mechanisms. J Neurosci 5:3379–3385

Mocchetti I, Naranjo JR, Costa E (1987) Regulation of striatal enkephalin turnover in rats receiving antagonists of specific dopamine receptor subtypes. J Pharmacol Exp Ther 241:1120–1124

Moneta ME, Höllt V (1990) Perforant path kindling induces differential alterations in the mRNA levels coding for prodynorphin and proenkephalin in the rat hippocampus. Neurosci Lett 110:273–278

Monstein HJ, Geijer T (1988) A highly sensitive Northern blot assay detects multiple proenkephalin A-like mRNAs in human caudate nucleus and pheochromocytoma. Biosci Rep 8:255–261

Monstein HJ, Folkesson R, Terenius L (1986) Proenkephalin A-like mRNA in human leukemia leukocytes and CNS-tissues. Life Sci 39:2237–2241

Morris B, Herz A, Höllt V (1989) Location of striatal opioid gene expression, and its modulation by the mesostriatal dopamine pathway: an in situ hybridization study. J Mol Neurosci 1:9–18

Morris BJ, Haarmann I, Kempter B, Höllt V, Herz A (1986) Localization of prodynorphin messenger RNA in rat brain by in situ hybridization using a synthetic oligonucleotide probe. Neurosci Lett 69:104–108

Morris BJ, Moneta ME, ten-Bruggencate G, Höllt V (1987) Levels of prodynorphin mRNA in rat dentate gyrus are decreased during hippocampal kindling. Neurosci Lett 80:298–302

Morris BJ, Feasey KJ, ten-Bruggencate G, Herz A, Höllt V (1988a) Electrical stimulation in vivo increases the expression of proenkephalin mRNA and decreases the expression of prodynorphin mRNA in rat hippocampal granule cells. Proc Natl Acad Sci USA 85:3226–3230

Morris BJ, Reimer S, Höllt V, Herz A (1988b) Regulation of striatal prodynorphin mRNA levels by the raphe-striatal pathway. Brain Res 464:15–22

Morris BJ, Höllt V, Herz A (1988c) Opioid gene expression in rat striatum is modulated via opioid receptors: evidence from localized receptor inactivation. Neurosci Lett 89:80–84

Morris BJ, Höllt V, Herz A (1988d) Dopaminergic regulation of striatal proenkephalin mRNA and prodynorphin mR. Neuroscience 25:525–532

Nakai Y, Usui T, Tsukuda T, Takahashi H, Fukata U, Fukushima M, Senoo K, Imura H (1991) Molecular mechanisms of glucocorticoid inhibition of human proopiomelanocortin gene transcription. J Steroid Biochem Molec Biol 40: 301–306

Nakamura M, Nakanishi S, Sueoka S, Imura H, Numa S (1978) Effects of steroid hormones on the level of corticotropin messenger RNA activity in cultured mouse-pituitary-tumor cells. Eur J Biochem 86:61–66

Nakanishi S, Inoue A, Kita T, Nakamura M, Chang AC, Cohen SN, Numa S (1979) Nucleotide sequence of cloned cDNA for bovine corticotropin-beta-lipotropin precursor. Nature 278:423–427

Nakanishi S, Teranishi Y, Watanabe Y, Notake M, Noda M, Kakidani H, Jingami H, Numa S (1981) Isolation and characterization of the bovine corticotropin/beta-lipotropin precursor gene. Eur J Biochem 115:429–438

Naranjo JR, Iadarola MJ, Costa E (1986a) Changes in the dynamic state of brain proenkephalin-derived peptides during amygdaloid kindling. J Neurosci Res 16:75–87

Naranjo JR, Mocchetti I, Schwartz JP, Costa E (1986b) Permissive effect of dexamethasone on the increase of proenkephalin mRNA induced by depolarization of chromaffin cells. Proc Natl Acad Sci USA 83:1513–1517

Naranjo JR, Wise BC, Mellstrom B, Costa E (1988) Negative feedback regulation of the content of proenkephalin mRNA in chromaffin cell cultures. Neuropharmacology 27:337–343

Naranjo JR, Mellström B, Achaval M, Sassone-Corsi P (1991) Molecular pathways of pain: fos/jun-mediated activation of a noncanonical AP-1 site in the prodynorphin gene. Neuron 6:606–617

Nishimori T, Moskowitz MA, Uhl GR (1988) Opioid peptide gene expression in rat trigeminal nucleus caudalis neurons: normal distribution and effects of trigeminal deafferentation. J Comp Neurol 274:142–150

Nishimori T, Buzzi MG, Moskowitz MA, Uhl GR (1989) Proenkephalin mRNA expression in nucleus caudalis neurons is enhanced by trigeminal stimulation. Mol Brain Res 6:203–210

Noble EP, Bommer M, Sincini E, Costa T, Herz A (1986) Hl-histaminergic activation stimulates inositol-1-phosphate accumulation in chromaffin cells. Biochem Biophys Res Commun 135:566–573

Noda M, Teranishi Y, Takahashi H, Toyosato M, Notake M, Nakanishi S, Numa S (1982) Isolation and structural organization of the human preproenkephalin gene. Nature 297:431–434

Noguchi K, Kowalski K, Traub R, Solodkin A, Iadarola MJ, Ruda MA (1991) Dynorphin expression and fos-like immunoreactivity following inflammation-induced hyperalgesia are colocalized in spinal cord neurones. Mol Brain Res 10:227–233

Normand E, Popovici T, Onteniente B, Fellmann D, Piatier-Tonneau D, Auffray C, Bloch B (1988) Dopaminergic neurons of the substantia nigra modulate preproenkephalin A gene expression in rat striatal neurons. Brain Res 439: 39–46

Notake M, Tobimatsu T, Watanabe Y, Takahashi H, Mishina M, Numa S (1983a) Isolation and characterization of the mouse corticotropin-beta-lipotropin precursor gene and a related pseudogene. FEBS Lett 156:67–71

Notake M, Kurosaki T, Yamamoto T, Handa H, Mishina M, Numa S (1983b) Sequence requirement for transcription in vitro of the human corticotropin/beta-lipotropin precursor gene. Eur J Biochem 133:599–605

Oates E, Herbert E (1984) 5' sequence of porcine and rat pro-opiomelanocortin mRNA. One porcine and two rat forms. J Biol Chem 259:7421–7425

Pintar JE, Schachter BS, Herman AB, Durgerian S, Krieger DT (1984) Characterization and localization of proopiomelanocortin messenger RNA in the adult rat testis. Science 225:632–634

Pittius CW, Kley N, Loeffler JP, Höllt V (1985) Quantitation of proenkephalin A messenger RNA in bovine brain, pituitary and adrenal medulla: correlation between mRNA and peptide levels. EMBO J 4:1257–1260

Pittius CW, Kley N, Loeffler JP, Höllt V (1987) Proenkephalin B messenger RNA in porcine tissues: characterization, quantification, and correlation with opioid peptides. J Neurochem 48:586–592

Pollack AE, Wooten GF (1992) Differential regulation of striatal preproenkephalin mRNA by D1 and D2 receptors. Mol Brain Res 12:111–119

Pritchett DB, Roberts JL (1987) Dopamine regulates expression of the glandular-type kallikrein gene at the transcriptional level in the pituitary. Proc Natl Acad Sci USA 84:5545–5549

Pruss RM, Stauderman KA (1988) Voltage-regulated calcium channels involved in the regulation of enkephalin synthesis are blocked by phorbol ester treatment. J Biol Chem 263:13173–13178

Przewlocki R, Haarmann I, Nikolarakis K, Herz A, Höllt V (1988) Prodynorphin gene expression in spinal cord is enhanced after traumatic injury in the rat. Brain Res 464:37–41

Quach TT, Tang F, Kageyama H, Mocchetti I, Guidotti A, Meek JL, Costa E, Schwartz JP (1984) Enkephalin biosynthesis in adrenal medulla. Modulation of proenkephalin mRNA content of cultured chromaffin cells by 8-bromoadenosine 3',5'-monophosphate. Mol Pharmacol 26:255–260

Rattner A, Korner M, Rosen H, Baenerle PA, Citri Y (1991) Nuclear factor KB activates proenkephalin transcription in T-lymphocytes. Mol Cell Biol 11: 1017–1022

Reimer S, Höllt V (1990a) Gabaergic regulation of striatal opioid gene expression. Mol Brain Res 10:49–54

Reimer S, Höllt V (1990b) Morphine increases proenkephalin gene expression in the adrenal medulla by a central mechanism. In: Quirion R, Jhamandas K, Giounalakis C (eds) The international narcotics research conference (IRNC) '89 Liss, New York, pp 215–218

Reimer S, Sirinathsinghji DJS, Nikolorakis KE, Höllt V (1992) Differential dopaminergic regulation of proenkephalin and prodynorphin mRNAs in the basal ganglia of rats. Mol Brain Res 12:259–266

Reisine T, Rougon G, Barbet J (1986) Liposome delivery of cAMP-dependent protein kinase inhibitor into intact cells: specific blockade of cAMP-mediated adrenocorticotropin release from mouse anterior pituitary cells. J Cell Biol 102:1630–1637

Riegel AT, Lu Y, Remenick J, Wolford RG, Berard DS, Hager GL (1991) Proopiomelanocortin gene promoter elements required for constitutive and glucocorticoid-repressed transcription. Mol Endocrinol 5:1973–1982

Roberts JL, Seeburg PH, Shine J, Herbert E, Baxter JD, Goodman HM (1979) Corticotropin and beta-endorphin: construction and analysis of recombinant DNA complementary to mRNA for the common precursor. Proc Natl Acad Sci USA 76:2153–2157

Roberts JL, Lundblad JR, Eberwine JH, Fremeau RT, Salton SR, Blum M (1987) Hormonal regulation of POMC gene expression in pituitary. Ann NY Acad Sci 512:275–285

Romano GJ, Shivers BD, Harlan RE, Howells RD, Pfaff DW (1987) Haloperidol increases proenkephalin mRNA levels in the caudate-putamen of the rat: a quantitative study at the cellular level using in situ hybridization. Brain Res 388:33–41

Romano GJ, Mobbs CV, Howells RD, Pfaff DW (1989) Estrogen regulation of proenkephalin gene expression in the ventromedial hypothalamus of the rat: temporal qualities and synergism with progesterone. Brain Res Mol Brain Res 5:51–58

Rosen H, Douglass J, Herbert E (1984) Isolation and characterization of the rat proenkephalin gene. J Biol Chem 259:14309–14313

Rosen H, Behar O, Abramsky O, Ovadia H (1989) Regulated expression of proenkephalin A in normal lymphocytes. J Immunol 143:3703–3707

Ruda MA, Iadarola MJ, Cohen LV, Young WS (1988) In situ hybridization histochemistry and immunocytochemistry reveal an increase in spinal dynorphin biosynthesis in a rat model of peripheral inflammation and hyperalgesia. Proc Natl Acad Sci USA 85:622–626

Schachter BS, Johnson LK, Baxter JD, Roberts JL (1982) Differential regulation by glucocorticoids of proopiomelanocortin mRNA levels in the anterior and intermediate lobes of the rat pituitary. Endocrinology 110:1442–1444

Schäfer MK-H, Day R, Herman JP, Kwasiborski V, Sladek CD, Akil H, Watson SJ (1989) Effects of electroconvulsive shock on dynorphin in the hypothalamic-neurohypophysial system of the rat. Adv Biosci 75:599–602

Schäfer MK-H, Day R, Akil H, Watson SJ (1990) Identification of prodynorphin and proenkephalin cells in the neurointermediate lobe of the rat pituitary gland. In: Quirion R, Jhamadas K, Giounalakis C (eds) The international narcotics research conference (IRNC) '89. Liss, New York, pp 231–234

Schwartz JP (1988) Chronic exposure to opiate agonists increases proenkephalin biosynthesis in NG108 cells. Brain Res 427:141–146

Schwartz JP, Simantov R (1988) Developmental expression of proenkephalin mRNA in rat striatum and in striatal cultures. Brain Res 468:311–314

Seger MA, van-Eekelen JA, Kiss JZ, Burbach JP, de-Kloet ER (1988) Stimulation of pro-opiomelanocortin gene expression by glucocorticoids in the denervated rat intermediate pituitary gland. Neuroendocrinology 47:350–357

Seizinger BR, Bovermann K, Höllt V, Herz A (1984a) Enhanced activity of the beta-endorphinergic system in the anterior and neurointermediate lobe of the rat pituitary after chronic treatment with ethanol liquid diet. J Pharmacol Exp Ther 230:455–461

Seizinger BR, Höllt V, Herz A (1984b) Effects of chronic ethanol treatment on the in vitro biosynthesis of pro-opiomelanocortin and its posttranslational processing to beta-endorphin in the intermediate lobe of the rat pituitary. J Neurochem 43:607–613

Sherman TG, Civelli O, Douglass J, Herbert E, Burke S, Watson SJ (1986) Hypothalamic dynorphin and vasopressin mRNA expression in normal and Brattleboro rats. Fed Proc 45:2323–2327

Shiomi H, Watson SJ, Kelsey JE, Akil H (1986) Pretranslational and post-translational mechanisms for regulating beta-endorphin-adrenocorticotropin of the anterior pituitary lobe. Endocrinology 119:1793–1799

Siegel RE, Eiden LE, Affolter HU (1985) Elevated potassium stimulates enkephalin biosynthesis in bovine chromaffin cells. Neuropeptides 6:543–552

Simantov R, Höllt V (1990) Regulation of proenkephalin A gene expression in aggregating fetal rat brain cells. Cell Mol Neurobiol 11:245–251

Simard J, Labrie F, Gossard F (1986) Regulation of growth hormone mRNA and pro-opiomelanocortin mRNA levels by cyclic AMP in rat anterior pituitary cells in culture. DNA 5:263–270

Sivam SP, Hong JS (1986) GABAergic regulation of enkephalin in rat striatum: alterations in Met5-enkephalin level, precursor content and preproenkephalin messenger RNA abundance. J Pharmacol Exp Ther 237:326–331

Sivam SP, Breese GR, Napier TC, Mueller RA, Hong JS (1986a) Dopaminergic regulation of proenkephalin-A gene expression in the basal ganglia. Natl Inst Drug Abuse Res Monogr Ser 75:389–392

Sivam SP, Strunk C, Smith DR, Hong JS (1986b) Proenkephalin-A gene regulation in the rat striatum: influence of lithium and haloperidol. Mol Pharmacol 30: 186–191

Sivam SP, Takeuchi K, Li S, Douglass J, Civelli O, Calvetta L, Herbert E, McGinty JF, Hong JS (1988) Lithium increases dynorphin A(1–8) and prodynorphin mRNA levels in the basal ganglia of rats. Brain Res 427:155–163

Sonnenberg JL, Rauscher FJ, Morgan JI, Curran T (1989) Regulation of proenkephalin by Fos and Jun. Science 246:1622–1625

Spampinato S, Bachetti T, Canossa M, Ferri S (1990) Prodynorphin messenger RNA expression in the rat anterior pituitary is regulated by estrogen. In: Quirion R, Jhamandas K, Giounalakis C (eds). Liss, New York, pp 211–214

Springhorn JP, Claycomb WC (1989) Preproenkephalin mRNA expression in developing rat heart and in cultured ventricular cardiac muscle cells. Biochem J 258:73–78

Stachowiak MK, Lee PH, Rigual RJ, Viveros OH, Hong JS (1988) Roles of the pituitary-adrenocortical axis in control of the native and cryptic enkephalin levels and proenkephalin mRNA in the sympathoadrenal system of the rat. Brain Res 427:263–273

Stalla GK, Stalla J, Huber M, Loeffler JP, Höllt V, von-Werder K, Müller OA (1988) Ketoconazole inhibits corticotropic cell function in vitro. Endocrinology 122:618–623

Stalla GK, Stalla J, von-Werder K, Müller OA, Gerzer R, Höllt V, Jakobs KH (1989a) Nitroimidaxzole derivatives inhibit anterior pituitary cell function apparently by a direct effect on the catalytic subunit of the adenylate cyclase holoenzyme. Endocrinology 125:699–706

Stalla GK, Stalla J, Mojto J, Oeckler R, Buchfelder M, Müller OA (1989b) Regulation of corticotrophic adenoma cells in vitro. Acta Endocrinol (Copenh) 120 [Suppl 1]:209–209

Suda T, Tozawa F, Yamada M, Ushiyama T, Tomori N, Sumitomo T, Nakagami Y, Demura H, Shizume K (1988a) Effects of corticotropin-releasing hormone and dexamethasone on proopiomelanocortin messenger RNA level in human corticotroph adenoma cells in vitro. J Clin Invest 82:110–114

Suda T, Tozawa F, Yamada M, Ushiyama T, Tomori N, Sumitomo T, Nakagami Y, Shizume K (1988b) In vitro study on proopiomelanocortin messenger RNA levels in cultured rat anterior pituitary cells. Life Sci 42:1147–1152

Suda T, Tozawa F, Ushiyama T, Tomori N, Sumitomo T, Nakagami Y, Yamada M, Demura H, Shizume K (1989) Effects of protein kinase-C-related adrenocorticotropin secretagogues and interleukin-1 on proopiomelanocortin gene expression in rat anterior pituitary cells. Endocrinology 124:1444–1449

Suda T, Tozawa F, Ushiyama T, Sumitomo T, Yamada M, Demura H (1990) Interleukin-1 stimulates corticotropin-releasing factor gene expression in rat hypothalamus. Endocrinology 126:1223–1228

Takahashi H, Hakamata Y, Watanabe Y, Kikuno R, Miyata T, Numa S (1983) Complete nucleotide sequence of the human corticotropin-beta-lipotropin precursor gene. Nucleic Acids Res 11:6847–6858

Tang F, Costa E, Schwartz JP (1983) Increase of proenkephalin mRNA and enkephalin content of rat striatum after daily injection of haloperidol for 2 to 3 weeks. Proc Natl Acad Sci USA 80:3841–3844

Tempel A (1990) Morphine-induced downregulation of mu opioid receptors and peptide synthesis in neonatal rat brain. In: Van Ree J, Mulder AH, Wiegant VM, van Wimersma Greidanus TB (eds) New leads in opioid research. Elseveier, Amsterdam, pp 99–101

Terao M, Watanabe Y, Mishina M, Numa S (1983) Sequence requirement for transcription in vivo of the human preproenkephalin A gene. EMBO J 2: 2223–2228

Therrien M, Drouin J (1991) Pituitary proopiomelanocortin gene expression requires synergistic interaction of several regulatory elements.Mol Cell Biol 11:3492–3503

Thiele EA, Eipper BA (1990) Effect of secretagogues on components of the secretory system in AtT-20 cells. Endocrinology 126:809–817

Tomiko SA, Taraskevich PS, Douglas WW (1983) GABA acts directly on cells of pituitary pars intermedia to alter hormone output. Nature 301:706–707

Tozawa F, Suda T, Yamada M, Ushiyama T, Tomori N, Sumitomo T, Nakagami Y, Demura H, Shizume K (1988) Insulin-induced hypoglycemia increases proopiomelanocortin messenger ribonucleic acid levels in rat anterior pituitary gland. Endocrinology 122:1231–1235

Tremblay Y, Tretjakoff I, Peterson A, Antakly T, Zhang CX, Drouin J (1988) Pituitary-specific expression and glucocorticoid regulation of a proopiomelanocortin fusion gene in transgenic mice. Proc Natl Acad Sci USA 85:8890–8894

Uhl GR, Ryan JP, Schwartz JP (1988) Morphine alters preproenkephalin gene expression. Brain Res 459:391–397

Uhler M, Herbert E, D'Eustachio P, Ruddle FD (1983) The mouse genome contains two nonallelic pro-opiomelanocortin genes. J Biol Chem 258:9444–9453

Vernier P, Julien JF, Rataboul P, Fourrier O, Feuerstein C, Mallet J (1988) Similar time course changes in striatal levels of glutamic acid decarboxylase and proenkephalin mRNA following dopaminergic deafferentation in the rat. J Neurochem 51:1375–1380

Vilijn MH, Vaysse PJ, Zukin RS, Kessler JA (1988) Expression of preproenkephalin mRNA by cultured astrocytes and neurons. Proc Natl Acad Sci USA 85: 6551–6555

Von Dreden G, Höllt V (1988) Vasopressin potentiates β-endorphin release but not the increase in the mRNA for proopiomelanocortin induced by corticotropin releasing factor in rat pituitary cells. Acta Endocrinol (Copenh) 117 [Suppl 287]:124–124

Von Dreden G, Loeffler JP, Grimm C, Höllt V (1988) Influence of calcium ions on proopiomelanocortin mRNA levels in clonal anterior pituitary cells. Neuroendocrinology 47:32–37

Vyas S, Bishop JF, Gehlert DR, Patel J (1990) Effects of protein kinase C downregulation on secretory events and proopiomelanocortin gene expression in anterior pituitary tumor (AtT-20) cells. J Neurochem 54:248–255

Wan DC, Livett BG (1989) Induction of phenylethanolamine N-methyltransferase mRNA expression by glucocorticoids in cultured bovine adrenal chromaffin cells. Eur J Pharmacol 172:107–115

Wan DC, Scanlon D, Choi CL, Bunn SJ, Howe PR, Livett BG (1989a) Colocalization of RNAs coding for phenylethanolamine N-methyltransferase and proenkephalin A in bovine and ovine adrenals. J Auton Nerv Syst 26:231–240

Wan DC, Marley PD, Livett BG (1989b) Histamine activates proenkephalin A mRNA but not phenylethanolamine N-methyltransferase mRNA expression in cultured bovine adrenal chromaffin cells. Eur J Pharmacol 172:117–129

Wand GS (1990) Differential regulation of anterior pituitary corticotrope function is observed in vivo but not in vitro in two lines of ethanol-sensitive mice. Alcoholism 14:100–106

Wand JA, Eiden LE (1988) Calcium requirements for barium stimulation of enkephalin and vasoactive intestinal peptide biosynthesis in adrenomedullary chromaffin cells. Neuropeptides 11:39–45

Waschek JA, Dave JR, Eskay RL, Eiden LE (1987) Barium distinguishes separate calcium targets for synthesis and secretion of peptides in neuroendocrine cells. Biochem Biophys Res Commun 146:495–501

Weihe E, Millan MJ, Höllt V, Nohr D, Herz A (1989) Induction of the gene encoding pro-dynorphin by experimentally induced arthritis enhances staining for dynorphin in the spinal cord of rats. Neuroscience 31:77–95

White JD, Gall CM, McKelvy JF (1987) Enkephalin biosynthesis and enkephalin gene expression are increased in hippocampal mossy fibers following a unilateral lesion of the hilus. J Neurosci 7:753–759

Wiemann JN, Clifton DK, Steiner RA (1989) Pubertal changes in gonadotropin-releasing hormone and proopiomelanocortin gene expression in the brain of the male rat. Endocrinology 124:1760–1767

Wilcox JN, Roberts JL (1985) Estrogen decreases rat hypothalamic proopiomelanocortin messenger ribonucleic acid levels. Endocrinology 117:2392–2396

Xie CW, Lee PH, Takeuchi K, Owyang V, Li SJ, Douglass J, Hong JS (1989) Single or repeated electroconvulsive shocks alter the levels of prodynorphin and proenkephalin mRNAs in rat brain. Brain Res Mol Brain Res 6:11–19

Xie C-W, McGinty JF, Lee PHK, Mitchell CL, Hong J-S (1991) A glutamate antagonist blocks perforant stimulation-induced reduction of dynorphin peptide and prodynorphin mRNA levels in rat hippocampus. Brain Res 562:243–250

Yoshikawa K, Sabol SL (1986) Expression of the enkephalin precursor gene in C6 rat glioma cells: regulation by beta-adrenergic agonists and glucocorticoids. Brain Res 387:75–83

Yoshikawa K, Hong JS, Sabol SL (1985) Electroconvulsive shock increases preproenkephalin messenger RNA abundance in rat hypothalamus. Proc Natl Acad Sci USA 82:589–593

Yoshikawa K, Maruyama M, Aizawa T, Yamamoto A (1989a) A new species of enkephalin precursor mRNA with a distinct 5′-untranslated region in haploid germ cells. FEBS Lett 246:193–196

Yoshikawa K, Aizawa T, Nozawa A (1989b) Phorbol ester regulates the abundance of enkephalin precursor mRNA but not of amyloid beta-protein precursor mRNA in rat testicular peritubular cells. Biochem Biophys Res Commun 161:568–575

Young WS, Bonner TI, Brann MR (1986) Mesencephalic dopamine neurons regulate the expression of neuropeptide mRNAs in the rat forebrain. Proc Natl Acad Sci USA 83:9827–9831

Zheng M, Yang SG, Zou G (1988) Electro-acupuncture markedly increases proenkephalin mRNA in rat striatum and pituitary. Sci sin [B] 31:81–86

Zurawski G, Benedik M, Kamb BJ, Abrams JS, Zurawski SM, Lee FD (1986) Activation of mouse T-helper cells induces abundant preproenkephalin mRNA synthesis. Science 232:772–775

CHAPTER 15
Regulation of Pituitary Proopiomelanocortin Gene Expression

J.L. Roberts, N. Levin, D. Lorang, J.R. Lundblad, S. Dermer, and M. Blum

A. Introduction

The proopiomelanocortin (POMC) gene encodes the complex precursor to a variety of biologically active, important neuroendocrine peptides. It is expressed in a variety of tissues in the mammal, but its main site of expression is the pituitary anterior lobe corticotroph and, in some species, the intermediate lobe melanotroph. The POMC molecule is posttranslationally processed to different biologically active peptides in these two cell types, with adrenocorticotropic hormone (ACTH), β-lipotrophic hormone (β-LPH), and β-endorphin being major products in the corticotroph and α-melanocyte-stimulating hormone (α-MSH), corticotropin-like intermediate lobe peptide (CLIP), and acetyl-β-endorphin in the melanotroph (Eipper and Mains 1980). This array of different biological activities derived from the POMC molecule possibly necessitates the complex regulation of POMC peptide secretion and POMC gene expression observed in the pituitary. Regulation of POMC peptide secretion has recently been reviewed in several places (Antoni 1986; Jones and Gillham 1988). This review will deal primarily with the regulation of POMC gene expression in rat and mouse pituitary tissues, the species in which the majority of the work has been done although examples of other mammalian systems will be used where appropriate (see also Chaps. 14 and 26).

I. The POMC Gene

Initially it was determined if there were multiple copies of the POMC gene in the genome which could explain the complexity of regulation in different expressing tissues. Possibly there were multiple genes, each with its own characteristic regulatory and tissue-specific expression pattern, or a single copy of the POMC gene capable of responding to many hormones. Genomic DNA fragments containing POMC-encoding sequences have been isolated and sequenced from several mammalian species including human (Takahashi et al. 1983), rat (Drouin and Goodman 1980; Drouin et al. 1985), cow (Nakanishi et al. 1981), and mouse (Uhler et al. 1983; Notake et al. 1983), and only one functional gene has been identified per haploid genome. The mouse contains a processed pseudogene, possibly a product of a reverse transposition event, that does not produce a functional mRNA, but possesses approximately 92% nucleotide sequence similarity to a portion of the coding region of its functional counterpart (UHLER et al. 1983; NOTAKE et al. 1983).

The overall arrangement of the introns and exons in the POMC gene is virtually identical between all mammalian species, with three exons separated by two relatively large introns. The first exon is approximately 100 nucleotides in length and comprises most of the 5' untranslated portion of the pituitary POMC mRNA. The second exon of about 150 nucleotides contains a small portion of 5' untranslated sequence and begins the protein-coding portion of the mRNA, including the signal peptide and a portion of the NH$_2$-terminal peptide. Exon 3 encodes all the peptides with known biological activity, including ACTH, β-endorphin, and the melanotropins. The introns are large compared to the exons, approximately 3.5–4 kb (kilobases) for the first intron and about 2–3 kb for the second intron.

Proopiomelanocortin-like mRNAs have been detected in a number of nonpituitary tissues, including the hypothalamus and other portions of the brain (amygdala, cerebral cortex, midbrain, cerebellum) (CIVELLI et al. 1982), adrenal medulla (CIVELLI et al. 1982), spleen and lung macrophages (LOLAIT et al. 1986; MECHANICK et al., to be published), and ovary, testes, and placenta (PINTAR et al. 1984; LACAZE-MASMONTEIL et al. 1987). The POMC mRNAs of the reproductive tissues and the adrenal medulla are smaller (about 850 and 1000 bases respectively), whereas the POMC mRNA detected in the hypothalamus and in spleen and lung macrophages is approximately the same size as the pituitary mRNA (approximately 1100 bases). Since only one POMC gene is present in the haploid genome, these different-sized mRNAs are either the product of differences in post-transcriptional processing of the POMC primary gene transcript or the product of transcription from alternative promoters within the POMC gene locus. Recently LACAZE-MASMONTEIL and coworkers (1987) showed by nuclease protection and primer extension that the shorter transcripts produced in human testes lack 5' coding sequences and thus may be the products of transcripts initiated from the 3' end of the second intron rather than alternative processing of RNA transcripts initiated from the pituitary promoter. They postulate that low levels of transcripts initiated at the pituitary promoter region may be the source of small amounts of POMC-derived peptides found in this tissue.

Alternative RNA splicing has, however, been demonstrated between exon 1 and exon 2 in the rat pituitary (OATES and HERBERT 1984) and in human pituitary (LACAZE-MASMONTEIL et al. 1987). Two forms of POMC mRNA are present in approximately the same ratios in anterior and intermediate lobes of the rat pituitary, a result of the use of two different splice acceptor sites, adding an additional 30 nucleotides within the 5' untranslated portion of the mRNA. The two mRNAs produced by this splice difference are not different in the protein-coding portion of the mRNA; however, it is not known whether there are functional differences between these two forms of POMC mRNA.

II. Intracellular Processes Regulating POMC Secretion

Only recently have the molecular mechanisms by which events at the cell surface are transduced to transcriptional signals in the nucleus become clearly delineated. The events occurring shortly after binding of a ligand to its cell surface receptor have received a great deal of attention in the past decade and the subject of second messenger generation and its relationship to POMC peptide release has received particular attention due to the existence of AtT20 cells, a clonal mouse anterior pituitary corticotroph tumor cell line. AtT20 cells have been exploited by a number of laboratories in correlation with perifusion culture systems and dispersed primary cultures of anterior and neurointermediate pituitary cells in the study of the receptors and cellular processes mediating the secretory response of POMC-producing cells (reviewed in AXELROD and REISINE 1984). Figure 1 schematically summarizes many of the processes involved in the secretory response, and subsequent gene regulation. The usefulness of the AtT20 cell

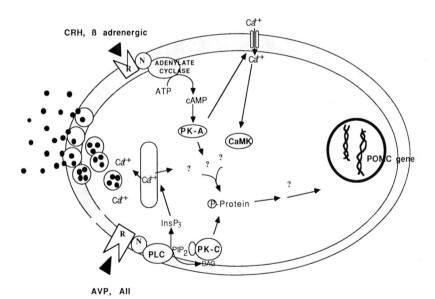

Fig. 1. Overview of corticotroph function. Schematic model of the anterior pituitary corticotroph indicating different plasma membrane G-protein (*N*) coupled receptors (*R*) and the intracellular second messenger systems implicated in mediating the actions of the various neurohormones as detailed in the text. *CRH*, corticotropin-releasing hormone; *AVP*, arginine vasopressin; *AII*, angiotensin II; *PKA*, protein kinase A; *PKC*, protein kinase C; *CaMK*, calmodulin-dependent protein kinase; *PLC*, phorpholipase C

line as a substrate for gene transfer studies and biochemical characterization of factors involved in tissue-specific and hormonal regulation of POMC gene transcription will be discussed below.

The major regulator of corticotroph POMC peptide secretion, hypothalamic corticotropin-releasing hormone (CRH), acts through a cytoplasmic membrane receptor coupled through a stimulatory guanine nucleotide-binding protein to adenylate cyclase (AGUILERA et al. 1983; PERRIN et al. 1986). CRH stimulates POMC peptide release by increasing intracellular cAMP levels in corticotrophs (BILEZIKJIAN and VALE 1983; GLGUERE et al. 1982). Long-term treatment of anterior lobe cells in culture with CRH increases total content of ACTH relative to control cells, which is suggestive of increased synthesis of ACTH, along with increased secretion of POMC-derived peptides (VALE et al. 1983).

Corticotropin-releasing hormone activation of cAMP-dependent protein kinase (PKA) has also been demonstrated in AtT20 cells (MIYAZKI et al. 1984; LITVIN et al. 1984) and intermediate lobe cells in vitro (COTE et al. 1985). The requirement for PKA in mediating the effects of CRH has recently been directly demonstrated by REISINE and coworkers (1985) by incorporation of PKA inhibitor (PKI, the Walsh inhibitor) into AtT20 cells by liposome fusion. Cells which received the PKA inhibitor did not respond to CRH or β-adrenergic agonists by increased ACTH secretion. In addition, PKA inhibitor blocked increases in the mRNA for POMC in response to 8-bromo-cAMP and CRH, indicating a role for PKA in regulation of POMC gene expression. However, PKA inhibitor did not block the ability of another POMC secretagogue, the phorbol ester PMA (phorbol 12-myristate 13-acetate), to stimulate POMC mRNA accumulation or POMC peptide secretion, suggesting that protein kinase C can also independently activate these events.

Vasopressin, oxytocin, angiotensin II, the cholecystokinin C-terminal octapeptide (CCK-8), and α-adrenergic agonists comprise another class of neurohormones which act on the anterior pituitary corticotroph through phosphatidylinositol (PIP_2) turnover, resulting in mobilization of intra-cellular calcium stores and activation of protein kinase C (ABOU-SAMARA et al. 1986a; SCHOENENBERG et al. 1987; RAYMOND et al. 1985). These substances alone may not be potent secretagogues, but act to potentiate the CRH-stimulated secretion of POMC-derived peptides in vitro (VALE et al. 1983). In fact, both vasopressin and angiotensin II act to facilitate CRH-stimulated cAMP formation in vitro (SCHOENENBERG et al. 1987; ABOU-SAMARA et al. 1987). The potential mechanisms involved are discussed below.

In corticotrophs, a cell type responsive to a number of secretagogues, the interrelationships between these pathways are complex. For example, CRH and other agents that increase intracellular cAMP levels also elevate cytosolic calcium levels in AtT20 cells (GUILD et al. 1986; LUINI et al. 1985) in part through the activation of protein kinase A (GUILD and REISINE

1987). Somatostatin blocks the stimulatory effects of CRH and β-adrenergic agonists in AtT20 cells by preventing cAMP formation (HEISLER et al. 1982; REISINE 1985). Somatostatin can also block POMC peptide release in response to 8-bromo-cAMP, suggesting a mechanism beyond the inhibition of adenylate cyclase. Somatostatin has been shown to decrease cytosolic calcium concentrations and to inhibit voltage-dependent calcium current in AtT20 cells independent of its ability to block cAMP formation (LUINI et al. 1986; REISINE and GUILD 1985). These studies underscore the complexity of interplay between intracellular signaling pathways within corticotrophs.

Genomic actions of glucocorticoids through transcriptional activation have been extensively described (RINGOLD 1985). However, details of how glucocorticoids at the cellular level act to rapidly inhibit POMC peptide secretion and expression of the POMC gene in the corticotroph are obscure (reviewed in KELLER-WOOD and DALLMAN 1984). Modulation of cAMP production in response to neurotransmitters and neurohormones by glucocorticoids has been described both in vivo and in vitro (reviewed in McEWEN et al. 1986). For example, glucocorticoids rapidly inhibit prolactin release and cAMP formation in response to vasoactive intestinal polypeptide (VIP) in anterior pituitary cultures (ROTSZTEJN et al. 1981). Thus second messenger pathways are potential targets for rapid glucocorticoid inhibition of stimulated peptide secretion in the pituitary.

Experiments performed with anterior pituitaries examined the role of corticosterone on CRH-stimulated POMC peptide release and found that there was a rapid inhibition of ACTH release with a latency of approximately 10–20 min (BUCKINGHAM 1979; GILLES and LOWRY 1978). Subsequent studies in similar cultures examining the effect of dexamethasone (DEX), a synthetic glucocorticoid, on ACTH secretion and cAMP accumulation reported conflicting results as to whether glucocorticoids could block CRH-stimulated cAMP accumulation (BILEZKIJIAN and VALE 1983; GIGUERE et al. 1982). WIDMAIER and DALLMAN (1984) showed a rapid inhibition by glucocorticoids of CRH-stimulated secretion in in vitro perfused intact pituitary, again with a latency of 10–20 min. The mechanisms involved in this rapid inhibition by glucocorticoids may also be involved in the rapid inhibition of CRH-stimulated POMC gene transcription by DEX (EBERWINE et al. 1987) as discussed below.

B. Proopiomelanocortin mRNA Levels in Pituitary

The pituitary POMC system is a major component in the physiological response to stress and a wealth of information is available as to what hormones, neurotransmitters, and behavioral states modulate release of POMC-derived peptides from the anterior lobe corticotroph and intermediate lobe melanotroph. Hence much of the work to date on regulation of POMC gene expression has focused on the effects of stress hormones such as glucocorticoids, adrenergic compounds, or CRH on POMC mRNA levels. Some studies have been done in whole animals to mimic normal physiological influences while other studies have used cell culture systems to try to tease apart the complex cellular and molecular mechanisms regulating POMC gene expression.

I. Whole Animal Studies

1. Adrenalectomy

Initial studies on the regulation of POMC mRNA levels used cell-free translation followed by immunoprecipitation to indirectly quantitate POMC mRNA. Using such techniques, NAKANISHI and colleagues (1977) were the first to show that adrenalectomy, a procedure known to stimulate ACTH release, was also accompanied by a time-dependent three fold increase in the amount of POMC mRNA activity isolated from the whole pituitary gland. Furthermore, glucocorticoid treatment of adrenalectomized rats caused a decrease in the level of translatable POMC mRNA to levels found in intact animals levels after several days. Subsequent studies by several research groups using POMC cDNA probes and hybridization assays showed that the sensitivity of POMC mRNA levels to glucocorticoids was displayed almost exclusively in the anterior lobe of the pituitary gland (SCHACHTER et al. 1982; JINGAMI et al. 1985; BIRNBERG et al. 1983; HÖLLT and HAARMAN 1984; BRUHN et al. 1984). Two of these studies also reported minor, but significant, inhibitory effects of glucocorticoids on neuro-intermediate lobe POMC mRNA (SCHACHTER et al. 1982; JINGAMI et al. 1985).

Similar observations of adrenalectomy and DEX replacement on pituitary POMC mRNA levels have been observed by a totally different method of assessing mRNA, namely that of in situ hybridization histochemistry. While this method is not absolutely quantitative, measurement of silver grain density has been shown to be a good indicator of relative changes in mRNA levels as well as for the identification of heterogeneous responses within a given population of cells (KELSEY et al. 1986). Using this approach, GEE and ROBERTS (1983) using a POMC cDNA probe were able to show that adrenalectomy for 10 days caused a marked increase in silver grains over the anterior lobe corticotrophs and that DEX replacement at the time of adrenalectomy caused a marked decrease relative to the intact animals in the anterior lobe corticotrophs. There were no detectable changes in silver grains localized over the intermediate lobe melanotrophs with any of the treatments. In a more recent study, FREMEAU et al. (1986) made a similar observation about the effect of 2 weeks of adrenalectomy on levels of silver grains detected over the anterior lobe corticotrophs. They found that short-term DEX replacement for 30 min to 2 h had no effect on reducing silver grain density over the corticotrophs, in agreement with the observations described above that glucocorticoids require many hours to elicit their inhibitory effect on POMC mRNA levels.

The variable magnitude of effects on POMC mRNA levels with adrenalectomy or glucocorticoid replacement are difficult to reconcile between all these studies because of the different periods of treatment and different methods of steroid replacement (drinking water versus i.p. injection versus s.c. injection). The one clear finding is that glucocorticoids have major effects on POMC mRNA in the anterior lobe with minimal effects on the neurointermediate lobe. The small but significant effects of glucocorticoids on intermediate lobe POMC mRNA in some studies are more difficult to explain, primarily because the melanotrophs normally do not contain detectable levels of glucocorticoid receptor (WAREMBOURG 1975; REES et al. 1977; ANTAKLY and EISEN 1984). This suggests that the glucocorticoid effects observed on POMC mRNA levels are mediated through indirect mechanisms, possibly through GABA, dopamine, CRH, or other inputs to the intermediate lobe. In addition, AUTELITANO and colleagues (1987) showed that DEX stimulates intermediate lobe POMC mRNA levels twofold in haloperidol-treated rats. Thus, while glucocorticoids can modulate POMC mRNA levels in the intermediate lobe, the mechanisms involved appear to be quite different in the animal from those involved in regulation of anterior pituitary POMC mRNA.

2. Hypothalamic Factors

As discussed above, glucocorticoids may directly inhibit POMC gene expression at the level of the corticotroph as well as modulate hypothalamic input to the corticotroph. By lesioning the paraventricular nucleus, a major site of CRH neurons which project to the median eminence, BRUHN and colleagues (1984) showed a decrease in the levels of POMC mRNA in the anterior pituitary in adrenalectomized rats, arguing that CRH and other hypothalamic factors are responsible for the increase in pituitary POMC gene expression in adrenalectomy. DALLMAN and colleagues (1985) have also shown the importance of hypothalamic input in maintaining high levels of POMC gene expression, demonstrating that the hypothalamus is the primary site in vivo of negative regulation of POMC gene expression by corticosterone. Using Halasz knife lesions to destroy CRH and vasopressin input to the anterior pituitary, they showed that POMC mRNA levels were decreased relative to those of sham-lesioned rats. More importantly, adding back increasing levels of corticosterone to lesioned adrenalectomized rats had no significant effect on the level of anterior pituitary POMC mRNA. These studies suggest that the inhibitory effects of glucocorticoids on anterior pituitary POMC mRNA levels observed in the intact animal are mediated through some region at or above the level of the hypothalamus. However, cell culture studies described in the next section show glucocorticoids do have direct inhibitory effects on POMC mRNA levels and transcription in the absence of any other stimulation, suggesting multiple levels of steroid control.

Several groups have examined the effects of CRH administration on POMC mRNA levels, pharmacologically mimicking chronic hypothalamic input to the pituitary. BRUHN et al. (1984) showed that 2-week administration of CRH by intravenous infusion to intact rats caused a two- to threefold increase in the level of POMC mRNA in the anterior pituitary but not the intermediate pituitary. DEX given immediately prior to CRH infusion prevented the increase in POMC mRNA seen with CRH alone. Chronic CRH administration to intact animals by subcutaneous implantation of osmotic minipumps results in stimulation of the level of POMC mRNA expression in the anterior pituitary relative to that in non-CRH-treated animals (HÖLLT and HAARMAN 1984). However, the surprising observation was made that intermediate pituitary POMC mRNA levels in these chronically CRH-treated animals were decreased to about 30% those of control animals, contrary to the findings by BRUHN et al. (1984). We made similar surprising observations using a multiple injection scheme for chronic administration of CRH to rats (AUTELITANO et al. 1990; LUNDBLAD and ROBERTS 1988). These data suggest that a secondary inhibitory system becomes dominant after chronic CRH administration or that secretion: transcription coupling downregulates quickly in the melanotroph. In a more detailed study (AUTELITANO et al. 1990), we observed that elevated POMC transcription in the melanotroph was not maintained after 30 min post-CRH injection despite the observation that plasma MSH levels were still elevated, as reported previously (PROULX-FERLAND et al. 1982).

3. Intermediate Lobe POMC mRNA Levels

A major regulator of POMC peptide secretion from intermediate lobe is dopamine, which inhibits secretion through an inhibition of the adenylate cyclase system. Dopamine has also been shown to be inhibitory to POMC gene expression in this tissue. HÖLLT and colleagues (1982) found that treatment of male rats with haloperidol, a dopamine antagonist, caused a reversible time-dependent increase in translatable POMC mRNA levels which was maximal at twofold above the saline-injected controls after 3 weeks. CHEN et al. (1984) found that haloperidol elicited a time-dependent increase which required 6 h to be detected (twofold above control), and that elevations in hybridizable POMC mRNA continued for up to 7 days of hormone treatment to levels of 700% of the control value. PRITCHETT and ROBERTS (1987) showed similar results by Northern blot analysis after 3 days of treatment. In several studies, dopamine agonists such as 8-bromo-ergocriptine or CB 154 were shown to have two- to fourfold inhibitory effects on POMC mRNA levels in the melanotrophs (MILLINGTON et al. 1986b; CHEN et al. 1984; PRITCHETT and ROBERTS 1987). Using the in situ hybridization technique, CHRONWALL and colleagues (1987) reported that essentially all of the melanotrophs in the intermediate pituitary were stimulated by haloperidol treatment and inhibited by bromocriptine treatment, again in a time-dependent fashion. Thus these studies show that stimulation of melanotroph POMC peptide secretion by blocking the inhibitory effect of the endogenous dopamine with haloperidol, or further suppressing release of POMC peptide by using a dopamine agonist, cause parallel changes in POMC peptide mRNA. Essentially no changes in anterior lobe POMC mRNA levels were observed with either haloperidol or bromocriptine treatment given acutely (CHEN et al. 1984), while more recent studies have demonstrated small but significant increases (AUTELITANO et al. 1987) or decreases (MEADOR-WOODRUFF et al. 1990) in anterior lobe POMC mRNA levels induced by chronic haloperidol treatment.

Changes in intermediate pituitary POMC mRNA have also been measured as a function of the time of day following a diurnal rhythm. MILLINGTON et al. (1986a) showed that the POMC mRNA levels varied twofold, with the highest levels being at 0200 hours, paralleling the levels of plasma β-endorphin, plasma α-MSH, and intermediate lobe β-endorphin content. These observations showed that even subtle diurnal variations in POMC peptide release from the pituitary are associated with parallel changes in POMC mRNA levels.

As can be seen from these examples of POMC gene expression in whole animals, changes in POMC mRNA levels parallel alterations in POMC peptide release from either lobe. This coupling of mRNA levels with release appears to be a major mechanism by which the pituitary POMC cells maintain the proper level of POMC biosynthesis to meet secretory needs for these peptides. In order to delve further into the molecular mechanisms involved in this phenomenon, it is necessary to determine exactly which neurohormones or neurotransmitters directly mediate this response at the pituitary level. While whole animal experiments demonstrate how the system functions as a whole, cell culture studies are necessary to determine which substances are acting directly on the pituitary cell and which are acting indirectly through other systems.

II. In Vitro Systems

In general, the studies on POMC gene expression using primary cultures of separated anterior and intermediate pituitary cells substantiate the earlier observations made in the intact animal and begin to identify the mechanisms by which POMC gene expression is regulated at the cellular level. Although important intact pituitary cell-cell interactions are destroyed in these cultures, observed changes in POMC mRNA levels in response to hormone or drug treatment can almost certainly be attributed to a direct effect on the corticotroph or melanotroph. Indeed, it is because of the extreme complexity of the in vivo POMC regulatory systems that many research groups have turned to culture systems to elucidate the molecular and cellular processes involved in regulation of POMC gene expression.

1. Glucocorticoids

The treatment of primary anterior pituitary cultures or AtT20 cells with either natural or synthetic glucocorticoids causes a decrease in the level of POMC mRNA. Early studies in the AtT20 cells showed that the decrease in POMC mRNA activity was detectable after 10 h of DEX treatment with maximal inhibition at 30%–40% of nontreated cultures after 48 h (ROBERTS et al. 1979; NAKAMURA et al. 1978). This was shown to be through the type II glucocorticoid receptor, since there are no type I receptors in the AtT20 cells (GANNON et al. 1990). Similar findings were made in anterior pituitary primary cultures, wherein DEX caused a time-dependent decrease in POMC mRNA levels which required several hours to be manifested and was maximal 2.5-fold below untreated cultures after 36 h (EBERWINE et al. 1987). Thus, it appears that at least part of the effects of glucocorticoid treatment in vivo on anterior pituitary POMC mRNA could be mediated by direct effects on the corticotroph. The magnitude of the glucocorticoid effect in vitro is only about half that observed in vivo, suggesting that glucocorticoids may be having effects on other systems that affect POMC mRNA levels, such as their inhibitory effects on hypothalamic CRH gene expression (JINGAMI et al. 1985) or alternatively that in vitro systems have lost some glucocorticoid responsiveness. There have been no studies reporting glucocorticoid effects on POMC mRNA levels in cultured neuro-intermediate lobe cells, despite the fact that the glucocorticoid receptor is expressed in melanotrophs after long-term culture (ANTAKLY et al. 1985; ANTAKLY et al. 1987).

2. cAMP- and Calcium-Dependent Processes

In addition to its in vivo effects, CRH has been demonstrated to have direct stimulatory effects on POMC mRNA accumulation in both AtT20 cells (AFFOLTER and REISINE 1985; REISINE et al. 1985) and on anterior and intermediate pituitary cells in dispersed primary cell culture (LOEFFLER et al. 1985). CRH-stimulated POMC mRNA levels two- to threefold in AtT20 cells in culture, an effect which is mimicked by the addition of 8-bromo-cAMP and phorbol ester (AFFOLTER and REISINE 1985). Maximal levels of POMC mRNA were observed after 8 h of continuous exposure to CRH, but were still elevated after 24 h of treatment. The effects on POMC mRNA of CRH and other agents that increased cAMP production (forskolin, isoproterenol, 8-bromo-cAMP), but not phorbol ester, could be blocked by fusion of AtT20 cells with liposomes containing protein kinase A inhibitor (PKI), demonstrating that the increase in POMC mRNA by cAMP analogues and CRH was due to direct activation of protein kinase A (REISINE et al. 1985). Thus protein kinase A activation is required for both stimulation of POMC mRNA production and peptide secretion in these cells in response to CRH or β-adrenergic activation, suggesting that protein kinase C activation increases POMC mRNA through its subsequent actions independent of protein kinase A activation.

LOEFFLER and coworkers (1985) showed that primary cultures of both rat anterior and intermediate pituitary respond to CRH to increase POMC mRNA. However, in this culture system (serum-free media) POMC mRNA showed an increase over 48 h of continuous CRH exposure in both anterior and intermediate lobe cells, to a final level of more than twofold the POMC mRNA content for control cultures. This time course differs from that of the accumulation of POMC mRNA in AtT20 cells (AFFOLTER and REISINE 1985) in response to CRH. Forskolin also stimulated POMC mRNA accumulation in both anterior and intermediate lobe cultures (LOEFFLER et al. 1985), again suggesting a common role for cAMP in regulating expression of the POMC gene in both pituitary cell types in culture. The cAMP analogue 8-bromo-cAMP increased POMC mRNA in primary cultures of anterior lobe cells (MAY et al. 1989; LOEFFLER et al. 1986) as well as in intermediate lobe cells (LOEFFLER et al. 1986) in further support of these findings.

Basal levels of POMC gene expression in vitro may be governed by cAMP-dependent processes. Treatment of anterior and intermediate lobe primary cultures with phosphodiesterase inhibitor elevated POMC mRNA levels (SIMARD et al. 1986; LOEFFLER et al. 1986). In addition, basal levels of POMC mRNA were reduced in AtT20 cells fused with liposomes containing PKI (REISINE et al. 1985). COTE and coworkers (1986) showed that bromocriptine (CB154), a dopaminergic agonist, decreased intermediate lobe POMC mRNA to half of control levels. Addition of CB154 and forskolin simultaneously still elevated POMC mRNA, but not to the same extent as forskolin alone. Cholera toxin also stimulated accumulation of POMC mRNA in both anterior and intermediate lobe cells (LOEFFLER et al. 1986). These results, along with the findings that pertussis toxin blocks the inhibition by dopamine agonists of the biosynthesis of POMC peptides in intermediate lobe cells, suggest that dopamine and CRH oppositely regulate POMC mRNA in the melanotroph via actions mediated through G proteins on basal adenylate cyclase activity.

The role of cAMP in modulating the intracellular levels of calcium ion in AtT20 cells and in intermediate lobe cells in vitro was briefly discussed in Sect. A. Because of the calcium dependence of stimulated peptide secretion from POMC-producing cells (GILLES and LOWRY 1978; ABOU-SAMRA et al. 1987; MURAKAMI et al. 1985), several groups have explored the calcium dependence of agents that stimulate POMC gene expression through cAMP-dependent processes. LOEFFLER and colleagues (1986) found that basal levels of POMC mRNA were inhibited by prolonged incubation with the calcium channel antagonists D600, verapamil, and nifedipine, and that nifedipine could partially block the stimulatory effects of forskolin on anterior and intermediate lobe POMC mRNA. The dihydropyridine calcium channel agonist BAYK 8644 stimulated POMC mRNA alone and augmented the stimulatory effects of forskolin in intermediate lobe cells. DAVE and coworkers (1987), however, did not detect differences in basal POMC mRNA levels in anterior lobe cultures treated with D600, although incubation in calcium-free medium did decrease basal levels significantly. In addition, D600 attenuated the increase in POMC mRNA elicited by CRH. EBERWINE et al. (1987) and LORANG et al. (1992) have shown that calcium ionophores stimulate POMC gene transcription directly, in vitro, as will be discussed below. Exactly how cAMP- and calcium-dependent processes interact to increase POMC gene expression remains an open area of investigation.

GABAergic innervation (OERTEL et al. 1982) and GABA receptor activation have also been implicated in negatively influencing POMC mRNA levels in vivo in the intermediate but not anterior pituitary (LOEFFLER et al. 1987). The decrease in POMC gene expression is also observed in primary cultures treated with GABA or GABAergic agonists (OERTEL et al. 1982; LOEFFLER et al. 1987). Whole cell calcium currents and secretion of POMC peptides were reduced by a specific GABA-B agonist in intermediate lobe cells (TALEB et al. 1986). Under the same conditions incubation in calcium-free media also decreases POMC mRNA. These results suggest that POMC gene expression is also under direct inhibitory control by GABA in this tissue and that calcium may play a role in the action of GABA on these cells.

III. Summary

A fundamental point derived from the experiments discussed above is that the lobe-specific stimulation or inhibition of POMC peptide release is accompanied by a subsequent increase or decrease in POMC mRNA levels in the same lobe-specific fashion. In both melanotrophs and corticotrophs, cAMP-dependent processes are important in regulation of POMC gene expression. The possible molecular mechanisms involved in these changes will be discussed in the next sections; however, the differences in regulation at the tissue level observed between the anterior and the intermediate lobes of the pituitary gland can be accounted for by the absence or presence of receptors for the specific neuropeptide or hormone-influencing secretion or biosynthesis. For example, glucocorticoids have little effect on POMC gene expression in the intermediate lobe and this can be attributed to the fact that, under normal physiological conditions, the melanotrophs do not express the glucocorticoid receptor. In contrast, but not as clearly characterized, dopaminergic compounds have little effect on POMC gene expression in the anterior pituitary apparently due to the lack of a dopamine receptor on anterior lobe corticotrophs, the known site of POMC gene expression in the anterior pituitary.

C. Proopiomelanocortin Gene Transcription

Many types of hormonal or neurotransmitter treatment alter the levels of POMC mRNA in the anterior and intermediate pituitary, explaining for the most part the observed changes in biosynthesis of the POMC molecule in these tissues. To determine the molecular mechanisms involved in modulation of POMC biosynthesis we need to understand what causes the changes in POMC mRNA levels. Basically there are two parameters that may change the level of mRNA, its synthesis and its degradation. The synthesis of a POMC mRNA molecule is a complex process involving the initial nuclear transcription of the POMC gene into primary transcript (i.e., the mRNA precursor), subsequent processing to the mature messenger mRNA, transport from the nucleus into the cytoplasm, and finally integration of the POMC mRNA into the actively translated mRNA pool on the rough endoplasmic reticulum. In principle, any of these steps could serve as points of regulation of POMC gene expression. Similarly, the degradation of the mRNA could also involve a complex process. However, very little is known about how mammalian mRNAs are degraded and there have been no reported studies of this type on POMC mRNA in any system. This section will focus on changes in synthesis and processing of the POMC mRNA precursor, the only aspect of mRNA synthesis that has been addressed.

I. Modulation of POMC hnRNA Levels

The POMC gene primary transcript contains two introns, and thus must undergo at least a two-step process of RNA maturation in which the two introns are spliced out prior to the production of the mature POMC mRNA. This process has been studied in detail in both anterior pituitary cultures and AtT20 cells with similar results. LEVIN et al. (1989), using intron-exon junctional probes in conjunction with solution hybridization assays on nuclear RNA from anterior pituitary cultures, proved that the second intron is spliced out first, followed by the first intron. Identical findings were made in AtT20 cells (LORANG et al. 1992). Our group's unpublished work shows the same pattern of splicing in nuclear RNA isolated from anterior or neurointermediate pituitary. Thus there appears to be only one basic pathway for the production of mature pituitary POMC mRNA.

Because the POMC primary transcript and the processing intermediate are rapidly processed to mature POMC mRNA, their levels should reflect changes in transcription of the POMC gene and thus provide an indirect assay for transcription. This parallelism was directly proven in AtT20 cells where identical effects were observed on POMC transcription and on levels of the primary transcript and processing intermediate for a variety of POMC gene modulators (LORANG et al. 1992). This parallelism was also observed in better established paradigms, such as adrenalectomy and glucocorticoid replacement (AUTELITANO et al. 1989) or CRH treatment of primary anterior pituitary cultures (LEVIN et al. 1989). Using the primary transcript assay as an indirect index of transcription LEVIN et al. (1989) showed that the synergistic effect of AVP with CRH on ACTH secretion was not accompanied by a similar synergy in POMC transcription. Indeed, there was a slight inhibition of POMC primary transcript level with AVP treatment alone. More recently, this approach has been used in the AtT20 cell to pharmacologically detail the mechanism by which calcium ion regulates POMC gene transcription (LORANG et al. 1992). In these studies, calcium ion from extracellular or intracellular sources was sufficient to elevate POMC primary transcript two- to threefold in the absence of cAMP elevation.

Using a unique sequence probe to the first intervening sequence (IVS-A) of the rat POMC gene, FREMEAU et al. (1986) have measured changes in the amounts of the nuclear mRNA precursor at the individual cell level by in situ hybridization histochemistry. A threefold increase in the number of silver grains over anterior pituitary cells in pituitary sections hybridized with an IVS-A probe was observed 2 weeks postadrenalectomy. Administration of DEX to 2-week adrenalectomized animals reduced the number of silver grains over the nuclei of anterior lobe cells below detection, within 30 min of injection. Thus, changes in levels of primary transcript occur well before changes in cytoplasmic mRNA are apparent.

II. Whole Animal Studies

Regulation of POMC gene transcription has been extensively studied using the nuclear run on assay. This assay indirectly quantitates the number of RNA polymerase II complexes transcribing the POMC gene in response to the in vivo manipulations. Using this approach it has been shown that adrenalectomy increased POMC gene transcription in the anterior pituitary within 1 h (BIRNBERG et al. 1983), and transcription remained elevated four- to eightfold for at least 2 weeks (EBERWINE and ROBERTS 1984; GAGNER and DROUIN 1985). FREMEAU et al. (1986) using an intervening sequence probe and in situ hybridization to detect the POMC mRNA precursor showed that these increases in the tissue as a whole may be due to increases both in the POMC transcription rate per cell and increases in the detectable number of cells transcribing the POMC gene. Adrenalectomy increased the auto-radiographic signal over each positive cell, implying an elevation in the primary transcript per nucleus, but also increased the number of positive cells in the anterior lobe from 3% to 10%. Thus the large increases in anterior pituitary POMC gene transcription after adrenalectomy may be due to both increases in transcription observed rate per individual cell and increases in the number of cells detectably transcribing the POMC gene.

Glucocorticoids have a rapid inhibitory effect upon anterior lobe POMC gene transcription in both intact and adrenalectomized animals (BIRNBERG et al. 1983; EBERWINE and ROBERTS 1984; GAGNER and DROUIN 1985). The effects of DEX are rapid, with a five- to sevenfold maximal inhibition observed within 15–30 min, as opposed to effects on POMC mRNA levels which required 36–48 h to be maximally inhibited. The endogenous glucocorticoid in the rat corticosterone had a slower time course with maximal inhibition of transcription after 45–120 min and, in addition, did not result in as large a magnitude of inhibitory effect (2.5-fold). It is not known whether the difference in effect between DEX and corticosterone is due to differences in renal clearance, or differences in affinities for type I and II glucocorticoid receptors. These observations suggest that the decreases in POMC mRNA levels observed in the anterior lobe of the intact animal with these hormonal treatments are, at least in part, due to inhibition of POMC mRNA synthesis.

Glucocorticoids were shown to have essentially no effect on intermediate lobe POMC gene transcription in intact animals (BIRNBERG et al. 1983; GAGNER and DROUIN 1985; EBERWINE and ROBERTS 1984). However, the dopamine antagonist haloperidol rapidly stimulates POMC gene transcription more than threefold (PRITCHETT and ROBERTS 1987), demonstrating the inhibitory influence of hypothalamic dopamine on POMC gene expression at the transcriptional level. Thus, in the intermediate lobe the small inhibitory effects of glucocorticoids on POMC mRNA levels discussed above may be attributed to secondary or indirect effects of glucocorticoids on other systems involved in pituitary regulation, possibly through hypothalamic dopaminergic or GABAergic inhibitory mechanisms.

III. Primary and AtT20 Cell Culture

Two groups (GAGNER and DROUIN 1987; EBERWINE et al. 1987) have shown a rapid stimulation, 2-fold and 4- to 13-fold, respectively, by physiological concentrations of CRH on POMC gene transcription in primary cultures of anterior pituitary cells. Similar observations were made in neurointermediate pituitary cultures. Despite the differences in magnitude between the two reports, it is clear that POMC gene transcription is rapidly stimulated by CRH, well prior to the observed CRH-induced increases in POMC mRNA described in Sect. B. CRH also causes a rise in POMC transcription in AtT20 cells (ROBERTS et al. 1987; LORANG et al. 1992).

Adrenergic influences on anterior lobe POMC gene transcription have also been tested in primary culture (EBERWINE et al. 1984). In these studies the β-adrenergic agonist, isoproterenol, was shown to stimulate POMC gene expression in anterior or neurointermediate pituitary cultures and was antagonized by propanolol. In neurointermediate lobe cells, EBERWINE et al. (1984) also reported that dopaminergic agonists such as bromocriptine are inhibitory to POMC gene transcription, whereas dopaminergic antagonists such as haloperidol stimulate POMC gene transcription, correlating with the rapid transcriptional effects observed in vivo. Thus as with peptide hormone stimulation, these studies shown that catecholamines can also influence POMC gene expression through transcriptional mechanisms.

Since the effects of adrenergic agonists and CRH are mediated through activation of adenylate cyclase, thus the cAMP analogue 8-bromo-cAMP was evaluated for the ability to mimic the stimulatory effects of these neurohormones on transcription of the POMC gene in primary culture. Transcription was stimulated in both anterior and neurointermediate lobe cell cultures (EBERWINE et al. 1987; GAGNER and DROUIN 1987), suggesting that the effects of the catecholamines and CRH on POMC gene transcription are mediated by cAMP-dependent processes as has been shown for mRNA accumulation.

The calcium ionophore A23187 stimulated POMC gene transcription seven- to tenfold in both anterior and intermediate lobe cells (EBERWINE et al. 1987); hence the processes mediating the stimulatory effects of these hormones on transcription may have a calcium component, as others have demonstrated for POMC gene expression at the mRNA level (LOEFFLER et al. 1986; DAVE et al. 1987). More recently, using AtT20 cells we have shown (LORANG et al. 1992) that various methods of elevating intracellular calcium cause an elevation in POMC gene transcription. It is not yet clear whether this calcium effect on POMC transcription is an integral part of the CRH signal transduction response, or a "permissive" effect, modulating the basal POMC gene activity.

Dexamethasone was also shown to have immediate direct inhibitory effects on POMC gene transcription in primary anterior pituitary cultures (EBERWINE et al. 1987; GAGNER and DROUIN 1987) and AtT20 cells (ROBERTS et al. 1987; LORANG et al. 1992). These inhibitory effects were maximal within 15–20 min of treatment at a level two- to fourfold below that of the control cultures. These effects were not quite as dramatic as those observed in the intact animal, but they have a time course that is similar to that observed in vivo. Simultaneous measurement of POMC peptide secretion in these same cultures showed that basal secretion of β-endorphin was not affected over this time course, as others have shown.

While both glucocorticoids and CRH have a direct effect on POMC gene transcription, the corticotroph is never exposed to only one of these hormones in the absence of the other. GAGNER and DROUIN (1985) measured POMC gene transcription in cultures simultaneously exposed both to CRH and DEX and found transcriptional levels to be intermediate between control levels and those of CRH alone. Because of the complex relationship between CRH and glucocorticoids in modulation of secretion of POMC-derived peptides in vitro (discussed above), EBERWINE et al. (1987) evaluated transcription of the POMC gene in primary culture in response to combinations of two hormones under different orders of addition. Treatment of corticotroph cultures with DEX for varying periods of time attenuated subsequent CRH-stimulated POMC gene transcription in a manner similar to be well-established inhibitory effects of glucocorticoids on subsequent CRH stimulation of POMC peptide release. The inhibitory effects of DEX were apparent after at least 15 min pretreatment, and were maximal within 40 min, paralleling the time course of inhibition of basal POMC transcription by DEX in vitro. The inhibitory effects of DEX pretreatment on CRH-stimulated transcription occurred before inhibition of CRH-stimulated secretion in the same cultures. If CRH was given first to the cultures, subsequent glucocorticoid addition had no effect at a time period (60 min) when CRH maximally stimulated POMC gene transcription, while DEX was fully inhibitory if added after only 10 min of CRH stimulation. Thus when POMC gene transcription was maximally activated by CRH, glucocorticoids could not inhibit transcription. Similar observations were made in AtT20 cells (LORANG et al. 1992). The molecular mechanism of this complex inter-action is obscure at this point; however, identification of the portions of the POMC gene responsive to the stimulatory effects of CRH and the negative effects of glucocorticoids may explain the hierarchy of this interaction. In addition, the recently evolving concepts between glucocorticoid and positive transcriptional systems, such as *fos/jun* (DIAMOND et al. 1990; YANG-YEN et al. 1990), may also play a role in this observation.

As discussed previously, functional glucocorticoid receptor may be expressed in melanotrophs after long-term culture. EBERWINE et al. (1987) demonstrated an inhibitory effect of glucocorticoids on basal POMC gene transcription as well as the inhibition of subsequent CRH-stimulated POMC gene expression in intermediate lobe cells after 3–4 days in culture. Assuming that the effect of glucocorticoids is due to the appearance of the glucocorticoid receptor in the melanotroph, this finding suggests that the glucocorticoid receptor, when expressed, is sufficient to mediate the inhibitory transcriptional response. This conclusion is supported by gene transfer studies described in the next section which demonstrate negative regulation of POMC-fusion genes transfected into heterologous, non-pituitary cells that contain glucocorticoid receptor.

IV. Summary

Alterations in transcription of the POMC gene in response to various hormonal manipulations in the animal or to hormonal additions in culture systems parallel and precede the changes observed in POMC mRNA levels. This suggests that the changes in mRNA levels are due to at least in part to changes in the rate of synthesis of POMC mRNA in the nucleus. The rapidity of the effects of stimulators or inhibitors of POMC peptide release on POMC gene transcription is sharply contrasted against the changes observed in mRNA levels in the cytoplasm. Previous calculations (EBERWINE and ROBERTS 1984) suggest that there is approximately half to one RNA polymerase molecule transcribing the POMC gene under basal conditions in both the corticotroph and melanotroph; this suggests that approximately 100–200 new POMC mRNA molecules are synthesized per hour. Since solution hybridization studies suggest that there are between 20 000 and 50 000 copies of POMC mRNA in individual melanotrophs and corticotrophs (LEVIN and ROBERTS 1991), even five- and tenfold changes up or down in the rate of transcription will require many hours to be mani-fested as measurable alterations in the relatively large pool of cytoplasmic mRNA.

While the addition of a single steroid, peptide hormone, or neuro-transmitter in isolation elicits clear effects on POMC gene transcription, the addition of combinations of stimulatory and inhibitory agents have more complex effects on POMC gene transcription. These paradigms may none-theless more closely resemble what happens in the intact animal where the pituitary corticotroph and melanotroph are exposed to a multitude of secretory modulators. It is possible that we will be able to decipher some of these complex interactions at the molecular level through the types of studies described in the next section where transcriptional regulatory regions of the POMC gene are dissected by molecular biological techniques.

D. Regulatory Elements in the POMC Gene

The identification of the gene sequences responsible for transcriptional regulation of the POMC gene is necessary for the ultimate biochemical characterization of the mediators of the hormonal regulation of POMC gene transcription. In the past few years, several laboratories have begun the characterization of the sequences responsible for CRH stimulation and glucocorticoid inhibition of POMC gene expression at the transcriptional level, as a first step in the identification of the nuclear factors and proteins which mediate that control.

I. Basal and Tissue-Specific Promoter Elements

The first characterization of the POMC promoter utilized transient expres-sion of the human POMC gene linked to a SV40 vector in COS cells (MISHINA et al. 1982). By linking an EcoRI fragment containing the entire human POMC gene to this SV40 vector, a high copy number of POMC trans- genes were generated in transfected COS cells. RNA analyzed by solution hybridization indicated POMC mRNA in the transfected cells was a product of proper initiation of transcription, utilizing the same initiation site as the anterior pituitary POMC mRNA. A hybrid gene was constructed to define the minimal sequences required for transcription of the POMC gene by linking the 5' flanking portion of the human POMC gene, including 680 nucleotides and about 65 nucleotides of exon 1, to the herpes simplex virus thymidine kinase structural gene (HSV tk). RNA produced in cells transfected with this construct and with progressive deletions of the 5' end to a position 95 nucleotides upstream of the transcription initiation site was initiated at the proper site and produced at approximately equal levels among all deletions. Deletion of bases past a −59 end point resulted in a threefold enhancement of RNA levels suggesting the deletion of a sequence possibly responsible for suppression of transcription. Deletion of sequences down to −35 still resulted in properly initiated transcription, although at a lower level. Deletion of sequences past −21 eliminated promoter activity, as expected since this included the TATA box (McKnight and Kingsbury 1982).

These gene transfer studies were extended with cell-free transcription using whole cell extracts from both HeLa cells and AtT20 cells, using essentially the same deletion mutants described above (Notake et al. 1983). Observed differences between extracts derived from HeLa and AtT20 cells are suggestive of the complexity of tissue-specific regulatory mechanisms of the POMC gene. Consistent with the results obtained in vivo, 5′ deletions to −52 and −41 end points directed synthesis of 2- and 1.5-fold enhanced levels of properly initiated transcripts relative to other deletions. Sequences between −59 and −53 may be part of a negative regulatory element which may bind a repressor-like protein. In the rat POMC gene, this region has been defined as a negative glucocorticoid regulatory element (nGRE) by Drouin and collegues (1989a,b, 1990). Interestingly, extracts prepared from AtT20 cells treated with DEX failed to demonstrate negative effects on transcription.

More recently, similar promoter studies have been done with the rat POMC gene using the AtT20 cells as the transfection host. Initial studies showed that only 480 bases of the rat POMC promoter were necessary to drive high level expression of the reporter (Jeannotte et al. 1987). Recently, Therrien and Drouin (1991) divided the POMC promoter into three functional elements – distal, central, and proximal – comprising regions from −480 to −323, −323 to −166, −166 to −34, respectively, and used them to drive a heterologus promoter/reporter gene. They identified a complex relationship between these three elements wherein the distal element had no basal activity but the central or proximal element alone maintained basal activity. When the distal and central elements were hooked together, basal activity was synergistically elevated and was equivalent to all three elements together. These studies suggest a complex interrelationship between different regions of the POMC gene necessary to maintain basal POMC transcription.

Riegel and colleagues (1990) identified another interesting region of the POMC promoter located between the TATA box and the start site of transcription which gave a strong footprint called PO-B. When this element was mutated, 75% of basal promoter activity was lost when studied in AtT20 cells. This cis-element shares sequence similarity to DNA elements involved in interleukin stimulated transcription and the authors proposed that the PO-B element may mediate POMC gene expression in the immune system.

Therrien and Drouin (1991) also presented an elegant set of studies with a set of linker scanner mutants throughout the −480 to +63 region of the rat POMC promoter fused to a luciferase reporter which defined numerous elements in the promoter involved in modulating basal expression. These were correlated with a set of DNAse footprint studies identifying protein factors which bound to the POMC promoter. In general, multiple

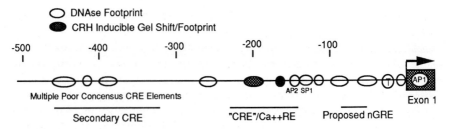

Fig. 2. Schematic structure of the rat POMC promoter. Protein binding sites identified by DNAse I footprint analysis of the rat POMC promoter are indicated. Sequences conforming to known *cis*-elements (CRE, AP2, SP1, AP1) are also identified, some of which correspond to footprints. *CRE*, cAMP regulatory element; *nGRE*, negative glucocorticoid regulatory element

protein binding elements were identified across the promoter region [similar to our observations (Fig. 2); ROBERTS et al. (to be published)], yet no crucial element was identified within the promoter which caused more than a two- to threefold change in basal transcriptional activity. Deletion analysis from the 5′ end starting at −480 (to +63) did identify several elements within the POMC promoter which were involved with basal gene expression, resulting in a progressive loss of promoter activity with progressive 3′ deletions which culminated in approximately 20-fold loss of promoter activity with the −34 promoter deletion. These studies suggest that there are multiple regions in the POMC promoter which are capable of maintaining basal POMC promoter expression, not unlike the conclusions derived from the study previously described. RIEGEL et al. (1991) also showed a loss of basal activity of a similar magnitude with progressive deletions from the 5′ end.

In contrast, recent studies from our laboratory do not agree with this observation (ROBERTS et al., to be published). Using the same promoter sequences, we have observed that deletions from the 5′ end of the POMC promoter result in, if anything, an enhanced level of basal gene expression and, similar to studies reported for the human gene (see above), deletion of the region between −134 and −37 results in a twofold elevation of basal activity. The reasons for these differences are not clear, but are possibly due to our use of the AtT20-D_{16-16} cells, a subclone of the AtT20 cells which show a greater CRH response and higher levels of POMC gene expression (SABOL 1980), since the method of transfection which we utilized is similar to that of the RIEGEL et al. (1991) study.

Proopiomelanocortin gene expression may in part be limited to the lobes of the pituitary and a limited number of additional cell types by the presence of specific transcription factors in these tissues and an absence of these tissue-specific factors in other cell types. If this is the case, portions of POMC promoter sequences may be responsible for mediating the tissue-specific expression of the POMC gene. TREMBLAY et al. (1988) observed that only −708 to +63 of the rat POMC gene was necessary to drive pituitary specific expression of a neomycin resistance reporter gene in transgenic mice. In situ hybridization studies clearly showed proper cell-type specific expression in the corticotrophs and melanotrophs. More recent studies by LIU and collegues (1991) suggest that only the rat POMC promoter region between −323 and −33 is required for this type of tissue-specific expression. Possibly some of the several DNA footprints in this region identified in the THERRIEN and DROUIN (1991) study or shown in Fig. 2 mediate this tissue specificity.

II. Glucocorticoid Regulatory Elements

As discussed above, the transcriptional effect of glucocorticoids on the POMC gene is negative, unlike the majority of genes where the effects are positive. In the case of positive transcriptional effects, clearly defined *cis*-acting GREs have been identified. However, in the case of negative regulation, the identification of specific nGREs has not been forthcoming. While sequences mediating the negative effects on several genes have been identified, there is no consensus between them, suggesting that there may be multiple mechanisms for negative glucocorticoid regulation of transcription. Indeed, recent developments in the field have proven this latter possibility to be the case. Glucocorticoids have been shown in some cases to elicit negative effects by blocking the ability of a positive transcription factor such as the CREB protein, to bind to the promoter as with the hCG-α gene (AKERBLOM et al. 1988). In other situations the glucocorticoid receptor has been shown to interact with the *fos/jun* oncogene products to inhibit its positive actions (DIAMOND et al. 1990; YANG-YEN et al. 1990). Thus, possibly the POMC gene will provide important information as to the mechanism of negative glucocorticoid regulation, since the negative effect of glucocorticoids on transcription of the POMC gene is more robust than on other genes.

ISRAEL and COHEN (1985) were the first to demonstrate glucocorticoid hormone regulation of a transfected POMC promoter using human POMC genomic sequences in mouse fibroblasts (Ltk⁻ cells). A *POMC-tk* fusion gene construct similar to that used by MISHINA and coworkers (1982) was expressed at low levels and was not detectably suppressed by DEX unless the SV40 enhancer was present on the same plasmid vector as the fusion transcription unit. The inhibition of expression observed in transfected L cells correlated well with the level of inhibition of expression of the mouse POMC gene in AtT20 cells (ROBERTS et al. 1979; NAKAMURA et al. 1978), and hence the molecular or cellular processes involved may not be tissue specific to the corticotroph. In addition, expression of a human POMC gene was inhibited in mouse cells, indicating that DNA sequences responsible for the inhibition may be conserved at least at the functional level between the human and mouse genes.

Charron and Drouin (1986) showed glucocorticoid negative regulatory sites within a similar fragment of the rat POMC gene, also in a heterologous cell line, mouse C127 cells, using a bovine papilloma virus vector. The rat POMC promoter from −706 to a position within exon 1 was linked to coding sequences for SV40 large T antigen as a marker gene. The rat promoter was active and hormonally responsive in the cells transfected with this vector as shown by RNA blot analysis and S1 and RNase protection mapping of the fusion transcripts. In order to better identify possible nGRE elements, Drouin et al. (1989b) defined five glucocorticoid receptor binding sites in the rat POMC gene, most notably one at −63 in a region already suggested to be involved in repression of basal activity (see discussion above). In the same study, this putative nGRE was further characterized by mutational analysis and a mutation that destroyed the negative regulation of promoter activity by DEX also destroyed the ability of the glucocorticoid receptor to bind to the DNA, implying that DNA binding of the receptor was necessary for negative regulation.

Riegel et al. (1991) have also addressed the issue of negative regulation of the rat POMC promoter. While they also define a region between −71 and −51 as being important in negative regulation, in addition they define a region from −480 to −320 as contributing to the negative regulation. Their studies also hint at the complexity of the −71/−51 nGRE since two different mutants in this region which lowered basal expression were not negatively regulated by DEX, even with the mutation of two bases previously shown by the Drouin group (1989b) to be crucial for negative regulation. The source of this discrepancy is not clear, but it serves to highlight the complexity of the regulatory mechanisms which modulate POMC transcription.

III. Promoter Elements and Second Messenger Pathways

As has been shown at the transcriptional level and at the level of mRNA accumulation, all of the signaling pathways activated by neurohormones that act at the cell surface have effects on POMC gene expression. CRH or other agents that increase intracellular cAMP increase POMC mRNA and transcription of the POMC gene in primary culture of anterior lobe cells and in AtT20 cells in culture. Phorbol esters increase POMC mRNA in AtT20 cells, although the effects of protein kinase C activators on transcription appear to be negative. Calcium ion clearly plays a role as well.

To address the question of whether these processes act through different nuclear transcription factors or whether they act through a final common pathway to increase transcription, Roberts and coworkers (1987) have identified a region within the 5′ flanking portion of the rat POMC gene that is responsible for CRH inducibility of a POMC-CAT fusion construct transfected transiently into AtT20 cells. A discrete fragment of the flanking sequence between −234 and −133 confers both CRH and forskolin inducibility on the *HSV tk* promoter in AtT20 cells when placed 5′ of this normally nonresponsive promoter. This region does not share similarity with the cAMP-responsive elements described for other genes, but does have several protein binding elements (see Fig. 2), including elements whose gel shifts appear to be induced by CRH treatment (ROBERTS et al., to be published). Sequence analysis of these regions suggest that the POMC gene may utilize a novel cAMP-inducible element to mediate at least part of the CRH transcriptional response. Although this ~100 base portion of the gene contains sufficient information to confer regulation by cAMP and CRH on a heterologous promoter, other regions of the gene may also participate in mediating the transcriptional response, and may work in synergy with this region of the promoter. Our studies suggest that the region between -37 and $+63$ is capable of mediating CRH induction, possibly through the AP-1 element at $+40/+50$ (THERRIEN and DROUIN 1991) since a recent study by BOUTILLIER et al. (1991) has shown that CRH induces c-*fos* gene expression in AtT20 cells.

IV. Summary

Characterization of the nucleotide sequences responsible for transcriptional regulation of the POMC gene both by hormonal influences and by tissue-specific factors may explain some of complexity of the transcriptional response of this gene. It appears that there are multiple elements present in the POMC promoter which are capable of driving basal POMC gene expression, even in the most minimal of promoters. Such redundancy was also observed in promoter regions capable of eliciting CRH(cAMP)-stimulated or glucocorticoid-inhibited POMC transcription. It is possible that these different elements come into play in different tissues of expression. For example, in the corticotroph one region of the promoter may mediate the cAMP response while in the hypothalamus another region would play the dominant role in this response. This redundancy may also explain some of the discrepancy between labs in the reported regions responsible for basal or hormonally modulated transcription. Different cell growth conditions, AtT20 subtypes, and/or transfection/reproter systems may cause differential usage of the multiple functional elements in the promoter.

The major goals of these studies are to identify the locations and relationships between sequence elements responsible for basal, tissue-specific, and hormonal regulation of transcription and determine whether the complexity of the transcriptional response to neurohormones, neurotransmitters, and glucocorticoids is reflected by interactions between transcription factors at the molecular level. In particular, since several second messenger pathways are implicated in controlling the transcriptional response of the POMC gene, it is of interest to determine whether these pathways each act through distinct transcriptional activator proteins or through a common final effector molecule.

E. Conclusions

Long utilized as a model for neuropeptide synthesis, the pituitary POMC system is also valuable as a model for the multihormonal regulation of neuroendocrine peptide gene expression at the molecular level. Peptide hormones, neurotransmitters, and corticosteroid hormones all influence release of POMC peptides and expression of the POMC gene in the pituitary in a coordinate fashion as we have described in this review. The coupling of gene expression and peptide secretion under physiologically relevant influences occurs at the level of gene transcription to alter mRNA levels; however, potentially any of the steps leading to accumulation of cytoplasmic mRNA could be points of regulation.

Glucocorticoids influence anterior lobe POMC gene expression in vivo both indirectly by alteration of modulatory inputs to the pituitary and directly by changing the responsiveness of the corticotroph itself to these inputs and interfering with intracellular signal transduction. In addition the glucocorticoid receptor complex itself may act directly at the genomic level through protein: DNA interactions, or induction of a repressor-like molecule to inhibit POMC gene transcription.

Glucocorticoids clearly have effects on pituitary intermediate lobe POMC mRNA levels; however, the physiological significance and the mechanisms involved are unknown. In particular, the possibility that glucocorticoids have direct effects on melanotroph POMC gene expression is especially exciting because of the complex regulation of glucocorticoid receptor gene expression in this cell type. It will be interesting to determine whether pharmacological or surgical manipulation of input to the melanotroph is permissive for glucocorticoid regulation of POMC gene expression in an anterior lobe fashion.

Studies of gene expression of hypothalamic factors involved in the release of POMC peptides, such as AVP and CRH, in conjunction with POMC gene expression will aid in interpretation of how these factors integrate the physiological response to stress. In addition, the effects of these factors on POMC gene expression at the molecular and cellular levels are only now being elucidated. Studies of transcriptional response of corticotrophs to activation of plasma membrane receptors linked to processes other than cAMP production will clarify the role of these factors in controlling POMC gene expression.

The molecular events mediating basal, cell-type specific, and hormonally regulated POMC gene expression are poorly understood. By analogy to the transcriptional control regions from better characterized genes, the POMC gene potentially has a complex arrangement of positive and negative transcriptional regulatory elements. More detailed analysis of the DNA sequences in the POMC gene responsible for controlling gene expression at all these levels, and identification of factors mediating effects through these promoter elements, is important for understanding stimulatory and inhibitory influences on POMC gene expression.

The basic lesson that can be learned from the POMC system, which holds true independent of the pituitary cell type or the hormone or neurotransmitter modulator regulating secretion of POMC peptides, is that when physiological means are used to modulate secretion of POMC peptides POMC gene expression changes in parallel. It is by this mechanism, which appears to be mediated by components of the intracellular metabolic cascade initiated by the secretagogue, that the corticotroph and melanotroph appropriately adjust their biosynthetic mechinery for POMC peptides to meet secretory demands.

Acknowledgments. We thank D. Carman for preparation of the manuscript.

References

Abou-Samra AB, Catt KJ, Aguilera G (1986a) Involvement of protein kinase C in the regulation of adrenocorticotropin release from rat anterior pituitary cells. Endocrinology 118:212–217

Abou-Samra A-B, Catt KJ, Aguilera G (1987) Calcium-dependent control of corticotropin release in rat anterior pituitary cell cultures. Endocrinology 121: 965–974

Affolter HU, Reisine T (1985) Corticotropin releasing factor increases proopiomelanocortin messenger RNA in mouse anterior pituitary tumor cells. J Biol Chem 260:15477–15481

Aguilera G, Harwood JP, Wilson JX, Morell J, Brown JH, Catt KJ (1983) Mechanisms of action of corticotropin releasing factor and other regulators of corticotropin release in rat pituitary cells. J Biol Chem 258:8039–8045

Akerblom IE, Slater EP, Beato M, Baxter JD, Mellon PL (1988) Negative regulation by glucocorticoids through intereference with a cAMP responsive enhancer. Science 241:992–994

Antakly T, Eisen HJ (1984) Immunocytochemical localization of glucocorticoid receptor in target cells. Endocrinology 115:1984–1989

Antakly T, Sasaki A, Liotta AS, Palkovits M, Krieger DT (1985) Induced expression of the glucocorticoid receptor in the rat intermediate pituitary lobe. Science 229:277–279

Antakly T, Mercille S, Cote JP (1987) Tissue-specific dopaminergic regulation of the glucocorticoid receptor in the rat pituitary. Endocrinology 120:1558–1562

Antoni FA (1986) Hypothalamic control of adrenocorticotropin secretion: advances since the discovery of 41-residue corticotropin-releasing factor. Endo Rev 7: 351–378

Autelitano DJ, Clements JA, Nikolaidis I, Canny BJ, Funder JW (1987) Concomitant dopaminergic and glucocorticoid control of pituitary proopiomelanocortin messenger ribonucleic acid and β-endorphin levels. Endocrinology 121:1689–1696

Autelitano DJ, Blum M, Roberts (1989) Changes in rat pituitary nuclear and cytoplasmic proopiomelanocortin RNAs associated with adrenalectomy and glucocorticoid replacement. Mol Cell Endocrinol 66:171–80

Autelitano DJ, Blum M, Lopingco M, Allen RG, Roberts JL (1990) Corticotropin-releasing factor differentially regulates anterior and intermediate pituitary lobe proopiomelanocortin gene transcription, nuclear precursor RNA and mature mRNA in vivo. Neuroendocrinology 51:123–130

Axelrod J, Reisine TD (1984) Stress hormones: their interaction and regulation. Science 224:452

Bilezikjian LM, Vale W (1983) Glucocorticoids inhibit CRF induced production of cAMP in cultured anterior pituitary cells. Endocrinology 113:657–669

Birnberg NC, Lissitzky JC, Hinman M, Herbert E (1983) Glucocorticoids regulate proopiomelanocortin gene expression in vivo at the levels of transcription and secretion. Proc Natl Acad Sci USA 80:6982–6986

Boutillier AL, Sassone-Corsi P, Loeffler JP (1991) The protooncogene c-*fos* is induced by corticotropin-releasing factor and stimulates proopiomelanocortin gene transcription in pituitary cells. Molec Endocrinol 5:1301–1310

Bruhn TA, Sutton RE, Rivier CL, Vale WW (1984) Corticotropin-releasing factor regulated proopiomelanocortin messenger ribonucleic acid levels in vivo. Neuroendocrinology 39:170–175

Buckingham JC (1979) The influence of corticosteroids on the secretion of corticotropin and its hypothalamic releasing hormone. J Physiol 286:331

Charron J, Drouin J (1986) Glucocorticoid inhibition of transcription from episomal proopiomelanocortin gene promoter. Proc Natl Acad Sci USA 83:8903

Chen CL, Dionne FT, Roberts JL (1984) Regulation of the pro-opiomelanocortin mRNA levels in rat pituitary by dopaminergic compounds. Proc Natl Sci USA 80:2211

Chronwall BM, Millington WR, Griffin WST, Unnerstall JR, O'Donohue TL (1987) Histological evaluation of the dopaminergic regulation of proopiomelanocortin gene expression in the intermediate lobe of the rat pituitary, involving in situ hybridization and [^{3}H] thymidine uptake measurement. Endocrinology 120: 1201–1208

Civelli O, Birnberg N, Herbert H (1982) Detection and quantitation of pro-opiomelanocortin mRNA in pituitary and brain tissues from different species. J Biol Chem 257:6783–6790

Cote TE, Frey EA, Sekura RD, Kebabian JW (1985) Dual regulation of adenylate cyclase activity and hormone release in the intermediate lobe of the rat pituitary gland: evidence for the involvement of membrane components of the stimulatory β-2-adrenergic system and of the inhibitory D-2 dopaminergic system. Adv Cyclic Nucleotide Res 19:151–168

Cote TE, Felder R, Kebabian JW, Sekura RD, Reisine T, Affolter HU (1986) D-2 dopamine receptor-mediated inhibition of pro-opiomelanocortin synthesis in rat intermediate lobe. J Biol Chem 261:4555–4561

Dallman MF, Makara GB, Roberts JL, Levin N, Blum M (1985) Corticotrope response to removal of releasing factors and corticosteroids in vivo. Endocrinology 117:2190–2197

Dave JR, Eiden LE, Lozovsky D, Waschek JA, Eskay RL (1987) Calcium-independent and calcium-dependent mechanisms regulate corticotropin-releasing factor-stimulated proopiomelanocortin peptide secretion and messenger ribonucleic acid production. Endocrinology 120:305–310

Diamond MI, Miner JN, Yoshinaga SK, Yamamoto KR (1990) Transcription factor interactions: selectors of positive or negative regulation from a single DNA element. Science 249:1266–1272

Drouin J, Goodman HM (1980) Most of the coding region of rat ACTH beta-LPH precursor gene lacks intervening sequences. Nature 288:610–614

Drouin J, Chamberland M, Charron J, Jeannotte L, Nemer M (1985) Structure of the rat pro-opiomelanocortin (POMC) gene. FEBS Lett 193:54–58

Drouin J, Nemer M, Charron J, Gagner JP, Jeannotte L, Sun YL, Therrein M, Tremblay Y (1989a) Tissue-specific activity of the pro-opiomelanocortin (POMC) gene and repression by glucocorticoids. Genome 31:510–519

Drouin J, Trifiro MA, Plante RK, Nemer M, Eriksson, Wrange O (1989b) Glucocorticoid receptor binding to a specific DNA sequence is required for hormone-dependent repression of pro-opiomelanocortin gene transcription. Mol Cell Biol 9:5302–5314

Drouin J, Sun YL, Nemer M (1990) Regulatory elements of the pro-opiomelanocortin gene: pituitary specificity and glucocorticoid repression. Trends Endocrinol Metab 2:219–225

Eberwine JH, Roberts JL (1984) Glucocorticoid regulation of pro-opiomelanocortin gene transcription in the rat pituitary. J Biol Chem 259:2166–2170

Eberwine JH, Jonassen J, Dionne FT, Blum M, Roberts JL (1984) Catecholamine regulation of POMC gene expression in primary cultures and intact rat anterior and intermediate pituitary lobes. Abstracts of the 7th International Congress of Endocrinology, Quebec City (abstract 1003)

Eberwine JH, Jonassen JA, Evinger MJQ, Roberts, JL (1987) Complex transcriptional regulation by glucocorticoids and corticotropin releasing hormone of proopiomelanocortin gene expression in rat pituitary cultures. DNA 6:483–492

Eipper BA, Mains RE (1980) Structure and biosynthesis of proadrenocorticotropin/endorphin and related peptides. Endo Rev 1:1–27

Fremeau RT, Lundblad JR, Pritchett DP, Wilcox JN, Roberts JL (1986) Regulation of POMC gene transcription in individual cell nuclei. Science 234:1265–1269

Gagner JP, Drouin J (1985) Opposite regulation of pro-opiomelanocortin gene transcription by glucocorticoids and CRH. Mol Cell Endocrinol 40:25–32

Gagner JP, Drouin J (1987) Tissue-specific regulation of pituitary proopiomelanocortin gene transcription by corticotropin-releasing hormone, 3′ 5′-cyclic adenosine monophosphate, and glucocorticoids. Mol Endocrinol 1:677–682

Gannon MN, Spencer R, Lundblad JR, McEwen BS, Roberts JL (1990) Pharmacological characterization of type II glucocorticoid binding sites in AtT20 pituitary cell culture. J Steroid Biochemistry 36:83–88

Gee CE, Roberts JL (1983) In situ hybridization histochemistry: a technique for study of gene expression in single cells. DNA 2:157–168

Giguere V, Labrie F, Cote J, Coy DH, Sueiras-Diaz J, Schally AV (1982) Stimulation of cyclic AMP accumulation and corticotropin release by synthetic ovine corticotropin-releasing factor in rat anterior pituitary cells; site of glucocorticoid action. Proc Natl Acad Sci USA 79:3466–3459

Gilles G, Lowry PJ (1978) Perfused rat isolated anterior pituitary cell column as bioassay for factor(s) controlling release of adrenocorticotropin: validation of a technique. Endocrinology 103:521–529

Guild S, Itoh Y, Kebabian JW, Luini A, Reisine T (1986) Forskolin enhances basal and potassium-evoked hormone release from normal and malignant pituitary tissue: the role of calcium. Endocrinology 118:268–277

Guild S, Reisine T (1987) Molecular mechanisms of corticotropin-releasing factor stimulation of calcium mobilization and adrenocorticotropin release from anterior pituitary tumor cells. J Pharm Exp Ther 241:12551–12558

Heisler S, Reisine TD, Hook VY, Axelrod J (1982) Somatostatin inhibits multireceptor stimulation of cyclic AMP formation and corticotropin secretion in mouse pituitary tumor cells. Proc Natl Acad Sci USA 79:6502–6506

Höllt V, Haarmann I, Seizinger BR, Herz A (1982) Chronic haloperidol treatment increases the level of in vitro translatable messenger ribonucleic acid coding for the β-endorphin/adrenocorticotropin precursor proopiomelanocortin in the pars intermedia of the rat pituitary. Endocrinology 110:1885–1891

Höllt V, Haarmann I (1984) Corticotropin-releasing factor differentially regulates proopiomelanocortin messenger ribonucleic acid levels in anterior as compared to intermediate pituitary lobes of rats. Biochem Biophys Res Commun 124:407–415

Israel A, Cohen SN (1985) Hormonally mediated negative regulation of human proopiomelanocortin gene expression after transfection into mouse L cells. Mol Cell Biol 5:2443–2454

Jeannotte L, Trifiro MA, Plante RK, Chamberland M, Drouin J (1987) Tissue-specific activity of the pro-opiomelanocortin gene promoter. Mol Cell Biol 7:4058–4069

Jingami H, Matsukura S, Numa S, Imura H (1985) Effects of adrenalectomy and dexamethasone administration on the level of prepro-corticotropin-releasing factor messenger ribonucleic acid (mRNA) in the hypothalamus and adrenocorticotropin/beta-lipotropin precursor mRNA in the pituitary in rats. Endocrinology 117:1314–1320

Jones MT, Gillham B (1988) Factors involved in the regulation of adreno-corticotropic hormone/β-lipotropic hormone. Physiol Rev 68:743–818

Keller-Wood ME, Dallman MF (1984) Corticosteroid inhibition of ACTH secretion. Endo Rev 5:1–36

Kelsey JE, Watson SJ, Burke S, Akil H, Roberts JL (1986) Characterization of POMC mRNA detected by in situ hybridization. J Neuroscience 6:38–49

Lacaze-Masmonteil T, de Ketzer Y, Luton J-P, Kahn A, Bertagna X (1987) Characterization of proopiomelanocortin transcripts in human nonpituitary tissues. Proc Natl Acad Sci USA 84:7261–7265

Levin N, Blum M, Roberts JL (1989) Modulation of basal and corticotropin-releasing factor-stimulated proopiomelanocortin gene expression by vasopressin in rat anterior pituitary. Endocrinology 125:2957–66

Levin N, Roberts JL (1991) Positive regulation of proopiomelanocortin gene expression in corticotropes and melanotropes. 12:1–22

Litvin Y, Pasmantier R, Fleischer N, Erlichman J (1984) Hormonal activation of the cAMP dependent protein kinases in AtT20 cells. J Biol Chem 259:10296–10304

Liu B, Hammer G, Low MJ (1991) Characterization of the rat POMC gene sequences responsible for pituitary specific expression. Proceedings of the 21st Annual Meeting of the Society for Neuroscience, New Orleans. LA (abstract 211.6)

Loeffler JP, Kley N, Pittius CW, Höllt V (1985) Corticotropin-releasing factor and forskolin increase proopiomelanocortin messenger RNA levels in rat anterior and intermediate cells in vitro. Neurosci Lett 62:383–387

Loeffler JP, Kley N, Pittius CW, Höllt V (1986) Calcium ion and cyclic adenosine 3′, 5′-monophosphate regulate proopiomelanocortin messenger ribonucleic acid levels in rat intermediate and anterior pituitary lobes. Endocrinology 119:2840–2847

Loeffler JP, Demeneix BA, Pittius CW, Kley N, Haegele KD, Höllt V (1987) GABA differentially regulates the gene expression of proopiomelanocortin in rat intermediate and anterior pituitary. Peptides 7:253–259

Lolait SJ, Clements JA, Markwick AJ, Cheng C, McNally M, Smith AI, Funder JW (1986) Pro-opiomelanocortin messenger ribonucleic acid and posttranslational processing of beta endorphin in spleen macrophages. J Clin Invest 77:1776–1787

Lorang D, Gillo B, Lundblad JR, Blum M, Roberts JL (1992) Calcium involvement in basal and CRH-stimulated POMC gene transcription. Mol Cell Biol (in press)

Luini A, Lewis D, Guild S, Corda D, Axelrod J (1985) Hormone secretagogues increase cytosolic calcium by increasing cAMP in corticotropin-secreting cells. Proc Natl Acad Sci USA 82:8034–8038

Luini A, Lewis D, Guild S, Schofield G, Weight F (1986) Somatostatin, an inhibitor of ACTH secretion, decreases cytosolic free calcium and voltage-dependent calcium current in a pituitary cell line. J Neurosci 6:3128–3137

Lundblad JR, Roberts JL (1988) Regulation of proopiomelanocortin gene expression in pituitary. Endocr Rev 9:135–158

May V, Stoffers DA, Eipper BA (1989) Proadrenoocorticotropin/endorphin production and messenger ribonucleic acid levels in primary intermediate pituitary cultures: effects of serum, isoproternol, and dibutyrl adenosine 3′, 5′-monophosphate. Endocrinology 124:157–166

McEwen BS, De Kloet ER, Rostene W (1986) Adrenal steroid receptors and actions in the nervous system. Physiol Rev 66:1121–1143

McKnight SL, Kingsbury R (1982) Transcriptional control signals of a eucaryotic protein-coding gene. Science 217:316–320

Meador-Woodruff JH, Pellerito B, Bronstein D, Lin HL, Ling N, Akil H (1990) Differential effects of haloperiodol on the rat pituitary: decreased biosynthesis, processing and release of anterior lobe pro-opiomelanocortin. Neuroendocrinology 51:294–303

Mechanick JI, Levin N, Roberts JL, Autelitano DJ (in press) Proopiomelanocortin (POMC) gene expression in a distinct population of rat spleen and lung leukocytes. Endocrinology

Millington WR, Blum M, Knight R, Mueller GP, Roberts JL, O'Donohue TL (1986a) Diurnal rhythm in proopiomelanocortin messenger ribonucleic acid that varies concomitantly with the content and secretion of β-endorphin in the intermediate lobe of the rat pituitary. Endocrinology 118:829–840

Millington WR, O'Donohue TL, Chappel MC, Roberts JL, Mueller GP (1986b) Coordinate regulation of peptide acetyltransferase activity and pro-opiomelanocortin gene expression in the intermediate lobe of the rat pituitary. Endocrinology 118:2024–33

Mishina M, Kurosaki T, Yamamoto T, Notake M, Masu M, Numa S (1982) DNA sequences required for transcription in vivo of the human corticotropin-β-lipotropin precursor gene. EMBO J 1:1533–1538

Miyazki K, Reisine T, Kebabian JW (1984) Adenosine 3', 5'-monophosphate (cAMP)-dependent protein kinase activity in rodent pituitary tissue: possible role in cAMP-dependent hormone secretion. Endocrinol 115:1933–1942

Murakami K, Hashimoto K, Ota Z (1985) The effect of nifedipine on CRF-41 and AVP-induced ACTH release in vitro. Acta Endocrinol 109:32–39

Nakamura N, Nakanishi S, Sueoka S, Imura H, Numa S (1978) Effects of steroid hormones on the level of corticotropin messenger RNA activity in cultured mouse-pituitary-tumor cells. Eur J Biochem 86:61–68

Nakanishi S, Kita T, Taii S, Imura H, Numa S (1977) Glucocorticoid effect on the level of corticotropin messenger RNA activity in rat pituitary. Proc Natl Acad Sci USA 74:3283–3286

Nakanishi S, Teranishi Y, Watanabe Notake M, Noda M, Kakidani H, Jingami H, Numa S (1981) Isolation and characterization of the bovine corticotropin/β-lipotropin precursor gene. Eur J Biochem 115:429–438

Notake M, Kurosaki T, Yamamoto T, Handa H, Mishina M (1983) Sequence requirement for transcription in vitro of the human corticotropin/β-lipotropin precursor gene. J Biochem 133:599–608

Oates E, Herbert E (1984) 5' Sequence of porcine and rat pro-opiomelanocortin mRNA. J Biol Chem 259:7421–7425

Oertel WH, Mugnaini E, Tappaz ML, Weise VK, Dahl AL, Schmechel DE, Kopin IJ (1982) Central GABAergic innervation of neurointermediate pituitary lobe: biochemical and immunocytochemical study in the rat. Neurobiology 79:675–688

Perrin MH, Haas Y, Rivier JE, Vale WW (1986) Corticotropin-releasing factor binding to the anterior pituitary receptor is modulated by divalent cations and guanyl nucleotides. Endocrinology 118:1171–1180

Pintar JE, Schacter BS, Herman AB, Durgerian S, Krieger DT (1984) Characterization and localization of proopiomelanocortin messenger RNA in the adult rat testes. Science 225:632–634

Pritchett DB, Roberts JL (1987) Dopamine regulates expression of glandular-type kallikrein gene at transcriptional level in pituitary. Proc Natl Acad Sci USA 84:5545–5549

Proulx-Ferland L, Labrie F, Dumont D, Cote J (1982) Corticotropin-releasing factor stimulates secretion of melanocyte-stimulating hormone from the rat pituitary. Science 217:62–63

Raymond V, Leung PCK, Veilleux R, Labrie F (1985) Vasopressin rapidly stimulates phosphatidic acid-phosphatidylinositol turnover in rat anterior pituitary cells. FEBS Lett 182:196–200

Rees H, Stumpf W, Sar M, Petrusz P (1977) Autoradiographic studies of ^{3}H-dexamethasone uptake by immunocytochemically characterized cells of the rat pituitary. Cell Tiss Res 182:347–359

Reisine T, Rougon G, Barbet J, Affolter HU (1985) Corticotropin-releasing factor-induced adrenocorticotropin hormone release and synthesis is blocked by incorporation of the inhibitor of cyclic AMP-dependent protein kinase into anterior pituitary tumor cells by liposomes. Proc Natl Acad Sci USA 82:8261–8265

Reisine TD (1985) Somatostatin inhibition of cyclic AMP accumulation and adrenocorticotropin release from mouse anterior pituitary tumor cells: mode of action and self-regulation. Adv Cyclic Nucleotide Res 19:169–184

Reisine T, Guild S (1985) Pertussis toxin blocks somatostatin inhibition of calcium mobilization and reduces the affinity of somatostatin receptors for agonists. J Pharm Exp Ther 235:551–558

Reisine T, Zhang Y-L, Sekura R (1985) Pertussis toxin treatment blocks the inhibition of somatostatin and increases the stimulation by forskolin of cyclic AMP accumulation and adrenocorticotropin secretion from mouse anterior pituitary tumor cells. J Pharm Exp Ther 232:275–280

Riegel AT, Remenick J, Wolford RG, Berard DS, Hager GL (1990) A novel transcriptional activator (PO-B) binds between the TATA box and cap site of the pro-opiomelanocortin gene. Nucleic Acids Res 18:4513–4521

Riegel AT, Yang L, Remenick J, Wolford RG, Berard DS, Hager GL (1991) Proopiomelanocortin gene promoter elements required for constitutive and glucocorticoid-repressed transcription. Mol Endocrinol 5:1973–1982

Ringold GM (1985) Steroid hormone regulation of gene expression. Ann Rev Pharmacol Toxicol 25:529–559

Roberts JL, Budarf MJ, Baxter JD, Herbert E (1979) Selective reduction of proadrenocorticotropin/endorphin protein and mRNA activity in mouse pituitary tumor cells by glucocorticoids. Biochemistry 18:4907

Roberts JL, Lundblad JR, Eberwine JH, Fremeau RT, Salton SRJ, Blum M (1987) Hormonal regulation of proopiomelanocortin gene expression in the pituitary. Ann NY Acad Sci 512:275–285

Roberts JL, Lorang D, Boutillier L, Lundblad JL, Dermer S, Salton SRJ, Loeffler JP (to be published) Characterization of the rat POMC promoter elements responsible for CRH stimulated transcription. J Biol Chem

Rotsztejn WH, Dussaillant M, Nobou F, Rosselin G (1981) Rapid glucocorticoid inhibition of vasoactive intestinal peptide-induced cyclic AMP accumulation and prolactin release in rat pituitary cells in culture. Proc Natl Acad Sci USA 78:7584–7588

Sabol SL (1980) Storage and secretion of β-endorphin and related peptides by mouse pituitary tumor cells: regulation by glucocorticoids. Arch Biochem Biophys 203:37

Schachter BS, Johnson LK, Baxter JD, Roberts JL (1982) Differential regulation by glucocorticoids of proopiomelanocortin mRNA levels in the anterior and intermediate lobes of the rat pituitary. Endocrinology 110:1442–1444

Schoenenberg P, Kehrer P, Muller AF, Gaillard RC (1987) Angiotensin II potentiates corticotropin-releasing activity of CRF_{41} in rat anterior pituitary cells: mechanism of action. Neuroendocrinology 45:86–96

Simard J, Labrie F, Gossard F (1986) Regulation of growth hormone mRNA and proopiomelanocortin mRNA levels by cyclic AMP in rat anterior pituitary cells in culture. DNA 5:263–270

Takakashi H, Hakamata Y, Watanabe Y, Kikuno R, Miyata T, Numa S (1983) Complete nucleotide sequence of the human corticotropin-β-lipotropin precursor gene. Nucleic Acids Res 11:6847–6856

Taleb O, Loeffler JP, Trousland J, Demeneix BA, Kley N, Höllt V, Feltz P (1986) Ionic conductances related to GABA action on secretory and biosynthetic activity of pars intermedia cells. Brain Res Bull 17:725–731

Therrien M, Drouin J (1991) Pituitary pro-opiomelanocortin gene expression requires synergistic interactions of several regulatory elements. Mol Cell Biol 11:3492–3503

Tremblay Y, Tretjakoff I, Peterson A, Atakly T, Zhang CX, Drouin J (1988) Pituitary-specific expression and glucocorticoid regulation of pro-opiomelanocortin (POMC) fusion gene in transgenic mice. Proc Natl Acad Sci USA 85:8890–8894

Uhler M, Herbert E, Deustachio P, Ruddle FD (1983) The mouse genome contains two nonallelic pro-opiomelanocortin genes. J Biol Chem 258:9444–9457

Vale W, Vaughn J, Smith M, Yamamoto G, Rivier J, Rivier C (1983) Effects of synthetic oCRF, glucocorticoids, catecholamines, neurohypophysial peptides and other substances on cultured corticotrophic cells. Endocrinology 113: 121–131

Warembourg M (1975) Radioautographic study of the rat brain and pituitary after injection of ^{3}H dexamethasone. Cell Tiss Res 161:183–197

Widmaier EP, Dallman MF (1984) The effects of corticotropin-releasing factor on adrenocorticotropin secretion from perifused pituitaries in vitro: rapid inhibition by glucocorticoids. Endocrinology 115:2368–2379

Yang-Yen HF, Chambard JC, Sun YL, Smeal T, Schmidt T, Drouin J, Karin J (1990) Transcriptional interference between c-*jun* and the glucocorticoid receptor: mutual inhibition of DNA binding due to direct protein-protein interaction. Cell 62:1189–1204

CHAPTER 16

Molecular Mechanisms in Proenkephalin Gene Regulation

N. KLEY and J.P. LOEFFLER

A. Introduction

Proenkephalin (PENK) belongs to a family of three genes encoding peptides possessing opiate-like activity. Expression of the PENK gene is developmentally regulated in a tissue-specific manner. Widely expressed during embryogenesis in mitotic cells (KESHET et al. 1989), its expression is progressively restricted upon terminal differentiation. The biological significance of this temporal regulated expression is as yet unclear. Although in the nervous system enkephalins are established neurotransmitters, one may also speculate on paracrine effects and growth factor properties of these peptides during development. In the adult organism PENK is expressed in tissues of different embryological origin: testis, adrenal medulla, and throughout the peripheral and central nervous system. In the latter, PENK is expressed in neurons and astrocytes (SPRUCE et al. 1990; SHINODA et al. 1989; MELNER et al. 1990).

The molecular mechanisms governing tissue-specific expression of PENK and its progressive restriction during development are not understood. However, regulatory mechanisms involved in adaptive changes in the expression of the PENK gene in terminally differentiated cells have been studied in detail and will be discussed in this review (see also Chap. 14).

Regulation of the expression of the PENK gene in response to extracellular stimuli is a complex, multistep process that ultimately leads to the production of bioactive PENK-derived peptides (for a recent review see KLEY et al. 1990). The cascade of events controlling gene expression include:

1. Reception and integration of extracellular signals (neurotransmitters, hormones, growth factors, etc.).
2. Subsequent activation of transducing mechanisms which generate second messengers (e.g., cAMP, Ca^{2+}, diacylglycerol inositol phosphates, arachidonic acid).
3. Activation of specific kinases that modulate DNA-binding proteins operating as transacting factors.

In this review we will report mainly on data obtained from simple "in vitro" models such as primary adrenal medullary chromaffin cells and established cell lines expressing the PENK gene.

B. Cellular Signaling Pathways Mediating PENK Gene Induction

I. Membrane-Associated Events and Second Messengers

1. Regulation of PENK Gene Expression by Electrical Activity and Ca^{2+} Metabolism in Excitable Cells

In adrenal medullary chromaffin cells membrane depolarization induced by low KCl concentrations or treatment with the alkaloid veratridine increases the bioelectrical activity by generating trains of action potentials. Chronic treatment with these agents results in elevated PENK mRNA levels (Siegel et al. 1985; Kley et al. 1986; Naranjo et al. 1986) and illustrates that PENK gene expression is linked to electrical cellular activity and is closely associated with secretory events.

Spiking activity is triggered by an initial increase in Na^+ permeability and is reduced by agents which specifically block voltage-sensitive Na^+ channels. Accordingly, treatment with tetrodotoxin (TTX) inhibits depolarization-induced PENK mRNA accumulation (Kley et al. 1986). A similar inhibition of depolarization-induced PENK gene expression is observed when Ca^{2+} flow into the cells is blocked with the Ca^{2+} channel blockers D600 and Co^{2+} (Kley et al. 1986; Washek et al. 1987). Thus Ca^{2+}, whose entry into the cells is enhanced as a consequence of increased electrical activity, appears to be the effective signaling molecule in this process of gene induction. That Ca^{2+} entry alone is sufficient to trigger PENK gene induction is indicated by studies showing that Ba^{2+}, which acts by increasing Ca^{2+} permeability (Hess and Tsien 1984), increases PENK mRNA levels (Kley et al. 1986). This effect is TTX resistant but, in contrast to secretory events where Ba^{2+} can substitute for Ca^{2+}, the effects on PENK gene expression are dependent on the presence of extracellular Ca^{2+} (Washek et al. 1987). Similarly, promoting Ca^{2+} entry by treatment with the Ca^{2+} ionophore A23187 leads to an increase in PENK mRNA accumulation (Kley et al. 1987a). These observations suggest that neurotransmitters or hormones which increase electrical activity and Ca^{2+} metabolism may lead to enhanced PENK gene expression.

Acetylcholine, originating from splanchnic nerve terminals located in the adrenal medulla, is the main physiological regulator of chromaffin cell activity. Early studies have shown that stimulation of nicotinic receptors increases PENK mRNA accumulation (Eiden et al. 1984) in a Ca^{2+}-dependent manner. Since acetylcholine increases electrical spiking activity in chromaffin cells (Douglas et al. 1967), the following model can be proposed: binding of acetylcholine to nicotinic receptors causes an influx of Na^+, membrane depolarization, and the subsequent opening of voltage-sensitive Ca^{2+} channels. The resulting increase in intracellular free Ca^{2+} then triggers PENK gene induction.

2. Cyclic AMP as a Regulator of PENK Gene Expression

The effects of cAMP on PENK gene expression have been evaluated by triggering an increase in intracellular cAMP levels by direct activation of the adenylate cyclase with forskolin or by mimicking such an increase using the stable and diffusible cAMP analogue 8-bromo-cAMP. Such treatments promote a strong rise in PENK mRNA levels (EIDEN and HOTCHKISS 1983; EIDEN et al. 1984; QUACH et al. 1984; KLEY et al. 1987). This induction appears to be mediated by a separate pathway than that used by Ca^{2+} since agents which promote Ca^{2+} entry (KCl and veratridine) do not increase cAMP levels in chromaffin cells (KLEY et al. 1987).

In the case of nicotinic stimulation of PENK gene expression, both pathways may operate. Although, compared with the level of cAMP generated by stimulation with forskolin, the rise in cAMP observed upon stimulation with nicotine appears rather marginal and is only transient in nature (EIDEN et al. 1984; KUROSAWA et al. 1976), it may be of physiological significance. In chromaffin cells cAMP promotes activation of Ca^{2+} channels (MORITA et al. 1987), increases Ca^{2+} entry, and may thus act to enhance and sustain the Ca^{2+} signal. The initial and transient increase in cAMP triggered by nicotinic receptor activation could mediate such an activation of Ca^{2+} channels. In such a scenario, distinct cAMP and Ca^{2+}-activated signaling pathways would have independent, additive effects on PENK gene expression on the one hand. On the other, early cross-talk at the level of the membrane would lead to a potentiation of Ca^{2+} entry and PENK gene induction.

3. Phosphoinositide Hydrolysis and PENK Gene Regulation

The role of phosphoinositide (PI) hydrolysis and stimulation of phospholipase C in PENK gene induction was first analyzed in the context of histaminergic receptors (H1-subtype) in chromaffin cells. Activation of such receptors produces a pronounced breakdown of phosphoinositides (NOBLE et al. 1986; KLEY 1988), thus generating two potential second messengers: inositoltrisphosphate (IP3) and diacylglycerol (DAG) (BERRIDGE and IRVINE 1984). Stimulation of histamine H1-receptors leads to a massive increase in PENK mRNA accumulation (KLEY et al. 1987b). This may result in part from an increase in intracellular free Ca^{2+} released from intracellular stores by IP3 (STOEHR et al. 1986). The signal generated by IP3 would then be relayed down to the PENK gene by mechanisms similar to those involved by an increase in extracellular Ca^{2+} influx as discussed above. In addition PENK gene induction may be mediated through DAG generated during phosphoinositide hydrolysis, a well-characterized activator of the Ca^{2+}/phospholipid-dependent protein kinase or protein kinase C (PKC, see below for further discussion).

In addition to mediating its effects through the direct activation of distinct intracellular targets (see below), Ca^{2+} may exert in part its effect via stimulation of the phospholipase C (PLC). It has recently been shown that an increase in Ca^{2+} influx through voltage-sensitive Ca^{2+} channels is associated with an increase in phosphoinositide hydrolysis (EBERHARD and HOLZ 1988). Thus multiple pathways may operate in the effects triggered by an increase in intracellular Ca^{2+}, which further extends the possible means of cross-talk among second messenger-activated pathways that play a role in gene induction.

II. Regulation of PENK Gene Expression by Third Messengers

Most of the physiological effects of cAMP are mediated by the cAMP-dependent kinase or protein kinase A (PKA). Gene regulation by PKA has been studied in great detail. It is now clear that cAMP acts by binding to the regulatory subunit of the PKA, thus promoting the subsequent release of the catalytic subunit in its active form (for a recent review see TAYLOR et al. 1990). As a consequence the catalytic subunit is translocated into the nucleus (NIGG et al. 1985), where it modulates the activity of cAMP-responsive genes through the activation of specific transacting nuclear DNA-binding proteins. In the case of the PENK gene it has been shown that introduction of a gene encoding a protein kinase inhibitor results in strong inhibition of cAMP-induced expression of chimeric genes containing the PENK gene promoter fused to a chloramphenicol-acetyl-transferase (CAT) reporter gene (GROVE et al. 1987; this strategy of analyzing gene activity will be discussed in more detail in the next section). In contrast direct activation of PENK-CAT fusion genes can be achieved by overexpression of the catalytic subunit of PKA. This has been observed for both chromaffin cells and primary striatal neurons (Barthel and Loeffler, unpublished observation). These studies directly demonstrate the fact that PKA regulates PENK gene expression and is probably responsible for the rise in PENK mRNA levels in response to physiological and pharmacological stimuli associated with an increase in cAMP levels.

The transducing mechanism by which Ca^{2+} leads to PENK gene induction is not as well understood. Two phosphorylating enzymes, the Ca^{2+}/calmodulin, and Ca^{2+}/phospholipid-dependent protein kinases have been dealt with as possible targets for Ca^{2+}-mediated effects. Little is known about the role of the Ca^{2+}/calmodulin-dependent kinase, the main reason being the lack of specific pharmacological tools to modulate its activity directly. It has, however, been shown that indirectly modulating its activity by using the calmodulin inhibitor W7 (the most appropriate agent available to date) results in a pronounced inhibition of depolarization-induced, but not basal, PENK gene expression in chromaffin cells (KLEY et al., unpublished observation) and PC12 cells (NGYUYEN et al. 1990). Though indirect, this suggests a possible role for Ca^{2+}/calmodulin-dependent kinase in mediating Ca^{2+} signals in electrically active cells.

More data are available on the role of protein kinase C (PKC) in the regulation of PENK gene expression. Treatment of chromaffin cells with the Ca^{2+} ionophore A23187 and the phorbol ester PMA has been shown to result in a synergistic activation of this enzyme (BROCKELHURST et al. 1985). Used at the same concentrations, A23187 and PMA result in a synergistic induction of PENK mRNA accumulation (KLEY 1988), suggesting a direct role for PKC in PENK gene regulation. As mentioned above, stimulation of chromaffin cells with histamine results in a stimulation of PI breakdown (NOBLE et al. 1986). Thus activation of PKC is likely to mediate this effect on PENK gene expression. This is supported by the findings that PKC inhibitor H7 and staurosporine prevent this induction (KLEY et al., unpublished observation). Similarly nicotinic stimulation has been reported to result in Ca^{2+}-mediated activation of PKC in chromaffin cells (TERBUSH et al. 1988), suggesting another role for PKC in relaying receptors mediating an increase in Ca^{2+} influx, in addition to the activation of PENK gene expression. However, in the latter case one may not exclude the operation of a coordinate parallel pathway mediated through Ca^{2+}/calmodulin protein kinase.

Although activation of PKC by phorbol esters in different cell types, including established cell lines, primary chromaffin cells, and striatal neurons, leads to a stimulation of the PENK gene, modulation of PENK gene expression by PKC may be more complex and include inhibitory effects. In chromaffin cells stimulatory or inhibitory effects of PKC on PENK gene expression depend on and vary with the state of cellular activity (KLEY 1988). Inhibitory effects of PKC could be traced down to an inhibition of voltage-sensitive Ca^{2+} channels and PLC. Treatment of chromaffin cells with phorbol esters was shown to inhibit depolarization-induced Ca^{2+} influx. This was associated with the ability of phorbol esters to inhibit KCl and Ca^{2+} channel agonist (BayK8644) induced rise in PENK mRNA levels. An inhibitory effect of PKC at the level of the PLC is supported by the observation that phorbol esters are able to abolish histamine-induced breakdown of phosphoinositides and increase in PENK mRNA levels (KLEY 1988). Thus, in addition to PKC playing a pivotal role as a stimulator of the PENK gene, it may function as an important feedback regulator in receptor- and depolarization-induced activation of PENK gene expression.

C. Mechanisms of PENK Gene Transcriptional Regulation

Two common processes are involved in regulating cellular mRNA levels: changes in specific gene transcription and/or alteration in the rate of degradation of the specific mRNA. Various approaches have been taken to study the role of such events in PENK gene expression and it is now well established that a major control point in the regulation of PENK expression occurs at the level of gene transcription. In the following section we will discuss several aspects involved in the coupling of cytoplasmic signaling events to the activation of specific transcription factors that associate with specific promoter elements mediating changes in PENK gene activity.

I. Transcriptional Regulation of the Endogenous PENK Gene

An initial indication of a possible involvement of transcriptional events regulating PENK mRNA levels came from studies by AFFOLTER et al. (1984) and SIEGEL et al. (1985) reporting a specific increase in nuclear PENK RNA precursor levels upon nicotinic stimulation and KCl-induced depolarization of adrenal medullary chromaffin cells in culture. However, in these studies only one major higher molecular weight band was observed on Northern blots, raising the question as to the nature of this effect. Indeed from these initial data it was not possible to rule out an effect on posttranscriptional events involved in the processing of nuclear PENK mRNA. However, in a later study a specific increase in multiple high molecular weight RNA species upon stimulation of chromaffin cells with the depolarizing agent veratridine was observed (FARIN et al. 1990). This overall increase in PENK mRNA precursor levels that are generated at different stages of hRNA processing indicates more strongly the involvement of a transcriptional effect.

A more direct approach to the study of transcriptional regulation of a gene is through the use of in vitro nuclear run-on experiments. This technique is based on the direct assessment of any changes in the levels of de novo synthesized RNA molecules. Using this approach it could be demonstrated that activation of PENK gene transcription in chromaffin cells is an early event in the response to nicotine and histamine stimulation as well as KCl- and veratridine-induced depolarization (FARIN et al. 1990). Following the decay of PENK mRNA levels in α-amanitin, an inhibitor of polymerase type II, treated cells revealed no apparent effect on the stability of the PENK mRNA (FARIN et al. 1990), indicating that increased gene activity is the major control point for the long-term induction of opioid peptide synthesis and release in chromaffin cells. It has recently been shown that in chromaffin cells induction of PENK mRNA levels by various stimuli is dependent on ongoing protein synthesis (FARIN et al. 1990). In this model this dependence is similarly manifest at the transcriptional level. Induction of PENK gene transcription by histamine is completely abolished by pretreatment with cycloheximide (FARIN et al. 1990), an efficient protein synthesis blocker. This indicates that de novo synthesized regulatory factors induced upon activation of the cells may be necessary for the subsequent PENK gene induction. Indeed the apparent start of PENK gene transcription is somewhat displaced in time compared with that of other genes induced under the same experimental conditions (FARIN et al. 1990). High levels of PENK gene transcription are reached after 2 h of continuous stimulation. In contrast transcriptional activation was readily observed after 30 min for the gene encoding tyrosine hydroxylase. Activation of the immediate early gene c-*fos* occurs even more rapidly, high levels being reached within 10 min of stimulation, an effect that also appears independent of de novo protein synthesis. This further underlines the specificity of the delayed induction of the PENK gene which requires the accumulation of critical factor(s) during a specific time window. In contrast, in a recent study GIRAUD et al. (1991) showed that PENK gene induction by cAMP and phorbol esters is independent of protein synthesis in cultured striatal neurons. A similar observation was made for C6-glioma cells (YOSHIKAVA and SABOL 1986). This difference may reflect tissue-specific differences in PENK gene regulation and suggests that the protein synthesis dependent induction of PENK in chromaffin cells may be rather an exception.

Using a different approach, WEISINGER et al. (1990) recently showed transcriptional regulation of the PENK gene in vivo. They showed that PENK gene expression may be regulated in a tissue-specific manner at the level of RNA start site usage. Determining PENK RNA start sites by using primer extension analysis, they identified four and two initiation sites in the rat brain striatum and adrenal medulla, respectively. A strong induction of start site usage was observed in adrenal medulla and striatum upon cholinergic and stress handling respectively. In addition a shift in specific start site usage in the striatum was suggested. Although these studies indicate a clear role for transcriptional events in PENK gene expression in vivo, the physiological significance of alternate PENK gene RNA start sites remains to be determined.

Another phenomenon of tissue-specific transcriptional regulation was reported recently by KILPATRICK et al. (1990), who showed that transcription of the rat and mouse proenkephalin genes is initiated at distinct sites in spermatogenic and somatic cells. In this instance, however, spermatogenic cell RNA transcription is initiated downstream of the well-characterized PENK somatic promoter in the first somatic intron. This region lacks TATA sequences and transcription may be directed by a second GC-rich promoter within the intron. This is reminiscent of previously described promoters that lack TATA sequences.

II. Gene Transfer Approach

Recent developments in molecular biology have made it possible to introduce foreign DNA into mammalian cells and to analyze the transcriptional regulation of specific genes, linking their promoters and regulatory sequences to reporter sequences encoding bacterial proteins such as -galactosidase and chloramphenicol acetyltransferase (CAT). Assay of the reporter gene products reflect the level of expression being directed by the regulatory sequences. CAT-vectors are the most commonly used, and levels of CAT activity are assessed by determining the degree of conversion of chloramphenicol into its acetylated derivatives (GORMAN et al. 1982). This approach has proven extremely useful in analyzing the cellular signaling mechanisms involved in gene regulation. Although one is not monitoring endogenous gene transcription by this approach, it is more practical and less time consuming than in vitro nuclear run-on assays and in addition provides the advantage of a possible delineation of the response DNA elements involved in signal transduction.

The first demonstration of PENK transcriptional regulation using chimeric constructs bearing 5'-flanking sequences of the human proenkephalin gene coupled to CAT was provided by elegant studies by COMB and collegues (COMB et al. 1986, 1988), who studied expression of the PENK gene either in transient transfection assays, while the DNA was still extrachromosomal (episomal), or after the PENK gene encoding plasmid was stably integrated into the chromosomal DNA. Using C6-glioma or CV1 cells they demonstrated a strong induction of PENK gene transcription by cAMP and phorbol esters. A similar induction by cAMP and phorbol esters was recently observed by GIRAUD et al. (1991) in cultured striatal neurons. In addition, VAN NGUYEN et al. (1990) showed that, in both transient and stable transfection of C6-glioma and PC12 cells, depolarization regulates expression of the PENK gene promoter. This induction was dependent on extracellular Ca^{2+} and inhibited by the Ca^{2+} channel blocker verapamil. These Ca^{2+}-mediated effects appear to be mediated by Ca^{2+}/calmodulin-dependent protein kinase as suggested by their sensitivity to the calmodulin inhibitor W7. These results are in line with studies discussed above concerning PENK mRNA and gene transcription in chromaffin cells. However, in both of the gene transfer studies (COMB et al. 1986; NGUYEN et al. 1990), induction of PENK transcription by phorbol esters and increase in intracellular Ca^{2+} levels were entirely dependent on the presence of agents that raise intracellular cAMP levels. In contrast, in cultured chromaffin cells no such requirement was observed (KLEY et al. 1986; WASHEK et al. 1987; KLEY 1988) at the PENK mRNA level. This difference between transformed PC12 or C6-glioma and primary chromaffin cells is unclear and may involve cell type specific differences in the activity of different components of the cAMP signal transduction pathway.

It would be interesting to test whether this difference indeed prevails in studies where the PENK-CAT fusion gene is transfected into primary chromaffin cells. Such a study has been much hampered by the lack of suitable transfection techniques applicable to postmitotic primary cells. BEHR et al. (1989) recently developed an efficient gene transfer protocol making use of lipopolyamine-coated DNA that is applicable to primary cells. The use of this transfection technique should offer an opportunity to analyze signal transduction events involving gene regulatory events in well-characterized primary cells that already express the endogenous PENK gene in a highly regulated manner. Indeed initial studies have proven this approach successful in cultured chromaffin cells (DEMENEIX et al. 1990; KLEY et al., manuscript in preparation).

In addition to the introduction of fusion genes to monitor transcription, the gene transfer approach may be used to address questions concerning intracellular regulators involved in signal transduction events leading to gene regulation. The feasibility of such an approach has recently proven successful in an analysis of the role of the c-*fos* oncogene in PENK gene regulation. In this study, expression of the c-FOS protein was specifically inhibited by the expression of c-*fos* antisense RNA (KLEY et al., in preparation).

A similar approach may be used to study second messenger pathways implicated in PENK gene regulation. Many pharmacological agents used today to inhibit protein kinase activities suffer from a lack of specificity. However, at least concerning the protein kinase A, the recent cloning of a full-length cDNA to the regulatory and catalytic subunits of protein kinase A offers the opportunity to directly test the role of this protein kinase in gene regulation. Thus, specific inhibition may be achieved by the introduction of mutated regulatory subunits that are able to bind to the endogenous catalytic subunit but are unresponsive to cAMP (MELLON et al. 1989). Such a scenario would result in a blockade of PKA-mediated stimuli. Indeed recent experiments using expression vectors encoding mutated regulatory subunit indicate a complete loss of PENK-CAT gene induction by cAMP in chromaffin cells and striatal neurons (GIRAUD et al., unpublished observation).

III. DNA-Responsive Elements

To understand in more detail the mechanisms underlying PENK gene regulation, COMB et al. (1986, 1988) studied in much detail the role for specific transcription factors and DNA sequences mediating transcriptional responses. Progressive deletions in the DNA extending through the control region mapped cAMP and phorbol ester regulatory elements to the region between -107 and -84. Further analysis defined two functionally distinct elements, ENKCRE1 (TGGCGTA) and ENKCRE2 (TGCGTCA), that are separated by one turn of the DNA helix within the enhancer.

Mutational analysis clearly demonstrated that both ENKCRE1 and ENKCRE2 elements are required for maximal cAMP and TPA transcriptional induction. Only very weak transcriptional activation is seen with ENKCRE2 alone. The cooperative interaction between ENKKCRE1 and ENKCRE2 may occur at the level of DNA binding or may be due to protein-protein interactions which enhance transcription. Several proteins bind to DNA in this region: AP1 (jun-A), AP2, AP4, and a novel factor ENKTF-1. ENKTF1 interacts with ENKCRE1 and is distinct from ATF/CREB transcription factors (known to be responsive to cAMP and phorbol esters and to bind to cAMP regulatory elements) as suggested by footprint competition experiments. In contrast, multiple factors bind to distinct DNA regions overlapping the ENKCRE2 element, AP1, AP2, and AP4. Analysis of mutants in vivo indicates that all these factors are likely to play major roles in the transcriptional regulation. In contrast to the ENKCRE1 element, ENKCRE2 oligonucleotide competes in vitro for binding of a factor binding to the VIP (vasoactive intestinal peptide) CRE. The VIP CRE also competes in vivo for transactivation of the PENK gene by cAMP (Hyman et al. 1988), suggesting that ATF/CREB transcription factors may be involved in ENKCRE2-mediated processes. Recently Van Nguyen et al. (1990) further extended the role for the ENKCRE2 element in mediating signal transduction events. They showed that depolarization-mediated activation on the PENK gene is conferred on the PENK gene by the ENKCRE2. Multiple ENKCRE2 elements conferred both cAMP and depolarization responsiveness on an inactive parent plasmid (pENKCAT 72). These experiments also indicate that multiple copies of one protein (or protein complex) bound in tandem can replace the protein/protein interaction between factors bound at ENKCRE1 and ENKCRE2 elements. Thus cAMP, phorbol ester, and Ca^{2+} responsiveness can converge on a single DNA element. This is reminiscent to the cAMP and Ca^{2+}-responsive element in the c-*fos* gene (Sheng et al. 1990). Interestingly c-FOS protein complexes with the product AP1 of the c-*jun* protooncogene, thereby potentially regulating promoters containing AP1-binding sites. Indeed, Sonnenberg et al. (1989) recently showed binding of FOS and AP1 complexes to oligonucleotides containing the ENK-CRE sequence and AP1 binding site. They suggest that FOS and AP1 may regulate transcriptional events at the PENK gene. These transacting factors may represent one set of proteins involved in protein synthesis dependent induction of the PENK gene. However, it appears that this is not a necessity. Indeed, Sonnenberg et al. (1989) were unable to find regulation of PENK by *fos/jun* expression constructs in fibroblasts where PENK has previously been shown to be efficiently regulated by cAMP an TPA (Comb et al. 1986). Furthermore, recent experiments using c-*fos* antisense expression vectors in chromaffin cells suggest that efficient downregulation of the c-FOS protein is not correlated with a significant decrease in PENK gene expression (Kley et al., unpublished observations).

Further upstream of the cAMP-responsive elements discussed above, Korner et al. (1989) recently identified a regulatory element that appears to bind the known transcription factor NF-kB and an apparently brain-specific transcriptional activator distinct from NF-kB, called BETA. At position 90 bp 5' to the TATA box the sequence GGGGACGTCCCC (E2) is found in the PENK promoter, which matches the classical NF-kB sequence (GGCGACTTTCC) in 9 of 11 nucleotides. Another similar sequence is found 40 bp further upstream (GGGGAGCCTCCG, E1). Both fragments bind BETA. Considerable amounts of BETA are present in brain extracts and appear to be gray-matter specific as suggested by comparative DNA-binding studies using BETA and NF-kB-binding oligonucleotide sequence GGGGACTTTCC. The findings that BETA-binding sites enhance brain-specific transcription suggest that these may be functionally important for neuronal regulation of the PENK gene. In contrast to BETA, NF-kB appears to play a role in lymphocyte-specific expression of the PENK gene. Upon activation with concanavalin A and TPA, T-helper cells have been shown to increase PENK mRNA synthesis (ZURAWASKI et al. 1986). Mutational analysis has shown that destruction of the B2 site (at −123 relative to cap site) results in a loss of PENK gene induction in these cells (RATTNER et al. 1991). The homodimeric form of NF-kB strongly binds to the B2 sequence in vitro, suggesting a direct role for NFkB in mediating PENK gene induction in T-helper cells. Whether NF-kB plays a role in other cell types remains to be established. Such a study is clearly of great interest as NF-kB is present in many cell types in an inactive form (exept in mature B lymphocytes) in which, upon a posttranslational activation step mediated by protein kinase C, it becomes active. The basis of this activation involves dissociation of an inhibitory subunit, termed IkB, from the DNA-binding subunit (BAEUERLE and BALTIMORE 1988, 1989). As PKC appears to be an important factor in the regulation of neuronally expressed genes, including the PENK gene, a role for NF-kB in the long-term induction of neuronal gene expression is of considerable interest.

D. Summary

In the course of studies performed in recent years, it has become clear that multiple-signaling pathways and tissue-specific transcription factors interact to fine-tune the expression of such highly regulated genes as the PENK gene. Interaction of these various systems enormously enhances the plasticity of gene regulation. Thus the specific regulation of a gene may not only be determined by the presence or absence of tissue-specific transcription factors, and their interaction, but also by the cell-specific interaction and cross-talk between second messenger signaling pathways. Application of classical molecular biological tools may further deepen our understanding of gene regulatory events. Thus DNA methylation at CpG dinucleotides may have profound effects on the binding of transcription factors and thus gene regulation. COMB and GOODMAN (1990) recently demonstrated this for the PENK gene. Methylation of CpG dinucleotide at an *HpaII* site in the AP2-binding site resulted in a strong inhibition of AP2 binding to the enhancer and inhibited both basal transcription and transcription induced by cAMP and phorbol esters. DNA methylation may represent a mechanism for introducing tissue-specific regulation of a gene, as tissue-specific methylation may result in displacement of a particular transcription factor and thus a variation in the combinatorial events involved in the regulation of the gene. A possible role of such events in developmental and tissue-specific expression of the PENK gene, however, remains to be determined.

References

Affolter HU, Giraud P, Hotchkiss AJ, Eiden LE (1984) Stimulus-secretion-synthesis coupling: a model for cholinergic regulation of enkephalin secretion and gene transcription in adrenomedullary chromaffin cells. In: Fraioli F (ed) Opiate peptides in the periphery. Elsevier, Amsterdam, pp 23–30

Baeuerle PA, Baltimore D (1988) IkB: a specific inhibitor of NF-kB transcription factor. Science 242:540–546

Baeuerle PA, Baltimore D (1989) A 65-kD subunit of active NF-kB is required for inhibition of NF-kB by IkB. Genes Dev 3:1689–1698

Behr JP, Demeneix BA, Loeffler JP, Perez-Mutul T (1989) Efficient gene transfer into mammalian primary endocrine cells with lipopolyamine-coated DNA. Proc Natl Acad Sci USA 86:6982–6986

Berridge MJ, Irvine RF (1984) Inositol trisphosphate; a novel second messenger in cellular signal transduction. Nature 312:315–321

Brockelhurst KW, Moritz K, Pollard HB (1985) Characterisation of protein kinase C and its role in catecholamine secretion from bovine adrenal-medullary cells. Biochem J 228:35–42

Comb M, Goodman HM (1990) CpG methylation inhibits proenkephalin gene expression and binding of the transcription factor AP2. Nucleic Acids Res 18: 3975–3982

Comb M, Birnberg NC, Seasholtz A, Herbert E, Goodman HM (1986) A cyclic AMP and phorbol ester-inducible DNA element. Nature 323:353–356

Comb M, Mermod N, Hyman SE, Pearlberg SE, Ross ME, Goodman HM (1988) Proteins bound at adjacent DNA elements act synergistically to regulate human proenkephalin cAMP inducible transcription. EMBO J 7:3793–3805

Demeneix BA, Kley N, Loeffler JP (1990) Differentiation to a neuronal phenotype in bovine chromaffin cells is repressed by protein kinase C and is not dependent on *cfos* oncoproteins. DNA Cell Biol 9:335–345

Douglas WW, Kanno T, Sampson SR (1967) Influence of the ionic environment on the membrane potential of adrenal chromaffin cells and on the depolarizing effect of acetylcholine. J Physiol (Lond) 262:743–753

Eberhard DA, Holz RW (1988) Intracellular Ca^{++} activates phospholipase C. Trends Neurosci 11:517–520

Eiden LE, Hotchkiss AJ (1983) Cyclic adenosine monophosphate regulates vaso-active intestinal polypeptide and enkephalin biosynthesis in cultured bovine chromaffin cells. Neuropeptides 4:1–9

Eiden LE, Giraud P, Dave JR, Hotchkiss AJ, Affolter HU (1984) Nicotinic receptor stimulation activates enkephalin release and biosynthesis in adrenal chromaffin cells. Nature 312:661–663

Farin CJ, Kley N, Hoellt V (1990) Transcriptional regulation of the proenkephalin gene in chromaffin cells. J Biol Chem 19116–19121

Giraud P, Rowalski C, Barthel F, Bequet D, Renard M, Grino M, Boudoure que F, Loeffler JP (1991) Striatal proenkephalin turn-over and gene transcription are regulated by c-AMP and protein kinase C related pathways. Neuroscience (in press)

Gorman CM, Moffat LM, Howard BH (1982) Recombinant genomes which express chloramphenicol acetyltransferase in mammalian cells. Mol Cell Biol 2: 1044–1051

Grove JR, Price DJ, Goodman HM, Avruch J (1987) Recombinant fragment of protein kinase inhibitor blocks cyclic AMP-dependent gene transcription. Science 238:530–533

Hess P, Tsien RW (1984) Mechanism of ion permeation through calcium channels. Nature 309:453–456

Hyman SE, Comb M, Lin YS, Pearlberg J, Green MR, Goodman HM (1988) A common *trans*-acting factor is involved in transcriptional regulation of neurotransmitter genes by cyclic AMP. Mol Cell Biol 8:4225–4233

Keshet E, Polakiewicz RD, Hin A, Ornoy A, Rosen H (1989) Proenkephalin A is expressed in mesodermal lineages during organogenesis. EMBO J 8:2917–2923

Kilpatrick DL, Zinn SA, Fitzgerald M, Higushi H, Sabol S, Meyerhardt J (1990) Transcription of the rat and mouse proenkephalin genes is initiated at distinct sites in spermatogenic and somatic cells. Mol Cell Biol 10:3717–3726

Kley N (1988) Multiple regulation of proenkephalin gene expression by protein kinase C. J Biol Chem 263:2003–2008

Kley N, Loeffler JP, Pittius CW, Hoellt V (1986) Proenkephalin A gene expression in bovine adrenal chromaffin cells is regulated by changes in electrical activity. EMBO J 5:967–970

Kley N, Loeffler JP, Pittius CW, Hoellt V (1987a) Involvement of ion channels in the induction of proenkephalin A gene expression by nicotine and cAMP in bovine chromaffin cells. J Biol Chem 262:4083–4089

Kley N, Loeffler JP, Hoellt V (1987b) Ca^{++} dependent histaminergic regulation of proenkephalin mRNA levels in cultured adrenal chromaffin cells. Neuroendocrinology 46:89–92

Kley N, Farin CJ, Loeffler JP (1990) Cellular signaling mechanisms regulating opioid peptide gene expression. In: Almeida OFX, Shippenberg T (eds) Neurobiology of opioids. Springer, Berlin Heidelberg New York

Korner M, Rattner A, Mauxion F, Sen R, Citri Y (1989) A brain-specific transcription activator. Neuron 3:563–572

Kurosawa A, Guidotti A, Costa E (1976) Induction of tyrosine 3-monooxygenase elicited by charbamylcholine in intact and denervated adrenal medulla: role of protein kinase activation and translocation. Mol Pharmacol 15:420–430

Morita K, Dohi T, Kitayama S, Koyama Y, Tsajimoto A (1987) Stimulation-evoked Ca^{++}-fluxes in cultured bovine adrenal chromaffin cells are enhanced by forskolin. J Neurochem 48:248–252

Mellon PM, Clegg CH, Correll LA, McKnight GS (1989) Regulation of transcription by cyclic AMP-dependent protein kinase. Proc Natl Acad Sci USA 86: 4887–4891

Melner MH, Low GK, Allen RG, Nielsen CP, Young SL, Saneto RP (1990) The regulation of proenkephalin expression in distinct population of glial cells. EMBO J 9:791–796

Naranjo JR, Mochetti I, Schwartz JP, Costa E (1986) Permissive effect of dexamethasone on the increase of proenkephalin mRNA induced by depolarization of chromaffin cells. Proc Natl Acad Sci USA 83:1513–1517

Nigg EA, Hilz H, Eppenberger HM, Dulty F (1985) Rapid and reversible translocation of the catalytic subunit of cAMP-dependent protein kinase type II from the golgi complex to the nucleus. EMBO J 4:2801–2806

Noble EP, Bommer M, Sincini E, Costa T, Herz A (1986) H1-histaminergic activation stimulates inositol-1-phosphate accumulation in chromaffin cells. Biochem Biophys Res Comm 135:566–573

Pruss RM, Stauderman KA (1988) Voltage-regulated calcium channels involved in the regulation of enkephalin synthesis are blocked by phorbolester treatment. J Biol Chem 263:13173–13178

Quach TT, Tang F, Kageyama H, Mocchetti I, Guidotti A, Meek JL, Costa E, Schwartz JP (1984) Enkephalin biosynthesis in adrenal medulla: modulation of proenkephalin mRNA content of cultured chromaffin cells by 8-bromo-adenosine 3'5'-monophoshate. Mol Pharmacol 26:255–260

Rattner A, Korner M, Rosen H, Baeuerle PA, Citri Y (1991) Nuclear factor kB activates proenkephalin transcription in T lymphocytes. Mol Cell Biol 11: 1017–1022

Sheng M, McFadden G, Greenberg ME (1990) Membrane depolarization and calcium induce c-*fos* transcription via phosphorylation of transcription factor CREB. Neuron 4:571–582

Shinoda H, Marini AM, Cosi C, Schwartz JP (1989) Brain region and gene specificity of neuropeptide gene expression in cultured astrocytes. Science 241:415–417

Siegel RE, Eiden LE, Affolter HU (1985) Elevated potassium stimulates enkephalin biosynthesis in bovine chromaffin cells. Neuropeptides 6:543–552

Sonnenberg JL, Rauscher FJ III, Morgan JL, Curran T (1989) Regulation of proenkephalin by *Fos* and *Jun*. Science 246:1622–1625

Spruce BA, Curtis R, Wilkin GP, Glover DM (1990) A neuropeptide precursor in cerebellum: proenkephalin exists in subpopulations of both neurons and astrocytes. EMBO J 9:1787–1795

Stoehr SJ, Smolen GE, Holz RW, Agranoff BW (1986) Inositol trisphosphate mobilizes intracellular calcium in permeabilized adrenal chromaffin cells. J Neurochem 46:637–640

Taylor SS, Buechler JA, Yonemoto W (1990) cAMP-dependent protein kinase: framework for a diverse family of regulatory enzymes. Annu Rev Biochem 59:971–1005

TerBush DR, Bittner MA, Holz RW (1988) Ca^{++}-influx causes rapid translocation of protein kinase C to membranes. J Biol Chem 263:18873–18879

Van Nguyen T, Kobierski L, Comb M, Hyman SE (1990) The effect of depolarization on expression of the human proenkephalin gene is synergistic with cAMP and dependent upon a cAMP inducible enhancer. J Neurosci 10:2825–2833

Washek JA, Dave JR, Eskay RL, Eiden LE (1987) Barium distinguishes separate calcium targets for synthesis and secretion of peptides in neuorendocrine cells. Biochem Biophys Res Commun 146:495–501

Weisinger G, DeCristofaro JD, LaGamma EF (1990) Multiple proenkephalin transcriptional start sites are induced by stress and cholinergic pathways. J Biol Chem 265:17389–17392

Yoshikawa K, Sabol SL (1986) Expression of the enkephalin precursor gene in C6 rat glioma cells: regulation by -adrenergic agonists and glucocorticoids. Mol Brain Res 1:75–83

Zurawaski G, Benedikt M, Komdb BJ, Abrams JS, Zurawaski SM, Lee FD (1986) Activation of mouse T-helper cells induces abundant proenkephalin mRNA synthesis. Science 232:772–775

CHAPTER 17

Proopiomelanocortin Biosynthesis, Processing, and Secretion: Functional Implications

E. Young, D. Bronstein, and H. Akil

A. Introduction

Peptide hormones and transmitters are synthesized as large molecular weight precursors, prohormones (Herbert and Uhler 1982; Steiner and Oyer 1967), which are processed intracellularly in neurotransmitter- or hormone-secreting cells to yield smaller active fragments. Within the structure of the hormone are processing "signals" that direct cellular enzymes to cut out or "cleave" the peptide hormones. Although the amino acid sequence of the prohormone determines the placement of processing signals, the particular signals recognized and consequently cleaved vary between types of cells. This cell-specific processing gives rise to different end products from the identical prohormone in different cells. It also results in biologically active sequences buried within the sequence of other end products in some tissues. In addition, different tissues can chemically modify the peptides posttranslationally, often producing substantial changes in the biological activity of the peptide products. All of the above variations can be combined to produce very different mixtures of biologically active products from different cell types. Finally, chronic activation of any cell may alter the mixture of secreted peptides, endowing these neurosecretory cells with a flexibility to meet the demands for one peptide hormone without shifting the homeostatic balance for its co-secreted peptide partner.

All of the above general principles are exemplified in the biosynthesis and processing of proopiomelanocortin (POMC). Of the three opioid peptide precursors, POMC is unique in that it contains only one copy of the opioid-defining amino acid sequence, Tyr-Gly-Gly-Phe-Met; this sequence is found at the NH_2-terminus of the opioid peptide, β-endorphin (βE) (Eipper and Mains 1980). POMC is also unique in containing other biologically active peptide hormones that are unrelated to opioid peptides. These other peptide hormones, adrenocorticotropin (ACTH), α-, γ-, and β-melanocyte stimulating hormone (α-, γ- and β-MSH), are part of the stress hormonal system (Mains et al. 1977; Nakanishi et al. 1979; Roberts and Herbert 1977). The presence of POMC-derived peptides in discrete CNS pathways related to antinociception as well as the pituitary gland, an integral component of the hypothalamo-pituitary-adrenal (HPA) stress axis, suggests that POMC may serve as a link between endogenous pain control and stress response systems in the body. Since POMC peptides are found in much greater abundance in the pituitary than in brain, and are present in two separate stress-responsive pituitary systems, i.e., anterior lobe corticotrophs and intermediate lobe melanotrophs, POMC systems in the pituitary have served as excellent model systems for studying POMC biosynthesis, tissue-specific processing, and posttranslational modifications (Eipper and Mains 1980, 1981; Mains et al. 1977; Zakarian and Smyth 1982a,b). The lessons learned from these peripheral model systems have been applied to brain systems, which appear to exhibit some of the features from both the corticotroph and melanotroph systems.

B. Tissue-Specific Processing

I. Anterior Lobe

Although structural similarities between ACTH and α-MSH were noted quite early (Orth et al. 1973), the isolation and characterization of pro-insulin was a leap forward in understanding that peptide hormones were synthesized in precursor forms which were processed to yield biologically active products (Steiner and Oyer 1967). In the case of POMC, the avail-ability of a mouse corticotroph tumor cell line (AtT 20) enabled several researchers to use both classical protein purification techniques (Mains et al. 1977) and molecular biological tools (Nakanishi et al. 1979; Roberts and Herbert 1977) to elucidate the structure of the mRNA for POMC and to demonstrate that ACTH, β-lipotropin (β-LPH), and βE were contained in the same prohormone precursor. By utilizing pulse labeling and pulse chase experiments in both AtT 20 cell lines and primary anterior pituitary cultures, Mains and Eipper were able to demonstrate a relatively rapid rate of synthesis (15–20 min for the precursor) and a rapid cleavage of this prohormonal molecule to β-LPH and a 22-kDa intermediate that con-tained ACTH (Eipper and Mains 1980; Mains and Eipper 1976). In normal anterior pituitary corticotrophs, the half-life ($t_{1/2}$) for this conversion is approximately 35 min (Shiomi et al. 1986). The work with the proinsulin model system had suggested that pairs of basic amino acids (lysine and arginine) served as the processing signal for a trypsin-like enzyme to liberate the biologically active peptide (Herbert and Uhler 1982; Steiner and Oyer 1967). This appeared to be the case with POMC as well, as production of β-LPH (the 93 amino acid peptide at the carboxy-terminal end of POMC) and a 22-kDa intermediate is the result of an initial cleavage at Lys-Arg residues at positions 170–171 in the precursor (see Fig. 1). Subsequently, cleavage at Lys-Arg pairs flanking both ends of the ACTH moiety results in the "liberation" of ACTH, the other principle active POMC product syn-thesized in anterior lobe corticotrophs. The N-terminal remainder of the precursor, a 16-kDa protein that contains the γ-MSH sequence, undergoes

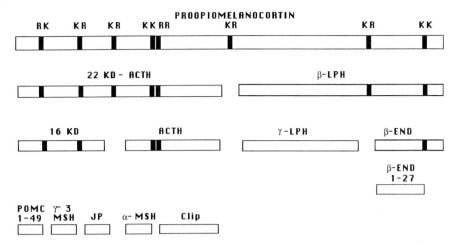

Fig. 1. Processing scheme for rat proopiomelanocortin. Processing of the prohormone occurs at paired basic residues of lysine (K) and arginine (R). In general, the anterior lobe corticotroph processes only the lysine-arginine pairs, while intermediate lobe melanotrophs and brain processes all the possible paired basic residues. See text for more complete description of tissue-specific processing. *LPH*, lipotropin; *ACTH*, adrenocorticotropin hormone; *END*, endorphin; *MSH*, melanocyte-stimulating hormone; *Clip*, corticotropin-like intermediate lobe peptide; *JP*, joining peptide

only limited further proteolysis, despite containing a Lys-Arg pair which, following cleavage, would produce a peptide of undetermined function known as "joining peptide" (EIPPER et al. 1986). In addition, a significant amount of βE is produced by cleavage of the Lys-Arg pair in β-LPH at amino acids positions 50 and 60 (EIPPER and MAINS 1980; ZAKARIAN and SMYTH 1982a,b). However, the conversion of β-LPH to βE is not complete, with rat anterior pituitary usually possessing β-LPH to βE ratios of 2:1 (EIPPER and MAINS 1980). Consequently, in corticotrophs of rodents, the principle end products of POMC processing are ACTH, β-LPH, βE, and a 16-kDa fragment. There are some species differences in the amino acid sequence of POMC, resulting in a second Lys-Arg pair within β-LPH that can give rise to β-MSH as well as βE in primate anterior pituitary (TAKAHASHI et al. 1983). It is important to note that describing these "final products" in the processing pathway does not necessarily imply that these are the preferred secreted end products of corticotroph activation. Since protein precursors are synthesized on the rough endoplasmic reticulum and then packaged into secretory granules for processing, estimates of the ratio of stored materials include the contents of a number of immature secretory granules which may not be representative of the products stored in the releasable pools of the corticotroph. In addition, these studies are carried out in vitro, removed from the influences of a number of stimulating factors such as corticotropin-releasing factor (CRF), arginine vasopressin (AVP), angiotensin II, and catecholamines, factors which activate both the cAMP and protein kinase C second messengers systems, which could impact upon biosynthesis and processing. Likewise, the inhibitory effects of glucocorticoids are absent in these in vitro systems. Thus, determining the peptides stored within a cell does not always reveal the peptide products which may be secreted from a cell. The interaction of processing with secretion, and the effects of stimulation and inhibition of corticotropin secretion on processing, will be discussed later in this chapter.

In addition to the typical cleavage of POMC at these Lys-Arg sequences, other chemical modifications are possible. In anterior pituitary, these main modifications are N- and O-glycosylation of the precursor, and phosphorylation of ACTH on the serine at position 31 (Bennett et al. 1981, 1983; Eipper and Mains 1982; Lennarz 1980; Seidah and Chrétien 1981). ACTH is also one of the sites of N-glycosylation within the POMC molecule (Eipper and Mains 1982). However, the functional significance of these modifications on the biological activity of ACTH is unclear. Finally, there is one other fragment of βE produced in the anterior lobe that does not involve cleavage between pairs of basic amino acids, but rather cleavage between Leu-Phe in positions 17–18 of βE. This cleavage produces γ-endorphin (βE_{1-17}), a weak opiate agonist. The terminal Leu of γ-endorphin can also be removed, giving rise to α-endorphin (βE_{1-16}) (Burbach 1984; Burbach et al. 1980, 1981; Burbach and Wiegant 1984; Smyth et al. 1979).

II. Intermediate Lobe

In the intermediate lobe melanotroph, additional modifications in POMC processing occur (Eipper and Mains 1981). In general, proteolysis is more complete than in the anterior lobe, i.e., smaller peptides are the result of POMC processing. In the anterior lobe, enzymatic proteolysis demonstrated a strong preference for Lys-Arg pairs, and failed to cleave the sequence of four basic amino acids (Lys-Lys-Arg-Arg) in the middle of ACTH. In the intermediate lobe, cleavage at the site of these four basic residues in ACTH liberates $ACTH_{1-14}$ and $ACTH_{19-39}$ (corticotropin-like intermediate lobe peptide; CLIP). $ACTH_{1-14}$ terminates with a Val-Gly sequence in positions 13 and 14 (Eipper and Mains 1980; Zakarian and Smyth 1982a); this sequence serves as the classic "signal" for amidation of the C-terminal Val, thereby converting $ACTH_{1-14}$ to $ACTH_{1-13}$ amide (Bardbury et al. 1982). Acetylation of this molecule ($ACTH_{1-13}$ amide) yields N-acetyl $ACTH_{1-13}$ amide (i.e., α-MSH) (Glembotski 1982b). These post-translational modifications appear critical for many of the biological properties characteristic of α-MSH. In addition to $ACTH_{1-14}$, the joining peptide found in the 16-kDa N-terminal region is also amidated (Eipper et al. 1986; Seidah et al. 1981). In the C-terminal region of the precursor, cleavage of the Lys-Arg site in β-LPH (positions 59–60) is virtually complete, releasing the 31 amino acid opioid peptide βE_{1-31}. In the intermediate lobe, βE_{1-31} is further processed by cleavage of the Lys-Lys sequence in positions 28 and 29, yielding βE_{1-27}, which in turn can be processed still further, to βE_{1-26} (ZAKARIAN and SMYTH 1982a). In addition to more complete processing at dibasic sites, cleavage of βE_{1-31} at the Leu-Phe residues (positions 17–18) is increased in intermediate lobe compared to the anterior pituitary, resulting in relatively more α- and γ-endorphin. C-terminal deletions of βE_{1-31} result in modifications of the opioid potency of the βE_{1-31} peptide. As will be discussed later, there is evidence to suggest that βE_{1-27} may function as an antagonist of βE_{1-31}, competing for binding sites at opiate receptors (AKIL et al. 1981a; SMYTH and ZAKARIAN 1980) and inhibiting a variety of behavioral and pharmacological effects induced by βE_{1-31} adminstration [e.g., (BALS-KUBIK et al. 1988; DEAKIN et al. 1980; HAMMONDS et al. 1984; NICOLAS et al. 1984)]. The same enzyme that acetylates α-MSH is believed to also act on βE fragments; thus, βE_{1-31}, βE_{1-27}, βE_{1-26} and α- and γ-endorphin all can serve as substrates for N-acetylation (BURBACH 1984; BURBACH and WIEGANT 1984). While acetylation increases the biological activity in the case of α-MSH, N-acetylation of any of the βE fragments renders them devoid of all opiate activity. The net result of all of the post-translational modifications which occur in the intermediate lobe is that very little authentic (opioid-active) βE_{1-31} is present in intermediate lobe melanotrophs (SMYTH et al. 1979; SMYTH and ZAKARIAN 1980, 1982; ZAKARIAN and SMYTH 1982a,b). Acetylated and nonacetylated forms of βE_{1-27} and βE_{1-26} are the predominant products synthesized from the C-terminal domain of POMC while α-MSH is the primary midportion product. In the NH_2-terminal, the 16-kDa fragment of POMC is processed into multiple forms of γ-MSH that have similar N-terminals but vary in the lengths of their C-terminal extensions (MEADOR-WOODRUFF et al. 1988).

III. Brain

The processing of POMC in the brain shows similarities to both the anterior and intermediate lobes of the pituitary. Region-specific differences in POMC peptide products may result, in part, from the existence of two separate POMC cell groups in the brain. Immunohistochemical and immunochemical studies have shown that the major POMC cell group is situated in the arcuate nucleus of the hypothalamus (BLOCH et al. 1978; BLOOM et al. 1978; WATSON et al. 1977, 1978a,b), with a much smaller cluster of POMC cell bodies localized in the nucleus tractus solitarius (NTS) region in the caudal medulla (JOSEPH et al. 1983; KHACHATURIAN et al. 1983, 1985; SCHWARTZBERG and NAKANE 1983). There is also recent data from our lab to suggest that some βE-containing cell bodies might be scattered caudally down the spinal cord (H.B. GUTSTEIN et al., in preparation). Lesion and deafferentation studies have helped to elucidate the nerve fiber projections of the arcuate and NTS POMC systems (AKIL et al. 1978a; JOSEPH and MICHAEL 1988; PALKOVITS and ESKAY 1987; PALKOVITS et al. 1987; PILCHER

and Joseph 1986). POMC soma in the arcuate project to a diverse number
of forebrain and midbrain structures including the amygdala, septum, periventricular nucleus of the thalamus, a number of hypothalamic nuclei, the
raphe nuclei, and the diencephalic and mesencephalic periaqueductal gray
(PAG). Presently, it is unclear whether there are subpopulations of POMC
cells within the arcuate which each project to distinct terminal fields or
whether some POMC soma send axon collaterals which reach all βE-ir nerve
terminal areas. The only study to address this question to date demonstrated
that there appeared to be a relatively selective innervation of the PAG by
POMC cells in the rostral portion of the arcuate (Yoshida and Taniguchi
1988). The caudal POMC system appears to have no ascending axonal
projections; rather, nerve fibers from the NTS project mostly within the
medulla itself and possibly into the spinal cord (Joseph and Michael 1988;
Khachaturian et al. 1985; Palkovits and Eskay 1987; Palkovits et al.
1987; Tsou et al. 1986). It should be noted that certain areas of the medulla
oblongata, including the NTS, probably receive some innervation from
POMC cells in the arcuate as well as the NTS.

The presence of POMC-derived peptides in the brain is not conclusive
evidence that these peptides are synthesized within CNS cells. Liotta et al.
(Liotta et al. 1980, 1984) first showed, using pulse-labeling techniques,
that de novo POMC biosynthesis took place in hypothalamic neurons. The
discovery of POMC mRNA in the hypothalamus provided further proof that
POMC peptides were synthesized within brain cells (Civelli et al. 1982;
Krieger et al. 1980; Pintar et al. 1984). More recently, POMC mRNA was
also detected in the NTS (Bronstein et al. 1990a), confirming the earlier
immunohistochemical data that POMC somata are localized in this brain
structure, and suggesting that de novo POMC biosynthesis also occurs
in the NTS. Interestingly, POMC mRNA has also been detected in a
number of brain regions (i.e., amygdala, midbrain central gray, cerebral
cortex, cerebellum) in which POMC cell bodies have not been immunohistochemically identified (Chen et al. 1984; Civelli et al. 1982; Pintar et
al. 1984). The size of the message in these areas appears to be 100–200
nucleotides shorter than that found in the pituitary, arcuate, or NTS, raising
the question of the nature of the protein that might be translated or whether
the shorter POMC mRNA species actually serves as a template for protein
translation. The possible functional significance of POMC message in these
brain regions remains speculative.

In general, the proteolytic cleavage of POMC precursor to smaller
peptides in the rostral arcuate system resembles the pattern observed in the
intermediate pituitary gland. Cleavage of β-LPH to βE_{1-31} is virtually complete in all rostral brain regions; furthermore, the presence of significant
amounts of βE_{1-27} and βE_{1-26} indicates that carboxy-terminal cleavage of
βE_{1-31} also takes place (Emeson and Eipper 1986; Gramsch et al. 1980;
Zakarian and Smyth 1982a,b). The extent of conversion of βE_{1-31} to βE_{1-27}
and βE_{1-26} is lower in regions such as the arcuate nucleus and PAG and

higher in the amygdala, hippocampus, and nucleus accumbens. Similar degrees of processing generally occur in the midportion and N-terminal domains of POMC. Thus, cleavage of $ACTH_{1-39}$ to $ACTH_{1-13}$ results in a predominance of α-MSH-like peptides (GRAMSCH et al. 1980), while the 16-kDa N-terminal region tends to be processed to 4-kDa γ3-MSH (MEADOR-WOODRUFF et al. 1988). In the caudal POMC system, cleavage of POMC tends to be less complete than in rostral brain regions (i.e., it increasingly resembles the anterior pituitary pattern of proteolysis). As one moves from the NTS down the spinal cord, the extent of processing is roughly inversely related to the distance caudal to the NTS. Thus, the relative proportions of high molecular weight forms of βE (e.g., POMC), β-LPH, and βE-sized molecules are $1:2.5:20$ in the NTS, $1:3:9$ in the cervical spinal cord, and $1:2:2$ in the thoracic spinal cord. In the lumbar and sacral regions of the spinal cord, there are approximately equal proportions of the three molecular weight forms of βE-immunoreactivity (βE-ir) (DORES et al. 1986; GIANOULAKIS and ANGELOGIANNI 1989; H.B. GUTSTEIN et al., in preparation). A possible explanation for the relative decrease in βE-size material as one moves caudally down the spinal cord may relate to the fact that some βE-containing nerve terminals in the NTS are derived from the arcuate cell group (JOSEPH and MICHAEL 1988; PALKOVITS et al. 1987). Since arcuate POMC neurons produce almost no POMC or β-LPH, they would strongly shift the relative amounts of different βE-ir species toward $βE_{1-31}$ size material. As one descends through the spinal cord, it is possible that the number of arcuate-derived fibers decreases and the observed pattern of POMC processing more accurately represents the population of NTS-derived POMC neurons. However, it is also possible that there are intrinsic POMC cells in the spinal cord which produce the unique set of βE-ir peptides observed in this tissue. We recently found preliminary support for this latter possibility; following spinal cord lesions, βE-ir was still detected in spinal tissue below the level of the lesion, suggesting that the peptides were not derived from cell bodies situated above the level of the lesion (H.B. GUTSTEIN et al., in preparation). In the NTS, α-MSH-sized peptides account for approximately 97% of the products of the midportion domain (i.e., $ACTH_{1-39}$ is a minor processing product in the NTS) (DORES et al. 1986). To date, there are no data available on the relative concentrations of ACTH and α-MSH peptides in the adult spinal cord.

While intermediate lobe-like POMC proteolysis is generally found throughout the extent of the rostral arcuate system, this is not always the case for post-translational modifications. For example, in some brain regions (e.g., the nucleus accumbens, hippocampus, dorsal colliculi), βE peptides are found primarily in acetylated states and α-MSH is either mono- or di-acetylated. In other areas, such as the hypothalamus, amygdala, or midbrain, only a small proportion of βE-ir peptides are acetylated; similarly, α-MSH is found predominantly in a nonacetylated state, i.e., $ACTH_{1-13}-NH_2$ (CHRÉTIEN et al. 1984; LOH et al. 1980; MILLINGTON et al. 1984; O'DONOHUE et al. 1979; TURNER et al. 1983; ZAKARIAN and SMYTH 1982a,b). Interestingly, in the NTS and spinal cord, acetylated forms of βE and α-MSH represent 50%–90% of the total immunoreactive content of these peptides (DORES et al. 1986; GIANOULAKIS and ANGELOGIANNI 1989; ZAKARIAN and SMYTH 1982a). Thus, within the same brain region, the pattern of precursor proteolysis resembles that found in the anterior pituitary while the extent of N-terminal acetylation parallels that observed in the intermediate lobe (CROMLISH et al. 1986).

C. Proopiomelanocortin Processing and Modifying Enzymes

One explanation for the existence of a variety of processing patterns is that different enzymes are responsible for cleavage of distinct dibasic sequences in POMC. Recent work by Dickerson and Mains (DICKERSON and MAINS 1990), using a simple peptide precursor with only one potential cleavage site, demonstrated clear differences between AtT 20 (a mouse corticotroph-derived cell line) and a growth hormone tumor cell line (GH3) in their preferences and completeness of processing different Lys-Arg combinations. Such simple model peptides can assist in understanding the basis of cell-specific processing; however, until the processing enzymes are isolated and cloned, it will be difficult to prove that different enzymes occur in different cell types. Several attempts have been made to isolate these processing enzymes. Loh's laboratory has isolated an aspartyl-protease from bovine intermediate lobe that processes POMC to produce a pattern characteristic of anterior lobe (Y.P. LOH 1986; Y.P. LOH et al. 1985) Cromlish has isolated a serine protease from porcine anterior pituitary, which processes POMC in vitro into a pattern resembling intermediate lobe processing (CROMLISH et al. 1986). Recently, Seidah and coworkers have cloned two closely related enzymes which are differentially distributed between anterior and intermediate lobe and appear to correctly process the midportion domain of POMC in a tissue-appropriate manner (SEIDAH et al. 1990, 1991; SMEEKENS and STEINER 1990; SMEEKENS et al. 1991). However, work with these enzymes is still at a very preliminary stage.

An enzyme responsible for the amidation of ACTH to α-MSH, peptidyl glycine α amidating monooxygenase (PAM), has been isolated (EIPPER et al. 1983; KIZER et al. 1986; MURTHY et al. 1986) and cloned (EIPPER et al. 1987; STOFFERS et al. 1989) by Eipper and coworkers. Although this enzyme is present in intermediate lobe and does succeed in amidating $ACTH_{1-14}$ in vitro, recent data suggest that the amidation of α-MSH is a two-step process involving enzyme activities from two different portions of the full-length PAM precursor (KATOPODIS et al. 1990; PERKINS et al. 1990; TAKAHASHI et al. 1990). The enzyme responsible for N-acetylation of α-MSH has not been isolated, nor is it clear if the same enzyme is responsible for acetylating both α-MSH and βE peptides in intermediate lobe (GLEMBOTSKI 1982a).

Cleavage of the N-terminal tyrosine destroys the activity of βE_{1-31} at opiate receptors (AKIL et al. 1981a); however, βE appears to be relatively resistant to amino-peptidase degradation (AUSTEN and SYMTH 1977; BURBACH et al. 1981). The major metabolic products of βE_{1-31} following incubation with brain synaptosomes are α- and γ-endorphin (βE_{1-16} and βE_{1-17}, respectively) (BURBACH et al. 1980, 1981). Both of these peptides still retain their opiate binding properties, but are less potent than βE_{1-31} itself (DE WIED and JOLLES 1990). A number of endopeptidase enzymes are capable of cleaving the Leu-Phe bond at positions 17–18 of βE, including cathepsin D, renin, endopeptidase 24.11, and a fourth enzyme described by Lebouille and colleagues as "γ-endorphin generating enzyme" (LEBOUILLE et al. 1984). Of the four enzymes which can cleave this bond, only cathepsin D and γ-endorphin generating enzyme are specific for this cleavage site. The distribution of γ-endorphin cleaving enzyme in the anterior and intermediate pituitary (LEBOUILLE et al. 1985) is consistent with it functioning as a catabolic enzyme for βE_{1-31}. However, the predominantly cytoplasmic localization of this enzyme is puzzling, given that βE processing and post-translational modifications take place within the secretory granules. Whether this enzyme is able to gain access to the secretory granule is unclear. The eventual isolation, cloning, characterization, and anatomical mapping of these putative dibasic cleavage enzymes, acetylating enzymes and amidating enzymes will contribute greatly to our understanding of the molecular basis of tissue-specific processing. It will also provide clues to how the cell can regulate end products that are secreted under ordinary circumstances and situations of increased demand.

D. Possible Functional Significance of Posttranslational Modifications to POMC-Derived Peptides

As described earlier, POMC cells in the pituitary and CNS process the POMC precursor in multiple ways to produce a variety of related POMC-derived peptides. While peptides from common domains may share immunoreactive features, their biochemical, behavioral, or pharmacological properties often are extremely different. For instance, there are at least six different βE-related peptides which are recognized by antibodies directed toward the midportion of βE_{1-31}; however, these peptides possess widely discrepant behavioral or physiological properties. These differences may be attributed in large part to the dramatic differences in the binding characteristics of various βE-ir peptides at opiate receptors – βE_{1-31} binds with high affinity, βE_{1-27} and βE_{1-26} have approximately tenfold lower affinities, and N-acetylated derivatives of βE bind with 1000-fold less affinities to opiate receptors (AKIL et al. 1981a). In addition, βE_{1-27} has been shown to be a more potent competitor of ^{3}H-βE_{1-31} binding, and a better antagonist of βE_{1-31}-induced analgesia than naloxone, the classical opiate antagonist (HAMMONDS et al. 1984; NICOLAS et al. 1984), suggesting that βE_{1-27} (and possibly other carboxy-terminal shortened forms of βE_{1-31}) may function as endogenous competitive antagonists of opioid activity. It has also been suggested that the selectivity for μ- and δ-receptors resides in different portions of the βE_{1-31} molecule, with the N-terminal enkephalin sequence having affinity for δ-sites and the C-terminal domain preferring μ-sites (LI et al. 1980b). The ability to proteolytically or chemically modify βE_{1-31} may function as a mechanism by which POMC cells physiologically regulate the amount and type (i.e., μ- or δ-selective) of opioid "message" released.

Despite our characterization of stored forms, defining the "true" end product in a POMC cell can be difficult. First, since the amino-, carboxy-, and mid-portion domains of POMC each contain at least one known biologically active peptide (i.e., γ-MSH, βE, and ACTH or α-MSH, respectively), one must decide whether one or more of the domains are producing the "true" end products. Furthermore, the same peptide may, under different conditions or in different tissues, be considered a precursor, an end product, or a degradation product (e.g., βE_{1-27} could alternately be viewed as a precursor for βE_{1-26}, a hormone or transmitter in its own right, or a degradative metabolite of βE_{1-31}). Should everything that is released from a cell be considered a transmitter or hormone or should that term only apply to substances with a known biological function? Is the most abundant stored form the "true" end product in a cell? Further complicating the task of defining the functional roles of POMC peptides is the possibility that the peptide products secreted may not always reflect what is stored within the cell, i.e., there may be peptide-selective release. This raises another set of questions, such as: Are there different types of releasable pools? Are there "rules" to judge which product will be released? Does processing take place before release, at release, or even following release? In brain, the nerve terminals containing synaptic vesicles which release the peptide products are anatomically distant from the cell body, the site of biosynthesis and processing, making it much more difficult to accurately define the relationship between peptide release and biosynthesis. In addition, one must keep in mind that the mix of peptides ultimately released depends upon the animal species, cell type, and physiological status of the cell (i.e., whether a cell has been recently activated or inhibited). All of these factors could greatly affect the ultimate message delivered to target receptors. The existence of multiple mechanisms to alter the mix of POMC peptide products released provides cells with a remarkable capacity to emit specific hormonal or transmitter information as a function of physiological demand. In the next sections, we shall describe selected examples which illustrate how regulation of POMC proteolysis and posttranslational modifications might be related to physiological functions.

I. Anterior Lobe

Studies on catecholamine systems demonstrated the existence of both releasable and nonreleasable pools from neurosecretory cells. While specific activation of these cells results in release of materials from the "releasable pools," nonspecific activation such as K^+ depolarization can result in the release of granules from both pools. If we examine the mixture of POMC peptides found circulating in plasma, we can gain some basic ideas of what products are released; however, some of the material present at rest may be "degraded" material carrying no specific information. Consequently, using specific challenges to the system to activate peptide secretion provides one means of examining the end products of prohormone processing.

In the rat and humans, acute stress or corticotropin-releasing hormone (CRH) activates POMC peptide release from anterior lobe corticotrophs (RIVIER and VALE 1983; WATSON et al. 1987; YOUNG and AKIL 1985). When we examined the released material in vivo, ACTH and β-LPH/βE were found in equimolar amounts. The ratio of β-LPH:βE was $1:2$, despite the predominance of β-LPH in the "stores" of anterior lobe corticotrophs. We then examined the anterior lobe corticotroph in vitro: at baseline the mixture of β-LPH:βE was $1:1$, but the addition of oCRH resulted in the release of less β-LPH relative to βE (i.e., β-LPH:βE ratio of $1:2$), the same as in vivo data with stress in rats or with CRH administration in humans (HAM and SMYTH 1985b; WATSON et al. 1987; YOUNG et al. 1986). Consequently, the evidence suggests that βE is the preferred POMC carboxy-terminal end product released from corticotrophs in response to specific challenges. However, not all investigators have replicated the in vivo rat data; at least one investigator reported more β-LPH than βE released following stress (DESOUZA and VAN LOON 1985). At the current time, there is no explanation for the discrepancy between these studies.

Are there different releasable pools for anterior lobe corticotrophs, i.e., an immediate release and then sustained release pool? Thus far, our comparisons between short and long stressors have not revealed differences in the ratio of β-LPH:βE released with 5 or 30 min of foot shock stress (YOUNG et al. 1986). Similarly when anterior lobes from rats which received footshock stress in vivo were challenged with CRH in vitro, the same ratio of β-LPH:βE release (i.e., $1:2$) was seen as in anterior lobe from unstressed rats (YOUNG et al. 1986). On the other hand, in frog intermediate lobe, different releasable pools have been shown for POMC products (Y.P. LOH and JENKS 1981). This underscores the tissue and species specificity of some peptide regulatory mechanisms. For example, in frog intermediate lobe, release-coupled processing has been demonstrated for α-MSH (VAUDRY et al. 1983). While this has not yet been demonstrated in mammals, we cannot exclude the possibility that a similar event occurs with βE release from anterior lobe corticotrophs.

What happens to the mixture of released materials with sustained demand? To examine the effects of chronic demand on processing, SHIOMI et al. (SHIOMI et al. 1986) conducted pulse-chase experiments in short-term anterior lobe cell cultures and determined the incorporation of radioactive leucine into the precursor POMC and the subsequent conversion of the precursor into β-LPH and βE. Following acute stress, the rate of processing of the precursor was increased in comparison to normal rats. However, following chronic stress, the rate of processing decreased in comparison to control rats, suggesting that the enzymes might be unable to keep pace with the increased rate of processing under situations of high demand. Do these changes in processing rates affect the products released from the anterior lobe? To examine this, we conducted studies with adrenalectomy as a model system of sustained corticotroph release (since removal of circulating glucocorticoids removes the inhibitory feedback signal which suppresses POMC peptide release). In adrenalectomized animals, the greatly elevated levels of β-LPH/βE immunoreactivity consisted predominantly of β-LPH (YOUNG 1989). In vitro data with anterior lobe corticotroph primary cultures that were exposed to continuous CRH led to similar conclusions: chronic CRH treatment resulted in proportionately more β-LPH release than "acute" treatment (HAM and SMYTH 1986; WAND et al. 1988), perhaps because the processing enzyme was not able to keep pace with the sustained demand for release or perhaps because sustained demand recruits a population of corticotrophs that, under basal conditions, are inactive. It is also possible that the biosynthesis of opiate-active βE_{1-31} must be maintained under tight regulation in order to protect organisms from potentially harmful or lethal amounts of this potent opioid. In any case, the cell or tissue appears to be able to select and change the preferred end product released under situations of high demand.

II. Intermediate Lobe

Are the lessons learned from anterior lobe applicable to intermediate lobe: Is the most processed form (i.e., βE in anterior lobe) the true end product? Can the end product change under situations of chronic demand? Do changes in end products result in changes in the messages encoded? As noted under the description of processing in the intermediate lobe, not only are smaller fragments produced, but chemically modified forms (in the case of βE, N-acytelated forms of βE) comprise most of the βE-ir. Although it is possible that a small amount of opiate-active nonacetylated βE is present and released from intermediate lobe, virtually all of the material released into plasma from the intermediate lobe is N-acetylated. In the intermediate lobe N-Ac βE_{1-27} comprises the majority of N-Ac βE-ir (50%–60%), N-Ac βE_{1-31} comprises about 30%–35%, and N-Ac γ-endorphin about 10%–15% (EIPPER and MAINS 1981; SMYTH and ZAKARIAN 1980). In vivo, certain stressors activate intermediate lobe release, with footshock and swim stress being two particularly good stressors for inducing intermediate lobe POMC peptide release (AKIL et al. 1985; PRZEWLOCKI et al. 1982; YOUNG 1990). Under basal conditions, N-Ac βE_{1-27} comprises the majority of N-Ac βE-ir in rat plasma. Following either footshock or swim stress, N-Ac βE_{1-31} is the primary species released (AKIL et al. 1985; YOUNG 1990). With repeated stress, N-Ac βE-ir increases by two- to threefold and N-Ac βE_{1-31} becomes the predominant molecular form stored in intermediate lobe. It also is the dominant form detected in plasma, even 24 h following the last stress session. With re-stress, N-Ac βE_{1-31} is again preferentially released into plasma (AKIL et al. 1985; YOUNG 1990). In this situation, it appears that the smallest products of processing (N-Ac βE_{1-27} and N-Ac βE_{1-26}) are not the preferred secreted end products. Although the accumulation in intermediate lobe and plasma of N-Ac βE_{1-31} may reflect an inability of the enzyme cleaving at amino acid positions 28–29 to keep pace with the demand for secretion, the preferential release of N-Ac βE_{1-31} with acute stress (e.g., swim stress) suggests that this form is somehow "selected for" among the various forms of N-Ac βE-ir present in the intermediate lobe. The physiological role of N-Ac βE_{1-31} is unknown, but, since it possesses an intact C-terminal, it may bind to nonopioid βE receptors (see HAZUM et al. 1979).

Another model to study the effects of increased demand on intermediate lobe functioning is chronic haloperidol treatment. Since the intermediate lobe is innervated by dopaminergic nerve terminals that exhibit a tonic inhibitory influence on N-Ac βE-ir release, administration of a dopamine antagonist, haloperidol, leads to increased secretion (BJORKLUND et al. 1973; HÖLLT and BERGMANN 1982; TILDERS and MULDER 1975). Chronic administration of haloperidol in rat leads to an increase in the larger molecular weight forms of N-Ac βE-ir according to some reports (HAM and SMYTH 1985a) although others have observed an increase in smaller peptide forms, i.e., N-Ac α- and γ-endorphin (AUTELITANO et al. 1985). It has been demonstrated that chronic haloperidol treatment leads to an increase in the *N*-acetyltransferase enzyme activity concomitant with the increase in peptide release and biosynthesis, suggesting that this enzyme is regulated in parallel with POMC biosynthesis (MILLINGTON et al. 1986; JENKS et al. 1985). Therefore, in the presence of haloperidol, chronic drive does not appear to alter the proportion of opiate active (i.e., nonacetylated) βE synthesized by intermediate lobe melanotrophs.

III. Brain

1. Central Analgesia, Tolerance and Dependence

In view of the dramatic and potent effects of exogenously administered opiates on pain perception in man, it is not surprising that endogenous opioid peptides have been implicated as modulators of nociceptive response (see also Chaps. 31, 41 in part II of this volume). While all three endogenous opioid families may ultimately be shown to be important antinociceptive agents, at this time the strongest case for an endogenous analgesic can be made for βE_{1-31}. First, administration of low doses of βE, either into the ventricles or directly into brain tissue, produces analgesia in a variety of nociceptive tests (i.e., tail-flick, hot-plate, writhing) (LI et al. 1980a; H. LOH et al. 1976). Second, focal electrical stimulation of specific brain sites, particularly the periaqueductal gray (PAG) region of the midbrain, produces an analgesic state in animals (MAYER and LIEBESKIND 1974; MAYER et al. 1971; REYNOLDS 1969). That endogenous opioids might be mediating this so-called stimulation-produced analgesia (SPA) was suggested by the finding that SPA was inhibited (though not completely blocked) by the opiate antagonist naloxone (AKIL et al. 1976a; M.H. MILLAN et al. 1986). Furthermore, tolerance to SPA's analgesic effects developed following repeated electrical stimulation (a phenomenon characteristic of chronic opiate treatment) and SPA and opiate adminstration exhibited cross-tolerance to each other, implying that both treatments acted via a common mechanism (MAYER and HAYES 1975; M.J. MILLAN et al. 1987). The discovery that βE-ir in CSF increased (AKIL et al. 1978b; HOSOBUCHI et al. 1979), while PAG concentrations of βE, but not other opioid peptides (i.e., dynorphin, enkephalin), declined following electrical stimulation (M.J. MILLAN et al. 1987) suggested that stimulation-induced βE release from POMC nerve terminals was involved in mediating analgesic responses. Further supporting this hypothesis are data showing that depletion of central βE-ir blocks SPA (M.H. MILLAN et al. 1986).

If βE-containing neurons are part of an endogenous antinociceptive system, an obvious question is: What are the physiological stimuli which engage this system? Available evidence indicates that stress may be an activator of central opioid pathways to produce analgesia (AKIL et al. 1976b; LEWIS et al. 1980; MADDEN et al. 1977). Following cold water swim or footshock stress, in vitro binding to opiate receptors was significantly reduced in a number of brain nuclei implicated in the modulation of pain sensitivity (CHRISTIE et al. 1981; SEEGER et al. 1984); presumably, this resulted from occupancy of receptors sites following stress-induced release of endogenous opioids. Some (AKIL et al. 1981b; M.J. MILLAN et al. 1981; PRZEWLOCKI et al. 1982; ROSSIER et al. 1977), but not all (BRONSTEIN et al. in press; MADDEN et al. 1977; PRZEWLOCKI et al. 1987), investigators have reported that βE-ir is reduced in the hypothalamus and the periventricular region of the diencephalon and mesencephalon immediately after acute exspoure to a stessor, consistent with the idea that stress-induced release of βE from nerve terminals might mediate opioid antinociception. Following repeated daily exposure to the stressor, POMC mRNA levels in the hypothalamus and midbrain levels of βE-ir increased significantly, reflecting adaptive changes in POMC biosynthetic activity in response to the recurring release of neuropeptide (BRONSTEIN et al., in press). The overall increase in βE production seems somewhat puzzling when one considers that re-exposing a previously stressed animal to another stressor no longer elicits analgesia (i.e., the animals have become tolerant). This paradox, of decreased analgesic response in the face of increased βE tone, can be explained by the fact that not all βE-ir species possess opioid properties. As mentioned earlier, there is good evidence to suggest that βE_{1-27} antagonizes the opioid analgesic effects of βE_{1-31} (DEAKIN et al. 1980; HAMMONDS et al. 1984; NICOLAS et al. 1984). Theoretically, there could be dramatic shifts in the relative amounts of opioid agonist (i.e., βE_{1-31}) and antagonist (i.e., βE_{1-27}) without any change in the concentration of total βE-ir. When we examined the different forms of βE-ir peptides in brains of stressed and control animals, we found that midbrains from repeatedly stressed rats contained approximately two to three times as much processed βE (i.e., $\beta E_{1-27}/\beta E_{1-26}$) as βE_{1-31}. When repeatedly stressed animals were restressed, the relative amounts of βE_{1-31} and $\beta E_{1-27}/\beta E_{1-26}$ returned to control levels, suggesting that the $\beta E_{1-27}/\beta E_{1-26}$ which had accumulated may have been selectively released following the new challenge. The parallel between the neurochemical data (showing that repeated stress exposure causes a large buildup of opioid anatagonist which gets preferentially released following acute stress rechallenge) and the behavioral data (tolerance develops to the analgesic effects of stress over time) suggests a possible role for βE processing events in the regulation of stress-induced effects.

We have recently discovered that alterations in βE_{1-31} processing may also be involved in mechanisms of morphine tolerance and/or dependence. The available evidence suggests that chronic morphine treatment inhibits βE release from hypothalamic neurons and negatively feeds-back upon endogenous POMC biosynthesis (BRONSTEIN et al. 1990b; MOCHETTI and COSTA 1986; MOCHETTI et al. 1989). Initially, βE-ir accumulates in the hypothalamus, presumably as a result of normal biosynthesis and decreased peptide release; with more prolonged opiate treatment, overall biosynthetic activity becomes downregulated, via reductions in POMC mRNA levels, to compensate for the reduced rate of βE release. Similar to the situation with repeated stress, the composition of βE-ir peptides which accumulates in the hypothalamus during the initial days of morphine treatment shows a shift toward more processed forms (i.e., there is proportionately more $\beta E_{1-27}/\beta E_{1-26}$ relative to βE_{1-31}). This may be due to a decrease in βE-ir release and, consequently, a longer period of storage in secretory granules, giving more time for the "slower" cleavage enzyme(s) to act at their appropriate sites. Thus, even though overall βE-ir peptide levels increase, there is a net decrease in the amount of opioid activity. The increase in the concentration $\beta E_{1-27}/\beta E_{1-26}$ could play a role in the development of tolerance to many of morphine's effects. It is possible that βE_{1-27}, which antagonizes opioid properties of $\beta E1-31$, also competitively antagonizes morphine's effects, which would result in decreased efficacy for a constant dose of morphine (i.e., tolerance). In addition, some withdrawal symptoms which develop with the cessation of morphine treatment may be related to a decrease in β-endorphinergic opioid tone. At early stages of opiate treatment, there is a relative increase in the endogenous antagonist βE_{1-27} while at later stages POMC mRNA levels decline. It is possible that reduced activation of opiate receptors at β-endorphinergic synapses contributes, in part, to the classical symptomology of the withdrawal syndrome.

2. Reinforcement

The idea that endogenous opioids might function as part of a reward or reinforcement system in brain arose shortly after the discovery of the enkephalins and has acquired considerable experimental support since that time (see also Chaps. 55, 56, in part II of this volume). The basic tenet of this hypothesis is that opioids are released under conditions of euphoria and well-being and act as positive reinforcers to reduce drive states. Evidence supporting this hypothesis comes from a variety of sources. Rats will self-administer βE (VAN REE et al. 1979) or enkephalins (BELLUZZI and STEIN 1977) directly into the ventricles and exhibit a conditioned place preference for environments associated with intraventricular βE injections (AMALRIC et al. 1987). Behaviors which are considered to be rewarding (e.g., intracranial electrical stimulation, appetitive behaviors) are increased by administration of opiate agonists and suppressed by opiate antagonists (BELLUZI and STEIN 1977; LOWY et al. 1980, 1981; TRUJILLO et al. 1989). A more direct role for central βE-ir peptides is suggested by the finding that, in rats given highly palatable food, hypothalamic concentrations of βE-ir, but not dynorphin-ir, decreased, at the same as the in vivo occupancy of opiate receptors appeared to increase (DUM et al. 1983). Thus, anticipation of highly palatable food appears to induce βE-ir release from nerve terminals in the hypothalamus which subsequently binds to opiate receptors.

Analogous to its effects on central analgesia, βE_{1-27} may function as an endogenous opioid antagonist of the reinforcing properties of opioid agonists. Whereas intraventricular administration of βE_{1-27} by itself had no effect on place preferences of animals, coinjection of βE_{1-27} with βE_{1-31} abolished the place preference produced by injection of βE_{1-31} alone (BALS-KUBIK et al. 1988). In addition, the place preference induced by intraventricular administration βE_{1-31} was completely blocked by co-administration of selective μ- or δ-receptor antagonists, suggesting that the reinforcing actions of βE_{1-31} might be mediated by μ- and δ-opioid receptors (BALS-KUBIK et al. 1990). Regardless of the receptor subtype with which βE_{1-31} interacts, C-terminal cleavage to βE_{1-27} may serve as a regulatory mechanism to alter opioid agonistic/antagonistic concentrations at neural synapses involved in motivational responses.

3. Autonomic Functions

The distribution of opioid peptides and receptors in the brainstem and hypothalamus suggests a key role in autonomic regulation, including cardiovascular, respiratory, and sympathetic responses (see Chap. 42, in part II of this volume). The effects of opioids on cardiovascular regulation are complex and depend on the specific brain region affected. For example, morphine or opioid peptide administration can either increase or decrease heart rate and blood pressure, depending on the injection site and the presence or absence of anesthetics (HOLADAY 1983). In addition, there are a number of cardiovascular reflexes such as the baroreceptor reflex which link blood pressure and heart rate and compensate for the effects of opiates on either system. This makes it difficult to use studies on exogenously administered opiates to understand the role of opioid peptides in normal physiology. Keeping in mind these limitations, there is some evidence to suggest that processing of βE_{1-31} to N-acetylated or C-terminal shortened forms may be a physiologically relevant mechanism involved in the regulation of autonomic function. Injections of βE_{1-27} into the cisterna magna of the brainstem reduced mean arterial blood pressure more potently than β_{1-31} while C-terminal proteolysis of βE_{1-27} (to βE_{1-26}), or N-acetylation of either βE_{1-31} or βE_{1-27}, abolished any hemodynamic effects (HIRSCH et al. 1988). Similarly, intraventricular injections of either βE_{1-31} or βE_{1-27} reversed physostigmine-induced increases in blood pressure (HONG and JHAMANDAS 1989). Intriguingly, these authours found that human, but not ovine, βE_{1-27} reversed physostigmine's effects, suggesting that the tyrosine in position 27 of human βE may be critical for cardiovascular function, since replacement of residue 27 with a histidine, as in the ovine βE sequence, seems to abolish its activity. Taken together, these results suggest that, whereas βE_{1-27} may function as an opioid antagonist in analgesic responses, it appears to act as a potent opioid agonist in brainstem autonomic responses. This discrepancy in functional effects may be related to a differential distribution of opiate receptors subtypes with which βE_{1-27} might interact. In this regard, it would be interesting to determine whether βE_{1-27} has agonist or antagonist properties on the opioid-mediated analgesia elicited by electrical stimulation in the NTS (see (LEWIS et al. 1987)).

βE-ir peptides in the caudal medulla may also be involved in regulating the sympathetic outflow to the adrenal medulla and peripheral sympathetic nerve terminals. Intracisternal injections of βE_{1-31} in conscious rats increased plasma concentrations of the three catecholamines, dopamine, norepinephrine, epinephrine, in a dose-dependent manner and these effects were blocked by pretreatment with naloxone (VAN LOON et al. 1981a,b). More detailed examination has revealed that βE_{1-31} elicits predominantly norepinephrine release whereas βE_{1-27} preferentially elevates epinephrine release (HIRSCH et al. 1990). This implies that βE_{1-31} may be more important in regulating release from sympathetic nerve terminals while βE_{1-27} may be more intimately involved in adrenal medullary responses. These data again illustrate how the conversion of βE_{1-31} to βE_{1-27} may produce a qualitatively different effect on autonomic function.

Classically, opiate alkaloids have been known to act as respiratory depressants, and opioid peptides injected intracisternally or peripherally mimic these respiratory depressant actions (HOLADAY and LOH 1981; Moss and FRIEDMAN 1978; SAPRU et al. 1981). There are speculations that endogenous opioids may be involved in the pathophysiology of respiratory diseases such as sudden infant death syndrome (SIDS), asthma, and chronic obstructive pulmonary disease in adults (HOLADAY 1985). However, it is not known whether opioid peptide concentrations increase in any of these diseases and consequently these speculations await supportive experimental data. The possible significance of βE_{1-31} proteolysis or acetylation vis-a-vis regulation of respiratory function also remains to be determined.

IV. Immune System

Opioid peptides may be involved in the regulation of the immune system. While the literature is confusing, there is evidence that opioids can modulate immune response by actions at central sites or by direct interaction with cells of the immune system (see Chaps. 34, 45, in part II of this volume). By using a morphine analogue which does not cross the blood-brain barrier, Shavit and coworkers (SHAVIT et al. 1986) showed that morphine acts at central opiate receptors to suppress natural killer cell (NK) activity. Endogenous opioids appear to have similar effects since exposure to inescapable footshock, which elicits opioid-mediated analgesia, suppresses NK activity and reduces the survival time of rats exposed to mammary ascites tumors (LEWIS et al. 1983, 1985) and this effect is blocked by administration of the opiate antagonist naltrexone (SHAVIT et al. 1984, 1985). Stressors which produced equipotent, but non-opioid-mediated, analgesia had no effect on NK activity. Data from lesion studies suggest that opioid-containing cells in the hypothalamus may be at least one brain site important for mediating stress-induced effects on NK activity (FORNI et al. 1983). At the present time, the possible role of βE-ir or other opioid peptides in stress-induced immunosuppression has not been established.

In addition to possible effects in the CNS, βE-ir peptides derived from the pituitary gland or immune system compartments may also modulate immune function. The detection of POMC mRNA and POMC-derived peptides in different components of the immune system (e.g., the thymus, spleen, leukocytes, lymphocytes) suggests that immune-related cells are capable of synthesizing βE-ir peptides (LAGAZE-MASMONTEI et al. 1987; LOLAIT et al. 1984, 1986; SMITH and BLALOCK 1981). However, the POMC mRNA found in B-cell lymphocytes resembles that found in reproductive organs, i.e., it is roughly 200 bases shorter than the POMC message in the pituitary gland or arcuate nucleus (OATES et al. 1988), raising doubts about whether this shortened mRNA species gets translated into functional POMC protein. It is also contentious whether POMC mRNA is expressed basally in splenocytes (LOLAIT et al. 1986) or is induced only following viral infection (WESTLY et al. 1986). The available data are consistent with a role for immune system-derived βE-ir peptides in the modulation of immune function, although the apparently low levels of POMC biosynthesis in immune-related cells would suggest a local, as opposed to hormonal, site of action.

There is evidence that βE-ir peptides affect immune responses via opiate- and non-opiate-receptor mechanisms. The potent opioid $βE_{1-31}$ is the major βE-ir species in the spleen (LOLAIT et al. 1986) and classical opioid receptors have been found on phagocytic leukocytes and lymphocytes (LOPKER et al. 1980; WYBRAN et al. 1979). In contrast to its purported suppressive effects in the CNS, several laboratories have reported that $βE_{1-31}$ enhances NK activity in vitro in a naloxone-reversible manner (MANDLER et al. 1986; MATHEWS et al. 1983). In addition, βE and the enkephalins have been shown to stimulate the mitogenic responses of T-cell lymphocytes (PLOTNIKOFF and MILLER 1983; WYBRAN et al. 1979). These data support a role for opioid receptor-mediated enhancement of immune responses. However, lymphocytes also possess nonopiate βE-specific receptors which recognize the C-terminus of $βE_{1-31}$ (HAZUM et al. 1979). It is tempting to contemplate the functional role of these receptors when one considers that approximately half of all βE-ir peptides in spleen are acetylated (LOLAIT et al. 1986) and do not bind to classical opioid receptors. βE has been shown to enhance the proliferative responses of rat T-lymphocytes to mitogens in a manner not reversible by naloxone and not mimicked by $βE_{1-16}$ (GILMAN et al. 1982), suggesting a possible functional role for the nonopioid, βE-specific receptor in modulating lymphocyte function. βE C-terminus-specific receptors have also been found in the terminal complexes of human complement (SCHWEIGERER et al. 1982) and several neuroblastoma cells (WESTPHAL and LI 1984a,b), although the possible significance of these findings in regard to immune function is at present unknown. In summary, βE-related peptides are capable of affecting various aspects of immune function through both classic opiate receptors and nonopiate, C-terminus-specific receptors. Modifications to $βE_{1-31}$ could alter functional effects in several ways: acetylation of the N-terminal tyrosine of βE would abolish binding to the opiate receptor but not affect binding to the C-terminal receptor; conversely, C-terminal cleavage of $βE_{1-31}$ would reduce affinity for the opiate receptor but would most likely eliminate binding at the nonopiate receptor. Thus, the net effect on immune function may depend on the precise mix of $βE_{1-31}$ processed products.

E. Conclusion

Polyprotein precursors can give rise to a number of different end products having different biological activities. In the case of POMC, these end products include both opioid (βE) and nonopioid (ACTH and α-MSH) peptides. Different mixtures of end products are produced and secreted, depending on the tissue examined and the physiological status of the cell. The present review focuses on changes in proteolysis and posttranslational modifications that affect the opioid portion of POMC, i.e., the βE_{1-31} molecule. Under normal circumstances, βE_{1-31} appears to be an important end product released from both the brain and the pituitary gland. In comparison to the other opioid peptides, βE is relatively resistant to degradation, either in the brain or in plasma. This stability accounts, in part, for its profound opioid effects in vivo. Findings reviewed in this chapter suggest that POMC systems may regulate the amount of opioid "signal" produced by altering the proteolysis and/or posttranslational modifications of βE-ir peptides. In three different POMC systems, we have shown that, following sustained demand, there appears to be a shift toward nonopioid forms of βE. In the anterior pituitary, this shift results in a greater release of β-LPH, which is opiate inactive. In the intermediate lobe, where the vast majority of βE peptides are N-acetylated, and therefore opioid-inactive, N-acetyltransferase activity increases under situations of chronic demand. In the hypothalamus and midbrain, βE_{1-27}, which is believed to act as an endogenous antagonist of βE_{1-31}-induced analgesia and reinforcement, appears to be preferentially synthesized and released under certain circumstances. The consistent effect of all these modifications, i.e., to proportionately decrease the amount of opioid-active product, suggests that the opioid properties of βE_{1-31} must be tightly controlled since pain and pain responsiveness serve as critical cues in preventing harm to an organism. For example, it is advantageous for an organism to closely regulate the opioid signal in cardiovascular systems since, if left unchecked, it would lead to death. It should be noted that alternations in βE processing may not always be driven by the need to maintain opioid levels within a narrow range. In different cells, the "true" end product of POMC processing may not be the opioid peptide βE_{1-31}. For example, βE_{1-27} has potent effect on cardiovascular responses, which in some cases are more potent, or qualitatively different than, βE_{1-31}'s effects. In the immune system, the presence of nonopiate, βE-specific receptors suggests that βE peptides other than βE_{1-31} may play important roles in modulating immune response. In these systems, regulating the processing of POMC to βE-ir peptide products may serve to produce a set of signals having different biological funcations. The ability to regulate POMC protelysis and posttranslational modifications, thereby altering the end products produced and secreted, imbues these cells with a remarkable capacity to adapt and respond to a diversity of challenges.

References

Akil H, Mayer DJ, Liebeskind JC (1976a) Antagonism of stimulation-produced analgesia by naloxone, a narcotic antagonist. Science 191:961

Akil H, Madden J, Patrick RL, Barchas JD (1976b) Stress-induced increase in endogenous opiate peptides: concurrent analgesia and its partial reversal by naloxone. In: Kosterlitz HW (ed) Opiates and endogenous opioid peptides. Elsevier, Amsterdam, p 63

Akil H, Watson SJ, Berger PA, Barchas JD (1978a) Endorphins, beta-lipotropin and ACTH: biochemical, pharmacological and anatomical studies. In: Trabucchi M, Costa E (eds) The endorphins: advances in biochemistry and psychopharmacology. Raven, New York, p 125

Akil H, Richardson DE, Barchas JD, Li CH (1978b) Appearance of beta-endorphin-like immunoreactivity in human ventricular cerebrospinal fluid upon analgesic electrical stimulation. Proc Natl Acad Sci USA 75:5170

Akil H, Young E, Watson SJ, Coy D (1981a) Opiate binding properties of naturally occurring N- and C-terminus modified beta-endorphin. Peptides 2:289

Akil H, Ueda Y, Lin H-L, Lewis JW, Walker JM, Shiomi H, Liebeskind JC, Watson SJ (1981b) Multiple forms of beta-endorphin (βE) in pituitary and brain: effects of stress. In: Takagi H, Simon E (eds) Advances in endogenous and exogenous opioids. Kodansha, Tokyo, p 116

Akil H, Shiomi H, Matthews J (1985) Induction of the intermediate pituitary by stress: synthesis and release of a nonopiod form of beta-endorphin. Science 227:424

Amalric M, Cline EJ, Martinez JL Jr, Bloom FE, Koob GF (1987) Rewarding properties of B-endorphin as measured by conditioned place preference. Psychopharmacology 91:14

Austen BM, Smyth DG (1977) The NH$_2$-terminus of C-fragment is resistant to the action of aminopeptidases. Biochem Biophys Res Commun 76:477

Autelitano DJ, Smith AI, Lolait SJ, Funder JW (1985) Dopaminergic agents differentially alter beta-endorphin processing patterns in the rat pituitary neurointermediate lobe. Neurosci Lett 59:141

Bals-Kubik R, Herz A, Shippenberg TS (1988) β-endorphin-(1–27) is a naturally occurring antagonist of the reinforcing effects of opioids. Naunyn Schmiedebergs Arch Pharmacol 338:392

Bals-Kubik R, Shippenberg TS, Herz A (1990) Involvement of central µ and δ opioid receptors in mediating the reinforcing effects of β-endorphin in the rat. Eur J Pharmacol 175:63

Belluzzi JD, Stein L (1977) Enkephalins may mediate euphoria and drive-reduction reward. Nature 266:556

Bennett HPJ, Browne CA, Solomon S (1981) Biosynthesis of phosphorylated forms of corticotropin related peptides. Proc Natl Acad Sci USA 78:4713

Bennett HPJ, Brubacker PL, Seger MA, Solomon S (1983) Human phosphoserine 31 corticotropin 1–39: isolation and characterization. J Biol Chem 258:8108

Bjorklund A, Moore RV, Nobin A, Stenevi U (1973) The organization of tubero-hypophyseal and reticulo-infundibular catecholamine neuron systems in the rat brain. Brain Res 51:171

Bloch B, Bugnon C, Fellman D, Lenys D (1978) Immunocytochemical evidence that the same neurons in the human infundibular nucleus are stained with anti-endorphins and antisera of other related peptides. Neurosci Lett 10:147

Bloom F, Battenberg E, Rossier J, Ling N, Guillemin R (1978) Neurons containing beta-endorphin in rat brain exist separately from those containing enkephalin: immunocytochemical studies. Proc Natl Acad Sci USA 75:1591

Bradbury AF, Finnie MDA, Smyth DG (1982) Mechanisms of C-terminal amide formation by pituitary enzymes. Nature 198:686

Bronstein DM, Schafer MKH, Trujillo KA, Watson SJ, Akil H (1990a) Pro-opiomelanocortin (POMC) mRNA in the nucleus tractus solitarius and other extrahypothalamic brain regions. Soc Neurosci Abstr 16:1026

Bronstein DM, Przewlocki R, Akil H (1990b) Effects of morphine treatment on proopiomelanocortin systems in rat brain. Brain Res 519:102

Bronstein DM, Kelsey JE, Akil H. Regulation of β-endorphin biosynthesis in the brain: different effects of morphine pelleting and repeated stress. In: Molecular approaches to drug abuse research. US Department of Health and Human Services (in press)

Burbach JPH (1984) Action of proteolytic enzymes on lipotropins and endorphins: biosynthesis, biotransformation and fate. Pharmacol Ther 24:321

Burbach JPH, Wiegant VM (1984) Isolation and characterization of α-endorphin and γ-endorphin from single human pituitary gland. FEBS Lett 166:267

Burbach JPH, Loeber JG, Verhoef J, Wiegant VM, De Kloet ER, De Wied D (1980) Selective conversion of β-endorphin into peptides related to γ- and α-endorphins. Nature 283:96

Burbach JPH, De Kloet ER, Schotman P, De Wied D (1981) Proteolytic conversion of β-endorphin by brain synaptic membranes: characterization of generated β-endorphin fragments and proposed metabolic pathway. J Biol Chem 256:12463

Chen C-LC, Mather JP, Morris PL, Bardin CW (1984) Expression of pro-opiomelanocortin-like gene in the testis and epididymis. Proc Natl Acad Sci USA 81:5672

Chrétien M, Seidah NG, Dennis M (1984) Processing of precursor polyproteins in rat brain: regional differences in acetylation of POMC peptides. In: Muller EE, Genazzani AR (eds) Central and peripheral endorphins: basic and clinical aspects. Raven, New York, p 27

Christie MJ, Chesher GB, Bird KD (1981) The correlation between swim-stress induced antinociception and [3H] leu-enkephalin binding to brain homogenates in mice. Pharmacol Biochem Behav 15:853

Civelli O, Brinberg N, Herbert E (1982) Detection and quantitation of pro-opiomelanocortin mRNA in pituitary and brain tissues from different species. J Biol Chem 257:6783

Cromlish JA, Seidah NG, Chrétien M (1986) Selective cleavage of human ACTH, beta-lipotropin, and the N-terminal glycopeptide at pairs of basic residues by IRCM-serine proteasel. Subcellular localization in small and large vesicles. J Biol Chem 261:10859

Deakin JF, Dostrovsky JO, Smyth D (1980) Influence of N-terminal acetylation and C-terminal proteolysis on the analgesic activity of beta-endorphin. Biochem J 189:501

DeSouza EB, Van Loon GR (1985) Differential plasma β-endorphin, β-lipotropin, and adrenocorticotropin responses to stress in rats. Endocrinology 116:1577

De Wied D, Jolles J (1990) Neuropeptides derived from pro-opiocortin: behavioral, physiological and neurochemical effects. Physiol Rev 72:976

Dickerson IM, Mains RE (1990) Cell-type specific post-transloational processing of peptides by different pituitary cell lines. Endocrinology 127:133

Dores RM, Jain M, Akil H (1986) Characterization of the forms of β-endorphin and α-MSH in the caudal medulla of the rat and guinea pig. Brain Res 377:251

Dum J, Gramsch C, Herz A (1983) Activation of hypothalamic β-endorphin pools by reward induced by highly palatable food. Pharmacol Biochem Behav 18:443

Eipper BA, Mains RE (1980) Structure and biosynthesis of proadrenocorticotropin/endorphin and related peptides. Endocr Rev 1:1

Eipper BA, Mains RE (1981) Further analysis of post-translational processing of beta-endorphin in rat intermediate pituitary. J Biol Chem 256:5689

Eipper BA, Mains RE (1982) Phosphorylation of pro-adrenocorticotroin/endorphin-derived peptides. J Biol Chem 257:4907

Eipper BA, Mains RE, Glembotski CC (1983) Identification in pituitary tissue of a peptide alpha-amidation activity that acts on glycine-extended peptides and requires molecular oxygen, copper and ascorbic acid. Proc Natl Acad Sci USA 80:5144

Eipper BA, Park L, Keutmann HT, Mains RE (1986) Amidation of joining peptide, a mauor pro-ACTH/endorphin-derived product peptide. J Biol Chem 261:8686

Eipper BA, Park LP, Dickerson IM, Keutmann HT, Thiele EA, Rodriguez H, Schoefield PR, Mains RE (1987) Structure of the precursor to an enzyme mediating COOH-terminal amidation in peptide biosynthesis. Mol Endocrinol 1:777

Emeson RB, Eipper BA (1986) Characterization of pro-ACTH/endorphin-derived peptides in rat hypothalamus. J Neurosci 6:837

Froni G, Bindoni M, Santoni A, Belluardo N, Marchese AE, Giovarelli M (1983) Radiofrequency destruction of the tuberoinfundibular region of the hypothalamus permanently abrogates NK cell activity in mice. Nature 306:181

Gianoulakis C, Angelogianni P (1989) Characterization of B-endorphin peptides in the spinal cord of the rat. Peptides 10:1049

Gilman SC, Schwartz JM, Milner AJ, Bloom FE, Feldman JD (1982) β-Endorphin enhances lymphocyte proliferative responses. Proc Natl Acad Sci USA 79:4226

Glembotski CC (1982a) Characterization of the peptide acetyl transferase activity in bovine and rat intermediate pituitaries responsible for the acetylation of beta-endorphin and alpha-melanotropin. J Biol Chem 257:10501

Glembotski CC (1982b) Acetylation of alpha-melanotropin and beta-endorphin in the rat intermediate pituitary. J Biol Chem 257:10493

Gramsch C, Kleber G,. Höllt V, Pasi A, Mehraein P, Herz A (1980) Pro-opiocortin fragments in human and rat brain: β-endorphin and α-MSH are the predominant peptides. Brain Res 192:109

Ham J, Smyth DG (1985a) β-Endorphin processing in pituitary and brain is sensitive to haloperidol. Neuropeptides 5:497

Ham J, Smyth DJ (1985b) β-Endorphin and ACTH related peptides in primary cultures of rat anterior pituitary cells: evidence for different intracellular pools. FEBS Lett 190:253

Ham J, Smyth DG (1986) Chronic stimulation of anterior pituitary cell cultures with CRF leads to the secretin of liptropin. Neuroendocrinology 44:533

Hammonds RG Jr, Nicolas P, Li CH (1984) β-Endorphin-(1–27) is an antagonist of β-endorphin analgesia. Proc Natl Acad Sci USA 81:1389

Hazum E, Chang KJ, Cuatrecasas P (1979) Specific nonopiate receptors for beta-endorphin. Science 205:1033

Herbert E, Uhler M (1982) Biosynthesis of polyprotein precursors to regulatory peptides. Cell 30:1

Hirsch MD, Millington WR, McKenzie JE, Mueller GP (1988) β-Endorphin-(1–27) is a potent endogenous hypotensive agent. Soc Neurosci Abstr 14:465

Hirsch MD, Villavicencio AE, McKenzie JE, Millington WR (1990) C-terminal proteolysis modifies cardioregulation by β-endorphin. Soc Neurosci Abstr 16:1025

Holaday JW (1983) Cardiovascular effects of endogenous opiate systems. Annu Rev Pharmacol Toxicol 23:541

Holaday JW (1985) Endogenous opioids and their receptors. Upjohn, Kalamazoo

Holaday JW, Loh HH (1981) Neurobiology of β-endorphin and related peptides. In: Li CH (ed) Hormonal proteins and peptides: β-endorphin. Academic, New York, p 204

Höllt V, Bergmann M (1982) Effects of acute and chronic haloperiodol treatment on the concentrations of immunoreactive beta-endorphin in plasma, pituitary and brain of rats. Neuropharmacology 21:147

Hong M, Jhamandas K (1989) Actions of β-endorphin and related peptide fragments on a pressor response induced by cholinergic stimulation. Prog Clin Biol Res 328:371

Hosobuchi Y, Rossier J, Bloom FE, Guillemin R (1979) Stimulation of human periaqueductal gray for pain relief increases immunoreactive B-endorphin in ventricular fluid. Science 203:279

Jenks BG, Verburg Van Kemenade BML, Tonon MC, Vaudry H (1985) Regulation of biosynthesis and release of pars intermedia peptides in *Rana ridibunda*: dopamine affects both acetylation and release of α-MSH. Peptides 6:913

Joseph SA, Michael GJ (1988) Efferent ACTH-IR opiocortin projections from nucleus tractus solitarius: a hypothalamic deafferentation study. Peptides 9:193

Joseph SA, Pilcher WH, Bennet-Clarke C (1983) Immunocytochemical localization of ACTH perikerya in nucleus tractus solitarius: evidence for a second opiocortin neuronal system. Neurosci Lett 38:221

Katopodis AG, Ping D, May SW (1990) A novel enzyme from bovine neuro-intermediate pituitary catalyzes dealkylation of a-hydroxyglycine derivatives, thereby functioning sequentially with peptidylglycine a-amidating monooxygenase in peptide amidation. Biochemistry 29:6115

Khachaturian H, Alessi NE, Munfakh N, Watson SJ (1983) Ontogeny of opioid and related peptides in the rat CNS and pituitary: an immunocytochemical study. Life Sci 33(Suppl I):61

Khachaturian H, Lewis ME, Tsou K, Watson SJ (1985) β-Endorphin, α-MSH, ACTH, and related peptides. In: Bjoorklund A, Hokfelt T (eds) Handbook of chemical neuroanatomy, vol 4: GABA and neuropeptides in the CNS, part I. Elsevier Science, Amsterdam, p 216

Kizer JS, Bateman RC Jr, Miller RC, Humm J, Busby WH Jr, Youngblood WW (1986) Purification and characterization of peptidyl glycine monooxygenase from porcine pituitary. Endocrinology 118:2262

Krieger DT, Liotta AS, Brownstein MJ, Zimmerman EA (1980) ACTH, β-lipotropin, and related peptides in brain, pituitary, and blood. Rec Prog Horm Res 36:277

Lagaze-Masmontei CT, De Keyser Y, Luton JP, Kahin A, Bertagna X (1987) Characterization of proopiomelanocortin transcripts in human non-pituitary tissues. Proc Natl Acad Sci USA 84:7261

Lebouille JLM, Burbach JPH, De Kloet ER (1984) Quantitation of the endopeptidase activity generating γ-endorphin from β-endorphin in rat brain synaptic membranes by a radiometric assay. Anal Biochem 141:1

Lebouille JLM, Burbach JPH, De Kloet ER (1985) γ-Endorphin generating endopeptidase in rat brain: subcellular and regional distribution. Biochem Biophys Res Commun 127:44

Lennarz WJ (1980) The biochemistry of glycoproteins and proteoglycans. Plenum, New York

Lewis JW, Cannon JT, Liebeskind JC (1980) Opioid and non-opioid mechanisms of stress analgesia. Science 208:623

Lewis JW, Shavit Y, Terman GW, Nelson LR, Gale RP, Liebeskind JC (1983) Apparent involvement of opioid peptides in stress-induced enhancement of tumor growth. Peptides 4:635

Lewis JW, Shavit Y, Terman GW, Nelson LR, Martin FC, Gale RP, Liebeskind JC (1985) Involvement of opioid peptides in the analgesic, immunoscuppressive, and tumor-enhancing effects of stress. Psychopharmacol Bull 21:479

Lewis JW, Baldrighi G, Akil H (1987) A possible interface between autonomic function and pain control: opioid analgesia and the nucleus tractus solitarius. Brain Res 424:65

Li CH, Tseng L-F, Ferrara P, Yamashiro D (1980a) β-Endorphin: dissociation of receptor binding activity from analgesic potency. Proc Natl Acad Sci USA 77:2303

Li CH, Yamashiro D, Tseng L-F, Chang W-C, Ferrara P (1980b) β-Endorphin omission analogs: dissociation of immunoreactivity from other biological activities. Proc Natl Acad Sci USA 77:3211

Liotta AS, Loudes C, McKelvy JF, Krieger DT (1980) Biosynthesis of precursor corticotropin/endorphin-, corticotropin-, α-melanotropin-, β-lipotropin-, and β-endorphin-loke material by cultured rat hypothalamic neurons. Proc Natl Acad Sci USA 77:1880

Liotta AS, Advis JP, Krause JE, McKelvy JF, Krieger DT (1984) Demonstration of in vivo synthesis of pro-opiomelanocortin-, β-endorphin, and α-melanotropin-like species in the adult rat brain. J Neurosci 4:956

Loh H, Tseng LF, Wei E, Li CH (1976) β-Endorphin is a potent analgesic agent. Proc Natl Acad Sci USA 73:2895

Loh YP (1986) Kinetic studies on the processing of human beta-lipotropin by bovine pituitary intermediate lobe pro-opiomelanocortin-converting enzyme. J Biol Chem 261:11949

Loh YP, Jenks BG (1981) Evidence for two different turnover pools of adrenocorticotropin, α-melanocyte stimulating hormone and endorphin-related peptides released by the frog pituitary neurointermediate lobe. Endocrinology 109:54

Loh YP, Eskay RL, Brownstein M (1980) α-MSH-like peptides in rat brain: identification and changes during development. Biochem Biophys Res Commun 94:916

Loh YP, Parish DC, Tuteja R (1985) Purification and characterization of a paired basic residue-specific pro-opiomelanocortin converting enzyme from bovine pituitary intermediate lobe secretory vesicle. J Biol Chem 260:7194

Lolait SJ, Lim ATW, Toh BH, Funder JW (1984) Immunoactive β-endorphin in a subpopulation of mouse spleen macrophages. J Clin Invest 73:277

Lolait SJ, Clements JA, Markwick AJ, Cheng MC, McNally M, Smith AI, Funder JW (1986) Pro-opiomelanocortin synthesis and post-translational processing of β-endorphin in spleen macrophages. J Clin Invest 77:1776

Lopker A, Abood LG, Hoss W, Lionetti FJ (1980) Stereoselective muscarinic acetylcholine and opiate receptors in human phagocytic leukocytes. Biochem Pharmacol 29:1361

Lowy MT, Maickel RP, Yim GK (1980) Naloxone reduction of stress-related feeding. Life Sci 26:2113

Lowy MT, Starkey C, Yim GK (1981) Stereoselective effects of opiate agonists and antagonists on ingestive behavior in rats. Pharmacol Biochem Behav 15:591

Madden J, Akil H, Tsou K, Watson SJ (1977) Stress-induced parallel changes in central opioid levels and pain responsiveness in the rat. Nature 265:358

Mains RE, Eipper BA (1976) Biosynthesis of ACTH in mouse pituitary tumor cells. J Biol Chem 251:4115

Mains RE, Eipper BA, Ling N (1977) Common precursor to corticotropins and endorphins. Proc Natl Acad Sci USA 74:3014

Mandler RN, Bididson WE, Mandler R, Serrate SA (1986) β-Endorphin augments the cytolytic activity and interferon production of natural killer cells. J Immunol 136:934

Mathews PM, Froelich CJ, Sibbit WL Jr, Bankhurst AD (1983) Enhancement of natural cytotoxicity by β-endorphin. J Immunol 130:1658

Mayer DJ, Hayes RL (1975) Stimulation-produced analgesia: development of tolerance and cross-tolerance. Science 188:941

Mayer DJ, Liebeskind JC (1974) Pain relief by focal electrical stimulation of the brain: anatomical and behavioral analysis. Brain Res 68:73

Mayer DJ, Wolfe TL, Akil H, Carder B, Liebeskind JC (1971) Analgesia from electrical stimulation in the brainstem of the rat. Science 174:1351

Meador-Woodruff JH, Pellerito B, Vaudry H, Jegou S, Seidah NG, Watson SJ, Akil H (1988) Regional processing of the N- and C-terminal domains of proopiomelanocortin in monkey pituitary and brain. Neuropeptides 11:111

Millan MJ, Millan MJ, Herz A (1986) Depletion of central β-endorphin blocks midbrain stimulation-produced analgesia in the freely-moving rat. Neuroscience 18:641

Millan MJ, Przewlocki R, Jerlicz M, Gramsch C, Hollt V, Herz A (1981) Stress-induced release of brain and pituitary β-endorphin: major role of endorphins in generation of hyperthermia, not analgesia. Brain Res 208:325

Millan MJ, Czlonkowski A, Millan MH, Herz A (1987) Activation of periaqueductal grey pools of β-endorphin by analgetic electrical stimulation in freely moving rats. Brain Res 407:199

Millington WR, Mueller GP, O'Donohue TL (1984) Regional heterogeneity in the ratio of α-MSH:β-endorphin in rat brain. Peptides 5:841

Millington WR, O'Donohue TL, Chappell MC, Roberts JL, Mueller GP (1986) Coordinate regulation of peptide acetyltransferase activity and pro-piomelanocortin gene expression in the intermediate lobe of the rat pituitary. Endocrinology 118:2024

Mochetti I, Costa E (1986) Down regulation of hypothalamic pro-opiomelanocortin system during morphine tolerance. Neuropharmacology 9(Suppl 1):125

Mochetti I, Ritter A, Costa E (1989) Down-regulation of pro-opiomelanocortin synthesis and beta-endorphin utilization in hypothalamus of morphine-tolerant rats. J Mol Neurosci 1:33

Moss IR, Friedman E (1978) β-Endorphin – effects on respiratory regulation. Life Sci 23:1271

Murthy ASN, Mains RE, Eipper BA (1986) Purification and characterizatioon of peptidylglycine α-amidating monooxygenase from bovine neurointermediate pituitary. J Biol Chem 261:1851

Nakanishi S, Inoue A, Kita T, Nakamura M, Chang ACY, Cohen SN, Numa S (1979) Nucleotide sequence of cloned cDNA for bovine corticotropin-beta-lipotropin precursor. Nature 278:423

Nicolas P, Hammonds RG Jr, Li CH (1984) β-Endorphin-induced analgesia is inhibited by synthetic analogs of B-endorphin. Proc Natl Acad Sci USA 81:3074

Oates EL, Allaway GP, Armstrong GR, Boyajian RA, Kehrl JH, Pranhakar BS (1988) Human lymphocytes produce pro-opiomelanocortin gene-related transcripts. J Biol Chem 263:10041

O'Donohue TL, Charlton CG, Helke CJ, Miller RJ, Jacobowitz DM (1979) Identification of α-MSH immunoreactivity in rat and human brain and CSF. In: Gross E, Meinhoffer J (eds) Peptide structure and biological functioning. Pierce Chemical, p 897

Orth DN, Nicholson WE, Mitchell WM, Island DP, Shapiro M, Byyny RL (1973) ACTH and MSH production by a single cloned mouse pituitary tumor cell line. Endocrinology 92:385

Palkovits M, Eskay RL (1987) Distribution and possible origin of β-endorphin and ACTH in discrete brainstem nuclei of rats. Neuropeptides 9:123

Palkovits M, Mezey E, Eskay RL (1987) Pro-opiomelanocortin-derived peptiddes (ACTH/β-endorphin/α-MSH) in brainstem baroreceptor areas of the rat. Brain Res 436:323

Perkins SN, Husten EJ, Eipper BA (1990) The 108-kDA peptidylglycine α-amidating monoxygenase precursor contains two separable enzymatic activities involved in peptide amidation. Biochem Biophys Res Commun 171:926

Pilcher WH, Joseph SA (1986) Differential sensitivity of hypothalamic and medullary opiocortin and tyrosine hydroxylase neurons to the neurotoxic effects of monsodium glutamate (MSG). Peptides 7:783

Pintar JE, Schacter BS, Herman AB, Durgerian S, Krieger DT (1984) Characterization and localization of proopiomelanocortin messenger RNA in the adult rat testis. Science 225:632

Plotnikoff NP, Miller GC (1983) Enkephalins as immunomodulators. J Immunopharmacol 5:437

Przewlocki R, Millan MJ, Gramsch C, Millan MH, Herz A (1982) The influence of selective adeno- and neurointermedio-hypophysectomy upon plasma and brain levels of β-endorphin and their response to stress in rats. Brain Res 242:107

Przewlocki R, Lason W, Hollt V, Silberring J, Herz A (1987) The influence of chronic stress on multiple opioid peptide systems in the rat: pronounced effects upon dynorphin in spinal cord. Brain Res 413:213

Reynolds DV (1969) Surgery in the rat during electrical analgesia induced by focal brain stimulation. Science 164:444

Rivier C, Vale W (1983) Modulation of stress-induced ACTH release by corticotropin-releasing factor, catecholamines and vasopressin. Nature 305:325

Roberts JL, Herbert E (1977) Characterization of a common precursor to corticotropin and beta-lipotropin: cell-free synthesis of the precursor and identification of corticotropin peptides in the molecule. Proc Natl Acad Sci USA 74:4826

Rossier J, French ED, Rivier C, Ling N, Guillemin R, Bloom FE (1977) Foot-shock induced stress increases B-endorphin levels in blood nut not brain. Nature 270:618

Sapru HN, Willette RN, Krieger AJ (1981) Stimulation of pulmonary J receptors by an enkephalin analog. J Pharmacol Exp Ther 217:228

Schwartzberg DG, Nakane PK (1983) ACTH-related peptide containing neurons within the medulla oblongata of the rat. Brain Res 276:351

Schweigerer L, Bhakdi S, Teschemacher H (1982) Specific non-opiate binding sites for human β-endorphin on the terminal complex of human complement. Nature 296:572

Seeger TF, Sforzo GA, Pert CB, Pert A (1984) In vivo autoradiography: visualization of stress-induced changes in opiate receptor occupancy in the rat brain. Brain Res 305:303

Seidah NG, Chrétien M (1981) Complete amino acid sequence of a human pituitary glycopeptide: an important maturation produce of pro-opiomelanocortin. Proc Natl Acad Sci USA 78:4236

Seidah NG, Rochemont J, Hamelin J, Benjannet S, Chrétien M (1981) The missing fragment of the pro-sequence of human proopiomelanocortin: sequence and evidence for C-terminal amidation. Biochem Biophys Res Commun 102:710

Seidah NG, Gaspar L, Mion P, Marcinkiewicz M, Mbikay M, Chrétien M (1990) cDNA sequence of two distinct pituitary proteins homologous to Kex2 and furin gene products: tissue-specific mRNAs encoding candidates for pro-hormone processing proteinases. DNA Cell Biol 9:415

Seidah NG, Marcinkiewicz M, Benjannet S, Gaspar L, Beaubien G, Mattei MG, Lazure C, Mbikay M, Chrétien M (1991) Cloning and primary sequence of a mouse candidate prohormone convertase PC1 homologous to PC2, furin, and kex2: distinct chromosomal localization and messenger RNA distribution in brain and pituitary compared to PC2. Mol Endocrinol 5:111

Shavit Y, Lewis JW, Terman GW, Gale RP, Liebeskind JC (1984) Opioid peptides mediate the suppressive effects of stress on natural killer cell cytotoxicity. Science 223:188

Shavit Y, Terman GW, Martin FC, Lewis JW, Liebeskind JC, Gale RP (1985) Stress, opioid-peptides, the immune system, and cancer. J Immunol (Suppl) 135:834

Shavit Y, Depaulis A, Martin FC, Terman GW, Pechnick RN, Zane CJ, Gale, RP, Liebeskind JC (1986) Involvement of brain opiate receptors in the immune-suppressive effect of morphine. Proc Natl Acad Sci USA 83:7114

Shiomi H, Watson SJ, Kelsey JE, Akil H (1986) Pretranslational and post-translational mechanisms for regulating β-endorphin-adrenocorticotropin of the anterior pituitary lobe. Endocrinology 119:1793

Smeekens SP, Steiner DF (1990) Identification of a human insulinoma cDNA encoding a novel mammalian protein structurally related to the yeast dibasic processing protease Kex2. J Biol Chem 265:2997

Smeekens SP, Avruch AS, LaMendola J, Chan SJ, Steiner DF (1991) Identification of a cDNA encoding a second putative prohormone convertase related to PC2 in AtT20 cells and islets of Langerhans. Proc Natl Acad Sci USA 88:340

Smith EM, Blalock EJ (1981) Human lymphocyte production of corticotropin and endorphin like substances: association with leukocyte interferon. Proc Natl Acad Sci USA 77:7530

Smyth DG, Zakarian Z (1980) Selective processing of β-endorphin in regions of porcine pituitary. Nature 288:613

Smyth DG, Massey DE, Zakarian S (1979) Endorphins are stored in biologically active and inactive forms: isolation of α-N-acetyl peptides. Nature 279:252

Smyth DG, Zakarian S (1982) α-N-Acetyl derivatives of β-endorphin in rat pituitary: chromatographic evidence for processed forms of beta-endorphin in pancreas and brain. Life Sci 31:1887

Steiner DF, Oyer PE (1967) The biosynthesis of insulin and a probable precursor of insulin by a human islet cell adenoma. Proc Natl Acad Sci USA 57:473

Stoffers DA, Green CB, Eipper BA (1989) Alternative mRNA splicing generates multiple forms of peptidyl-glycine alpha-amidating monooxygenase in rat atrium. Proc Natl Acad Sci USA 86:735

Takahashi H, Hakamata Y, Watanabe Y, Kikuno R, Miyata T, Numa S (1983) Complete nucleotide sequence of the human corticotropin-beta-lipotropin precursor gene. Nucleic Acids Res 11:6847

Takahashi K, Okamoto H, Seino H, Noguchi M (1990) Peptidylglycine α-amidating reaction: evidence for a two-step mechanism involving a stable intermediate at neutral pH. Biochem Biophys Res Commun 169:524

Tilders FJH, Mulder AH (1975) In vitro demonstration of melanocyte-stimulating hormone release inhibiting action of dopaminergic nerve fibres. J Endocrinol 64:63

Trujillo KA, Belluzzi JD, Stein L (1989) Opiate antagonists and self-stimulation: extinction-like response patterns suggest selective reward deficit. Brain Res 492:15

Tsou K, Khachaturian H, Akil H, Watson SJ (1986) Immunocytochemical localization of proopiomelanocortin-derived peptides in the adult rat spinal cord. Brain Res 378:28

Turner JD, Keith AB, Smith AI, Mcdermott JR, Biggins JA, Edwardson JA (1983) Studies on the characterization of α-MSH-like immunoreactivity in rat hypothalamus. Regul Pept 5:283

Van Loon GR, Appel NM, Ho D (1981a) β-Endorphin-induced increases in plasma epinephrine, norepinephrine and dopamine in rats: inhibition of adreno-medullary response by intracisternal somatostatin. Brain Res 212:207

Van Loon GR, Appel NM, Ho D (1981b) β-Endorphin-induced stimulation of central sympathetic outflow: β-endorphin increases plasma concentrations of epinephrine, norepinephrine and dopamine in rats. Endocrinology 109:46

Van Ree JM, Smyth DG, Colpaert FC (1979) Dependence creating properties of lipotropin C-fragment (β-endorphin): evidence for its internal control of behavior. Life Sci 24:495

Vaudry H, Jenks BG, van Overbeeke AP (1983) The frog pars intermedia contains only the non-acetylated form of α-MSH: acetylation to generate α-MSH occurs during the release process. Life Sci 33(Suppl 1):97

Wand GS, May V, Eipper BA (1988) Comparison of acute and chronic secretagogue regulation of proadrenocorticotropin/endorphin synthesis, secretion and messenger ribonucleic acid production in primary cultures of rat anterior pituitary. Endocrinology 123:1153

Watson SJ, Barchas JD, Li CH (1977) Beta-lipotropin: localization in cells and axons in rat brain by immunocytochemistry. Proc Natl Acad Sci USA 74:5155

Watson SJ, Akil H, Richard CW, Barchas JD (1978a) Evidence for two separate opiate peptide neuronal systems and the coexistence of beta-lipotropin, beta-endorphin and ACTH immunoreactivities in the same hypothalamic neurons. Nature 275:226

Watson SJ, Richard CW, Barchas JD (1978b) Adrenocorticotropin in rat brain: immunocytochemical localization in the cells and axons. Science 200:1180

Watson SJ, Lopez J, Young EA, Vale W, Rivier J, Akil H (1987) Effects of low
    dose α-CRF in humans: endocrine relationships and β-endorphin/β-lipotropin
    response. J Clin Endocrinol Metab 66:10
Westly HJ, Kleiss AJ, Kelley KW, Wong PK, Yuen P-H (1986) Newcastle disease
    virus-infected splenocytes express the pro-opiomelanocortin gene. J Exp Med
    163:1589
Westphal M, Li CH (1984a) β-Endorphin: evidence for the existence of opioid and
    non-opioid binding components for the tritiated human hormone in NG108–15
    cells. Biochem Biophys Res Commun 122:428
Westphal M, Li CH (1984b) β-Endorphin: demonstration of binding sites in three
    human neuroblastoma cell lines specific for the COOH-terminal segment of the
    human hormone. Biochem Biophys Res Commun 120:873
Wybran J, Appelboom T, Famaly JP, Govaerts A (1979) Suggestive evidence for
    receptors for morphine and methionine-enkephalin on normal human blood T
    lymphocytes. J Immunol 123:1068
Yoshida M, Taniguchi Y (1988) Projection of pro-opiomelanocortin neurons from
    the rat arcuate nucleus to the midbrain central gray as demonstrated by double
    staining with retrograde labeling and immunohistochemistry. Arch Histol Cytol
    51:175
Young EA (1989) Adrenalectomy increases β-lipotropin secretion over β-endorphin
    secretion from anterior pituitary corticotrophs. Life Sci 45:2233
Young EA (1990) Induction of the intermediate lobe POMC system with chronic
    swim stress and B-adrenergic modulation of this induction. Neuroendocrinology
    52:405
Young EA, Akil H (1985) Corticotropin-releasing factor stimulation of adreno-
    corticotropin and β-endorphin release: effects of acute and chronic stress.
    Endocrinology 117:23
Young EA, Lewis J, Akil H (1986) The preferential release of β-endorphin from the
    anterior pituitary lobe by corticotropin releasing factor (CRF). Peptides 7:603
Zakarian S, Smyth DG (1982a) Distribution of β-endorphin-related peptides in rat
    pituitary and brain. Biochem J 202:561
Zakarian S, Smyth DG (1982b) β-Endorphin is processed differently in specific
    regions of rat pituitary and brain. Nature 296:250

CHAPTER 18

Biosynthesis of Enkephalins
and Proenkephalin-Derived Peptides

J. ROSSIER

A. Introduction

The enkephalins [Met^5]- and [Leu^5]enkephalin were isolated in 1975 by HUGHES et al. Since then, numerous other opioid peptides have been characterized although none of these are found in levels comparable to [Met^5]enkephalin in brain tissue (see Table 1). Brain levels of prodynorphin and proopiomelanocortin-derived peptides, for example, are at least one order of magnitude lower than those of [Met^5]enkephalin. When compared to other nonopioid peptides, the levels of [Met^5]enkephalin are of the same order as two other widely distributed peptides, CCK8 and somatostatin (see review in CRAWLEY 1985).

Tissue levels are not always of physiological significance. They do, however, give an indication of the importance of the neurohormone in the tissue. In homogenates of the globus pallidus, for example, the final tissue concentration of [Met^5]enkephalin has been calculated to be $10\,\mu M$ (STELL et al. 1990), assuming that the peptide is distributed equally between all cells. However, if it is assumed that enkephalin is restricted to enkephalinergic neurons and that this compartment represents between 1% and 10% of the total tissue, the final neuronal concentration of [Met^5]enkephalin lies between 1 and $0.1\,mM$, which is far from negligible. Neuronal cytoplasmic concentrations of a classical neurotransmitter such as acetylcholine have been estimated at around $20\,mM$.

Studies have shown that enkephalins are released and can be assayed in fluid and extracellular space after stimulation of neuronal pathways (CHAMINADE et al. 1984; FAYADA et al. 1987; ROSSIER et al. 1988). These studies have far more physiological relevance than assaying levels in tissue. Unfortunately, release studies are always complicated by the rapid degradation of enkephalin by numerous peptidases and by the difficulties in sampling fluids in relevant areas. No specific biocaptor or biosensor for enkephalins has been engineered. It is not impossible that such a device could one day be made available to the physiologist, who, for the moment, can only dream that a biosensor as tiny as a microelectrode could be used to monitor on-line the levels of enkephalinergic release.

This review deals with proenkephalin-derived peptides and mainly the opioid peptides [Met^5]enkephalin, [Leu^5]enkephalin, the octapeptide

Table 1. Regional distribution of [Met⁵]enkephalin and α-neoendorphin in the rat brain. (Giraud et al. 1983)

Region	[Met⁵]enkephalin	α-Neoendorphin
Cortex	302 ± 64	15 ± 2.4
Striatum	3656 ± 496	127 ± 15
Hippocampus	469 ± 46	91 ± 15
Hypothalamus	2169 ± 426	91 ± 9
Medulla/pons	986 ± 214	24.8 ± 4.5
Cerebellum	66 ± 17	3 ± 0.6
Spinal cord	752 ± 64	22.9 ± 1.6

Results are expressed as picomoles per gram tissue, wet weight. All values (radioimmunoassay) are means $\pm$ SEM for five animals.

[Met⁵]enkephalin-Arg⁶-Gly⁷-Leu⁸, and the heptapeptide [Met⁵]enkephalin-Arg⁶-Phe⁷. Other potent opioid peptides such as peptides E, F, and BAM P 22, 20, 12 are also described. The importance of nonopioid peptides such as synenkephalin, peptide I, and peptide B, also derived from proenkephalin, is discussed. These nonopioid peptides do not have a N-terminal starting with the sequence Tyr-Gly-Gly-Phe and they do not bind to opiate receptors. Their physiological role is as yet unknown.

B. History

Soon after the enkephalins were discovered, it was observed that the 91 amino acid long peptide β-lipotropin contains the sequence of [Met⁵]enkephalin at residues 61–65. This sequence homology was pointed out during a discussion in 1975 between Howard Morris, who had just sequenced the enkephalins (by mass spectrometry), and Derek Smyth, then working on what was known as fragment C of β-lipotropin. Fragment C is β-lipotropin 61–91, rechristened β-endorphin after the observation that this fragment was a very potent opioid peptide.

It was then proposed that β-endorphin was the precursor of [Met⁵]enkephalin. This proposal was a little heterodox considering that in 1976 the work of Steiner et al. (1974) on proinsulin and the idea that active peptides in precursors should be sandwiched between pairs of basic amino acids was already well accepted. This was not the case for [Met⁵]enkephalin since, although in β-lipotropin the amino acids in front of Tyr are indeed a pair of basic amino acid residues, the amino acid after methionine is a serine.

In any case, β-lipotropin could not possibly be considered a precursor for Leu-enkephalin. However, in those early days of opioid peptide research, any wild hypothesis was acceptable and for several months [Leu⁵] β-endorphin was a rising star in biological psychiatry. The idea was proposed that in schizophrenia too many peptides, including [Leu^5] β-endorphin, were accumulated in the blood and that they should be removed by dialysis (PALMOUR et al. 1979). Psychiatric wards were soon equipped with dialysis units. Fortunately, after 2 years of misjudgment, the episode came to an end, and, to my knowledge, [Leu^5] β-endorphin was never isolated in mammals.

In 1977 at the Salk Institute, we observed that the distributions of β-endorphin and [Leu^5]enkephalin were not at all parallel in extracts of various tissues. Anterior pituitary contains large amounts of β-endorphin and virtually no enkephalins, while the reverse is seen in the globus pallidus (ROSSIER et al. 1977). The anatomical distribution of β-endorphinergic and enkephalinergic pathways was also a good indication that enkephalins and β-endorphin were unrelated molecules (BLOOM et al. 1978). The definitive proof came from studies carried out at the Roche Institute, when we were able to isolate and fully characterize from the adrenals molecules bearing both the sequence of [Met^5]enkephalin and [Leu^5]enkephalin. Proenkephalin was then discovered in 1979, and in 1981 three groups isolated clones of proenkephalin with no homology with proopiomelanocortin. The origin of [Leu^5]enkephalin, however, was not completely resolved by the identification of proenkephalin since in 1979 a leucine-enkephalin C-terminally extended peptide, dynorphin, was characterized by Avram GOLDSTEIN et al. (1981). The fact that in dynorphin the [Leu^5]enkephalin sequence is followed by a pair of basic amino acids led to the proposal the [Leu^5]enkephalin was the active peptide and dynorphin a mere precursor. This is of course possible, as advocated by ZAMIR et al. (1984), but then it could equally be argued that [Leu^5]enkephalin is a degradation product of the inactivation process of dynorphin.

The structure of proenkephalin in various species is given in Fig. 1. Proenkephalin contains seven copies of enkephalins bracketed between pairs of basic amino acids: four copies of [Met^5]enkephalin, one copy each of [Leu^5]enkephalin, [Met^5]enkephalin-Arg^6-Gly^6-Leu^8, also known as the octapeptide, and [Met^5]enkephalin-Arg^6-Phe^7. This latter enkephalin, also known as the heptapeptide, constitutes the C-terminus of proenkephalin. The main characteristics of the proenkephalin molecule were obtained from numerous pluridisciplinary studies conducted between 1978 and 1985. One of the key points in the elucidation of the complete structure of the molecule came in 1982 with the sequencing of the cDNA clones. I will now describe the characterization of proenkephalin from an historical viewpoint.

C. Enkephalin Biosynthesis in the Adrenal Medulla

The studies on enkephalin biosynthesis would have taken much longer without the work of SCHULTZBERG et al. (1978), who, using immunofluorescence techniques, visualized [Met^5]enkephalin-like immunoreactivity in the cells of

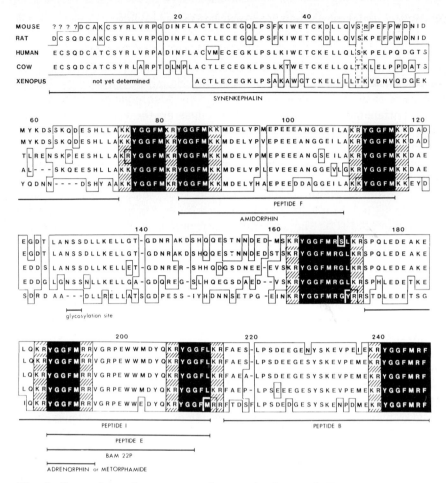

Fig. 1. Comparison of mouse, rat, human, bovine, and *Xenopus* proenkephalin
sequences. This figure represents the amino acid sequences (expressed according to
the one-letter code) of the five proenkephalin molecules known at the present time.
The sequence of *Xenopus* and mouse proenkephalin is not yet completely known, as
shown by the space in the first line. The sequences have been aligned to obtain the
maximum homologies. The sequences of the opioid peptides ([Met⁵]enkephalin,
[Leu⁵]enkephalin, the octapeptide [Met⁵]enkephalin-Arg⁶-Gly⁷-Leu⁸, and the
heptapeptide [Met⁵]enkephalin-Arg⁶-Phe⁷ are shown *on a black background*. Note
that, in the *Xenopus* proenkephalin, the sequence of [Leu⁵]enkephalin is replaced by
a sequence of [Met⁵]enkephalin and the last amino acid of the octapeptide is a
tyrosine, whereas the corresponding amino acid in the four other species is a leucine.
Note also in the case of the mouse the presence of Ser⁷ instead of Gly⁷ in the
octapeptide sequence. The most important homologies between the sequences are
found in three regions. The first region is constituted by the amino-terminal half of
synenkephalin. Synenkephalin is the amino-terminal part of proenkephalin, which
extends to the first basic amino acid pair in front of the first [Met⁵]enkephalin
sequence. A marked homology between the proenkephalin sequences is also found
in the region comprising the first three [Met⁵]enkephalin sequences. Finally, starting
from the octapeptide sequence, the carboxy-terminal parts of the four proenkephalin
sequences are almost identical. It is worth noting that certain regions in the sequences
from species as far apart phylogenetically as man and *Xenopus* are identical, suggesting that these regions may play a major role in the structure and/or function of this
protein

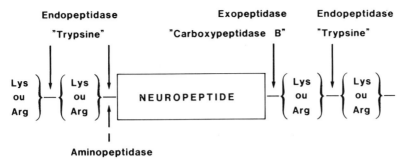

Fig. 2. Model of the maturation of neuropeptide precursors, involving two peptidases with substrate specificities close to those of trypsin and carboxypeptidase B, and possibly an aminopeptidase

guinea pig adrenal medulla. The presence of enkephalin-like peptides and putative enkephalin precursors in bovine adrenal medulla was established by LEWIS et al. (1979). At the same time, it was shown that opioid material was stored and cosecreted with catecholamines from adrenal chromaffin granules (VIVEROS et al. 1979; LIVETT et al. 1981; ROSSIER et al. 1981). When chromaffin granules were separated on self-generating Percoll gradients, enkephalin-like material was found to be associated with the adrenergic, and not with the denser, nonadrenergic vesicules (ROISIN et al. 1983). The relative concentration of enkephalin in the adrenergic vesicle is high. Indeed, the molar ratio of adrenalin to total [Met^5]enkephalin is around 100 (ROISIN et al. 1983). Other studies using immunocytochemical methods have also indicated that enkephalins are located in adrenergic and not in the nonadrenergic cells in the bovine adrenal medulla (LIVETT et al. 1982).

Chromatography of extracts from bovine adrenal medulla or chromaffin granule acid yielded several peptides in a molecular weight range up to 20 000 from which peptides with opioid activity could be liberated after sequential digestion with trypsin and carboxypeptidase B (see Fig. 2 for rationale). The absence of proopiomelanocortin and related peptides in the bovine adrenal medulla (LEWIS et al. 1979) and the high concentration of opioids and opioid-containing peptides present made this an ideal tissue with which to study enkephalin biosynthesis. Investigators should, however, be aware of important species differences in the levels of enkephalins in adrenal as rat and guinea pig adrenal contain little material, compared to bovine adrenal (METTERS et al. 1985).

Evidence for the hypothesis that [Met^5]enkephalin and [Leu^5]enkephalin were synthesized via a larger precursor came from the following series of experiments. Pulse-chase studies demonstrated that [^{35}S]methionine, incubated with cultured bovine chromaffin cells, was incorporated into an approximately 22-kDa enkephalin-containing peptide before being detected in free [Met^5]enkephalin (ROSSIER et al. 1980b).

Denervation of the rat adrenal gland was found to stimulate a large increase in the concentration of enkephalin and enkephalin-containing peptides in this tissue. The initial increase, occurring only in the region of a >20-kDa species, was replaced over a time course of 96h by increasing concentrations of intermediate-size enkephalin-containing peptides and finally free enkephalin (LEWIS et al. 1981).

Many biologically active peptide sequences are located between pairs of basic residues within their precursors. Where this arrangement occurs these peptides can be liberated by treating the precursor with trypsin, which cleaves to the carboxyl side of basic residues, followed by carboxypeptidase B, which specifically removes remaining basic amino acids from the COOH-terminus (Fig. 2). Putative precursors can then be detected by assaying for released biological activity or immunoreactivity. This approach was used to identify putative opioid precursors. Gel filtration chromatography of bovine chromaffin granule extracts yielded various peptides containing the enkephalin sequence. The high molecular weight region was digested by trypsin and carboxypeptidase B. These digests were shown to contain enkephalins with an approximate ratio of 7:1 for [Met^5]enkephalin: [Leu^5]enkephalin (LEWIS et al. 1980a).

The strategy adopted most successfully in 1979 by Sidney Udenfriend's group at the Roche Institute was to purify the putative intermediates in the biosynthesis of enkephalin in order to build up a structure for the precursor (UDENFRIEND and KILPATRICK 1983). The peptides were first isolated from an initial crude separation of bovine adrenal medulla chromaffin granule extract (LEWIS et al. 1979) and then sequenced. In addition to both [Met^5]enkephalin and [Leu^5]enkephalin, several COOH-terminally extended small enkephalin congeners were purified. Two of these, the hetapeptide [Met^5]enkephalin-Arg^6-Phe^7 (STERN et al. 1979; ROSSIER et al. 1980a) and the octapeptide [Met^5]enkephalin-Arg^6-Gly^7-Leu^8 (KILPATRICK et al. 1981b), showed that the precursor may produce two other opioid peptides known also as the hepta- and octapeptide.

The complete proenkephalin protein with the C-terminus of [Met^5]enkephalin-Arg^6-Phe^7 was never isolated from bovine adrenal although this protein was characterized in guinea pig brain by BEAUMONT et al. (1985). The structure of the higher molecular weight enkephalin-containing peptides and their interrelationship is shown schematically in Fig. 3. The largest enkephalin-containing peptide isolated from the adrenal medulla is the 23.3-kDa peptide. This peptide starts with the N-terminal of proenkephalin and terminates with the Leu of [Leu^5]enkephalin. It was first detected by PATEY et al. (1984) and purified to homogeneity by immunoaffinity by METTERS and ROSSIER (1987). The 18.2-kDa peptide starts at the N-terminal of proenkephalin and finishes with the sequence of the octapeptide [Met^5]enkephalin-Arg^6-Gly^7-Leu^8. The 12.6-kDa and 8.6-kDa peptides finish with Met-enkephalin sequences.

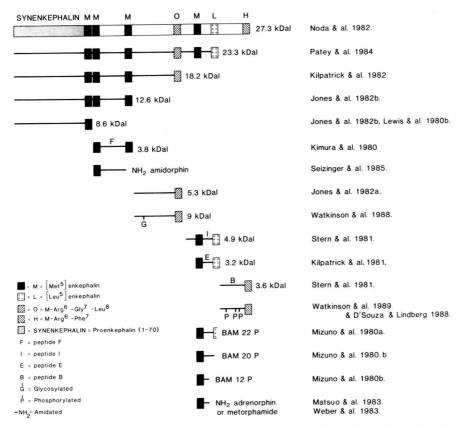

Fig. 3. Proenkephalin and the enkephalin-containing peptides in the bovine adrenal medulla

The first sequencing data on isolated peptides were made on peptides F (3.8 kDa) and I (4.7 kDa). The former contains two copies of [Met^5]enkephalin and the presence of both [Met^5]enkephalin and [Leu^5]enkephalin in the latter indicated a common precursor for both pentapeptides (Kimura et al. 1980; Jones et al. 1980; Stern et al. 1981). The work of Kimura et al. (1980) was the first to indicate that [Met^5] and [Leu^5]enkephalin were synthesized together by the same proenkephalin molecule.

These intermediates had several other interesting features. Peptide E, with an enkephalin sequence at each terminus, was found to be an extremely potent opioid agonist on the guinea pig ileum (Kilpatrick et al. 1981a).

A 5.3-kDa peptide (Jones et al. 1982a) was also characterized in several species corresponding to the C-terminal of the 18.2-kDa peptide. Both of these peptides contain the sequence -Asn-Ser-Ser-, known to act as an attachment site for asparagine-linked oligosaccharide chains (MARSHALL 1972). Only a small percentage of the 5.3- and 18-kDa peptides are glycosylated in the adrenal, but those that are migrate with anomalously high molecular weights of 11 and 22 k respectively on SDS-PAGE, a phenomenon associated with glycoproteins (KILPATRICK et al. 1982; PATEY et al. 1984; METTERS et al. 1988). WATKINSON et al. (1988) used enzymatic digestion with endoglycosidase F in order to demonstrate that the 11-kDa form (identified as 9 kDa in their publication) was a glycosylated form of the 5.3 kDa form.

The 18.2-kDa and a 12.6-kDa species both contained multiple copies of Met[5]-enkephalin, the 18.2-kDa peptide proving a common precursor for Met[5]-enkephalin and the octapeptide. An antibody against the octapeptide was used to purify the 18.2-kDa peptide by immunoaffinity (METTERS and ROSSIER 1987). Peptide B was the only species found containing Met[5]-enkephalin-Arg[6]-Phe[7]. This peptide contains three serine residues that can be phosphorylated and several phosphorylated forms have been isolated from bovine adrenal medulla by WATKINSON et al. (1989) and by D'SOUZA and LINDBERG (1988).

A shorter amidated form of peptide F, called amidorphin, was isolated from bovine adrenal (SEIZINGER et al. 1985). This peptide has 26 amino acid residues. The sequence of peptide F contains in position 27 a glycyl residue followed by LysArg and the sequence of [Met[5]]enkephalin (see Fig. 1). It is known that a C-terminal glycyl residue may serve as a nitrogen donor for the amidation of the preceding amino acid residue in a reaction catalyzed by a specific amidation enzyme (BRADBURY et al. 1982).

Amidorphin had so far only been found in bovine adrenal, with low amounts also detected in bovine hypothalamus and posterior pituitary. In other species, the glycyl residue of peptide F is substituted by an alanyl residue and amidorphin was not detected.

The opioid peptides BAM 12P, BAM 20P, and BAM 22P were purified from acid extracts of crude adrenal medulla and found to correspond to parts of peptide I or E (MIZUNO et al. 1980a,b). The C-terminal of BAM 12P and BAM 22P would need uncommon cleavages at the COOH-terminus to be released in vivo.

These BAM peptides could be considered as precursors for another amidated octapeptide discovered simultaneously by WEBER et al. (1983) and MATSUO et al. (1983) and named metorphamide by the former and adrenorphin by the latter. The sequence of this octapeptide is Tyr-Gly-Gly-Phe-Met-Arg-Arg-Val-amide. The glycyl residue following Val in proenkephalin is essential for C-terminal amidation. This amidated peptide was found in all species examined (rat, human, guinea pig, bovine). The levels of the peptide in bovine brain are quite low. The absolute value in bovine caudate nucleus was 12–15 pmol/g as compared to 700 pmol/g for [Leu[5]]enkephalin.

D. Molecular Biology

GIRAUD and EIDEN (1981) were the first to show that a cell-free translation of human pheochromocytoma mRNA synthesized putative opioid precursors which liberated authentic [Met^5]enkephalin following sequential digestion with trypsin and carboxypeptidase B. Using a similar approach, DANDEKAR and SABOL (1982a) showed that cell-free synthesis of [Met^5]enkephalin-containing proteins could also be directed by bovine adrenal medulla mRNA.

An oligodeoxynucleotide probe of defined sequence complementary to the codons specifying the amino acid sequence NH_2-Trp-Trp-Met-Asp-Tyr-Gln-COOH found within peptide E was synthesized by GUBLER et al. (1981). This probe was found to hybridize to bovine adrenal medullary mRNA, which was long enough to code for the proposed size of the enkephalin precursor (circa 1500 nucleotides). Similar results were obtained with both bovine adrenal medulla (NODA et al. 1982a) and human pheochromocytoma (COMB et al. 1982a), using oligodeoxynucleotide probes coding for [Met^5]enkephalin. These probes also hybridized with pro-opiomelanocortin mRNA from mouse pituitary tumor cells and bovine pituitary. However, the mRNA detected in adrenal tissues did not hybridize with a cDNA sequence complementary to mRNA coding for β-lipotropin, another demonstration that the adrenal mRNA was not related to pro-opiomelanocortin (COMB et al. 1982a).

The predicted amino acid sequence of bovine adrenal medulla proenkephalin was simultaneously reported by two groups using the recombinant DNA approach. GUBLER et al. (1982) used their peptide E derived probe to identify positive clones whose nucleotide sequences were then aligned with those coding for known enkephalin-containing peptides. The cDNA sequence formed was almost complete but terminated within known protein sequences. NODA et al. (1982a) reported the complete mRNA sequence coding for preproenkephalin. The deduced amino acid structure (29.786 kDa) contained a 24 amino acid signal peptide and the sequences of all known adrenal enkephalin-containing species (Fig. 1). At the same time preproenkephalin was also cloned from human pheochromocytoma (COMB et al. 1982b).

The cDNA of rat brain preproenkephalin has also been reported (YOSHIKAWA et al. 1984; ROSEN et al. 1984; HOWELLS et al. 1984) and rat preproenkephalin has a high degree of homology with the bovine and human forms (see Fig. 1). The enkephalin, heptapeptide, octapeptide, and peptide E sequences are all conserved, as are the paired basic amino acid residues, the glycosylation site at position 152–154, and the cysteine residues located in the N-terminal region.

The gene for human proenkephalin was first characterized by NODA (NODA et al. 1982b) (Fig. 4). It contains three introns and has some homology with proopiomelanocortin and prodynorphin (see Fig. 5). The chromosomal

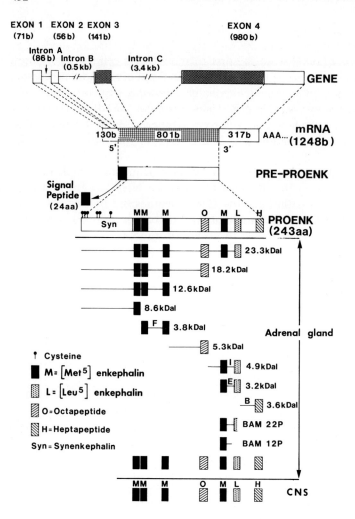

Fig. 4. Biosynthesis and maturation of proenkephalin. The upper part of the figure describes the biosynthesis of human proenkephalin from the corresponding gene. For practical reasons, the 5′ end of the gene upstream from the first exon and the 3′ end of the gene downstream from the fourth exon have not been represented on the figure. The gene is composed of four exons containing respectively 71, 56, 141, and 980 base pairs, separated by three introns of 86 base pairs, and 0.5 and 3.4 kilobase pairs. The four exons are transcribed into a messenger RNA (mRNA) 1248 bases long, to the 3′ end of which is added a polyadenylated tail (AAA . . .). This messenger RNA possesses a 5′ noncoding region 130 bases long and a 3′ noncoding region 317 bases long, which are not translated. Translation of the coding part of the messenger RNA (801 bases) gives rise to pre-proenkephalin (*PRE-PROENK*). Like other precursors of secreted peptides, its amino-terminus is constituted by a short sequence of hydrophobic amino acids, the signal peptide. In the case of human pre-proenkephalin, this peptide comprises the first 24 amino acids of the precursor. The

localization of the human proenkephalin gene was assigned to the distal half of the long arm of chromosome 8 (q23–q24) (LITT et al. 1988). The nucleotide sequence of the cloned rat preproenkephalin gene has also been determined and found to be similar in structural organization to the human gene (ROSEN et al. 1984), although it contains only two introns.

The proenkephalin from *Xenopus laevis* has been partially sequenced by MARTENS and HERBERT (1984) and the proenkephalin cDNA sequence from mouse was found by serendipity by ZURAWSKI et al. (1986) from a cDNA library of activated T-helper cells. In these activated T cells, 0.5% of the mRNA coded for proenkephalin (see extraneuronal enkephalin below).

E. Enkephalin Biosynthesis in the CNS

The hypothesis that enkephalin biosynthesis in the CNS follows a similar pathway to that in the adrenal medulla developed more slowly from biochemical and immunohistochemical investigations. Many groups have raised specific antisera to adrenal peptides, known to be derived from proenkephalin, identified the presence of immunologically related peptides in the brain, and compared their distribution in different brain regions. Most of these investigations have used gel filtration and/or HPLC to further characterize observed immunoreactivity. More often HPLC retention time is the criterion to identify the immunoreactivity as the authentic peptide.

[Met^5]enkephalin-Arg^6-Phe^7 is present in striatal extracts from human, rat, cattle, and guinea pig (ROSSIER et al. 1980a; KOJIMA et al. 1982). The distribution of Met^5-enkephalin-Arg^6-Phe^7 in rat brain extracts parallels that of [Met^5]enkephalin, with the highest levels in globus pallidus, intermediate levels in caudate putamen and hypothalamus, and low levels in the cortex and cerebellum (BOARDER et al. 1982; GIRAUD et al. 1983). Reports have shown that the molar ratio of [Met^5]enkephalin, [Leu^5]enkephalin, [Met^5]enkephalin-Arg^6-Phe^7, and [Met^5]enkephalin-Arg^6-Gly^7-Leu^8 in guinea pig, rat, and golden hamster brain is similar to their ratio within proenkephalin (IKEDA et al. 1982).

← signal peptide is cleaved by the signal peptidase during the transfer of the precursor across the membrane of the endoplasmic reticulum. Proenkephalin (*PROENK*), which results from this cleavage, undergoes proteolytic maturation and gives rise to biologically active peptides. Human proenkephalin is a 243 amino acid long protein. Its amino terminal part is rich in cysteine residues and devoid of opioid activity, and has been called synenkephalin (LISTON et al. 1983). The sequences of opioid peptides are grouped in the carboxy-terminal part of the protein. In the lower part of the figure are schematically represented all the peptides derived from proenkephalin which have been purified or characterized from bovine adrenal medulla, as well as the opioid peptides [Met^5]enkephalin, [Leu^5]enkephalin, [Met^5]-enk-Arg^6-Phe^7, and [Met^5]-enk-Arg^6-Gly^7-Leu^8; which are also present in this tissue. These four opioid peptides have been found also in the central nervous system of several species

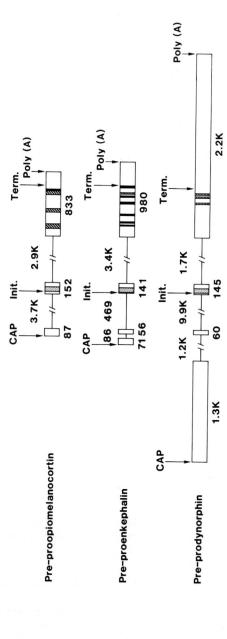

Fig. 5. Comparison of the structures of the human genes coding for the three precursors of opioid peptides. The figure represents the genes coding for human pre-proopiomelanocortin, pre-proenkephalin, and pre-prodynorphin. The 5′ end of the genes upstream from the first exons and the 3′ end of the genes downstream from the last exons are not represented on the figure. The exons are represented by *rectangles*. The length of each exon is indicated under the corresponding exon in base pairs or kilobase pairs (*K*). Introns are represented by *the lines between the exons*. Their lengths are indicated above each one. The sites of initiation (*Init.*) and termination (*Term.*) of translation into protein of the messenger RNA coded for by each gene are indicated above the corresponding gene. The *shaded area* in each gene represents the region of the gene coding for the signal peptide. The *cross-hatched areas* in the third exon of the pre-proopiomelanocortin gene code for the sequences of MSH and the *thick black bar after the last cross-hatched area* represents the [Met⁵]enkephalin sequence of β-endorphin. The *thick black bars* in the fourth exon of the pre-proenkephalin gene code for the sequences of [Met⁵]enkephalin or related opioid peptides (heptapeptide and octapeptide), and the *area containing horizontal bars* codes for the [Leu⁵]enkephalin sequence. In the fourth exon of the pre-prodynorphin gene, the *areas containing horizontal bars* code for [Leu⁵]enkephalin sequences. *CAP*, site of capping of messenger RNA; *Poly(A)*, site of polyadenylation of messenger RNA

IKEDA et al. (1983) have also reported a parallel distribution for these four opioid peptides in human and bovine brain with regional levels of the same order as described by GIRAUD et al. (1983). PITTIUS et al. (1983) found that BAM 12P distribution in human brain was similar to that of [Met^5]enkephalin-Arg^6-Phe^7 and [Met^5]enkephalin-Arg^6-Gly^7-Leu^8 but that this peptide was present in much lower concentrations.

A [Met^5]enkephalin-Arg^6-Gly^7-Leu^8 immunoreactive species with a molecular weight of approximately 8 k has been detected in rat brain and bovine adrenal chromaffin granules (LINDBERG et al. 1983), which has similar chromatographic characteristics to the 5.3-kDa adrenal intermediated isolated by JONES et al. (1982a).

It was thought that if proenkephalin was the precursor for [Met^5]enkephalin and [Leu^5]enkephalin in the central nervous system then high molecular weight forms of these peptides, similar to those purified from adrenal medulla, may exist in the brain. In many distribution studies the antisera that were used failed to cross-react with any higher molecular weight forms of the antigen in the brain (BOARDER et al. 1982; IKEDA et al. 1982, 1983; PITTIUS et al. 1983). However, groups using the sequential trypsin and carboxypeptidase B digest to liberate enkephalin prior to radioreceptor assays, radioimmunoassays, or bioassays reported the presence of putative opioid precursors with estimated molecular weights of up to or greater than 60000 in striatal extracts from cow, guinea pig, and rat (LEWIS et al. 1978; BEAUMONT et al. 1980; KOJIMA et al. 1982).

Evidence that the precursor identified in adrenal was present in brain came unambiguously from a study performed on guinea pig brain. It appeared that striatum of guinea pig (in high levels in that species only) accumulated the unprocessed proenkephalin precursor. BEAUMONT et al. (1985) isolated from a 6 M urea homogenate of striatum a fraction with an apparent molecular weight of 29 k. After digestion with trypsin and carboxypeptidase, this fraction represented approximately 9% of the total [Met^5]enkephalin immunoreactivity. After chromatofocusing and SDS polyacrylamide gel electrophoresis, the precursor was digested and found to contain [Met^5]enkephalin, [Leu^5]enkephalin, and [Met^5]enkephalin-Arg^6-Phe^7 in a proper ratio. Moreover, the heptapeptide was found to constitute the C-terminal. In brain from rat, bovine, and human tissue, this demonstration was never as conclusive.

Other convincing evidence that the same proenkephalin gene is expressed in both adrenal medulla and brain was initially obtained from cell-free translation and cross-hybridization experiments. Using a cell-free translation system, DANDEKAR and SABOL (1982b) identified a putative primary gene product from bovine striatum which had a molecular weight of 31 ± 1 k and was similar to that produced from adrenal medulla using the same technique. This protein liberated [Met^5]enkephalin, [Leu^5]enkephalin, and [Met^5]enkephalin-Arg^6-Phe^7 in a ratio of 4.7:1 after trypsin and carboxypeptidase B treatment. Antiserum directed against [Met^5]enkephalin-Arg^6-

Phe[7] cross-reacted with a $30 \pm 0.5\,\text{kDa}$ protein which was synthesized by translation of mRNA extracted from bovine and guinea pig striata, rat brain, and bovine adrenal medulla. This protein also liberated [Met[5]]enkephalin sequences after digestion (SABOL et al. 1983). Cross-hybridization experiments using cloned cDNA from human pheochromocytoma detected proenkephalin mRNA in rat striatum, hypothalamus, cortex, cerebellum, hippocampus, midbrain, and brainstem as well as rat and bovine adrenal. The mRNA ratio between regions paralleled that of [Met[5]]enkephalin (TANG et al. 1983; LEGON et al. 1982).

F. Synenkephalin

When analyzing the sequences of the proenkephalin molecules available from five different species, it appears that they share a great homology not only in their general organization, but also in the sequences of the non-opioid peptides (see Fig. 1). This is more obvious for the N-terminal region (called synenkephalin), peptide F, peptide E, and peptide B. Synenkephalin in particular contains six Cys residues with identical locations in all five species. This molecule accumulates in brain (LISTON et al. 1983) and is not destroyed during the processing of proenkephalin (LISTON et al. 1984a,b). The molar ratio of synenkephalin to [Met[5]]enkephalin in tissue is close to their stoichiometry in proenkephalin (LISTON and ROSSIER 1984; STELL et al. 1990). The prefix "syn" comes from the Greek, meaning "with." Synenkephalin is always associated with the enkephalins during biosynthesis and secretion. When released in physiological fluid, synenkephalin is not destroyed (LISTON and ROSSIER 1984) in contrast to [Met[5]]enkephalin, [Leu[5]]enkephalin, [Met[5]]enkephalin-Arg[6]-Phe[7], and [Met[5]]enkephalin-Arg[6]-Gly[7]-Leu[8], which are readily hydrolyzed by a variety of peptidases including aminopeptidases and neutral endopeptidase 24.11 (PATEY et al. 1985).

Synenkephalin is not the only case where a large fragment of a prophormone survives the processing of the precursor into the active hormone. Other examples include the N-terminal fragment of proopiomelanocortin (CHAN et al. 1983), peptide C derived from proinsulin (STEINER et al. 1974), and the neurophysins associated with vasopressin and oxytocin (BROWNSTEIN et al. 1980). This phenomenon may thus represent a general feature of peptide hormone biosynthesis.

Synenkephalin is easily measured by radioimmunoassay and in a recent study STELL et al. (1990) validated a new antibody against the C-terminal of synenkephalin. As this part of the molecule is similar in all species, the assay was used with success to analyze human samples (STELL et al. 1990; CORDER et al. 1987). This antibody is available free on request to the author.

For immunohistochemical studies the antisera against synenkephalin have been proven to be superior for localization of enkephalinergic cell bodies than against [Met[5]]enkephalin. Oocytocinergic magnocellular nuclei from bovine brain were visualized by VANDERHAEGHEN et al. (1983), who also detected strong immunoreactivity in the neurohypophyseal terminals. CHARNAY et al. (1985) colocalized synenkephalin immunoreactivity with monoamines in pontobulbar neurons of the cat. EYBALIN et al. (1985) were able to localize the fine localization of synenkephalin in the organ of Corti of the guinea pig at the electron microscopic level. In human tissue, SCHOENEN et al. (1986) localized synenkephalin immunoreactivity in the spinal cord and DE LAET et al. (1989) in the autonomic nervous system of the infant gastrointestinal tract.

In immunocytology, one of the main problems resides in the cross-reactivity of serum. It is almost impossible to obtain monoclonal antibodies to [Met^5]enkephalin that will not show some cross-reactivity with [Leu^5]enkephalin. It was stated earlier in this review that dynorphin neurons contain [Leu^5]enkephalin (ZAMIR et al. 1984). Therefore an antiserum against [Met^5]enkephalin showing immunoreactivity for [Leu^5]enkephalin could also label dynorphin-containing neurons. The use of an antiserum against synenkephalin is therefore an elegant way to overcome these problems associated with cross-reactivity as it allows the specific localization of proenkephalin-containing neurons and excludes the prodynorphin-containing neurons. The importance of the specific labeling of proenkephalin neurons with synenkephalin immunoserum and the absence of the labeling of prodynorphin neurons was stressed recently by SONG et al. (1990).

G. Molecular Evolution of Proenkephalin

Figure 1 shows the primary sequence of proenkephalin from five species. The main difference is the absence of [Leu^5]enkephalin in *Xenopus*. This could mean that the [Leu^5]enkephalin sequence appeared after amphibians and reptiles diverged. However, as pointed out by DORES et al. (1990), [Leu^5]enkephalin is found in fish (DORES et al. 1989; DORES and GORBMAN 1990) and reptiles (LINDBERG and WHITE 1986) and the current hypothesis is that the [Leu^5]enkephalin sequence in proenkephalin appeared early in evolution and has been lost in amphibians.

The presence of proenkephalin-derived peptides in invertebrates has been described by several groups from imunocytochemical evidence. A chemical identification has also been performed in extracts of pedal ganglia of *Mytilus edulis* (the common mussel) by LEUNG and STEFANO (1984). [Met^5] and [Leu^5]enkephalin were identified by their retention times on HPLC. Based on this observation, the proenkephalin molecule seems to have appeared quite early in evolution.

Figure 1 also shows that the sequence of the octapeptide varies between species: mouse with [Met^5]enkephalin-Arg^6-Ser^7-Leu^8 and *Xenopus* with [Met^5]enkephalin-Arg^6-Gly^7-Tyr^8. A recent report from CUPO et al. (1990) showed that in the cat the octapeptide, if it exists in that species, is also

different from the sequence [Met^5]enkephalin-Arg^6-Gly^7-Leu^8 as they were
unable to detect this peptide in the brain or adrenal using a highly specific
and sensitive radioimmunoassay (Cupo et al. 1984).

H. Extraneuronal Proenkephalin

I. Reproductive Tissue

In 1985, Kilpatrick et al. reported that proenkephalin mRNA and its
peptide products were found in mammalian testis and ovary. Since then
proenkephalinergic material (mRNA or enkephalin immunoreactivity) has
been localized in numerous components of the male reproductive system:
in Sertoli cells (Kew and Kilpatrick 1989), in Leydig cells (Garret and
Douglass 1989), and in epididymis (Garret et al. 1990).

In the primate female reproductive system proenkephalinergic material
was found in endometrial cells of the uterus, where it varies with menstrual
cycle (Low et al. 1989), with increasing levels during the follicular phase and
suppression with progesterone during the luteal phase. In the rodent the
regulation of proenkephalin materials seems to be completely different from
the primate as progesterone increases proenkephalin mRNA levels (Jin et
al. 1988; Muffly et al. 1988).

II. Glial Cells

In 1985, Zagon et al. made the observation that germinative cells of
developing cerebellum contained immunoreactive [Met^5]enkephalinergic
material. This observation was followed by the detection of high levels of
proenkephalin mRNA in C6 rat glioma cell line (Yoshikawa and Sabol
1986) and also in primary cultures of astrocytes (Vilijn et al. 1988). In a
similar culture of astrocytes, [Met^5]enkephalin and [Met^5]enkephalin-Arg^6-
Phe^7 were identified by Shinoda et al. (1989) and by Melner et al. (1990).

The levels of the peptidergic material are never very impressive, being
only about 1/50 of the values found for [Met^5]enkephalin in extracts of
corresponding brain regions. Nevertheless, the presence of proenkephalin-
derived material in glial cells has been proven and deserves more attention.

In a study on the cerebellum, Spruce et al. (1990) detected proenkephalin mRNA and protein in subpopulations of both gray and white
matter astrocytes but not Bergmann glia. The general idea evolving from
this work is that proenkephalin-derived peptides are secreted by astrocytes
and play an important role during neural development, as earlier proposed by Zagon et al. (1985), or trauma-induced gliosis. Even if it is
not [Met^5]enkephalin which plays such a role, other good candidates exist
among the nonopioid peptides derived from proenkephalin. Figure 1 shows
that in the proenkephalin sequence some nonopioid peptides are conserved

among different species: peptides I, B and synenkephalin. These have been isolated from various tissues and could have some physiological function in neural development.

III. Immune System

In Chap. 45 in part II of this volume, H.V. BRYANT and J.W. HOLADAY have described the role of the opioid system in the immune response. Proenkephalin is indeed an important actor in this process. In 1986, ZURAWESKI et al. found that up to 0.5% of mRNA of stimulated T-helper cells was proenkephalin mRNA. At that time, immunologists were looking for new lymphokines. ZURAWSKI et al. prepared a subtracted cDNA library from mouse T cells activated by concanavalin A and isolated several clones that contained proenkephalin cDNA. [Met^5]enkephalin immunoreactivity was also found in media of T-helper cells stimulated for 24 h with concanavalin A with levels of 1 pmol/ml, levels which are of the same order as those found in the media of bovine chromaffin cells in culture (ROSSIER et al. 1980b). In bovine adrenals, proenkephalin mRNA frequency is about 1/1000 and in brain less than 1/3000 (HOWELLS et al. 1984), thus making the frequency of 1/200 in stimulated T cells startling. Are enkephalins important lymphokines? Yes, if their levels are compared with those of other lymphokines, although I would like to point out that, as for the glial cells, the enkephalins themselves might *not* be the physiologically important peptides. Processing of proenkephalin leads to several other compounds, peptides I, E, B, F, and synenkephalin, all of which are putative lymphokines.

I. Processing of Proenkephalin

The role of enzymes in prohormone processing is reviewed in Chap. 20 by L. FRICKER. I wish only to emphasize that proenkephalin processing is not the same in all tissues, including the extraneuronal tissues discussed in the preceding paragraphs. LISTON et al. (1984b) have demonstrated that proenkephalin enters different processing pathways in adrenal and brain. The peptides I, E, F, and B accumulate in adrenals and not in brain tissue. By alternate processing, proenkephalin could generate a variety of different peptides, some devoid of the N-terminal YGGF, and consequently with no opioid activity. It is thus possible, but not yet proven, that several nonopioid peptides obtained by partial digestion of proenkephalin are important physiological messengers.

J. Regulation

The regulation of the opioid genes and the mechanisms of this regulation are reviewed in Chaps. 14, 15 and 16. I will thus just briefly summarize the major features.

The initial observation was that adrenal denervation led to a large increase of proenkephalin (Lewis et al. 1981) and proenkephalin mRNA (Kilpatrick et al. 1984). In contrast, a strong depolarization of the adrenal led to a decrease in proenkephalin mRNA (La Gamma et al. 1985). The general idea was thus that enkephalin biosynthesis, as opposed to catecholamines, was increased by denervation and decreased by transynaptic activation. This simple view of the situation lasted only until it was observed that various stimuli known to increase catecholamine synthesis also increase proenkephalin synthesis (Kanamatsu et al. 1986c; La Gamma et al. 1989; DeCristofaro and La Gamma 1990).

The regulation of proenkephalin is complex, with numerous transcriptional regulators already characterized. In glial C6 glioma cells, Comb et al. (1988) have shown that the increase in proenkephalin mRNA seen after treatment with cAMP or phorbol ester is mediated by at least four transcription factors, AP-1, AP-2, AP-4, and ENKTF-1. One of these transcription factors, AP-1, is so far known to consist of the products of *fos* and *jun* oncogenes. Phorbol ester, following a cascade of events, induces phosphorylation of the hetero dimer Fos/Jun that will bind, after phosphorylation, to the DNA (Auwerx and Sassone-Corsi 1991). Comb et al. (1988) have shown that a sequence of DNA located in the 5′ region of the enkephalin gene will bind AP-1. This sequence called ENKCRE-2 acts in a synergistic fashion with another promoter element ENKCRE-1. The nuclear protein ENKTF-1 will bind specifically to ENKCRE-1. Comb et al. (1988) have thus identified at least two *cis*-acting elements upstream of the proenkephalin gene.

These DNA responsive elements have also been studied by Sonnenberg et al. (1989) in an in vivo model. Following seizure with pentylenetetrazol, proenkephalin materials increase markedly in the dentate gyrus of hippocampus. A similar increase in the hippocampus is also seen after seizure induced by kainic acid injection (Kanamatsu et al. 1986b), electroconvulsive shock (Kanamatsu et al. 1986a), kindling (McGinty et al. 1986), and lesion of the hilus (White et al. 1987). Sonnenberg et al. (1989) have observed that c-*fos* and c-*jun* mRNA are markedly increased in the minute following seizure induction. This increase is followed by an increase in proenkephalin mRNA. Once again, this could indicate that the transactivating factor AP-1, formed by the heterodimeric complex Fos/jun, functions as a transcriptional regulator in enkephalinergic neurons.

Another transcriptional regulator in enkephalinergic neurons could be the estrogen receptor. Romano et al. (1989) have found that the proenkephalin gene contains a putative estrogen regulatory element whose activation could be directly involved in the ventromedial hypothalamus, where an increase in proenkephalin mRNA was seen after treatment with estrogen.

K. Conclusion

This story began with the discovery of two opioid peptides, [Met^5]enkephalin and [Leu^5]enkephalin, by HUGHES et al. in 1975. Later, β-endorphin was discovered, followed by the prodynorphin-derived peptides. The increase in the number of opioid peptides characterized has shown that the endogenous opioid systems are much more complex than we might have thought at first. To add to the multitude of different opioid peptides, the nonopioid peptides known to be derived from the opioid peptide precursors have only further complicated matters. Today, the search for new opioid peptides is almost over apart from peptides being isolated from frog's skin (dermorphin and deltorphin) and from other nonnervous tissues (see Chap. 21). The mystery of the apparent redundancy of all these opioid systems have yet to be solved, although one day the roles of all these peptides in physiological control at several levels will no doubt become clearer. Once brain mechanisms are better understood, we will certainly be in a better position to comprehend the purpose of the opioid systems.

References

Auwerx J, Sassone-Corsi P (1991) IP-1: a dominant inhibitor of FOS/Jun whose activity is modulated by phosphorylation. Cell 64:983–993

Beaumont A, Fuentes JA, Hughes J, Metters KM (1980) Opioid peptide precursors in striatum. FEBS Lett 122:135–137

Beaumont A, Metters KM, Rossier J, Hughes J (1985) Identification of a pro-enkephalin precursor in striatal tissue. J Neurochem 44:934–940

Bloom F, Battenberg E, Rossier J, Ling N, Guillemin R (1978) Neurons containing β-endorphin in rat brain exist separately from those containing enkephalin: immunohistochemical studies. Proc Natl Acad Sci USA 75:1591–1595

Boarder MR, Lockfeld AJ, Barchas JD (1982) Measurement of methionine-enkephalin (Arg^6, Phe^7) in rat brain by specific radioimmunoassay directed at methionine sulphoxide enkephalin (Arg^6, Phe^7). J Neurochem 38:299–304

Bradbury AF, Finnie MD, Smyth DG (1982) Mechanism of C-terminal amide formation by pituitary enzymes. Nature 298:686–688

Brownstein MJ, Russell JT, Gainer H (1980) Synthesis, transport and release of posterior pituitary hormones. Science 207:373–378

Chaminade M, Foutz AS, Rossier J (1984) Co-release of enkephalins and precursors with catecholamines from the perfused cat adrenal gland in situ. J Physiol 353:157–169

Chan JSD, Seidah NG, Chrétien M (1983) Measurement of N-terminal (1–76) of human proopiomelancocortin in human plasma: correlation with adreno-corticotropin. J Clin Endocrinol Metab 56:791–796

Charnay Y, Leger L, Rossier J, Jouvet M, Dubois PM (1985) Evidence for synenkephalin-like immunoreactivity in pontobulbar monoaminergic neurons of the cat. Brain Res 335:160–164

Comb M, Herbert E, Crea R (1982a) Partial characterization of the mRNA that codes for enkephalins in bovine adrenal medulla and human pheochromocytoma. Proc Natl Acad Sci USA 79:360–364

Comb M, Seebury PH, Adelman J, Eiden L, Herbert E (1982b) Primary structure of the human Met- and Leu-enkephalin precursor and its mRNA. Nature 295: 663–666

Comb M, Mermod N, Hyman SE, Pearlberg J, Ross ME, Goodman HM (1988) Proteins bound at adjacent DNA elements act synergistically to regulate human proenkephalin cAMP inducible transcription. EMBO J 7:3793–3805

Corder R, Gaillard RC, Rossier J (1987) Indentification of human synenkephalin-like immunoreactivity in phaeochromocytoma tissue using a novel carboxy-terminal radioimmunoassay. Neurosci Lett 82:308–314

Crawley JN (1985) Comparative distribution of cholecystokinin and other neuro-peptides. Why is this peptide different from all other peptides? Ann NY Acad Sci 448:1–8

Cupo A, Eybalin M, Patey G, Rossier J, Jarry T (1984) Quantitation and localiza-tion of met-enkephalin Arg-Gly-Leu in rat brain using highly sensitive anti-bodies. Neuropeptides 4:389–401

Cupo A, Leger L, Charnay Y, Fourrier O, Jarry T, Masmejean F (1990) The proenkephalin-A-derivative Met-enkephalin-Arg-Gly-Leu is not present in the feline species. Neuropeptides 17:171–176

Dandekar S, Sabol SL (1982a) Cell-free translation and partial characterization of mRNA coding for enkephalin-precursor protein. Proc Natl Acad Sci USA 79:1017–1021

Dandekar S, Sabol SL (1982b) Cell-free translation and partial characterization of proenkephalin messenger RNA from bovine striatum. Biochem Biophys Res Commun 105:67–74

DeCristofaro JD, La Gamma EF (1990) Bimodal regulation of adrenal opiate peptides by cholinergic mechanisms. Neuroscience 35:203–210

De Laet M-H, Dassonville M, Lotstra F, Vierendeels G, Rossier J, Vanderhaeghen J-J (1989) Proenkephalin A associated peptides in the autonomic nervous system of the human infant gastrointestinal tract. Neurochem Int 14:129–134

Dores RM, Gorbman A (1990) Detection of Met-enkephalin and Leu-enkephalin in the brain of the hagfish, Eptatretus stouti, and the lamprey, Petromyzon marinus. Gen Comp Endocrinol 77:489–499

Dores RM, McDonald LK, Crim JW (1989) Detection of Met-enkephalin and Leu-enkephalin in the posterior pituitary of the holostean fish, Amia calva. Peptides 10:951–956

Dores RM, McDonald LK, Tami CS, Sei CA (1990) The molecular evolution of neuropeptides: prospects for the '90s. Brain Behav Evol 36:80–99

D'Souza NB, Lindberg I (1988) Evidence for the phosphorylation of a proenkephalin-derived peptide, peptide B. J Biol Chem 263:2548–2552

Eybalin M, Abou-Madi L, Rossier J, Pujol R (1985) Electron microscopic localiza-tion of N-terminal proenkephalin (synenkephalin) immunostaining in the guinea pig organ of Corti. Brain Res 358:354–359

Fayada C, Guibert B, Patey G, Cupo A, Chaminade M, Rossier J, Leviel V (1987) Release of [Met^5]enkephalin in the central nucleus of the amygdala is increased by application of potassium in the substantia nigra. Neuropeptides 9:9–17

Garrett JE, Douglass JO (1989) Human chorionic gonadotropin regulates expression of the proenkephalin gene in adult rat Leydig cells. Mol Endocrinol 3: 2093–2100

Garrett JE, Garrett SH, Douglass JO (1990) A spermatozoa-associated factor regulates proenkephalin gene expression in the rat epididymis. Mol Endocrinol 4:108–118

Giraud P, Eiden LE (1981) Cell-free translation of human pheochromocytoma messenger RNA yields protein(s) containing methionine-enkephalin. Biochem Biophys Res Comm 99:969–975

Giraud P, Castanas E, Patey G, Oliver C, Rossier J (1983) Regional distribution of methionine-enkephalin-Arg^6-Phe^7 in the rat brain: comparative study with the distribution of other opioid peptides. J Neurochem 41:154–160

Goldstein A, Fischli A, Lowney LI, Hunkapille M, Hood L (1981) Porcine pituitary dynorphin: Complete amino acid sequence of the biologically active heptade-capeptide. Proc Natl Acad Sci USA 78:7218–7223

Gubler U, Kilpatrick DL, Seeburg PH, Gage LP, Udenfriend S (1981) Detection and partial characterization of proenkephalin mRNA. Proc Natl Acad Sci USA 78:5484–5487

Gubler U, Seeburg P, Hoffman BJ, Gage LP, Udenfriend S (1982) Molecular cloning establishes proenkephalin as precursor of enkephalin-containing peptides. Nature 295:206–208

Howells RD, Kilpatrick DL, Bhatt R, Monahan JJ, Poonian M, Udenfriend S (1984) Molecular cloning and sequence determination of rat preproenkephalin cDNA: sensitive probe for studying transcriptional changes in rat tissues. Proc Natl Acad Sci USA 81:7651–7655

Hughes J, Smith TW, Kosterlitz HW, Fothergill LA, Morgan BA, Morris HR (1975) Identification of two related pentapeptides from the brain with potent opiate agonist activity. Nature 258:577–579

Ikeda Y, Nakao K, Yoshimasa T, Yanaihara N, Numa S, Imura H (1982) Existence of Met-enkephalin-Arg^6-Gly^7-Leu^8 with Met-enkephalin, Leu-enkephalin and Met-enkephalin-Arg^6-Phe^7 in the brain of guinea pig, rat and golden hamster. Biochem Biophys Res Commun 107:656–662

Ikeda Y, Nakao K, Yoshimasa T, Sakamoto M, Suda M, Yanaihara N, Imura H (1983) Parallel distribution of methionine-enkephalin-Arg^6-Gly^7-Leu^8 with methionine-enkephalin, leucine-enkephalin and methionine-enkephalin-Arg^6-Phe^7 in human and bovine brains. Life Sci 33(Suppl 1):65–68

Jin DF, Muffly KE, Okulicz WC, Kilpatrick DL (1988) Estrous cycle- and pregnancy-related differences in expression of the proenkephalin and pro-opiomelanocortin genes in the ovary and uterus. Endocrinology 122:1466–1471

Jones BN, Stern AS, Lewis RV, Kimura S, Stein S, Udenfriend S, Shively JE (1980) Structure of two adrenal polypeptides containing multiple enkephalin sequences. Arch Biochem Biophys 204:392–395

Jones BN, Shively JE, Kilpatrick DL, Kojima K, Udenfriend S (1982a) Enkephalin biosynthetic pathway: a 5300-dalton adrenal polypeptide that terminates at its COOH end with the sequence (Met)enkephalin-Arg-Gly-Leu-COOH. Proc Natl Acad Sci USA 79:1313–1315

Jones BN, Shively JE, Kilpatrick DL, Stern AS, Lewis RV, Kojima K, Udenfriend S (1982b) Adrenal opioid proteins of 8600 and 12 600 daltons: intermediates in proenkephalin processing. Proc Natl Acad Sci USA 79:2096–2100

Kanamatsu T, McGinty JF, Mitchell CL, Hong JS (1986a) Dynorphin- and enkephalin-like immunoreactivity is altered in limbic-basal ganglia regions of rat brain after repeated electroconvulsive shock. J Neurosci 6:644–649

Kanamatsu T, Obie J, Grimes L, McGinty JF, Yoshikawa K, Sabol SL, Hong JS (1986b) Kainic acid alters the metabolism of Met^5-enkephalin and the level of dynorphin A in the rat hippocampus. J Neurosci 6:3094–3102

Kanamatsu T, Unsworth CD, Diliberto EJ, Jr, Viveros OH, Hong JS (1986c) Reflex splanchnic nerve stimulation increases levels of proenkephalin A mRNA and proenkephalin A-related peptides in the rat adrenal medulla. Proc Natl Acad Sci USA 83:9245–9249

Kew D, Kilpatrick DL (1989) Expression and regulation of the proenkephalin gene in rat Sertoli cells. Mol Endocrinol 3:179–184

Kilpatrick DL, Taniguchi T, Jones BN, Stern AS, Shively JE, Hullihan J, Kimura S, Stein S, Udenfriend S (1981a) A highly potent 3200-dalton adrenal opioid peptide that contains both a (Met)- and (Leu)enkephalin sequence. Proc Natl Acad Sci USA 78:3265–3268

Kilpatrick DL, Jones BN, Kojima K, Udenfriend S (1981b) Identification of the octapeptide (Met)enkephalin-Arg[6]-Gly[7]-Leu[8] in extracts of bovine adrenal medulla. Biochem Biophys Res Commun 103:698–705

Kilpatrick DL, Jones BN, Lewis RV, Stern AS, Kojima K, Shively JE, Udenfriend S (1982) An 18 200-dalton adrenal protein that contains four (Met)enkephalin sequences. Proc Natl Acad Sci USA 79:3057–3061

Kilpatrick DL, Howells RD, Fleminger G, Udenfriend S (1984) Denervation of rat adrenal glands markedly increases proenkephalin mRNA. Proc Natl Acad Sci USA 81:7221–7223

Kilpatrick DL, Howells RD, Noe M, Bailey LC, Udenfriend S (1985) Expression of preproenkephalin-like mRNA and its peptide products in mammalian testis and ovary. Proc Natl Acad Sci USA 82:7467–7469

Kimura S, Lewis RV, Stern AS, Rossier J, Stein S, Udenfriend S (1980) Probable precursors of (Leu)enkephalin and (Met)enkephalin in adrenal medulla: peptides of 3–5 kilodaltons. Proc Natl Acad Sci USA 77:1681–1685

Kojima K, Kilpatrick DL, Stern AS, Jones BN, Udenfriend S (1982) Proenkephalin: a general pathway for enkephalin biosynthesis in animal tissues. Arch Biochem Biophys 215:638–643

La Gamma EF, White JD, Adler JE, Krause JE, McKelvy JF, Black IB (1985) Depolarization regulates adrenal proenkephalin mRNA. Proc Natl Acad Sci USA 82:8252–8255

La Gamma EF, De Cristofaro JE, Agarwel BL, Weisinger G (1989) Ontogeny of the opiate phenotype: an approach to defining transsynaptic mechanisms at the molecular level in the rat adrenal medulla. Int J Dev Neurosci 7:499–511

Legon S, Glover DM, Hughes J, Lowry PJ, Rigby PWJ, Watson CJ (1982) The structure and expression of the preproenkephalin gene. Nucleic Acid Res 10:7905–7918

Leung MK, Stefano GB (1984) Isolation and identification of enkephalins in pedal ganglia of Mytilus edulis (Mollusca). Proc Natl Acad Sci USA 81:955–958

Lewis RV, Stein S, Gerber LD, Rubinstein M, Udenfriend S (1978) High molecular weight opioid-containing proteins in striatum. Proc Natl Acad Sci USA 75:4021–4023

Lewis RV, Stern AS, Rossier J, Stein S, Udenfriend S (1979) Putative enkephalin precursors in bovine adrenal medulla. Biochem Biophys Res Commun 89:822–829

Lewis RV, Stern AS, Kimura S, Stein S, Udenfriend S (1980a) Enkephalin biosynthetic pathways: proteins of 8000 and 14000 daltons in bovine adrenal medulla. Proc Natl Acad Sci USA 77:5018–5020

Lewis RV, Stern AS, Kimura S, Rossier J, Stein S, Udenfriend S (1980b) An about 50 000-dalton protein in adrenal medulla: a common precursor of (Met)- and (Leu)-enkephalin. Science 208:1459–1461

Lewis RV, Stern AS, Kilpatrick DL, Gerber LD, Rossier J, Stein S, Udenfriend S (1981) Marked increases in large enkephalin-containing polypeptides in the rat adrenal gland following denervation. J Neurosci 1:80–82

Lindberg I, White L (1986) Reptilian enkephalins: implications for the evolution of proenkephalin. Arch Biochem Biophys 245:1–7

Lindberg I, Yang H-YT, Costa E (1983) A high molecular weight form of Met[5]-enkephalin-Arg[6]-Gly[7]-Leu[8] in rat brain and bovine adrenal chromaffin granules. Life Sci 33(Suppl):5–8

Liston D, Rossier J (1984) Synenkephalin is coreleased with Met-enkephalin from neuronal terminals in vitro. Neurosci Lett 48:211–216

Liston DR, Vanderhaeghen J-J, Rossier J (1983) Presence in brain of synenkephalin, a proenkephalin-immunoreactive protein which does not contain enkephalin. Nature 302:335–341

Liston D, Bohlen P, Rossier J (1984a) Purification from brain of synenkephalin, the N-terminal fragment of proenkephalin. J Neurochem 43:335–341

Liston D, Patey G, Rossier J, Verbanck P, Vanderhaeghen J-J (1984b) Processing of proenkephalin is tissue-specific. Science 225:734–737

Litt M, Buroker NE, Kondoleon S, Douglass J, Liston D, Sheehy R (1988) Chromosomal localization of the human proenkephalin and prodynorphin genes. Am J Hum Genet 42:327–334

Livett BG, Dean DM, Whelan LG, Udenfriend S, Rossier J (1981) Co-release of enkephalin and catecholamines from cultured adrenal chromaffin cells. Nature 289:317–319

Livett BG, Day R, Elde RP, Howe PRC (1982) Co-storage of enkephalins and adrenaline in the bovine adrenal medulla. Neuroscience 7:1323–1332

Low KG, Nielsen CP, West NB, Douglass J, Brenner RM, Maslar IA, Melner MH (1989) Proenkephalin gene expression in the primate uterus: regulation by estradiol in the endometrium. Mol Endocrinol 3:852–857

Marshall RD (1972) Glycoproteins. Annu Rev Biochem 41:673–702

Martens GJM, Herbert E (1984) Polymorphism and absence of leu-enkephalin sequences in proenkephalin genes in Xenopus laevis. Nature 310:251–254

Matsuo H, Miyata A, Mizuno K (1983) Novel C-terminally amidated opioid peptide in human phaeochromocytoma tumour. Nature 305:721–723

McGinty JF, Kanamatsu T, Obie J, Dyer RS, Mitchell CL, Hong JS (1986) Amygdaloid kindling increases enkephalin-like immunoreactivity but decreases dynorphin A-like immunoreactivity in rat hippocampus. Neurosci Lett 71:31–36

Melner MH, Low KG, Allen RG, Nielsen CP, Young SL, Saneto RP (1990) The regulation of proenkephalin expression in a distinct population of glial cells. EMBO J 9:791–796

Metters KM, Rossier J (1987) Affinity purification of synenkephalin-containing peptides, including a novel 23.3-kilodalton species. J Neurochem 49:721–728

Metters KM, Beaumont A, Rossier J, Hughes J (1985) A comparison of opioid peptide precursors in guinea pig, rat and bovine striata and guinea pig adrenal. Neuropeptides 5:521–524

Metters KM, Rossier J, Paquin J, Chrétien M, Seidah NG (1988) Selective cleavage of proenkephalin-derived peptides (<23 300 Daltons) by plasma kallikrein. J Biol Chem 263:12543–12553

Mizuno K, Minamino N, Kangawa K, Matsuo H (1980a) A new family of endogenous "big" Met-enkephalins from bovine adrenal medulla purification and structure of docosa-(BAM-22P) and eicosapeptide (BAM-20P) with very potent opioid activity. Biochem Biophys Res Comm 97:1283–1290

Mizuno K, Minamino N, Kangawa K, Matsuo H (1980b) A new endogenous opioid peptide from bovine adrenal medulla: isolation and amino acid sequence of a dodecapeptide (BAM-12P). Biochem Biophys Res Comm 95:1482–1488

Muffly KE, Jin DF, Okulicz WC, Kilpatrick DL (1988) Gonadal steroids regulate proenkephalin gene expression in a tissue-specific manner within the female reproductive system. Mol Endocrinol 2:979–985

Noda M, Furutani Y, Takahashi H, Toyosato M, Hirose T, Inayama S, Nakanishi S, Numa S (1982a) Cloning and sequence analysis of cDNA for bovine adrenal preproenkephalin. Nature 295:202–206

Noda M, Teranishi Y, Takahashi M, Toyosato M, Notake M, Nakanishi S, Numa S (1982b) Isolation and structural organization of the human preproenkephalin gene. Nature 297:431–434

Palmour RM, Ervin FR, Wagemaker H, Cade R (1979) Characterization of a peptide derived from the serum of psychotic patients. In: Udsin E, Bunney WE, Kline NS (eds) Endorphins in mental health research. MacMillian, London, pp 581–593

Patey G, Liston D, Rossier J (1984) Characterization of new enkephalin-containing peptides in the adrenal medulla by immunoblotting. FEBS Lett 172:303–308

Patey G, Cupo A, Mazarguil H, Morgat JL, Rossier J (1985) Release of proenkephalin-derived opioid peptides from rat striatum in vitro and their rapid degradation. Neuroscience 15:1035–1044

Pittius CW, Seizinger BR, Mehraein P, Pasi A, Herz A (1983) Proenkephalin-A-
    derived peptides are present in human brain. Life Sci 33(Suppl 1):41–44
Roisin MP, Artola A, Henry JP, Rossier J (1983) Enkephalins are associated with
    adrenergic granules in bovine adrenal medulla. Neuroscience 10:83–88
Romano GJ, Mobbs CV, Howells RD, Pfaff DW (1989) Estrogen regulation of
    proenkephalin gene expression in the ventromedial hypothalamus of the rat:
    temporal qualities and synergism with progesterone. Mol Brain Res 5:51–58
Rosen H, Douglass J, Herbert E (1984) Isolation and characterisation of the rat
    preproenkephalin gene. J Biol Chem 259:14309–14313
Rossier J, Vargo TM, Minick S, Ling N, Bloom FE, Guillemin R (1977) Regional
    dissociation of β-endorphin and enkephalin contents in rat brain and pituitary.
    Proc Natl Acad Sci USA 74:5162–5165
Rossier J, Audigier Y, Ling N, Cros J, Udenfriend S (1980a) Met-enkephalin-Arg[6]-
    Phe[7], present in high amounts in brain of rat, cattle and man, is an opioid
    agonist. Nature 288:88–90
Rossier J, Trifaro JM, Lewis RV, Lee RWH, Stern AS, Kimura S, Stein S,
    Udenfriend S (1980b) Studies with (^{35}S)methionine indicate that the 22 000-
    dalton (Met)enkephalin-containing protein in chromaffin cells is a precursor of
    (Met)enkephalin. Proc Natl Acad Sci USA 77:6889–6891
Rossier J, Dean D, Livett BG, Udenfriend S (1981) Enkephalin congeners and
    precursors are synthesized and released by primary cultures of adrenal
    chromaffin cells. Life Sci 28:781–789
Rossier J, Barrès E, Cupo A, Edwards AV (1988) The release of enkephalin-
    containing peptides from the adrenal gland in conscious calves. In: Pickering
    BT, Wakerley JB, Summerlee AJS (eds) Neurosecretion cellular aspects of the
    production and release of neuropeptides. Proceedings of the 10th international
    symposium on neurosecretion. Plenum, London, pp 53–59
Sabol SL, Liang C-M, Dandekar S, Kranzler LS (1983) In vitro biosynthesis and
    processing of immunologically identified methionine-enkephalin precursor
    protein. J Biol Chem 258:2697–2704
Schoenen J, Lotstra F, Liston D, Rossier J, Vanderhaeghen J-J (1986)
    Synenkephalin in bovine and human spinal cord. Cell Tissue Res 246:641–645
Schultzberg M, Lundberg JM, Hokfelt T, Terenius L, Brandt J, Elde RP, Goldstein
    A (1978) Enkephalin-like immunoreactivity in gland cells and nerve terminals of
    the adrenal medulla. Neuroscience 3:1169–1186
Seizinger BR, Liebisch DC, Gramsch C, Herz A, Weber E, Evans CJ, Esch FS,
    Böhlen P (1985) Isolation and structure of a novel C-terminally amidated opioid
    peptide, amidorphin, from bovine adrenal. Nature 313:57–59.
Shinoda H, Marini AM, Cosi C, Schwartz JP (1989) Brain region and gene specificity
    of neuropeptide gene expression in cultured astrocytes. Science 245:415–417
Song DD, Rossier J, Harlan RE (1990) Comparison of synenkephalin and
    methionine enkephalin immunocytochemistry in rat brain. Peptides 10:1239–
    1246
Sonnenberg JL, Rauscher JR III, Morgan JI, Curran T (1989) Regulation of
    proenkephalin by Fos and Jun. Science 246:1622–1625
Spruce BA, Curtis R, Wilkin GP, Glover DM (1990) A neuropeptide precursor in
    cerebellum: proenkephalin exists in subpopulations of both neurons and
    astrocytes. EMBO J 9:3790–3798
Steiner DF, Kemmler W, Tager HS, Peterson JD (1974) Proteolytic processing in
    the biosynthesis of insulin and other proteins. Federation Proc 33:2105–2115
Stell WK, Chaminade M, Metter KM, Rougeot C, Dray F, Rossier J (1990)
    Detection of synenkephalin, the amino-terminal portion of proenkephalin, by
    antisera directed against its carboxyl terminus. J Neurochem 54:434–443
Stern AS, Lewis RV, Kimura S, Rossier J, Gerber LD, Brink L, Stein S, Udenfriend
    S (1979) Isolation of the opioid heptapeptide Met-enkephalin(Arg[6], Phe[7]) from
    bovine adrenal medullary granules and striatum. Proc Natl Acad Sci USA
    76:6680–6683

Stern AS, Jones BN, Shively JE, Stein S, Udenfriend S (1981) Two adrenal opioid polypeptides: proposed intermediates in the processing of proenkephalin. Proc Natl Acad Sci USA 78:1962–1966

Tang F, Costa E, Schwartz JP (1983) Increase of proenkephalin mRNA and enkephalin content of rat striatum after daily injection of holoperidol for 2 to 3 weeks. Proc Natl Acad Sci USA 80:3841–3844

Udenfriend S, Kilpatrick DL (1983) Biochemistry of the enkephalins and enkephalin-containing peptides. Arch Biochem Biophys 221:309–323

Vanderhaeghen JJ, Lotstra F, Liston DR, Rossier J (1983) Proenkephalin, [Met]enkephalin, and oxytocin immunoreactivities are colocalized in bovine hypothalamic magnocellular neurons. Proc Natl Acad Sci USA 80:5139–5143

Vilijn M-H, Vaysse PJ-J, Zukin RS, Kessler JA (1988) Expression of pre-proenkephalin mRNA by cultured astrocytes and neurons. Proc Natl Acad Sci USA 85:6551–6555

Viveros OH, Diliberto EJ, Hazum E, Chang K-J (1979) Opiate-like materials in the adrenal-medulla: evidence for storage and secretion with catecholamines. Mol Pharmacol 16:1101–1108.

Watkinson A, Dockray GJ, Young J (1988) N-linked glycosylation of a proenkephalin A-derived peptide. Evidence for the glycosylation of an NH_2-terminally extended Met-enkephalin Arg[6]-Gly[7]-Leu[8] variant. J Biol Chem 263:7147–7152

Watkinson A, Young J, Varro A, Dockray GJ (1989) The isolation and chemical characterization of phosphorylated enkephalin-containing peptides from bovine adrenal medulla. J Biol Chem 264:3061–3065

Weber E, Esch FS, Bohlen P, Paterson S, Corbett AD, McKnight AS, Kosterlitz HW, Barchas JD, Evans CJ (1983) Metorphamide: isolation, structure and biologic activity of an amidated opioid octapeptide from bovine brain. Proc Natl Acad Sci USA 80:7362–7366

White JD, Gall CM, McKelvy JF (1987) Enkephalin biosynthesis and enkephalin gene expression are increased in hippocampal mossy fibers following a unilateral lesion of the hilus. J Neurosci 7:753–759

Yoshikawa K, Sabol SL (1986) Expression of the enkephalin precursor gene in C6 rat glioma cells: regulation by β-adrenergic agonists and glucocorticoids. Mol Brain Res 1:75–83

Yoshikawa K, Williams C, Sabol SL (1984) Rat brain preproenkephalin mRNA: cDNA cloning, primary structure, and distribution in the central nervous system. J Biol Chem 259:14301–14308

Zagon IS, Rhodes RE, McLaughlin PJ (1985) Distribution of enkephalin immunoreactivity in germinative cells of developing rat cerebellum. Science 227:1049–1051

Zamir N, Palkovits M, Weber E, Mezey E, Brownstein M (1984) A dynorphinergic pathway of Leu-enkephalin production in the rat substantia nigra. Nature 307:643–645

Zurawski G, Benedik M, Kamb BJ, Abrams JS, Zurawski SM, Lee FD (1986) Activation of mouse T-helper cells induces abundant preproenkephalin mRNA synthesis. Science 232:772–776

CHAPTER 19

Prodynorphin Biosynthesis
and Posttranslational Processing

R. Day, K.A. Trujillo, and H. Akil

A. History of Dynorphin

In 1979 Goldstein and colleagues (GOLDSTEIN et al. 1979) reported the
characterization and partial sequence of a highly potent endogenous
opioid peptide, obtained from pituitary extracts, that contained the
amino acid sequence for leu-enkephalin at its amino-terminus (this
peptide was found to be 17 amino acids in length when sequencing
was completed; GOLDSTEIN et al. 1981). They were so impressed with the
potency of the peptide that they named it dynorphin, from the Greek prefix
dyn-, signifying strength or power. The same year, Kangawa and colleagues
(KANGAWA and MATSUO 1979) reported the partial sequence of another
highly potent opioid peptide, obtained from hypothalamic extracts, containing the sequence for leu-enkephalin at its amino-terminus (this peptide,
which they named α-neo-endorphin, was found to be ten amino acids
in length when sequencing was completed; KANGAWA et al. 1981). Subsequently, several other leu-enkephalin-extended peptides were isolated
from brain and pituitary, including dynorphin A 1–8 (MINAMINO et al.
1980), β-neo-endorphin (MINAMINO et al. 1981), and dynorphin B (also
known as rimorphin; FISCHLI et al. 1982a,b; KILPATRICK et al. 1982a).
Immunohistochemical distribution studies showed a colocalization of these
leucine-enkephalin extended peptides, particularly in the hypothalamus
and posterior pituitary, and it was predicted that a common precursor
molecule was biosynthesized (WATSON et al. 1982, 1983). This hypothsis was
proven correct by the cloning of the prodynorphin (ProDyn) cDNA from a
hypothalamic library (KAKIDANI et al. 1982), demonstrating that dynorphin
A, α-neo-endorphin, and dynorphin B are all contained within the same
protein precursor structure. The numerous other opioid peptide sequences
which had been isolated were quickly sorted into what is now known as the
three families of opioid peptide genes (AKIL et al. 1984). ProDyn (sometimes called proenkephalin B) and its biosynthetically derived peptides
constitute one of these three distinct gene families of endogenous opioids
found in the central and peripheral nervous systems, the other two being
proenkephalin and proopiomelanocortin (POMC). Figure 1 is a schematic of
the ProDyn precursor and the peptide products derived from this precursor
are shown in Table 1. Like most precursors, the pro-hormone in its entirety

Table 1. Peptide products of the ProDyn precursor

Neo-endorphin domain
　α-Neo-endorphin (ProDyn 175–184)
　　Tyr-Gly-Gly-Phe-Leu-Arg-Lys-Tyr-Pro-Lys
　β-Neo-endorphin (ProDyn 175–183)
　　Tyr-Gly-Gly-Phe-Leu-Arg-Lys-Tyr-Pro
Bridge peptide domain
　Bridge peptide (ProDyn 186–206; nonopioid)
　　Ser-Ser-Glu-Val-Ala-Gly-Glu-Gly-Asp-Gly-Asp-Arg-Asp-Lys-Val-Gly-His-Glu-
　　Asp-Leu-Tyr
Dynorphin A domain
　Dynorphin A 1–17 (ProDyn 209–225)
　　Tyr-Gly-Gly-Phe-Leu-Arg-Arg-Ile-Arg-Pro-Lys-Leu-Lys-Trp-Asp-Asn-Gln
　Dynorphin A 1–8 (ProDyn 209–216)
　　Tyr-Gly-Gly-Phe-Leu-Arg-Arg-Ile
Dynorphin B domain
　Leumorphin (ProDyn 228–256; dynorphin B-29)
　　Tyr-Gly-Gly-Phe-Leu-Arg-Arg-Gln-Phe-Lys-Val-Val-Thr-Arg-Ser-Gln-Glu-
　　Asp-Pro-Asn-Ala-Tyr-Tyr-Glu-Glu-Leu-Phe-Asp-Val
　Dynorphin B 1–13 (ProDyn 228–240)
　　Tyr-Gly-Gly-Phe-Leu-Arg-Arg-Gln-Phe-Lys-Val-Val-Thr
　C-Terminal peptide (ProDyn 242–256; nonopioid)
　　Ser-Gln-Glu-Asp-Pro-Asn-Ala-Tyr-Tyr-Glu-Glu-Leu-Phe-Asp-Val

In addition to these peptide products, the opioid domains of the precursor may produce the five amino acid peptide leucine-enkephalin (shown in italics to emphasize the opioid core sequence), as well as nonopioid des-tyrosine derivatives of the above opioid pepides. Large molecular weight products containing combinations of the above molecules may also be produced. Sequences derived from KAKIDANI et al. (1982). See text for further discussion.

is inactive, and requires posttranslational processing to produce biologically functional peptides.

B. Posttranslational Processing Signals

Limited proteolysis of prohormones or proproteins was first proposed as a mechanism of activation and release of bioactive peptides over 25 years ago (CHRÉTIEN and LI 1967). With the elucidation of the amino acid sequences for many precursors, it is not generally accepted that biologically active peptides are first synthesized as part of large inactive precursors, and are subsequently generated by cleavage at basic residues (i.e., mono-, di-, tri-, and tetra-basic) within these molecules. Among these processing signal sequences, the most common is the dibasic lysine-arginine (KR) sequence. Other dibasic sequences are also recognized, such as lysine-lysine (KK), or arginine-arginine (RR) as well as single basic residues such as arginine (R). It has become increasingly clear that these signal sequences are not equally cleaved, even when comparing apparently identical Lys-Arg dibasic residues within the same precursor. More than likely, the amino acids surrounding these signal sequences confer the selectivity or specificity that makes two Lys-Arg sequences different.

In general, as with other protein precursors, ProDyn must be cleaved at appropriate sites through a cascade of events resulting in final active end products. Dibasic recognition sites are cleaved on the carboxyl side of the basic amino acids and followed by removal of the carboxyl-terminal basic residues by the action of carboxypeptidase E (CPE). The carboxyl-terminal end can then be amidated by the peptidyl α-mono-oxygenase enzyme (PAM). In the case of ProDyn, carboxyl-terminal amidation has not been shown to ensue processing. Only dibasic and monobasic sequences are known to occur in ProDyn, and of the disbasic sequences none is of the Lys-Lys type; Lys-Arg sites are the principal sequence responsible for the formation of the ProDyn-derived peptides. While Arg-Arg sites are also found, and if cleaved would result in the formation of leucine-enkephalin, these sites appear to be rarely used. Evidence for this selectivity derives mainly from immunocytochemical studies which show extensive distribution of ProDyn products in the brain, but rarely localize leucine enkephalin with dynorphin peptides such as dynorphin A or dynorphin B (see Chap. 20); rather, leucine-enkephalin immunoreactivity appears colocalized with methione enkephalin. The conclusion is that, although this is a potential cleavage site, leucine enkephalin is not a major intracellular storage product of ProDyn.

There are four Lys-Arg residues which, when cleaved, result in a number of opioid peptides, including dynorphin A 1-17, leumorphin, α-neo-endorphin, and bridge peptide (see Fig. 1, Table 2). Each of these theoretical cleavage products has been demonstrated to exist as free peptide end product (GOLDSTEIN et al. 1981; KANGAWA et al. 1981; SUDA et al. 1983; DAY and AKIL 1986). While dibasic cleavage at Lys-Arg sites plays a critical role in the maturation of ProDyn, this precursor is remarkable because it also relies extensively on another type of endoproteolytic-cleavage at single arginine residues. Thus, other ProDyn-related end products have been isolated, such as dynorphin AB 1-32 ("big dynorphin"), dynorphin B 1-13, and dynorphin A 1-8, which can only be obtained by the processing of ProDyn at several single Arg residues strategically located throughout the molecule (MINAMINO et al. 1980; SEIZINGER et al. 1981a; FISCHLI et al. 1982a; KILPATRICK et al. 1982b).

C. Prodynorphin Biosynthesis and Processing in Peripheral Tissues

While the initial study of ProDyn expression and processing focussed on the brain, there are other sites which have been recently reported to express ProDyn. In the periphery, two tissues have drawn particular attention for their capacity to biosynthesize the ProDyn molecule: the adrenal gland (DAY

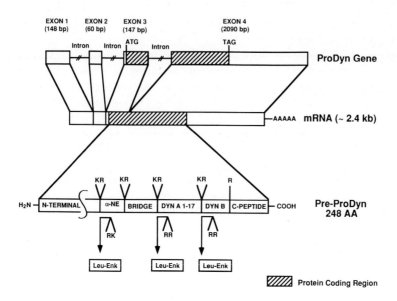

Fig. 1. Prodynorphin gene, messenger RNA, and precursor protein structure. The precursor protein is encoded in exons 3 and 4 of the ProDyn gene. Basic amino aicd cleavage sites in the precursor are denoted by their single letter codes: *K*, lysine; *R*, arginine

et al. 1991) and the testis (COLLARD et al. 1990). In the adrenal gland, the ProDyn was demonstrated to be most abundant in the adrenocortical cells of the zona fasciculata and reticularis. These cells do not contain typical storage granules found in most neuropeptide-producing endocrine and neuronal cells; however, the correctly processed ProDyn end product Dyn A 1-17 can be demonstrated in this tissue. Unusual ProDyn end products have also been detected in the adrenal, such as extended and trimmed forms of Dyn A 1-17. In the testis, ProDyn products, possibly corresponding to Dyn AB 32, were detected, indicating that processing was also occurring in this tissue. Sertoli cells were shown to be the site of ProDyn biosynthesis. Although the characterization of ProDyn processing in both the testis and the adrenal has begun, it is far from complete. The major obstacle in completing these studies is the low abundance of intracellular ProDyn storage products in Sertoli cells and corticosteroid cells. These tissues represent important areas for future studies in ProDyn processing, since it is very likely that they utilize different mechanisms of processing as compared to the typical neuropeptide-producing neuron or endocrine cell.

Table 2. Known and putative dibasic and monobasic cleavage sites in the ProDyn precursor

Cleavage sites						Comments
Prodynorphin dibasic cleavage sites						
P 4	P 3	P 2	P 1	P 0	P-1	
Gln	Ala	*Lys*	*Arg* ↓ Tyr		Gly	Junction of N-terminal and α-neo-endorphin, first cleavage of "major" pathway
Tyr	Pro	*Lys*	*Arg* ↓ Ser		Ser	Junction between α-neo-endorphin and bridge peptide, first cleavage "minor" pathway
Leu	Tyr	*Lys*	*Arg* ↓ Tyr		Gly	Junction between bridge peptide dynorphin A
Asn	Gln	*Lys*	*Arg* ↓ Tyr		Gly	Junction between dynorphin A dynorphin B. Most resistant of dibasic cleavage sites
Other significant dibasic cleavage sites						
Phe	Leu	*Arg*	*Arg* ↓ Ile		Arg	Dibasic site in dynorphin A which if cleaved would produce leucine-enkephalin
Phe	Leu	*Arg*	*Arg* ↓ Gln		Phe	Dibasic site in dynorphin B which if cleaved would produce leucine-enkephalin
Phe	Leu	*Arg*	*Lys* ↓ Tyr		Pro	Dibasic site in α-neo-endorphin which if cleaved would produce leucine-enkephalin. Most likely not a preferred cleavage site because of P1 lysine
Monobasic cleavage sites						
Val	Val	Thr	*Arg* ↓ Ser		Gln	Monobasic cleavage required to generate dynorphin B
Gly	Asn	Gly	*Arg* ↓ Glu		Ser	Putative monobasic site required to generate the 3.5-kDa α-neo-endorphin-containing intermediate of the "minor" pathway

D. Processing Pathway of Prodynorphin

As discussed above, the structure of the ProDyn precursor has been elucidated, as well as the final products that can be obtained in pituitary and brain. However, the specific processing pathway(s) leading to the known dynorphin peptide end products is inadequately defined. To achieve this objective will require a systematic assessment of the precursor-product relationship, such as can be obtained with pulse-chase labeling studies. This approach has been used successfully in the study of other precursor molecules such as POMC (see Chap. 17). For ProDyn, pulse-chase studies have been unsuccessful, largely due to the lower levels of biosynthesis for this precursor (100 times less than POMC in the anterior pituitary), and the lack of an available cell line producing a high abundance of ProDyn. There are a number of potential solutions to this problem. For example, the stable transfection of cell lines, such as AtT-20 and GH4C1 cells, with ProDyn may provide useful systems to carry out such studies (DEVI and GUPTA 1989; DEVI et al. 1989). In these transfected cell lines, differential processing patterns of ProDyn have been demonstrated. For example, GH4C1 cells have been observed to incompletely process ProDyn while AtT-20 cells processed this molecule to known end products. However, as discussed below, most of the data regarding the *initial* processing events of ProDyn to date have been deduced from steady state studies and the isolation of ProDyn processing intermediates in the spinal cord and anterior pituitary.

The initial outcome of studies isolating ProDyn-derived peptides was the characterization of small fragments or so-called final products of ProDyn precursor processing. However, using antibodies to the final product ProDyn peptides, such as Dyn A 1-17 or Dyn B, analysis of gel-fractionated immunoreactivity revealed that in certain tissues large molecular weight processing intermediates were present. The first of these to be identified was a 4-kDa molecule containing Dyn A 1-17 and Dyn B, now known as Dyn AB 1-32 (Fischli et al. 1982a). Other larger molecular weight intermediates were subsequently discovered and characterized. The anterior pituitary was shown to be a rich source of ProDyn processing intermediates (Seizinger et al. 1981b, 1984b). A 6-kDa intermediate was described in the anterior pituitary, having both Dyn A 1-17 and Dyn B immunoreactivity. The larger mass of this 6-kDa ProDyn product as compared to the 4-kDa Dyn AB 1-32 peptide, suggested an N-terminal or C-terminal extension to Dyn AB 1-32. Independently, an 8-kDa molecule, spanning α-neo-endorphin at the N-terminal to Dyn B at the C-terminal, was characterized in the spinal cord (Xie and Goldstein 1987). More detailed studies in the anterior pituitary subsequently demonstrated the presence and high abundance of other processing intermediates of the ProDyn precursor, including 10-kDa and 8-kDa intermediates containing α-neo-endorphin, Dyn A 1-17, and Dyn B in their structures, as well as 16-kDa and 3.5-kDa intermediates containing only α-neo-endorphin. Based on the combination of overlapping elements and the relative abundance of each of these intermediates, a scheme was proposed for the pathways of ProDyn posttranslational processing (Fig. 2; Day and Akil 1989).

The processing of ProDyn, as determined in rat anterior pituitary, occurs in two distinct pathways, a "major" and "minor" pathway. This designation is based on the estimate of relative abundance of the processing intermediates that are generated in each of the pathways. As shown in Fig. 2, the "major" pathway begins at the Lys-Arg dibasic site N-terminal to α-neo-endorphin, which appears to be the primary cleavage site of the ProDyn molecule (Table 2). In the anterior pituitary, it is thought that this is the first processing site for 80%–90% of the ProDyn precursor molecules. This cleavage is responsible for generating the 10-kDa molecule noted above. The C-terminal portion of the 10-kDa intermediate can then be cleaved to yield an 8-kDa molecule. These two intermediates, 8 kDa and 10 kDa, are the major ProDyn products found in the anterior pituitary. In this tissue, final processed products such as Dyn A 1-17, Dyn B, or Dyn A 1-8 occur in low concentration. With further processing, the final products would

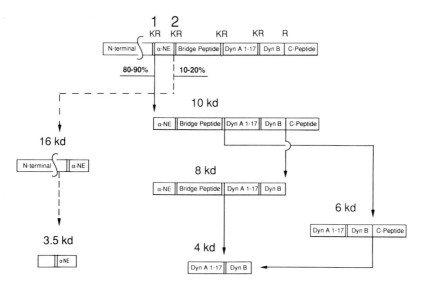

Fig. 2. Prodynorphin processing pathways. *1* and *2* indicate the initial cleavage sites in the ProDyn precursor. Note that site *1* represents the initial cut of the major pathway, occurring 80%–90% in rat anterior pituitary, while site *2* represents the initial cut of the minor pathway, occurring only 10%–20% in this tissue. See text for further discussion

presumably eventually be generated from the 8-kDa and 10-kDa molecules, via the formation of the other two known intermediates, the 6-kDa and 4-kDa fragments. Other tissues, such as the hypothalamus or the spinal cord, which tend to process ProDyn more efficiently, also contain low levels of the 8-kDa and 10-kDa molecules, suggesting that ProDyn precursor may be processed, at least in the initial phases, in a similar manner across tissues (DAY and AKIL 1989).

A "minor" pathway of processing has been postulated to account for the presence of the 16-kDa and 3.5-kDa α-neo-endorphin-containing intermediates. This processing pathway begins with the cleavage of the Lys-Arg dibasic site C-terminal to α-neo-endorphin, and occurs in only 10%–20% of the ProDyn precursor molecules (Fig. 2; Table 2). This results in the formation of a 16-kDa intermediate that contains α-neo-endorphin at its C-terminal. Theoretically, α-neo-endorphin could then be directly cleaved from this 16-kDa molecule. However, the observation of a 3.5-kDa intermediate also containing α-neo-endorphin at its C-terminal suggests another step before the final cleavage of α-neo-endorphin. In this respect, it is interesting to note that there is no dibasic cleavage site in the N-terminal region of ProDyn. Based on the observed mass of 3.5 kDa, a cleavage site should be present some 25–30 amino acids N-terminal to α-neo-endorphin (DAY and AKIL 1989). Careful examination of the N-terminal region adjacent to α-neo-endorphin reveals the presence of at least three potential single Arg cleavage sites. In a recent report (DEVI 1991), a consensus sequence was hypothesized for the processing of peptide precursors at monobasic sites. Application of the rules and tendencies of this consensus sequence to the ProDyn N-terminal region reveals that an Arg residue exactly 34 amino acids upstream from the N-terminal Tyr of α-neo-endorphin is an ideal candidate for monobasic cleavage (Table 2). Cleavage of the 16-kDa intermediate at this site would explain the formation of the 3.5-kDa intermediate. Furthermore if cleavage did occur at this monobasic site, a ProDyn N-terminal molecule containing a Gly at its C-terminal would be generated (see Table 2). Gly residues such as this are ideal sites for amidation by the C-terminal amidating enzyme, PAM. Although there has never been a reported function for the ProDyn N-terminal molecule, C-terminal amidation would suggest a possible physiological role; however, this is still hypothetical and remains to be investigated.

The four known dibasic sequences of ProDyn are not always equally processed, as evidenced by the presence of various ProDyn intermediates. One common product found is the so-called big dynorphin, or Dyn AB 1-32. The presence of such a peptide indicates that the linking Lys-Arg bond (between Dyn A 1-17 and Dyn B 1-13) is more resistant to proteolysis relative to other similar bonds in the ProDyn precursor. In fact, evidence suggests that proteolysis at the monobasic site, resulting in the excision of the C-terminal ProDyn peptide, is a more likely event (DEVI and GOLDSTEIN 1984, 1986). While a Dyn B 1-13-extended molecule (leumorphin) has been described, it appears to be a rarer product.

The products of the "major" and "minor" pathways described above are highly abundant only in the anterior pituitary, since in this tissue ProDyn is incompletely processed. In other ProDyn-synthesizing tissues, such as the hypothalamus or striatum, these intermediates are present only in trace amounts. This suggests that although the processing pathway of ProDyn may be similar in these tissues, processing is more complete in the hypothalamus and striatum, perhaps because of a differential tissue-specific expression of the required processing enzymes.

As can be seen from the above description, our understanding of the posttranslational processing of ProDyn remains relatively sketchy. This is likely due to two reasons. The first is the above-mentioned lack of a dynorphin-expressing cell line that would offer a convenient model for studying the maturation events. The second may be due to a distinct intrinsic feature of the molecule, the presence of several types of processing signals. The presence of these signals, particularly Lys-Arg and single Arg, contrasts with other precursors, such as POMC, which rely primarily on dibasic cleavage. This multiplicity of signals suggests that ProDyn is a substrate for more than one type of processing enzyme. Thus, both the *extent* and the *nature* of the processing will depend on the exact mix of endoproteases expressed in a given cell type. For example, if a cell expresses a high level of single Arg cleaving enzyme and low levels of dibasic enzymes, the appearance of Dyn AB 1-32 would be more likely than the appearance of leumorphin. While the processing of precursors, such as POMC, appears to begin in an identical manner across tissues (e.g., anterior and inter-mediate lobe) and simply proceed further with the addition of specialized enzymes (e.g., in intermediate lobe), dynorphin processing exhibits mutu-ally exclusive end products (e.g., leumorphin versus DynAB) which likely reflects the interaction between multiple processing signals and differential tissue-specific expression of the enzymes capable of recognizing them.

To fully understand the processing and regulation of ProDyn, it will be important to identify the specific enzymes involved in the maturation. The dibasic cleavage may be mediated by the recently cloned enzymes PC_1/PC_3 (SEIDAH et al. 1990, 1991; SMEEKENS et al. 1991) and PC_2 (SEIDAH et al. 1990, 1991; SMEEKENS et al. 1991), which have been shown to recognize Lys-Arg and Arg-Arg sequences (BENJANNET et al. 1991). That PC_1 is capable of cleaving ProDyn is supported by the studies in AtT_{20} in which ProDyn cDNA was introduced into this PC_1-expressing cell line (SEIDAH et al. 1990, 1991; SMEEKENS et al. 1991) and shown to be fully processed (DEVI et al. 1989). Interestingly, AtT_{20} cells also produced leucine-enkephalin from ProDyn, most likely because PC_1 recognizes the Arg-Arg sequence very well. In brain, these Arg-Arg sites appear to be spared, and the coexpression of leucine-enkephalin with dynorphin, while documented (TRAYNOR 1987), is not common. Thus, either a different enzyme(s) which specifically avoids Arg-Arg sites is responsible for the Lys-Arg cleavage in ProDyn, or specific sequences surrounding Arg-Arg sites in ProDyn serve to inhibit processing at these sites.

The cleavage at single arginine residues is even less well understood, as no enzymes have yet been identified with this recognition specificity. Work by Devi and coworkers (DEVI and GOLDSTEIN 1984, 1986; DEVI 1991) has characterized the potential structure requirements for such cleavage. This characterization is a critical prelude to the isolation of such an enzyme, which appears to play a key role in the maturation of this complex precursor.

The postulated interplay between multiple processing signals, embedded in specific sequences, and multiple enzymes that may be differentially ex-pressed in various cell types, yields a wide range of regulatory options. Activation or inhibition of one of these steps can result in altering the nature of the end products from a given domain of the precursor, its stability postsecretion, and its receptor selectivity. This leaves a great deal of leeway for biological regulation based on relatively subtle changes in enzyme ex-pression or enzyme activity. Such regulation can occur across tissues, through developmental stages, or as a function of cellular activity elicited by various demands placed on a neuronal circuit.

E. Functional Significance
of Prodynorphin Peptide Processing

It is apparent from the preceding discussion that the processing of the
ProDyn precursor can yield a number of neuroactive peptides. To briefly
summarize, processing of the neo-endorphin domain can yield the 10 amino
acid peptide α-neo-endorphin or the 9 amino acid β-neo-endorphin; processing of the dynorphin A domain can result in dynorphin A 1-17 or dynorphin
A 1-8; and processing of the dynorphin B domain can produce the 29 amino
acid peptide leumorphin or dynorphin B 1-13 (Table 1). Further processing
of either of these domains has the potential to produce the 5 amino acid
opioid peptide leu-enkephalin. In addition to the opioid peptides, the
ProDyn precursor has the potential to give rise to nonopioid peptides,
including the putative "bridge peptide," and the carboxy-terminal peptide
(adjacent to dynorphin B on the ProDyn molecule). Finally, postsecretory
events can lead to the removal of the amino-terminal tyrosine, resulting in
des-tyrosine derivatives of each of the above opioid peptides. These may be
biologically active but are inactive at the opioid receptors, as the N-terminal
tyrosine is a requirement for opioid receptor recognition. The ProDyn
precursor can therefore yield peptides that interact with a number of receptors, both opioid and nonopioid.

As a general rule it is important to remember that there is no pharmacological or anatomical correspondence of any opioid peptide, or peptide
family, with a particular receptor – each known opioid peptide will bind
to each of the three recognized opioid receptors with varying affinities.
Although each opioid peptide will show a selectivity for the μ-, δ-, or
κ-receptor, no peptide will show specificity for a particular receptor. Both
convergence and divergence are seen in opioid peptide-receptor interactions; convergence, in that several peptides have the ability to act at a
chosen receptor type, and divergence, in that a chosen peptide has the
ability to interact with several receptor types. A physiological consequence
of the ability of opioid peptides to potently stimulate each of the three
opioid receptor types is that the functional expression of activation of
endogenous opioid neurons is dependent not only on which peptides are
released, and in what proportion, but also on which receptors are present at
the synapse of interest. This is particularly true for ProDyn peptides, which
tend to bind with high affinity to all three opioid receptor types. In fact,
examination of opioid receptor binding affinities reveals that although
ProDyn opioid peptides tend to be selective for κ-receptors, dynorphin A
(1-17), dynorphin B, and α-neo-endorphin are more potent than β-endorphin
at μ-receptors, and α-neo-endorphin is more potent than leu-enkephalin at
δ-receptors (see Table 3). The fact that ProDyn opioid peptides bind with
high affinity to μ- and δ-receptors is emphasized because of the common
misconception that these peptides act specifically at κ-receptors. However,
ProDyn opioid peptides show at best a relatively modest selectivity for
κ-receptors (see Table 3).

Table 3. Relative affinities of selected opioid peptides for
μ-, δ-, and κ-receptors

	μ	δ	κ
Leu-enkephalin	158.3	10.0	68 416.7
Dyn A 1-8	31.7	41.7	10.8
Dyn A 1-17	5.8	20.0	1.0
Dyn B 1-13	5.8	26.7	1.0
α-Neo-endorphin	10.8	4.8	1.7
β-Endorphin	16.7	22.5	475.0

Relative affinities were derived from K_i values for peptide binding to guinea pig brain membranes (CORBETT et al. 1982; LESLIE 1987). Values were calculated relative to dynorphin A 1-17 binding to κ-receptors.

Since ProDyn neurons (and perhaps most other peptidergic neurons as well) have the ability to release several neuroactive peptides, with differing receptor profiles, there is the opportunity for a number of complex actions and interactions. In a very real sense, release of ProDyn peptides from a neuron can be looked upon as an example of cotransmission (see Chap. 22). Although neuroscientists are more familiar with the concept of cotransmission from the perspective of interactions between a classical neurotransmitter and a peptide, the fact that several peptides can be coreleased from a single neuron raises the possibility that these peptides can interact in complicated ways. For example, there are suggestion in the literature that μ and δ-receptors may interact allosterically under certain circumstances (ROTHMAN et al. 1988, 1991; QI et al. 1990; SCHOFFELMEER et al. 1990), and that dynorphin analogues can functionally antagonize classical opioid effects (FRIEDMAN et al. 1981; TULUNAY et al. 1981a, 1981b; WALKER et al. 1982c, 1985; WOO et al. 1983; TRUJILLO and AKIL 1990a). Such interactions would be expected to produce dramatically different effects than activation of a single receptor type by a single peptide. As a result, when considering the physiological or functional effects of peptide release from a ProDyn neuron, one must keep in mind several factors, including the relative amounts of the different peptides that might be released from the neuron of interest, the different receptor types available for these peptides to interact with, and the potential interactions between the different receptors.

Although the above discussion makes it seem as if the events at even a single synapse are hopelessly complex, if we step back and examine function from a more integrated level there are some general concepts that can be recognized. First is the recognition that longer forms of dynorphin peptides tend to have a higher selectivity for κ-receptors (see Table 3). The consequence of this is that in neural systems where there is less processing of ProDyn peptides, and the availability of an adequate concentration of κ-receptors, one would expect greater κ-activity than in systems where processing was more complete or κ-receptors were few. The functional consequences of κ-receptor activation would be expected to be quite different from μ- or δ-receptor activation. At the second messenger level, activation of μ- or δ-receptors produces an increase in potassium conductance via a G-protein-mediated mechanism, leading to hyperpolarization, decreased calcium flux, and inhibition of action potential discharge, while activation of κ-receptors causes a direct inhibition of calcium conductance and inhibition of action potential discharge (WERZ and MACDONALD 1983a,b, 1984a,b, 1985; CHERUBINI and NORTH 1985; NORTH 1986; NORTH et al. 1987). At the behavioral level, while μ- or δ-selective drugs tend to produce effects typical of opiate compounds, such as analgesia and reward, the most prominent effects of κ-selective drugs are dysphoria and diuresis (HERZ and SHIPPENBERG 1989; WATSON et al. 1989).

A second general observation is that ProDyn peptides often produce effects that are not antagonized by opioid receptor antagonists, such as naloxone, and that can be mimicked by des-tyrosine analogues of the peptides (HERMAN et al. 1980; WALKER et al. 1980, 1982a,b,c, 1985; PETRIE et al. 1982; PRZEWLOCKI et al. 1983; FADEN and JACOBS 1984; HERRERA-MARSCHITZ et al. 1984; HERMAN and GOLDSTEIN 1985; STEVENS and YAKSH 1986; FRIEDERICH et al. 1987; LONG et al. 1987, 1988a,b,c,d, 1989; ROBERTSON et al. 1987; FADEN 1990; TRUJILLO and AKIL 1990a). Since the amino-terminal tyrosine is required for peptide binding to opioid receptors, the des-tyrosine ProDyn peptides have no ability to activate these receptors (WALKER et al. 1982a, 1985). Moreover, since naloxone reversibility is the critical pharmacological test for opiate receptor involvement in a particular function, the results suggest that ProDyn peptides produce nonopioid actions. In the brain, aminopeptidase activity rapidly cleaves the amino-terminal tyrosine from ProDyn peptides (presumably in the synapse, following release of the peptides from a neuron) leading to the liberation of des-tyrosine derivatives of these peptides (LESLIE and GOLDSTEIN 1982; ROBSON et al. 1983; YOUNG et al. 1987). Although the cleavage of tyrosine from the peptides might be viewed as simply the first step in the degradation of ProDyn peptides, evidence suggests that these des-tyrosine derivatives are functionally significant – these peptides produce dramatic motor effects, alterations in electroencephalogram, changes in neuronal firing, and antagonize some opioid effects, and these actions appear to be mediated by a nonopioid receptor (WALKER et al. 1982a, 1985; TRUJILLO and AKIL 1990a). The functional domain for the nonopioid actions of ProDyn peptides appears to reside in residues 3–7, or 3–8 (LONG et al. 1988a). Although the receptor, or receptors, responsible for the nonopioid actions of ProDyn peptides have yet to be identified, intriguing evidence suggests that excitatory amino acid receptors may be involved (CAUDLE and ISAAC 1988; MASSARDIER and HUNT 1989). The relevance of these nonopioid ProDyn effects to a specific neural system would depend on the presence of appropriate aminopeptidase action, and the appropriate nonopioid receptor sites.

The above discussion provides an introduction to both the complexities and the generalities of functional consideration in ProDyn peptide processing. This introduction brings up important questions related to the functional consequences of ProDyn processing in specific neural and hormonal systems. How does the processing of these peptides in specific systems relate to function and behavior? How does altering the processing in these systems alter the functional and behavioral roles of these peptides? In the following section we will attempt to approach these questions by briefly examining selected physiological systems, focussing our discussion on the striatonigral ProDyn pathway. From the outset, it is important to keep in mind that very few studies have specifically addressed these questions, so much of what will be discussed has been inferred by applying the general principles discussed above to what is known about the specific systems. For more complete discussion of specific opioid-related functions and behaviors the reader is referred to other chapters in this volume.

I. Striatonigral System

A dense ProDyn projection has been identified, with cell bodies in the striatum and terminals in the substantia nigra pars reticulata (Vincent et al. 1982a,b; Fallon et al. 1985; McLean et al. 1985). This pathway has been studied extensively with a variety of techniques, including behavioral, anatomical, biochemical, and electrophysiological, and has been suggested to be an excellent model system for understanding opioid peptide function (Thompson et al. 1990). ProDyn peptides are found in medium spiny projection neurons in the striatum, and are colocalized virtually 100% with γ-aminobutyric acid (GABA) and from 70% to 100% with tachykinins (Anderson and Reiner 1990). Dynorphin A 1-8, dynorphin A 1-17, dynorphin B, α-neo-endorphin, and β-neo-endorphin have all been found in the striatum and the substantia nigra. Dynorphin A 1-17 and β-neo-endorphin are relatively low in concentration, while dynorphin A 1-8, dynorphin B, and α-neo-endorphin are considerably higher (Seizinger et al. 1984a; Dores and Akil 1985; Dores et al. 1985; Trujillo et al. 1990). Leu-enkephalin has also been suggested to be a product of the ProDyn precursor in this projection (Zamir et al. 1984a; Zamir 1985). Thus, ProDyn neurons in this pathway produce peptides that have the ability to potently interact with each of the three opioid receptor types. Correspondingly, the striatum and the substantia nigra each contain μ-, δ-, and κ-opioid receptors (Mansour et al. 1987).

When injected unilaterally into the substantia nigra pars reticulata, ProDyn peptides produce circling behavior contralateral to the side of the injection, indicating that these peptides induce locomotor activation in this system (Herrera-Marschitz et al. 1983, 1984, 1986; Morelli and Di Chiara 1985; Friederich et al. 1987; Matsumoto et al. 1988b). Similar results have been obtained by injecting a number of different opioids into this region, including μ-, δ-, and κ-agonists (MATSUMOTO et al. 1988a). While the μ- and δ-receptor agonists appear to produce locomotor activation via disinhibition of nigrostriatal dopamine neurons, κ-agonists appear to act by inhibition of nigrotectal or nigrothalamic GABAergic efferents (MATSUMOTO et al. 1988a; THOMPSON et al. 1990). It is presently unclear whether the actions of ProDyn peptides on this system are mediated by μ-, δ-, or κ-receptors; however it is possible that all three subtypes are involved.

Both opioid and nonopioid mechanisms have been observed for the effects of ProDyn peptides in this system – while some studies have found the effects of these peptides to be antagonized by naloxone (HERRERA-MARSCHITZ et al. 1984; MORELLI and DI CHIARA 1985; MATSUMOTO et al. 1988b), others have found them to be unaffected by opioid antagonists (FRIEDERICH et al. 1987). In addition, contralateral circling behavior has been observed following administration of nonopioid des-tyrosine analogues of ProDyn peptides (HERRERA-MARSCHITZ et al. 1984; FRIEDERICH et al. 1987). It therefore appears that ProDyn peptides may produce behavioral effects in the substantia nigra either through opioid or nonopioid actions.

It is apparent that the striatonigral ProDyn projection, like most brain systems, is a dynamic system. Dramatic changes in this system occur during development (SEI and DORES 1990), and evidence suggests that this system may be involved in several neuropathalogical states (ZAMIR et al. 1984b; TAQUET et al. 1985; HABER et al. 1986; SEIZINGER et al. 1986). This system has been found to be profoundly altered by a variety of pharmacological and behavioral manipulations. Increases in striatonigral ProDyn peptides have been observed following treatment with dopaminergic drugs, including amphetamine (PETERSON and ROBERTSON 1984; HANSON et al. 1987, 1988; LI et al. 1990; TRUJILLO et al. 1990), cocaine (SIVAM 1989; SMILEY et al. 1990), and apomorphine (LI et al. 1986, 1988, 1990), as well as by other drugs, such as opiates (WEISSMAN and ZAMIR 1987; TRUJILLO and AKIL 1989, 1990b), phencyclidine (HANSON et al. 1989), and lithium (SIVAM et al. 1988). Alterations in these peptides have also been observed following dopamine antagonists (QUIRION et al. 1985; NYLANDER and TERENIUS 1986, 1987; TRUJILLO et al. 1990), following 6-hydroxydopamine lesions of the nigrostriatal dopamine pathway (LI et al. 1990), and following stress (VASWANI et al. 1988). In addition to altering the absolute concentration of ProDyn peptides, various treatments have been observed to change the relative ratios of the different peptide products of the ProDyn precursor (TRUJILLO et al. 1990). It therefore appears that a variety of manipulations have the ability to dramatically affect the functional "tone" of the striatonigral ProDyn system, altering both the absolute concentration and the relative proportions of the stored peptide products. The consequence of this is that the striatonigral ProDyn system represents a very dynamic system, with the ability to change dramatically from day to day, or even from moment to moment.

II. Other Systems

ProDyn peptides are found in several other areas in the brain and periphery, including the hippocampus, hypothalamus, spinal cord, pituitary, adrenal, and testis. Studies are consistent in suggesting that the processing of these peptides differs across the different neural and hormonal systems (WEBER et al. 1982a,b; CONE et al. 1983; SEIZINGER et al. 1984b; ZAMIR et al. 1984c; XIE and GOLDSTEIN 1987). In addition, the ProDyn peptides in several of these systems have been found to change during development, and to be modified by a variety of pharmacological, physiological, and behavioral manipulations. Thus, as discussed above for the striatonigral system, the processing of ProDyn peptides throughout the central nervous system and periphery is a very important factor in determining function. Minor changes in the proportions of the peptide products resulting from changes in processing have the ability to produce significant functional consequences.

F. Conclusions

It is probably evident from the above discussion that ProDyn is unique among the opioid peptide families from a number of points of view. The precursor is processed in a complex fashion to give rise to multiple opioid peptides, each with a unique pharmacological profile. This processing is both tissue specific and regulatable. Within a given domain of some of the products, multiple active cores exist, with both opioid and nonopioid actions. The opioid activity itself encompasses the potential to interact with all three members of the opioid receptor family – μ, σ, or κ. In turn, activation of one or the other of these receptors can lead to very different, sometimes antagonistic effects. Thus, in order to understand the role of ProDyn, it is critical to determine which peptides are being elaborated by the posttranslational machinery, which are being secreted, what modifications can be generated in the synaptic cleft, and which receptors are encountered by the peptides. While it may be difficult to determine these features at every site, studying a number of systems at a cellular, integrative, and behavioral level can allow us to elaborate some general principles of this rich and complex mode of communication.

References

Akil H, Watson SJ, Young E, Lewis ME, Khachaturian H, Walker JM (1984) Endogenous opioids: biology and function. Annu Rev Neurosci 7:223–255

Anderson KD, Reiner A (1990) Extensive co-occurrence of substance P and dynorphin in striatal projection neurons: an evolutionarily conserved feature of basal ganglia organization. J Comp Neurol 295:339–369

Benjannet S, Rondeau N, Day R, Chrétien M, Seidah NG (1991) PC1 and PC2 are proprotein convertases capable of cleaving proopiomelanocortin at distinct pairs of basic residues. Proc Natl Acad Sci USA 88:3564

Caudle RM, Isaac L (1988) A novel interaction between dynorphin (1-13) and an
    N-methyl-D-aspartate site. Brain Res 443:329–332.
Cherubini E, North RA (1985) μ and κ opioids inhibit transmitter release by
    different mechanisms. Proc Natl Acad Sci USA 82:1860–1863
Chrétien M, Li CH (1967) Isolation and purification of γ lipotropic hormone from
    sheep pituitary glands. Can J Biochem 45:1163
Collard MW, Day R, Akil H, Uhler MD, Douglass JO (1990) Sertoli cells are the
    primary site of prodynorphin gene expression in rat testis: regulation of mRNA
    synthesis and peptide secretion by cAMP analogs in cultured cells. Mol
    Endocrinol 4:1488
Cone RI, Weber E, Barchas JD, Goldstein A (1983) Regional distribution of
    dynorphin and neo-endorphin peptides in rat brain, spinal cord, and pituitary.
    J Neurosci 3:2146–2152
Corbett AD, Paterson SJ, McKnight AT, Magnan J, Kosterlitz HW (1982)
    Dynorphin 1-8 and dynorphin 1-9 are ligands for the kappa-subtype of opiate
    receptor. Nature 299:79–81
Day R, Akil H (1986) Bridge peptide is a cleavage product of pro-dynorphin
    processing in the rat anterior pituitary. Natl Inst Drug Abuse Res Monogr Ser
    75:244–246
Day R, Akil H (1989) The posttranslational processing of prodynorphin in the rat
    anterior pituitary. Endocrinology 124:2392–2405
Day R, Schäfer MK-H, Collard MW, Watson SJ, Akil H (1991) Atypical
    prodynorphin gene expression in corticosteroid producing cells of the rat adrenal
    gland. Proc Natl Acad Sci USA 88:1320
Devi L (1991) Consensus sequence for processing of peptide precursors at monobasic
    sites. FEBS Lett 280:189
Devi L, Goldstein A (1984) Dynorphin converting enzyme with unusual specificity
    from rat brain. Proc Natl Acad Sci USA 81:1892–1896
Devi L, Goldstein A (1986) Conversion of leumorphin (dynorphin B-29) to
    dynorphin B and dynorphin B-14 by thiol protease activity. J Neurochem
    47:154–157
Devi L, Gupta P (1989) Expression and posttranslational processing of pre-
    prodynorphin in the rat anterior pituitary cell line GH4C1. J Neuroendocrinol
    1:363
Devi L, Gupta P, Douglass J (1989) Expression and posttranslational processing of
    preprodynorphin complementary DNA in the mouse anterior pituitary cell line
    AtT-20. Mol Endocrinol 3:1852–1860
Dores RM, Akil H (1985) Steady state levels of pro-dynorphin-related end products
    in the striatum and substantia nigra of the adult rhesus monkey. Peptides
    2:143–148
Dores RM, Lewis ME, Khachaturian H, Watson SJ, Akil H (1985) Analysis of
    opioid and non-opioid end products of pro-dynorphin in the substantia nigra of
    the rat. Neuropeptides 5:501–504
Faden AI (1990) Opioid and nonopioid mechanisms may contribute to dynorphin's
    pathophysiological actions in spinal cord injury. Ann Neurol 27:67–74
Faden AI, Jacobs TP (1984) Dynorphin-related peptides cause motor dysfunction in
    the rat through a non-opiate action. Br J Pharmacol 81:271–276
Fallon JH, Leslie FM, Cone RI (1985) Dynorphin-containing pathways in the
    substantia nigra and ventral tegmentum: a double labeling study using com-
    bined immunofluorescence and retrograde tracing. Neuropeptides 5:457–
    460
Fischli W, Goldstein A, Hunkapiller MW, Hood LE (1982a) Isolation and amino
    acid sequence analysis of a 4000-dalton dynorphin from porcine pituitary. Proc
    Natl Acad Sci USA 79:5435–5437
Fischli W, Goldstein A, Hunkapiller MW, Hood LE (1982b) Two "big" dynorphins
    from porcine pituitary. Life Sci 31:1769–1772

Friederich MW, Friederich DP, Walker JM (1987) Effects of dynorphin (1-8) on movement: non-opiate effects and structure-activity relationship. Peptides 8:837–840

Friedman HJ, Jen MF, Chang JK, Lee NM, Loh HH (1981) Dynorphin: a possible modulatory peptide on morphine or beta-endorphin analgesia in mouse. Eur J Pharmacol 69:357–360

Goldstein A, Tachibana S, Lowney LI, Hunkapiller M, Hood L (1979) Dynorphin-(1-13), an extraordinarily potent opioid peptide. Proc Natl Acad Sci USA 76:6666–6670

Goldstein A, Fischli W, Lowney LI, Hunkapiller M, Hood L (1981) Porcine pituitary dynorphin: complete amino acid sequence of the biologically active heptadecapeptide. Proc Natl Acad Sci USA 78:7219–7223

Haber SN, Kowall NW, Vonsattel JP, Bird ED, Richardson EJ (1986) Gilles de la Tourette's syndrome. A postmortem neuropathological and immuno-histochemical study. J Neurol Sci 75:225–241

Hanson GR, Merchant KM, Letter AA, Bush L, Gibb JW (1987) Methamphetamine-induced changes in the striatal-nigral dynorphin system: role of D-1 and D-2 receptors. Eur J Pharmacol 144:245–246

Hanson GR, Merchant KM, Letter AA, Bush L, Gibb JW (1988) Characterization of methamphetamine effects on the striatal-nigral dynorphin system. Eur J Pharmacol 155:11–18

Hanson GR, Midgley LP, Bush LG, Johnson M, Gibb JW (1989) Comparison of responses by neuropeptide systems in rat to the psychotropic drugs, methamphetamine, cocaine and PCP. Natl Inst Drug Abuse Res Mongr Ser 95:348

Herman BH, Goldstein A (1985) Antinociception and paralysis induced by intrathecal dynorphin A. J Pharmacol Exp Ther 232:27–32

Herman BH, Leslie F, Goldstein A (1980) Behavioral effects and in vivo degradation of intraventricularly administered dynorphin-(1-13) and D-Ala2-dynorphin-(1-11) in rats. Life Sci 27:883–892

Herrera-Marschitz M, Hokfelt T, Ungerstedt U, Terenius L (1983) Functional studies with the opioid peptide dynorphin: acute effects of injections into the substantia nigra reticulata of naive rats. Life Sci 33 (Suppl 1):555–558

Herrera-Marschitz M, Hokfelt T, Ungerstedt U, Terenius L, Goldstein M (1984) Effect of intranigar injections of dynorphin, dynorphin fragments and alpha-neoendorphin on rotational behavior in the rat. Eur J Pharmacol 102:213–227

Herrera-Marschitz M, Christensson-Nylander I, Sharp T, Staines W, Reid M, Hokfelt T, Terenius L, Ungerstedt U (1986) Striato-nigral dynorphin and substance P pathways in the rat: II. Functional analysis. Exp Brain Res 64:193–207

Herz A, Shippenberg TS (1989) Neurochemical aspects of addiction: opioids and other drugs of abuse. In: Goldstein A (ed) Molecular and cellular aspects of the addictions. Springer, Berlin Heidelberg New York, pp 111–141

Kakidani H, Furutani Y, Takahashi H, Noda M, Morimoto Y, Hirose T, Asai M, Inayama S, Nakanishi S, Numa S (1982) Cloning and sequence analysis of cDNA for porcine beta-neo- endorphin/dynorphin precursor. Nature 298:245–249

Kangawa K, Matsuo H (1979) Alpha-Neo-endorphin: a "big" Leu-enkephalin with potent opiate activity from porcine hypothalami. Biochem Biophys Res Commun 86:153–160

Kangawa K, Minamino N, Chino N, Sakakibara S, Matsuo H (1981) The complete amino acid sequence of alpha-neo-endorphin. Biochem Biophys Res Commun 99:871–878

Kilpatrick DL, Wahlstrom A, Lahm HW, Blacher R, Ezra E, Fleminger G, Udenfriend S (1982a) Characterization of rimorphin, a new [leu]enkephalin-containing peptide from bovine posterior pituitary glands. Life Sci 31:1849–1852

Kilpatrick DL, Wahlstrom A, Lahm HW, Blacher R, Udenfriend S (1982b) Rimorphin, a unique, naturally occurring [Leu]enkephalin-containing peptide found in association with dynorphin and alpha-neo-endorphin. Proc Natl Acad Sci USA 79:6480–6483

Leslie FM (1987) Methods used for the study of opioid receptors. Pharmacol Rev 39:197–249

Leslie FM, Goldstein A (1982) Degradation of dynorphin-(1-13) by membrane-bound rat brain enzymes. Neuropeptides 2:185–196

Li S, Sivam SP, Hong JS (1986) Regulation of the concentration of dynorphin A1-8 in the striatonigral pathway by the dopaminergic system. Brain Res 398:390–392

Li SJ, Sivam SP, McGinty JF, Jiang HK, Douglass J, Calavetta L, Hong JS (1988) Regulation of the metabolism of striatal dynorphin by the dopaminergic system. J Pharmacol Exp Ther 246:403–408

Li SJ, Jiang HK, Stachowiak MS, Hudson PM, Owyang V, Nanry K, Tilson HA, Hong JS (1990) Influence of nigrostriatal dopaminergic tone on the biosynthesis of dynorphin and enkephalin in rat striatum. Mol Brain Res 8:219–225

Long JB, Kinney RC, Malcolm DS, Graeber GM, Holaday JW (1987) Intrathecal dynorphin A1-13 and dynorphin A3-13 reduce rat spinal cord blood flow by non-opioid mechanisms. Brain Res 436:374–379

Long JB, Martińez AA, Echevarria EE, Tidwell RE, Holaday JW (1988a) Hindlimb paralytic effects of prodynorphin-derived peptides following spinal subarachnoid injection in rats. Eur J Pharmacol 153:45–54

Long JB, Mobley WC, Holaday JW (1988b) Neurological dysfunction after intrathecal injection of dynorphin A (1-13) in the rat: I. Injection procedures modify pharmacological responses. J Pharmacol Exp Ther 246:1158–1166

Long JB, Petras JM, Holaday JW (1988c) Neurologic deficits and neuronal injury in rats resulting from nonopioid actions of the delta opioid receptor antagonist ICI 174864. J Pharmacol Exp Ther 244:1169–1177

Long JB, Petras JM, Mobley WC, Holaday JW (1988d) Neurological dysfunction after intrathecal injection of dynorphin A (1–13) in the rat: II. Nonopioid mechanisms mediate loss of motor, sensory and autonomic function. J Pharmacol Exp Ther 246:1167–1174

Long JB, Rigamonti DD, de Costa B, Rice KC, Martinez Arizala A (1989) Dynorphin A-induced rat hindlimb paralysis and spinal cord injury are not altered by the kappa opioid antagonist nor-binaltorphimine. Brain Res 497:155–162

Mansour A, Khachaturian H, Lewis ME, Akil H, Watson SJ (1987) Autoradiographic differentiation of mu, delta, and kappa opioid receptors in the rat forebrain and midbrain. J Neurosci 7:2445–2464

Massardier D, Hunt PF (1989) A direct non-opiate interaction of dynorphin-(1–13) with the N-methyl-D-aspartate (NMDA) receptor. Eur J Pharmacol 170:125–126

Matsumoto RR, Brinsfield KH, Patrick RL, Walker JM (1988a) Rotational behavior mediated by dopaminergic and non-dopaminergic mechanisms following intranigral microinjection of specific mu, delta and kappa opiate agonists. J Pharmacol Exp Ther 246:196–203

Matsumoto RR, Lohof AM, Patrick RL, Walker JM (1988b) Dopamine-independent motor behavior following microinjection of rimorphin in the substantia nigra. Brain Res 444:67–74

McLean S, Bannon MJ, Zamir N, Pert CB (1985) Comparison of the substance P- and dynorphin-containing projections to the substantia nigra: a radioimmunocytochemical and biochemical study. Brain Res 361:185–192

Minamino N, Kangawa K, Fukuda A, Matsuo H, Lagarashi M (1980) A new opioid octapeptide related to dynorphin from porcine hypothalamus. Biochem Biophys Res Commun 95:1475–1481

Minamino N, Kangawa K, Chino N, Sakakibara S, Matsuo H (1981) Beta-neo-endorphin, a new hypothalamic "big" Leu-enkephalin of porcine origin: its purification and the complete amino acid sequence. Biochem Biophys Res Commun 99:864–870

Morelli M, Di Chiara CG (1985) Non-dopaminergic mechanisms in the turning behavior evoked by intranigral opiates. Brain Res 341:350–359

North RA (1986) Membrane conductances and opioid receptor subtypes. Natl Inst Drug Abuse Res Monogr Ser 71:81–88

North RA, Williams JT, Surprenant A, Christie MJ (1987) μ and δ receptors belong to a family of receptors that are coupled to potassium channels. Proc Natl Acad Sci USA 84:5487–5491

Nylander I, Terenius L (1986) Chronic haloperidol and clozapine differentially affect dynorphin peptides and substance P in basal ganglia of the rat. Brain Res 380:34–41

Nylander I, Terenius LH (1987) Dopamine receptors mediate alterations in striato-nigral dynorphin and substance P pathways. Neuropharmacology 26:1295–1302

Peterson MR, Robertson HA (1984) Effect of dopaminergic agents on levels of dynorphin 1–8 in rat striatum. Prog Neuropsychopharmacol Biol Psychiatry 8:725–728

Petrie EC, Tiffany ST, Baker TB, Dahl JL (1982) Dynorphin (1–13): analgesia, hypothermia, cross-tolerance with morphine and beta-endorphin. Peptides 3:41–47

Przewlocki R, Shearman GT, Herz A (1983) Mixed opioid/nonopioid effects of dynorphin and dynorphin related peptides after their intrathecal injection in rats. Neuropeptides 3:233–240

Qi JA, Bowen WD, Mosberg HI, Rothman RB, Porreca F (1990) Opioid agonist and antagonist antinociceptive properties of [D-Ala2,Leu5,Cys6]enkephalin: selective actions at the deltanoncomplexed site. J Pharmacol Exp Ther 255:636–641

Quirion R, Gaudreau P, Martel JC, St Pierre S, Zamir N (1985) Possible interactions between dynorphin and dopaminergic systems in rat basal ganglia and substantia nigra. Brain Res 331:358–362

Robertson BC, Hommer DW, Skirboll LR (1987) Electrophysiological evidence for a non-opioid interaction between dynorphin and GABA in the substantia nigra of the rat. Neuroscience 23:483–490

Robson LE, Gillan MG, McKnight AT, Kosterlitz HW (1983) [3H]dynorphin A (1–9): binding characteristics and degradation profile in brain homogenates. Life Sci 33(Suppl 1):283–286

Rothman RB, Long JB, Bykov V, Jacobson AE, Rice KC, Holaday JW (1988) Beta-FNA binds irreversibly to the opiate receptor complex: in vivo and in vitro evidence. J Pharmacol Exp Ther 247:405–416

Rothman RB, Mahboubi A, Bykov V, Kim CH, Jacobson AE, Rice KC (1991) Probing the opioid receptor complex with (+)-trans-superfit: I. Evidence that [D-Pen2,D-Pen5]enkephalin interacts with high affinity at the delta cx binding site. Peptides 12:359–364

Schoffelmeer AN, Yao YK, Gioannini TL, Hiller JM, Ofri D, Roques BP, Simon EJ (1990) Cross-linking of human [125I]beta-endorphin to opioid receptors in rat striatal membranes: biochemical evidence for the existence of a mu/delta opioid receptor complex. J Pharmacol Exp Ther 253:419–426

Sei CA, Dores RM (1990) Changes in the processing of pro-dynorphin end products in the substantia nigra during neonatal development. Peptides 11:89–94

Seidah NG, Gaspar L, Mion P, Marcinkiewicz M, Mbikay M, Chrétien M (1990) cDNA sequence of two distinct pituitary proteins homologous to kex2 and furin gene products: tissue specific mRNAs encoding candidates for prohormone processing proteinases. DNA 9:415

Seidah NG, Marcinkiewicz M, Benjannet S, Gaspar L, Beaubien G, Mattei MG, Lazure C, Mbikay M, Chrétien M (1991) Cloning and primary sequence of a mouse candidate prohormone convertase PC1 homologous to PC2, furin, and kex2: distinct chromosomal localization and messenger RNA distribution in brain and pituitary compared to PC2. Mol Endocrinol 5:111

Seizinger BR, Hollt V, Herz A (1981a) Evidence for the occurrence of the opioid octapeptide dynorphin-(1–8) in the neurointermediate pituitary of rats. Biochem Biophys Res Commun 102:197–205

Seizinger BR, Hollt V, Herz A (1981b) Immunoreactive dynorphin in the rat adenohypophysis consists exclusively of 6000 dalton species. Biochem Biophys Res Commun 103:256–263

Seizinger BR, Grimm C, Höllt V, Herz A (1984a) Evidence for a selective processing of proenkephalin B into different opioid peptide forms in particular regions of rat brain and pituitary. J. Neurochem 42:447–457

Seizinger BR, Hollt V, Herz A (1984b) Proenkephalin B (prodynorphin)-derived opioid peptides: evidence for a differential processing in lobes of the pituitary. Endocrinology 115:662–671

Seizinger BR, Liebisch DC, Kish SJ, Arendt RM, Hornykiewicz O, Herz A (1986) Opioid peptides in Huntington's disease: alterations in prodynorphin and proenkephalin system. Brain Res 378:405–408

Sivam SP (1989) Cocaine selectively increases striatonigral dynorphin levels by a dopaminergic mechanism. J Pharmacol Exp Ther 250:818–824

Sivam SP, Takeuchi K, Li S, Douglass J, Civelli O, Calvetta L, Herbert E, McGinty JF, Hong JS (1988) Lithium increases dynorphin A(1–8) and prodynorphin mRNA levels in the basal ganglia of rats. Brain Res 427:155–163

Smeekens SP, Avruch AS, Lemendola J, Chan SJ, Steiner DF (1991) Identification of a cDNA encoding a second putative prohormone convertase related to PC2 in AtT20 cells and islets of Langerhans. Proc Natl Acad Sci USA 88:340–344

Smiley PL, Johnson M, Bush L, Gibb JW, Hanson GR (1990) Effects of cocaine on extrapyramidal and limbic dynorphin systems. J Pharmacol Exp Ther 253:938–943

Stevens CW, Yaksh TL (1986) Dynorphin A and related peptides administered intrathecally in the rat: a search for putative kappa opiate receptor activity. J Pharmacol Exp Ther 238:833–838

Suda M, Nakao K, Yoshimasa T, Ikeda Y, Sakamoto M, Yanaihara N, Numa S, Imura H (1983) A novel opioid peptide, leumorphin, acts as an agonist at the kappa opiate receptor. Life Sci 32:2769–2775

Taquet H, Javoy AF, Giraud P, Legrand JC, Agid Y, Cesselin F (1985) Dynorphin levels in parkinsonian patients: Leu5-enkephalin production from either proenkephalin A or prodynorphin in human brain. Brain Res 341:390–392

Thompson LA, Matsumoto RR, Hohmann AG, Walker JM (1990) Striatonigral prodynorphin: a model system for understanding opioid peptide function. Ann NY Acad Sci 579:192–203

Traynor JR (1987) Prodynorphin as a source of [Leu] enkephalin. Trends Pharmacol Sci 8:47–48

Trujillo KA, Akil H (1989) Changes in prodynorphin peptide content following treatment with morphine or amphetamine: possible role in mechanisms of action of drug of abuse. Natl Inst Drug Abuse Res Monogr Ser 95:550–551

Trujillo KA, Akil H (1990a) Opioid and non-opioid behavioral actions of dynorphin A and the dynorphin analogue DAKLI. Natl Inst Drug Abuse Res Monogr Ser 105:397–398

Trujillo KA, Akil H (1990b) Pharmacological regulation of striatal prodynorphin peptides. Prog Clin Biol Res 328:223–226

Trujillo KA, Day R, Akil H (1990) Regulation of striatonigral prodynorphin peptides by dopaminergic agents. Brain Res 518:244–256

Tulunay FC, Jen MF, Chang JK, Loh HH, Lee NM (1981a) Possible regulatory role of dynorphin on morphine- and beta-endorphin-induced analgesia. J Pharmacol Exp Ther 219:296–298

Tulunay FC, Jen MF, Chang JK, Loh HH, Lee NM (1981b) Possible regulatory role of dynorphin-(1-13) on narcotic-induced changes in naloxone efficacy. Eur J Pharmacol 76:235–239

Vaswani KK, Richard CW, Tejwani GA (1988) Cold swim stress-induced changes in the levels of opioid peptides in the rat CNS and peripheral tissues. Pharmacol Biochem Behav 29:163–168

Vincent S, Hokfelt T, Christensson I, Terenius L (1982a) Immunohistochemical evidence for a dynorphin immunoreactive striato- nigral pathway. Eur J Pharmacol 85:251–252

Vincent SR, Hokfelt T, Christensson I, Terenius L (1982b) Dynorphin-immunoreactive neurons in the central nervous system of the rat. Neurosci Lett 33:185–190

Walker JM, Katz RJ, Akil H (1980) Behavioral effects of dynorphin 1-13 in the mouse and rat: initial observations. Peptides 1:341–345

Walker JM, Moises HC, Coy DH, Baldrighi G, Akil H (1982a) Nonopiate effects of dynorphin and des-Tyr-dynorphin. Science 218:1136–1138

Walker JM, Moises HC, Coy DH, Young EA, Watson SJ, Akil H (1982b) Dynorphin (1-17): lack of analgesia but evidence for non-opiate electrophysiological and motor effects. Life Sci 31:1821–1824

Walker JM, Tucker DE, Coy DH, Walker BB, Akil H (1982c) Des-tyrosine-dynorphin antagonizes morphine analgesia. Eur J Pharmacol 85:121–122

Walker JM, Moises HC, Friederich MW (1985) A review of some nonopioid actions of dynorphin. Prog Clin Biol Res 192:309–312

Watson SJ, Khachaturian H, Akil H, Coy DH, Goldstein A (1982) Comparison of the distribution of dynorphin systems and enkephalin systems in brain. Science 218:1134–1136

Watson SJ, Khachaturian H, Taylor L, Fischli W, Goldstein A, Akil H (1983) Prodynorphin peptides are found in the same neurons throughout rat brain: immunocytochemical study. Proc Natl Acad Sci USA 80:891–894

Watson SJ, Trujillo KA, Herman JP, Akil H (1989) Neuroanatomical and neurochemical substrates of drug-seeking behavior: overview and future directions. In: Goldstein A (ed) Molecular and cellular aspects of the addictions. Springer, Berlin Heidelberg New York, pp 29–91

Weber E, Evans CJ, Barchas JD (1982a) Predominance of the amino-terminal octapeptide fragment of dynorphin in rat brain regions. Nature 299:77–79

Weber E, Evans CJ, Chang JK, Barchas JD (1982b) Brain distribution of a-neo-endorphin and b-neo-endorphin: evidence for regional processing differences. Biochem Biophys Res Comm 108:81–88

Weissman BA, Zamir N (1987) Differential effects of heroin on opioid levels in the rat brain. Eur J Pharmacol 139:121–123

Werz MA, Macdonald RL (1983a) Opioid peptides selective for mu and delta receptors reduce calcium dependent action potentials by increasing potassium conductance. Neurosci Lett 42:173–178

Werz MA, Macdonald RL (1983b) Opioid peptides with differential affinity for mu and delta receptors decrease sensory neuron calcium-dependent action potentials. J Pharmacol Exp Ther 227:394–402

Werz MA, Macdonald RL (1984a) Dynorphin reduces calcium-dependent action potential duration by decreasing voltage-dependent calcium conductance. Neurosci Lett 46:185–190

Werz MA, Macdonald RL (1984b) Dynorphin reduces voltage-dependent calcium conductance of mouse dorsal root ganglion neurons. Neuropeptides 5:253–256

Werz MA, Macdonald RL (1985) Dynorphin and neoendorphin peptides decrease dorsal root ganglion neuron calcium-dependent action potential duration. J Pharmacol Exp Ther 234:49–56

Woo SK, Tulunay FC, Loh HH, Lee NM (1983) Effect of dynorphin-(1–13) and related peptides on respiratory rate and morphine-induced respiratory rate depression. Eur J Pharmacol 96:117–122

Xie GX, Goldstein A (1987) Characterization of big dynorphins from rat brain and spinal cord. J Neurosci 7:2049–2055

Young EA, Walker JM, Houghten R, Akil H (1987) The degradation of dynorphin A in brain tissue in vivo and in vitro. Peptides 8:701–707

Zamir N (1985) On the origin of Leu-enkephalin and Met-enkephalin in the rat neurohypophysis. Endocrinology 117:1687–1692

Zamir N, Palkovits M, Weber E, Mezey E, Brownstein MJ (1984a) A dynorphinergic pathway of Leu-enkephalin production in rat substantia nigra. Nature 307: 643–645

Zamir N, Skofitsch G, Bannon MJ, Helke CJ, Kopin IJ, Jacobowitz DM (1984b) Primate model of Parkinson's disease: alterations in multiple opioid systems in the basal ganglia. Brain Res 322:356–360

Zamir N, Weber E, Palkovits M, Brownstein M (1984c) Differential processing of prodynorphin and proenkephalin in specific regions of the rat brain. Proc Natl Acad Sci USA 81:6886–6889

CHAPTER 20

Anatomy and Function
of the Endogenous Opioid Systems

H. Khachaturian, M.K.H. Schaefer, and M.E. Lewis

A. Introduction

The endogenous opioid systems constitute three distinct neuronal systems
that are widely distributed throughout the central nervous system (CNS).
The three opioid precursors found in these neurons, proopiomelanocortin
(POMC), proenkephalin (PENK), and prodynorphin (PDYN), each contain
numerous biologically active products that are released at the synaptic
terminals of opioidergic neurons. These peptides exert their physiological
actions by interacting with various classes of opioid receptor types (μ, δ, κ)
present on both pre- and postsynaptic membranes of opioid and opioid-
target neurons. Opioid neurotransmission appears to influence many CNS
functions, including nociception, cardiovascular regulation, respiration,
neuroendocrine and neuroimmune activity, thermoregulation, and consum-
matory, sexual, aggressive, locomotor, and hedonic behavior, as well
as learning and memory (Adler et al. 1988; Herz and Millan 1988;
Khachaturian et al. 1988; Martinez et al. 1988; Pasternak 1988; Stefano
1989). Opioid peptides have also been implicated either directly or indirectly
in the pathophysiology of several neurological, addictive, or psychiatric
disorders, including Alzheimer's, Parkinson's, Huntington's disease, stroke,
epilepsy, brain and spinal cord injury, drug and alcohol addiction, eating
disorders, manic-depressive illness, anxiety disorders, and schizophrenia
(Nemeroff and Bissette 1986; Watson et al. 1986; Topel 1988; Kaye et al.
1989; Gulya 1990).

In this chapter, we describe the anatomical distribution of these
neuronal systems as elucidated with immunocytochemical and in situ hybridization techniques, and as well the distribution of the opioid receptor
types using autoradiography, and their functional significance. Since many
previous review articles have dealt extensively with the distribution of the
central opioid systems, opioid receptors, and their functional implications,
we have limited the present review to the most pertinent and when possible
the most recent findings, and the reader is referred to the following reviews
for details about specific topics covered in this chapter (Khachaturian et al.
1985b; Petrusz et al. 1985; Fallon and Leslie 1986; Mansour et al. 1988;
Weihe et al. 1988a; Illes 1989; Stengaard-Pedersen 1989; Loh and Smith
1990), as well as the numerous specific reviews appearing in this volume.

B. Immunocytochemical Anatomy of Opioid Systems

I. Proopiomelanocortin

The major products of this precursor include the biologically active peptides β-endorphin (β-END), adrenocorticotrophic hormone (ACTH), and α-melanocyte-stimulating hormone (α-MSH). Proopiomelanocortin (POMC) is synthesized in the brain as well as the anterior and intermediate lobes of the pituitary gland in a number of species including the rat, monkey, and man (KHACHATURIAN et al. 1984, 1985a; IBUKI et al. 1989). The pituitary is the major organ of POMC biosynthesis. In fact, β-END was first isolated and characterized in this gland (see LI and CHUNG 1976). This discovery was soon followed by the immunocytochemical localization of β-END in anterior lobe corticotrophs (co-stored with ACTH) and intermediate lobe melanotrophs (co-stored with α-MSH) (BLOOM et al. 1977). Biochemical studies soon followed the anatomical ones in elucidating the protein struc- ture of the POMC precursor and its various bioactive peptides (MAINS et al. 1977; ROBERTS and HERBERT 1977). Soon thereafter, the complete structure of POMC was deduced through molecular biological techniques using cDNA clones of POMC mRNA (NAKANISHI et al. 1979).

The brain sites of POMC synthesis include the arcuate nucleus of hypothalamus and the medullary nucleus tractus solitarius (KHACHATURIAN et al. 1985c). The early immunocytochemical work demonstrated the coexistence of β-END and ACTH in the same neurons of the arcuate nucleus (BLOOM et al. 1978; WATSON et al. 1978a,b). Similarly, β-END has been shown to coexist with α-MSH within the same arcuate neurons, in- dicating that the processing of POMC in the brain and pituitary intermediate lobe follow a similar course (WATSON and AKIL 1980). The second POMC neuronal system resides in the nucleus tractus solitarius (SCHWARTZBERG and NAKANE 1983). This neuronal group has been shown to costore β-END, ACTH, and an N-terminal POMC precursor fragment known as 16K peptide. The projections of the latter system appear to be local within the medulla oblongata, with possible projections rostrally to the parabrachial nuclei, and also to the spinal cord (TSOU et al. 1986).

The projections of arcuate POMC neurons are extensive (KHACHATURIAN et al. 1985c). Main rostral target areas include the periventricular diencephalon and telencephalon, including several hypothalamic nuclei, medial preoptic area, medial septum, and bed nucleus of stria terminalis. The main lateral projection of arcuate POMC neurons courses through the medial-basal hypothalamus, and innervates several amygdaloid nuclei, including the densely innervated central and medial nuclei. Other pro- jections enter the thalamus and course through the periventricular regions. Caudal projections of arcuate neurons enter the mesencephalon to innervate many autonomic and nociceptive areas including the periaqueductal gray and raphe nuclei. Recently, retrograde tract-tracing techniques using horseradish peroxidase-wheat germ agglutinin have demonstrated that the major source of POMC fibers within the rat periaqueductal gray are neurons located in the rostral three-fifths of the hypothalamic arcuate nucleus (YOSHIDA and TANIGUCHI 1988). More caudally located arcuate neurons are thought to contribute fibers to the caudal brainstem. For example, the pontine and medullary sites of innervation include the parabrachial nuclei, nuclei reticularis gigantocellularis and raphe magnus, nucleus tractus solitarius, dorsal motor nucleus of the vagus nerve, and other nuclei involved with cardiovascular and respiratory function.

II. Proenkephalin

The precursor proenkephalin (PENK), unlike its opioid counterpart POMC, codes for several opioid peptides, namely [Leu]enkephalin (L-ENK), [Met]enkephalin (M-ENK), M-ENK-Arg-Phe, M-ENK-Arg-Gly-Leu, and other larger peptides such as peptide E. L-ENK and M-ENK were first isolated from the brain and shown to be opiate active (HUGHES et al. 1975). Numerous immunocytochemical studies soon followed demonstrating the similar anatomical distribution pattern of these two peptides (ELDE et al. 1976), which was distinct from the distribution of the POMC-derived peptides (BLOOM et al. 1978; WATSON et al. 1978a). Later, the full structure of the PENK precursor was deduced through molecular cloning and sequencing of cDNA from PENK mRNA (COMB et al. 1982; GUBLER et al. 1982; NODA et al. 1982).

The neuronal perikarya which synthesize PENK are distributed widely throughout the neuraxis in a number of species including the rat, monkey, and man (HABER and ELDE 1982; KHACHATURIAN et al. 1983a,b,c; McGINTY et al. 1984; HABER and WATSON 1985; FALLON and LESLIE 1986; ROUGEOT et al. 1988; SIMERLY et al. 1988; CASSELL and GRAY 1989; CHUNG et al. 1989; IBUKI et al. 1989; WALKER et al. 1989). Many enkephalinergic neuronal systems form local circuits, while others have long tract projections either rostrally or caudally (NAHIN 1988). The use of the neurotoxin colchicine has been instrumental in localizing many of the smaller neuronal perikarya which contain enkephalin peptides, particularly in the cerebral cortex and other brain areas which contain small neurons synthesizing relatively low amounts of PENK. For example, the initial observation of L-ENK and M-ENK in hypothalamus, striatum, and globus pallidus was later amended to include such diverse neuroanatomical structures as specific cerebral cortical layers, hippocampus, amygdala, septum, bed nucleus of stria terminalis, preoptic area, numerous pontine and medullary nuclei, and the spinal cord nociceptive regions. Within diencephalon, PENK is found in most hypothalamic nuclei, periventricular thalamus, and lateral geniculate nucleus. In mesencephalon, PENK containing perikarya are localized throughout the periaqueductal gray, the superior and inferior colliculi, interpeduncular nucleus, and substantia nigra. In the pons and medulla, cells are found in the parabrachial nuclei, dorsal tegmental nuclei, raphe magnus, nucleus reticularis gigantocellularis, vestibular nuclei, nucleus tractus solitarius, lateral reticular nucleus, spinal trigeminal nucleus, as well as in the spinal cord dorsal gray laminae. All of the above regions mentioned also contain enkephalin fibers and terminals, making these peptides strategically situated to influence a wide variety of CNS functions. Indeed, PENK peptides are often found to coexist and/or have synaptic interactions with other neurotransmitters (e.g., acetylcholine, epinephrine, norepinephrine, serotonin, GABA, and substance P) in the same neurons, and thus might function as a cotransmitter or neuromodulator in these areas (Khachaturian and Watson 1982; Hoekfelt et al. 1986; Ibuki et al. 1988; Senba et al. 1988; Shinoda et al. 1988; Weihe et al. 1988a; Milner et al. 1989; Murakami et al. 1989; Pickel et al. 1989; see also Chap. 22, this volume).

III. Prodynorphin

Prodynorphin (PDYN), like PENK, contains multiple biologically active opioid peptides, including dynorphin-A (DYN-A), dynorphin-B (DYN-B or rimorphin), and α-neo-endorphin or β-neo-endorphin. PDYN is synthesized in many neuronal systems throughout the brain and spinal cord. Additionally, PDYN is also synthesized in the anterior lobe of the pituitary gland (Seizinger et al. 1983), colocalized with luteinizing hormone (LH) and follicle-stimulating hormone (FSH) in a subset of gonadotrophs (Khachaturian et al. 1986). The first 13 residues of DYN-A were sequenced from extracts of the pituitary gland, and the peptide was shown to contain L-ENK at its N-terminus (Goldstein et al. 1979). Soon a second L-ENK-containing peptide was also characterized from hypothalamic extracts and named α-neo-endorphin (Kangawa et al. 1981). Finally, a third peptide was also identified which contained L-ENK, and was shown to be a C-terminally extended DYN-A; this peptide was termed rimorphin or DYN-B (Fischli et al. 1982; Kilpatrick et al. 1982). The immunocytochemical studies that followed demonstrated the coexistence of these three peptides within the same neuronal perikarya (Watson et al. 1983; Weber and Barchas 1983). These results pointed to the potential for the existence of a common precursor to all dynorphin peptides, i.e., PDYN, the complete sequence of which was deduced from cloning and sequence analysis of PDYN cDNA (Kakidani et al. 1982).

The initial immunocytochemical studies of dynorphin peptides were carried out in the hypothalamus, where it was demonstrated that DYN-A(1–13) peptide is colocalized with arginine-vasopressin in magnocellular neurons of the supraoptic (SON) and paraventricular (PVN) nuclei (Watson et al. 1981, 1982a,b). Subsequent immunocytochemical observations showed another widespread peptidergic neuronal system that is found in virtually all levels of the neuraxis in a number of species including the rat, monkey, and man (Khachaturian et al. 1982, 1985a; Vincent et al. 1982; Weber and

BARCHAS 1983; McGINTY et al. 1984; HABER and WATSON 1985; FALLON and LESLIE 1986; ABE et al. 1988; CHO and BASBAUM 1988; IBUKI et al. 1989; MILLER and SEYBOLD 1989). Again, the application of the neurotoxin colchicine proved essential in the demonstration of smaller neuronal perikarya that were otherwise undetectable with conventional immuno-cytochemistry (KHACHATURIAN et al. 1982). Perikarya-containing PDYN products are seen in the cerebral cortex, striatum, amygdala, hippocampus, several hypothalamic nuclei, mesencephalic periaqueductal gray, pontine parabrachial nuclei, medullary spinal trigeminal nuclei, nucleus tractus solitarius, lateral reticular nucleus, as well as in the spinal cord dorsal gray laminae. Fibers and terminals containing PDYN peptides are further found in the globus pallidus, substantia nigra, and raphe nuclei, to name a few. Many of these dynorphinergic systems form local circuits while others con-stitute long-tract projections in the spinal cord and brain (NAHIN 1988; ZARDETTO-SMITH et al. 1988). Thus, both PENK and PDYN products have a wide distribution throughout the brain and spinal cord, and their dis-tribution is often in parallel. These observations point to the potential for collaborative participation of these two opioidergic neuronal systems in many similar regulatory functions, but most probably through different receptor mechanisms. In addition, as mentioned for PENK, the PDYN peptides are also often found colocalized with other neurotransmitters (e.g., substance P, enkephalin), and thus might function as a cotransmitter or neuromodulator in a variety of CNS functions (SASEK and ELDE 1986; TUCHSCHERER and SEYBOLD 1989).

C. In Situ Hybridization Histochemical Studies

While the above-described immunocytochemical studies on opioid peptidergic systems have generated a detailed picture of the distribution of all three opioid families in the CNS, the introduction of molecular biological tech-niques to the neuroanatomical repertoire has added another dimension, namely the examination of opioid gene expression at the single cell level. Thus, in situ hybridization histochemistry has emerged as a powerful tech-nique for the localization of the mRNA encoded by many neuropeptide genes, including those of the opioids (for review see UHL 1986; VALENTINO et al. 1987; M.E. LEWIS et al. 1988; CHESSELET 1990). Immunocytochemistry provides a measure of peptide content, and thus yields a somewhat static picture of gene expression. By contrast, in situ hybridization analysis of mRNA levels allows insight into the dynamic events of gene expression, since the cellular levels of mRNA are generally regarded as a measure of the biosynthetic activity of a given gene (WATSON et al. 1988; McCABE et al. 1989; W.S. YOUNG 1990; SCHAEFER et al. 1990a). Furthermore, the high degree of spatial resolution, the great sensitivity of this technique to detect even minute amounts of mRNA, and the quantifiability of the autoradiographic signal, makes it the method of choice for the examination of gene expression and regulation in heterogeneous and complex tissues such as the brain.

One of the pioneering studies which established the technique of in situ localization of mRNA in the CNS was the demonstration of POMC mRNA within the hypothalamic ACTH-containing neurons of the arcuate nucleus (GEE et al. 1983). While immunocytochemical studies often required colchicine in order to visualize POMC-derived peptides in neuronal perikarya (KHACHATURIAN et al. 1985c), in situ hybridization readily demonstrated POMC mRNA in neurons of the arcuate nucleus in normal, untreated tissue. Therefore, the latter technique presents a clear advantage for physiological and pharmacological studies which aim to examine opioid gene expression, since the effect of colchicine treatment on gene expression and other possible unwanted side effects can be eliminated.

I. Proopiomelanocortin mRNA

Proopiomelanocortin mRNA has been detected in extracts of several brain regions including the basal ganglia, cortex, and amygdala (CIVELLI et al. 1982). In general, in situ hybridization studies have confirmed the previous immunocytochemical findings regarding the major site of POMC synthesis in the brain, namely the arcuate nucleus of the hypothalamus. In addition, in situ hybridization studies have confirmed the previous immunocytochemical findings of the existence of POMC-synthesizing cells in the caudal portion of the nucleus tractus solitarius (SCHAEFER et al. 1990b, 1991). Compared to the arcuate POMC neurons, the nucleus tractus solitarius cells contain much lower levels of POMC mRNA and can only be visualized following long autoradiographic exposure times. Whether or not other, yet undiscovered, CNS neurons express the POMC gene requires careful reevaluation using in situ hybridization analysis.

As anatomical studies have progressed, several groups have begun to examine the physiology of the arcuate POMC system by making measurements of the changes in cellular content of POMC mRNA. A role for POMC peptides in the regulation of reproductive physiology has been suggested in studies which have demonstrated that gonadal steroids can regulate POMC gene expression. For example, estrogen treatment of ovariectomized rats caused a decrease in POMC mRNA levels in the arcuate neurons (WILCOX and ROBERTS 1985). Furthermore, castration resulted in a testosterone-reversible decrease in POMC mRNA levels in a select group of cells in the most rostral areas of the arcuate nucleus (CHOWEN-BREED et al. 1989a,b). The latter experiment raises the possibility that POMC gene expression might be differentially regulated in different subpopulations of arcuate neurons. Whether androgens upregulate POMC mRNA levels or have an inhibitory effect, as proposed by others (BLUM et al. 1989), remains to be resolved. Nevertheless, the potential role of

POMC peptides in reproductive physiology has been bolstered by the recent observation of an increase in POMC mRNA levels at the onset of puberty, indicating a potential role for POMC peptides in the regulation of gonadotrophin-releasing hormone (GnRH) secretion (WIEMANN et al. 1989).

A role in pain modulation of the central POMC system has been proposed based on the potent analgesic properties of β-END and noxious stimulation studies (described elsewhere in this chapter). While biochemical evidence exists that peptide content in projection areas of the arcuate region is changed in response to noxious stimuli (cf. MILLAN et al. 1991), POMC mRNA levels following acute or chronic noxious stimulation have not been examined with in situ hybridization, which could also address the question of functional arcuate subgroups. The effect of opiate treatment on POMC gene expression also needs a more careful examination with in situ hybridization at the subregional level. Following chronic morphine administration, decreased levels of POMC mRNA have been reported in hypothalamic tissue extracts (MOCCHETTI et al. 1989; BRONSTEIN et al. 1990), while others have observed no changes in POMC mRNA (HÖLLT et al. 1989).

To examine rapid changes in POMC gene transcription at the single cell level, a variation of in situ hybridization has been applied using intervening sequence specific probes (FREMEAU et al. 1986, 1989). Nuclear precursor RNA, still containing intronic sequences, rather than cytoplasmic mRNA, was analyzed with this technique in pituitary and brain. Using these specific probes for the measurement of primary RNA transcripts allows the analysis of acute or small changes in gene transcription (due to the short half-life of the primary RNA transcripts) and presents an alternative to the in vitro run on transcription assay (EBERWINE and ROBERTS 1984) to study transcription at the single cell level. POMC primary transcript levels in the pituitary were found to increase threefold within 15 min after removal of the negative glucocorticoid feedback, while cytoplasmic mRNA levels remained unchanged (SCHAEFER et al. 1990b). On the other hand, injection of a single dose of the glucocorticoid dexamethasone rapidly decreased POMC primary RNA transcript levels, while leaving cytoplasmic mRNA levels unaffected. The potential of nuclear precursor RNA in situ hybridization for pharmacological and physiological studies examining stimulus-transcription coupling is obvious, but depends at present largely on the availability of genomic clones and sequence information on introns in the three opioid genes.

II. Proenkephalin and Prodynorphin mRNA

While the expression of the POMC gene is restricted to just a few brain areas, PENK and PDYN mRNA appear to be widely expressed in neurons throughout the CNS. In general, although cells containing PENK mRNA are more numerous and are found in many more areas than those containing PDYN mRNA, the distribution pattern of neurons synthesizing these transcripts is overlapping (see Fig. 1). Therefore, the localization and

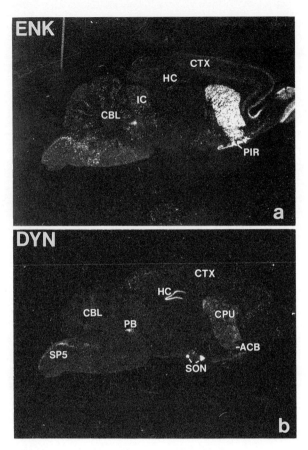

Fig. 1a,b. Localization of proenkephalin (*ENK*) mRNA (**a**) and prodynorphin (*DYN*) mRNA (**b**) in the rat CNS. Adjacent frozen 20-μm-thick sagittal sections (2 mm lateral of the midline) were hybridized with ^{35}S-labeled RNA probes complementary to ENK mRNA and DYN mRNA, respectively. In general, ENK mRNA-expressing cells are more widely distributed throughout the CNS when compared to DYN mRNA-containing neurons (see text). Note the abundance of ENK mRNA in the caudate-putamen (*CPU*) and piriform cortex (*PIR*) (**a**) and the strong labeling in the supraoptic nucleus (*SON*), hippocampus (*HC*), and parabrachial nucleus (*PB*) with the DYN cRNA probe (**b**). Exposure times of X-rays were 48 h. (*ACB*, nucleus accumbens; *CBL*, cerebellum; *CTX*, cortex; *IC*, inferior colliculus; *SP5*, spinal trigeminal nucleus)

regulation of PENK and PDYN mRNA will be discussed together. The extent to which PENK and PDYN are coexpressed can be addressed in future studies using in situ hybridization. Given the presence of sequence homologies in PENK and PDYN (the Leu-enkephalin sequence is present in both protein precursors), immunocytochemical studies were carefully designed using highly specific antisera for each precursor. However, cross-reactivities were often difficult to rule out. The application of in situ hybridization to the study of opioid precursor coexistence could overcome this limitation due to the highly specific nature of probe-mRNA hybrid formation.

Of the three known opioid genes, PENK appears to be the most abundantly expressed, both in cell number and in brain regions. Recently, in situ hybridization was used to map the cellular distribution of PENK mRNA throughout the rat brain and spinal cord (HARLAN et al. 1987). Although good agreement existed with previous immunocytochemical results (e.g., KHACHATURIAN et al. 1983a,b), even more PENK mRNA containing perikarya were observed. This was particularly obvious in regions of the neocortex, the olfactory tubercle, the piriform cortex, the nucleus accumbens, the striatum, and the cerebellum. The presence of PENK mRNA in all Golgi type II cells of the cerebellar cortex was discovered. This observation has led to the suggestion that PENK products may be involved in the classical conditioning of certain motor patterns (for review see ITO 1984). Interestingly, PENK immunoreactivity was detected only in some Golgi type II cells, whereas PENK immunoreactivity in these cells seemed to be more easily detectable during specific developmental stages (ZAGON et al. 1985).

The expression of the PDYN gene in the CNS is intermediate to POMC and PENK, with PDYN-containing cells relatively widespread throughout many regions, but significantly less in number than PENK. In contrast to PENK mRNA, the cellular distribution of PDYN mRNA in the CNS has only been investigated in certain key areas of physiological interest. These include the hypothalamic magnocellular neurons, where PDYN is coexpressed with vasopressin (MORRIS et al. 1986; SHERMAN et al. 1986), the basal ganglia, where PDYN mRNA is expressed at high levels in the nucleus accumbens and to a lesser degree in the caudate-putamen (W.S. YOUNG et al. 1986; MORRIS et al. 1986, 1989), the dentate gyrus of the hippocampal formation (MORRIS et al. 1986), the cerebral cortex (ALVEREZ et al. 1990), and the spinal cord (IADAROLA et al. 1986).

In rat brain, the highest levels of PENK mRNA are found in the striatum. About 50%–60% of all medium spiny neurons, which project in their majority to the pallidum, express PENK mRNA. Another set of neurons, expressing mainly PDYN and substance P and intermingled with the former, project to the substantia nigra (GERFEN and YOUNG 1988). To what extent coexpression of PENK and PDYN mRNA occurs in the same medium spiny neurons needs further investigation using double labeling techniques at the mRNA level. The regulation of striatal opioid gene expression by dopamine has been a particularly active area of research and is discussed elsewhere in this chapter. However, in brief, whereas PENK mRNA levels dramatically increase in striatum following dopamine antagonist treatment (haloperidol) or removal of the dopaminergic input

(6-OHDA), PDYN mRNA levels appear unaffected or show even a slight decrease (Tang et al. 1983; Sivam et al. 1986; Morris et al. 1989). Dopamine has the opposite effect on PDYN expression in the nigrostriatonigral loop, which participates in motor behavior. PDYN synthesis seems to be stimulated after chronic application of dopamine against apomorphine (S.J. Li et al. 1988). Recently, it was suggested, combining in situ hybridization and retrograde tracing, that the differential effects of dopamine on striatal projection neurons are transmitted through different dopamine receptor subtypes. The D2 receptor seems to be preferentially expressed by PENK mRNA-containing neurons, whereas PDYN-containing cells express mainly the D1 receptor (Gerfen et al. 1990; Morris et al. 1988b). A parallel regulation pattern appears to exist in the nucleus accumbens, where opioids seem to play a role in reward mechanisms and possibly schizophrenia (Morris et al. 1988b). These functional issues are further addressed later in this chapter.

In hypothalamus, high levels of PDYN mRNA are present in the magnocellular neurons of the SON and PVN. Salt loading and dehydration studies have shown that chronic osmotic challenge increases PDYN mRNA levels over several days concomitantly with vasopressin mRNA levels, suggesting possible coregulation of expression of these coexisting neuro-peptides. While magnocellular neurons in both the SON and the PVN respond the same to osmotic challenge in terms of PDYN expression, in situ hybridization studies have demonstrated that the same mRNAs are increased following repeated electroconvulsive shocks in the SON, but not the PVN (Schafer et al. 1989). In the PVN, the coregulated expression of PENK mRNA and oxytocin mRNA has been reported following stress induced by hypertonic saline injection (Lightman and Young 1987).

Gonadal steroids seem to regulate, in addition to POMC, also the expression of PENK and PDYN in the hypothalamus. In the ventromedial nucleus of the hypothalamus, the expression of PENK mRNA is changed by both estrogen and progesterone treatment, suggesting altered activity of PENK neurons in the hormonal regulation of the estrous cycle (Romano et al. 1989, 1990; Lauber et al. 1990).

In the hippocampal formation, a great deal of attention has been paid to the effects of induced epileptiform and seizure activities on the expression of opioid mRNA. Both PENK and PDYN mRNAs are expressed in the granule cell layer of dentate gyrus, with PDYN mRNA being more abundant in normal rats (see Fig. 1). Induction of acute seizure activity in the hippocampus causes depletion of both PENK- and PDYN-derived peptides. However, at the mRNA level, PDYN and PENK appear to be regulated in opposite directions. Kindling seizures decrease rapidly the levels of PDYN mRNA in the dentate gyrus, while PENK mRNA is markedly increased at the stimulated site (Gall et al. 1990; Hong et al. 1987, 1988; Morris et al. 1988a).

III. Expression of Opioids in Nonneuronal Cells

For many years, opioid gene expression in the CNS was believed to occur in neurons and neuroendocrine cells only (for review see KHACHATURIAN et al. 1985b). However, recent evidence from in vitro studies of neuronal/glial cell cultures and from localization of opioids in the periphery have clearly demonstrated that this is not the case. For example, the PENK gene, but not the PDYN gene, was found to be expressed in astroglia in neonatal brain tissue cultures (VILIJN et al. 1988; H. SHINODA et al. 1989; MELNER et al. 1990; HAUSER et al. 1990). More recently, PENK mRNA was discovered in pituicytes of adult rat brain in situ and in the cerebellum in both neurons and a subset of neuroglia (SPRUCE et al. 1990). While the function of PENK expression in astroglia remains to be elucidated, preliminary biochemical data obtained from cultures suggest that, in contrast to neurons, the posttranslational processing of the PENK precursor seems to yield larger protein precursor fragments and less of the smaller peptides such as Met-enkephalin (H. SHINODA et al. 1989; MELNER et al. 1990). Interestingly, the presence of PENK mRNA in astroglia seems to be region specific and higher in developing animals than in adults. In addition, the high expression of PENK mRNA during ontogenic development in mesenchymal-derived tissues (POLAKIEWICZ and ROSEN 1990) has raised the possibility that the expression of the PENK gene may play an important role in cell growth and cell differentiation. The extent to which PENK gene expression is induced in nonneuronal cells in the adult CNS following brain lesions, degenerative and regenerative processes, and infections such as encephalitis, needs further examination in double-labeling experiments combining specific glial cell markers with specific opioid gene probes.

Another area of opioid research demanding increased attention is the expression of opioid genes in the immune system and its interrelationship to the nervous system (WEIHE et al. 1992). The POMC peptides ACTH and β-endorphin were detected in leukocytes and macrophages (E.M. SMITH et al. 1986), and, more recently, POMC mRNA was found in human mononuclear cells (BUZZETTI et al. 1989). PENK mRNA is expressed at high levels by T-helper cells (ZURAWSKI et al. 1986), but is also present in normal B-lymphocytes (ROSEN et al. 1989) and expressed at low levels in thymus and spleen. In contrast, the expression of the PDYN gene has not yet been detected in immune cells. However, it is now well established that the expression of PDYN mRNA is markedly increased in the dorsal horn of the spinal cord by acute and chronic inflammation (IADAROLA et al. 1986, 1988; HÖLLT et al. 1987; WEIHE et al. 1989). Dramatic increases in PDYN mRNA were observed in monoarthritic rats in the ipsilateral cord segments receiving sensory inputs from the affected limb. These changes occurred rapidly within a few hours and, using in situ hybridization, could be localized to lamina I and II and the deep layers V and VI (RUDA et al.

1988). The increase in PENK mRNA was less pronounced and more localized to lamina I and II of the superficial dorsal horn (IADAROLA et al. 1988). Furthermore, a subset of inflammation-responsive neurons in lamina IV and V were reported to coexpress PDYN- and PENK-derived peptides (WEIHE et al. 1988b). Whether immune cells themselves in the spinal cord or the brain can express opioids under normal conditions, during inflammatory processes, or in response to noxious stimuli needs further examination at the cellular level.

D. Opioid Receptors and Functional Systems

I. Problems in the Functional Analysis of Endogenous Opioid Systems

What can be deduced about the functions of the endogenous opioid systems? There are, on the one hand, well-defined maps of the distribution of opioid peptidergic systems and multiple receptor types, and on the other hand numerous pharmacological studies investigating the functional consequences of administering diverse opiate agonists or antagonists. The task of integrating these two areas of work is difficult because of striking discrepancies in the anatomical distribution of opioid neuronal systems and receptor types, as well as considerable uncertainties in relating pharmacological effects of agonists or antagonists, acting on one or more particular receptor types, to the potential actions of specific opioid neuronal systems which generally have a poorly defined relationship to these receptors. To make matters even more confusing, it appears that opioid precursors are differentially processed in different opioid neuronal systems (WEBER et al. 1982; SEIZINGER et al. 1983; WHITE et al. 1986), resulting in peptide products with varying selectivities for the multiple types of opioid receptors (CORBETT et al. 1982; QUIRION and WEISS 1983). Even for peptides with relatively high selectivity for a particular receptor type (e.g., DYN-A for the κ-receptor; CHAVKIN et al. 1982), it is likely that "crossover" to other opioid receptor types will occur if there is a relative paucity of the "preferred" receptor type in a given brain region or species (E.A. YOUNG et al. 1986). To add further complexity, there is evidence for species differences in the processing of opioid peptide precursor proteins (DORES et al. 1984) and in the relative abundance to different opioid receptor types (MOON EDLEY et al. 1982). Finally, some neurons appear to express both the PENK and PDYN precursor proteins (MULCAHY et al. 1983). Thus, for any particular opioid system, there is likely to be considerable uncertainty over which opioid peptides are actually being released, which receptor types these peptides are contacting, and where these activated receptors are localized. This uncertainty complicates pharmacological analyses of endogenous opioid neuronal function.

The distribution of multiple opioid receptor types has been well characterized (e.g., Mansour et al. 1988) and is reviewed elsewhere in this volume (Chap. 5). In the following section, prior to considering opioid neuronal functions, we attempt to give some perspective on the issue of opioid peptide-receptor anatomical relationships.

II. Opioid Peptide-Receptor Relationships

The anatomical relationship between opioid peptidergic neuronal systems and multiple opioid receptors has been discussed elsewhere (Khachaturian et al. 1985b; Herkenham 1987; Pilapil et al. 1987; Mansour et al. 1988), and need not be reviewed here in detail. We and other investigators have noted that the anatomical distribution of the multiple opioid receptor systems is very similar across mammalian species as divergent as the rat and the rhesus monkey, but that the distribution and relative abundance of each opioid receptor subtype varies dramatically across species. What is the significance of the differential conservation of the distributions of the multiple opioid peptide neuronal systems and receptors? If phylogenetic differences reflect divergence in the evolution of the nervous system, these differences in receptor distribution may reflect evolutionary specializations of the multiple opioid systems. Rather than a restructuring of the opioid neuronal pathways, evolutionary specialization has favored differential neuronal expression of the multiple opioid receptors as a more efficient means for modifying central opioid peptide neuronal functions. Thus, not surprisingly, the opioid neuronal systems per se are fixed; it is the receptors through which they act that are evolutionarily plastic. This type of plasticity, involving only an up- or down-regulation of receptor expression, is much simpler to encode genomically than a fundamental restructuring of neuronal connections. This view also provides another perspective from which to contemplate so-called neurotransmitter-receptor "mismatches" (Herkenham 1987). In addition, superimposed on receptor plasticity are species differences in the processing of opioid peptide precursors within fixed neuronal pathways (Dores et al. 1984). This presynaptic form of plasticity may again be simpler to encode genomically, involving only an up- or down-regulation of the precursor processing enzymes. Given the evidence that differential processing of opioid precursors gives rise to peptides with varying affinities for the multiple opioid receptor subtypes (Corbett et al. 1982; Quirion and Weiss 1983), it is important to discriminate between "mismatches" at the anatomical level and those at molecular level. Although there are a number of "mismatches" at both levels (Mansour et al. 1988), it is perhaps too extreme to conclude that "the opiate receptors show . . . no relationship to the opioid peptide distribution patterns" (Herkenham 1987), implying that all opioid peptides act extrasynaptically, diffusing over very long distances. A final set of "mismatches," though perhaps more properly regarded as a physiological form of regulating endogenous opioid activity, are generated

by developmental changes in the expression of opioid peptides and receptors
(McDowell and Kitchen 1987). These changes can be quite dramatic. For
example, β-END immunoreactivity can be detected histochemically in spinal
cord at embryonic day 14, but disappears later in development (Haynes
et al. 1982; Tsou et al. 1986). In contrast, [^{3}H]naloxone binding sites appear
prenatally but do not appear to peak until postnatal day 6, and are still
present later in life (Kirby and Mattio 1982). Such "mismatches," whether
detected in a phylogenetic or ontogenetic context, should be regarded as
alluring signals for opportunities to further explore incompletely characterized neuronal systems. Given our level of ignorance, it may be premature
to conclude that there is a physiological "mismatch" when further investigation could reveal a "missed match."

E. Functional Roles of Opioid Systems

As noted before (Mansour et al. 1988), there is a plethora of studies on
the physiological and behavioral effects of administering diverse opioid
peptides, or nonpeptidergic opiate agonists or antagonists (e.g., Olson
et al. 1989), but it has still been difficult to draw firm conclusions regarding
the functional roles of different opioid receptor types in any neuronal
system. While this is also true for attempts to characterize the functions of
the opioid systems in development, ontogenetic studies do provide a unique
opportunity to attempt to correlate anatomical and biochemical changes
with possible functional roles of these systems (McDowell and Kitchen
1987). Below, we highlight some features of the literature which point to
possible functional roles of the multiple opioid peptide/receptor systems in
the CNS. Although there is a massive literature in this general area, we have
chosen to focus briefly on some developments in better-characterized
systems (i.e., the endogenous pain control system and extrapyramidal motor
system) where there is more promise of achieving a more thorough
understanding.

I. Endogenous Pain Control Systems

The role of endogenous opioids in regulating nociception has been widely
investigated. The existence of endogenous pain control systems was first
provided by studies using electrical stimulation of the brain to produce a
reduction in pain responsiveness in humans and other species (Mayer
et al. 1971; Hosobuchi et al. 1977; Richardson and Akil 1977a,b). This
stimulation-produced analgesia was suggested to be mediated by endogenous
opioid systems when the analgesia was found to be naloxone-reversible and
cross-tolerant with morphine (Akil et al. 1972, 1978; Mayer and Hayes
1975). The anatomical sites for effective stimulation coincide with the
presence of β-END immunoreactive fibers in the periaqueductal gray and

elsewhere (BASBAUM and FIELDS 1984), and such stimulation increases cerebrospinal fluid levels of β-END (AKIL et al. 1978; HOSOBUCHI et al. 1979). Nevertheless, there is evidence for involvement of other opioid systems as well as nonopioid systems in the regulation of nociception (for reviews, see AKIL et al. 1984; BASBAUM and FIELDS 1984).

One of the most interesting trends in the recent study of the role of endogenous opioids in endogenous pain control mechanisms has been an increased appreciation of the possible role of interactions with κ-opioid receptors (MILLAN 1990). Earlier investigations had emphasized the role of μ-receptors since prototypical opiate analgesics exhibit the greatest affinity for this class of receptors. However, in the hope of reducing the undesirable effects associated with μ-receptor agonists, e.g., high abuse potential, dependence, tolerance, respiratory depression, and nausea, investigators have recently turned to κ-agonists as potentially useful analgesic agents. Selective κ-agonists, such as the arylacetamides U50488H and PD117302, are antinociceptive at the level of the brain and spinal cord, with efficacy diminishing as a function of increasing stimulus intensity (MILLAN 1990). Unfortunately, it appears that κ-agonists induce dysphoric and psycho-tomimetic effects which are likely to limit the clinical utility of these compounds. Nevertheless, κ-agonists have been useful in demonstrating both spinal and supraspinal loci of κ-receptor-mediated antinociception, and the development of the selective κ-antagonist, nor-binaltorphine, should permit studies of the role of κ-receptors in the mediation of physiological (e.g., stress-induced) antinociception. Similarly, the development of selective δ-receptor agonists and antagonists should permit further testing of the possible role of δ-receptors in mediating antinociception (MATHIASEN and VAUGHT 1987; see also Chap. 32, in part II of this volume).

One novel approach to the problem of defining the involvement of multiple systems in endogenous pain control mechanisms has been to explore the effects of antinociceptive treatments on the activity of these systems. At the simplest level, one might suppose that increased activation of one of these systems, coincident with the induction of analgesia, might begin to tie the two together. Fortunately, due to the advent of recombinant DNA technology, it is now possible to measure specific opioid precursor mRNA levels, either biochemically (with Northern or dot blot analysis) or anatomically (with in situ hybridization histochemistry, as shown earlier in this chapter). The underlying rationale of this approach is that increased neuropeptide utilization will create an increased demand for biosynthesis, which will be reflected in increased levels of the neuropeptide precursor mRNA. The validity of this rationale, as well as details of the mRNA measurement technologies, has been discussed elsewhere (M.E. LEWIS et al. 1988; BALDINO et al. 1989). Following this logic, then, it has already been reported that electroconvulsive shock (ECS) induces a profound analgesia which is naloxone reversible (J.W. LEWIS et al. 1981; see HOLADAY et al. 1986 for review) and, more recently, that ECS results in dramatic time- and structure-dependent changes in PENK and PDYN mRNA in rats (XIE et al. 1989). This study was not designed to attempt to relate changes in opioid precursor protein gene expression to the induction of analgesia, which might be a fruitful area for future research.

II. Extrapyramidal Motor Systems

Long before the discovery of endogenous opioid systems, administration of opiates was known to alter motor function. The first hints in defining the interaction of opiates with a chemically defined pathway within the extrapyramidal system, the nigrostriatal dopamine pathway, came in 1970 with dopamine metabolism studies (CLOUET and RATNER 1970; REIS et al. 1970; C.B. SMITH et al. 1970). Supporting previous findings is the report that administration of morphine (or β-END) into the region of the A10 dopaminergic neurons in the mesencephalon produces locomotor activation (JOYCE and IVERSEN 1979). In contrast, microinjection of morphine into the nucleus accumbens (which is innervated by A10 dopaminergic neurons) results in a dose-dependent biphasic locomotor response, with catalepsy followed by locomotor activation (COSTALL et al. 1978). Administration of κ-agonists (tifluadom, bremazocine, and ethylketocyclazocine) decreases locomotor activity in rats (JACKSON and COOPER 1988), which appears to be consistent with electrophysiological studies showing that μ- and κ-opiates have opposite actions on A9 cellular firing rates (J.M. WALKER et al. 1987). The inhibitory effects of these agonists on dopaminergic A9 neurons appear to be mediated at the level of the striatum rather than the substantia nigra (J.M. WALKER et al. 1987), which is consistent with the much higher density of κ-receptors in striatum compared to the substantia nigra (MANSOUR et al. 1988). In addition, these results are supported by dialysis studies in freely moving rats, showing that μ-agonists increase (while κ-agonists decrease) the release of dopamine in the striatum (DICHIARA and IMPERATO 1988). These findings confirm and extend earlier in vivo studies in cats showing that morphine enhances the striatal release of newly synthesized [^{3}H]dopamine (CHESSELET et al. 1981).

It is important to note that the effects of opioids on locomotor activity depend critically on the stage of development (McDOWELL and KITCHEN 1987), although it is uncertain whether these differences are due to developmental changes in opioid metabolism and distribution or to changes in opioid receptors. Not only do opioid receptor subtypes in different regions show different temporal patterns of maturation (McDOWELL and KITCHEN 1987), but the physical state of μ-receptors also appears to change during maturation (McLEAN et al. 1989), which may have functional consequences. In this context, it is interesting to note that the maturational profile of striatal opioid receptors labeled by [^{3}H]naloxone is altered by prenatal haloperidol treatment (MOON 1984).

A different approach to the analysis of opioid interactions with the extrapyramidal dopamine system has been taken by investigators who study the effects of dopamine agonist or antagonist drug treatments on measures of opioid neuronal activity, as measured by changes in levels of opioid peptides or their precursor mRNAs. Following the report that chronic administration of the dopamine receptor antagonist haloperidol results in a significant increase in the level of M-ENK in the striatum (HONG et al. 1985), several investigators reported that this treatment also results in an elevation in striatal PENK mRNA (SABOL et al. 1983; HONG et al. 1985; ANGULO et al. 1986; SIVAM et al. 1986; ROMANO et al. 1987). In contrast, administration of dopaminergic agonists, such as apomorphine, amphetamine, or cocaine, results in an increase in PDYN peptide levels in the striatum and substantia nigra (S.J. LI et al. 1986; HANSON et al. 1990; TRUJILLO and AKIL 1990). This increase appears to be due to increased biosynthesis (S.J. LI et al. 1988; GERFEN et al. 1991), possibly coupled to the acute agonist-induced release of PDYN peptides, particularly DYN-A(1–8) (TRUJILLO and AKIL 1990), which has substantial affinity for both μ- and κ-receptor types (CORBETT et al. 1982; QUIRION and WEISS 1983). These results, taken together, indicate that striatal PENK and PDYN systems are regulated oppositely by dopaminergic neurotransmission. In addition, there is recent evidence that dopamine actions on striatopallidal enkephalin neurons and striatonigral dynorphin neurons are mediated by D2 and D1 dopamine receptor subtypes, respectively (GERFEN et al. 1990; JIANG et al. 1990). Based on these findings, it is tempting to hypothesize that increases in dopamine activity are followed, "downstream," by increased dynorphin-mediated κ- and μ-receptor activation in substantia nigra, while decreases in dopamine activity are followed by increased enkephalin-mediated δ-receptor activation in the globus pallidus/striatum.

To summarize, it appears that the multiple opioid systems in the striatum can be differentially influenced by dopaminergic activity, and that the nigrostriatal dopamine system can, in turn, be differentially influenced by the activation of different opioid receptor types. For reasons reviewed by THOMPSON et al. (1990), the striatonigral DYN pathway is a particularly attractive target for functional studies. Further attention to this pathway, particularly by combining systems approaches with molecular approaches, should allow investigators to more fully understand the complex relationships between dopaminergic and opioid neuronal activity, opioid precursor protein gene expression, and opioid receptor activation.

Acknowledgements. The authors wish to thank Mrs. Mary Lou Prince for manuscript preparation.

References

Abe J, Okamura H, Kitamura T, Ibata Y, Minamino N, Matsuo H, Paull WK (1988) Immunocytochemical demonstration of dynorphin(PH-8P)-like immunoreactive elements in the human hypothalamus. J Comp Neurol 276:508–513

Adler MW, Geller EB, Rosow CE, Cochin J (1988) The opioid system and temperature regulation. Annu Rev Pharmacol Toxicol 28:429–49

Akil H, Mayer DJ, Liebeskind JC (1972) Comparison chez le rat entre l'analgesie induite par stimulation de la substance grise peri-aqueducale et l'analgesie morphinique. CR Acad Sci (Paris) 274:3603–3605

Akil H, Richardson DE, Barcgas JD, Li CH (1978) Appearance of beta-endorphin-like immunoreactivity in human ventricular cerebrospinal fluid upon analgesic electrical stimulation. Proc Natl Acad Sci USA 75:5170–5172

Akil H, Watson SJ, Young E, Lewis ME, Khachaturian H, Walker JM (1984) Endogenous opioids: biology and function. Annu Rev Neurosci 7:223–255

Alvarez BG, Fairen A, Dougless J, Naranjo JR (1990) Expression of the pro-dynorphin gene in the developing and adult cerebral cortex of the rat: an in situ hybridization study. J Comp Neurol 300:287–300

Angulo JA, Davis LG, Burkhart BA, Christoph GR (1986) Reduction of striatal dopaminergic neurotransmission elevates striatal pro-enkephalin mRNA. Eur J Pharmacol 130:341–343

Baldino F, Chesselet MF, Lewis ME (1989) High resolution in situ hybridization histochemistry. Methods Enzymol 168:761–777

Basbaum AI, Fields HL (1984) Endogenous pain control systems: brainstem spinal pathways and endorphin circuitry. Annu Rev Neurosci 7:309–234

Bloom FE, Battenberg E, Rossier J, Ling N, Leppaluoto J, Vargo TM, Guillemin R (1977) Endorphins are located in the intermediate and anterior lobes of the pituitary gland, not in the neurohypophysis. Life Sci 20:43–48

Bloom FE, Battenberg E, Rossier J, Ling N, Guillemin R (1978) Neurons containing beta-endorphin exist separately from those containing enkephalin: immunocytochemical studies. Proc Natl Acad Sci USA 75:1591–1595

Blum M, Roberts JL, Wardlaw SL (1989) Androgen regulation of proopiomelanocortin expression and peptide content in the basal hypothalamus. Endocrinology 124:2283–2288

Bronstein DM, Przewlocki R, Akil H (1990) Effects of morphine treatment of proopiomelanocortin systems in rat brain. Brain Res 519:102–111

Buzzetti R, McLoughling R, Lavender PM, Clark AJ, Rees L (1989) Expression of proopiomelanocortin gene and quantification of adrenocorticotropic hormone-like immunoreactivity in human normal peripheral mononuclear cels and lymphois and myeloid malignancies. J Clin Invest 83:733–7838

Cassell MD, Gray TS (1989) Morphology of peptide-immunoreactive neurons in the rat central nucleus of the amygdala. J Comp Neurol 281:320–333

Chavkin C, James I, Goldstein A (1982) Dynorphin is a specific endogenous ligand of the kappa opioid receptor. Science 215:413–415

Chesselet MF (1990) In situ hybridization histochemistry. CRC Press, Boca Raton

Chesselet MF, Cheramy A, Reisine TD, Glowinski J (1981) Morphine and delta-opiate agonists locally stimulate in vivo dopamine release in cat caudate nucleus. Nature 291:320–322

Cho HJ, Basbaum AI (1988) Increased staining of immunoreactive dynorphin cell bodies in the deafferented spinal cord of the rat. Neurosci Lett 84:125–130

Chowen-Breed JA, Clifton DK, Steiner RA (1989a) Regional specificity of testosterone regulation of proopiomelanocortin gene expression in the arcuate nucleus of the male rat brain. Endocrinology 124:2875–2881

Chowen-Breed JA, Fraser HM, Vician L, Damassa DJ, Clifton DK, Steiner RA (1989b) Testosterone regulation of proopiomelanocortin messenger ribonucleic acid in the arcuate nucleus of the male rat. Endocrinology 124:1697–1702

Chung K, Briner RP, Carlton SM, Westlund KN (1989) Immunohistochemical localization of seven different peptides in the human spinal cord. J Comp Neurol 280:158–170

Civelli O, Birnberg N, Herbert E (1982) Detection and quantitation of proopiomelanocortin mRNA in pituitary and brain tissues from different species. J Biol Chem 257:6783–6887

Clouet DH, Ratner M (1970) Catecholamine biosynthesis in rats treated with morphine. Science 168:854–856

Comb M, Seeburg PH, Adelman J, Eiden L, Herbert E (1982) Primary structure of human Met- and Leu-enkephalin Precursor and its mRNA. Nature 295:663–666

Corbett AD, Peterson SJ, McKnight AT, Magnan J, Kosterlitz H (1982) Dynorphin (1–8) and dynorphin(1–9) are ligands for the kappa subtype of opiate receptor. Nature 299:79–81

Costall B, Fortune DH, Naylor RJ (1978) The induction of catalepsy and hyperactivity by morphine administered directly into the nucleus accumbens of rats. Eur J Pharmacol 49:49–64

Di Chiara G, Imperato A (1988) Opposite effects of mu and kappa opiate agonists on dopamine release in the nucleus accumbens and in the dorsal caudate of freely moving rats. J Pharmacol Exp Ther 244:1067–1080

Dores RM, Akil H, Watson SJ (1984) Strategies for studying opioid peptide regulation at the gene, message, and protein levels. Peptides 5(Suppl 1):9–17

Eberwine JH, Roberts JL (1984) Glucocorticoid regulation of proopiomelanocrotin gene transcription in the rat pituitary. J Biol Chem 259:2166–2170

Elde R, Hokfelt T, Johansson O, Terenius L (1976) Immunohistochemical studies using antibodies to leucine enkephalin: initial observations on the nervous system of the rat. Neuroscience 1:349–351

Fallon JH, Leslie FM (1986) Distribution of dynorphin and enkephalin peptides in the rat brain. J Comp Neurol 249:293–336

Fischli W, Goldstein A, Hunkapiller M, Hood L (1982) Two "big" dynorphins from porcine pituitary. Life Sci 31:1769–1772

Fremeau RT, Lundblad JR, Pritchett DB, Wilcox JN, Roberts JL (1986) Regulation of pro-opiomelanocortin gene transcription in individual cell nuclei. Science 234:1265–1269

Fremeau RT, Autelitano DJ, Blum M, Wilcox J, Roberts JL (1989) Intervening sequence-specific in situ hybridization: detection of the proopiomelanocortin gene primary transcript in individual neurons. Mol Brain Res 6:197–201

Gall C, Lauterborn J, Isackson P, White J (1990) Seizures, neuropeptide regulation, and mRNA expression in the hippocampus. Prog Brain Res 83:371–390

Gee C, Chen CLC, Roberts J, Thompson RC, Watson SJ (1983) Identification of proopiomelanocortin neurons in rat hypothalamus by in situ cDNA mRNA hybridization. Nature 374–376

Goldstein A, Tachibana S, Lowney LI, Hunkapiller M, Hood L (1979) Dynorphin-(1–13), an extraordinarily potent opioid peptide. Proc Natl Acad Sci USA 76:6666–6670

Gerfen CR, Young WS (1988) Distribution of striatonigral and striatopallidal peptidergic neurons in both patch and matrix compartments: an in situ hybridization histochemistry and fluorescent retrograde tracing study. Brain Res 460:161–167

Gerfen CR, Engber TM, Mahan LC, Susel Z, Chase TN, Monsma FJ, Sibley DR (1990) D1 and D2 dopamine receptor-regulated gene expression of striatonigral and striatopallidal neurons. Science 250:1429–1432

Gerfen CR, McGinty JF, Young WS III (1991) Dopamine differentially regulates dynorphin, substance P, and enkephalin expression in striatal neurons: in situ hybridization histochemical analysis. J Neurosci 11:1016–1031

Gubler U, Seeburg P, Hoffman BJ, Gage LP, Udenfriend S (1982) Molecular cloning establishes pro-enkephalin as precursor of enkephalin-containing peptides. Nature 295:206–208

Gulya K (1990) The opioid system in neurologic and psychiatric disorders and in their experimental models. Pharmacol Ther 46:395–428

Haber SN, Elde R (1982) The distribution of enkephalin immunoreactive fibers and minals in the monkey central nervous system. Neuroscience 7:1049–1095

Haber SN, Watson SJ (1985) The comparative distribution of enkephalin, dynorphin and substance P in the human globus pallidus and basal forebrain. Neuroscience 14:1011–1024

Hanson GR, Midgley LP, Bush LG, Johnson M, Gibb JW (1990) Comparison of responses by neuropeptide systems in rat to the psychotropic drugs, methamphetamine, cocaine and PCP. NIDA Res Monogr 95:348

Harlan RE, Shivers BD, Romano GJ, Howells RD, Pfaff DW (1987) Localization of proenkephaline mRNA in the rat brain and spinal cord by in situ hybridization. J Comp Neurol 258:159–184

Hauser KF, Osborne JG, Stiene MA, Melner MH (1990) Cellular localization of proenkephaline mRNA and enkephalin peptide products in cultured astrocytes. Brain Res 522:347–353

Haynes LW, Smyth DG, Zakarian S (1982) Immunocytochemical localization of β-endorphin (lipotropin C fragment) in the developing rat spinal cord and hypothalamus. Brain Res 232:115–128

Herkenham M (1987) Mismatches between neurotransmitter and receptor localizations in brain: observations and implications. Neuroscience 23:1–38

Herz A, Millan MJ (1988) Endogenous opioid peptides in the descending control of nociceptive responses of spinal dorsal horn neurons. Prog Brain Res 77:263–273

Hökfelt T, Holets VR, Staines W, Meister B, Melander T, Schalling M, Schultzberg M, Freedman J, Bjorklund H, Olson L, Lindh B, Elfvin L-G, Lundberg JM, Lindgren JA, Samuelsson B, Pernow B, Terenius L, Post C, Everitt B, Goldstein M (1986) Coexistence of neuronal messengers – an overview. Prog Brain Res 68:33–70

Holaday JW, Tortella FC, Meyerhoff JL, Belenky GL, Hitzenmann RJ (1986) Electroconvulsive shock activates endogenous opioid systems: behavioral and biochemical correlates. Ann N Y Acad Sci 467:249–255

Höllt V, Haarmann I, Millan MJ, Herz A (1987) Prodynorphine gene expression is enhanced in the spinal cord of chronic arthritic rats. Neurosci Lett 73:90–94

Höllt V, Haarmann I, Reimer S (1989) Opioid gene expression in rats after chronic morphine treatment. Adv Biosci 75:711–714

Hong JS, Yoshikawa K, Kanamatsu T, Sabol SL (1985) Modulation of striatal enkephalinergic neurons by antipsychotic drugs. Fed Proc 44:1535–2539

Hong JS, Grimes L, Kanamatsu T, McGinty JF (1987) Kainic acid as a tool to study the regulation and function of opioid peptides in the hippocampus. Toxicology 46:141–157

Hong JS, McGinty JF, Grimes L, Kanamatsu T, Obie J, Mitchell CL (1988) Seizure induced alterations in the metabolism of hippocampal opioid peptides suggest opioid modulation of seizure related behavior. NIDA Res Monogr Ser 82: 48–46

Hosobuchi Y, Adams JE, Linchitz R (1977) Pain relief by electrical stimulation of the central grey matter in humans and its reversal by naloxone. Science 197: 183–186

Hosobuchi Y, Rossier J, Bloom FE, Guillemin R (1979) Stimulation of human periaqueductal grey for pain relief increases immunoreactive beta-endorphin in ventricular fluid. Science 203:279–281

Hughes J, Smith TW, Kosterlitz HW, Fothergill LA, Morgan BA, Morris HR (1975) Identification of two related pentapeptides from the brain with potent opiate agonist activity. Nature 258:577–579

Iadarola MJ, Douglas J, Civelli O, Naranjo JR (1986) Increased spinal cord dynorphin mRNA during peripheral inflammation. NIDA Res Monogr Ser 75:406–409

Iadarola MJ, Douglass J, Civelli O, Naranjo JR (1988) Differential activation of spinal cord dynorphin and enkephalin neurons during hyperalgesia: evidence using cDNA hybridization. Brain Res 455:205–212

Ibuki T, Okamura H, Miyazaki M, Kimura H, Yanaihara N, Ibata Y (1988) Colocalization of GABA and [Met]enkephalin-Arg6-Gly7-Leu8 in the rat cerebellum. Neurosci Lett 91:131–135

Ibuki T, Okamura H, Miyazaki M, Yanaihara N, Zimmerman EA, Ibata Y (1989) Comparative distribution of three opioid systems in the lower brainstem of the monkey (*Macaca fasciculata*). J Comp Neurol 279:445–456

Illes P (1989) Modulation of transmitter and hormone release by multiple neuronal opioid receptors. Rev Physiol Biochem Pharmacol 112:139–233

Ito M (1984) The cerebellum and neural control. Raven, New York

Jackson A, Cooper SJ (1988) Observational analysis of the effects of kappa opioid agonists on open field behaviour in the rat. Psychopharmacology (Berl) 94: 248–253

Jiang H-K, McGinty JF, Hong JS (1990) Differential modulation of striatonigral dynorphin and enkephalin by dopamine receptor subtypes. Brain Res 507:57–64

Joyce EM, Iversen SD (1979) The effect of morphine applied locally to mesencephalic dopamine cell bodies on spontaneous motor activity in the rat. Neurosci Lett 14:207–212

Kakidani H, Furutani Y, Takahashi H, Noda M, Morimoto Y, Hirose T, Asai M, Inayama S, Nakanishi S, Numa S (1982) Cloning and sequence analysis of cDNA for porcine beta-neo-endorphin/dynorphin precursor. Nature 298:245–249

Kangawa K, Minamino N, Chino N, Sakakibara S, Matsuo H (1981) The complete amino acid sequence of alpha-neo-endorphin. Biochem Biophys Res Commun 99:871–878

Kaye WH, Berrettini WH, Gwirtsman HE, Gold PW, George DT, Jimerson DC, Ebert MH (1989) Contribution of CNS neuropeptide (NPY, CRH, and beta-endorphin) alterations to psychophysiological abnormalities in anorexia nervosa. Psychopharmacol Bull 25:433–438

Khachaturian H, Watson SJ (1982) Some perspectives on monoamine-opioid peptide interactions in rat central nervous system. Brain Res Bull 9:441–462

Khachaturian H, Watson SJ, Lewis ME, Coy DH, Goldstein A, Akil H (1982) Dynorphin peptide immunocytochemistry in the rat central nervous system. Peptides 3:941–954

Khachaturian H, Lewis ME, Höllt V, Watson SJ (1983a) Telencephalic enkephalinergic systems in the rat brain. J Neurosci 3:844–855

Khachaturian H, Lewis ME, Watson SJ (1983b) Enkephalin systems in diencephalon and brainstem of the rat. J Comp Neurol 220:310–320

Khachaturian H, Lewis ME, Watson SJ (1983c) Colocalization of pro-enkephalin peptides in rat brain neurons. Brain Res 279:369–373

Khachaturian H, Lewis ME, Haber SN, Akil H, Watson SJ (1984) Pro-opiomelanocortin peptide immunocytochemistry in rhesus monkey brain. Brain Res Bull 13:785–800

Khachaturian H, Lewis ME, Haber SN, Houghten RA, Akil H, Watson SJ (1985a) Pro-dynorphin peptide immunocytochemistry in rhesus monkey brain. Peptides 6(Suppl 2):155–166

Khachaturian H, Lewis ME, Schäfer M-KH, Watson SJ (1985b) Anatomy of CNS opioid systems. Trends Neurosci 8:111–119

Khachaturian H, Lewis ME, Tsou K, Watson SJ (1985c) β-Endorphin α-MSH, ACTH, and related peptides. In: Bjorklund A, Hokfelt T (eds) GABA and neuropeptides in CNS, part I. Elsevier, Amsterdam, pp 216–272 (Handbook of chemical neuroanatomy, vol 4)

Khachaturian H, Sherman TG, Lloyd RV, Civelli O, Douglas J, Herbert E, Akil H, Watson SJ (1986) Pro-dynorphin is endogenous to the anterior pituitary and is co-localized with LH and FSH in the gonadotrophs. Endocrinology 119: 1409–1411

Khachaturian H, Day R, Watson SJ, Akil H (1988) Opioid peptides in the hypothalamus-pituitary-adrenal axis: neuroendocrine anatomy. In: Barchas JD, Bunney WE (ed) Perspectives in psychopharmacology: a collection of papers in honor of Earl Usdin. Liss, New York, pp 233–247

Kilpatrick DL, Wahlstrom A, Lahm HW, Blacher R, Udenfriend S (1982) Rimorphin, a unique, naturally occurring [Leu]enkephalin-containing peptide found in association with dynorphin and alpha-neo-endorphin. Proc Natl Acad Sci USA 79:6480–6483

Kirby ML, Mattio TG (1982) Developmental changes in serotonin and 5-hydroxyindolacetic acid concentrations and opiate receptor binding in rat spinal cord following neonatal 5,7-dihydroxytryptamine treatment. Dev Neurosci 5: 394–402

Lauber AH, Romano GJ, Mobbs CV, Howells RD, Pfaff DW (1990) Estradiol induction of proenkephalin messenger RNA in hypothalamus: dose-response and relation to reproductive behavior in the female rat. Brain Res Mol Brain Res 8:47–54

Lewis JW, Canno JT, Chudler EH, Liebeskind JC (1981) Effects of naloxone and hypophysectomy on electroconvulsive shock-induced analgesia. Brain Res 208: 230–233

Lewis ME, Krause RG II, Roberts-Lewis JM (1988) Recent developments in the use of synthetic oligonucleotides for in situ hybridization histochemistry. Synapse 2:308–316

Li CH, Chung D (1976) Isolation and structure of a triakontapeptide with opiate activity from camel pituitary glands. Proc Natl Acad Sci USA 73:1145–1148

Li SJ, Sivam SP, Hong JS (1986) Regulation of the concentration of dynorphin A(1–8) in the striatonigral pathway by the dopaminergic system. Brain Res 398:390–392

Li SJ, Sivam SP, McGinty JF, Jiang HK, Douglass J, Calavetta L, Hong JS (1988) Regulation of the metabolism of striatal dynorphin by the dopaminergic system. J Pharmacol Exp Therap 246:403–408

Lightman SL, Young WS (1987) Changes in hypothalamic preproenkephalin A mRNA following stress and opiate withdrawal. Nature 328:643–645

Loh HH, Smith AP (1990) Molecular characterization of opioid receptors. Annu Rev Pharmacol Toxicol 30:123–147

Mains RE, Eipper EA, Ling N (1977) Common precursor to corticotropins and endorphins. Proc Natl Acad Sci USA 74:3014–3018

Mansour A, Khachaturian H, Lewis ME, Akil H, Watson SJ (1988) Anatomy of CNS opioid receptors. Trends Neurosci 11:308–314

Martinez JL Jr, Weinberger SB, Schulteis G (1988) Enkephalins and learning and memory: a review of evidence for a site of action outside the blood-brain barrier. Behav Neural Biol 49:192–221

Mathiasen JR, Vaught JL (1987) [D-Pen2, L-Pen5]enkephalin induced analgesia in the jimpy mouse: in vivo evidence for delta-receptor mediated analgesia. Eur J Pharmacol 136:405–407

Mayer DJ, Hayes RL (1975) Stimulation-produced analgesia: development of tolerance and cross-tolerance to morphine. Science 188:941–943

Mayer DJ, Wolfle TL, Akil H, Carder B, Liebeskind JC (1971) Analgesia from electrical stimulation in the brainstem of the rat. Science 174:1351–1354

McCabe JT, Desharnais RA, Pfaff DW (1989) Graphical and statistical approaches to data analysis for in situ hybridization. Methods Enzymol 168:822–848

McDowell J, Kitchen I (1987) Development of opioid systems: peptides, receptors and pharmacology. Brain Res Rev 12:397–421

McGinty JF, van der Kooy D, Bloom FE (1984) The distribution and morphology of opioid peptide immunoreactive neurons in the cerebral cortex of rats. J Neurosci 4:1104–1117

McLean S, Rothman RB, Chuang DM, Rice KC, Spain JW, Coscia CJ, Roth BL (1989) Cross-linking of [^{125}I]beta-endorphin to mu-opioid receptors during development. Dev Brain Res 45:283–289

Melner MH, Low KG, Allen RG, Nielsen CP, Young SL, Saneto RP (1990) The regulation of proenkephalin expression in a distinct population of glial cells. EMBO J 9:791–796

Millan MJ (1990) Kappa-opioid receptors and analgesia. Trends Pharmacol Sci 11:7076

Millan MJ, Weihe E, Czlonkowski AC (1991) Endogenous opioid systems in the control of pain. In: Almeida OF, Shippenberg TS (eds) Neurobiology of opioids. Springer, Berlin Heidelberg New York, pp 245–260

Miller KE, Seybold VM (1989) Comparison of Met-enkephalin, dynorphin A, and neurotensin immunoreactive neurons in the cat and rat spinal cords: II. Segmental differences in the marginal zone. J Comp Neurol 279:619–628

Milner TA, Pickel VM, Reis DJ (1989) Ultrastructural basis for interactions between central opioids and catecholamines: I. Rostral ventrolateral medulla. J Neurosci 9:2114–2130

Mocchetti I, Ritter A, Costa E (1989) Down-regulation of proopiomelanocortin synthesis and beta-endorphin utilization in hypthalamus of morphine-tolerant rats. J Mol Neurosci 1:33–38

Moon SL (1984) Prenatal haloperidol alters striatal dopamine and opiate receptors. Brain Res 323:109–113

Moon Edley S, Hall SL, Herkenham M, Pert CB (1982) Evolution of striatal opiate receptors. Brain Res 249:184–188

Morris BJ, Haarmann I, Kempter B, Höllt V, Herz A (1986) Localization of prodynorphin messenger RNA in rat brain by in situ hybridization using a synthetic oligonucleotide probe. Neurosci Lett 69:104–108

Morris BJ, Feasey KJ, Ten BG, Herz A, Höllt V (1988a) Electrical stimulation in vivo increases the expression of proenkephalin mRNA and decreases the expression of prodynorphin mRNA in rat hippocampal granule cells. Proc Natl Acd Sci USA 85:3226–3230

Morris BJ, Höllt V, Herz A (1988b) Dopaminergic regulation of striatal proenkephalin mRNA and prodynorphin mRNA: contrasting effects of D1 and D2 anatgonists. Neuroscience 25:525–532

Morris BJ, Herz A, Höllt V (1989) Localization of striatal opioid gene expression, and its modulation by the mesostriatal dopamine pathway; an in situ hybridization study. J Mol Neurosci 1:9–18

Mulcahy J, Lee HS, Basbaum AI (1983) Coexistence of immunoreactive enkephalin (I-Enk) and dynorphin (I-Dyn) in the nucleus of the solitary tract of the rat. Soc Neurosci Abstr 9:439

Murakami S, Okamura H, Pelletier G, Ibata Y (1989) Differential colocalization of neuropeptide Y- and methionine-enkephalin-Arg6-Gly7-Leu8-like immunoreactivity in catecholaminergic neurons in the rat brain stem. J Comp Neurol 281:532–544

Nahin RL (1988) Immunocytochemical identification of long ascending, peptidergic lumbar spinal neurons terminating in either the medial or lateral thalamus in the rat. Brain Res 443:345–349

Nakanishi S, Inoue A, Kita T, Nakamura M, Chang ACY, Cohen S, Numa S (1979) Nucleotide sequence of cloned cDNA for bovine corticotropin-beta-lipotropin precursor. Nature 278:423–427

Nemeroff CB, Bissette G (1986) Neuropeptides in psychiatric disorders. In: Berger PA, Brodie KH (eds) American handbook of psychiatry, 2nd edn. Basic Books, New York, pp 64–110

Noda M, Furutani Y, Takahashi H, Toyosato M, Hirose T, Inayama S, Numa S (1982) Cloning and sequence analysis of cDNA for bovine adrenal pre-pro-enkephalin. Nature 295:202–206

Olson GA, Olson RD, Kastin AJ (1989) Endogenous opiates: 1988. Peptides 10: 1253–1280

Pasternak GW (1988) Multiple morphine and enkephalin receptors and the relief of pain. JAMA 259:1362–1367

Petrusz P, Merchenthaler I, Maderdrut JL (1985) Distribution of enkephalin-containing neurons in the central nervous system. In: Bjorklund A, Hokfelt T (eds) GABA and neuropeptides in CNS, part I. Elsevier, Amsterdam, pp 273–334 (Handbook of chemical neuroanatomy, vol 4)

Pickel VM, Chan J, Milner TA (1989) Ultrastructural basis for interactions between central opioids and catecholamines: II. Nuclei of the solitary tract. J Neurosci 9:2519–2535

Pilapil C, Welner S, Magnan J, Gauthier S, Quirion R (1987) Autoradiographic distribution of multiple classes of opioid receptor binding sites in human forebrain. Brain Res Bull 19:611–615

Polakiewicz RD, Rosen H (1990) Regulated expression of proenkephalin A during ontogenic development of mesenchymal derivative tissues. Mol Cell Biol 10: 736–742

Quirion R, Weiss AS (1983) Peptide E and other pro-enkephalin-derived peptides are kappa opiate receptor agonists. Peptides 4:445–449

Reis DJ, Hess P, Azmitia E (1970) Changes in enzymes subserving catecholamine metabolism in morphine tolerance and withdrawal in rat. Brain Res 20:309–312

Richardson DE, Akil H (1977a) Pain reduction by electrical brain stimulation in man: 1. Acute administration in periaqueductal and periventricular sites. J Neurosurg 47:184–194

Richardson DE, Akil H (1977b) Pain reduction by electrical brain stimulation in man: 2. Chronic self-administration in the periventricular grey matter. J Neurosurg 47:184–194

Roberts JL, Herbert E (1977) Characterization of a common precursor to corticotropin and beta-lipotropin: identification of beta-lipotropin peptides and their arrangement relative to corticotropin in the precursor synthesized in a cell-free system. Proc Natl Acad Sci USA 74:5300–5304

Romano GJ, Shivers BD, Harlan RE, Howells RD, Pfaff DW (1987) Haloperidol increases pro-enkephalin mRNA levels in the caudate-putamen of the rat: a quantitative study at the cellular level using in situ hybridization. Mol Brain Res 2:33–41

Romano GJ, Mobbs CV, Howells RD, Pfaff DW (1989) Estrogen regulation of proenkephalin gene expression the ventromedial hypothalamus of the rat: temporal qualities and synergism with progesterone. Brain Res Mol Brain Res 5:51–58

Romano GJ, Mobbs CV, Lauber A, Howells RD, Pfaff DW (1990) Differential regulation of proenkephalin gene expression by estrogen in the ventromedial hypthalamus of male and female rats: implications for the molecular basis of a sexually differentiated behavior. Brain Res 536:63–68

Rosen H, Behar O, Abramsky O, Ovadia H (1989) Regulated expression of proenkephalin A in normal lymphocytes. J Immunol 143:3703–3707

Rougeot C, Charnay Y, Dray F, Dubois PM (1988) Chromatographic identification of Met- and Leu-enkephalin in the human fetal spinal cord. Peptides 9:125–131

Ruda MA, Iadarola MJ, Cohen LV, Young WS (1988) In situ hybridization histochemistry and immunocytochemistry reveal an increase in spinal dynorphin biosynthesis in a rat model of peripheral inflammation and hyperalgesia. Proc Natl Acad Sci USA 85:622–626

Sabol SL, Yoshikawa K, Hong JS (1983) Regulation of methionine-enkephalin precursor messenger RNA in rat striatum by haloperidol and lithium. Biochem Biophys Res Commun 113: 391–399

Sasek CA, Elde RP (1986) Coexistence of enkephalin and dynorphin immunoreactivities in neurons in the dorsal gray commissure of the sixth lumbar and first sacral spinal cord segments in rat. Brain Res 381:8–14

Schäfer MK-H, Day R, Herman JP, Kwasiborski V, Sladek CD, Akil H, Watson SJ (1989) Effect of electroconvulsive shock on dynorphin in the hypothalamic-neurohypophysial system of the rat. Adv Biosci 75:599–602

Schäfer MK-H, Day R, Ortega MR, Akil H, Watson SJ (1990a) Proenkephalin messenger RNA is expressed both in the rat anterior and posterior pituitary. Neuroendocrinology 51:444–448

Schäfer MK-H, Herman JP, Thompson RC, Watson SJ (1990b) In situ detection of POMC heteronuclear RNA in individual nuclei in rat brain and pituitary. Soc Neurosci Abstr 20:1276

Schäfer MK-H, Day R, Watson SJ, Akil H (1991) Distribution of opioids in brain and peripheral tissues. In: Almeida OF, Shippenberg TS (eds) Neurobiology of opioids. Springer, Berlin Heidelberg New York, pp 53–71

Schwartzberg DG, Nakane PK (1983) ACTH-related peptide containing neurons within the medulla oblongata of the rat. Brain Res 276:351–356

Seizinger BR, Grimm C, Höllt V, Herz A (1983) Evidence for a selective processing of pro-enkephalin B into different opioid peptide forms in particular regions of rat brain and pituitary. J Neurochem 42:447–457

Senba E, Yanaihara C, Yanaihara N, Tohyama M (1988) Co-localization of substance P and Met-enkephalin-Arg6-Gly7-Leu8 in the intraspinal neurons of the rat, with special reference to the neurons in the substantia gelatinosa. Brain Res 453:110–116

Sherman TG, Civelli O, Douglass J, Herbert E, Burke S, Watson SJ (1986) Hypothalamic dynorphin and vasopressin mRNA expression in normal and Brattelboro rats. Fed Proc 45:2323–2327

Shinoda H, Marini AM, Cosi C, Schwartz JP (1989) Brain region and gene specificity of neuropeptide gene expression in cultured astrocytes. Science 245:415–417

Shinoda K, Michigami T, Awanr K, Shiotani Y (1988) Analysis of the rat inter-peduncular subnuclei by immunocytochemical double-staining for enkephalin and substance P, with reference to the coexistence of both peptides. J Comp Neurol 271:243–256

Simerly RB, McCall LD, Watson SJ (1988) Distribution of opioid peptides in the preoptic region: immunohistochemical evidence for a steroid-sensitive enkephalin sexual dimorphism. J Comp Neurol 276:442–459

Sivam SP, Strunk C, Smith DR, Hong JS (1986) Pro-enkephalin-A gene regulation in the rat striatum: influence of lithium and haloperidol. Mol Pharmacol 30:186–191

Smith CB, Villarreal JE, Bednarczyk JH, Sheldon MI (1970) Tolerance to morphine-induced increases in (11C) catecholamine synthesis in mouse brain. Science 170:1106–1108

Smith EM, Morill AC, Meyer WJ, Blalock JE (1986) Corticotropin releasing factor induction of leucocyte-derived immunoreactive ACTH and endorphins. Nature 321:881–882

Spruce BA, Curtis R, Wilkin GP, Glover DM (1990) A neuropeptide precursor in cerebellum: proenkephalin exists in subpopulations of both neurons and astrocytes. EMBO J 9:1787–1795

Stefano GB (1989) Role of opioid neuropeptides in immunoregulation. Prog Neurobiol 33:149–159

Stengaard-Pedersen K (1989) Opioid peptides and receptors. Localization, inter-actions and relationships to other molecules in the rodent brain, especially the hippocampal formation. Prog Histochem Cytochem 20:1–119

Tang F, Costa E, Schwartz JP (1983) Increase of proenkephalin mRNA and enkephalin content of rat striatum after daily injection of haloperidol for 2 to 3 weeks. Proc Natl Acad Sci USA 80:3841–3844

Thompson LA, Matsumoto RR, Hohmann AG, Walker JM (1990) Striatonigral pro-dynorphin: a model system for understanding opioid peptide function. Ann NY Acad Sci 579:192–203

Topel H (1988) Beta-endorphin genetics in the etiology of alcoholism. Alcohol
    5:159–165
Trujillo KA, Akil H (1990) Changes in pro-dynorphin peptide content following
    treatment with morphine or amphetamine: possible role in mechanisms of action
    of drug of abuse. NIDA Res Monogr 95:550–551
Tsou K, Khachaturian H, Akil H, Watson SJ (1986) Immunocytochemical local-
    ization of pro-opiomelanocortin-derived peptides in the adult rat spinal cord.
    Brain Res 378:28–35
Tuchscherer MM, Seybold VM (1989) A quantitative study of the coexistence of
    peptides in varicosities within the superficial laminae of the dorsal horn of the
    rat spinal cord. J Neurosci 9:195–205
Uhl G (1986) In situ hybridization in brain. Plenum, New York
Valentino KL, Eberwine JH, Barchas JD (1987) In situ hybridization: applications to
    neurobiology. Oxford University Press, Oxford
Vilijn MH, Vaysse PJ, Zukin RS, Kessler JA (1988) Expression of preproenkephalin
    mRNA by cultured astrocytes and neurons. Proc Natl Acad Sci USA 85:
    6551–6555
Vincent SR, Hokfelt T, Christensson I, Terenius L (1982) Dynorphin immuno-
    reactive neurons in the central nervous system of the rat. Neurosci Lett 33:
    185–190
Walker JM, Thompson LA, Frascella J, Friederich MW (1987) Opposite effects of
    mu and kappa opiate on the firing rate of dopamine cells in the substantia nigra
    of the rat. Eur J Pharmacol 134:53–59
Walker LC, Koliatsos VE, Kitt CA, Richardson RT, Rokaeus A, Price DL (1989)
    Peptidergic neurons in the basal forebrain magnocellular complex of the rhesus
    monkey. J Comp Neurol 280:272–282
Watson SJ, Akil H (1980) Alpha-MSH in rat brain: occurrence within and outside
    brain beta-endorphin neurons. Brain Res 182:217–223
Watson SJ, Akil H, Richard CW, Barchas JD (1978a) Evidence for two separate
    opiate peptide neuronal systems. Nature 275:226–228
Watson SJ, Richard CW, Barchas JD (1978b) Adrenocorticotropin in rat brain:
    immunocytochemical localization in cells and axons. Science 200:1180–1182
Watson SJ, Akil H, Ghazarossian VE, Goldstein A (1981) Dynorphin immunocyto-
    chemical localization in brain and peripheral nervous system. Proc Natl Acad Sci
    USA 78:1260–1263
Watson SJ, Akil H, Fischli W, Goldstein A, Zimmerman E, Nilaver G, van
    Wimersma Greidanus TB (1982a) Dynorphin and vasopressin: common local-
    ization in magnocellular neurons. Science 216:85–87
Watson SJ, Khachaturian H, Akil H, Coy DH, Goldstein A (1982b) Comparison of
    the distribution of dynorphin systems and enkephalin systems in brain. Science
    218:1134–1136
Watson SJ, Khachaturian H, Taylor L, Fischli W, Goldstein A, Akil H (1983)
    Pro-dynorphin peptides are found in the same neurons throughout rat brain:
    immunocytochemical study. Proc Natl Acad Sci USA 80:891–894
Watson SJ, Khachaturian H, Lewis ME, Akil H (1986) Chemical neuroanatomy as a
    basis for biological psychiatry. In: Berger PA, Brodie KH (eds) American
    handbook of psychiatry, 2nd edn. Basic Books, New York, pp 3–33
Watson SJ, Sherman TG, Schäfer MK-H, Patel P, Herman JP, Akil H (1988)
    Regulation of mRNA in peptidergic systems: quantitative and in situ studies.
    In: Chretien M, McKerns KW (eds) Molecular biology of brain and endocrine
    peptidergic systems. Plenum, New York, pp 225–241
Weber E, Barchas JD (1983) Immunocytochemical distribution of dynorphin B in
    rat brain: relation to dynorphin A and alpha-neo-endorphin. Proc Natl Acad
    Sci USA 80:1125–1129
Weber E, Evans CJ, Barchas JD (1982) Predominance of the amino-terminal beta-
    peptide fragment of dynorphin in rat brain regions. Nature 299:77–79

Weihe E, Nohr D, Hartschuh W (1988a) Immunohistochemical evidence for a co-transmitter role of opioid peptides in primary sensory neurons. Prog Brain Res 74:189–199

Weihe E, Nohr D, Millan MJ, Stein C, Mueller S, Gramsch C, Herz A (1988b) Peptide neuroanatomy of adjuvant-induced arthritic inflammation in rat. Agents Actions 25:255–259

Weihe E, Milan MJ, Höllt V, Nohr D, Herz A (1989) Induction of the gene encoding prodynorphin by experimentally induced arthritis enhances staining for dynorphin in the spinal cord of rats. Neuroscience 31:77–95

Weihe E, Nohr D, Michel S, Muller S, Zentel H-H, Fink T, Krekel J (1992) Molecular anatomy of the neuro-immune connection. Int J Neurosci (in press)

White JD, Gall CM, McKelvy JF (1986) Pro-enkephalin is processed in a projection-specific manner in the rat central nervous system. Proc Natl Acad Sci USA 83:7099–7103

Wiemann JN, Clifton DK, Steiner RA (1989) Pubertal changes in gonadotropin-releasing hormone and proopiomelanocortin gene expression in the brain of the male rat. Endocrinology 124:1760–1767

Wilcox JN, Roberts JL (1985) Estrogen decreases rat hypothalamic proopiomelanocortin messenger ribonucleic acid levels. Endocrinology 117: 2392–2396

Xie CW, Lee PHK, Takeuchi K, Owyang V, Li SJ, Douglass J, Hong JS (1989) Single or repeated electroconvulsive shocks alter the levels of pro-dynorphin and pro-enkephalin mRNAs in rat brain. Mol Brain Res 6:11–19

Yoshida M, Taniguchi Y (1988) Projection of pro-opiomelanocortin neurons from the rat arcuate nucleus to the midbrain central gray as demonstrated by double label staining with retrograde labeling and immunohistochemistry. Arch Histol Cytol 51:175–183

Young EA, Walker JM, Lewis ME, Houghten RA, Woods JH, Akil H (1986) [3H]Dynorphin A binding and selectivity of pro-dynorphin peptides in rat, guinea-pig and monkey brain. Eur J Pharmacol 121:355–365

Young WS (1990) In situ hybridization histochemistry. In: Hokfelt T (ed) Handbook of chemical neuroanatomy, vol 7. Elsevier, Amsterdam, pp 481–512

Young WS, Bonner TI, Brann MR (1986) Mesencephalic dopamine neurons regulate the expression of neuropeptide mRNAs in the rat forebrain. Proc Natl Acad Sci USA 83:9827–9831

Zagon DS, Rhodes RE, McLaughlin PJ (1985) Distribution of enkephalin immuno-reactivity in germinativa cells of developing rat cerebellum. Science 227: 1049–1051

Zardetto-Smith AM, Moga MM, Magnuson DJ, Gray TS (1988) Lateral hypo-thalamic dynorphinergic efferents to the amygdala and brainstem in rat. Peptides 9:1121–1127

Zurawski G, Benedik M, Kamb BJ, Abrams JS, Zurawski SM, Lee FD (1986) Activation of mouse T-helper cells induces abundant preproenkephalin mRNA synthesis. Science 232:772–775

CHAPTER 21

Atypical Opioid Peptides

H. Teschemacher

A. Introduction

I. Atypical Opioid Peptides: Atypical Representatives of Natural Opioid Peptides

The term "atypical opioid peptides" as used in this article requires definition.

Opioid activity may be displayed by compounds with alkaloid or with peptide structure. Opioids with peptide structure may be of natural origin or they may be synthetic derivatives of the natural compounds. The natural opioid peptides may be subdivided again in "typical" and "atypical" opioid peptides; their synthetic derivatives thus may be subdivided in "typical" and "atypical" opioid peptide analogues.

The accurate terms, of course, would be "typical" or "atypical" *natural* opioid peptides and "typical" or "atypical" *natural* opioid peptide analogues respectively. Since a sequence like "atypical natural", so far never used, might rather provide confusion than information, in this article a reduced version "atypical opioid peptides" has been favored; for future use, the complete (since correct!) term may be recommended, however.

Separation of "typical" from "atypical" opioid peptides is based on the following differences: "Typical" opioid peptides are derived from three precursor molecules only: proenkephalin (PENK), prodynorphin (PDYN), and proopiomelanocortin (POMC); they all have the same N-terminal amino acid sequence, Tyr-Gly-Gly-Phe. In contrast, "atypical" opioid peptides are derived from a variety of parent proteins; only a Tyr residue is obligatory for their N-terminal amino acid sequence and, in further contrast to "typical" opioid peptides, N-terminal extensions of the sequence beyond the Tyr residue occur. The properties and positions of these peptide groups within the opioid group may be seen from Table 1.

II. Peptides with Indirect Opioid or Opioid Antagonist Activity

Although closely related in some cases to atypical opioid peptides, compounds with "indirect" opioid agonist or antagonist activity (Table 1) have to be regarded as an entirely different group of compounds. Well-known

Table 1. Compounds with "direct" or "indirect" opioid or opioid antagonist activity (for representative compounds, see Tables 2 and 3)

Compounds able to elicit opioid effects	Compounds able to antagonize opioid effects (including agonists-antagonists)
A. Compounds with "direct" opioid activity: opioid receptor ligands with agonistic activity = opioid agonists = *opioids*	A. Compounds with "direct" opioid antagonist activity: opioid receptor ligands with antagonistic activity = *opioid antagonists*

I. Opioids with alkaloid structure: opioid alkaloids = "opiates"
    1. Naturally occurring compounds (e.g., morphine)
    2. Synthetic compounds (e.g., sufentanyl[a])
	I. Opioid antagonists with alkaloid structure
	    1. Naturally occurring compounds
	    2. Synthetic compounds (e.g., naltrindole[a])

II. Opioids with peptide structure: *opioid peptides*
    1. Naturally occurring compounds = *natural opioid peptides*: amino acid sequences contained in naturally occurring (precursor) proteins, natural modification of certain amino acid residues possible
      a) *"Typical" (natural) opioid peptides*:
      N-terminal amino acid sequence: *H*-Tyr-Gly-Gly-Phe-; precursor proteins: PENK, PDYN, POMC only (e.g., enkephalins)
      b) *"Atypical" (natural) opioid peptides*:
      N-terminal amino acid sequence: *H*-Tyr-X-X-X-; (precursor) proteins: casein, hemoglobin, etc.; (e.g., β-casomorphins)
	II. Opioid antagonists with peptide structure
	    1. Natural or modified natural compounds sharing characteristics of structure and origin with atypical opioid peptides (e.g., casoxins)

2. Synthetic compounds structurally related to natural opioid peptides: *natural opioid peptide analogues*
      a) *"Typical" (natural) opioid peptide analogues*: typical opioid peptide amino acid sequence modified (e.g., DPDPE)
      b) *"Atypical" (natural) opioid peptide analogues*: respective atypical opioid peptide amino acid sequence modified (e.g., PL017)
    3. Further synthetic opioid peptides
	2. Synthetic compounds (e.g., CTAP[a])

B. Compounds with "indirect" opioid activity (e.g., kyotorphin)	B. Compounds with "indirect" opioid antagonist activity (e.g., cholecystokinin)

[a] See WATSON and ABBOTT, 1989.

compounds with "indirect" opioid agonist activity are inhibitors of opioid peptide degrading enzymes (which are discussed elsewhere in this volume) and an opioid peptide releaser, kyotorphin (TAKAGI et al. 1979). Mechanisms of biosynthesis (UEDA et al. 1987b; YOSHIHARA et al. 1988) and opioid effects at the cellular level (UEDA et al. 1987a) of kyotorphin as mediated by specific G protein-coupled receptors (UEDA et al. 1989) have been demonstrated. Further compounds with "indirect" opioid activity have been reported, e.g., kentsin (BUENO et al. 1985), NAGA (KOSAKA et al. 1985), or so-called morphine-modulating peptides (RAFFA and JACOBY 1989); their mechanisms of action are still unclear. "Gliadorphins", as well, appear to interact rather indirectly than directly with opioid receptors (PAYAN et al. 1987; GRAF et al. 1987).

An arbitrary selection from a number of peptides with "indirect" opioid antagonist activity is as follows: cholecystokinin (FARIS et al. 1983), MIF-1 (KASTIN et al. 1979), FMRF-amide (TANG et al. 1984), or morphine-modulating peptides again (YANG et al. 1985). Although binding of Tyr-MIF-1 to opioid receptors has been reported (ZADINA and KASTIN 1986), Tyr-MIF-1 has been classified as an indirectly acting opioid antagonist (ZADINA et al. 1990). Further compounds of this type are referred to in a minireview on the significance and mechanisms of action of these compounds (GALINA and KASTIN 1986), focussing on Tyr-MIF-1 and MIF-1 as prototypes.

B. Atypical Opioid Peptides

Details on the structure and origin of various atypical opioid peptide groups or subgroups are listed in Table 2. Due to limitations of space, only a few characteristics can be added in the text, based on an arbitrary selection of references.

I. Structure and Activity

A number of naturally occurring proteins have been shown to contain fragments with opioid activity; some of these peptide fragments have been demonstrated to be released from their precursors under in vivo or in vitro conditions; other fragments have only been synthesized (Table 2). Amino acid sequences of representative peptide fragments and their amino acid residue positions in the parent proteins are listed in Table 2 for various atypical opioid peptide groups or subgroups. Some natural amino acid sequences just slightly modified at the C-terminal residue by synthesis or isolation procedures have been listed in Table 2 as well, although, in a strict sense, they are analogues.

Table 2. Characteristics of "atypical" opioid peptides, i.e., atypical representatives of natural opioid peptides. These peptides are opioid receptor ligands behaving like opioid agonists and have amino acid sequences, which represent segments of naturally occurring proteins *not* identical with POMC, PDYN, or PENK. For comparison, "typical" opioid peptides are also listed as well as peptides which display characteristics of "atypical" opioid

Type
Group (classification by
      parent protein
      and name)
Subgroup
representative i.e.,
peptide with the longest
AAS observed so far
within the respective
group or subgroup*)
	Amino acid sequence (of representative)	Species,
		genus, etc.
		(of group or
		subgroup)

Typical opioid peptides		
Proenkephalin-derived opioid peptides: enkephalins, etc.		
[Met]enkephalin	*H*-Tyr-Gly-Gly-Phe–Met-OH	Bovine, etc.
Prodynorphin-derived opioid peptides: dynorphins, etc.		
Dynorphin A (1–9)	*H*-Tyr-Gly-Gly-Phe–Leu-Arg-Arg-Ile-Arg-OH	Porcine, etc.
Proopiomelanocortin-derived opioid peptides: endorphins		

β-Endorphin (1–31)	*H*-Tyr-Gly-Gly-Phe–Met-Thr-Ser-Glu-Lys-Ser-
	      –Gln-Thr-Pro-Leu-Val-Thr-
	      –Leu-Phe-Lys-Asn-Ala-Ile-
	      –Ile-Lys-Asn-Ala-His-Lys-
	      –Lys-Gly-Gln-OH
		Bovine, etc.

Atypical opioid peptides		
α-Casein-derived opioid peptides: α-casein exorphins		
α-Casein exorphin (1–7)	*H*-Arg-Tyr-Leu-Gly-Tyr–Leu-Glu-OH	Bovine
β-Casein-derived opioid peptides: β-casomorphins and β-casorphin		
Human β-casomorphins		
β$_H$-Casomorphin (1–8)	*H*-Tyr-Pro-Phe-Val–Glu-Pro-Ile-Pro-OH	Human
Bovine β-casomorphins		
β$_B$-Casomorphin (1–11)	*H*-Tyr-Pro-Phe-Pro-Gly-Pro-Ile-Pro-Asn-Ser –Leu-OH	Bovine

peptides, but have been reported to behave like opioid antagonists. For distinct groups or subgroups, a representative, i.e., the peptide with the longest amino acid sequence within the respective group or subgroup so far studied is given. Information about the prediction of peptide expression or about peptide isolation was considered as far as based on cDNA or protein sequencing and/or amino acid analysis, respectively

Parent protein: proven or potential precursor (of group or subgroup)[‡]	[Ref.] (parent protein AAS)	Amino acid residue positions in the parent protein (of representative)	Modification of C-terminal residue (of representative)	Opioid activities of representatives or fragments thereof demonstrated for: A. Peptides formed under in vivo conditions B. Peptides formed under in vitro conditions C. Peptides just synthesized A and B: structure of isolated peptide usually confirmed by synthesis
PENK		(136–140)		See respective chapters in this volume
PDYN		(209–217)		
POMC		(235–265)		
α-Casein	[1]	(90–96)		α-*Casein exorphins* B. α-Casein exorphin (1–7) and (1–6) found in a peptic α$_B$-casein digest [2, 3]. C. Synthetic α-casein exorphin (2–7) and (2–6) [3]
β-Casein	[4] [5]	(51–58) (50–57)		β-*Casomorphins and β-casorphin* C. Synthetic human β-casomorphin (1–4), (1–5) [6, 7, 8], (1–6) [7], (1–7) [8] and (1–8) [7, 8] as derived from the AAS of human β-casein
β-Casein A2	[9]	(60–70)		A. Bovine β-casomorphin (1–11) formed in the gastrointestinal tract of minipigs [12]

Table 2 (continued)

Type Group (classification by parent protein and name) Subgroup representative i.e., peptide with the longest AAS observed so far within the respective group or subgroup*)	Amino acid sequence (of representative)	Species, genus, etc. (of group or subgroup)
β_B-Casomorphin (1–4) amide = morphiceptin	H-Tyr-Pro-Phe-Pro–NH$_2$	Bovine
Ovine β-casomorphins β_O-Casomorphin (1–8)	H-Tyr-Pro-Phe-Pro–Gly-Pro-Ile-Ala-OH H-Tyr-Pro-Phe-Thr–Gly-Pro-Ile-Pro-OH	Ovine Ovine
Buffalo β-casomorphins β_{WB}-Casomorphin (1–8)	H-Tyr-Pro-Phe-Pro–Gly-Pro-Ile-Pro-OH	Water buffalo
β-Casorphin β_H-Casorphin (1–4)	H-Tyr-Pro-Ser-Phe-NH$_2$	Human
Further β-casein fragments NN	H-Tyr-Gly-Phe-Leu–Pro-OH	Human
α-Lactalbumin-derived opioid peptides: α-lactorphins *Human α-lactorphin* α_H-Lactorphin (1–4)	H-Tyr-Gly-Leu-Phe–NH$_2$	Human
Bovine α-lactorphin α_B-Lactorphin (1–4)	H-Tyr-Gly-Leu-Phe–NH$_2$	Bovine

Table 2 (continued)

Parent protein: proven or potential precursor (of group or subgroup)[‡]	[Ref.] (parent protein AAS)	Amino acid residue positions in the parent protein (of representative)	Modification of C-terminal residue (of representative)	Opioid activities of representatives or fragments thereof demonstrated for: A. Peptides formed under in vivo conditions B. Peptides formed under in vitro conditions C. Peptides just synthesized A and B: structure of isolated peptide usually confirmed by synthesis
β-Casein A2	[9]	(60–63)	–NH$_2$	B. Bovine β-casomorphin (1–7) [10], (1–8) [11] and (1–4) amide, i.e., morphiceptin [11] isolated from bovine casein digests C. Synthetic bovine β-casomorphin (1–4), (1–5), (1–6) [13], and (1–4) amide, i.e., morphiceptin [16]
β$_1$-Casein β-Casein	[14] [15]	(60–67) (60–67)		No data about ovine β-casomorphins as far as different from bovine β-casomorphin sequences
β-Casein	[17]	(60–67)		B. Water buffalo β-casomorphin (1–8) proven identical with bovine β-casomorphin (1–8), formed upon water buffalo β-casein digestion with gastrointestinal enzymes [18]
β-Casein	[4] [5]	(41–44) (40–43)	–NH$_2$ –NH$_2$	C. Synthetic human β-casorphin (1–4) [19, 22]
β-Casein	[4] [5]	(59–63) (58–62)		C. Synthetic peptide (NN) [19, 22]
				α-Lactorphins
α-Lactalbumin	[20]	(50–53)	–NH$_2$	C. Synthetic human α-lactorphin (1–4) [19, 22], identical with
α-Lactalbumin	[21]	(50–53)	–NH$_2$	C. Synthetic bovine α-lactorphin (1–4) [19, 22]

Table 2 (continued)

Type
Group (classification by
        parent protein
        and name)
Subgroup
representative i.e.,
peptide with the longest
AAS observed so far
within the respective
group or subgroup*)
	Amino acid sequence (of representative)	Species,
		genus, etc.
		(of group or
		subgroup)

β-*Lactoglobulin–derived opioid peptides:* β-*lactorphin* β$_B$-Lactorphin (1–4)	*H*-Tyr-Leu-Leu-Phe–NH$_2$	Bovine
Hemoglobin–derived opioid peptides: hemorphins Hemorphin (1–5)	*H*-Tyr-Pro-Trp-Thr–Gln-OH	Human, etc. Many further vertebrates
Cytochrome B–derived opioid peptides: cytochrophins Cytochrophin (1–5)	*H*-Tyr-Pro-Phe-Thr–Ile-OH	Human, etc. Eukaryotes

Dermorphin and deltorphin precursor–derived opioid peptides: dermorphins and deltorphins
Dermorphins
Dermorphin (1–7)
[Hyp^6]Dermorphin (1–7)
Dermorphin (1–7)-OH
[Hyp^6]Dermorphin
(1–7)-OH
	
	H-Tyr-D-Ala-Phe-Gly–Tyr-Pro-Ser-NH$_2$
	H-Tyr-D-Ala-Phe-Gly–Tyr-Hyp-Ser-NH$_2$
	H-Tyr-D-Ala-Phe-Gly–Tyr-Pro-Ser-OH
	H-Tyr-D-Ala-Phe-Gly–Tyr-Hyp-Ser-OH
		
		} Frog (genus
		  *Phyllo
		  medusarum*):
		  P. sauvagei
		  P. rhodei,
		  etc.

[Lys^7]Dermorphin
(1–7)-OH
[Trp^4,Asn^7]Dermorphin
(1–7)-OH
[Trp^4,Asn^5]Dermorphin
(1–5)-OH
	H-Tyr-D-Ala-Phe-Gly–Tyr-Pro-Lys-OH
	
	H-Tyr-D-Ala-Phe-Trp–Tyr-Pro-Asn-OH
	
	H-Tyr-D-Ala-Phe-Trp–Asn-OH
		} Frog (genus
		  *Phyllome-
		  dusarum*):
		  P. bicolor

Table 2 (continued)

Parent protein: proven or potential precursor (of group or subgroup)[‡]	[Ref.,] (parent protein AAS)	Amino acid residue positions in the parent protein (of representative)	Modification of C-terminal residue (of representative)	Opioid activities of representatives or fragments thereof demonstrated for: A. Peptides formed under in vivo conditions B. Peptides formed under in vitro conditions C. Peptides just synthesized A and B: structure of isolated peptide usually confirmed by synthesis
β-Lacto-globulin	[23]	(102–105)	–NH$_2$	β-*Lactorphin* C. Synthetic bovine β-lactorphin (1–4) [19, 22]
Hemoglobin β-[24], γ-[25], δ-[26], ε-[27] chain) Hemoglobin (β-, γ-, δ-, ε-, ρ-chains.)		(35–39) (var.)		*Hemorphins* B. Hemorphin (1–4) isolated from a bovine blood digest (gastrointestinal enzyme treatment) [28] C. Synthetic hemorphin (1–4) [32] and (1–5) [28]
Cytochrome b Cytochrome b	[30]	(345–349)		*Cytochrophins* B. Cytochrophin (1–4) isolated from a bovine blood digest (gastrointestinal enzyme treatment) [29] C. Synthetic cytochrophin (1–4) [32] and (1–5) [29]
Var., N.N. ? Var., N.N.	[31] [37]	(?) (?) (?)	–NH$_2$ –NH$_2$	*Dermorphins and deltorphins* A. Dermorphin (1–7), [Hyp^6]dermorphin (1–7), dermorphin (1–7)-OH and [Hyp^6]dermorphin (1–7)-OH isolated from the skin of *P. sauvagei* [33, 35], *P. rhodei* [34, 35] and further *P.* [36] C. Synthetic dermorphin (1–4)amide, (1–5)amide and (1–6)amide [35] C. [Lys^7] and [Trp^4, Asn^7] dermorphin (1–7)-OH as well as [Trp^4, Asn^5] dermorphin (1–5)-OH predicted from precursor cDNA sequences and then synthesized [37]

Table 2 (continued)

Type
Group (classification by
  parent protein
  and name
Subgroup
representative (i.e.,
peptide with the longest
AAS observed so far
within the respective
group or subgroup*)
	Amino acid sequence (of representative)	Species,
		genus, etc.
		(of group or
		subgroup)

Deltorphins Deltorphin (1–7) = dermenkephalin (1–7) = dermorphin gene- associated peptide (1–7)	H-Tyr-D-Met-Phe-His–Leu-Met-Asp-NH$_2$	Frog (genus *Phyllome- dusarum*): *P. sauvagei*
[D-Ala$_2$] Deltorphin I (1–7) [D-Ala^2] Deltorphin II (1–7)	H-Tyr-D-Ala-Phe-Asp–Val-Val-Gly-NH$_2$ H-Tyr-D-Ala-Phe-Glu–Val-Val-Gly-NH$_2$	Frog (genus *Phyllome- dusarum*): *P. bicolor*

Opioid antagonists sharing characteristics with atypical opioid peptides

κ-*Casein–derived peptides: casoxins*
| Casoxin (1–6) | H-Ser-Arg-Tyr-Pro-Ser-Tyr–OCH$_3$ | Bovine |
| Casoxin C (1–10) | H-Tyr-Ile-Pro-Ile–Gln-Tyr-Val-Leu-Ser-Arg-OH | Bovine |

Table 2 (continued)

Parent protein: proven or potential precursor (of group or subgroup)‡	[Ref.] (parent protein AAS)	Amino acid residue positions in the parent protein (of representative)	Modification of C-terminal residue (of representative)	Opioid activities of representatives or fragments thereof demonstrated for: A. Peptides formed under in vivo conditions B. Peptides formed under in vitro conditions C. Peptides just synthesized A and B: structure of isolated peptide usually confirmed by synthesis
Var., N.N.	[31]	(?)	−NH$_2$	A. Deltorphin (1−7) (= dermenkephalin, dermorphin gene-associated peptide) predicted from precursor cDNA sequences [31] and subsequently isolated from the skin of *P. sauvagei* [38, 39] C. Deltorphin (1−7) (= dermenkephalin, dermorphin gene-associated peptide) predicted from precursor cDNA sequences [31] and subsequently synthesized [38, 40, 41]
Var., N.N.	[37]	(?)	−NH$_2$ −NH$_2$	A. [D-Ala^2] deltorphin I and II (1−7) isolated from the skin of *P. bicolor* [42]
κ-casein κ-casein	[43] [43]	(33−38) (25−34)	−OCH$_3$	*Casoxins* B. Casoxin (1−6) isolated from a peptic digest of bovine κ-casein and methylated during the isolation procedure [19, 44]; casoxin C (1−10) isolated from a tryptic digest of bovine κ-casein [45] C. Synthetic casoxin (1−6), (2−6) and (3−6) as well as (1−6)-OH, (2−6)-OH (3−6)-OH, (3−6)-[Gly^7], and (3−6)-NH$_2$ [19, 45]

Table 2 (continued)

Type
Group (classification by
    parent protein
    and name)
Subgroup
representative i.e.,
peptide with the longest
AAS observed so far
within the respective
group or subgroup*)
	Amino acid sequence (of representative)	Species,
		genus, etc.
		(of group or
		subgroup)

Lactoferrin–derived peptides: lactoferroxins		
Lactoferroxin A (1–6)	H-Tyr-Leu-Gly-Ser-Gly-Tyr-OCH$_3$	Human
Lactoferroxin B (1–5)	H-Arg-Tyr-Tyr-Gly-Tyr-OCH$_3$	Human
Lactoferroxin C (1–7)	H-Lys-Tyr-Leu-Gly-Pro–Gln-Tyr-OCH$_3$	Human

References: [1] Mercier et al. 1971; [2] Zioudrou et al. 1979; [3] Loukas et al. 1983; [4] Greenberg et al. 1984; [5] Lönnerdal et al. 1990; [6] Brantl 1984; [7] Yoshikawa et al. 1984; [8] Koch et al. 1985; [9] Ribadeau-Dumas et al. 1972; [10] Henschen et al. 1979; [11] Chang et al. 1985; [12] Meisel 1986; [13] Brantl et al. 1981; [14] Richardson and Mercier 1979; [15] Provot et al. 1989; [16] Chang et al. 1981; [17] Petrilli et al. 1983; [18] Petrilli et al. 1984; [19] Chiba and Yoshikawa 1986; [20] Findlay and Brew 1972; [21] Brew et al. 1970; [22] Yoshikawa et al. 1986a; [23] Braunitzer et al. 1973; [24] Lawn et al. 1980; [25] Slightom et al. 1980; [26] Spritz et al. 1980; [27] Baralle et al. 1980; [28] Brantl et al. 1986; [29] Brantl et al. 1985; [30] Anderson et al. 1981; [31] Richter et al. 1987; [32] Liebmann et al. 1989; [33] Montecucchi et al. 1981a; [34] Montecucchi et al. 1981b; [35] Broccardo et al. 1981; [36] Erspamer et al. 1981; [37] Richter et al. 1990; [38] Kreil et al. 1989; [39] Mor et al. 1989; [40] Lazarus et al. 1989b; [41] Amiche et al. 1989; [42] Erspamer et al. 1989; [43] Mercier et al. 1973; [44] Yoshikawa et al. 1986b; [45] Chiba et al. 1989; [46] Metz-Boutigue et al. 1984; [47] Yoshikawa et al. 1988.

Table 2 (continued)

Parent protein: proven or potential precursor (of group or subgroup)[‡]	[Ref.] (parent protein AAS)	Amino acid residue positions in the parent protein (of representative)	Modification of C-terminal residue (of representative)	Opioid activities of representatives or fragments thereof demonstrated for: A. Peptides formed under in vivo conditions B. Peptides formed under in vitro conditions C. Peptides just synthesized A and B: structure of isolated peptide usually confirmed by synthesis
				Lactoferroxins
Lactoferrin	[46]	(318–323)	–OCH$_3$	B. Lactoferroxin A, B and C
Lactoferrin	[46]	(536–540)	–OCH$_3$	isolated from a peptic digest
Lactoferrin	[46]	(673–679)	–OCH$_3$	of human lactoferrin and apparently methoxylated during the isolation procedure [47]

Abbreviations: ND, not determined; NN, not named by the authors; AAS, amino acid sequence; PENK, proenkephalin; PDYN, prodynorphin; POMC, proopiomelanocortin
Footnotes: *) Applies to "atypical opioid peptides"! Arbitrary choice for other types of peptide groups! ‡) For location or source of proven or potential precursor see section B II of this chapter!

1. α-Casein Exorphins

Certain bovine α-casein fragments, named α-casein exorphins, have been shown to bind to opioid receptors in brain homogenates (apparently with relatively low affinity); they have been demonstrated to induce a naloxone-reversible inhibition of adenylate cyclase activity in neuroblastoma × glioma hybrid cells and, in addition, an inhibition of electrically stimulated contractions in the mouse vas deferens. In contrast to all other typical or atypical opioid peptides, the N-terminal Tyr residue is preceded by an Arg residue with two of the α-casein exorphins; the Arg-α-casein exorphins were reported to display even higher opioid activities than the des-Arg-α-casein exorphins (LOUKAS et al. 1983).

2. β-Casomorphins

About β-Casomorphins more information has been collected than about any other of the atypical opioid peptide groups. Details on their detection, structure, absorption, distribution, degradation, as well as their opioid or nonopioid activities have been reviewed (TESCHEMACHER 1987a; PAROLI 1988; RAMABADRAN and BANSINATH 1989; KOCH and BRANTL 1990; TESCHEMACHER et al. 1990).

In brief, β-casein molecules of several species have been shown to contain fragments with opioid activity. They were named "β-casomorphins," and, as a characteristic, they carry the amino acid sequence Tyr-Pro-Phe- in N-terminal position. Details on the steric conformation of β-casomorphins are presented elsewhere in this volume. Studies have proven β-casomorphins to be μ-selective opioid receptor ligands with some affinity to δ- and almost no affinity to κ-type opioid receptors (BRANTL et al. 1981; KOCH et al. 1985; KOCH and BRANTL 1990).

In contrast to several of their synthetic analogues, natural β-casomorphins display affinities to opioid receptors, which are one to two or two to three orders of magnitude below that of normorphine or morphine, respectively; therefore, their opioid potencies in isolated organ preparations, i.e., guinea pig ileum or mouse vas deferens, are relatively low. In addition to these in vitro activities, opioid effects in the intact animal have been demonstrated also, e.g., effects on the central nervous system, on the endocrine system, or on the gastrointestinal tract; in some test systems, their potencies as compared to those of morphine were considerably higher than observed in the in vitro assays (for reviews see TESCHEMACHER 1987a; PAROLI 1988; RAMABADRAN and BANSINATH 1989).

Besides many data about "pharmacodynamic" properties, some information about the "pharmacokinetic" behavior of β-casomorphins is available. Apparently natural β-casomorphins do not penetrate from the gastrointestinal lumen into the cardiovascular compartment beyond the liver barrier in adult mammals (TESCHEMACHER et al. 1986; TOMÉ et al. 1987; READ et al. 1990). Permeation from blood into brain tissue appears to be restricted for β-casomorphins except for certain blood-brain barrier-free areas (ERMISCH et al. 1983). Although β-casomorphins in general are very stable against enzymatic attack, they are highly susceptible to enzymatic degradation by dipeptidylpeptidase IV (DPIV); DPIV cleaves dipeptide fragments from the N-terminal portion of the β-casomorphin sequence as long as the second residue is proline (HARTRODT et al. 1982b). Proline-specific endopeptidase (PSE) and post-proline-cleaving enzyme (PPCE) are β-casomorphin-degrading enzymes as well, but of minor importance (HARTRODT et al. 1982a).

3. β-Casorphin, α- and β-Lactorphins

Little information has been available so far about a human β-casein fragment with opioid activity, named "β-casorphin," and opiate-like acting fragments from human or bovine α-lactalbumin and bovine β-lactoglobulin, called "α-lactorphins" or "β-lactorphin," respectively. As a characteristic, C-terminal amidation is common to all four of these protein fragments; although amidated by means of synthesis and not by nature, they have not been regarded as analogues here in view of the minimal deviations from the respective atypical opioid peptide structures. Like β-casomorphins, they are μ-selective opioid receptor ligands but their receptor affinities and their potencies in the guinea pig ileum preparation are lower than those of the β-casomorphins (YOSHIKAWA et al. 1986a; CHIBA and YOSHIKAWA 1986).

4. Hemorphins and Cytochrophins

Hemorphins occur as fragments of β-, γ-, δ-, or ε-chains of hemoglobin, and cytochrophins as fragments of cytochrome b (BRANTL et al. 1985, 1986). Hemorphin or cytochrophin (1–4) amino acid sequences are contained in further vertebrate proteins and in a series of bacterial or viral proteins. The affinities of hemorphins and cytochrophins to μ- and δ-opioid receptors do not differ very much and are in the range of β-casomorphin affinities to μ-receptors; their affinities to κ-receptors are somewhat lower, but not as low as observed for β-casomorphins (LIEBMANN et al. 1989). The potencies in the guinea pig ileum preparation proved to be lower than the potencies of β-casomorphins (BRANTL et al. 1986). For hemorphins, opioid effects on the central nervous system, e.g., antinociceptive effects, have been demonstrated (DAVIS et al. 1989).

5. Dermorphins and Deltorphins

In 1981, a novel opioid peptide was demonstrated to occur in the skin of a South American frog, *Phyllomedusa sauvagei*; in view of its origin and opioid activity it was named "dermorphin" (MONTECUCCHI et al. 1981a). In addition, three analogues thereof were also found in this tissue (BROCCARDO et al. 1981) and very soon the skin of further *Phyllomedusa* species was shown to contain the dermorphin family as well (MONTECUCCHI et al. 1981b; ERSPAMER et al. 1981). The dermorphins contained a D-amino acid residue in their sequence, which had so far never been found with natural opioid peptides. Dermorphin displayed a very high selectivity *and* affinity for μ-type opioid receptors and proved to be very potent in the guinea pig ileum preparation (Table 3); its pharmacological profile has been characterized (ERSPAMER et al. 1981; BROCCARDO et al. 1981).

Despite of additional interesting findings about the South American frog products, the scene remained quiet for more than half a decade until in 1987 the publication of a paper by RICHTER and colleagues changed the perspective from *exotic* to *dramatic* apparently overnight. In this paper, the amino acid sequences of several dermorphin precursors from the skin of P. *sauvagei* were presented; they had been derived from cDNA libraries constructed from frog skin mRNA, screened with dermorphin oligonucleotide codons. In one of the precursor molecules one dermorphin sequence was found to be replaced by a different peptide sequence: the N-terminal Tyr residue indicated opioid properties (see "Introduction") and the second residue could be speculated to appear in the D-form after posttranslational L-/ D-conversion as also shown for dermorphin in this paper (RICHTER et al. 1987).

The peptide thus predicted by RICHTER et al. (1987) was synthesized and tested for opioid activity by the same group (KREIL et al. 1989) as well as by two further groups (AMICHE et al. 1989; LAZARUS et al. 1989b). Harmoniously, it was demonstrated to be the natural opioid peptide with the highest affinity *and* selectivity for δ-opioid receptors known at that time (Table 3); less harmoniously, it was named "deltorphin" (KREIL et al. 1989), "dermenkephalin" (AMICHE et al. 1989), and "dermorphin gene-associated peptide" or "DGAP" (LAZARUS et al. 1989b). Attempts to demonstrate the peptide now in the skin of P. *sauvagei* have been successful (KREIL et al. 1989; MOR et al. 1989). Molecular determinants for μ- or δ-opioid receptor affinity and selectivity of dermorphin or deltorphin = dermenkephalin = DGAP, respectively, have been evaluated (SAGAN et al. 1989).

In parallel, ERSPAMER et al. (1989) succeeded in isolating two further peptides from the skin of P. *bicolor* which showed even higher affinity and selectivity for δ-receptors than deltorphin (Table 3); they were named [D-Ala^2] deltorphin I and II (ERSPAMER et al. 1989). Subsequently, the same group presented the structures of four precursors for [D-Ala^2] deltorphin I and II derived from cDNAs cloned from skin of P. *bicolor* (RICHTER et al. 1990). In addition, further dermorphin-like peptides could be predicted from the sequences of these precursors; they were synthesized and their μ-selectivities and μ-affinities, in fact, proved to be in the same range as observed for dermorphin (RICHTER et al. 1990); they are listed in Table 3 as [Trp^4, Asn^7] dermorphin-OH and [Lys^7] dermorphin-OH.

II. Origin and Destination

Do atypical opioid peptides play a physiological or even a pathophysiological role? Is their presence essential or accidental? If they do play such a
role, one would expect it to become manifest by atypical opioid peptide
interaction with endogenous opioid receptors; this again would indicate that
atypical opioid peptide systems are supplements of typical, i.e., endogenous,
opioid systems. Thus, the search for a functional role for atypical opioid
peptides involves finding out whether the respective peptide or its parent
protein is present at potential sites of opioid action in the organism in
functionally relevant situations. Further, it is important to know whether
there is any indication of the peptide being released from its parent protein
(which could then be called its "precursor") under in vivo or, at least,
in vitro conditions. Furthermore, a functional role for an *atypical* opioid
peptide could be suggested if the location and function of its parent protein
within the respective organism fitted into certain functions of the *typical*
opioid peptide systems of the organism.

1. Milk Protein-Derived Opioid Peptides

Milk protein-derived opioid peptides appear very likely to have a functional
role: The milk is known to contain many bioactive compounds (SCHAMS and
KARG 1986; KOLDOVSKY and THORNBURG 1987; MEISEL and SCHLIMME 1990)
and the well-known nutritive and reproductive significance of milk con-
stitutents appears to match nutritive and reproductive functions, wherein
certain endogenous opioid systems appear to be involved (see chapters V
and VI). The information collected so far about a functional role varies
considerably for the various milk protein-derived opioid peptide groups,
however.

a) α-Casein Exorphins, β-Casorphin, α- and β-Lactorphins

β-Casorphin as well as α- or β-lactorphins are only synthetic compounds;
there is no evidence so far that their amino acid sequences can be released
from their parent proteins unter in vitro or in vivo conditions to elicit any
functionally relevant effects. For α-casein exorphins, release from their precursor protein, α-casein, has been demonstrated under in vitro conditions
(Table 2); however, such a release under in vivo conditions has not been
shown. Although similar roles as postulated for β-casomorphins (see below)
are possible for these peptides, at the moment evidence for this is lacking.

b) β-Casomorphins

β-Casomorphins have been shown to be released under in vivo conditions
from their precursor in functionally relevant situations. The evidence so far
raised in favor of a functional significance of β-casomorphins in the mamma-

lian organism has been reviewed (Teschemacher 1987a,b; Teschemacher and Koch 1990, 1991).

Very briefly, β-casomorphins might be of reproductive significance in the female or in the neonate's organism and of nutritive importance in the milk consumer's gastrointestinal tract.

α) *Female Organism.* In pregnant or lactating women, β-casein cleavage products were found in the plasma (Koch et al. 1988; Nyberg et al. 1989) and a peptide apparently identical with β-casomorphin(1–8) was found in cerebrospinal fluid of such women (Nyberg et al. 1989). β-Casomorphins could play a physiological role within a feedback loop between mammary tissue and the neuroendocrine axis, modulating prolactin release and thus mammary function. The presence of a β-casomorphin in the cerebrospinal fluid of puerperal women has also provoked the hypothesis of a pathophysiological role for β-casomorphins in relation to postpartum psychosis (Lindström et al. 1984).

β) *Neonate's Organism.* After milk feeding in newborn calves (Umbach et al. 1985) or dogs (Singh et al. 1989), a β-casomorphin-immunoreactive material was found in the plasma, which apparently could represent a precursor, from which β-casomorphins could be released to elicit effects at any site in the newborn organism. Depending on the situation, the presence of β-casomorphins in the neonate's central nervous system could gain pathophysiological significance: Recently, a role for β-casomorphins in the sudden infant death syndrome (SIDS) has been proposed (Hedner and Hedner 1987; Ramabadran and Moore 1988; Ramabadran and Bansinath 1988).

γ) *Milk Consumer's Gastrointestinal Tract.* If β-casomorphins are released from β-casein into the gastrointestinal lumen after milk intake, they could be expected to interact with endogenous opioid systems in the gastrointestinal wall, in neonates as well as in adult milk consumers. In fact, β-casomorphins have been shown to be released from β-casein upon milk digestion in vitro (Petrilli et al. 1984; Svedberg et al. 1985) or upon milk (Svedberg et al. 1985) or casein (Meisel 1986) ingestion in vivo. Thus, the naloxone-antagonizable inhibition of gastrointestinal transit in rats fed with bovine casein (Daniel et al. 1990a) would be compatible with an opioid effect elicited by β-casomorphins at the gastrointestinal wall upon their release from β-casein. In fact, β-casomorphins have been shown to inhibit intestinal propulsion (De Ponti et al. 1988). Thus, β-casomorphins might fit into the concept of "food hormones," nutrients postulated to modulate gastrointestinal functions (Morley 1982).

2. Hemoglobin- or Cytochrome b-Derived Opioid Peptides

A physiological or pathophysiological role of hemorphins or cytochrophins would be very important, since the parent proteins are not only present in mammals, but also in other vertebrates and, in the case of cytochrome b, even at a very low evolutionary level; in their respective organisms they may be widespread or even ubiquitous. Unfortunately, so far, there is no information about any release of hemorphins or cytochrophins from their parent proteins in vivo under physiological or pathophysiological conditions. Hemorphin (1–4), however, was shown to release opioid peptide immunoreactive materials from pituitary tissue in vitro (SCHEFFLER et al. 1990); thus, hemorphins could play a modulatory role in the activation of neuroendocrine systems upon their liberation from hemoglobin, e.g., in the case of hemolysis.

3. Amphibian Skin Protein-Derived Opioid Peptides

Dermorphins and deltorphins, opioid peptides of extremely high affinities and selectivities for μ-type or δ-type opioid receptors, respectively, have been detected in the skin of several South American frogs. Thus, in contrast to other atypical opioid peptides, *a priori*, there is no question at all as to their liberation from the respective precursors and their presence in the skin in active form. However, apparently, there is no evidence for a functional role of these peptides in the amphibian organism. It even remains to be clarified whether they are destined to interact with intracorporal opioid systems or whether they are destined to have extracorporal effects, e.g., for protection or signalling.

Interestingly, in agreement with the "brain-gut-skin-triangle" concept [focussing mainly on the presence of peptides with high bioactivity in amphibian skin and mammalian gut and central nervous system; ERSPAMER et al. (1981)], evidence has recently been presented for the presence of dermorphin precursor processing products in rat brain and intestine (MOR et al. 1990). The identity and function of these compounds remain to be clarified.

C. Opioid Antagonists Sharing Characteristics with Atypical Opioid Peptides

From in vitro digests of bovine κ-casein or human lactoferrin, peptide fragments of these proteins have been isolated which were shown to behave like opioid antagonists; some of them had been modified at their C-terminus by the isolation procedure (Table 2). These opioid receptor ligands share characteristics with "atypical" opioid peptides insofar as their N-terminal amino acid sequences and their parent proteins are not identical with those of the "typical" opioid peptides (see "Introduction").

I. Structure and Activity

1. Casoxins

Casoxin(1–6) (Table 2) binds (with relatively low affinity) to μ- and κ-receptors, but apparently not to δ-receptors. It has been reported to have no agonistic opioid activity in the guinea pig ileum or in vas deferens preparations of the mouse or the rabbit. However, casoxin(1–6) antagonized the (opioid) morphiceptin effect in the guinea pig ileum, the (opioid) dynorphin A (1–13) effect in the rabbit vas deferens, but not the (opioid) [Leu]enkephalin effect in the mouse vas deferens. The antagonistic activity was about two orders of magnitude lower than that of naloxone; the pA_2 value for reduction of morphiceptin activity in the guinea pig ileum preparation was about 5.5 (YOSHIKAWA et al. 1986b, 1988).

The antagonistic activities of casoxin(2–6) and (3–6) appear to be in the same range as observed for casoxin(1–6). Nonmethoxylated casoxin(1–6) fragments showed lower activities, as did further nonmethoxylated κ-casein fragments – with the exception of casoxin C(1–10) (CHIBA and YOSHIKAWA 1986; CHIBA et al. 1989).

2. Lactoferroxins

Lactoferroxins A, B, and C (Table 2) have been reported to antagonize the opioid effect of morphiceptin in the guinea pig ileum preparation, showing low opioid receptor affinities and, as far as determined, pA_2 values in a range as observed for casoxin(1–6) (YOSHIKAWA et al. 1988).

II. Origin and Destination

Although liberation of at least one fragment with noteworthy opioid antagonist activity upon κ-casein digestion in vitro has been shown (CHIBA et al. 1989), no evidence has been provided so far for its functional role under in vivo conditions. One might consider, however, that the presence of agonists as well as antagonists in the same foodstuff, i.e., milk, provides the possibility of a balance of effects which might be useful or even necessary for a subtle control of the respective target functions.

D. Atypical Opioid Peptide Analogues with Agonist or Antagonist Activity

"Atypical" opioid peptides and their analogues, by definition and quantity, are "borderliners" of the opioid peptide field. However, this peptide group has provided opioid peptide agonists with extremely high affinity and selectivity for μ- or δ-opioid receptors, some of which have been used as tools in many studies. Table 3 shows representatives of atypical opioid peptides and analogues thereof. Due to lack of space, a very brief and arbitrary selection of analogues is referred to here; these analogues have been developed for improvement of certain characteristics such as stability against enzymatic degradation, μ- or δ-opioid receptor selectivity, analgesic potency, etc.

I. Agonists

1. μ-Selective Opioid Receptor Ligands

Opioid peptides with high affinity and selectivity for μ-type opioid receptors were obtained by development of β-casomorphin (CHANG et al. 1981, 1983; BRANTL et al. 1982; LIEBMANN et al. 1986; NEUBERT et al. 1990) or dermorphin analogues (SCHILLER et al. 1989; LAZARUS et al. 1989a). β-Casomorphin (BRANTL et al. 1982; CHANG et al. 1983; MATTHIES et al. 1984; NEUBERT et al. 1990) and dermorphin analogues (KISARA et al. 1986) have been shown to display high antinociceptive potencies. Certain β-casomorphin analogues appear to be appropriate for clinical application (HAUTEFEUILLE et al. 1986; DANIEL et al. 1990b; MANSFELD et al. 1990). Morphiceptin and PLO17 are regarded as standard μ-selective opioid receptor ligands (WATSON and ABBOTT 1989); morphiceptin, in particular, has been used in many studies.

2. δ-Selective Opioid Receptor Ligands

Opioid receptor ligands with high affinity and selectivity for δ-type opioid receptors were obtained by synthesis of deltorphin (identical with dermenkephalin or DGAP; see Sect. B.I.5) (SAGAN et al. 1989) or [D-Ala^2] deltorphin I analogues (SCHILLER et al. 1990). δ-Selective α-casein exorphin analogues were used to characterize δ-type opioid receptors in rat brain membranes (LOUKAS et al. 1990).

II. Antagonists

Lactoferroxin analogues have been synthesized to obtain information about the structural requirements for antagonistic activity of atypical opioid peptide analogues. Methoxylation or equivalent modification of a Tyr residue in the C-terminal position were reported to be important for antagonistic activity of the respective peptides (YOSHIKAWA et al. 1988).

E. Concluding Remarks

Typical opioid peptides, i.e., the bulk of endogenous opioids so far identified, originate from three precursor molecules only, proenkephalin, prodynorphin, and proopiomelanocortin; *atypical* opioid peptides are

Table 3. Opioid receptor selectivities and potencies in isolated organ preparations for some "typical" or "atypical" natural opioid peptides or analogues thereof as well as of morphine for comparison. Mean values of data from references as listed. The deviations of the individual values from the mean values were remarkably small; in a few cases only, e.g., for GPI IC$_{50}$ values of morphiceptin [1, 7] or for μ/δ-opioid receptor selectivities of dermorphin [6, 9], the differences were in the range of one order of magnitude

Opioid	Amino acid sequence	Opioid potency in isolated organ preparations:			Opioid receptor selectivity Binding assays: IC$_{50}$ (δ)/IC$_{50}$ (μ) or K_i (δ)/K_i (μ) (μ/δ selectivity)	[Ref.]
		MVD IC$_{50}$ (nM)	GPI IC$_{50}$ (nM)	IC$_{50}$ (MVD)/IC$_{50}$ (GPI) (GPI/MVD potency)		
μ-Selective opioid receptor ligands						
Morphine		1257.0	142.0	8.9	87.5	[1, 2]
[D-Ala^2, MePhe^4, Gly-ol^5] enkephalin = DAGO = DAMGO	H-Tyr-D-Ala-Gly-MePhe-Gly-ol	32.8	4.5	7.3	185.0	[3, 4, 5, 12]
β$_B$-Casomorphin (1–4) amide = morphiceptin	H-Tyr-Pro-Phe-Pro-NH$_2$	3400.0	884.0	3.84	1237.0	[1, 7, 8]
[MePhe^3, D-Pro^4]β$_B$-Casomorphin (1–4) amide = PLO17	H-Tyr-Pro-MePhe-D-Pro-NH$_2$	240.0	34.0	7.1	1818.0	[1]
[D-Pro^4]β$_B$-Casomorphin (1–4) amide = PLO32	H-Tyr-Pro-Phe-D-Pro-NH$_2$	359.0	61.0	5.9	4825.0	[1, 11]
[Trp^4, Asn^7] Dermorphin-OH	H-Tyr-D-Ala-Phe-Trp-Tyr-Pro-Asn-OH	7.4	1.3	5.7	357.0	[9]
Dermorphin	H-Tyr-D-Ala-Phe-Gly-Tyr-Pro-Ser-NH$_2$	23.4	2.18	10.8	107.0	[2, 3, 5, 9]
[Lys^7]Dermorphin-OH	H-Tyr-D-Ala-Phe-Gly-Tyr-Pro-Lys-OH	52.0	1.72	30.2	30.3	[9]

Table 3. *Continued*

Opioid	Amino acid sequence	Opioid potency in isolated organ preparations			Opioid receptor selectivity Binding assays (IC_{50} (δ)/IC_{50} (μ) or (K_i (δ)/K_i (μ) (μ/δ selectivity))	[Ref.]
		MVD IC_{50} (nM)	GPI IC_{50} (nM)	$\frac{IC_{50}\ (MVD)}{IC_{50}\ (GPI)}$ (GPI/MVD potency)		
δ-Selective Opioid Receptor Ligands						
[D-Ala², D-Leu⁵] Enkephalin = DADLE	H-Tyr-D-Ala-Gly-Phe-D-Leu-OH	0.70	14.7	0.048	0.2	[1, 3, 4, 6, 12]
[D-Pen², D-Pen⁵] Enkephalin = DPDPE	H-Tyr-D-Pen-Gly-Phe-D-Pen-OH	3.69	4209.0	0.0009	0.007	[3, 4, 5, 6, 12]
Deltorphin = dermenkephalin = dermorphin gene-associated peptide	H-Tyr-D-Met-Phe-His-Leu-Met-Asp-NH₂	1.58	2967.0	0.0005	0.011	[4, 5, 6]
[D-Ala²]Deltorphin I	H-Tyr-D-Ala-Phe-Asp-Val-Val-Gly-NH₂	0.15	854.0	0.0002	0.00005	[3, 10]
[D-Ala²]Deltorphin II	H-Tyr-D-Ala-Phe-Glu-Val-Val-Gly-NH₂	0.37	>3000.0	<0.0001	0.0003	[3]

MVD, mouse vas deferens preparation; GPI, guinea pig ileum longitudinal muscle-myenteric plexus preparation. IC_{50}, opioid concentration inhibiting the electrically induced contractions of the MVD or GPI preparations or the binding of μ- or δ-radioligands to opioid receptors by 50%. K_i, inhibitory constant;

References: [1] CHANG et al. 1983; [2] BROCCARDO et al. 1981; [3] ERSPAMER et al. 1989; [4] LAZARUS et al. 1989b; [5] AMICHE et al. 1989; [6] KREIL et al. 1989; [7] BRANTL et al. 1982; [8] LIEBMANN et al. 1989; [9] RICHTER et al. 1990; [10] SCHILLER et al. 1990; [11] LIEBMANN et al. 1986; [12] CORBETT et al. 1984.

derived from a variety of proteins, e.g., β-casein. All *typical* opioid peptides have the same N-terminal amino acid sequence, Tyr-Gly-Gly-Phe; for *atypical* opioid peptides only the N-terminal Tyr residue is obligatory (however, N-terminal extensions of the sequence beyond the Tyr residue occur). Much information has been collected about *typical* opioid peptides; in comparison, there is little information about *atypical* opioid peptides.

The physiological significance of *atypical opioid peptides* as derived from hemoglobin, from cytochrome b, from milk proteins, or from amphibian skin proteins is still not clear; nevertheless, there is indication that they represent essential supplements of the typical opioid systems. Efficient peptide interaction with opioid receptors would be a prerequisite for this: In fact, amphibian skin protein-derived peptides display very high opioid receptor affinities; the other peptides do not, but their parent proteins occur in high amounts which, in the case of atypical opioid peptide liberation, could compensate for their low affinities to opioid receptors.

The pharmacological profile of *atypical opioid peptides* or their analogues in general is of moderate interest; some representatives, however, show outstanding properties. Dermorphins and deltorphins, in fact, do have extremely high μ- or δ-opioid receptor affinities and selectivities. Further, certain analogues of β-casomorphins display high affinities and selectivities for μ-type opioid receptors; they have been chosen as standard μ-selective ligands and have been used in many studies.

Generally, by definition and quantity, atypical opioid peptides may be regarded as "borderliners" of the opioid peptide field. However, some earned broad interest.

Acknowledgement. The excellent secretarial aid of Sigrid Burghart is gratefully appreciated.

References

Amiche M, Sagan S, Mor A, Delfour A, Nicolas P (1989) Dermenkephalin (Tyr-D-Met-Phe-His-Leu-Met-Asp-NH$_2$): a potent and fully specific agonist for the δ opioid receptor. Mol Pharmacol 35:774–779

Anderson S, Bankier AT, Barrell BG, de Bruijn MHL, Coulson AR, Drouin J, Eperon IC, Nierlich DP, Roe BA, Sanger F, Schreier PH, Smith AJH, Staden R, Young IG (1981) Sequence and organization of the human mitochondrial genome. Nature 290:457–465

Baralle FE, Shoulders CC, Proudfoot NJ (1980) The primary structure of the human ε-globin gene. Cell 21:621–626

Brantl V (1984) Novel opioid peptides derived from human β-casein: Human β-casomorphins. Eur J Pharmacol 106:213–214

Brantl V, Teschemacher H, Bläsig J, Henschen A, Lottspeich F (1981) Opioid activities of β-casomorphins. Life Sci 28:1903–1909

Brantl V, Pfeiffer A, Herz A, Henschen A, Lottspeich F (1982) Antinociceptive potencies of β-casomorphin analogs as compared to their affinities towards μ and δ opiate receptor sites in brain and periphery. Peptides 3:793–797

Brantl V, Gramsch C, Lottspeich F, Henschen A, Jaeger KH, Herz A (1985) Novel opioid peptides derived from mitochondrial cytochrome b: cytochrophins. Eur J Pharmacol 111:293–294

Brantl V, Gramsch C, Lottspeich F, Mertz R, Jaeger KH, Herz A (1986) Novel opioid peptides derived from hemoglobin: hemorphins. Eur J Pharmacol 125: 309–310

Braunitzer G, Chen R, Schrank B, Stangl A (1973) Die Sequenzanalyse des β-Lactoglobulins. Hoppe-Seylers Z Physiol Chem 354:867–878

Brew K, Castellino FJ, Vanaman TC, Hill RL (1970) The complete amino acid sequence of bovine α-lactalbumin. J Biol Chem 245:4570–4582

Broccardo M, Erspamer V, Falconieri Erspamer G, Improta G, Linari G, Melchiorri P, Montecucchi PC (1981) Pharmacological data on dermorphins, a new class of potent opioid peptides from amphibian skin. Br J Pharmacol 73:625–631

Bueno L, Fioramonti J, Menezo Y (1985) Central opioid-like influence of a tetrapeptide from hamster embryo (kentsin) on gastrointestinal motility in dogs. Eur J Pharmacol 114:67–70

Chang KJ, Killian A, Hazum E, Cuatrecasas P, Chang JK (1981) Morphiceptin (NH_2-Tyr-Pro-Phe-Pro-$CONH_2$): a potent and specific agonist for morphine (μ) receptors. Science 212:75–77

Chang KJ, Wei ET, Killian A, Chang JK (1983) Potent morphiceptin analogs: structure, activity relationships and morphine-like activities. J Pharmacol Exp Ther 227:403–408

Chang KJ, Su YF, Brent DA, Chang JK (1985) Isolation of a specific μ-opiate receptor peptide, morphiceptin, from an enzymatic digest of milk protein. J Biol Chem 260:9706–9712

Chiba H, Yoshikawa M (1986) Biologically functional peptides from food proteins: new opioid peptides from milk proteins. In: Feeney RE, Whitaker JR (eds) Protein tailoring for food and medical uses. Dekker, New York, pp 123–153

Chiba H, Tani F, Yoshikawa M (1989) Opioid antagonist peptides derived from κ-casein. J Dairy Res 56:363–366

Corbett AD, Gillan MGC, Kosterlitz HW, McKnight AT, Paterson SJ, Robson LE (1984) Selectivities of opioid peptide analogues as agonists and antagonists at the δ-receptor. Br J Pharmacol 83:271–279

Daniel H, Vohwinkel M, Rehner G (1990a) Effect of casein and β-casomorphins on gastrointestinal motility in rats. J Nutr 120:252–257

Daniel H, Wessendorf A, Vohwinkel M, Brantl V (1990b) Effect of D-Ala^{2,4}, Tyr^5-β-casomorphin-5-amide on gastrointestinal functions. In: Nyberg F, Brantl V (eds) β-casomorphins and related peptides. Fyris-Tryck, Uppsala, pp 95–104

Davis TP, Gillespie TJ, Porreca F (1989) Peptide fragments derived from the β-chain of hemoglobin (hemorphins) are centrally active in vivo. Peptides 10:747–751

De Ponti F, Marcoli M, Lecchini S, Manzo L, Frigo GM, Crema A (1988) Effect of β-casomorphins on intestinal propulsion in the guinea-pig colon. J Pharm Pharmacol 41:302–305

Ermisch A, Rühle HJ, Neubert K, Hartrodt B, Landgraf R (1983) On the blood-brain barrier to peptides: [^{3}H]β-casomorphin-5 uptake by eighteen brain regions in vivo. J Neurochem 41:1229–1233

Erspamer V, Melchiorri P, Broccardo M, Falconieri Erspamer G, Falaschi P, Improta G, Negri L, Renda T (1981) The brain-gut-skin triangle: new peptides. Peptides 2:7–16

Erspamer V, Melchiorri P, Falconieri-Erspamer G, Negri L, Corsi R, Severini C, Barra D, Simmaco M, Kreil G (1989) Deltorphins: a family of naturally occurring peptides with high affinity and selectivity for δ opioid binding sites. Proc Natl Acad Sci USA 86:5188–5192

Faris PL, Komisaruk BR, Watkins LR, Mayer DJ (1983) Evidence for the neuropeptide cholecystokinin as an antagonist of opiate analgesia. Science 219: 310–312

Findlay JBC, Brew K (1972) The complete amino-acid sequence of human α-lactalbumin. Eur J Biochem 27:65–86

Galina ZH, Kastin AJ (1986) Existence of antiopiate systems as illustrated by MIF-1/Tyr-MIF-1. Life Sci 39:2153–2159

Graf L, Horvath K, Walcz E, Berzetei I, Burnier J (1987) Effect of two synthetic α-gliadin peptides on lymphocytes in celiac disease: identification of a novel class of opioid receptors. Neuropeptides 9:113–122

Greenberg R, Groves ML, Dower HJ (1984) Human β-casein. Amino acid sequence and identification of phosphorylation sites. J Biol Chem 259:5132–5138

Hartrodt B, Neubert K, Fischer G, Demuth U, Yoshimoto T, Barth A (1982a) Degradation of β-casomorphin-5 by proline-specific endopeptidase (PSE) and post-proline cleaving enzyme (PPCE). Pharmazie 37:72–73

Hartrodt B, Neubert K, Fischer G, Schulz H, Barth A (1982b) Synthese und enzymatischer Abbau von β-Casomorphin-5. Pharmazie 37:165–169

Hautefeuille M, Brantl V, Dumontier AM, Desjeux JF (1986) In vitro effects of β-casomorphins on ion transport in rabbit ileum. Am J Physiol 250:G92–G97

Hedner J, Hedner T (1987) β-Casomorphins induce apnea and irregular breathing in adult rats and new-born rabbits. Life Sci 41:2303–2312

Henschen A, Lottspeich F, Brantl V, Teschemacher H (1979) Novel opioid peptides derived from casein (β-casomorphins). II. Structure of active components from bovine casein peptone. Hoppe-Seylers Z Physiol Chem 360:1217–1224

Kastin AJ, Olson RD, Ehrensing RH, Berzas MC, Schally A, Coy DH (1979) MIF-1's differential actions as an opiate antagonist. Pharmacol Biochem Behav 11:721–723

Kisara K, Sakurada S, Sakurada T, Sasaki Y, Sato T, Suzuki K, Watanabe H (1986) Dermorphin analogues containing D-kyotorphin: structure-antinociceptive relationships in mice. Br J Pharmacol 87:183–189

Koch G, Brantl V (1990) Binding of β-casomorphins to opioid receptors. In: Nyberg F, Brantl V (eds) β-Casomorphins and related peptides, Fyris-Tryck, Uppsala, pp 43–52

Koch G, Wiedemann K, Teschemacher H (1985) Opioid activities of human β-casomorphins. Naunyn-Schmiedebergs Arch Pharmacol 331:351–354

Koch G, Wiedemann K, Drebes E, Zimmermann W, Link G, Teschemacher H (1988) Human β-casomorphin-8 immunoreactive material in the plasma of women during pregnancy and after delivery. Regul Peptides 20:107–117

Koldovsky O, Thornburg W (1987) Hormones in milk. A review. J Pediatr Gastroenterol Nutr 6:172–196

Kosaka T, Sakurada S, Sakurada T, Sato T, Kisara K, Hosono M, Sasaki Y, Suzuki K (1985) Antinociceptive properties of a new tetrapeptide, Asn-Ala-Gly-Ala, in mice. Arch Int Pharmacodyn 277:280–288

Kreil G, Barra D, Simmaco M, Erspamer V, Falconieri Erspamer G, Negri L, Severini C, Corsi R, Melchiorri P (1989) Deltorphin, a novel amphibian skin peptide with high selectivity and affinity for δ opioid receptors. Eur J Pharmacol 162:123–128

Lawn RM, Efstratiadis A, O'Connell C, Maniatis T (1980) The nucleotide sequence of the human β-globin gene. Cell 21:647–651

Lazarus LH, Guglietta A, Wilson WE, Irons BJ, de Castiglione R (1989a) Dimeric dermorphin analogues as μ-receptor probes on rat brain membranes. J Biol Chem 264:354–362

Lazarus LH, Wilson WE, de Castiglione R, Guglietta A (1989b) Dermorphin gene sequence peptide with high affinity and selectivity for δ-opioid receptors. J Biol Chem 264:3047–3050

Liebmann C, Szücs M, Neubert K, Hartrodt B, Arold H, Barth A (1986) Opiate receptor binding affinities of some D-amino acids substituted β-casomorphin analogs. Peptides 7:195–199

Liebmann C, Schrader U, Brantl V (1989) Opioid receptor affinities of the blood-derived tetrapeptides hemorphin and cytochrophin. Eur J Pharmacol 166: 523–526

Lindström LH, Nyberg F, Terenius L, Bauer K, Besev G, Gunne LM, Lyrenäs S, Willdeck-Lund G, Lindberg B (1984) CSF and plasma β-casomorphin-like opioid peptides in post-partum psychosis. Am J Psychiatry 141:1059–1066

Lönnerdal B, Bergström S, Andersson Y, Hjalmarsson K, Sundqvist AK, Hernell O (1990) Cloning and sequencing of a cDNA encoding human milk β-casein. FEBS Lett 269:153–156

Loukas S, Varoucha D, Zioudrou C, Streaty RA, Klee WA (1983) Opioid activities and structures of α-casein-derived exorphins. Biochemistry 22:4567–4573

Loukas S, Panetsos F, Donga E, Zioudrou C (1990) Selective δ-antagonist peptides, analogs of α-casein exorphin, as probes for the opioid receptor. In: Nyberg F, Brantl V (eds) β-Casomorphins and related peptides. Fyris-Tryck, Uppsala, pp 65–75

Mansfeld R, Kautni J, Grunert E, Brantl V, Jöchle W (1990) Clinical application of bovine β-casomorphins for treatment of calf diarrhea. In: Nyberg F, Brantl V (eds) β-Casomorphins and related peptides. Fyris-Tryck, Uppsala, pp 105–108

Matthies H, Stark H, Hartrodt B, Rüthrich HL, Spieler HT, Barth A, Neubert K (1984) Derivatives of β-casomorphins with high analgesic potency. Peptides 5:463–470

Meisel H (1986) Chemical characterization and opioid activity of an exorphin isolated from in vivo digests of casein. FEBS Lett 196:223–227

Meisel H, Schlimme E (1990) Milk proteins: precursors of bioactive peptides. Trends Food Sci Technol 1:41–43

Mercier JC, Grosclaude F, Ribadeau-Dumas B (1971) Structure primaire de la caseine α_{s1}-bovine: séquence complète. Eur J Biochem 23:41–51

Mercier JC, Brignon G, Ribadeau-Dumas B (1973) Structure primaire de la casein kB bovine: séquence complète. Eur J Biochem 35:222–235

Metz-Boutigue MH, Jollès J, Mazurier J, Schoentgen F, Legrand D, Spik G, Montreuil J, Jollès P (1984) Human lactotransferrin: amino acid sequence and structural comparisons with other transferrins. Eur J Biochem 145:659–676

Montecucchi PC, de Castiglione R, Piani S, Gozzini L, Erspamer V (1981a) Amino acid composition and sequence of dermorphin, a novel opiate-like peptide from the skin of *Phyllomedusa sauvagei*. Int J Pept Protein Res 17:275–283

Montecucchi PC, de Castiglione R, Erspamer V (1981b) Identification of dermorphin and Hyp⁶-dermorphin in skin extracts of the Brazilian frog *Phyllomedusa rhodei*. Int J Pept Protein Res 17:316–321

Mor A, Delfour A, Sagan S, Amiche M, Pradelles P, Rossier J, Nicolas P (1989) Isolation of dermenkephalin from amphibian skin, a high-affinity δ-selective opioid heptapeptide containing a D-amino acid residue. FEBS Lett 255:269–274

Mor A, Pradelles P, Delfour A, Montagne JJ, Quintero FL, Conrath M, Nicolas P (1990) Evidence for pro-dermorphin processing products in rat tissues. Biochem Biophys Res Commun 170:30–38

Morley JE (1982) Food peptides: a new class of hormones? J Am Med Assoc 247:2379–2380

Neubert K, Hartrodt B, Born I, Barth A, Ruethrich HL, Grecksch G, Schrader U, Liebmann C (1990) Structural modifications of β-casomorphin-5 and related peptides. In: Nyberg F, Brantl V (eds) β-Casomorphins and related peptides. Fyris-Tryck, Uppsala, pp 15–20

Nyberg F, Lieberman H, Lindström LH, Lyrenäs S, Koch G, Terenius L (1989) Immunoreactive β-casomorphin-8 in cerebrospinal fluid from pregnant and lactating women: a positive correlation with plasma levels. J Clin Endocrinol Metab 68:283–289

Paroli E (1988) Opioid peptides from food (the exorphins). World Rev Nutr Diet 55:58–97

Payan DG, Horváth K, Gráf L (1987) Specific high-affinity binding sites for a
     synthetic gliadin heptapeptide on human peripheral blood lymphocytes. Life Sci
     40:1229–1236
Petrilli P, Addeo F, Chianese L (1983) Primary structure of water buffalo β-casein:
     tryptic and CNBr peptides. Ital J Biochem 32:336–344
Petrilli P, Picone D, Caporale C, Addeo F, Auricchio S, Marino G (1984) Does
     casomorphin have a functional role? FEBS Lett 169:53–56
Provot C, Persuy MA, Mercier JC (1989) Complete nucleotide sequence of ovine β-
     casein cDNA: inter-species comparison. Biochimie 71:827–832
Raffa RB, Jacoby HI (1989) A-18-famide and F-8-famide, endogenous mammalian
     equivalents of the molluscan neuropeptide FMRF amide (Phe-Met-Arg-Phe-
     NH_2), inhibit colonic bead expulsion time in mice. Peptides 10:873–875
Ramabadran K, Bansinath M (1988) Opioid peptides from milk as a possible cause
     of sudden infant death syndrome. Med Hypotheses 27:181–187
Ramabadran K, Bansinath M (1989) Pharmacology of β-casomorphins, opioid
     peptides derived from milk protein. Asia Pac J Pharmacol 4:45–58
Ramabadran K, Moore BE (1988) Sudden infant death syndrome and opioid
     peptides from milk. Am J Dis Child 142:12–13
Read LC, Lord APD, Brantl V, Koch G (1990) Absorption of β-casomorphins from
     autoperfused lamb and piglet small intestine. Am J Physiol 259:G443–452
Ribadeau-Dumas B, Brignon G, Grosclaude F, Mercier JC (1972) Structure primaire
     de la caséine β bovine. Séquence complète. Eur J Biochem 25:505–514
Richardson BC, Mercier JC (1979) The primary structure of the ovine β-caseins. Eur
     J Biochem 99:285–297
Richter K, Egger R, Kreil G (1987) D-Alanine in the frog skin peptide dermorphin is
     derived from L-alanine in the precursor. Science 238:200–202
Richter K, Egger R, Negri L, Corsi R, Severini C, Kreil G (1990) cDNAs encoding
     [D-Ala²]deltorphin precursors from skin of *Phyllomedusa bicolor* also contain
     genetic information for three dermorphin-related opioid peptides. Proc Natl
     Acad Sci USA 87:4836–4839
Sagan S, Amiche M, Delfour A, Mor A, Camus A, Nicolas P (1989) Molecular
     determinants of receptor affinity and selectivity of the natural δ-opioid agonist,
     dermenkephalin. J Biol Chem 264:17100–17106
Schams D, Karg H (1986) Hormones in milk. Ann N Y Acad Sci 464:75–86
Scheffler H, Koch G, Brantl V, Teschemacher H (1990) Release of opioid peptide
     immunoreactive materials from pituitary tissue upon stimulation with a
     hemoglobin fragment, hemorphin-4, in vitro. In: van Ree JM, Mulder AH,
     Wiegant VM, van Wimersma Greidanus TB (eds) New leads in opioid research.
     Excerpta Medica, Amsterdam, pp 379–380
Schiller PW, Nguyen TMD, Chung NN, Lemieux C (1989) Dermorphin analogues
     carrying an increased positive net charge in their "message" domain display
     extremely high μ opioid receptor selectivity. J Med Chem 32:698–703
Schiller PW, Nguyen TMD, Weltrowska G, Lemieux C, Chung NN (1990) Develop-
     ment of [D-Ala²]deltorphin I analogs with extraordinary delta receptor selectivity.
     In: van Ree JM, Mulder AH, Wiegant VM, van Wimersma Greidanus TB (eds)
     New leads in opioid research. Excerpta Medica, Amsterdam, pp 288–290
Singh M, Rosen CL, Chang KJ, Haddad GG (1989) Plasma β-casomorphin-7
     immunoreactive peptide increases after milk intake in newborn but not in adult
     dogs. Pediatr Res 26:34–38
Slightom JL, Blechl AE, Smithies O (1980) Human fetal $^G\gamma$ and $^A\gamma$-globin genes:
     complete nucleotide sequences suggest that DNA can be exchanged between
     these duplicated genes. Cell 21:627–638
Spritz RA, DeRiel JK, Forget BG, Weissman SM (1980) Complete nucleotide
     sequence of the human δ-globin gene. Cell 21:639–646
Svedberg J, de Haas J, Leimenstoll G, Paul F, Teschemacher H (1985) Demon-
     stration of β-casomorphin immunoreactive materials in in vitro digests of bovine

milk and in small intestine contents after bovine milk ingestion in adult humans. Peptides 6:825–830

Tang J, Yang HYT, Costa E (1984) Inhibition of spontaneous and opiate-modified nociception by an endogeneous neuropeptide with Phe-Met-Arg-Phe-NH$_2$-like immunoreactivity. Proc Natl Acad Sci USA 81:5002–5005

Takagi H, Shiomi H, Ueda H, Amano H (1979) A novel analgesic dipeptide from bovine brain is a possible Met-enkephalin releaser. Nature 282:410–412

Teschemacher H (1987a) Casein-derived opioid peptides: physiological significance? Adv Biosci 65:41–48

Teschemacher H (1987b) β-Casomorphins: do they have physiological significance? In: Goldman AS, Atkinson SA, Hanson LA (eds) Human lactation 3. Plenum, New York, pp 213–225

Teschemacher H, Koch G (1990) β-Casomorphins: possible physiological significance. In: Nyberg F, Brantl V (eds) β-Casomorphins and related peptides. Fyris-Tryck, Uppsala, pp 143–149

Teschemacher H, Koch G (1991) Opioids in the milk. Endocrine Regul 25:147–150

Teschemacher H, Umbach M, Hamel U, Praetorius K, Ahnert-Hilger G, Brantl V, Lottspeich F, Henschen A (1986) No evidence for the presence of β-casomorphins in human plasma after ingestion of cows' milk or milk products. J Dairy Res 53:135–138

Teschemacher H, Brantl V, Henschen A, Lottspeich F (1990) β-Casomorphins – β-casein fragments with opioid activity: detection and structure. In: Nyberg F, Brantl V (eds) β-Casomorphins and related peptides. Fyris-Tryck, Uppsala, pp 9–14

Tomé D, Dumontier AM, Hautefeuille M, Desjeux JF (1987) Opiate activity and transepithelial passage of intact β-casomorphins in rabbit ileum. Am J Physiol 253:G737–744

Ueda H, Yoshihara Y, Fukushima N, Shiomi H, Nakamura A, Takagi H (1987a) Kyotorphin (tyrosine-arginine) synthetase in rat brain synaptosomes. J Biol Chem 262:8165–8173

Ueda H, Fukushima N, Yoshihara Y, Takagi H (1987b) A Met-enkephalin releaser (kyotorphin)-induced release of plasma membrane-bound Ca^{2+} from rat brain synaptosomes. Brain Res 419:197–200

Ueda H, Yoshihara Y, Misawa H, Fukushima N, Katada T, Ui M, Takagi H, Satoh M (1989) The kyotorphin (tyrosine-arginine) receptor and a selective reconstitution with purified G$_i$, measured with GTPase and phospholipase C assays. J Biol Chem 264:3732–3741

Umbach M, Teschemacher H, Praetorius K, Hirschhäuser R, Bostedt H (1985) Demonstration of a β-casomorphin immunoreactive material in the plasma of newborn calves after milk intake. Regul Pept 12:223–230

Watson, S, Abbott A (1989) Opioid receptors. Trends Pharmacol Sci 10, Receptor Nomenclature Supplement, p 21

Yang HYT, Fratta W, Majane EA, Costa E (1985) Isolation, sequencing, synthesis, and pharmacological characterization of two brain neuropeptides that modulate the action of morphine. Proc Natl Acad Sci USA 82:7757–7761

Yoshihara Y, Ueda H, Imajoh S, Takagi H, Satoh M (1988) Calcium-activated neutral protease (CANP), a putative processing enzyme of the neuropeptide, kyotorphin, in the brain. Biochem Biophys Res Commun 155:546–553

Yoshikawa M, Yoshimura T, Chiba H (1984) Opioid peptides from human β-casein. Agric Biol Chem 48:3185–3187

Yoshikawa M, Tani F, Yoshimura T, Chiba H (1986a) Opioid peptides from milk proteins. Agric Biol Chem 50:2419–2421

Yoshikawa M, Tani F, Ashikaga T, Yoshimura T, Chiba H (1986b) Purification and characterization of an opioid antagonist from a peptic digest of bovine κ-casein. Agric Biol Chem 50:2951–2954

Yoshikawa M, Tani F, Chiba H (1988) Structure-activity relationship of opioid antagonist peptides derived from milk proteins. In: Shiba S, Sakakibara S (eds) Peptide chemistry. Protein Research Foundation, Osaka, pp 473–476

Zadina JE, Kastin AJ (1986) Interactions of Tyr-MIF-1 at opiate receptor sites. Pharmacol Biochem Behav 25:1303–1305

Zadina JE, Kastin AJ, Ge LJ, Brantl V (1990) Casomorphin-related peptides bind to non-opiate (Tyr-MIF-1) sites as well as opiate receptors in brain. In: Nyberg F, Brantl V (eds) β-Casomorphins and related peptides. Fyris-Tryck, Uppsala, pp 61–63

Zioudrou C, Streaty RA, Klee WA (1979) Opioid peptides derived from food proteins. J Biol Chem 254:2446–2449

CHAPTER 22
Opioid Peptide Processing Enzymes

L.D. FRICKER

A. Introduction

The biosynthesis of the opioid peptides is generally similar to the bio-synthesis of many other peptide hormones and neurotransmitters. The bioactive peptides are initially produced as larger precursors which require posttranslational processing by several enzymes (Table 1). A necessary step for the production of most bioactive peptides is the limited proteolytic cleavage of the precursor by one or more endopeptidases which selectively cleave the precursor at specific sites, usually pairs of basic amino acids. In some cases, these cleavage sites are single basic amino acids. Following the endopeptidase action, a carboxypeptidase is required to remove the cleavage site residues from the C-terminus of the peptides. In addition to these proteolytic steps, some opioid peptides undergo other posttranslational modifications including sulfation, phosphorylation, glycosylation, N-terminal acetylation, and C-terminal amidation. Some of these modifications appear to be required for biological activity and/or stability of the peptide. All of these posttranslational modifications are performed inside the cell, prior to secretion. Once the peptides are secreted, they are exposed to extracellular enzymes. Some of the extracellular enzymes inactivate the opioid peptides, while other enzymes cleave the peptides into smaller fragments which retain opioid activity. In many cases, the differential processing, both intracellular and extracellular, leads to peptides with distinct biological activities. Thus, the enzymes that process opioid peptides play a key role in the generation of specific messengers.

This review focusses on enzymes that produce bioactive opioid peptides, including both intracellular and extracellular enzymes. In many cases, enzymes that process opioid peptides are also involved with processing other peptides, and so the enzymes described for the opioid system should not be regarded as being specific for the opioid peptides. While some of the enzymes are well characterized, little is known about others, and this review represents a brief overview of the field.

Table 1. Summary of intracellular posttranslational peptide processing steps

Posttranslational processing step	Number (names) of enzymes	Subcellular location	Modification site/consensus sequence
Cleavage of signal peptide	1 (signal peptidase)	ER	Enzyme cleaves after Ala, Ser, Gly or Cys, usually 20–25 amino acids from N-terminus of precursor.
N-Glycosylation	1 enzyme adds sugar in ER Many process sugar in Golgi		Asparagine is modified. Asn-X-Ser/Thr (X = any amino acid)
O-Glycosylation	? Many	Golgi	Ser or Thr are modified. No consensus site is known.
Phosphorylation	1 (casein kinase I)	"	Ser or Thr are modified. Ser/Thr-X-Acidic (Acidic = Asp, Glu)
Sulfation	1 (tyrosylprotein sulfotransferase)	"	Tyr is modified. Surrounding region is acidic, with few basic or hydrophobic residues, or disulfide bonds nearby.
Cleavage at dibasic sites	? 5–15	Secretory Pathway	Lys-Arg and Arg-Arg best. (better than Arg-Lys or Lys-Lys)
Cleavage at monobasic sites	? 1–5	"	A second basic residue (Arg, Lys, His) is present in either −3, −5, or −7 positions. Leu, Ile, Val, Met never occur in +1, and Trp, Tyr, Phe never occur in −1 positions. Cleavage site usually Arg-Ser/Ala.
Removal of C-terminal basic residues	1 (many names: carboxypeptidase E, H, enkephalin convertase)	"	Requires C-terminal basic residue. Preference Arg ≥ Lys ≫ His
C-terminal amidation	2 enzymes required (peptidylglycine-α-amidating-monooxygenase and α-hydroxyglycine amidating dealkylase)	"	Requires C-terminal Gly (N of Gly becomes amide, remainder removed by concerted action of two enzymes.

B. Enzymes in the Endoplasmic Reticulum and Golgi Apparatus

I. Signal Peptidase

The first step in the biosynthesis of opioid peptides and virtually all other proteins that are present in the secretory pathway is the removal of an N-terminal "signal peptide." This peptide functions to direct translocation of newly synthesized protein into the lumen of the endoplasmic reticulum (SHIELDS 1991). Although there is little homology between the amino acid sequences of the signal peptides from different precursors, all signal peptides share certain characteristics (VON HEIJNE 1985). A single enzyme, referred to as a "signal peptidase," appears to be capable of cleaving many different signal peptides from a variety of precursors. This enzyme has been partially purified and characterized; it is an integral membrane protein that cleaves signal peptides after amino acids with small side chains (Ala, Ser, Cys, Gly) (LIVELY and WALSH 1983; BAKER and LIVELY 1987).

Little is known regarding the regulation of the signal peptidase. Although it is generally considered that all proteins that pass through the secretory pathway have cleavable signal peptides, there are a few cases where proteins are not completely processed by the signal peptidase. This results in two forms of the protein: the form with the signal peptide attached is usually membrane associated, and the form without the signal peptide is usually soluble (TALJANIDISZ et al. 1990). One of the opioid peptide precursors, proopiomelanocortin (POMC), has been found to exist in both forms, although the form with the uncleaved signal peptide is only a small percentage of the total (H. AKIL, personal communication). The functional consequences of this are not known.

II. Glycosylation, Sulfation, and Phosphorylation

Opioid peptides have been isolated which contain carbohydrates, sulfates, and/or phosphates. There is considerable variation between the extent of these modifications from one tissue to another. In general, these modifications of opioid peptides have unknown functions; possibilities that have been suggested include altered specificity for the various opiate receptors, altered susceptibility to degradation, and altered proteolytic processing within the cell. In support of this latter possibility, carbohydrate attachment to the γ_3-MSH region of POMC alters the proteolytic processing of this precursor (BENNETT 1991). However, other modifications of POMC, such as the attachment of carbohydrates or phosphates to the ACTH region, do not substantially alter the proteolytic processing at nearby sites (BENNETT 1991).

The attachment of carbohydrates, sulfates, and/or phosphates to the opioid peptide precursor occurs in the endoplasmic reticulum and Golgi apparatus. The enzymes responsible for these modifications are not specific for peptide precursors, and are involved with the modification of other proteins that pass through the Golgi apparatus. However, some modifications are uniquely associated with proteins that are in a specific pathway. An example of this is the carbohydrate side chain mannose-6-phosphate, which is only found on proteins that pass through the Golgi apparatus into the lysosomal vesicles. No modifications have been found that are specific for proteins sorted into the regulated secretory pathway, which includes peptide precursors and the proteolytic processing enzymes.

Carbohydrates can be attached either to the nitrogen present on asparagine residues ("N-linked sugars") or to the oxygen on serine or threonine residues ("O-linked sugars"). Not all asparagine residues can serve as glycosylation sites: only those with the sequence Asn-X-Ser or Asn-X-Thr, where X is any amino acid, are potential sites. In contrast to N-linked glycosylation, there is no consensus site for O-linked glycosylation. Both N-linked and O-linked carbohydrates have been found on some of the opioid peptide precursors, although there is considerable variation in the extent of these modifications between tissues (WATKINSON et al. 1988; EIPPER and MAINS 1980; BENNETT 1991). N-linked carbohydrates are usually added in a single step by an enzyme within the endoplasmic reticulum. Further processing of the core sugars into complex carbohydrate chains occurs in the Golgi apparatus. The addition of O-linked sugars initially occurs in the Golgi apparatus. In general, O-linked carbohydrates are less complex than N-linked carbohydrates. It has been estimated that more than 100 enzymes are involved in carbohydrate attachment and processing in various tissues; only a few of these have been well characterized (PAULSON and COLLEY 1989).

Sulfation of peptides occurs primarily on tyrosine residues and on the sugar side chains. The enzyme responsible for the sulfation of tyrosine, tyrosylprotein sulfotransferase, uses 3'-phosphoadenosine-5'-phosphosulfate as a cofactor (HUTTNER 1988). This enzyme is present as an integral membrane protein in the Golgi apparatus of a variety of tissues and cell lines (HUTTNER 1988). Enzyme activity is optimal at pH 6, and is stimulated by Mg^{2+} and Mn^{2+} and inhibited by metal chelating agents. A consensus sequence for tyrosine sulfation has been described (HUTTNER 1988). In general, the amino acids near the sulfated tyrosine are usually acidic residues, and rarely basic or hydrophobic residues. Disulfide bonds and residues that are glycosylated are never present nearby sulfated tyrosine residues.

Opioid peptides that have been reported to undergo tyrosine sulfation include β-lipotropin and Leu-enkephalin. Approximately 50% of the β-lipotropin in bovine neurointermediate pituitary was found to exist with a sulfate on Tyr^{28}, as determined by fast atom bombardment mass spectrometry (BENNETT 1991). The presence of sulfated Leu-enkephalin was less rigorously demonstrated, using only chromatographic comparison of synthetic O-sulfated Leu-enkephalin with the endogenous opioid peptide (UNSWORTH and HUGHES 1982). Interestingly, the synthetic O-sulfated Leu-enkephalin was devoid of opioid activity. If this modification does occur in vivo, it would play an important role in the modulation of bioactivity.

Phosphorylation also occurs in the Golgi apparatus, and is usually limited to the modification of serine or threonine residues (BENNETT 1991). The consensus site for attachment of phosphate groups is Ser/Thr-X-acidic, where X is any amino acid and the acidic residue is usually aspartic or glutamic acid (BENNETT 1991). In the case of peptide B, a proenkephalin-derived peptide, the site Ser^{13}-Tyr-Ser^{15}-Lys-Glu is phosphorylated on both serine residues. Phosphorylation of Ser^{15} makes this residue acidic, which then serves as a consensus site for phosphorylation of Ser^{13} (D'SOUZA and LINDBERG 1988). The enzyme responsible for the phosphorylation of secreted peptides and proteins is casein kinase I (BENNETT 1991). This enzyme, which is located in the endoplasmic reticulum and Golgi apparatus, utilizes ATP as the source of phosphate groups. Many tissues contain casein kinase I activity, including lactating mammary gland where the enzyme is involved with the phosphorylation of the milk protein casein.

The function of peptide phosphorylation is not known. Several phosphorylation sites are found in POMC, and the degree of phosphorylation varies between tissues (BENNETT 1991). One of the phosphorylation sites within POMC is Ser^{31} of ACTH. The addition of phosphate to this site does not alter the potency of ACTH in a variety of physiological assays (BENNETT 1991). Furthermore, phosphorylation of this site does not alter the proteolytic processing of POMC, or the degree of N-glycosylation of a nearby residue, Asn^{29}. It is likely that phosphorylation of some peptides has a large influence on their bioactivity and/or stability, and further studies are needed.

C. Enzymes in the Secretory Granules

The proteolytic processing of peptide precursors is thought to begin in the trans Golgi network, as the secretory granules are forming, and to continue in the newly formed secretory granules. Several lines of evidence support this. First, studies examining the time course of the incorporation of radio-labeled amino acids into peptides have determined that incubation times of 30–60 min are required before any of the radiolabel is incorporated into the fully processed peptides (STEINER 1991). Since transit of proteins through the endoplasmic reticulum and Golgi apparatus requires 30–60 min, this finding is consistent with proteolytic processing occurring in the secretory granules. Recent electron microscopic studies using antisera that are specific for the processed forms of the peptides have found that processing of proinsulin (ORCI et al. 1986), POMC (SCHNABEL et al. 1989), and prosomatostatin (BOURDAIS et al. 1990) does not occur in the Golgi apparatus. Processing of these precursors begins in the secretory granules as they form within the trans Golgi network, and continues as the granules mature. Factors that regulate enzymatic activity so that processing begins only in the trans Golgi network are not yet known, but possible candidates include pH and Ca^{2+}. The internal pH of the trans Golgi network is more acidic than the endoplasmic reticulum and Golgi apparatus (ANDERSON and PATHAK 1985). Some of the endoproteases described below are activated by low pH and/or Ca^{2+}. Other enzymes described below have been reported to be maximally active at neutral pH. It is possible that the pH optimum of these enzymes is different in the environment within secretory granules, or that factors other than pH activate the enzymes in the trans Golgi network, and so these enzymes cannot be excluded as potential peptide-processing enzymes based on their pH optimum.

I. Endopeptidases Selective for Paired Basic Residues

A variety of enzymes have been reported to cleave opioid and other peptide precursors at paired basic amino acid cleavage sites (LINDBERG and HUTTON 1991). These endopeptidases are difficult to study for several reasons. First, the substrates for the endopeptidases are difficult to obtain since the full-length precursors are usually not very abundant in tissues. Small synthetic substrates that resemble the cleavage site are often used, but these substrates may not accurately reflect the structure of the cleavage site within the larger precursor. For some peptide precursors, it has been shown that mutation of residues located at a considerable distance from the cleavage site can inhibit proteolysis (DOCHERTY et al. 1989). Thus, small synthetic peptides may not be good substrates for peptide-processing enzymes. Recently, molecular biological techniques have been used to express high levels of the opioid peptide precursors in cell lines that do not process the protein; this will be extremely useful for studies on the processing enzymes. Another difficulty encountered with studies on peptide-processing enzymes is the abundance of other proteases in the cell that are capable of cleaving most substrates. This problem can be reduced by using purified secretory granules, rather than tissue homogenates. However, even highly purified bovine adrenal chromaffin granules have been found to contain high levels of lysosomal enzymes, relative to the enzymes that appear to be selectively enriched in the chromaffin granules (LASLOP et al. 1990). For these reasons, studies on the opioid-processing endoproteases have lagged behind studies on other enzymes that process peptides within the secretory granules. Recently, a great deal of interest has been generated by the cloning of several endopeptidases which have homology to the yeast peptide processing enzyme "KEX2". These enzymes are discussed after a brief review of opioid peptide processing enzymes.

An enzyme that cleaves POMC has been identified in secretory granules from bovine and rat pituitary (LOH and GAINER 1982; LOH et al. 1985;

PARISH et al. 1986). This enzyme, named prohormone converting enzyme (PCE), has an acidic pH optimum. Initial reports described the enzyme as a cysteine protease (LOH and GAINER 1982), but later work from the same researchers indicated that the enzyme is an aspartyl protease (LOH et al. 1985). PCE cleaves POMC at the pairs of basic residues, liberating β-endorphin 1–31, ACTH, and other peptides (LOH et al. 1985).

Another enzyme has been described as a POMC-processing enzyme in bovine pituitary (CROMLISH et al. 1986). This enzyme, named "IRCM-1" after the research institute where the work was performed, was later identified as plasma kallikrein (SEIDAH et al. 1988). It is unclear whether this enzyme is produced in the pituitary, or is only present in the blood within the pituitary. Interestingly, purified IRCM-1 is able to correctly process intermediates derived from POMC, proenkephalin, prodynorphin, and other peptide precursors at the pairs of basic amino acids; this specificity is not expected for plasma kallikrein (SEIDAH et al. 1988). IRCM-1 and other kallikreins are serine proteases with neutral pH optima.

An enzyme with a specificity for paired basic residues has been identified in bovine adrenal chromaffin granules (LINDBERG et al. 1982), and has been named "adrenal trypsin-like enzyme," or ATLE (SHEN et al. 1989). This enzyme is a serine protease with a molecular weight of 31 kDa (SHEN et al. 1989). Purified ATLE cleaves proenkephalin at the pairs of basic amino acids, and, after carboxypeptidase treatment of the ATLE reaction products, these two enzymes produce Met-enkephalin, Leu-enkephalin, and the octapeptide Met-enkephalin-Arg^6-Gly^7-Leu^8 (LINDBERG and THOMAS 1990). ATLE also cleaves proenkephalin-derived peptides, such as peptide B, at the pairs of basic amino acids. The pH optimum of ATLE is in the 8.5–9 range.

Other opioid peptide processing endopeptidases have been detected in bovine adrenal medulla chromaffin granules. Using small peptides as substrates, an enzyme with an unusual specificity was found (SUPATTAPONE et al. 1988). This enzyme cleaves either at pairs of basic residues or at single basic sites, depending on the peptide. Large peptides are less efficiently cleaved than peptides smaller than 20 amino acids, even if the same cleavage site residues are present in both peptides. The specificity of this enzyme is similar, but not identical, to two other enzymes that have been reported to process opioid peptides: "soluble metalloendopeptidase" or "endopeptidase 24.15" (CHU and ORLOWSKI 1985) and "endo-oligopeptidase A" (CAMARGO et al. 1987; OLIVEIRA et al. 1990). Neither of these other enzymes is detectable in bovine adrenal chromaffin granules. The bovine adrenal chromaffin granule endopeptidase, as well as soluble metalloendopeptidase and endo-oligopeptidase A, are maximally active in the neutral pH range.

Several endopeptidases have been characterized for nonopioid peptide precursors, and it is possible that these enzymes also function in processing opioid peptides. In a recent study using chromogranin as a substrate, two activities were detected in bovine adrenal chromaffin granules (LASLOP et al.

1990). One of these activities is similar to the enzyme designated ATLE, the other activity being similar to insulin-processing activities previously found in pancreatic islets (DAVIDSON et al. 1988). The insulin-processing activities exist in two forms, named types 1 and 2. Both are serine proteases that are activated by Ca^{2+} and are maximally active in the pH 5–6 range. The two forms differ in their specificity for pairs of basic residues: type 1 prefers the Arg-Arg site, and type 2 prefers the Lys-Arg site of proinsulin (DAVIDSON et al. 1988). It is not known if either of these activities cleaves opioid peptide precursors, or if the chromaffin granule activities are identical to the pancreatic enzymes.

The only endopeptidase that has been definitively shown to be involved in prohormone processing is the yeast enzyme designated Kex-2. This activity functions in the processing of α-mating factor and killer toxin at pairs of basic amino acids (JULIUS et al. 1984). When introduced into mammalian cells using a vaccinia viral vector, Kex-2 is able to cleave POMC and liberate β-endorphin (THOMAS et al. 1988). Recently, several groups have identified mammalian proteins that are homologous to the yeast Kex-2. Three of these homologous proteins are furin (ROEBROEK et al. 1986), PC-2 (SMEEKENS and STEINER 1990), and another protein designated both PC-1 and PC-3 (SEIDAH et al. 1990). All of these proteins appear to be serine proteases which are evolutionarily related to subtilisin, a bacterial serine endopeptidase. When introduced into mammalian cells using a vaccinia viral vector, Kex-2, furin, PC-1, and PC-2 are able to cleave POMC into smaller fragments (THOMAS et al. 1988; LEDUC et al. 1990; BENJANNET et al. 1991). Interestingly, although all of these enzymes process POMC at pairs of basic amino acids, the enzymes differ in their specificity for individual cleavage sites, generating distinct sets of products. The regulation of PC-1 and PC-2 has been examined in several cell culture systems; in general these enzymes appear to be co-regulated along with peptide hormones (BLOOMQUIST et al. 1991). Further evidence that PC-1 is a physiological neuropeptide-processing enzyme was obtained by stable expression of antisense PC-1 RNA in the AtT-20 cell line in order to lower the endogenous level of PC-1 protein; the resulting cell lines did not process POMC as well as wild type AtT-20 cells (BLOOMQUIST et al. 1991). It is possible that these Kex-2-like proteins are identical to some of the enzyme activities described above; likely candidates are the type-1 and type-2 insulin processing enzymes described by DAVIDSON and colleagues (1988).

II. Opioid Peptide Processing Endopeptidases Selective for Single Basic Residues

Although the majority of cleavage sites used in the processing of opioid peptides are pairs of basic amino acids, there are several cleavages that occur at single basic sites (usually Arg). Examples of opioid peptides that require processing at single basic sites include dynorphin B-13, dynorphin

A-8, and metorphamide (adrenorphin). All of these single basic cleavage sites fit specific rules based on the analysis of known cleavage sites for many different bioactive peptides (DEVI 1991). Since most of the enzymes described above have been reported to be specific for pairs of basic amino acids, it is likely that a distinct enzyme (or enzymes) is involved with the processing of opioid peptides at single basic sites.

An enzyme capable of processing dynorphin B-29 into dynorphin B-13 has been identified in rat brain and bovine pituitary (DEVI and GOLDSTEIN 1984; DEVI et al. 1991). This activity, designated "dynorphin-converting enzyme" (DCE), is enriched in purified bovine pituitary secretory granules (DEVI et al. 1991). DCE is a thiol protease with a pH optimum in the neutral range, although this enzyme retains considerable activity at low pH. Partially purified DCE is able to process both dynorphin A-17 and B-29 at the single basic cleavage site. The specificity of DCE was studied using a variety of dynorphin-related peptides as inhibitors of the conversion of dynorphin B-29 to dynorphin B-13. The enzyme binds peptides that contain the consensus sequence for single basic processing, but does not bind peptides without this consensus sequence (DEVI and GOLDSTEIN 1986; DEVI 1991). It is possible that this dynorphin-processing enzyme is also involved with the processing of other peptides at single basic cleavage sites.

III. Carboxypeptidase E

Most of the endopeptidases described above cleave the precursor on the C-terminal side of the basic residues, generating peptides containing basic residues on the C-terminus. Since most of the bioactive opioid peptides do not contain C-terminal basic residues, these residues must be removed by a carboxypeptidase. A single carboxypeptidase appears to be involved with the processing of many different bioactive peptides, although this one enzyme has several names: carboxypeptidase E (CPE), enkephalin convertase, and carboxypeptidase H.

Carboxypeptidase E activity is present in all tissues that are known to produce peptide hormones or neurotransmitters (FRICKER 1991). The enzyme has been purified to homogeneity from bovine brain, pituitary, adrenal medulla (FRICKER and SNYDER 1983), and other tissues (DAVIDSON and HUTTON 1987; FRICKER 1991). No differences are apparent between the enzyme isolated from the different tissues. Several forms of CPE are present in each tissue, including both soluble and membrane-bound forms (SUPATTAPONE et al. 1984; FRICKER et al. 1990a). All forms presumably arise from posttranslational processing of a single protein precursor and not from distinct genes or differential mRNA splicing, based on analysis of cDNA clones and genomic DNA (FRICKER et al. 1986; JUNG et al. 1991). The C-terminal region of CPE has been identified as the membrane anchor (FRICKER et al. 1990a). This region presumably forms an amphiphilic α-helix which "floats" on the surface of the lipid bilayer. The soluble form of CPE lacks this C-terminal region due to proteolytic cleavage.

The substrate specificity of CPE has been extensively studied (FRICKER 1991). This enzyme removes only basic C-terminal amino acids, with a slight preference for arginine over lysine. C-terminal histidine residues are removed very slowly (SMYTH et al. 1989). The penultimate amino acid has an influence on enzymatic activity: substrates containing alanine are hydrolyzed the most rapidly, and those containing proline are cleaved the least rapidly of the peptides examined (FRICKER and SNYDER 1983). Multiple basic residues on the C-terminus are removed sequentially. There is no evidence that CPE cleaves non-basic residues from the C-terminus, although high concentrations of peptides without basic C-terminal residues (such as Met-enkephalin) are competitive inhibitors of CPE (HOOK and LAGAMMA 1987). The inhibition of CPE by millimolar concentrations of enkephalin, and other peptides, has been proposed to be an important mechanism for regulating CPE in vivo, although it is not clear if significant inhibition would occur with typical concentrations of these peptides inside the secretory granules (HOOK and LAGAMMA 1987).

The most important factor in the regulation of CPE activity is pH. CPE is maximally active at an acidic pH (5.0–5.5), corresponding to the intra-granular pH of mature secretory granules. In contrast, at the neutral internal pH of the endoplasmic reticulum and Golgi apparatus, CPE is several hundred fold less active (FRICKER 1991). Thus, the acidification of the secretory granules that begins in the trans Golgi network activates CPE. As the secretory granules continue to mature, the additional acidification further increases CPE activity. Finally, after the secretion of the contents of the secretory granules, which includes both peptides and the processing enzymes (MAINS and EIPPER 1984), CPE is largely inactivated by the neutral extracellular pH.

The regulation of CPE activity and mRNA have been studied in several in vivo systems and in cell culture (MAINS and EIPPER 1984; HOOK et al. 1985; STRITTMATTER et al. 1985; BONDY et al. 1989; FRICKER et al. 1990b,c). In general, treatments that alter the rate of peptide biosynthesis tend to similarly affect CPE activity and/or mRNA, although the magnitude of the change in CPE is usually much smaller than the change in peptide levels. The time course also appears to be different: changes in CPE activity and/or mRNA levels occur more slowly than changes in peptide levels. These results are consistent with the proposal that CPE is not a rate-limiting enzyme in the production of most peptides. Two peptides for which CPE is presumably the rate-limiting enzyme are β-neoendorphin and β-endorphin 1–26 (SMYTH et al. 1989). β-Neoendorphin is produced from α-neoendorphin by cleavage at the Pro-Lys bond, and β-endorphin 1–26 is derived from β-endorphin 1–27 by removal of His^{27} (except for human β-endorphin, which contains a Tyr in place of His^{27}). CPE removes the basic C-terminal residues (Lys, His) from these peptides extremely slowly (SMYTH et al.

1989). Small changes in CPE activity would therefore have a large influence on the production of β-neoendorphin and β-endorphin 1–26.

IV. Aminopeptidase B-Like Enzyme

A few of the endopeptidases described above cleave the precursor between pairs of basic amino acids, generating products with both N- and C-terminal basic residues. The peptides with the N-terminal basic amino acids could be converted into the bioactive peptides by an aminopeptidase. Alternatively, further action of the endopeptidase could remove these N-terminal residues. An example of this is trypsin, an endopeptidase that can slowly remove N-terminal basic residues. Thus, it is not clear if an aminopeptidase is required for peptide biosynthesis.

An aminopeptidase that removes the arginine residue from Arg^0-Met^5-enkephalin has been reported to be present in bovine pituitary secretory granules (GAINER et al. 1984). This enzyme is a metallopeptidase with a pH optimum of 6. Although the enzyme removes basic N-terminal residues, the highest activity was reported for substrates containing N-terminal leucine residues (GAINER et al. 1984). However, these studies were performed on crude secretory granule homogenates, and it is not clear if a single activity cleaves substrates with both N-terminal leucine and arginine residues.

V. Amidation

Although there are only a few opioid peptides that are known to have amide groups on their C-termini, many other peptides undergo this modification (MAINS and EIPPER 1988; BRADBURY and SMYTH 1991). In all cases, the precursor contains a glycine immediately preceding the basic amino acids of the endopeptidase cleavage site. Following endopeptidase and carboxypeptidase action, the glycine residue is exposed on the C-terminus. This glycine is then converted into a NH_2 group by two enzymes. The first enzyme has been named peptidyl-α-amidating monooxygenase (PAM) (MAINS and EIPPER 1988). This enzyme uses molecular oxygen to hydroxylate the CH_2-group of the glycine residue, forming the α-hydroxyglycine intermediate. Ascorbate is a cofactor for this reaction. The second enzyme then facilitates the dissociation of the hydroxyglycine intermediate into glyoxylate and the amidated peptide (KATOPODIS et al. 1990). Several names for this enzyme have been proposed, including "α-hydroxyglycine amidating dealkylase" (KATOPODIS et al. 1990) and "peptidylhydroxyglycine N-C lyase" (BRADBURY and SMYTH 1991). This second step can occur at high pH without an enzyme, but at the acidic pH of the mature secretory granules the second enzyme is required. Most of the research has focussed on the first enzyme, which for many years was thought to be the only enzyme required for amidation.

The tissue distribution of PAM activity and mRNA is fairly broad (BRAAS et al. 1989). Detectable levels of PAM are found in most tissues, including those that are not known to produce amidated peptides. As with CPE, multiple forms of PAM activity are found in most tissues, including soluble and membrane-bound forms (MAY et al. 1988). In contrast to CPE, the membrane-binding region of PAM appears to be a conventional membrane-spanning hydrophobic region located near the C-terminus (EIPPER et al. 1987). The soluble forms of PAM are considerably smaller (30–40 kDa) than the membrane-bound form (approximately 90–110 kDa); the size of both varies between tissues and species (BRADBURY and SMYTH 1991).

The substrate specificity of PAM is consistent with the proposal that this one enzyme is involved with the modification of all peptides with C-terminal amide groups. Any peptide with a C-terminal glycine residue can serve as a substrate for PAM (BRADBURY and SMYTH 1991). Interestingly, synthetic peptides with a C-terminal D-alanine, but not L-alanine, are slowly amidated by PAM (LANDYMORE-LIM et al. 1983). The penultimate amino acid influences the rate of enzymatic activity, although this varies with pH (MAINS and EIPPER 1988).

The regulation of PAM activity and mRNA has been examined in several systems (MAINS and EIPPER 1988; BRADBURY and SYMTH 1991). Both PAM activity and mRNA are regulated by treatments that alter peptide production in cultured cells and in tissues. The magnitude of the changes in PAM levels generally correlate with the changes in peptide levels. This is surprising since PAM is not thought to be a rate-limiting enzyme for the production of amidated peptides.

VI. Acetylation

The N-terminal acetylation of peptides is not very common, and little is known regarding the enzymes responsible for this modification. Two POMC-derived peptides, α-MSH and β-endorphin, are acetylated in some tissues, but not in others. Whereas acetylation is necessary for the bioactivity of α-MSH, this modification destroys the opioid activity of β-endorphin (BRADBURY and SMYTH 1991). The acetylated form of β-endorphin is predominant in the intermediate lobe of the pituitary (SMYTH et al. 1979). Low levels of acetylated β-endorphin are detectable in the hypothalamus (ZAKARIAN and SMYTH 1982).

Several acetyl transferase activities have been described in anterior and intermediate pituitary (GLEMBOTSKI 1982). The enzyme activity present in secretory granules from the intermediate lobe of the pituitary is able to acetylate both ACTH and β-endorphin, which is consistent with the tissue distribution of these acetylated peptides. A cDNA clone was obtained from an expression library that was screened for acetyl transferase activity (EBERWINE et al. 1987). The enzyme encoded by the cDNA was capable of acetylating Leu-enkephalin, although it is not clear if this activity is physiologically involved with peptide acetylation, or if Leu-enkephalin is acetylated in vivo.

D. Extracellular Opioid Peptide Processing Enzymes

The classic view of neurotransmission is that the messenger molecules are produced inside the cell, and that, once secreted, all further processing destroys the biological activity. While this view still holds for classic neurotransmitters, such as acetylcholine, it is clearly not the case for bioactive peptides. Many of the processing steps that occur in the extracellular environment do not destroy all of the biological activities of the peptide. In some cases, extracellular processing of a peptide produces fragments that display lower affinity for one receptor, but greater affinity for another receptor (MOLINEAUX and WILK 1991).

Extracellular enzymes that have been proposed to be involved with the processing of opioid peptides into biologically active fragments include angiotensin converting enzyme, endopeptidase 24.15, a dynorphin converting enzyme present in spinal cord, and several other enzymes (MOLINEAUX and WILK 1991). Angiotensin converting enzyme is present in several opioid peptide-containing brain regions (STRITTMATTER and SNYDER 1987). This enzyme converts Met-enkephalin-Arg^6-Phe^7 into Met-enkephalin, and inhibitors of angiotensin converting enzyme are able to block this conversion in crude particulate fractions of rat brain (YANG et al. 1981). Endopeptidase 24.15 has been shown to process several precursors of Met- and Leu-enkephalin into the pentapeptides: examples include adrenorphin, Met-enkephalin-Arg^6-Gly^7-Leu^8, and several dynorphin-related peptides (CHU and ORLOWSKI 1985). An enzyme activity has been described in spinal cord that is able to convert dynorphin B-13 into Leu-enkephalin-Arg^6 (SILBERRING and NYBERG 1989). In all cases, these enzyme activities generate smaller peptides that bind to the various opiate receptors with affinities that are substantially different than the affinities of the larger peptides. These examples of extracellular processing are modulatory, rather than degradative.

References

Anderson RGW, Pathak RK (1985) Vesicles and cisternae in the trans Golgi apparatus of human fibroblasts are acidic compartments. Cell 40:635–643
Baker RK, Lively MO (1987) Purification and characterization of hen oviduct microsomal signal peptidase. Biochemistry 26:8561–8567
Benjannet S, Rondeau N, Day R, Chretien M, Seidah NG (1991) PC1 and PC2 are proprotein convertases capable of cleaving proopiomelanocortin at distinct pairs of basic residues. Proc Natl Acad Sci USA 88:3564–3568
Bennett HPJ (1991) Glycosylation, phosphorylation, and sulfation of peptide hormones and their precursors. In: Fricker LD (ed) Peptide biosynthesis and processing. CRC Press, Boca Raton
Bloomquist BT, Eipper BA, Mains RE (1991) Prohormone converting enzymes: regulation and evaluation of function using antisense RNA. Molec Endocrinol 5:2014–2024

Bondy CA, Whitnall MH, Brady LS (1989) Regulation of carboxypeptidase H gene expression in magnocellular neurons: response to osmotic stimulation. Mol Endocrinol 3:2086–2092

Bourdais J, Devilliers G, Girard R, Morel A, Bennedetti L, Cohen P (1990) Prosomatostatin II processing is initiated in the trans Golgi network of anglerfish pancreatic cells. Biochem Biophys Res Commun 170:1263–1272

Braas KM, Stoffers DA, Eipper BA, May V (1989) Tissue specific expression of rat peptidylglycine α-amidating monooxygenase activity and mRNA. Mol Endocrinol 89:1387–1398

Bradbury AF, Smyth DG (1991) Modification of the N- and C-termini of bioactive peptides: amidation and acetylation. In: Fricker LD (ed) Peptide biosynthesis and processing. CRC Press, Boca Raton

Camargo ACM, Oliveira EB, Toffoletto O, Metters KM, Rossier J (1987) Brain endo-oligopeptidase A, a putative enkephalin converting enzyme. J Neurochem 48:1258–1263

Chu TG, Orlowski M (1985) Soluble metalloendopeptidase from rat brain: action on enkephalin-containing peptides and other bioactive peptides. Endocrinology 116:1418–1425

Cromlish JA, Seidah NG, Chretien M (1986) A novel serine protease (IRCM-serine protease 1) from porcine neurointermediate and anterior pituitary lobes. J Biol Chem 261:859–867

Davidson HW, Hutton JC (1987) The insulin secretory granule carboxypeptidase H: purification and demonstration of involvement in proinsulin processing. Biochem J 245:575–582

Davidson HW, Rhodes CJ, Hutton JC (1988) Intraorganellar Ca^{2+} and pH control proinsulin cleavage in the pancreatic a cell via Arg-Arg and Lys-Arg specific endopeptidases. Nature 333:93–96

Devi L (1991) Peptide processing at monobasic sites. In: Fricker LD (ed) Peptide biosynthesis and processing. CRC Press, Boca Raton

Devi L, Goldstein A (1984) Dynorphin converting enzyme with unusual specificity from rat brain. Proc Natl Acad Sci USA 81:1892–1896

Devi L, Goldstein A (1986) Opioid and other peptides as inhibitors of leumorphin (dynorphin B-29) converting activity. Peptides 7:87–90

Devi L, Gupta P, Fricker LD (1991) Purification and characterization of a dynorphin processing endoprotease from bovine pituitary. J Neurochem 56:320–329

Docherty K, Rhodes CJ, Shennan KIJ, Taylor NA, Hutton JC (1989) Proinsulin endopeptidase substrate specificities defined by site directed mutagenesis of proinsulin. J Biol Chem 264:18335–18341

D'Souza NB, Lindberg I (1988) Evidence for the phosphorylation of a proenkephalin-derived peptide, peptide B. J Biol Chem 263:2548–2552

Eberwine JH, Barchas JD, Hewlett WA, Evans CJ (1987) Isolation of enzyme cDNA clones by enzyme immunodetection assay: isolation of a peptide acetyl-transferase. Proc Natl Acad Sci USA 84:1449–1453

Eipper BA, Mains RE (1980) Structure and biosynthesis of pro-adrenocorticotropin/ β-endorphin and related peptides. Endocr Rev 1:1–27.

Eipper BA, Park LP, Dickerson IM, Keutmann HT, Thiele EA, Rodriguez H, Schofield PR, Mains RE (1987) Structure of the precursor to an enzyme mediating COOH-terminal amidation in peptide biosynthesis. Mol Endocrinol 1:777–790

Fricker LD (1991) Peptide processing exopeptidases: amino- and carboxy-peptidases involved with peptide biosynthesis. In: Fricker LD (ed) Peptide biosynthesis and processing. CRC Press, Boca Raton

Fricker LD, Snyder SH (1983) Purification and characterization of enkephalin convertase, an enkephalin-synthesizing carboxypeptidase. J Biol Chem 258: 10950–10955

Fricker LD, Evans CJ, Esch FS, Herbert E (1986) Cloning and sequence analysis of cDNA for bovine carboxypeptidase E. Nature 323:461–464

Fricker LD, Das B, Angeletti RH (1990a) Identification of the pH-dependent membrane anchor of carboxypeptidase E (EC 3.4.17.10). J Biol Chem 265: 2476–2482

Fricker LD, Reaves BJ, Das B, Dannies PS (1990b) Comparison of the regulation of carboxypeptidase E and prolactin in GH_4C_1 cells, a rat pituitary cell line. Neuroendocrinology 51:658–663

Fricker LD, Rigual RJ, Diliberto EJ, Viveros OH (1990c) Reflex splanchnic nerve stimulation increases levels of carboxypeptidase E mRNA and enzymatic activity in the rat adrenal medulla. J Neurochem 55:461–467

Gainer H, Russell JT, Loh YP (1984) An aminopeptidase activity in bovine pituitary secretory vesicles that cleaves the N-terminal arginine from β-lipotropin 60–65. FEBS Lett 175:135–139

Glembotski CC (1982) Characterization of the peptide acetyltransferase activity in bovine and rat intermediate pituitaries responsible for the acetylation of β-endorphin and α-melanotropin. J Biol Chem 257:10501–10509

Hook VYH, LaGamma EF (1987) Product inhibition of carboxypeptidase H. J Biol Chem 262:12583–12588

Hook VYH, Eiden LE, Pruss RM (1985) Selective regulation of carboxypeptidase peptide hormone-processing enzyme during enkephalin biosynthesis in cultured bovine adrenomedullary chromaffin cells. J Biol Chem 260:5991–5997

Huttner WB (1988) Tyrosine sulfation and the secretory pathway. Annu Rev Physiol 50:363–376

Julius D, Brake A, Blair L, Kunisawa R, Thorner J (1984) Isolation of the putative structural gene for the lysine-arginine-cleaving endopeptidase required for processing of yeast prepro-α-factor. Cell 37:1075–1089

Jung YK, Kunczt CJ, Pearson RK, Dixon JE, Fricker LD (1991) Structural characterization of the rat carboxypeptidase E gene. Molec Endocrinol 5:1257–1268

Katopodis AG, Ping D, May SW (1990) A novel enzyme from bovine neurointermediate pituitary catalyzes dealkylation of α-hydroxyglycine derivatives, thereby functioning sequentially with peptidylglycine α-amidating monooxygenase in peptide action. Biochemistry 29:6115–6120

Landymore-Lim A, Bradbury AF, Smyth DG (1983) The amidating enzyme in pituitary will accept a peptide with C-terminal D-alanine as substrate. Biochem Biophys Res Commun 117:289–293

Laslop A, Fischer-Colbrie R, Kirschke H, Angeletti RH, Winkler H (1990) Chromogranin A-processing proteases in purified chromaffin granules – contaminant or endogenous enzymes? Biochim Biophys Acta 1033:65–72

Leduc R, Thorne B, Thomas L, Smeekens S, Steiner D, Thomas G (1990) POMC is cleaved in vivo by two mammalian proteases structurally related to the yeast Kex2 endoprotease. J Cell Biol 111:1873–1903

Lindberg I, Hutton JC (1991) Peptide processing proteinases with selectivity for paired basic residues. In: Fricker LD (ed) Peptide biosynthesis and processing. CRC Press, Boca Raton

Lindberg I, Thomas G (1990) Cleavage of proenkephalin by a chromaffin granule processing enzyme. Endocrinology 126:480–487

Lindberg I, Yang H-YT, Costa E (1982) An enkephalin-generating enzyme in bovine adrenal medulla. Biochem Biophys Res Commun 106:186–193

Lively MO, Walsh KA (1983) Hen oviduct signal peptidase is an integral membrane protein. J Biol Chem 258:9488–9495

Loh YP, Gainer H (1982) Characterization of pro-opiocortin-converting activity in purified secretory granules from rat pituitary neurointermediate lobe. Proc Natl Acad Sci USA 79:108–112

Loh YP, Parish DC, Tuteja R (1985) Purification and characterization of a paired basic residue-specific pro-opiomelanocortin converting enzyme from bovine pituitary intermediate lobe secretory vesicles. J Biol Chem 260:7194–7205

Mains RE, Eipper BA (1984) Secretion and regulation of two biosynthetic enzyme activities, peptidyl-glycine alpha-amidating monooxygenase and a carboxypeptidase, by mouse pituitary corticotropic tumor cells. Endocrinology 115: 1683–1690

Mains RE, Eipper BA (1988) Peptide α-amidation. Annu Rev Physiol 50:333–344

May V, Cullen EI, Braas KM, Eipper BA (1988) Membrane-associated forms of peptidylglycine α-amidating monooxygenase activity in rat pituitary. J Biol Chem 262:7550–7554

Molineaux CJ, Wilk S (1991) Extracellular processing of neuropeptides. In: Fricker LD (ed) Peptide biosynthesis and processing. CRC Press, Boca Raton

Oliveira ES, Leite PEP, Spillantini MG, Camargo ACM, Hunt SP (1990) Localization of endo-oligopeptidase (EC 3.4.22.19) in the rat nervous tissue. J Neurochem 55:1114–1121

Orci L, Ravazzola M, Amherdt M, Madsen O, Perrelet A, Vassalli J-D, Anderson RGW (1986) Conversion of proinsulin to insulin occurs coordinately with acidification of maturing secretory vesicles. J Cell Biol 103:2273–2281

Parish DC, Tuteja R, Altstein M, Gainer H, Loh YP (1986) Purification and characterization of a paired basic residue specific prohormone converting enzyme from bovine pituitary neural lobe secretory vesicles. J Biol Chem 261: 14393–14398

Paulson JC, Colley KJ (1989) Glycosyltransferases: structure, localization, and control of cell type-specific glycosylation. J Biol Chem 264:17615–17618

Roebroek AJM, Schalken JA, Leunissen JAM, Onnekink C, Bloemers HPJ, van de Ven WMJ (1986) Evolutionary conserved close linkage of the c-*fes/fps* proto-oncogene and genetic sequences encoding a receptor-like protein. EMBO J 5:2197–2202

Schnabel E, Mains RE, Farquhar MG (1989) Proteolytic processing of pro-ACTH/endorphin begins in the Golgi complex of pituitary corticotropes and AtT-20 cells. Mol Endocrinol 3:1223–1235

Seidah NG, Paquin J, Hamelin J, Benjannet S, Chretien M (1988) Structural and immunological homology of human and porcine pituitary and plasma IRCM-serine protease 1 to plasma kallikrein: marked selectivity for pairs of basic residues suggests a widespread role in pro-hormone and pro-enzyme processing. Biochimie 70:33–46

Seidah NG, Gaspar L, Mion P, Marcinkiewics M, Mbikay M, Chretien M (1990) cDNA sequence of two distinct pituitary proteins homologous to Kex2 and furin gene products: tissue-specific mRNAs encoding candidates for pro-hormone processing proteinases. DNA Cell Biol 9:415–424

Shen FS, Roberts SF, Lindberg I (1989) A putative processing enzyme for proenkephalin in bovine adrenal chromaffin granule membranes. J Biol Chem 264:15600–15605

Shields D (1991) Signals for intracellular protein sorting: implications for peptide hormone precursor processing and secretion. In: Fricker LD (ed) Peptide biosynthesis and processing. CRC Press, Boca Raton

Silberring J, Nyberg F (1989) A novel bovine spinal cord endoprotease with high specificity for dynorphin B. J Biol Chem 264:11082–11086

Smeekens SP, Steiner DF (1990) Identification of a human insulinoma cDNA encoding a novel mammalian protein structurally related to the yeast dibasic processing protease Kex2. J Biol Chem 265:2997–3000

Smyth DG, Massey DE, Zakarian S, Finnie MDA (1979) Endorphins are stored in active and inactive forms; isolation of α-N-acetyl peptides. Nature 279:252–254

Smyth DG, Maruthainar K, Darby NJ, Fricker LD (1989) C-terminal processing of neuropeptides: involvement of carboxypeptidase H. J Neurochem 53:489–493

Steiner DF (1991) The biosynthesis of biologically active peptides: a perspective. In: Fricker LD (ed) Peptide biosynthesis and processing. CRC Press, Boca Raton

Strittmatter SM, Snyder SH (1987) Angiotensin converting enzyme immunohisto-chemistry in rat brain and pituitary gland: correlation of isozyme type with cellular localization. Neuroscience 21:407–420

Strittmatter SM, Lynch DR, De Souza EB, Snyder SH (1985) Enkephalin convertase demonstrated in the pituitary and adrenal gland by [3H]guanidinoethylmer-captosuccinic acid autoradiography: dehydration decreases neurohypophyseal levels. Endocrinology 117:1667–1674

Supattapone S, Fricker LD, Snyder SH (1984) Purification and characterization of a membrane-bound enkephalin-forming carboxypeptidase, "enkephalin con-vertase". J Neurochem 42:1017–1023

Supattapone S, Strittmatter SM, Fricker LD, Snyder SH (1988) Characterization of a neutral, divalent cation-sensitive endopeptidase: a possible role in neuropeptide processing. Mol Brain Res 3:173–182

Taljanidisz J, Stewart L, Smith AJ, Klinman JP (1990) Structure of bovine adrenal dopamine beta-monooxygenase, as deduced from cDNA and protein sequencing: evidence that the membrane-bound form of the enzyme is anchored by an uncleaved signal peptide. Biochemistry 28:10054–10061

Thomas G, Thorne BA, Thomas L, Allen RG, Hruby DE, Fuller R, Thorner J (1988) Yeast Kex2 endopeptidase correctly cleaves a neuroendocrine pro-hormone in mammalian cells. Science 241:226–229

Unsworth CD, Hughes J (1982) O-sulphates leu-enkephalin in brain. Nature 295: 519–522

Von Heijne G (1985) Signal sequences: the limits of variation. J Mol Biol 184: 99–105

Watkinson A, Dockray GJ, Young J (1988) N-linked glycosylation of a pro-enkephalin A-derived peptide. J Biol Chem 263:7141–7147

Yang H-YT, Majane E, Costa E (1981) Conversion of [Met5]-enkephalin-Arg6-Phe7 to [Met5]-enkephalin by dipeptidyl carboxypeptidase. Neuropharmacology 20: 891–894

Zakarian S, Smyth DG (1982) β-Endorphin is processed differently in specific regions of rat pituitary and brain. Nature 296:250–252

Peptidase Inactivation of Enkephalins: Design of Inhibitors and Biochemical, Pharmacological, and Clinical Applications

B.P. Roques, A. Beaumont, V. Daugé, and M.-C. Fournié-Zaluski

A. Introduction

Because of their critical role in various adaptational processes, extensive pharmacological studies have been devoted to the neuropeptides, a family of chemical messengers acting in the central nervous system as neuro-transmitters and/or neuromodulators. This is particularly true for the opioid peptides, which are involved in the control of pain and modulation of mood through their interaction with different classes of binding sites.

In contrast to the amine and amino acid transmitters, which are mainly removed from the extracellular space by reuptake mechanisms, the message conveyed by neuropeptides (such as the enkephalins) appears to be inter-rupted by peptidases which cleave the biologically active peptide into inactive fragments, although a role for putative peptidergic autoreceptors (Ueda et al. 1986) cannot be completely excluded. This was clearly demon-strated for the enkephalins with the characterization of a discretely dis-tributed "enkephalinase" (Malfroy et al. 1978) in brain regions enriched in opioid receptors (Waksman et al. 1986) and enkephalins and by the demonstration of naloxone-reversible antinociceptive responses elicited by inhibitors of this enzyme, such as thiorphan (Roques et al. 1980). Amino-peptidases, especially aminopeptidase-N (APN), have also been shown to be critically involved in enkephalin inactivation (Hambrook et al. 1976; Pert et al. 1976).

The demonstration that "enkephalinase" was identical to the neutral endopeptidase-24.11 (NEP), purified from rabbit kidney (Kerr and Kenny 1974) and subsequently found in many other tissues, argued against the existence of specific "neuropeptidases" (Schwartz 1983; Kenny 1986). It now appears that in both nervous and peripheral tissue peptides are degraded extracellularly by a limited number of ectoenzymes with relatively broad specificities, a great number of them belonging to the group of Zn-metallopeptidases (review in Kenny et al. 1987). Peripheral NEP, for example, has been clearly shown to be involved in the inactivation of the atrial natriuretic peptide (review in Roques and Beaumont 1990). However, in spite of the wide distribution of NEP, the "opioid" activity of thiorphan has initiated numerous studies to investigate the reasonable assumption that inhibitors of enkephalin degradation produce their physiological effects by increasing the extracellular levels of endogenous opioid peptides, released either tonically or following stimuli-evoked depolarization. Under these conditions, the effects of the inhibitors will depend upon: (1) the magnitude and duration of the enkephalin release evoked by a particular stimulus, which probably varies in the different enkephalinergic pathways, and (2) the efficiency of the inhibition (selective inhibition of NEP or APN or inhibition of both). The relative occupancy of μ- and δ-receptors and the associated pharmacological responses will therefore be modulated by the levels of extracellular opioid peptides and by the local concentrations of opioid receptors (review in ROQUES et al. 1991). It was hoped that increasing the levels of endogenous opioid peptides, by inhibiting their inactivating enzymes, would eliminate or minimize serious drawbacks inasmuch as they could be related to an overstimulation of tonically or phasically activated opioid receptors in all brain areas.

This chapter is devoted to the molecular biology and structural characterization of NEP and APN, the design of either selective or mixed inhibitors, their in vivo actions, and various possible clinical applications such as new analgesics, antidepressants, or antihypertensive drugs (reviews in DICKENSON 1985; ROQUES and FOURNIE-ZALUSKI 1985, 1986; SCHWARTZ et al. 1985; CHIPKIN 1986; ROQUES and BEAUMONT 1990).

B. Enkephalin Degrading Enzymes

I. Metabolism of Opioid Peptides

Early studies on the enkephalins showed that they had a very short half-life in both in vivo and in vitro preparations. Complete disappearance of [³H]Leu-enkephalin, with the concomitant appearance of [³H]Tyr, was shown to take place within 1 min at 37°C when the peptide was incubated with rat brain membranes or plasma (HAMBROOK et al. 1976; VOGEL and ALTSTEIN 1977; DUPONT et al. 1977) and [³H]Tyr was found to be the main metabolite after intracerebroventricular injection (i.c.v.) of [³H]Leu-enkephalin (MEEK et al. 1977). An additional fragment was identified as Tyr-Gly-Gly after in vivo (CRAVES et al. 1978) and in vitro (MALFROY et al. 1978) studies whereas Tyr-Gly appeared as a minor metabolite. These results accounted for the weak and transient analgesia obtained only with high doses (0.1 mg) of i.c.v. administered Met-enkephalin in mice (BELLUZI et al. 1976) and the higher potency of enkephalin analogues protected from peptidase inactivation by replacement of Gly² by an amino acid with a D-configuration, amidation or reduction of the free carboxyl group, N-methylation of the Gly³-Phe⁴ bond, or replacement of Phe⁴ by its D-isomer (PERT et al. 1976; FOURNIE-ZALUSKI et al. 1979). Owing to the inability of enkephalins to enter the cells, the presence of Tyr, Tyr-Gly-Gly, and Tyr-Gly following i.c.v. administration of Leu-enkephalin supported the occurrence of aminopeptidase, dipeptidylaminopeptidase, and peptidyldipeptidase activities located at the cell surface and acting therefore as ectoenzymes; studies were therefore carried out to purify and characterize these peptidases. A Tyr-Gly-Gly-releasing enzyme was detected in rat striatal membranes and designated "enkephalinase" (MALFROY et al. 1978), and its presence in brain was confirmed by SULLIVAN et al. (1978). In addition it was shown that the tripeptide was not produced by the sequential action of a carboxypeptidase (GUYON et al. 1979). Although the K_m of the enkephalins for "enkephalinase" was subsequently shown to be higher ($\sim 20\,\mu M$) (GORESTEIN and SNYDER 1979; FOURNIE-ZALUSKI et al. 1979; GUYON et al. 1979) than previously thought ($\sim 90\,nM$) (MALFROY et al. 1978), the physiological relevance of the enzyme in enkephalin metabolism was firmly established by the naloxone-reversible antinociceptive properties elicited by the synthetic inhibitor thiorphan (ROQUES et al. 1980).

The Zn-metallopeptidase angiotensin-converting enzyme (ACE) was also found to cleave the Gly^3-Phe^4 bond of the enkephalins (ERDÖS et al. 1978) and although initially suggested to be identical (SWERTS et al. 1979; BENUCK and MARK 1979), "enkephalinase" and ACE were shown to correspond to two distinct enzymes and the enkephalins were found to have a low affinity for ACE ($K_m \sim 10^{-3}\,M$), excluding a major role for this enzyme in their in vivo metabolism. Enkephalinase was in fact shown to be neutral endopeptidase 24.11 (NEP) (RELTON et al. 1983; MATSAS et al. 1983), an already well-characterized Zn-metallopeptidase, known to be present in the brush border cells of the proximal tubes of the kidney (KERR and KENNY 1974). Subsequently NEP was also shown to be identical to the common acute lymphoblastic leukemia antigen (CALLA) expressed transiently at the surface of lymphohematopoietic cells (review in LEBIEN and McCORMACK 1989).

Due to their rather homogeneous distribution, a physiological role for aminopeptidases as enkephalin-metabolizing enzymes was initially questioned (SCHWARTZ et al. 1981). Nevertheless, two aminopeptidases, differing by their sensitivity to the natural inhibitors puromycin and bestatin, were purified (HERSH 1981; HUI et al. 1983), both capable of cutting the Tyr^1-Gly^2 bond of enkephalins. Bestatin, but not puromycin however, was shown to potentiate the analgesic effect of i.c.v. injected Met-enkephalin (CARENZI et al. 1981) and the membrane-bound bestatin-sensitive aminopeptidase was finally shown to be identical to aminopeptidase-N (APN) by using antibodies directed toward the kidney enzyme (MATSAS et al. 1985; GROS et al. 1985). The preferential involvement of APN in the physiological inactivation of enkephalins was demonstrated by the increased analgesic potency of inhibitors more selective toward APN than bestatin (WAKSMAN et al. 1985). A membrane-bound dipeptidyl aminopeptidase (DAP), able to cleave the Gly^2-Gly^3 bond of the enkephalins, was also identified in rat brain (GORENSTEIN and SNYDER 1979). Pig kidney DAP was purified to characterize its active site and to design specific inhibitors (CHÉROT et al. 1986a,b), which suggested a minor role of this enzyme in in vivo enkephalin in-activation. Interestingly, all the enzymes susceptible to participation in enkephalin degradation belong to the group of Zn-metallopeptidase, offering the possibility of designing mixed inhibitors able to completely block enkephalin metabolism.

II. Substrate Specificity of NEP and APN

Neutral endopeptidase-24.11, like the bacterial Zn-endopeptidase ther-molysin (TLN), preferentially cleaves peptides on the amino size of hydro-phobic residues such as Phe, Met, and Leu (Kerr and Kenny 1974), suggesting the occurrence of a lipophilic S_1' subsite similar to that found in TLN.

Neutral endopeptidase-24.11 has a broad selectivity and can cleave various short linear or cyclic peptides as well as polypeptides of intermediate or large length such as insulin-B chain (~3000 daltons) (Kerr and Kenny 1974) or interleukin IL-α1 (17000 daltons) (Pierart et al. 1988), although it sometimes acts more efficiently as a dipeptidylcarboxypeptidase than as a true endopeptidase. This was interpreted as being due to a favorable ionic interaction between the free C-terminal carboxyl group of Leu-enkephalin and a well-positioned, positively charged amino acid in the active site (Fournié-Zaluski et al. 1979, 1981), leading NEP to be considered as more closely structurally related to a carboxypeptidase than to an endopeptidase (Malfroy and Schwartz 1982; Herch and Morihara 1986). However, the enzyme also behaves as a very efficient endopeptidase cleaving in vitro peptides such as substance P (SP) and neurokinins (Matsas et al. 1983), gastrin and cholecystokinin (CCK_8) (Matsas et al. 1984; Zuzel et al. 1985; Durieux et al. 1985, 1986), neurotensin (Checler et al. 1983), Met-enkephalin-Arg-Phe, and the cyclic atrial natriuretic peptide SLRRSSCFGGRMDRIGAQSGLGCNSFRY (ANP) at the Cys^7-Phe^8 bond (review in Stephenson and Kenny 1987). The chemotactic peptide fMet-Leu-Phe has also been shown to be hydrolyzed by NEP (review in Erdös and Skidgel 1989). It is interesting to observe that TLN is also able to cleave the enkephalins and ANP at the same bonds as NEP (unpublished results) and that the TLN inhibitor phosphoramidon also behaves as a good NEP inhibitor, emphasizing the close correspondence between the active sites of these two peptidases.

Like NEP, with which it is often found colocalized, the membrane-bound APN also has a broad specificity (reviews in Thorsett and Wyvratt 1987; Rich 1990) although hydrophobic residues, preferentially aromatic, in the N-terminal position are more rapidly removed. Moreover the S_1' and S_2' subsites of APN also seem to prefer hydrophobic residues (Hernandez et al. 1988; Xie et al. 1989a,b). Apart from the enkephalins and Met-enkephalin-Arg-Phe, NEP and to a lesser degree APN show little activity toward other opioid peptides. Thus, probably for conformational reasons, dynorphin 1-9, 1-13, α- and β-neo-endorphin, and β-endorphin are poor substrates. This indicates that the "opioid" effects induced by NEP and NEP/APN inhibitors are mainly due to the protection of the two endogenous enkephalins and perhaps partially to that of the extended heptapeptide Met-enkephalin-Arg-Phe.

The possible involvement of NEP in the degradation of a peptide in a crude tissue preparation, contaminated by other peptidases, is usually demonstrated by using either thiorphan or phosphoramidon as selective inhibitors. Nevertheless, this does not necessarily mean that the peptidase is responsible for its metabolism in vivo. Thiorphan for example has little effect on the in vivo degradation of spinal SP (YAKSH and CHIPKIN 1989) or CCK_8 released from striatum (BUTCHER et al. 1989) in spite of the presence of NEP in these tissues.

III. Assays of NEP and APN Activities

Current methods for studying the kinetic properties of NEP include measuring the tripeptide fragments [³H]Tyr-Gly-Gly or [³H]Tyr-D-Ala-Gly formed by cleavage of the Gly-Phe bond of [³H]Leu-enkephalin or [³H]D-Ala²-Leu-enkephalin, respectively (VOGEL and ALTSTEIN 1977; LLORENS et al. 1982). [³H]Leu-enkephalin is also currently used to study APN activity. Internally quenched fluorogenic substrates such as the NEP-selective, commercially available Dansyl-D-Ala-Gly-Phe(pNO_2)-Gly (DAGNPG) (FLORENTIN et al. 1984) allow continuous recording of NEP activity. Activity can also be detected using a two-step reaction catalyzed sequentially by NEP and APN. The substrate Bz-Gly-Arg-Arg-Leu-2NA (2-NA = 2-naphtylamine) is cleaved by NEP at the Arg-Leu bond, leading, after addition of APN, to the formation of the 2-NA by removal of the N-terminal Leu-amino-acid. The 2-Na can then be quantified by fluorescence after diazotation (ALMENOFF and ORLOWSKI 1984). The recently developped highly potent ($K_I \sim 3^{-11}$ M) radiolabeled NEP inhibitor [¹²⁵I] RB104 allows NEP to be quantified directly after gel electrophoresis (FOURNIÉ-ZALUSKI et al. 1992).

C. Structure and Molecular Biology of NEP

I. Structure of NEP

The primary structure of NEP, cloned from rabbit kidney (DEVAULT et al. 1987), consists of 749 amino acids and contains 5 glycosylation sites and 12 cysteine residues involved in disulfide bridges. NEP has a short N-terminal cytoplasmic domain (27 amino acids), followed by a 23-residue hydrophobic domain, anchoring the protein in the plasma membrane, and a large extracellular domain containing the active site. The rat kidney and

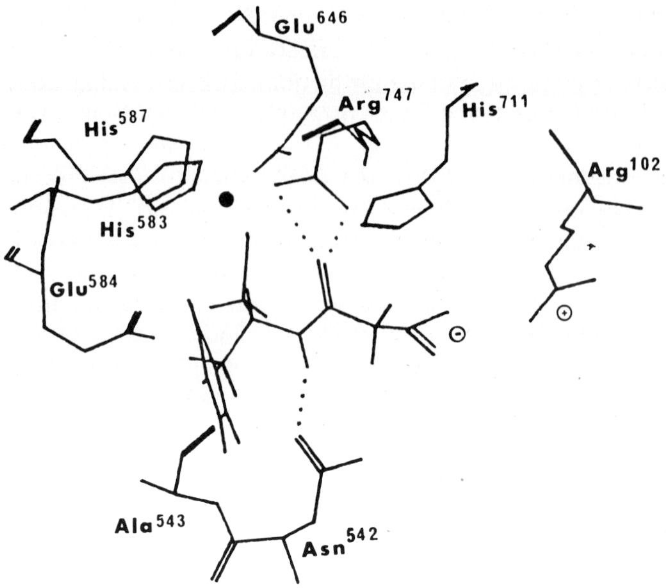

Fig. 1. Active site of endopeptidase 24.11, derived from that of the bacterial Zn metalloendopeptidase thermolysin. The NEP inhibitor thiorphan is schematically located inside the active site

brain or human placenta enzyme have more than 90% homology with the rabbit enzyme (MALFROY et al. 1987). NEP contains a consensus sequence [508]VxxHExxH[587], also found in the catalytic site of numerous other Zn endopeptidases including TLN, human collagenase, human ACE, and the exopeptidase APN, but not in the Zn carboxypeptidases so far sequenced (JONGENEEL et al. 1989). In TLN the two histidines are Zn-binding residues and the glutamate plays a role in catalysis by polarizing a water molecule. The assignment and the role of these and other putative active site residues of NEP has been tested by site-directed mutagenesis and expression of the recombinant enzyme at the cell surface of COS-1 cells (DEVAULT et al. 1988). Thus replacing Glu[584] by Asp[584] did not change the affinity of the inhibitor [^{3}H]HACBO-Gly but abolished the enzymatic properties of the mutated NEP, showing that shortening the side chain of Glu[584] by a single methylene group is sufficient to suppress the polarization of the water molecule. In addition, replacement of Arg[102] or Arg[747] or both indicates that they could both play a role in substrate binding. Arg[102] interacting with the free carboxyl group of the P_2' residue of some substrates, and Arg[747] with the carbonyl amide group of the P_1' residue. The localization of these two arginines could explain why NEP has both endopeptidase and dipeptidylcarboxypeptidase activities (BEAUMONT et al. 1991; BATEMAN et al. 1989). The model of the NEP active-site derived from these findings (Fig. 1) emphasizes the previously proposed close correspondence between TLN and NEP regarding the location and function of amino acids crucially involved in binding and substrate hydrolysis (ROQUES et al. 1983; ROQUES and FOURNIE-ZALUSKI 1986; RODERICK et al. 1989). Recombinant, fully active soluble NEP has also been obtained (DEVAULT et al. 1988) and could be used as a pharmacological tool (KOROGI et al. 1989) or for crystallization studies. APN has also been cloned from different tissue sources (OLSEN et al. 1988) and has large sequence homologies. Interestingly, this exopeptidase also possesses the consensus sequence VxxHExxH, suggesting that, in some aspects, the active site structure and mechanism of action of APN may be closer to a Zn endopeptidase than to that of classical exopeptidases (HÉLÈNE et al. 1991).

II. Human NEP (CALLA) Gene

The human NEP/CALLA gene spans more than 80 kilobases and contains 24 mini-exons. NEP gene transcription could be controlled by alternative splicing of a common or distinct pre-mRNAs leading of differentially controlled gene expression in a tissue-specific and/or developmentally regulated manner (D'ADAMIO et al. 1989). The NEP gene has been shown to be located on human chromosome 3, which also encodes somatostatin, transferrin and its receptor, enzymes such as acetylcholinesterase and β galactosidase, and the oncogenes c-raf-1 and c-erb-A-B. As the gene for human APN has been located on chromosome 15q 13q ter (KRUSE et al. 1988) and that of another ectoenzyme, γ-glutamyl transpeptidase, is on chromosome 22, it appears that the genes of these ectoenzymes are not under a common regulatory DNA control (KRUSE et al. 1988).

D. Localization of Neutral Endopeptidase 24.11

I. Central Nervous System

The first precise localization of NEP in the CNS was obtained by quantitative autoradiography using the tritiated inhibitor [^{3}H]HACBO-Gly (WAKSMAN et al. 1984, 1986, 1987). NEP was found to be discretely distributed in rat brain: choroid plexus, substantia nigra, caudate putamen, globus pallidus, olfactory tubercle, nucleus accumbens, the substantia gelatinosa of the spinal cord, the amygdala, the periaqueductal gray matter, the hippocampus, and more generally in regions known to correspond to sites of morphine actions. A relatively good correspondence was found between the distribution of the enzyme, the opioid receptors (WAKSMAN et al. 1986), and the enkephalins (POLLARD et al. 1989). High levels of NEP has been found in the choroid plexus. Large amounts of NEP, ACE, and aminopeptidases have also been detected in the meninges of rat and human spinal cord, where they could maintain the homeostatic concentration of neuropeptides in the central nervous system (Zajac et al. 1987). Similar NEP localizations were observed in the pig central nervous system using a polyclonal antibody and immunoperoxidase staining (Matsas et al. 1986) and in rat brain using a [125I]iodinated monoclonal antibody (Pollard et al. 1989) or a fluorescent histochemical method (Back and Gorenstein 1989). In human brain a high density of NEP, overlapping that of μ- and δ-opioid receptors, was found in the caudate putamen, globus pallidus, substantia nigra, and substantia gelatinosa, whereas lower levels were found in the periaqueductal gray and cortical layers (Zajac and Roques 1989). In the fetus, NEP and μ- and δ-opioid receptors have been shown to appear in the superficial layer of the dorsal horn at an early stage of development (14 weeks) (Sales et al. 1989), suggesting a possible role in developmental activity. Initially thought to be present on glial cells and not on neurons from studies with cultured cells (Horsthemke et al. 1983), the neuronal localization of neutral endopeptidase 24.11 in brain was demonstrated by the time-dependent large reduction in striatal [3H]HACBO-Gly binding following local injection of kainic acid (Waksman et al. 1987). The associated distant and large decrease in NEP (70%) and in μ- and δ (50%)-binding sites in the globus pallidus and substantia nigra support a major presynaptic localization of NEP and opioid receptors, possibly on the major opioidergic pathway connecting the neostriatum to the pallidum (Del Fiacco et al. 1982) and on striatonigral projection containing GABA or SP and/or dynorphin (Cuello 1983). In contrast to μ- and δ-opioid receptors, 6-OHDA-induced lesions of the DA nigrostriatal or mesolimbic pathways did not induce any significant changes in NEP labeling (Waksman et al. 1987), although a decrease in NEP activity after this treatment was initially reported (Malfroy et al. 1979). A large depletion in both NEP and opioid receptors has been observed in the caudate putamen, globus pallidus, and substantia nigra in Huntington's disease, which is characterized by a severe loss of neurons (Zajac and Roques 1989) but not in Parkinson's disease (Delay-Goyet et al. 1987).

In rats, unilateral dorsal root rhizotomy produced a 60%–70% decrease in μ- and δ-opioid receptors, whereas NEP levels were unaltered (Zajac et al. 1989). This indicates that, unlike NEP, most of the opioid μ- and δ-binding sites are presynaptically located on afferent fibers. Accordingly, the enkephalin action revealed by iontophoretic (Morton et al. 1987) or intrathecal (Dickenson et al. 1987, 1988; Sullivan et al. 1989) infusion of kelatorphan could be both postsynaptic, by hyperpolarization of the target neurons via an increased potassium conductance (Yoshimura and North 1983), and presynaptic, by regulation of the release of other messengers especially peptides such as SP, CCK, and calcitonin gene-releasing peptide, from afferent terminals (Jessel and Yversen 1977).

An electron microscopic study also supports a neuronal localization for the enzyme in the globus pallidus (Barnes et al. 1988) and showed that NEP is not strictly synaptosomal, in agreement with its distribution all along the nigrostriatal pathway (WAKSMAN et al. 1986), suggesting that endogenous opioid peptides, sparsely localized at the synaptic level (COULTER 1988), primarily act nonjunctionally on the plasma membranes of dendrites, axons, and probably perikarya of neurons, where the majority of opioid receptors are found (HAMEL and BEAUDET 1987). NEP could also be present on oligodendrocytes and on Schwann cells in the peripheral nervous system (MATSAS et al. 1986). APN in the brain appears to be mainly located on microvessels (HERSH et al. 1987; SOLHONNE et al. 1987). In contrast to the kidney (unpublished results) and except for the striatum (WILCOX et al. 1989), the brain levels of NEP mRNA in rats were found to be low, even in regions (choroid plexus) rich in enzyme activity. The lack of a direct relationship between the amount of NEP expressed at the cell surface and the levels of its mRNA would suggest tissue-specific regulation of the multi-exon NEP gene.

II. Localization of NEP in Peripheral Tissues

As shown using an enzymatic assay (LLORENS and SCHWARTZ 1981), immunological methods (GEE et al. 1985; RONCO et al. 1988), or in vivo binding studies (ROQUES and BEAUMONT 1990), NEP is largely distributed in peripheral organs: brush border epithelial cells of intestine and kidney, prostate, lymph nodes, placenta, lung, testis, fibroblast neutrophils, exocrine glands, and various epithelial and endocrine cells (review in KENNY et al. 1987) and in the bones including the marrow and the joint, suggesting multiple possible physiological functions for this peptidase (review in SALES et al. 1991). The transient, high expression of NEP on pre-B cells suggests a role for the enzyme in hematopoieisis. As NEP generally seems to function as an inactivating enzyme, this could be to temporarily protect the developing cell from a peptidergic signal, although an activation process cannot be ruled out. Low levels of NEP have also been found on some normal B and T cells and macrophages (BEAUMONT et al. 1989). Recently [^{125}I]RB104 has been used to show the presence of NEP in the endothelium of vascular tissue (SOLEILHAC et al. 1992).

III. In Vitro and In Vivo Studies of Enkephalin Degradation by NEP and APN

The protection of exogenous or endogenous opioid peptides has been studied using slices of brain (PATEY et al. 1981; ALTSTEIN et al. 1983; WILLIAMS et al. 1987; WAKSMAN et al. 1985; MAUBORGNE et al. 1987a) or spinal cord (BOURGOIN et al. 1986), from which the enkephalins can be released by depolarization and the metabolites measured in the superfusion medium. Under these conditions, the NEP inhibitor thiorphan was found to reduce the formation of [^{3}H]Tyr-Gly-Gly but enhance [^{3}H]Tyr levels formed from exogenously added [^{3}H]Met-enkephalin whereas the opposite effect was observed with the APN inhibitor bestatin, showing that a blockade of both enzymes by a mixed NEP/APN inhibitor such as kelatorphan is required to obtain a major increase in the extracellular level of exogenous (WAKSMAN et al. 1985) or endogenous enkephalins (BOURGOIN et al. 1986).

Nociceptive stimuli have been shown to enhance Met-enkephalin levels in the spinal cord (CESSELIN et al. 1982). When the spontaneous outflow of endogenous Met-enkephalin was measured, in the CSF of halothane-anesthetized rat, there was a twofold better recovery in the presence of kelatorphan and a fivefold enhancement during noxious stimulation (muzzle pinching), with no apparent change in the release process itself. Similar results were obtained with a carboxyl-containing inhibitor (OSHITA et al. 1990). Kelatorphan-induced elevated levels of endogenous enkephalins in the extracellular domain were shown to stimulate δ-opioid receptors and thus increase brain CCK_8 overflow (CESSELIN et al. 1989; RUIZ-GAYO et al. 1992) or reduce SP release from substantia nigra or spinal cord (MAUBORGNE et al. 1987b). The reduction in spinal SP could explain the strong antinociceptive effects of kelatorphan or δ-agonists and their dissociation from those resulting from μ-receptor activation (DICKENSON et al. 1988; PORRECA et al. 1984; ROQUES 1990).

A direct demonstration of the increase in "synaptic" levels of enkephalins following protection of endogenous enkephalins was recently shown by in vivo maximum inhibition (~60%) of [3H]DAGO binding following to i.c.v. coinjection of the tritiated μ-agonist with the mixed inhibitor RB38A (MEUCCI et al. 1989). Moreover, the inhibitor RB101 (Sect. E.VII) blocked 15% of [^{3}H]diprenorphine binding after i.v. injection in normal mouse and about 32% in stressed animals (RUIZ-GAYO et al. 1992). Changes in enkephalin release induced by noxious stimuli and the effects of inhibitors have also been studied by measuring, by radioimmunoassay, the turnover rate of Tyr-Gly-Gly, expected to reflect the activity of enkephalinergic neurons (LLORENS-CORTES et al. 1985). This yielded results generally similar to those obtained by measuring Met-enkephalin levels in the spinal cord (BOURGOIN et al. 1986) although there were some apparent discrepancies between the low changes in spinal Tyr-Gly-Gly and Met-E levels induced by i.v. acetorphan and carbaphethiol (LLORENS-CORTES et al. 1989) and the tenfold increase in spinal enkephalins induced by oral administration of SCH-34,826 or thiorphan (YAKSH and CHIPKIN 1989).

E. Inhibitor Design and Synthesis

I. Design of Selective and Mixed Inhibitors of Neutral Endopeptidase 24.11 and Aminopeptidase N

As shown from the crystallographic analysis of carboxypeptidase A (CPA) and TLN, all the Zn metalloproteases have similarities in their active sites and in their respective mechanisms of action (review in Matthews 1988). Schematically, the hydrolysis of a peptide bond by these enzymes involves: (1) the coordination of the oxygen of the scissile bond to the Zn atom; (2) a glutamate-promoted nucleophic attack by a water molecule on the carbonyl carbon polarized by the Zn ion; (3) the protonation of the nitrogen of the peptide bond to be cleaved, leading to a breakdown of the weakened linkage betweeen the tetrahedral carbon and the protonated nitrogen atoms, with subsequent release of the two peptide fragments.

The specificity of the Zn metallopeptidases is essentially ensured by Van der Waals and ionic interactions between their S_2, S_1, S_1', and S_2' subsites and the lateral chains of the corresponding P_2, P_1, P_1', and P_2' moieties of the substrate (defined using the nomenclature of Schechter and Berger 1967), and several well-positioned hydrogen bonds between donor and acceptor groups of the bound molecule and polar residues of the peptidases, such as Asn^{112}, Arg^{203} in TLN. The rational design of potent and selective NEP inhibitors and mixed inhibitors of NEP and APN (or NEP and ACE) was therefore based on the synthesis of molecules, bearing a strong metal-coordinating group, and able to satisfy all the possible energetically favorable interactions with at least one of the subsites surrounding the catalytic site (review in Roques and Fournie-Zaluski 1986).

As ACE is also able to cleave the enkephalins at their Gly^3-Phe^4 bonds, showing that its active site has some similarities to that of NEP, a comparison of the inhibitory potencies of some inhibitors will be given for both enzymes, to illustrate how selective or mixed inhibitors can be obtained (Fournie-Zaluski 1984a; Roques et al. 1982; Roques 1985). Only the most representative compounds in each series of inhibitors, characterized by the nature of the Zn-coordinating group, are reported. The thiol inhibitors can be considered as by-products while carboxyl-, phosphoryl-, and bidentate-containing NEP blockers probably act as transition state analogues.

II. Thiol Inhibitors

The specificity of NEP is essentially ensured by the S_1' subsite, which interacts preferentially with aromatic or large hydrophobic moieties whereas the S_2' subsite has a poor specificity, although in contrast to ACE, but like TLN, it will not accept a proline (Fournié-Zaluski et al. 1979, 1981, 1984a; Llorens et al. 1980). In contrast a proline in the P_2' position was advantageously incorporated in captopril [(S)-2-methyl-3-mercaptopropionyl]-L-proline (Ondetti et al. 1977) and then in almost all subsequent synthetic ACE inhibitors (Thorsett and Vywratt 1987). These observations were used to design the first described synthetic potent NEP inhibitor, thiorphan (1) (Table 1) (Roques et al. 1980).

The similar affinities of R and S thiorphan for NEP contrast with the 100-fold better inhibitory potency of L-Phe-L-Ala (IC_{50} ~1 μM) as compared to D-Phe-L-Ala (IC_{50} ~100 μM), showing the energetically greater

Table 1. Structure and inhibitory potencies toward endopeptidase 24.11 (NEP) and angiotensin-converting enzyme (ACE) of the main thiol-containing inhibitors

	S_1 Zn^{2+} S_1' S_2' (+)	K_i (nM) NEP	ACE
1	CH_2 above: $^-S-CH_2-CH-CONH-CH_2-COO^-$ (R, S)	4	140
2	$CH_2\phi$ and $CH_2\phi$ above: $^-S-CH_2-CH-CONH-CH-COO^-$ (S, R)	1.5	400
3	$CH_2\phi$ and $CH_2OCH_2\phi$ above: $^-S-CH_2-CH-CONH-CH-COO^-$	4	12
4	$CH_2\phi$ above: $^-S-CH_2-CH-NHCO-CH_2-COO^-$	4	>10 000
5	$CH_2\phi$ and $CH_2\phi$ above: $^-S-CH_2-CH-CONH-CH-CH_2-COO^-$	1.5	>10 000
6	$CH_2\phi$ above: $^-S-CH_2-CH-CONH-(CH_2)_6-COO^-$	26	ND
7	$CH_2\phi$ above: $^-S-CH_2-CH-CONH-CH-CH-COO^-$ (cyclopropane)	3	400

importance of the binding of the coordinating group (thiol) with the Zn atom, than the stereochemically dependent Van der Waals interactions governing subsite recognition. This shows that caution must be taken in directly extrapolating the results of peptide inhibition to the design of potent and selective inhibitors. Introduction of an aromatic side chain in the P_2' position improves NEP affinity (compound 2).

   To try to increase NEP selectivity, various structural modifications of the P_1' and/or P_2' moieties of thiorphan were made (Roques et al. 1982; Roques 1985; Gordon et al. 1983; Fournié-Zaluski et al. 1982, 1984a; Thorsett and Wyvratt 1987). However, this generally led to potent mixed inhibitors of NEP and ACE, such as compound 3 (Fournié-Zaluski et al. 1984a). A clear increased selectivity for NEP was observed by replacing the benzyl group of thiorphan with a cyclohexyl residue but this was also associated with a decreased affinity (IC$_{50}$, 31 nM for NEP; IC$_{50}$ > 10 000 nM for ACE).

Taking into account that modifying the P_1' and P_2' residues cannot ensure a complete differentiation of NEP and ACE inhibition, modification of the amide P_1'-P_2' bond of the inhibitors was considered as the most promising discriminating factor. Thus the compound resulting from retroinversion of the amide bond of thiorphan, retrothiorphan, compound 4, is almost as potent as thiorphan, with a K_I of 6 nM, but displays a drastic loss of potency for ACE (Roques et al. 1983). This successful approach was based on the assumption that the retroinversion of the natural amide bond of thiorphan would allow the respective groups of (R)-retrothiorphan to maintain similar interactions, including hydrogen bonding, with NEP but not with ACE, given the stringent stereochemical requirements of the S_1'-S_2' subsites of the latter. As hypothesized, (R)retrothiorphan (K_I = 2.3 nM) is a better NEP inhibitor than its S-isomer (K_I = 210 nM). Since inhibition experiments, using separated R- and S-isomers of thiorphan and retrothiorphan, indicated that the specificity of NEP and TLN was very similar, computer studies and crystallographic determination of the three-dimensional structures of (S)thiorphan and (R)retro-thiorphan bound to TLN were undertaken showing that, as anticipated, the carbonyl oxygen and amide hydrogen display very similar hydrogen bonding despite the inversion of the -CONH- linkage. The good agreement between the computer modeling results (Benchetrit et al. 1987) and crystallographic analysis (Roderick et al. 1989) suggest that docking experiments, using a reconstructed active site of NEP, may soon be feasible.

An increased selectivity was also recently obtained by replacing the glycine moiety of thiorphan by substituted β-alanyl residues (compound 5) or by longer amino-alkyl carboxylic acids as in compound 6 (SQ 29,072), by a heterocyclic hydrazide as in RU (R,S)HS-CH_2-CH(CH_2φ)-CONH-N$C_4$$H_8$O, or by introduction of a cyclic moiety in P_2' position (compound 7) (unpublished result).

Another class of mercapto inhibitors, N-mercaptoacetyldipeptides, were found to have inhibitory potencies in the 30–70 nM range (Altstein et al. 1982, 1983; Van Amsterdam et al. 1987). In these compounds the mercaptoacetyl function is assumed to act as a bidentate ligand for the zinc ion.

An improvement in the bioavailability of thiorphan has been obtained by protecting its thiol and carboxyl hydrophilic groups. The resulting prodrugs, such as acetorphan [CH_3COS-CH_2-CH(CH_2φ)-CONH-CH_2-$CO_2$$CH_2$φ] (Roques et al. 1980), are rapidly transformed to thiorphan by esterases in the brain and blood.

III. Carboxyl Inhibitors

Introducing a carboxyl group at the N-terminus of pseudodipeptides, capable of interacting with the S_1' and S_2' subsites (compound 8, Table 2), led to modest NEP inhibitors with IC_{50}s in the micromolar range, and,

Table 2. Structure and inhibitory potencies toward endopeptidase 24.11 (NEP) and angiotensin-converting enzyme (ACE) of the main carboxyl-containing inhibitors

S_1	Zn^{2+}	S_1'	S_2' (+)	K_1 (nM) NEP	ACE
8	COO^-, CH_2—NH—CH—CONH—CH—COO$^-$	CH_2 (phenyl)	CH_3 CH_3 \ / CH, CH_2	2000	2000
9	(phenyl) CH_2—CH_2—CH—NH—CH—CONH—CH_2—COO$^-$	COO^-, $CH_2\phi$		450[a]	ND
10	(phenyl) CH_2—CH_2—CH—NH—CH—CONH—CH_2—CH_2—COO$^-$	COO^-, $CH_2\phi$		320[a]	ND
11	(phenyl) CH_2—CH_2—CH—NH—CH—CONH—CH_2—CH—COO$^-$	COO^-, $CH_2\phi$	OH	11	ND
12	(phenyl) CH_2—CH—CH_2—CH—CONH—CH—COO$^-$	COO^-, $CH_2\phi$	$CH_2OCH_2\phi$	8	ND
13	(phenyl) CH_2—CH—CH_2—CH—*NHCO*—CH_2—CH2—COO$^-$	COO^-, $CH_2\phi$		2	ND
14	OCH_3, CH_2—CH_2, O—CH_2—CH—NH—C—CONH—(phenyl)—COO$^-$	COO^- (cyclopentyl)		52	ND

[a] With IC_{50} thiorphan, 200 nM (Mumford et al. 1982).

unlike ACE inhibitors, the affinities were not modulated by the relative positions of the carboxyl group and the phenyl moiety, supporting the idea of a larger catalytic site in NEP (Fournié-Zaluski et al. 1982, 1983). Consequently, some of these molecules are relatively potent, mixed inhibitors of NEP and ACE. The design and synthesis in 1980 of the highly potent ACE inhibitor enalapril (review in Thorsett and Wyvratt 1987), a tripeptide analogue which interacts with the S_1, S_1', and S_2' subsites of the enzyme, stimulated a reinvestigation of carboxyl-derived inhibitors of NEP; and various *N*-carboxyl alkyl dipeptides, bearing a hydrophobic chain on the carboxylalkyl group, were synthesized, such as compounds 9, 10 (SCH 34,826), 11 (SCH 39,370) in Table 2 (MUMFORD et al. 1982; CHIPKIN 1986; NORTHRIDGE et al. 1989). The significant increased potency obtained with these compounds and the influence of the chirality of the P_1 side chains (S-isomer 100-fold better than R-isomer) suggested the existence in NEP of either a hydrophobic S_1 subsite, or at least stereoselective nonspecific Van Der Waals interactions with the peptidase surface (ROQUES et al. 1982). The results of substituting lipophilic moieties on the N-terminus of the peptide phenylalanyl-*p*-aminobenzoic acid (ALMENOFF and ORLOWSKI 1983) also support these hypotheses.

In compound 14, UK 69,578, a cyclopentyl group and a *p*-amino cyclohexane carboxyl moiety were introduced in the P_1' and P_2' positions, respectively, to improve the selectivity for NEP as described (FOURNIÉ-ZALUSKI et al. 1984a). Prodrugs of all these molecules can be easily obtained by esterifying the carboxyl function with more or less lipophilic alcohols. Shortening the P_1 residue by a methylene group or introducing a retro-inversion at the P_1'-P_2' level in glutaramic-derived tripeptides 12 and 13 led also to highly potent NEP inhibitors (KSANDER et al. 1989) (Table 2).

IV. Hydroxamic Acids and Derivatives

The tripeptide-derived hydroxamates originally synthesized as TLN inhibitors were also found to be very efficient NEP inhibitors with IC_{50}s in the nanomolar range (HUDGIN et al. 1981). The increased inhibitory potencies of N-protected (D) amino acid hydroxamates such as Z(D)Phe-NHOH ($IC_{50} = 0.2 \mu M$) compared with their natural isomers (BLUMBERG et al. 1981) suggest that these compounds could bind backwards in the active site of NEP.

A detailed analysis of NEP inhibition by N-terminal hydroxamates was performed by BOUBOUTOU et al. (1984), using four series of novel dipeptides analogues. This study showed that: (1) hydroxamates are more efficient than *N*-formyl-*N*-hydroxy amino derivatives, a result identical to that obtained for TLN; (2) the insertion of a methylene spacer between the zinc-chelating group and the benzyl-bearing carbon increases the inhibitory potency of the molecules; (3) all the inhibitors have poor affinities for ACE ($IC_{50} > 10\,000$ nM). Among these derivatives, HACBO-Gly, $(R,S)HONH-CO-CH_2-CH(CH_2\phi)-CONH-CH_2-COOH$ was developed as a tritiated probe for binding studies and in vitro or in vivo visualization of NEP by autoradiography (WAKSMAN et al. 1984).

The optimization of the interactions of hydroxamate inhibitors belonging to the HACBO-Gly series, in the active site of NEP (FOURNIÉ-ZALUSKI et al. 1985; XIE et al. 1989a,b), has shown that the absolute configuration of the P_1' residue, as well as the size and the hydrophobicity of the P_2' residue,

Table 3. Structure and inhibitory potencies toward endopeptidase 24.11 (NEP) and aminopeptidase (APN) and dipeptidylaminopeptidase (DAP) of selective or mixed peptidase inhibitors

	S_1 $\quad$ Zn^{2+} $\quad$ S_1' $\quad$ S_2'	NEP	$K_i(nM)$ APN	DAP
	$(-)$ $\qquad\qquad\qquad\qquad$ $(+)$			
15	CH₃ CH₃ (CH), ring ONH; O⁻, CH₂, CH₂; Rh—O—P(=O)—NH—CH—CONH—CH—COO⁻	2	>1000	ND
16	CH₂(⟨phenyl⟩) OH O; CH₃ CH₃ (CH), CH₂; ⁺H₃N—CH—CH—C—NH—CH—COO⁻	>10000	3500	ND
17	CH₂(⟨phenyl⟩); ⁺H₃N—CH—CH₂—S⁻	>10000	20	ND
18	⁻O O CH₂(⟨phenyl⟩) CH₃; HN—C—CH₂—CH—CONH—CH—COO⁻ (R, 5)	1.8	380	0.9
19	⁻O O CH₂φ CH₃; HN—C—CH₂—CH—NHCO—CH₂—CH—COO⁻	0.2	2000	900
20	⁻O O CH₂φ CH₂φ; HN—C—CH₂—CH—CONH—CH—COO⁻ (R, S)	0.9	120	2.5
21	⁻O O CH₂φ; HN—C—CH₂—CH—CONH—CH—CH—COO⁻	3.8	74	ND
22	SCH₃; (CH₂)₂; ⁺H₃N—CH—CH₂—S⁻	>10000	4	ND
6	CH₂φ CH₂φ; S⁻—CH₂—CH—CONH—CH—COO⁻	1.5	>10000	ND

does not greatly influence enzyme recognition (Table 3). However, these two parameters have played an important role in the design of selective or mixed inhibitors of NEP, APN, and DAP as discussed later. The retro-inversion of the amide bond in dipeptide hydroxamates led to very efficient (IC_{50} ~0.15 nM) and highly selective NEP (HERNANDEZ et al. 1988).

V. Phosphorus-Containing Inhibitors

Another interesting series of inhibitors are phosphorus-containing dipeptides (Table 3), among which is the competitive inhibitor of NEP, phosphoramidon (15), initially described as a TLN inhibitor. Various phosphorylated inhibitors of NEP were described (ALGERI et al. 1981; ALTSTEIN et al. 1982), the most potent being N-phosphoryl leucylphenylalanine, with an IC_{50} of 0.3 nM. More recently, phosphoramidate derivatives have also been reported (ELLIOT et al. 1985). However, these compounds, although potentially able to interact with the S_1, S_1', and S_2' subsites of NEP, are less efficient than the phosphorylated dipeptide. Nevertheless this series of inhibitors deserves further investigation.

VI. Aminopeptidase-N and Dipeptidyl Peptidase Inhibitors

Various natural aminopeptidase inhibitors (review in RICH 1990), such as the weakly active puromycin and the more potent peptide analogues bestatin (16) and amastatin, $H_2N-CH[CH_2CH(CH_3)_2-CH(OH)CO-Val-Val-Asp$, which act as bidentates, have little selectivity for APN.

Substituted aminoethanethiols such as compound 17 (Table 3) were found to be highly potent APN inhibitors (CHAN 1983; ROQUES 1988a), which recognize only the S_1 subsite and interact with both the Zn atom and a negatively charged group of the enzyme in front of the N-terminal (HELENE et al. 1991). Recently, α-thiolbestatin analogues (OCAIN and RICH 1988) and sulfur-containing modified di- or tripeptides (GORDON et al. 1988) were shown to exhibit high inhibitory potencies on various aminopeptidases but poor affinities for APN (IC_{50} >10 μM). The bioavailability of phenylalanine (IC_{50} ~20 nM) was improved by the introduction of a hydrophobic phenyl carbamate group leading to carbaphethiol, a compound reported to elicit antinociceptive activity after i.v. administration in mice (GROS et al. 1988).

Inhibitors of DAP were designed by taking into account the requirement for a charged amino group in the P_2 position and the hydrophobicity of the extended S_1, S_1', S_2' active site. The most potent DAP inhibitor Tyr-Phe-NHOH (K_I ~10 nM) is also highly selective with an IC_{50} >10 000 nM, for NEP, APN, and ACE (CHÉROT et al. 1986b).

VII. Development of Mixed Inhibitors
of Enkephalin-Degrading Enzymes

As the enkephalins are degraded in vivo by more than one enzyme, NEP, APN, and possibly DAP, mixed inhibitors of these enzymes have been designed. This was achieved using hydroxamate- or thiol-containing inhibitors. In the case of the hydroxamates, it was hypothesized that the strength of the coordination to the zinc atom would be able to counterbalance a less than perfect fit of the inhibitor side chains to the active sites of the three metallopeptidases. Accordingly, kelatorphan (18) was shown to strongly inhibit NEP, APN, and DAP (Table 3) while its S,S-stereoisomer is a highly potent and selective NEP inhibitor with IC_{50}s of $1.8\,nM$ for NEP, $29\,000\,nM$ for APN, and $100\,nM$ for DAP (FOURNIÉ-ZALUSKI et al. 1985).

Using this new concept of mixed inhibition, a large number of analogues have been synthesized, all of them having a pseudodipeptide structure. RB 38A (compound 20, Table 3) is as active as kelatorphan on DAP and NEP but more potent on APN ($IC_{50} = 120\,nM$) (SCHMIDT et al. 1991), while the (S,S)-stereoisomer RB38B behaves as one of the most selective NEP blockers reported to date. It was interesting to observe that a hydrophobic, large residue in the P_2' position significantly increased APN recognition without affecting NEP (compound 21, Table 3), and that retroinversion of the amide bond in compound 19 also led to highly efficient mixed inhibitors (FOURNIÉ-ZALUSKI et al. 1985; HERNANDEZ et al. 1988).

At the present time, kelatorphan- and retrokelatorphan-related bidentates are the only mixed inhibitors with nanomolar affinities for both NEP and APN. However, their high water solubility, although favorable for binding studies and inhibiting enzymes easily accessible from the circulation, prevents them from crossing the blood-brain barrier. Efforts to improve their bioavailability have met with little success. Another strategy was therefore employed, which consisted of linking highly potent thiol-containing APN and NEP inhibitors by a disulfide bond. In addition to the easy modulation of their hydrophobicity, one of the main advantages of these mixed inhibitors is the stability of the disulfide bond in plasma, contrasting with its relatively rapid breakdown in brain. Among the various compounds synthesized, RB101 $H_2N\text{-}CH(CH_2\text{-}CH_2\text{-}S\text{-}CH_3)\text{-}CH_2\text{-}S\text{-}S\text{-}CH_2\text{-}CH(CH_2\phi)\text{-}CONH\text{-}CH(CH_2\phi)\text{-}COOH$, an association of compounds 22 and 6, has been shown to be very active in antinociceptive tests after i.v. or s.c. administration at low doses (NOBLE et al. 1990, 1992).

Compared with ACE, relatively few NEP inhibitors and NEP/APN or NEP/ACE mixed inhibitors have so far been synthesized but this number will probably grow in the near future and attention must be paid to the introduction of pharmacokinetically favorable cyclic moieties in the structure of these compounds, taking advantage of the now well-established structural characteristics of the active site of NEP.

F. Pharmacological Studies of Enkephalin-Degrading-Enzyme Inhibitors

Given their potency in increasing the extracellular levels of enkephalins, the pharmacological action of selective and mixed inhibitors has been studied using various morphine-sensitive tests.

I. Inhibitor-Induced Analgesia

Neutral endopeptidase-24.11 and/or APN inhibitors are able to potentiate
the analgesic effects of exogenous enkephalins or enkephalin analogues and,
more interestingly, possess intrinsic opioidergic action after i.c.v. injection.
This has been established for thiorphan or bestatin alone, or in association
(Roques et al. 1980; Zhang et al. 1982; Chipkin et al. 1982a,b; Carenzi
et al. 1981, 1983; Chaillet et al. 1983), retrothiorphan (Roques et al.
1983), and phosphoryl (Altstein et al. 1982; Rupreht et al. 1983) or
carboxyl-containing inhibitors (Fournié-Zaluski et al. 1981, 1982, 1983;
Murthy et al. 1984; Chipkin et al. 1988). Different analgesic tests have been
employed, such as the hot-plate test in mice (Roques et al. 1980; Hachisu
et al. 1985; Lecomte et al. 1986) or the tail flick test in mice (Roques
et al. 1980) and rat (Chipkin et al. 1982a,b; Hachisu et al. 1985), and the
writhing test (Hachisu et al. 1985); and different routes of administration
have also been used (reviews in Roques and Fournié-Zaluski 1986;
Chipkin 1986). All the responses observed were antagonized by prior
administration of naloxone.

The N-carboxyalkyldipeptide SCH 34826 was found to be active at
100 mg/kg in the mouse low-temperature hot-plate test, the mouse acetic
acid-induced writhing test, and the rat yeast-paw test (Chipkin et al. 1988);
and the more lipophilic prodrug of thiorphan, acetorphan (also designated
ES 52 or GN 52), was reported to be active after i.v. administration in the
writhing and the hot-plate test in mice (Lecomte et al. 1986) although it was
unable to modify the nociceptive activities of dorsal horn neurons in the
anesthetized rat (Villanueva et al. 1985). Carbaphethiol (Gros et al. 1988),
a prodrug of the APN inhibitor phenylalaninethiol, was found to be weakly
active in the hot-plate test after i.v. injection in mice.

As expected, mixed inhibitors (Fournié-Zaluski et al. 1984b; Van
Amsterdam and Llorens-Cortes 1988; Xie et al. 1989a,b; Noble et al.
1990; Schmidt et al. 1991) or coadministered NEP and APN inhibitors
produce stronger analgesic responses than those achieved by inhibiting only
one enzyme. Thus, kelatorphan was shown to decrease the dose of Met-
enkephalin required to obtain 50% analgesia (ED_{50}) by a factor of 50000
(Fournié-Zaluski et al. 1984b). Under these conditions the ED_{50} of
Met-enkephalin was not very different from that of the μ-agonist DAGO,
in agreement with the similar in vitro affinities of both compounds for
the opioid receptors. However, the inability of thiorphan plus bestatin to
produce significant antinociception in the tail flick, tail withdrawal, and
hot-plate (paw-licking) tests in either mouse or rat (Chaillet et al. 1983;
Chipkin et al. 1982a; Chipkin 1986) led to the proposal that the ability of
the inhibitors to induce analgesia is restricted to tests in which naloxone has
intrinsic activity (Schwartz 1983; Costentin et al. 1986). However, stress-
induced analgesia (SIA) is sensitive to inhibitors and thiorphan potentiates
footshock SIA in rats, immobilization SIA in mice, warm water swim SIA in
mice (review in Chipkin 1986), and transcranial electrostimulation analgesia

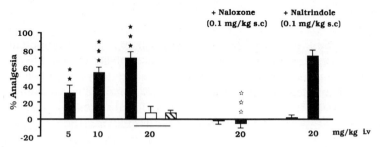

Fig. 2. Comparison of analgesic potencies (hot plate test) of selective and mixed inhibitors of enkephalin degrading enzymes after i.v. injection in mice. Acetorphan (NEP inhibitor, *open column*) and carbaphetiol (aminopeptidase inhibitor, *hatched columns*) were administered i.v. 15 min, and RB101 (*filled column*) 10 min, before testing, i.e., at the time corresponding to their maximum effects. Naloxone or NTI (δ-selective antagonist) were s.c. injected 20 min before testing. The plate was heated to 55° ± 0.5°C and antinociceptive effects evaluated by measuring the jump latencies (cutoff time, 240s)

(MALIN et al. 1989) measured by the tail flick test. This is probably due to an increased release of enkephalins in regions involved in pain control. In addition, the complete inhibition of enkephalin metabolism by i.c.v. RB38A or i.v. RB101 induced naloxone-antagonized antinociceptive responses on all the various assays commonly used to select analgesics: mouse hot-plate test, tail flick test in mice and rats, electrical stimulation of the tail in rats, paw pressure test in rats, and phenylbenzoquinone-induced writhing in mice (SCHMIDT et al. 1991; NOBLE et al. 1990, 1992) (Fig. 2). This suggests that, given their comparable affinities for opioid-binding sites, similar analgesic responses could theoretically be obtained with morphine and endogenous enkephalins if a synaptic concentration of these compounds leading to a similar related opioid receptor occupancy could be achieved (ROQUES and FOURNIÉ-ZALUSKI 1986). Moreover, using s.c. naloxone as antagonist, the pA2 value (7.53) of i.v. RB101 was similar to that of i.v. DAGO (7.38) in the hot-plate test in mice (NOBLE et al. 1992), supporting the proposed preferential interaction of endogenous enkephalins with supraspinal μ-receptors (GACEL et al. 1981; CHAILLET et al. 1984).

II. Inhibitor-Induced Spinal Antinociception

Electrophoretic administration of kelatorphan in the substantia gelatinosa of anesthetized spinal cats led to naloxone-reversible inhibition of nociceptive responses and marked potentiation of coadministered Met-enkephalin (MORTON et al. 1987).

The antinociceptive properties of kelatorphan, locally infused onto the spinal cord, were inhibited by the selective δ-opioid antagonist ICI 174,864

(DICKENSON et al. 1986) and were shown to be additive with those of the μ-selective agonist DAGO, but not with those of the selective δ-agonist DSTBULET (DICKENSON et al. 1988), confirming that endogenous enkephalins and δ-selective agonists act on a common binding site to produce spinal antinociception. Kelatorphan (i.t.) was also efficient in reducing the more prolonged noxious stimulation induced by s.c. formalin (SULLIVAN et al. 1989). The mechanism of action of the δ-induced reduction in nociceptive responses could involve a presynaptic inhibition of SP release (MAUBORGNE et al. 1987b). Thiorphan and SCH 32615 displayed strong analgesia after intrathecal administration (YAKSH and HARTY 1982; OSHITA et al. 1990).

III. Peptidase Inhibitors in Chronic Pain

In the Freund's adjuvant-induced arthritic rat, a widely used model of chronic pain, kelatorphan, at doses as low as 2.5 mg/kg i.v., at which acetorphan was ineffective (KAYSER et al. 1984), produced potent naloxone-reversible antinociceptive responses in normal rats, comparable to those induced by 1 mg/kg i.v. morphine, although at higher doses (5, 10, 15 mg/kg i.v.) the effects of kelatorphan were no more pronounced than those of acetorphan (KAYSER et al. 1989). Unlike acetorphan, kelatorphan was found to be much more effective in arthritic than in normal rats, in raising the vocalization threshold, even at 2.5 mg/kg i.v.: 244% in arthritic vs. 144% in normal rats. Given the very weak passage of kelatorphan into the brain, its strong antinociceptive effects in inflammatory pain raise the intriguing question of a possible action at the level of peripheral nociceptors, where all opioid targets including NEP seem to be present (STEIN et al. 1989).

IV. Tolerance, Dependence, and Side Effects of Selective and Mixed Inhibitors of NEP and APN

Apotropin and bacitracin, or the NEP inhibitors phosphoramidon, thiorphan, and acetorphan and the mixed inhibitor phelorphan have been shown to minimize the severity of the naloxone-precipitated morphine withdrawal syndrome in rats (review in HAFFMANS and DZOLJIC 1987). In another study, RB38A was found to be more effective than kelatorphan and thiorphan (MALDONADO et al. 1989), suggesting that attenuation of the narcotic withdrawal syndrome is related to the level of opioid receptor occupancy by exogenous or endogenous agonists. Some physical dependence effects were observed after naloxone administration to rats chronically treated i.c.v. with thiorphan, while no sign of withdrawal syndrome was observed in mice challenged with naloxone, after chronic i.v. administration of acetorphan (LECOMTE et al. 1986). Nevertheless at the concentration used (50 mg/kg i.p. twice daily, 10 days) no clear antinociceptive responses can be obtained in the hot-plate test in mouse (Noble et al. 1990, 1992), which is in agreement with acute studies (Fig. 2). In contrast to DAGO, the δ-selective agonist DSTBULET and the mixed inhibitor RB38A produced a weak physical dependence at comparable antinociceptive doses (Maldonado et al. 1990a). Chronic i.c.v. administration of DAGO, DSTBULET, and RB38A resulted in a time-dependent reduction in their analgesic effects, and after 120 h continuous infusion only RB38A was still able to induce a significant antinociceptive effect. These data suggest that, even under the drastic conditions of chronic i.c.v. infusion of a mixed inhibitor, long-term complete inhibition of enkephalin catabolism induces only a weak tolerance and a moderate physical dependence, similar to that produced by δ-opioid agonists. This has been recently confirmed by chronic administration of RB101 (40 mg i.v. twice daily for 8 days), which was unable to induce tolerance and, even more interestingly, cross-tolerance to morphine (Noble et al. 1992; Noble et al., in press).

The weak tolerance and the minimized dependence effects induced by chronic stimulation of opioid receptors by endogenous enkephalins could result from differences in adaptative changes of the opioidergic system, when stimulated by either native or synthetic enkephalins. In the latter case the local concentration of the opioid substances probably largely exceeds the concentration of endogenous enkephalins in brain regions such as the periaqueductal gray or the locus coeruleus of rats, which are rich in μ-receptors and where local injection of morphine or enkephalin analogues has been shown to cause exceptionally pronounced pharmacological effects and a high degree of physical dependence. It is interesting to observe that, in slices of rat pons, kelatorphan was able to potentiate strongly the firing of the locus coeruleus, induced by exogenous Met-enkephalin, but had no intrinsic effect, indicating that there is little or no tonic endogenous opioid action in this region (Williams et al. 1987). Moreover, neither physical nor psychic dependence was observed after 8 days chronic i.p. administration of RB101 at doses (twice daily) inducing strong analgesic responses (Noble et al., in press).

A major side effect of opiate analgesia is a central respiratory depression, which is mainly due to the inhibition of bulbar respiratory neurons. After i.v. injection in freely moving rats, at concentrations which give analgesic responses in the vocalization test, kelatorphan had no significant effect on respiratory frequency and tidal volume (Boudinot et al. 1988). Likewise the NEP inhibitors acetorphan (Lecomte et al. 1986) and SCH 34826 (Chipkin et al. 1988) have also been reported to be devoid of respiratory effects.

V. Gastrointestinal Effects

Numerous studies have shown that inhibition of NEP, APN, and ACE, which are codistributed all along the gastrointestinal tract, potentiates the inhibitory effects of exogenously administered enkephalins on the electrically stimulated contractions of the guinea pig ileum (AOKI et al. 1984).

The antidiarrheal effects of thiorphan and acetorphan have been compared with those of loperamide, a clinically used μ-agonist unable to enter the brain, in a model of castor oil-induced diarrhea in rats (MARCAIS-COLLADO et al. 1987). Both compounds, but not SCH 34826 (CHIPKIN et al. 1988), delayed the onset of diarrhea with no reduction in gastrointestinal transit, in contrast to loperamide. The naloxone-antagonized antidiarrheal effect of thiorphan and its prodrug seems to result from an antisecretory effect, possibly due to the stimulation of peripheral δ-opioid receptors. The localization of both enkephalins and NEP in the wall of the cat gallbladder could explain the decrease in fluid secretion in the inflamed and distended gallbladder elicited by 3 mg/kg i.v. acetorphan (JIVEGARD et al. 1989). This suggests that inhibitors could be of clinical interest in the treatment of acute cholecystitis. A weak inhibition (12% maximum) of the lower oesophageal sphincter was observed in humans after perfusion of acetorphan (2.5 mg/kg i.v. in 20 min) (CHAUSSADE et al. 1988).

The type and localization of opioid receptors involved in controlling gastrointestinal function, including food intake (BADO et al. 1989), also deserves further study, since, as previously discussed, μ- or δ-agonists could differentially modulate the release of other neuropeptides such as SP or CCK also involved in gastrointestinal functioning.

VI. Role of Neutral Endopeptidase-24.11 in Airways

In airways, removal of the epithelium, which is enriched in NEP, or administration of thiorphan or phosphoramidon has been shown to potentiate SP-induced contractions of airway smooth muscle (DZOLJIC et al. 1989). NEP activity was also found to be decreased by 40% in viral respiratory infection, suggesting that the resulting enhanced asthma and bronchoconstrictor responses (cough) could be due to increased levels of SP (DUSSER et al. 1989). In agreement with this, recombinant NEP, administered by aerosol to guinea pigs, reduced the drastic cough induced by SP inhalation (KOHROGI et al. 1989).

VII. Behavioral Effects of Inhibitors

Opioids are involved in emotional, cognitive, and motor functions through modulation of the limbic (mesocorticolimbic) and motor (nigrostriatal) dopaminergic systems (review in KALIVAS 1985).

Foot-shock stress or local infusion of thiorphan (GLIMCHER et al. 1984; KALIVAS et al. 1986) or kelatorphan into the ventral tegmental area (CALENCO-CHOUKROUN et al. 1991) both increases the level of dopamine in projection areas and potentiates its effects, suggesting a phasic control of the dopamine mesocorticolimbic pathway by endogenous enkephalins (Algeri et al. 1981; Wood and Richard 1982; Llorens-Cortes and Schwartz 1984; De Witte et al. 1989). The similar psychostimulant responses induced by selective δ-agonists (DSTBULET, DPDPE, BUBU) and kelatorphan locally injected in the ventral tegmental area (Calenco-Choukroun et al. 1991) or in the nucleus accumbens (Daugé et al. 1988) support a preferential role for δ-receptors in opioid-induced euphorogenic and disinhibitory effects. In contrast, DAGO seems to increase emotionality and fear when injected into the same regions (Daugé et al. 1989; Calenco-Choukroun et al. 1991).

An interaction between dopaminergic and opioidergic terminals in the nucleus accumbens has been clearly demonstrated by 6-OHDA-induced lesions of the dopamine neurons of the ventral tegmental area and chronic neuroleptic treatment, both of which potentiate the behavioral effects of exogenous opioid or kelatorphan infusion into the nucleus accumbens (Stinus et al. 1985; Maldonado et al. 1990b). In agreement with the presence of dopamine receptors on enkephalin neurons of the nucleus accumbens, chronically administered sulpiride (D_2-receptor antagonist), but not the D_1 antagonist SCH23390, has been found to facilitate the opioid behavioral effects induced by kelatorphan. This effect was maximal after 2–3 weeks, a delay corresponding to the first appearance of the antipsychotic effects of neuroleptics (Maldonado et al. 1990b). This could be related to the observed disinhibition of the enkephalinergic neuron, normally negatively controlled by the dopaminergic input, with an increase in preproenkephalin expression. Therefore, alterations in the opioidergic system, very likely through its interrelations with the dopaminergic pathway, could be taking place in a neuronal system which is critically involved in the control of mood (Roques et al. 1985; MacLennan and Mayer 1983).

More generally, a link between opioidergic and dopaminergic systems has also been suggested from the results of experiments used to study antidepressant drugs (Ben Natan et al. 1984; Dzoljic et al. 1985; Nabeshima et al. 1987; De Felipe et al. 1989; Gibert-Rahola et al. 1990). Thus systemic administration of RB101 was shown to induce antidepressant-like effects resulting from activation of the DA striatal pathway (Baamonde et al. 1992).

The increased locomotor activity induced by intrastriatal injection of DTLET or kelatorphan (Roques et al. 1985; Daugé et al. 1989) could be related to a specific δ-induced increase in the spontaneous and K^+-induced release of newly synthesized dopamine (Petit et al. 1986; Dourmap et al. 1990).

G. Inhibition of NEP Inactivation of Atrial Natriuretic Peptide: Pharmacological and Clinical Implications

The circulating atrial natriuretic peptide (ANP) SLRRSSCFGGRMDRI-GAQSGLGCNSFRY[126] is rapidly inactivated by NEP, which cleaves the

Cys[7]-Phe[8] bond (KENNY and STEPHENSON 1988; KOEHN et al. 1987). Accordingly i.v. administered NEP inhibitors such as thiorphan, the SS-isomer of kelatorphan, SQ 29,072, SCH 39,070, and UK 69,578 (Tables 1, 2 and 3) have been found to increase the magnitudes and especially the durations of the depressor, natriuretic, and cGMP responses induced by exogenous ANP in the conscious spontaneously hypertensive rat (SHR) and to exhibit proper weak diuretic and natriuretic effects in normal animals. In a volume-based model of hypertension (DOCA salt rat), thiorphan and retrothiorphan (PHAM et al. 1990) lowered blood pressure for at least 4 h after i.v. injection. In the human, UK 69,578 (NORTHRIDGE et al. 1989) and acetorphan (GROS et al. 1989) orally administered increased diuresis and natriuresis without significant changes in blood pressure. UK 69,578 had beneficial effects in six patients with heart failure where the basal levels of ANP were already increased.

It should be noted that, although the role of NEP in degrading ANP in vivo seems to be firmly established, its site(s) of action remain to be determined. It has recently been shown, however, that the enzyme is present in the endothelial cells of vascular tissue (SOLEILHAC et al. 1992). For a fuller review of the potential of NEP inhibitors as diuretics and antihypertensives (see ROQUES and BEAUMONT (1990)).

H. Clinical Applications of Selective and Mixed Zn Metallopeptidase Inhibitors

The thiorphan prodrug acetorphan was the first NEP inhibitor used in clinical investigations and was found to have no effect on flexion reflexes or pain sensation (WILLER et al. 1986). Likewise, in a double-blind study using 84 patients requiring myelography, an i.v. infusion of thiorphan (150 mg in 30 min), although producing a reduction in the post myelographic side effects (headache nausea and vomiting) did not reduce lumbar puncture pain (FLORAS et al. 1983), emphasizing the necessity of completely inhibiting NEP and APN to obtain a significant morphine-like analgesia (FOURNIE-ZALUSKI et al. 1984b; NOBLE et al. 1990, 1992).

Owing to the independent modulation of pain following stimulation of μ- or δ-receptors, mixed inhibitors may be of clinical interest in patients insensitive or tolerant to morphine and could avoid, or at least minimize, the unwanted side effects mediated by μ-receptors (DICKENSON et al. 1986). This novel approach to analgesia has provided promising preliminary clinical results after intrathecal administration of either kelatorphan (MEYNADIER et al., personal communication) in morphine-tolerant patients or for the association of bestatin and thiorphan in normal patients (MEYNADIER et al. 1988). Mixed inhibitors, such as RB101, unable to modify ANP levels and shown to exhibit strong antinociceptive properties in animals and to be devoid of tolerance effect and physical or psychic dependence (NOBLE et al.

1992) after chronic i.v. administration, are promising compounds with which to tackle the challenging problem of obtaining a highly potent analgesic, devoid of morphine-associated drawbacks.

The strategy used to synthesize mixed inhibitors such as RB101 could be extended to selective NEP inhibitors able to act almost exclusively in the brain. These inhibitors may have potential as new antidepressant agents by stimulating δ-opioid receptors and subsequent DA activation of the mesocorticolimbic pathways.

Acetorphan has been recently introduced in the marked as an anti-diarrheal agent in humans, and the interesting antisecretory effects observed raise the question of the different role of gastrointestinal opioid receptors and their possible stimulation by orally active selective δ-agonists unable to enter the brain. Finally the recent discovery of the involvement of NEP in ANP degradation led to preliminary clinical investigations on the possible use of NEP inhibitors as new anti-hypertensive agents (review in Roques and Beaumont 1990). However, owing to the rather weak hypotensive effect of selective NEP blockers and taking into account the opposed pharmacological effects of ANP and angiotensin II, we have proposed that mixed inhibitors of NEP and ACE could be of greatest clinical interest (Roques and Beaumont 1990).

Other possible clinical uses of NEP and mixed inhibitors could appear when the role of the peptidases in different tissues is defined. Nevertheless it can be noted that, despite a distribution of ACE as wide as that of NEP, ACE inhibitors exhibit a pharmacological activity almost exclusively limited to blood pressure control. This situation might be due to an important tonic release of putative substrates of ACE almost exclusively restricted to AI, a situation which could also occur in the case of NEP for enkephalins and ANP (Roques 1988b).

References

Algeri S, Altstein M, Blumberg S, de Simoni GM, Guardabasso V (1981) In vivo potentiation of [D-Ala²] Met-enkephalin amide central effects of the administration of an enkephalinase inhibitor. Eur J Pharmacol 74:261–262

Almenoff J, Orlowski M (1983) Membrane-bound kidney neutral metalloendopeptidase: Interaction with synthetic substrates, natural peptides and inhibitors. Biochemistry 22:590–599

Almenoff J, Orlowski M (1984) Biochemical and immunological properties of a membrane-bound brain metalloendopeptidase: comparison with thermolysin-like kidney neutral metalloendopeptidase. J Neurochem 42:151–157

Altstein M, Blumberg S, Vogel Z (1982) Phosphoryl-Leu-Phe: a potent inhibitor of the degradation of enkephalin by enkephalinase. Eur J Pharmacol 76:299–300

Altstein M, Bacher E, Vogel Z, Blumberg S (1983) Protection of enkephalins from enzymatic degradation utilizing selective metal-chelating inhibitors. Eur J Pharmacol 91:353–361

Aoki K, Kajiwara M, Oka T (1984) The role of bestatin sensitive aminopeptidase, angiotensin converting enzyme and thiorphan sensitive "enkephalinase" in the potency of enkephalins in the guinea-pig ileum. Jpn J Pharmacol 36:59–65

Baamonde A, Daugé V, Ruiz-Gayo M, Fulga IG, Turcaud S, Fournié-Zaluski MC, Roques BP (1992) Antidepressant-type effects of endogenous enkephalins protected by systemic RB101 are mediated by opioid δ and D₁ dopamine receptor stimulation. Eur J Pharmacol (in press)

Back SA, Gorenstein C (1989) Histochemical visualization of neutral endopeptidase-24.11 (enkephalinase) activity in rat brain: cellular localization and codistribution with enkephalins in the globus pallidus. J Neurosci 9:4439–4455

Bado A, Roze C, Lewin JM, Dubrasquet M (1989) Endogenous opioid peptides in the control of food intake in cats. Peptide 10:967–971

Barnes K, Turner AJ, Kenny AJ (1988) Electronmicroscopic immunocytochemistry of pig brain shows that endopeptidase-24.11 is localized in neuronal membranes. Neurosci Lett 94:64–69

Bateman RC, Jackson D, Slaughter CA, Unnithan S, Chai YG, Moomaw C, Hersh LB (1989) Identification of the active-site arginine in rat neutral endopeptidase 24.11 (enkephalinase) as arginine 102 and analysis of a glutamine 102 mutant. J Biol Chem 264:6151–6157

Beaumont A, Brouet JC, Roques BP (1989) Neutral endopeptidase 24.11 and angiotensin converting enzyme like activity in CALLA positive and CALLA negative lymphocytes. Biochem Biophys Res Commun 160:1323–1329

Beaumont A, Le Moual H, Boileau G, Crine P, Roques BP (1991) Evidence that both arginine 102 and arginine 747 are involved in substrate binding to neutral endopeptidase-24.11. J Biol Chem 266:214–220

Belluzi JD, Grant N, Garsky V, Sarantakis D, Wise CD, Stein D (1976) Analgesia induced in vivo by central administration of enkephalin in rat. Nature 260:625–626

Ben Natan L, Chaillet P, Lecomte JM, Marçais H, Uchida G, Costentin J (1984) Involvement of endogenous enkephalins in the mouse "behavioral despair" test. Eur J Pharmacol 97:301–304

Benchetrit T, Fournié-Zaluski MC, Roques BP (1987) Relationship between the inhibitory potencies of thiorphan and retrothiorphan enantiomers on thermolysin and neutral endopeptidase 24.11 and their interactions with the thermolysin active site by computer modelling. Biochem Biophys Res Commun 147:1034–1040

Benuck M, Mark N (1979) Co-identity of brain angiotensin converting enzyme with a membrane bound dipeptidyl carboxypeptidase inactivating met-enkephalin. Biochem Biophys Res Commun 88:215–221

Blumberg S, Vogel Z, Altstein M (1981) Inhibition of enkephalin-degrading enzymes from rat brain and of thermolysin by amino acid hydroxamates. Life Sci 28:301–306

Bouboutou R, Waksman G, Devin J, Fournié-Zaluski MC, Roques BP (1984) Bidentate peptides: highly potent new inhibitors of enkephalin degrading enzymes. Life Sci 35:1023–1030

Boudinot E, Denavit-Saubié M, Fournié-Zaluski MC, Morin-Surun MP, Roques BP (1988) Respiratory consequences in cats and rats of inhibition of enkephalin-degrading enzymes by kelatorphan. J Physiol 406:169P

Bourgoin S, Le Bars D, Artaud F, Clot AM, Bouboutou R, Fournié-Zaluski MC, Roques BP, Hamon M, Cesselin F (1986) Effects of kelatorphan and other peptidase inhibitors on the in vitro and in vivo release of methionine-enkephalin-like material from the rat spinal cord. J Pharmacol Exp Ther 238:360–366

Butcher SP, Varro A, Kelly JS, Dockray GJ (1989) In vivo studies on the enhancement of cholecystokinin release in the rat striatum by dopamine depletion. Brain Res 505:119–122

Calenco-Choukroun G, Daugé V, Gacel G, Féger J, Roques BP (1991) Opioid δ-agonists and endogenous enkephalins induce different emotional reactivity than μ-agonists after injection in the rat ventral tegmental area. Psychopharmacology 103:493–502

Carenzi A, Frigeni V, Della-Bella D (1981) Strong analgesic effect of Leu-enkephalin after inhibition of brain aminopeptidases: a pharmacological study. In: Takagi

H, Simon EF (eds) Advances in endogenous and exogenous opioids, proceedings of the international Narcotic Research Conference, Kyoto, p 267

Carenzi A, Frigeni V, Reggiani A, Della-Bella D (1983) Effect of inhibition of neuropeptidases on the pain threshold of mice and rats. Neuropharmacology 22:1315–1319

Cesselin F, Oliveras JL, Bourgoin S, Sierralta F, Michelot R, Besson JM, Hamon M (1982) Increased levels of Met-enkephalin like material in the CSF of anesthetized cats after tooth pulp stimulation. Brain Res 237:325–338

Cesselin F, Benoleil JJ, Bourgoin S, Mauborgne A, Hamon M (1989) Effects of opioid receptor agonists on the in vitro release of CCK-8 like material from the rat substantia nigra and spinal cord. Adv Biosc 75:205–208

Chaillet P, Marçais-Collado H, Costentin J, Yi CC, de la Baume S, Schwartz JC (1983) Inhibition of enkephalin metabolism and antinociceptive activity of, bestatin, an aminopeptidase inhibitor. Eur J Pharmacol 86:329–336

Chaillet P, Coulaud A, Zajac JM, Fournié-Zaluski MC, Costentin J, Roques BP (1984) The mu rather than the delta subtype of opioid receptors appears to be involved in enkephalin induced analgesia. Eur J Pharmacol 101:83–90

Chan WWC (1983) L-Leucinethiol – a potent inhibitor of leucine aminopeptidase. Biochem Biophys Res Commun 116:297–302

Chaussade S, Hamm R, Lecomte JM, Couturier D, Guerre J (1988) Effects of an enkephalinase inhibitor on oesophageal motility in man. Gastroenterol Clin Biol 12:793–796

Checler F, Vincent JP, Kitabgi P (1983) Degradation of neurotensin by rat brain synaptic membranes involvement of a thermolysin like metalloendopeptidase (enkephalinase), angiotensin converting enzyme, and other unidentified peptides. J Neurochem 41:375–384

Chérot P, Devin J, Fournié-Zaluski MC, Roques BP (1986a) Enkephalin degrading dipeptidylaminopeptidase: characterization of the active site and selective inhibition. Mol Pharmacol 30:338–344

Chérot P, Fournié-Zaluski MC, Laval J (1986b) Purification and characterization of an enkephalin-degrading dipeptidyl-aminopeptidase from porcine brain. Biochemistry 25:8184–8191

Chipkin RE (1986) Inhibitors of enkephalinase: the next generation of analgesics. In: Drug of the future, vol 11, pp 593–607

Chipkin RE, Latranyi MZ, Iorio LC (1982a) Potentiation of stress-induced analgesia (SIA) by thiorphan and its block by naloxone. Life Sci 31:1189–1192

Chipkin RE, Latranyi MZ, Iorio LC, Barnett A (1982b) Potentiation of [D-Ala^2] enkephalinamide analgesia in rats by thiorphan. Eur J Pharmacol 83:283–288

Chipkin RE, Berger JG, Billard W, Iorio LC, Chapman R, Barnett A (1988) Pharmacology of SCH 34826, an orally active enkephalinase inhibitor analgesic. J Pharmacol Exp Ther 245:829–838

Costentin J, Valiculescu A, Chaillet P, Ben Natan L, Aveaux D, Schwartz JC (1986) Dissociated effects of inhibitors of enkephalin-metabolising peptidases or naloxone on various nociceptive responses. Eur J Pharmacol 123:37–44

Coulter HD (1988) Vesicular localisation immunoreactive [Met5]enkephalin in the globus pallidus. Proc Natl Acad Sci USA 85:7028–7032

Craves FB, Law PY, Hunt CA, Loh HH (1978) The metabolic disposition of radiolabeled enkephalins in vitro and in situ. J Pharmacol Exp Ther 206: 492–506

Cuello AC (1983) Central distribution of opioid peptides. Br Med Bull 33:11–17

D'Adamio L, Shipp MA, Masteller EL, Reinherz EI (1989) Organization of the gene encoding common acute lymphoblastic leukemia antigen (neutral endopeptidase 24.11): multiple miniexons and separate 5' untranslated regions. Proc Natl Acad Sci USA 86:7103–7107

Daugé V, Rossignol P, Roques BP (1988) Comparison of the behavioural effects induced by administration in rat nucleus accumbens or nucleus caudatus of selective μ and δ opioid peptides or kelatorphan, an inhibitor of enkephalin-degrading enzymes. Psychopharmacology 96:343–352

Daugé V, Rossignol P, Roques BP (1989) Blockade of dopamine receptors reverse the behavioral effects of endogenous enkephalins in the nucleus caudatus but not in the nucleus accumbens: differential involvement of δ and μ opioid receptors. Psychopharmacology 99:168–175

Del Carmen de Felipe M, Jimenez I, Castro A, Fuentes JA (1989) Antidepressant action of imipramine and iprindole in mice is enhanced by inhibitors of enkephalin-degrading peptidases. Eur J Pharmacol 159:175–180

Del Fiacco M, Paxinos G, Cuello AC (1982) Neostriatal enkephalin-immmunoreactive neurons project to the globus pallidus. Brain Res 231:1–17

Delay-Goyet P, Zajac JM, Javoy-Agid F, Agid Y, Roques BP (1987) Regional distribution of μ, ∂ and κ opioid receptors in human brain from controls and parkinsonian subjects. Brain Res 414:8–14

Devault A, Lazure C, Nault C, Le Moual H, Seidah NG, Chrétien M, Kahn P, Powell J, Mallet J, Beaumont A, Roques BP, Crine P, Boileau C (1987) Amino acid sequence of rabbit kidney neutral endopeptidase 24.11 (enkephalinase) deduced from a complementary DNA. EMBO J 6:1317–1322

Devault A, Nault C, Zollinger M, Fournié-Zaluski MC, Roques BP, Crine P, Boileau G (1988) Expression of neutral endopeptidase (enkephalinase) in heterologous cos-1 cells: characterization of the recombinant enzyme and evidence for a glutamic acid residue at the active site. J Biol Chem 263:4033–4040

De Witte P, Heidbreder C, Roques BP (1989) Kelatorphan, a potent enkephalinase inhibitor, and opioid receptor agonists DAGO and DTLET, differentially modulate self-stimulation behaviour depending on the site of administration. Neuropharmacology 28:667–676

Dickenson AH (1986) Enkephalins. A new approach to pain relief? Nature 320: 681–682

Dickenson AH, Sullivan A, Feeney C, Fournie-Zaluski MC, Roques BP (1986) Evidence that endogenous enkephalins produce δ-opiate receptor mediated neuronal inhibitions in rat dorsal horn. Neurosci Lett 72:179–182

Dickenson AH, Sullivan AF, Fournié-Zaluski MC, Roques BP (1987) Prevention of degradation of endogenous enkephalins produces inhibition of nociceptive neurones in rat spinal cord. Brain Res 408:185–191

Dickenson AH, Sullivan AF, Roques BP (1988) Evidence that endogenous enkephalins and a ∂ opioid receptor agonist have a common site of action in spinal antinociception. Eur J Pharmacol 148:437–439

Dzoljic MR, Ukponmwan OE, Rupreht J, Haffman J (1985) Role of the enkephalinergic system in sleep studies by an enkephalinase inhibitor. In: Vauquier A (ed) Sleep: neurotransmitters and neuromodulators. Raven, New York, p 251

Dzoljic TD, Nadel JA, Dusser DJ, Sekizawa K, Graf PD, Borson DB (1989) Inhibitors of neutral endopeptidase potentiate electrically and capsaicin-induced noncholinergic contraction in guinea pig bronchi. J Pharmacol Exp Ther 248: 7–11

Dourmap N, Michael-Titus A, Costentin J (1990) Local enkephalins tonically modulate dopamine release in the striatum: a microdialysis study. Brain Res 524:153–155

Dupont A, Cusan L, Garon M, Alvarado-Urbina G, Labrie F (1977) Extremely rapid degradation of [^{3}H]-methionine enkephalin by various rat tissues in vivo and in vitro. Life Sci 21:907–914

Durieux C, Charpentier B, Fellion E, Gacel G, Pélaprat D, Roques BP (1985) Multiple cleavage sites of cholecystokinin heptapeptides by enkephalinase. Peptides 6:495–501

Durieux C, Charpentier D, Pélaprat D, Roques BP (1986) Investigation on the metabolism of CCK$_8$ analogues by rat brain slices. Neuropeptides 7:1–9

Dusser DJ, Jocoby DB, Djokil TD, Rubinstein F, Borson DB, Nadel JA (1989) Virus induces airway hyperresponsiveness to tachykinins: role of neutral endopeptidase. J Appl Physiol 67:1504–1511

Elliot RL, Marks N, Berg MJ, Portoghese PS (1985) Synthesis and biological evaluation of phosphonomidate peptide inhibitors of enkephalinase and angiotensin converting enzyme. J Med Chem 28:1208–1216

Erdös EG, Skidgel RA (1989) Neutral endopeptidase 24.11 (enkephalinase) and related regulators of peptide hormones. FASEB J 3:145–151

Erdös EG, Johnson AR, Boyden NT (1978) Hydrolysis of enkephalin by cultured human endothelial cells and by purified peptidyl dipeptidase. Biochem Pharmacol 27:843–845

Floras P, Bidabe AM, Vaille JM, Simonnet G, Lecomte JM, Sabathie M (1983) Double-blind study of effects of enkephalinase inhibitor on adverse reactions to myelography. Am J Neuroradiol 4:653–655

Florentin D, Sassi A, Roques BP (1984) A highly sensitive fluorimetric assay for "enkephalinase", a neutral metalloendopeptidase that releases Tyr-Gly-Gly from enkephalins. Anal Biochem 141:62–69

Fournié-Zaluski MC, Perdrisot R, Gacel G, Swerts JP, Roques BP, Schwartz JC (1979) Inhibitory potency of various peptides on enkephalinase activity from mouse striatum. Biochem Biophys Res Commun 91:130–135

Fournié-Zaluski MC, Llorens C, Gacel G, Malfroy B, Swerts JP, Lecomte JM, Schwartz JC, Roques BP (1981) Synthesis and biological properties of highly potent enkephalinase inhibitors. In: Brunfeld K (ed) Peptides 1980. Scriptor, Copenhagen, pp 476–481

Fournié-Zaluski MC, Soroca-Lucas E, Waksman G, Llorens C, Schwartz JC, Roques BP (1982) Differential recognition of "enkephalinase" and angiotensin-converting-enzyme by new carboxyalkyl inhibitors. Life Sci 31:2947–2954

Fournié-Zaluski MC, Chaillet P, Soroca-Lucas E, Costentin J, Roques BP (1983) New carboxyalkyl inhibitors of brain "enkephalinase": synthesis, biological activity and analgesic properties. J Med Chem 26:60–65

Fournié-Zaluski MC, Lucas E, Waksman G, Roques BP (1984a) Differences in the structural requirements for selective interaction with neutral metallo-endopeptidase (enkephalinase) or angiotensin converting enzyme: molecular investigation by use of new thiol inhibitors. Eur J Biochem 139:267–274

Fournié-Zaluski MC, Chaillet P, Bouboutou R, Coulaud A, Chérot P, Waksman G, Costentin J, Roques BP (1984b) Analgesic effects of kelatorphan, a new highly potent inhibitor of multiple enkephalin degrading enzymes. Eur J Pharmacol 102:525–528

Fournié-Zaluski MC, Coulaud A, Bouboutou R, Chaillet P, Devin J, Waksman G, Costentin J, Roques BP (1985) New bidentates as full inhibitors of enkephalin degrading enzymes: synthesis and analgesic properties. J Med Chem 28:1158–1169

Fournié-Zaluski MC, Soleihac JM, Turcaud S, Lai-Kuen R, Crine P, Beaumont A, Roques BP (1992) Development of [125I]RB104, a new potent inhibitor of neutral endopeptidase-24,11 and its use in detecting nanogram quantities of the enzyme by "Inhibitor Gel Electrophoresis." Proc Natl Acad Sci USA (in press)

Gacel G, Fournié-Zaluski MC, Fellion E, Roques BP (1981) Evidence of the preferential involvement of μ-receptors in analgesia using enkephalins highly selective for peripheral μ or ∂ receptors. J Med Chem 24:1119–1124

Gee NS, Bowes MA, Buck P, Kenny AJ (1985) An immunoradiometric assay for endopeptidase 24-11 shows it to be a widely distributed enzyme in pig tissues. Biochem J 228:119–126

Gibert-Rahola J, Tejedor P, Chover AJ, Puyana M, Rodriguez MM, Leonsegui I, Mellado M, Mico JA, Maldonado R, Roques BP (1990) RB38B, a selective neutral endopeptidase inhibitor, induced reversal of escape deficits caused by inescapable shocks pretreatment in rats. In: Van Ree JM, Mulder AH, Wiegant

VM, Van Wimersma Greidanus TB (eds) New leads in opioid research. Excerpta Medica, Amsterdam, p 2317

Glimcher PW, Giovino AA, Margolin DH, Hoebel BG (1984) Endogenous opiate reward induced by an enkephalinergic inhibitor, thiorphan, injected into the ventral midbrain. Behav Neurosci 98:262–268

Gordon EM, Cushman DW, Tung R, Cheung HS, Wang FL, Delaney NG (1983) Rat brain enkephalinase: characterization of the active site using mercapto-propanoyl amino acid inhibitors and comparison with angiotensin-converting enzyme. Life Sci 33:113–116

Gordon EM, Godfrey JD, Delaney NG, Asaad MM, Von Langen D, Cushman DW (1988) Design of novel inhibitors of aminopeptidases, synthesis of peptide-derived diamino thiols and sulfur replacement analogues of bestatin. J Med Chem 31:2199–2211

Gorenstein C, Snyder SH (1979) Two distinct enkephalinases: solubilization, partial purification and separation from angiotensin converting enzyme. Life Sci 25:2065–2070

Gros C, Giros B, Schwartz JC (1985) Identification of aminopeptidase M as an enkephalin-inactivating enzyme in rat cerebral membranes. Biochemistry 24:2179–2186

Gros C, Giros B, Schwartz JC, Vlaiculescu A, Costentin J, Lecomte JM (1988) Potent inhibition of cerebral aminopeptidases by carbaphethiol, a parenterally active compound. Neuropeptides 12:111–118

Gros C, Souque A, Schwartz JC, Duchier J, Cournot A, Baumer P, Lecomte JM (1989) Protection of atrial natriuretic factor against degradation: diuretic and natriuretic responses after in vivo inhibition of enkephalinase (EC 3.4.24.11) by acetorphan. Proc Natl Acad Sci USA 86:7580–7584

Guyon A, Roques BP, Foucaud A, Guyon F, Caude M, Perdrisot R, Schwartz JC (1979) Enkephalin degradation in mouse brain studied by a new HPLC method: further evidence for the involvement of a carboxypeptidase. Life Sci 25:1605–1612

Hachisu M, Takahashi H, Hiranuma T, Shibazaki Y, Murata S (1985) Relationship between enkephalinase inhibition of thiorphan in vivo and its analgesic activity. J Pharmacobiodyn 8:701–710

Haffmans J, Dzoljic MR (1987) Inhibition of enkephalinase activity attenuates naloxone-precipitated withdrawal symptoms. Gen Pharmacol 18:103–105

Hambrook JM, Morgan BA, Rance MJ, Smith CFC (1976) Mode of deactivation of the enkephalins by rat and human plasma and rat brain homogenates. Nature 262:782–783

Hamel E, Beaudet A (1987) Opioid receptors in rat neostriatum: radioautographic distribution at the electron microscopic level. Brain Res 401:239–257

Hélène A, Beaumont A, Roques BP (1991) Functional residues at the active site of aminopeptidase N. Eur J Biochem 196:385–393

Hernandez JF, Soleihac JM, Roques BP, Fournié-Zaluski MC (1988) Retro-inverso concept applied to the mixed inhibitors of enkephalin-degrading enzymes. J Med Chem 31:1825–1831

Hersh LB (1981) Solubilization and characterization of two rat brain amino-peptidases active on Met-enkephalin. Biochemistry 20:2345–2350

Hersh LB, Morihara K (1986) Comparison of the subsite specificity of the mammalian neutral endopeptidase 24-11 (enkephalinase) to the bacterial neutral endo-peptidase thermolysin. J Biol Chem 261:6433–6437

Hersh LB, Aboukhair N, Watson S (1987) Immunohistochemical localization of aminopeptidase M in rat brain and periphery: relationship of enzyme local-ization and enkephalin metabolism. Peptides 8:523–532

Horsthemke B, Hamprecht B, Bauer K (1983) Heterogenous distribution of enkephalin-degrading peptidases between neuronal and glial cells. Biochem Biophys Res Commun 115:423–429

Hudgin RL, Charlson SE, Zimmerman M, Mumford R, Wood PL (1981) Enkephalinase: selective peptide inhibitors. Life Sci 29:2593–2601

Hui KS, Wang YJ, Lajtha A (1983) Purification and characterization of an enkephalin aminopeptidase from rat brain membranes. Biochemistry 22:1062–1067

Jessell TM, Iversen LL (1977) Opiates analgesic inhibit substance P release from rat trigeminal nucleus. Nature 268:549–551

Jivegard L, Pollard H, Moreau J, Schwartz JC, Thune A, Svanik J (1989) Naloxone-reversible inhibition of gall-bladder mucosa fluid secretion in experimental cholecystities in the cat by acetorphan, an enkephalinase inhibitor. Clin Sci 77:49–54

Jongeneel CV, Bouvier J, Bairoch A (1989) A unique signature identifies a family of zinc-dependent metallopeptidase. FEBS Lett 242:211–214

Kalivas PW (1985) Interactions between neuropeptides and dopamine neurons in the ventro-medial mesencephalon. Neurosci Behav Rev 9:573–587

Kalivas PW, Richardson-Carlson R, Van Orden G (1986) Cross-sensitization between foot shock stress and enkephalin-induced motor activity. Biol Psychiatry 21:939–950

Kayser V, Benoist JM, Gautron M, Guilbaud G, Roques BP (1984) Effects of ES52 an enkephalinase inhibitor, on responses of ventrobasal thalamic neurons in rat. Peptides 5:1159–1164

Kayser V, Fournié-Zaluski MC, Guilbaud G, Roques BP (1989) Potent anti-nociceptive effects of kelatorphan (a highly efficient inhibitor of multiple enkephalin degrading enzymes) systemically administered in normal and arthritic rats. Brain Res 497:94–101

Kenny AJ (1986) Cell surface peptidases are neither peptide- nor organ-specific. Trends Biochem Sci 11:40–42

Kenny AJ, Stephenson SL (1988) Role of endopeptidase-24.11 in the inactivation of atrial natriuretic peptide. FEBS Lett 232(1):1–8

Kenny AJ, Stephenson SL, Turner AJ (1987) Cell surface peptidases. In: Kenny AJ, Turner AJ (eds) Mammalian ectoenzymes, Elsevier. Amsterdam, p 169

Kerr MA, Kenny AJ (1974) The purification and specificity of a neutral endo-peptidase from rabbit kidney brush border. Biochem J 137:477–488

Koehn JA, Norman JA, Jones BN, Le Sueur L, Sakane Y, Ghai RD (1987) Degradation of atrial natriuretic factor by kidney cortex membranes. Isolation and characterization of the primary proteolytic product. J Biol Chem 262: 11623–11627

Kohrogi H, Nadel JA, Malfroy B, Gorman C, Bridenbaugh R, Patton JS, Borson DB (1989) Recombinant human enkephalinase (neutral endopeptidase) prevents cough induced by tachikinins in awake guinea pigs. J Clin Invest 84: 781–786

Kruse TA, Bolund L, Grzeschik KH, Ropers SC (1988) Assignment of the human aminopeptidase N (peptidase E) gene to chromosome 15p13-qter. FEBS Lett 239:305–308

Ksander GM, Diefenbacher CG, Yuan AM, Clark F, Sakane Y, Ghai RD (1989) Enkephalinase inhibitors 1-2,4-dibenzylglutaric acid derivatives. J Med Chem 32:2519–2526

Lebien TW, McCormack RT (1989) The common acute lymphoblastic leucemia antigen (CD10) – emancipation from a functional enigma. Blood 73(3):625–634

Lecomte JM, Costentin J, Vlaiculescu A, Chaillet P, Marçais-Collado H, Llorens-Cortes C, Leboyer M, Schwartz JC (1986) Pharmacological properties of acetorphan, a parenterally active "enkephalinase" inhibitor. J Pharmacol Exp Ther 237:937–944

Llorens C, Schwartz JC (1981) Enkephalinase activity in rat peripheral organs. Eur J Pharmacol 69:113–116

Llorens C, Gacel G, Swerts JP, Perdrisot R, Fournié-Zaluski MC, Schwartz JC, Roques BP (1980) Rational design of enkephalinase inhibitors: substrate specificity of enkephalinase studied from inhibitory potency of various peptides. Biochem Biophys Res Commun 96:1710–1715

Llorens C, Malfroy B, Schwartz JC, Gacel G, Roques BP, Roy J, Morgat JL, Javoy-Agid F, Agid Y (1982) Enkephalin dipeptidyl carboxypeptidase (enkephalinase) activity: selective radioassay, properties and regional distribution in human brain. J Neurochem 39:1081–1089

Llorens-Cortes C, Schwartz JC (1984) Changes in turnover of cerebral monoamines following inhibition of enkephalin metabolism by thiorphan and bestatin. Eur J Pharmacol 104:369–374

Llorens-Cortes C, Gros C, Schwartz JC (1985) Study of endogenous Tyr-Gly-Gly a putative enkephalin metabolite in mouse brain: validation of a radio-immunoassay, localisation and effects of peptidase inhibitors. Eur J Pharmacol 119:183–191

Llorens-Cortes C, Gros C, Schwartz JC, Clot AM, Le Bars D (1989) Changes in levels of the tripeptide Tyr-Gly-Gly as an index of enkephalin release in the spinal cord: effects of noxious stimuli and parenterally active peptidase inhibitors. Peptides 10:609–614

Mac Lennan AJ, Maier SF (1983) Coping and the stress-induced potentiation of stimulant stereotypy in the rat. Science 219:1091–1093

Maldonado R, Daugé V, Callebert J, Villette JM, Fournié-Zaluski MC, Féger J, Roques BP (1989) Comparison of selective and complete inhibitors of enkephalins degrading enzymes on morphine withdrawal syndrome. Eur J Pharmacol 165:199–207

Maldonado R, Féger J, Fournié-Zaluski MC, Roques BP (1990a) Differences in physical dependence induced by selective μ or ∂ opioid agonists and by endogenous enkephalins protected by peptidase inhibitors. Brain Res 520: 247–254

Maldonado R, Daugé V, Féger J, Roques BP (1990b) Chronic blockade of D2 but not D1-dopamine receptors facilitates behavioural responses to endogenous enkephalins, protected by kelatorphan administered in the accumbens in rats. Neuropharmacol 29:215–223

Malfroy B, Schwartz JC (1982) Properties of enkephalinase from rat kidney: comparison of dipeptidyl-carboxypeptidase and endopeptidase activities. Biochem Biophys Res Commun 106:276–285

Malfroy B, Swerts JP, Guyon A, Roques BP, Schwartz JC (1978) High-affinity enkephalin-degrading peptidase in mouse brain and its enhanced activity following morphine. Nature 276:523–526

Malfroy B, Swerts JP, Llorens C, Schwartz JC (1979) Regional distribution of a high-affinity enkephalin-degrading peptidase (enkephalinase) and effects of lesions suggest localization in the vicinity of opiate receptors in brain. Neurosci Lett 11:329–334

Malfroy B, Schofield PR, Kuang WJ, Seeburg PM, Mason AJ, Heurd WJ (1987) Molecular cloning and amino acid sequence of rat enkephalinase. Biochem Biophys Res Commun 144:59–66

Malin DH, Lake JR, Hamilton RF, Skolnick MH (1989) Augmentated analgesic effects of enkephalinase inhibitors combined with transcranial electrostimulation. Life Sci 44:1371–1376

Marçais-Collado H, Uchida G, Costentin J, Schwartz JC, Lecomte JM (1987) Naloxone reversible antidiarrheal effects of enkephalinase inhibitors. Eur J Pharmacol 144:125–132

Matsas R, Fulcher IS, Kenny AJ, Turner AJ (1983) Subtance P and Leu-enkephalin are hydrolyzed by an enzyme in pig caudate synaptic membranes that is identical with the endopeptidase of kidney microvilli. Proc Natl Acad Sci USA 80:3111–3115

Matsas R, Turner AJ, Kenny AJ (1984) The metabolism of neuropeptides: the hydrolysis of peptides including enkephalins, tachykinins and their analogues by endopeptidase 24.11. Biochem J 223:433–440

Matsas R, Stephenson SL, Hryszko J, Kenny AJ, Turner AJ (1985) The metabolism of neuropeptides: phase separation of synaptic membrane preparations with Triton X-114 reveals the presence of aminopeptidase N. Biochem J 231:445–449

Matsas R, Kenny AJ, Turner AJ (1986) An immunohistochemical study of endopeptidase 24-11 ("enkephalinase") in the pig nervous system. Neuroscience 18:991–1012

Matthews BW (1988) Structural basis of the action of thermolysin and related zinc peptidases. Acc Chem Res 21:333–340

Mauborgne A, Bourgoin S, Benoleil JJ, Hirsh H, Berthier JL, Hamon M, Cesselin F (1987a) Enkephalinase is involved in the degradation of endogenous substance P released from slices of rat substantia nigra. J Pharmacol Exp Ther 243:674–680

Mauborgne A, Lutz O, Legrand JC, Hamon M, Cesselin F (1987b) Opposite effects of ∂ and μ opioid receptor agonists on the in vitro release of substance P-like material from the rat spinal cord. J Neurochem 48:529–537

Meek JL, Yang HYT, Costa E (1977) Enkephalin catabolism in vitro and in vivo. Neuropharmacology 16:151–154

Meucci E, Delay-Goyet P, Roques BP, Zajac JM (1989) Binding in vivo of selective μ and ∂ opioid agonists: opioid receptors occupancy by endogenous enkephalins. Eur J Pharmacol 171:167–178

Meynadier J, Dalmas S, Lecomte JM, Gros C, Schwartz JC (1988) Potent analgesic effects of inhibitors of enkephalin metabolism administered intrathecally to cancer patients. Pain Clinic 2:201–206

Morton CR, Zhao ZQ, Duggan AW (1987) Kelatorphan potentiates the effect of Met^5-enkephalin in the substantia gelatinosa of the cat spinal cord. Eur J Pharmacol 140:195–201

Mumford RA, Zimmerman M, Broeke JT, Taub D, Joshua H, Rothrock JW, Hirshfield JM, Springer JP, Patchett AA (1982) Inhibition of porcine kidney "enkephalinase" by substituted N-carboxymethyl dipeptides. Biochem Biophys Res Commun 109:1303–1309

Murthy LR, Glick SD, Almenoff J, Wilk S, Orlowski M (1984) Inhibitors of an enkephalin degrading membrane bound metalloendopeptidase: analgesic properties and effects on striatal enkephalin levels. Eur J Pharmacol 102:305–313

Nabeshima T, Katoh A, Hiramatsu M, Kameyama T (1987) A role played by dopamine and opioid neuronal systems in stress-induced motor suppression (conditioned suppression of mobility) in mice. Brain Res 398:354–360

Noble F, Coric P, Soleihac JM, Turcaud S, Daugé V, Fournié-Zaluski MC, Roques BP (1990) Analgesic properties of systematically active mixed enkephalin-degrading enzyme inhibitors. In: Van Ree JM, Mulder AH, Wiegant VM, Van Wimersma Greidanus TB (eds) New leads in opioid research. Excepta Medica, Amsterdam, pp 83–86

Noble F, Soleihac JM, Lucas-Soroca E, Turcaud S, Fournié-Zaluski MC and Roques BP (1992) Inhibition of the enkephalin metabolizing enzymes by the first systemically active mixed inhibitor prodrug, RB101 induces potent analgesic responses in mice and rats. J Pharm Exp Ther 261:181–190

Noble F, Fournié-Zaluski MC, Roques BP (1992) Unlike morphine, the endogenous enkephalins protected by the systemically active mixed inhibitor prodrug RB101 are unable to establish a conditioned place preference in mice. Eur J Pharmacol (in press)

Noble F, Coric P, Fournié-Zaluski MC, Roques BP (1992) Lack of physical dependence development in mice following repeated systemic administration of the mixed inhibitor prodrug of enkephalin-degrading enzymes, RB101. Eur J Pharmacol (in press)

Noble F, Turcaud S, Fournié-Zaluski MC, Roques BP (1992) Repeated systemic administration of the mixed inhibitor of enkephalin-degrading enzymes, RB101, did not induce either antinociceptive tolerance or cross tolerance with morphine. Eur J Pharmacol (in press)

Northridge DB, Jardine AG, Alabaster CT, Barclay PL, Connell JMC, Dargie HJ, Dilly SG, Findlay IN, Lever AF, Samuels GMR (1989) Effects of UK 69578: a novel atriopeptidase inhibitor. Lancet II: 591–593

Ocain ID, Rich DM (1988) Synthesis of sulfur containing analogues of Bestatin. Inhibitors of amino peptidases by α-thiobestatin analogues. J Med Chem 31: 2193–2199

Olsen J, Corvell GM, Konigshofer FG, Danielsen EM, Moller J, Laustsen L, Hausen OC, Welinder FG, Engberg J, Hunziber W, Spiers M, Sjostrom H, Noren (1988) Complete amino acid sequence of human intestinal aminopeptidase N as deduced from cloned cDNA. FEBS Lett 238:307–314

Ondetti MA, Rubin B, Cushman DW (1977) Design of specific inhibitors of angiotensin-converting enzyme: new class of orally active antihypertensive agents. Science 196:441–444

Oshita S, Yaksh TL, Chipkin R (1990) The antinociceptive effects of intrathecally administered SCH 32615, an enkephalinase inhibitor in the rat. Brain Res 515:143–148

Patey G, de la Baume S, Schwartz JC, Gros C, Fournié-Zaluski MC, Lucas-Soroca E, Roques BP (1981) Selective protection of methionine enkephaline released from brain slices by thiorphan, a potent enkephalinase inhibitors. Science 212: 1153–1155

Pert C, Pert A, Chang JK, Fong BTW (1976) [D-Ala^2]-Met-enkephalinamide: a potent, long-lasting synthetic pentapeptide analgesic. Science 194:330–332

Petit F, Hamon M, Fournié-Zaluski MC, Roques BP, Glowinski J (1986) Further evidence for a role of delta opiate receptors in the presynaptic regulation of newly synthesized dopamine release. Eur J Pharmacol 126:1–9

Pham I, Fournié-Zaluski MC, Corvol P, Roques BP, Michel JB (1990) Effects hypotenseur et diurétique du rétrothiorphan chez le rat normal et le docasel. Arch Malad Coeur et des Vaisseaux 83:50

Pierart ME, Najidovski T, Appelboom TE, Deschodt-Lanckman MM (1988) Effect of human endopeptidase 24.11 ("enkephalinase") on IL-1-induced thymocyte proliferation activity. J Immunol 140:3808–3811

Pollard M, Bouthenet ML, Moreau J, Souil E, Verroust P, Ronco P, Schwartz JC (1989) Detailed immunoautoradiographic mapping system comparison with enkephalins and SP. Neuroscience 30:339–376

Porréca F, Mosberg HI, Hurst R, Hruby VJ, Burks TF (1984) Roles of mu, delta and kappa opioid receptors in spinal and supraspinal mediation of gastrointestinal transit effects and hot-plate analgesia in the mouse. J Pharmacol Exp Ther 230:341–348

Relton JM, Gee NS, Matsas R, Turner AJ, Kenny AJ (1983) Purification of endopeptidase 24-11 (enkephalinase) from pig brain by immunoadsorbent chromatography. Biochem J 215:519–523

Rich DH (1990) Peptidase inhibitors. In: Sammes PG, Taylor JB (eds) Comprehensive medicinal chemistry. The rational design, mechanistic study and therapeutic application of chemical compounds, vol. 2. Pergamon, Oxford, p 391

Roderick SL, Fournié-Zaluski MC, Roques BP, Matthews BW (1989) Thiorphan and retrothiorphan display equivalent interactions when bound to crystalline thermolysin. Biochemistry 28:1493–1497

Ronco P, Pollard H, Galceran M, Delauche M, Schwartz JC, Verroust P (1988) Distribution of enkephalinase (membrane metalloendopeptidase, E.C.3.4.24.11) in rat organs. Detection using a monoclonal antibody. Lab Invest 58:210–217

Roques BP (1985) Inhibiteurs d'enképhalinase et exploration moléculaire des différences entre sites actifs de l'enképhalinase et de l'enzyme de conversion de l'angiotensine. J Pharmacol (Paris) 16:5–31

Roques BP (1988a) Novel approaches to the pharmacological modification of peptidergic neurotransmission. In: Leeming PR (ed) Proceedings of the IVth SCI-RSC medicinal chemistry symposium, topics in medicinal chemistry. Royal Society of Chemistry, Cambridge, pp 22–42

Roques BP (1988b) Physiological role of endogenous peptide effectors studied with peptidase inhibitors. Kidney Int 34:27–33

Roques BP (1991) What are the relevant features of the distribution, selective binding and metabolism of opioid peptides and how can these be applied to drug design? In: Basbaum A, Besson JM (eds) Towards a new pharmacotherapy of pain. Wiley, New York, pp 257–277

Roques BP, Beaumont A (1990) Neutral endopeptidase-24,11 inhibitors: from analgesics to antihypertensives. Trends Pharmacol Sci 11:245–249

Roques BP, Fournié-Zaluski MC (1985) A new way to antinociceptive compounds through rational design of enkephalin degrading enzyme inhibitors. In: Dalhbom R, Nilsson JLG (ed) Proceeding of international symposium on medicinal chemistry. Swedish Pharmaceutical Press, Stockholm, pp 134–146

Roques BP, Fournié-Zaluski MC (1986) Enkephalin degrading enzyme inhibitors: a physiological way to new analgesics and psychoactive agents. In: Rapaka RS, Hawks RL (eds) Opioid peptides: molecular, pharmacology, biosynthesis and analysis. NIDA Res Monogr 70:128ᵇ–154

Roques BP, Fournié-Zaluski MC, Soroca E, Lecomte JM, Malfroy B', Llorens C, Schwartz JC (1980) The enkephalinase inhibitor thiorphan shows antinociceptive activity in mice. Nature 288:286–288

Roques BP, Fournié-Zaluski MC, Florentin D, Waksman G, Sassi A, Chaillet P, Collado H, Costentin J (1982) New enkephalinase inhibitors as probes to differentiate "enkephalinase" and angiotensin-converting-enzyme active sites. Life Sci 31:1749–1752

Roques BP, Lucas-Soroca E, Chaillet P, Costentin J, Fournié-Zaluski MC (1983) Complete differentiation between "enkephalinase" and angiotensin converting enzyme inhibition by retro-thiorphan. Proc Natl Acad Sci USA 80:3178–3182

Roques BP, Daugé V, Gacel G, Fournié-Zaluski MC (1985) Selective agonists and antagonists of delta opioid receptors and inhibitors of enkephalin metabolism. Potential use in treatment of mental illness. In: Shagass C, Josiassen RC, Bridger WH, Weiss KJ, Stoff D, Simpon GM (eds) Biological psychiatry. Developments in psychiatry, vol. 7. Elsevier, New York, pp 287–289

Roques BP, Beaumont A, Fournié-Zaluski MC (1991) Structure, localization and inhibition of endopeptidase 24.11; pharmacological studies and possible clinical applications. Pharmacol Rev (in press)

Ruiz-Gayo M, Baamonde A, Turcaud S, Fournié-Zaluski MC, Roques BP (1992) in vivo occupation of mouse brain opioid receptors by endogenous enkephalins: blockade of enkephalin degrading enzymes by RB101 inhibits [3H]-diprenorphine binding. Brain Res 511:306–312

Ruiz-Gayo M, Durieux C, Fournié-Zaluski MC, Roques BP (1992) Stimulation of δ opioid receptors reduces the in vivo binding of the CCK-B selective agonist [3H]pBC264: evidence for a physiological regulation of CCKergic systems by endogenous enkephalins. J Neurochem (in press)

Rupreht J, Ukponmwan OE, Admiral PV, Dzoljic MR (1983) Effect of phosphoramidon, a selective enkephalinase inhibitor on nociception and behaviour. Neurosci Lett 41:331–335

Sales N, Charnay Y, Zajac JM, Dubois PM, Roques BP (1989) Ontogeny of μ and ∂ opioid receptors and of neutral endopeptidase "enkephalinase" in human spinal cord: an autoradiographic study. J Chem Neuroanat 2:179–188

Sales N, Dutriez I, Maziére B, Ottaviani M, Roques BP (1991) Neutral endopeptidase 24.11 in rat peripheral tissues: comparative localization by "ex vivo" and "in vitro" autoradiography. Regul Pept 33:209–222

Schechter I, Berger A (1967) On the site of the active site in proteases. I. Papain. Biochem Biophys Res Commun 27:157–162

Schmidt C, Peyroux J, Noble F, Fournié-Zaluski MC, Roques BP (1991) A comparison of the analgesia produced by morphine and by endogenous enkephalins (protected by mixed peptidase inhibitors) using a variety of antinociceptive tests. Eur J Pharmacol 192:253–262

Schwartz JC (1983) Metabolism of enkephalins and the inactivating neuropeptidase concept. Trends Neurosci 6:45–48

Schwartz JC, Malfroy B, de la Baume S (1981) Biological inactivation of enkephalins and the role of enkephalin-dipeptidyl-carboxypeptidase ("enkephalinase") as neuropeptidase. Life Sci 29:1715–1740

Schwartz JC, Costentin J, Lecomte JM (1985) Pharmacology of enkephalinase inhibitors. TIPS 472–476

Soleilhac JM, Lucas E, Beaumont A, Turcaud S, Michel JB, Crine P, Fournie-Zaluski MC, Roques BP (1992) A 94 Kdalton protein, identified as neutral endopeptidase-24.11, can inactivate atrial natriuretic peptide in the vascular endothelium. Mol Pharmacol 41:609–614

Solhonne B, Gros C, Pollard H, Schwartz JC (1987) Major localization of aminopeptidase M in rat brain microvessels. Neuroscience 22:225–232

Stein C, Millan MJ, Shippenberg TS, Peter K, Herz A (1989) Peripheral opioid receptors mediating antinociception in inflammation. Evidence for involvement of mu, delta and kappa receptors. J Pharmacol Exp Ther 248:1269–1275

Stephenson SL, Kenny AJ (1987) The hydrolysis of α-human atrial natriuretic peptide by pig kidney microvillar membranes is initiated by endopeptidase-24.11. Biochem J 243:183–187

Stinus L, Winnock MR, Kelley AE (1985) Chronic neuroleptic treatment and mesolimbic dopamine denervation induce behavioral supersensitivity to opiates. Psychopharmacology 85:323–328

Sullivan AF, Akil H, Barchas JD (1978) In vitro degradation of enkephalin: evidence for cleavage at the Gly-Phe bond. Psychopharmacology 2:525–531

Sullivan AF, Dickenson AH, Roques BP (1989) δ-Opioid mediated inhibitions of acute and prolonged noxious-evoked responses in rat dorsal horn neurones. Br J Pharmacol 98:1039–1049

Swerts JP, Perdrisot R, Malfroy B, Schwartz JC (1979) Is "enkephalinase" identical with angiotensin converting enzyme? Eur J Pharmacol 53:209–210

Thorsett ED, Wyvratt MJ (1987) Inhibition of zinc peptidases that hydrolyse neuropeptides. In: Turner AJ (ed) Neuropeptides and their peptidases. Horwood, Chichester, p 229

Ueda H, Fukashima N, Kitao T, Ge M, Takagi H (1986) Low doses of naloxone produce analgesia in the mouse brain by blocking presynaptic autoinhibition of enkephalin release. Neurosci Lett 65:247–252

Van Amsterdam JGC, Llorens-Cortes C (1988) Inhibition of enkephalin degradation by phelorphan: effects on striatal [Met^5-enkephalin levels and jump latency in mouse hot plate test. Eur J Pharmacol 154:319–324

Van Amsterdam JGC, Van Buren KJM, Blod MWH, Soujikn W (1987) Synthesis of enkephalinase B inhibitors, and their activity on isolated enkephalin-degrading enzymes. Eur J Pharmacol 135:411–418

Villanueva L, Cadden S, Chitour D, Le Bars D (1985) Failure of ES52, a highly potent enkephalinase inhibitor, to affect nociceptive transmission by rat dorsal horn convergent neurones. Brain Res 333:156–160

Vogel Z, Altstein M (1977) The adsorption of enkephalin to porous polystyrene beads: a simple assay for enkephalin hydrolysis. FEBS Lett 80:332–336

Waksman G, Hamel E, Bouboutou R, Besselièvre R, Fournié-Zaluski MC, Roques BP (1984) Distribution regionale de l'enképhalinase dans le cerveau du rat par autoradiographie. C R Acad Sci [III] 299:613–616

Waksman G, Bouboutou R, Devin J, Bourgoin S, Cesselin F, Hamon M, Fournié-Zaluski MC, Roques BP (1985) In vitro and in vivo effects of kelatorphan on enkephalin metabolism in rodent brain. Eur J Pharmacol 117:233–243

Waksman G, Hamel E, Fournié-Zaluski MC, Roques BP (1986) Comparative distribution of the neutral endopeptidase "enkephalinase" and mu and delta opioid receptors in rat brain by autoradiography. Proc Natl Acad Sci USA 83:1523–1527

Waksman G, Hamel E, Delay-Goyet P, Roques BP (1987) Neutral endopeptidase 24.11 mu and delta opioid receptors after selective brain lesions: an autoradiographic study. Brain Res 436:205–216

Wilcox JN, Pollard H, Moreau J, Schwartz JC, Malfroy B (1989) Localization of enkephalinase mRNA in rat brain by in situ hybridization: comparison with immunohistochemical localization of the protein. Neuropeptides 14:77–83

Willer JC, Roby A, Ernst M (1986) The enkephalinase inhibitor GB52, does not effect nociceptive flexion reflexes nor pain sensation in humans. Neuropharmacology 25:819–822

Williams JT, Macdonald JC, Christie J, North RA, Roques BP (1987) Potentiation of enkephalin action by peptidase inhibitors in rat locus coeruleus in vitro. J Pharmacol Exp Ther 243:397–401

Wood PL, Richard SW (1982) Morphine and nigrostriatal function in the rat and mouse: the role of nigral and striatal opiate receptors. Neuropharmacology 21:1305–1310

Xie J, Soleilhac JM, Renwart N, Peyroux J, Roques BP, Fournié-Zaluski MC (1989a) Inhibitors of the enkephalin degrading enzymes: modulation of the activity of hydroxamate containing compounds by modification of the C-terminal residue. Int J Pep Protein Res 34:246–255

Xie J, Soleilhac JM, Schmidt C, Peyroux J, Roques BP, Fournié-Zaluski MC (1989b) New kelatorphan related inhibitors of enkephalin metabolism: improved antinociceptive properties. J Med Chem 32:1497–1503

Yaksh TL, Chipkin RE (1989) Studies on the effect of SCH-34826 and thiorphan on [Met^5]enkephalin levels and release in rat spinal cord. Eur J Pharmacol 167:367–373

Yaksh TL, Harty GJ (1982) Effects of thiorphan on the antinociceptive actions of intrathecal D-Ala^2-Met^5-enkephalin. Eur J Pharmacol 79:293–300

Yoshimura M, North RA (1983) Substantia gelatinosa neurones in vitro hyperpolarized by enkephalin. Nature 305:529–530

Zajac JM, Roques BP (1989) Properties required for reversible and irreversible radiolabeled probes for selective characterization of brain receptors and peptidases by autoradiography. In: Sharif NA, Lewis ME (eds) Brain imaging, techniques and applications. Wiley, New York, pp 18–35

Zajac JM, Charnay Y, Soleilhac JM, Salès N, Roques BP (1987) Enkephalin-degrading enzymes and angiotensin-converting enzyme in human and rat meninges. FEBS Lett 216:118–122

Zajac JM, Lombard MC, Peschanski M, Besson JM, Roques BP (1989) Autoradiographic study of μ and ∂ opioid binding sites and neutral endoepeptidase 24-11 in rat after dorsal root rhizotomy. Brain Res 477:400–403

Zhang AZ, Yang HYT, Costa E (1982) Nociception, enkephalin content and dipeptidyl carboxypeptidase activity in brain of mice treated with exopeptidase inhibitors. Neuropharmacology 21:625–630.

Zuzel KA, Rose C, Schwartz JC (1985) Assessment of the role of "enkephalinase" in cholecystokinin inactivation. Neuroscience 15:149–158

CHAPTER 24

Coexistence of Opioid Peptides with Other Neurotransmitters

R. Elde and T. Hökfelt

A. Principles

I. Introduction

The opioid peptides were discovered during the early, explosive period of neuropeptide research. A great deal of excitement surrounded this research, in part because the path that led to the discovery of the opioids was, and remains, unique. Opioids have been the only neuropeptides isolated for their ability to bind to and act at an already well-characterized receptor. In addition, the function of these receptors was known in several neuronal systems, and the effects caused by either the alkaloid opiates or the newly characterized opioid peptides could be blocked by existing antagonists, such as naloxone. Thus, even at its birth, the field of opioid peptide research was more advanced than for any other neuropeptide.

The discovery of the endogenous opioids brought the long-distinguished field of opiate pharmacology into the new domain of the neurobiology of putative peptide transmitters. An important concept that emerged from this period of research was the idea that neuropeptides are produced by neurons which also produce classical transmitters, and that between the time of synthesis and release of neuropeptides, they coexist with classical trans-mitters within neurons. A functional consequence of this concept is that individual neurons can release a mixture of transmitters, consisting of one or more classical, low-molecular-weight neurotransmitters and one or more specific neuropeptides. The purpose of this review is to emphasize some of the findings that led to these concepts, the extent to which opioids are now known to coexist with other transmitters, and the implications of these cellular features for understanding the role that opioids and their receptors play in neurotransmission and neural communication.

By the late 1960s Pearse and colleagues (PEARSE 1969) had presented arguments suggesting that many peptide-producing endocrine cells possess (at least transiently) uptake mechanisms for monoamine precursors (the *a*mine *p*recursor *u*ptake and *d*ecarboxylation concept of Pearse; see also OWMAN et al. 1973). In addition, studies of large, single neurons from invertebrates established that they produce more than one neurotransmitter (BROWNSTEIN et al. 1974). Soon after this, we discovered that somatostatin

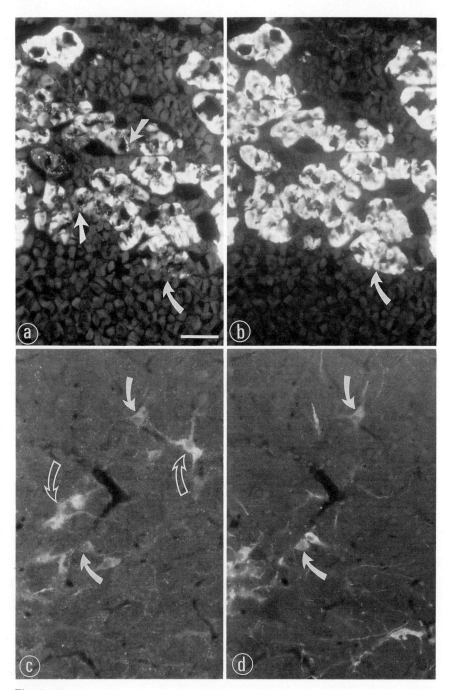

Fig. 1a–d.

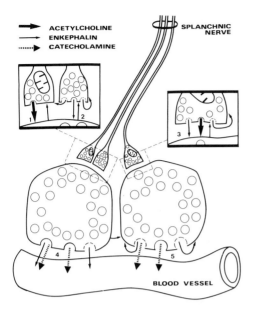

ACETYLCHOLINE
ENKEPHALIN
CATECHOLAMINE

SPLANCHNIC
NERVE

BLOOD VESSEL

Fig. 2. Schematic illustration of the coexistence and release of ENK-ir peptides and catecholamines from adrenal chromaffin cells and the occurrence of enkephalin immunoreactivity in the cholinergic fibers of the splanchnic nerve. *Arrows* indicate possible sites of release and action of ENK, acetylcholine, and catecholamines. (From SCHULTZBERG et al. 1978)

immunoreactivity (ir) occurs within guinea pig sympathetic neurons which produce the classical transmitter norepinephrine (HÖKFELT et al. 1977b). Within a short period of time, we also found that enkephalin (ENK)-ir occurs in the catecholamine-producing chromaffin cells of the adrenal medulla (Figs. 1, 2), and in presumed cholinergic nerve fibers which innervate the adrenal gland (Fig. 2; SCHULTZBERG et al. 1979). Thus, opioids were important in the expansion of the concept of coexistence of peptides with classical neurotransmitters, a concept that suggests that opioids, just like other peptides, have auxiliary roles in neuronal communication.

Fig. 1a–d. Immunofluorescence photomicrographs of guinea pig adrenal gland (**a,b**) and rat caudal medulla oblongata (**c,d**) after incubation with a mixture of mouse antiserum to met-ENK and rabbit antiserum to dopamine β-hydroxylase (**a,b**) or rabbit antiserum to met-ENK and mouse antiserum to tyrosine hydroxylase (**c,d**) followed by species-specific secondary antibodies labeled with fluorescein (**a,c**) and lissamine rhodamine (**b,d**). Most dopamine β-hydroxylase-ir chromaffin cells in the adrenal medulla of guinea pig exhibit ENK-ir (**b** and **a** respectively: *curved arrow* indicates a group of dopamine β-hydroxylase-ir cells which contain little, if any, ENK-ir). In addition, ENK-ir is observed in varicose nerve fibers (**a**, *straight arrows*). Many of the tyrosine hydroxylase-ir neurons in the A1/C1 cell group of the caudal medulla are also ENK-ir (**c,d**, *closed arrows*; *open arrows* indicate neurons in which such coexistence does not occur). *Bar* = 50 µm (all four figure parts)

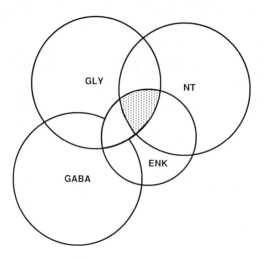

Fig. 3. Set diagram illustrating the combinations of coexisting transmitters with ENK-ir in amacrine cells in chick retina. Five subpopulations of ENK-ir amacrine cells have been characterized: those which take up either GABA or glycine (GLY), or contain neurotensin (NT)-ir, or take up GLY and contain NT-ir (*stippled area*) and those which only contain ENK-ir. (Based on WATT et al. 1988)

Since the time of the initial discovery of the coexistence of opioids and other neuropeptides with classical neurotransmitters, it has become apparent that this is a widespread phenomenon which occurs throughout the central and peripheral nervous systems of all vertebrates investigated. Attempts have been made to generalize and predict the combinations of coexisting neuropeptides and classical transmitters (LUNDBERG et al. 1982), but these principles have been difficult to apply except within limited regions of the nervous sytem (i.e., the sympathetic system). At this time it is possible to say that the patterns of coexistence are very complex, as exemplified by the work of Lam and colleagues on the coexistence of putative transmitters in amacrine cells of the chick retina. The set diagram which summarizes their work on ENK coexistence (Fig. 3; WATT et al. 1988) demonstrates that even within this single cell population the pattern of coexistence is highly varied. Several investigators have speculated on the possibility that the patterns of coexistence or "chemical coding" within an otherwise homogeneous population of neurons may disclose functional subsets of these neurons (LAM et al. 1985; COSTA et al. 1986; HÖKFELT et al. 1986, 1988; FURNESS and COSTA 1987).

II. Subcellular Features

Classical transmitters and neuropeptides are stored in different types of vesicles. Thus, early electron microscopic studies demonstrated that catecholamines and serotonin are stored in both small synaptic vesicles

(SSVs) and large dense granular vesicles (LGVs), both in the peripheral (WOLFE et al. 1962) and central (HÖKFELT 1968) nervous systems (see KLEIN and THURESON-KLEIN 1990). A number of more recent immunocytochemical investigations at the fine structural level (see PICKEL 1985), as well as subcellular fractionation studies (LUNDBERG et al. 1981; FRIED et al. 1985; KLEIN and THURESON-KLEIN 1990), suggest that peptides are exclusively stored in the LGVs (see LUNDBERG and HÖKFELT 1983). Since neurons simultaneously possess and independently control two distinct regulated exocytic pathways, one for SSVs and one for LGVs (CUTLER and CRAMER 1990; DE CAMILLI and JAHN 1990; KELLEY 1988; KLEIN and THURESON-KLEIN 1990; POW and MORRIS 1991; SÜDHOF and JAHN 1991; TRIMBLE et al. 1991), the intracellular trafficking of classical transmitters and neuropeptides differs.

1. Classical Neurotransmitters and Small Synaptic Vesicles

Putative neurotransmitters are generally thought to be stored within and released from membrane-bound vesicles.[1] Classical, low-molecular-weight neurotransmitters (such as acetylcholine, monoamines, and the amino acid transmitters) are sequestered within SSVs which measure approximately 30–50 nm in diameter (KLEIN and THURESON-KLEIN 1990). This sequestration is the result of the presence in the membrane of SSVs of transporters selective for particular classes of neurotransmitters, as well as proton pumps which enable the transmitters to be transported against a concentration gradient (SÜDHOF and JAHN 1991; TRIMBLE et al. 1991). Under normal circumstances the sequestration of classical neurotransmitters into SSVs does not occur to any great extent in neural perikarya or preterminal axons, but occurs primarily where large numbers of SSVs are clustered, i.e. within synaptic boutons. Release of the neurotransmitters contained within SSVs usually occurs by Ca^{2+}-dependent fusion (see DOUGLAS 1968; KATZ 1969; AUGUSTINE et al. 1987) of SSVs with highly specialized regions of the axon terminal membrane – the active zone. The crucial event – fusion of membranes – has been postulated to involve proteins residing on the outer surface of SSVs, particularly synaptophysins, synapsins and synaptotagmins (VALTORTA et al. 1989; DE CAMILLI and JAHN 1990; SÜDHOF and JAHN 1991), as well as their interaction with docking proteins on the cytoplasmic face of the active zone of the terminal membrane. At least two putative docking proteins; physophilin, identified by its binding of synaptophysin, and the α-latrotoxin receptor, identified for its binding of synaptotagmin, have been characterized (THOMAS and BETZ 1990; PETRENKO et al. 1991).

---

[1] Exceptions to this statement include nitric oxide (see SNYDER and BREDT 1991), and possibly, under some circumstances, amino acid neurotransmitters, such as GABA (see SCHWARTZ 1987).

2. Neuropeptides and Large Granular Vesicles

In contrast, releasable stores of neuropeptides such as the opioids are contained, perhaps exclusively, within LGVs approximately 75–100 nm in diameter (Klein and Thureson-Klein 1990). The occurrence of neuropeptides within this particular subcellular compartment is the consequence of synthesis of the neuropeptide as a pre-pro-peptide on the rough endoplasmic reticulum, and subsequent trafficking of the maturing peptide into the Golgi network and then into a regulated exocytic pathway (Kelley 1988; Trimble et al. 1991). In neurons the regulated exocytic pathway for peptides entails anterograde axonal transport from the cell body toward the nerve terminal. In analogy to SSVs, it is presumed that specialized sites for the fusion of peptide-laden LGVs exist on the membrane of peptidergic axons. However, the "machine" responsible for docking, fusion and release of peptides from LGVs does not appear to utilize the same molecules (e.g., synaptophysins, physophilin, or rab3a) as in the case of SSVs (Navone et al. 1984; Burgoyne and Morgan 1990; De Camilli and Jahn 1990; Südhof and Jahn 1991). LGVs apparently do not compete with SSVs for docking sites, since ultrastructural studies show that LGVs do not accumulate at the active zone where SSVs accumulate and undergo exocytosis (Verhage et al. 1991). In fact, a strong case has been made for the existence of two, independent pathways of regulated exocytosis; one for SSVs and another for LGVs (Cutler and Cramer 1990; Klein and Thureson-Klein 1990; Pow and Morris 1991). Most neurons appear to utilize both pathways simultaneously.

III. Methods for Establishing Coexistence

Initially, the coexistence of opioids and other peptides with classical transmitters became obvious on arithmetical grounds. For example, in the first work which established coexistence in mammalian neurons (Hökfelt et al. 1977b), it was determined that approximately 60% of the principal ganglion cells in the inferior mesenteric ganglion of guinea pig were somatostatin positive, whereas on adjacent sections it could be shown that nearly all of the principal cells in this ganglion contained the noradrenaline-synthesizing enzyme dopamine β-hydroxylase. Thus, it became obvious that many of these neurons must produce both a catecholamine and a somatostatin-like peptide. Also staining of adjacent tissue sections with antisera for each phenotype revealed instances when cells were split and occurred in both sections. A formal, statistical method has been developed which validates this approach (Agnati et al. 1982).

A second method, widely used to establish coexistence is the so-called elution-restaining method developed by Tramu and colleagues (1978). In this case, a routine immunofluorescence procedure for one transmitter is conducted and photomicrographs are taken. Subsequently, the coverslips are removed, previously bound antibodies are eluted by incubation of the section in a solution containing potassium permanganate or high salt at low pH. After rinsing, a second immunofluorescence procedure is conducted for the other transmitter, and after photomicrography, the localizations are compared.

A third approach, now in frequent use, allows for simultaneous or nearly simultaneous visualization of markers for two or more antigens in the same tissue section. These approaches capitalize upon multiple-color/multiple-antigen immunofluorescence (NAIRN 1969; ERICHSEN et al. 1982; WESSENDORF and ELDE 1985; COSTA et al. 1986; STAINES et al. 1988; WESSENDORF 1990; WESSENDORF et al. 1990) or multiple-chromophore immunoenzymatic methods (NAKANE 1968; HANCOCK 1986; JOSEPH and PIEKUT 1986). In these cases individual transmitters are represented by different colored markers, and thereby coexistence of transmitters, even at the level of single nerve varicosities and nerve terminals, can be determined. In some cases, investigators have used computerized image processing to quantify the extent of coexistence (TUCHSCHERER et al. 1987; MOSSBERG et al. 1990). An alternative, ultrastructural approach is the use of two different sizes of colloidal gold at the electron-microscopic level in order to reveal simultaneously the distribution of pairs of antigens (ROTH et al. 1978; GEUZE et al. 1981). An additional variation of this approach was described by CUELLO et al. (1982) in which a monoclonal antibody can be internally radiolabeled in vitro and then detected by autoradiographic methods in combination with another antibody detected by more traditional immunocytochemical methods.

It should be noted that in many cases coexistence of peptides and classical transmitters has been established in tissue from animals treated with colchicine. This manipulation has been used in order to reduce the exit of newly synthesized neuropeptides from neuronal cell bodies by exploiting colchicine's ability to block axonal transport (DAHLSTRÖM 1968; KREUTZBERG 1969) and cause accumulation of transmitter-containing vesicles in the cell body (HÖKFELT and DAHLSTRÖM 1971). Recent studies have demonstrated that colchicine may act through additional mechanisms to increase the expression of at least some peptide transmitters (CORTÉS et al. 1990).

In other cases it has been useful to study the coexistence of neuropeptides and classical transmitters in nerve fibers and terminals. Firstly, it can be argued that the coexistence observed in nerve fibers and terminals is likely to be physiologically relevant, since it is expected that it is this mixture of transmitters that can be released upon depolarization of a neuron. Secondly, neuropeptides are more abundant in nerve fibers and terminals than in neuronal cell bodies, and thus the use of colchicine can be avoided. Thus, the multicolor fluorescence methods have been a productive approach to the study of coexistence at the level of nerve fibers and terminals (WESSENDORF and ELDE 1985; WESSENDORF 1990).

In some cases the coexistence of neuropeptides with classical transmitters could be inferred by using selective lesioning methods. For example,
the serotonergic neurotoxin 5,7-dihydroxytryptamine causes the degeneration
of nerve fibers and terminals containing serotonin and the neuropeptides
which coexist within these fibers and terminals (Hökfelt et al. 1978;
Johansson et al. 1981; Gilbert et al. 1981, 1982).

With the advent of molecular cloning of precursors for neuropeptides as
well as enzymes responsible for synthesis of classical neurotransmitters, it
has been possible to use in situ hybridization to confirm and extend the
immunohistochemically established profile of coexisting neurotransmitters.
In some cases this has been possible by combining immunocytochemistry
and in situ hybridization (Young et al. 1986; see also Young 1990), and in
other cases it has been possible to conduct in situ hybridization procedures
for two transmitter candidates on the same tissue section (Kiyama et al.
1990; Young 1990; Dagerlind et al. 1992). Although immunocytochemistry
has been used for the most part to establish coexistence of neuropeptides
and classical transmitters, in situ hybridization studies have confirmed many
of the individual immunocytochemical localizations.

B. Coexistence Within Areas of the Nervous System

In general the opioids have been found to be widely distributed in neurons
in both the central and peripheral nervous system of a variety of vertebrates.
The exception to the wide occurrence of opioids is for β-endorphin, which is
a product of pro-opiomelanocortin (POMC) and appears to be expressed by
only two groups of neurons within the vertebrate CNS. The production of
β-endorphin was described first in the hypothalamic arcuate nucleus
(Watson et al. 1977; Bloch et al. 1978; Bloom et al. 1978) and more
recently in a portion of the nucleus of the solitary tract in the medulla
oblongata (see Khachaturian et al. 1985b). Thus far, other transmitters
which coexist with β-endorphin in arcuate neurons have not been identified,
although this has been investigated rather thoroughly (Pilcher and Joseph
1986; Everitt et al. 1986; Meister and Hökfelt 1988; Meister et al. 1989).
Similarly, little is know about possible substances coexisting with β-endorphin
in the neurons of the nucleus of the solitary tract.

The following sections review the coexistence of opioids (mainly
products of the proenkephalin (PENK) and prodynorphin (PDYN) genes)
with both classical transmitters and other neuropeptide families. The studies
reviewed are selected only from the intact nervous systems of vertebrates.
As a consequence, we have not reviewed coexistence in either cultured
neurons nor in endocrine cells. Furthermore, the studies chosen for citation
have provided histological evidence of *coexistence* within individual neurons
or their axons, not just the *codistribution* of immunostaining within a region.

Moreover, the instances of coexistence discussed within this chapter are cases in which the coexisting substances are products of different genes. Thus, we have not included studies of, for example, the coexistence of differently processed fragments of PENK in neurons (LEHTOSALO et al. 1984; WANG and WYATT 1987). Similarly, the coexistence of various products of the POMC gene, such as ACTH, β-endorphin, and MSH (O'DONOHUE et al. 1982; McGINTY and BLOOM 1983; WOLTER 1985; YOSHIDA and TANIGUCHI 1988; VALLARINO et al. 1989), is not considered further in this chapter. However, there are several instances in which products of PENK and PDYN do, in fact, coexist, and these cases are considered. According to FALLON and CIOFI (1990), a small number of nerve fibers in many brain regions contain both PENK and PDYN products, although the amount is a very small fraction of the total that contain products of either PENK or PDYN.

The schematic maps of brain and spinal cord in this chapter (Fig. 4) record only the coexistence reported for opioids in neuronal cell bodies in rat brain, although instances of coexistence in other species are described in the text and in Tables 1 and 2. For more details on the distribution of the individual opioids the reader is referred to reviews on the enkephalins (KHACHATURIAN et al. 1985b; PETRUSZ et al. 1985), dynorphins (KHACHATURIAN et al. 1985b; FALLON and CIOFI 1990), and β-endorphin (KHACHATURIAN et al. 1985a,b). An extensive mapping of mRNA encoding PENK has also been reported (HARLAN et al. 1987). The coexistence of monoamines and PENK-ir has been previously reviewed (CHARNAY et al. 1984). More general reviews on the coexistence of neuropeptides with classical transmitters (HÖKFELT et al. 1980, 1986, 1988; OSBORNE 1983; CHAN-PALAY and PALAY 1984) provide a broader view of this field.

I. Retina

The retina of the chick has been thoroughly examined for the coexistence of peptides and classical transmitters. The amacrine cells, interneurons without axons, are striking for the variety of neuropeptides and classical transmitters they produce. More than 90% of the ENK-ir amacrine cells also contain somatostatin-ir, and vice versa (HAMANO et al. 1989; LI et al. 1990). A small fraction of these cells (18%) is also likely to be GABAergic, based upon their ability to take up [^{3}H]GABA (LI et al. 1990). Other studies have found that ENK-ir amacrine cells also produce neurotensin-ir (LI et al. 1985) and glycine-ir (WU and LAM 1988). Quantitative estimates suggest that of the ENK-ir amacrine cells in chick retina 28% are GABAergic and 53% are glycinergic, and of the latter 26% are predicted to be neurotensin-ir (WATT et al. 1984, 1988). This complex pattern of substances which coexist with ENK-ir in this single population of cells has been summarized as a set diagram in the work of WATT and colleagues (1988; Fig. 3).

Table 1. Coexistence of opioids and other transmitters: central nervous system

Area	Cell [species]	Opioid[a]	Classical transmitter[a]	Peptide[a]	Reference(s)
Retina	Amacrine [chick]	ENK	GABA	SOM	Hamano et al. 1989; Li et al. 1990
	Amacrine [chick]	ENK	GLY	NT	Li et al. 1985; Wu and Lam 1988; Watt et al. 1984, 1988
Telencephalon	Neocortex (layers II and III); Allocortex [rat]	ENK		CCK	Gall et al. 1987
	Caudate, medium sized [rat, cat, pigeon, turtle]	ENK	GAD	SP	Aronin et al. 1984; Penny et al. 1986; Anderson and Reiner 1990
	Caudate [rat, pigeon, turtle]	DYN		SP	Anderson and Reiner 1990
	Caudate, accumbens [cat]	ENK	GABA	NT	Sugimoto and Mizuno 1987
	Olfactory nuc, amygdala [rat]	ENK		CCK	Gall et al. 1987
	Amygdala, bed nuc stria terminalis, med preoptic area [hamster]	DYN		SP	Neal et al. 1989; Neal and Newman 1991
Diencephalon	Supraoptic/paraventricular nuc [rat]	DYN	TH[b]	VP + GAL[b]	Watson et al. 1982; Whitnall et al. 1983; Gayman and Martin 1987, 1989; Meister et al. 1990a,b
	Paraventricular [rat]	ENK		CRF + VIP; TRH	Sawchenko and Swanson 1985; Everitt et al. 1986; Hökfelt et al. 1987; Ceccatelli et al. 1989a; Pretel and Piekut 1990
	Perifornical [rat]	ENK		DYN; TRH	Tsuruo et al. 1988; Fallon and Ciofi 1990

Region	Location	Opioid	Transmitter	Other	References
	Arcuate [rat]	DYN			Everitt et al. 1986
	Hypothalamus, scattered [rat]	ENK	TH	SP	Shimada et al. 1987
	Med preoptic area [hamster]	DYN		SP	Neal et al. 1989
	Fibers, median eminence [guinea pig]	ENK		SOM	Beauvillain et al. 1984
Mesencephalon	Fibers, thalamic nuclei [rat]	ENK		CCK; GAL	Gall et al. 1987; Ju et al. 1987
	Edinger-Westphal nuc [chick]	ENK	c	SP	Erichsen et al. 1982
	Interpeduncular nuc [rat]	ENK		SP	Shinoda et al. 1988
	Sup colliculus [cat]	ENK	GABA		Mize 1989
	Fibers, periaqueductal gray [rat]	ENK		CCK	Gall et al. 1987
Pons and medulla	Raphe nuc, nuc paragigantocellularis [cat]	ENK	5-HT		Glazer et al. 1981; Léger et al. 1986; Arvidsson et al. 1992
	Bulbospinal [guinea pig]	ENK	5-HT	SOM + SP	Chiba and Masuko 1989b
	Bulbospinal [rat]	ENK	5-HT	SP	Millhorn et al. 1989; Sasek and Helke 1989; Wessendorf et al. 1990
	Fibers, area postrema [rat]	ENK	5-HT		Armstrong et al. 1984
	Medullary raphe [rat]	ENK + DYN			Fallon and Ciofi 1990
	Lat sup olive [guinea pig, rat]	ENK + DYN	ChAT	CGRP	Altschuler et al. 1983, 1984; Abou-Madi et al. 1987; Tohyama et al. 1990
	Locus coeruleus [cat]	ENK	TH		Charnay et al. 1982
	A1/C1 cell group [rat]	ENK	TH/PNMT	NPY	Ceccatelli et al. 1989b; Murakami et al. 1989; Okamura et al. 1989
	Nuc solitary tract; medullary raphe and reticular formation [rat]	ENK + DYN		SOM; Iβ	Guthrie and Basbaum 1984; Millhorn et al. 1987a,b; Sawchenko et al. 1990
	Inf olivary complex [opossum]	ENK		CRF	Cummings and King 1990

Table 1. *Continued*

Area	Cell [species]	Opioid[a]	Classical transmitter[a]	Peptide[a]	Reference(s)
Cerebellum	Stellate cells [rat]	ENK	GABA		IBUKI et al. 1988
	Fibers, cortex [opossum]	ENK			CUMMINGS and KING 1990
Spinal cord	Thoracic intermediolateral cell column [rat]	ENK	ChAT	CRF	KONDO et al. 1985
	Thoracic intermediolateral cell column [rat]	ENK		SP	KRUKOFF 1987
	Fibers, thoracic intermediolateral cell column [guinea pig]	ENK	5-HT	SOM	CHIBA and MASUKO 1987
	Sacral intermediolateral cell column [rat]	ENK		APP	HUNT et al. 1981
	Dorsal gray commissure (lumbosacral) [rat]	ENK + DYN			SASEK and ELDE 1986
	Dorsal horn [rat]	ENK		SP	KATOH et al. 1988; SENBA et al. 1988
	Dorsal horn [arthritic rat]	ENK + DYN			WEIHE et al. 1988
	Fibers, dorsal horn [rat]	DYN		SP	TUCHSCHERER and SEYBOLD 1989
	Fibers, ventral horn [cat]	ENK		SP	TASHIRO et al. 1987

Abbreviations: 5-HT, serotonin; APP, avian pancreatic polypeptide; CCK, cholecystokinin; CGRP, calcitonin gene-related peptide; ChAT, choline acetyltransferase; CRF, corticotropin-releasing factor; GABA, γ-aminobutyric acid; GAD, glutamate decarboxylase; GAL, galanin; GLY, glycine; Iβ, inhibin β; NPY, neuropeptide Y; NT, neurotensin; PNMT, phenylethanolamine N-methyltransferase; SOM, somatostatin; SP, substance P; TH, tyrosine hydroxylase; TRH, thyrotropin-releasing hormone; VIP, vasoactive intestinal polypeptide; VP, vasopressin.
inf, inferior; lat, lateral; med, medial; nuc, nucleus; sup, superior.
[a] Substance used to elicit antisera used for localization.
[b] May be produced upon osmotic stimulation.
[c] Presumed to be cholinergic.

Table 2. Coexistence of opioids and other transmitters: peripheral nervous system

Area	Cell [species]	Opioid[a]	Classical transmitter[a]	Peptide[a]	Reference(s)
Doral root ganglia	Primary afferent neurons [cat]	ENK		VIP; SP; CCK	DE GROAT 1987
	Primary afferent neurons [cat]	ENK		SP + CGRP + SOM	GARRY et al. 1989
	Primary afferent neurons [guinea pig]	DYN		SP + CGRP	GIBBINS et al. 1987
	Primary afferent neurons [guinea pig]	DYN		SP + CGRP + CCK	GIBBINS et al. 1987
Superior cervical ganglion	Principal cells [guinea pig]	ENK + DYN	TH/DBH	NPY	SCHULTZBERG et al. 1979; GIBBINS and MORRIS 1987 KANAGAWA et al. 1986
	Small intensely fluorescent cells [guinea pig]	ENK	5-HT		
Carotid body and paraganglia	Glomus cells [several species]	ENK +/or DYN	Monoamine	SP	HEYM and KUMMER 1989
	Preaortic paraganglion cells [fetal guinea pig and newborn pig]	ENK	TH/DBH	NPY or GAL	FRIED et al. 1989
Prevertebral ganglia	Small intensely fluorescent cells (inf mesenteric and celiac-sup mesenteric ganglia) [guinea pig]	ENK + DYN	DBH	VIP; SOM; NPY	SCHULTZBERG et al. 1979; CHIBA and MASUKO 1989
	Principal cells, celiac ganglion [bovine]	ENK	TH/DBH	NPY	FRIED et al. 1986
Other ganglia	Parasympathetic ganglion cells (tongue) [guinea pig]	ENK		CCK	ICHIKAWA et al. 1990

Table 2. *Continued*

Area	Cell [species]	Opioid[a]	Classical transmitter[a]	Peptide[a]	Reference(s)
Postganglionic nerve fibers	Splenic nerve [bovine]	ENK	TH/DBH	NPY	FRIED et al. 1986
	Nerve to vas deferens [bovine]	ENK	Norepinephrine[b]		DE POTTER et al. 1987
	Nerve to uterus [guinea pig]	DYN		NPY; VIP	
Adrenal medulla	Chromaffin cells [cat, guinea pig, rat, bovine, hamster, frog, human]	ENK	TH and/or DBH and/or PNMT	NPY; CGA; GAL	SCHULTZBERG et al. 1978; LIVETT et al. 1982; LANG et al. 1982; PELTO-HUIKKO et al. 1985; PRUSS et al. 1986; RÖKAEUS et al. 1990; VIVEROS et al. 1983; WINKLER et al. 1986; LEBOULENGER et al. 1983a,b; LUNDBERG et al. 1979
	Chromaffin cells [human]	POMC	PNMT		BJARTELL et al. 1990
Enteric nervous system	Myenteric plexus [guinea pig]	DYN + ENK		NPY; VIP	VINCENT et al. 1984; FURNESS and COSTA 1987
	Myenteric plexus [guinea pig]	DYN		GRP; VIP	VINCENT et al. 1984; FURNESS and COSTA 1987
	Submucous plexus [guinea pig]	DYN		VIP	FURNESS and COSTA 1987

Myenteric plexus [cat]	ENK	SP	Domoto et al. 1984
Fibers, ext muscle layer [human]	ENK	SP	Wattchow et al. 1988
Fibers, celiac-sup mesenteric ganglion (originate from gut and preganglionic sources) [rat]	ENK	BOM	Järvi 1989

Abbreviations: 5-HT, serotonin; BOM, bombesin; CCK, cholecystokinin; CGA, chromogranin A; CGRP, calcitonin gene-related peptide; CRF, corticotropin-releasing factor; DBH, dopamine β-hydroxylase; GAL, galanin; GRP, gastrin-releasing peptide; NPY, neuropeptide Y; PNMT, phenylethanolamine N-methyltransferase; SOM, somatostatin; SP, substance P; TH, tyrosine hydroxylase; TRH, thyrotropin-releasing hormone; VIP, vasoactive intestinal polypeptide. ext, external; inf, inferior; sup, superior.

[a] Substance used to elicit antisera used for localization.

[b] Coexistence determined by differential centrifugation, ENK by immunocytochemistry.

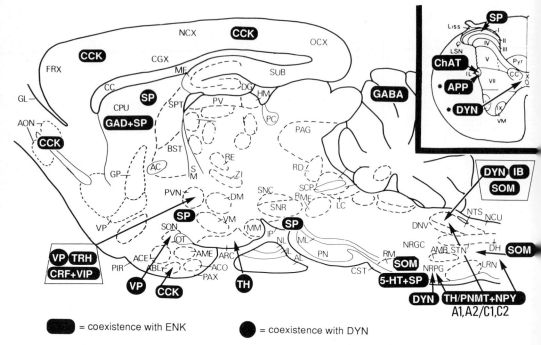

Fig. 4. Schematic representation of some instances of the coexistence of classical transmitters and neuropeptides with opioid peptides in rat brain and spinal cord (*inset*). Further examples, especially in other species, may be found in the text and in Tables 1 and 2. The form of schematics was derived from Khachaturian et al. 1985a (brain) and Molander et al. 1984 (spinal cord)

Abbreviations

Substances which coexist with ENK or DYN (white letters, dark surround): *5-HT*, serotonin; *APP*, avian pancreatic polypeptide; *CCK*, cholecystokinin; *ChAT*, choline acetyltransferase; *CRF*, corticotropin-releasing factor; *GABA*, γ-aminobutyric acid; *GAD*, glutamate decarboxylase; *IB*, inhibin-β; *NPY*, neuropeptide Y; *PNMT*, phenylethanolamine N-methyl transferase; *SOM*, somatostatin; *SP*, substance P; *TH*, tyrosine hydroxylase; *TRH*, thyrotropin-releasing hormone; *VIP*, vasoactive intestinal polypeptide; *VP*, vasopressin. Brain map: *A1,A2*, noradrenaline-producing neurons; *ABL*, basolateral nucleus of amygdala; *AC*, anterior commissure; *ACE*, central nucleus of amygdala; *ACO*, cortical nucleus of amygdala; *AL*, anterior lobe of pituitary; *AMB*, nucleus ambiguus; *AME*, medial nucleus of amygdala; *AON*, anterior olfactory nucleus; *ARC*, arcuate nucleus; *BST*, bed nucleus of stria ter-minalis; *C1,C2*, adrenaline-producing neurons; *CC*, corpus collosum; *CGX*, cingulate cortex; *CPU*, caudate-putamen; *CST*, corticospinal tract; *DH*, dorsal horn of spinal cord; *DG*, dentate gyrus; *DM*, dorsomedial nucleus of hypothalamus; *DNV*, dorsal motor nucleus of vagus; *FRX*, frontal cortex; *GL*, glomerular layer of olfactory bulb; *GP*, globus pallidus; *HM*, medial habenular nucleus; *IL*, inter-mediate lobe of pituitary; *IP*, interpeduncular nuclear complex; *LC*, nucleus locus coeruleus; *LRN*, lateral reticular nucleus; *MF*, mossy fibers of hippocampus; *ML*, medial lemniscus; *MM*, medial mammillary nucleus; *NCU*, nucleus cuneatus; *NCX*, neocortex; *NL*, neural lobe of pituitary; *NRGC*, nucleus reticularis gigantocellularis; *NRPG*, nucleus reticularis paragigantocellularis; *NTS*, nucleus tractus solitarius; *OCX*, occipital cortex; *OT*, optic tract; *PAG*, periaqueductal gray; *PAX*, peri-

II. Telencephalon

In the neocortex of rat, ENK-ir neurons are found in layers II and III (PETRUSZ et al. 1985), and a large proportion of these neurons also contain cholecystokinin-ir (Fig. 4; GALL et al. 1987). These authors also found coexistence of these two peptides, although somewhat less frequently, in perirhinal and piriform portions of the allocortex. ARONIN and colleagues (1984) reported the coexistence of ENK-ir and GAD-ir in medium-sized neurons in the caudate nucleus of rat (Fig. 4). Further studies demonstrated that ENK-ir coexists not only with GAD-ir, but also with substance P-ir in both rat and cat (Fig. 4; PENNY et al. 1986). They revealed instances where combinations of two of the above coexisted as well as all three. However, ANDERSON and REINER (1990) found that ENK-ir coexists in 5% or less of the substance P-ir striatal neurons of pigeon, turtle, and rat. In contrast, they found that 70% or more of the DYN-ir striatal neurons in these three species also produce substance P-ir (Fig. 4). Approximately half of the neurotensin-ir neurons in the caudate and accumbens of cat are also ENK-ir (SUGIMOTO and MIZUNO 1986), and 5% of the neurotensin-ir neurons in these areas are positive for both ENK- and GABA-ir (SUGIMOTO and MIZUNO 1987). The projections of some of these striatal neurons which produce coexisting transmitters have been described (ANDERSON and REINER 1990; REINER and ANDERSON 1990; see also ZAHM et al. 1985).

In other deep nuclei of the telencephalon, e.g., the anterior olfactory nucleus and the basolateral nucleus of the amygdala, ENK-ir and cholecystokinin-ir coexist (Fig. 4; GALL et al. 1987). DYN-ir coexists with substance P-ir in the caudal portion of the medial nucleus of the amygdala and the dorsocaudal aspect of the bed nucleus of stria terminalis of the hamster (NEAL et al. 1989). In addition, some of these neurons in which DYN-ir and substance P-ir coexist have been demonstrated to project to the medial preoptic area (NEAL and NEWMAN 1991).

---

amygdaloid cortex; *PC*, posterior commissure; *PIR*, piriform cortex; *PN*, pons; *PV*, periventricular nucleus of thalamus; *PVN*, paraventricular nucleus; *RD*, nucleus raphe dorsalis; *RE*, nucleus reuniens of thalamus; *RM*, nucleus raphe magnus; *RME*, nucleus raphe medianus; *SCP*, superior cerebellar peduncle; *SM*, stria medullaris thalami; *SNC*, substantia nigra (pars compacta); *SNR*, substantia nigra (pars reticulata); *SON*, supraoptic nucleus; *SPT*, septal nuclei; *STN*, spinal nucleus of trigeminal nerve; *SUB*, subiculum; *VM*, ventromedial nucleus of hypothalamus; *VP*, ventral pallidum; *ZI*, zona incerta. Spinal cord map (inset): *CC*, central canal; *I-X*, laminae, after Rexed; *IL*, intermediolateral cell column; *Liss*, Lissauer's tract; *LSN*, lateral spinal nucleus; *Pyr*, pyramidal (corticospinal) tract; *VM*, ventral medial motor group; *, found at lumbosacral levels

III. Diencephalon

The most prominent coexistence of opioids with other transmitters in the diencephalon is seen in the magnocellular neurons of the hypothalamo-neurohypophyseal system. In rat, peptides derived from PDYN are produced in a large number of vasopressin neurons (Fig. 4; WATSON et al. 1982; WHITNALL et al. 1983; GAYMAN and MARTIN 1987; MEISTER et al. 1990b), and the expression of DYN is upregulated by stimuli, such as hyperosmolarity, which also upregulate vasopressin expression (SHERMAN et al. 1986; MEISTER et al. 1990a). These PDYN-producing magnocelluar neurons are also capable of producing other neuropeptides, such as galanin (GAYMAN and MARTIN 1989; MEISTER et al. 1990b), as well as tyrosine hydroxylase (MEISTER et al. 1990b). It has been demonstrated that opioids, in all probability DYN, which are coreleased with vasopressin from terminals in the neural lobe of the pituitary act to inhibit the release of oxytocin from nearby terminals (SUMMY-LONG et al. 1984; BONDY et al. 1988).

The occurrence of PENK-derived peptides in vasopressin- and oxytocin-producing neurons is more controversial. It has been claimed that ENK-ir appears within vasopressin neurons (MARTIN and VOIGT 1981; MARTIN et al. 1983) and within oxytocin-ir neurons of the rat (MARTIN and VOIGT 1981; MARTIN et al. 1983; ADACHI et al. 1985; GAYMAN and MARTIN 1987). However, these claims have not been substantiated by in situ hybridization studies or by immunocytochemical localizations with antisera directed against cryptic portions of PENK, so these results may have been the consequence of cross-reactions of the antibodies with peptides derived from PDYN.

Some parvocellular neurons in the hypothalamic paraventricular nucleus of rat produce ENK-ir (HÖKFELT et al. 1977a), and most of these neurons also produce corticotropin-releasing factor (Fig. 4; SAWCHENKO and SWANSON 1985; HÖKFELT et al. 1987; CECCATELLI et al. 1989a; PRETEL and PIEKUT 1990) and peptide HI/vasoactive intestinal polypeptide (HÖKFELT et al. 1987), whereas a small fraction of the ENK-producing cells also produce thyrotropin-releasing hormone-ir (Fig. 4; CECCATELLI et al. 1989). Some of the ENK-ir parvocellular neurons have also been noted to produce PDYN-derived peptides (Fig. 4), as have neurons in the perifornical region (FALLON and CIOFI 1990), and in this area coexistence of ENK-ir and thyrotropin-releasing hormone-ir is common (Fig. 4; TSURUO et al. 1988).

Several other instances of coexistence of opioids with other transmitters in the hypothalamus have been noted. The A12 group of dopamine neurons is found within the hypothalamic arcuate nucleus, and small proportion of these tyrosine hydroxylase-ir neurons contain DYN-ir (Fig. 4; EVERITT et al. 1986). ENK-ir and substance P-ir were observed in single neurons in many hypothalamic nuclei, although the total number of such neurons is not great (SHIMADA et al. 1987). DYN-ir was found within substance P-ir neurons in the medial preopticarea of the hamster (NEAL et al. 1989). In the median eminence of the guinea pig, ENK-ir and somatostatin-ir have been observed within the same vesicles within nerve terminals (BEAUVILLAIN et al. 1984).

Nerve fibers and terminals in which ENK-ir and cholecystokinin-ir coexist have been reported in several thalamic nuclei, including the central medial, paracentral, and ventral anterior nucleus and the intralaminar nuclei (GALL et al. 1987). At least some of these fibers may also contain galanin-ir and originate in the lumbar spinal cord (JU et al. 1987).

IV. Mesencephalon

Neurons within three mesencephalic regions have been reported to contain opioids which coexist with other transmitters. Preganglionic parasympathetic neurons within the Edinger-Westphal nucleus of the chick (presumed to be cholinergic) contain both ENK-ir and substance P-ir, as do their axons and terminals in the ciliary ganglion (ERICHSEN et al. 1982). Interestingly, it has been suggest that the axons of these Edinger-Westphal neurons release ENK during development which prevents the death of neurons in the ciliary ganglion (MERINEY et al. 1992). In rat, some small spherical cells in the rostral subdivision of the interpeduncular nucleus contain both ENK-ir and substance P-ir (Fig. 4; SHINODA et al. 1988). Several neuronal types in the superficial aspect of the superior colliculus of cat contain ENK-ir, and 18% of these neurons are also GABA-ir (MIZE 1989). Finally, fibers and terminals containing both ENK-ir and cholecystokinin-ir in the periaqueductal gray matter have been reported (GALL et al. 1987).

V. Pons and Medulla

At several levels of the brainstem, serotonergic neurons of the raphe system have been reported to contain ENK-ir. This coexistence appears to be most prominent in the colchicine-treated cat. Originally, GLAZER and colleagues (1981) reported the coexistence of ENK-ir and serotonin-ir in nucleus raphe dorsalis and paragigantocellularis of cat. LÉGER et al. (1986) reported that approximately half of the cells in nucleus raphe magnus and obscurus were positive for both ENK-ir and serotonin-ir. They found that approximately one third of the cells in raphe magnus coexpress these transmitters, whereas virtually no coexistence of these transmitters was found in nucleus raphe dorsalis, in contrast to the findings of GLAZER et al. (1981). ARVIDSSON and colleagues (1992) have confirmed the extensive coexistence of ENK-ir and serotonin-ir in the pons and medulla of cat and have commented further on the paradox that the axons and terminals of these neurons within the spinal cord only occasionally contain both ENK-ir and serotonin-ir. The reason behind this paradox is not apparent, but they have suggested that it may be a consequence of colchicine's ability to induce the expression of some transmitters and peptides in neurons which under normal conditions fail to produce detectable quantities of transmitter or peptide (see also Cortés et al. 1990). In guinea pig bulbospinal serotonin neurons, ENK-ir, somatostatin-ir and substance P-ir have been reported to all coexist (Chiba and Masuko 1989b).

In contrast, bulbospinal neurons containing serotonin in rat often contain substance P-ir and/or thyrotropin-releasing hormone-ir, but only rarely contain ENK-ir (Wessendorf et al. 1990), but they can be observed in the midline and adjacent areas, especially at the level of the facial nucleus, and some project to the spinal cord (Fig. 4; Millhorn et al. 1989). Similarly, ENK-ir and substance P-ir have been reported to coexist, but only rarely, in bulbospinal neurons which project to the intermediolateral cell column of the thoracic spinal cord (Sasek and Helke 1989). A small number (approximately 5%) of the ENK-ir terminals in area postrema of rat take up radiolabeled serotonin and are therefore likely to be serotonergic (Armstrong et al. 1984). Some of the ENK-ir neurons in the medullary raphe were also found to be DYN-ir (Fallon and Ciofi 1990).

Some brainstem cholinergic neurons have also been shown to produce opioids. Altschuler and colleagues (1983, 1984) reported the occurrence of ENK-ir in the cholinergic neurons of the lateral superior olive of guinea pig which project to the cochlea as the olivo-cochlear bundle. ENK-ir neurons in the lateral superior olive of guinea pig also produce calcitonin gene-related peptide-ir (Tohyama et al. 1990). In rat, Abou-Madi and colleagues (1987) found that all neurons in the lateral superior olive which are either ENK-ir or DYN-ir are also stained with antisera to choline acetyltransferase and project to the cochlea. Furthermore, they found that all DYN-ir neurons are also ENK-ir, although the converse is not always true.

Catecholamine-producing neurons in the brainstem also produce opioids. The first evidence for coexistence of opioids in catecholamine-producing neurons of the CNS was reported by Charnay and colleagues (1982) who found that most tyrosine hydroxylase-ir neurons in the locus coeruleus of colchicine-treated cats also produce ENK-ir (Charnay et al. 1982). In the more caudal catecholamine-producing cell groups of the brainstem substantial numbers of neurons produce opioids. Many tyrosine hydroxylase-ir neurons (or catecholamine-fluorescent neurons, in the case of Okamura et al. 1989) in the A1/C1 cell group of rat were found to contain ENK-ir (Fig. 5; approximately 30%, Ceccatelli et al. 1989b; 47%, Murakami et al. 1989; 33%, Okamura et al. 1989), and many of these cells also contain neuropeptide Y-ir (Fig. 4; Ceccatelli et al. 1989b; Murakami et al. 1989). However, Milner and colleagues (1989) found coexistence of ENK-ir and tyrosine hydroxylase-ir to be less common. A somewhat smaller fraction of the tyrosine hydroxylase-positive cells of the A2 group (Fig. 5) and the adrenaline-producing, PNMT-ir cells of the associated C1 and C2 cell groups produce ENK-ir (Ceccatelli et al. 1989b; Murakami et al. 1989).

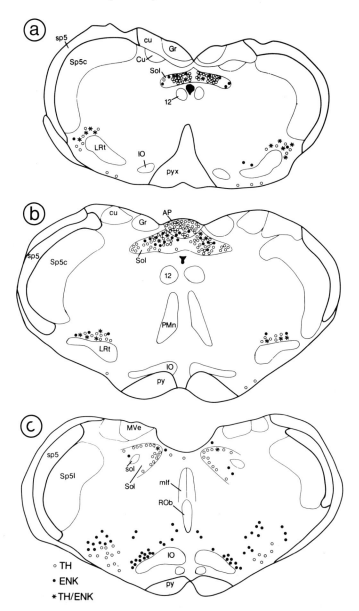

Fig. 5a–c. Schematic representation of the distribution of tyrosine hydroxylase-ir and ENK-ir neurons, and their coexistence, at three levels of the medulla oblongata, where *a* represents the most caudal level and *c* represents the most rostral level. *AP*, area postrema; *Cu*, cuneate nucleus; *cu*, cuneate fasciculus; *Gr*, gracile nucleus; *IO*, inferior olive; *LRt*, lateral reticular nucleus; *mlf*, medial longitudinal fasciculus; *PMn*, paramedian reticular nucleus; *py*, pyramidal tract; *pyx*, pyramidal decussation; *ROb*, raphe obscurus nucleus; *Sol*, nucleus of the solitary tract; *sol*, solitary tract; *Sp5c*, spinal trigeminal nucleus, caudal part; *Sp5I*, spinal trigeminal nucleus, interpositus part; *sp5*, spinal tract of the trigeminal nerve; *12*, hypoglossal nucleus. (from CECCATELLI et al. 1989b)

The nucleus of the solitary tract contains substantial numbers of opioid-producing neuronal cell bodies, in addition to the A2/C2 neurons mentioned above. Most neurons in the caudal ventrolateral nucleus of the solitary tract of rat which contain ENK-ir also contain DYN-ir, as do some neurons in the medullary raphe and nucleus reticularis paragigantocellularis (Guthrie and Basbaum 1984). ENK-ir and somatostatin-ir coexist in neurons in caudal brainstem of rats, especially in the nucleus of the solitary tract, the caudal medullary reticular formation, along the ventrolateral surface of the medulla, and in nucleus raphe magnus (Fig. 4; Millhorn et al. 1987a,b), and some of these neurons project to the nucleus of the solitary tract and to the spinal cord (Millhorn et al. 1987b). More than 25% of the neurons in the caudal portion of the nucleus of the solitary tract which contain inhibin β-ir also contain ENK-ir and somatostatin-ir (Fig. 4; Sawchenko et al. 1990). Many of these neurons also project to oxytocinergic compartments of the magnocellular neurosecretory system.

Neurons in the medial accessory olive and dorsal cap of Kooy in opossum, which project as climbing fibers to cerebellum, produce both ENK-ir and corticotropin-releasing factor-ir (Cummings and King 1990). A similar pattern of coexistence was found in neurons in nucleus prepositus hypoglossi, the subtrigeminal reticular nucleus, and the reticular formation – sites which are also likely to provide climbing fiber input to cerebellum.

VI. Cerebellum

Medium-sized, rounded neurons containing ENK-ir have been reported in the granule cell layer of the cerebellar cortex (Petrusz et al. 1985), but only occasional DYN-ir cells have been observed in the cerebellum (Fallon and Ciofi 1990). Ibuki and colleagues (1988) reported coexistence of PENK-ir and GABA-ir in stellate cells within the granule cell layer in rat cerebellum (Fig. 4). In opossum (as noted above) some olivary neurons which project as climbing fibers to the cerebellar cortex have been observed which contain both ENK-ir and corticotropin-releasing factor-ir (Cummings and King 1990).

VII. Spinal Cord

Several populations of neurons in the spinal cord produce opioid peptides (Miller and Seybold 1987, 1989; Petrusz et al. 1985; Fallon and Ciofi 1990). Thus far, coexistence has been demonstrated in two general groups of opioid-producing spinal cord neurons. Firstly, neurons of the inter-mediolateral cell column in several species contain ENK-ir (Glazer and Basbaum 1980; Dalsgaard et al. 1982; Krukoff 1987), and in one case, the ENK-ir neurons in the intermediolateral cell column in the lower thoracic spinal cord of rat have been demonstrated to be cholinergic (Fig. 4; Kondo et al. 1985), as expected for preganglionic autonomic neurons. In addition, some ENK-ir preganglionic sympathetic neurons in cat have been demonstrated to also produce substance P-ir (KRUKOFF 1987). In the sacral parasympathetic system ENK-ir coexists with an immunoreactive peptide of the pancreatic polypeptide/neuropeptide Y family (Fig. 4; HUNT et al. 1981) A high percentage of neurons in the dorsal gray commissure of the lumbosacral spinal cord of rats are both ENK-ir and DYN-ir (Fig. 4; SASEK and ELDE 1986). This group of neurons has been suggested to act as interneurons in certain autonomic reflexes.

ENK-ir nerve fibers and terminals are prominent in the intermediolateral cell column of the thoracic spinal cord of guinea pig. CHIBA and MASUKO (1987) found that ENK-ir and serotonin-ir coexist in some fibers in this region, as do somatostatin-ir and serotonin-ir. Thus, ENK-ir, somatostatin-ir, and serotonin-ir may all coexist in at least some of the fibers which provide supraspinal input to preganglionic sympathetic neurons. However, in the intermediolateral cell column of rat, coexistence of ENK-ir and serotonin-ir is rare (SASEK and HELKE 1989).

A great deal of attention has been paid to opioidergic neurons in the dorsal horn of the spinal cord, because of the role that opioids at this site may play in regulating nociceptive thresholds. Here, ENK-ir has been shown to coexist with substance P-ir in local neurons (Fig. 4; KATOH et al. 1988; SENBA et al. 1988). Interestingly, both ENK and DYN expression is upregulated in animal models of inflammation and hyperalgesia (IADAROLA et al. 1988a,b; RUDA et al. 1988). WEIHE and colleagues (1988) not only found upregulation of opioids in the dorsal horn of rats with experimental arthritis, but also observed coexistence of PENK-ir and PDYN-ir in large, multipolar neurons in laminae IV and V of the dorsal horn of arthritic, but not normal animals.

Some varicosities in the superficial laminae of the dorsal horn of the spinal cord of rat are DYN-ir, and some of these also contain substance P-ir and probably represent spinal or supraspinal neurons, rather than primary afferent neurons (TUCHSCHERER and SEYBOLD 1989). ENK-ir and substance P-ir coexist in nerve fibers and terminals in the ventral horn of the lumbar spinal cord of cat; far less coexistence was observed in the dorsal horn (TASHIRO et al. 1987).

VIII. Peripheral Nervous System

1. Primary Afferent Neurons

Small and intermediate diameter neurons in sensory ganglia prominently express a variety of neuropeptides, such as substance P, somatostatin, and calcitonin gene-related peptide. Generally, only low levels of opioid expression have been reported in sensory ganglia in rat. However, primary afferent neurons which innervate the pelvic viscera, especially in cat, contain ENK-ir which coexists with several other peptides, including vasoactive intestinal polypeptide, substance P, and cholecystokinin (DE GROAT 1987). In addition, lumbar dorsal root ganglion cells in cat produce leu-ENK-ir; in one group ENK-ir coexists with substance P and calcitonin gene-related peptide, and in the other group ENK-ir coexists with substance P, calcitonin gene-related peptide, and somatostatin (GARRY et al. 1989). In guinea pig, axons of primary afferent neurons containing DYN-ir, substance P-ir and calcitonin gene-related peptide-ir are found which innervate the ureter, bladder, vas deferens, uterus, the airways of the lung and the skin, the latter also contain cholecystokinin-ir (GIBBINS et al. 1987).

2. Autonomic Ganglion Cells and Their Fibers

Opioid peptides are prominent in the autonomic nervous system. Noradrenergic cell bodies of the superior cervical ganglion and their fibers in guinea pig also contain ENK-ir (SCHULTZBERG et al. 1979), DYN-ir, and neuropeptide Y-ir (GIBBINS and MORRIS 1987). In addition, "small intensely fluorescent" (SIF) interneurons in this ganglion and species produce both serotonin-ir and ENK-ir (KANAGAWA et al. 1986).

Glomus cells in the carotid body of a variety of species contain either ENK-ir or DYN-ir which coexists with substance P and typically a monoamine (HEYM and KUMMER 1989). Paraganglia, in analogy to the carotid body, are highly vascularized collections of neuron-like cells which often produce catecholamines and may serve a sensory function (see FRIED et al. 1989). Most preaortal paraganglionic neurons from fetal guinea pig are tyrosine hydroxylase and dopamine β-hydroxylase positive, and many of these contain ENK or ENK in combination with neuropeptide Y or galanin (FRIED et al. 1989). In newborn pig the carotid body-like paraganglia cells were tyrosine hydroxylase positive, but not dopamine β-hydroxylase positive, and contained several peptides, including ENK-ir.

In more caudal aspects of the sympathetic system it has been found that ENK-ir coexists in some dopamine β-hydroxylase-ir SIF cells of the inferior mesenteric and celiac-superior mesenteric ganglion of guinea pig (SCHULTZBERG et al. 1979). ENK-ir and neuropeptide Y-ir are stored with norepinephrine in LGVs in bovine splenic nerve and are found in tyrosine hydroxylase-positive and dopamine β-hydroxylase-positive ganglion cells in the celiac ganglia (FRIED et al. 1986). Several peptides coexist in the adrenergic SIF cells in the inferior mesenteric ganglion of the guinea pig, where ENK-ir was the most prominent of the peptides examined (the others being vasoactive intestinal polypeptide, somatostatin, neuropeptide Y, and DYN) (CHIBA and MASUKO 1989a). ENK-ir is found in varicose adrenergic fibers of bovine vas deferens, in LGVs which also contain norepinephrine. The electrically stimulated release of ENK-ir is accompanied by the release of norepinephrine (DE POTTER et al. 1987). Most nonadrenergic axons along the uterine artery in guinea pig contain neuropeptide Y-ir, vasoactive intestinal polypeptide-ir, and DYN-ir (MORRIS et al. 1985). Finally, ENK-ir coexists with cholecystokinin-ir in presumed parasympathetic ganglion cells and fibers in guinea pig tongue (ICHIKAWA et al. 1990).

3. Adrenal Medulla

SCHULTZBERG and colleagues (1978) reported the first example of co-existence of an opioid peptide with a classical transmitter (see Figs. 1 and 2). In these studies, ENK-ir was found in most catecholamine-containing chromaffin cells in the adrenal of cat and in a large fraction of chromaffin cells in guinea pig, but in only a few cells in the normal rat, with the highest concentrations in norepinephrine cells. However, after transection of the splanchnic nerve, many chromaffin cells (both epinephrine and norepinephrine containing) in the rat adrenal contain detectable quantities of ENK-ir. In addition, ENK-ir in nerve fibers was found within the adrenal, which probably represents preganglionic input via the splanchnic nerve.

LIVETT and colleagues (1982) found that ENK-ir is contained exclu-sively within the epinephrine-producing chromaffin cells of bovine adrenal medulla. Differential centrifugation studies in bovine adrenal medulla established that ENK-ir cofractionates with epinephrine-containing granules, not norepinephrine granules (LANG et al. 1982). PELTO-HUIKKO and col-leagues (1985) in a study of the hamster and rat adrenal medulla, found that ENK-ir coexists preferentially in epinephrine-producing chromaffin cells, and that it is also found in ganglion cells within the adrenal medulla and in nerve fibers which innervate the epinephrine-producing chromaffin cells. Additionally, it has been found that ENK-ir coexists not only with epinephrine in bovine chromaffin cells, but also with neuropeptide Y (PRUSS et al. 1986), chromogranin A, and galanin (RÖKAEUS et al. 1990; see also VIVEROS et al. 1983; WINKLER et al. 1986).

In the frog, ENK-ir was found to coexist with vasoactive intestinal polypeptide in dopamine β-hydroxylase-ir dense-cored vesicles in chromaffin cells from adrenal gland (LEBOULENGER et al. 1983a,b). Finally, POMC-derived peptides have been described in epinephrine-containing cells of human adrenal medulla (BJARTELL et al. 1990), and ENK-ir was found in the catecholamine-producing cells in human adrenal medulla and pheochromocytoma (LUNDBERG et al. 1979).

4. Enteric Nervous System

Opioidergic neurons and opioid receptors within the wall of the gastro-intestinal tract have played an important role in the development of con-cepts of opioid function. Soon after the initial localization of ENK-ir in nerve fibers and terminals in the myenteric plexus (ELDE et al. 1976), SCHULZ and colleagues (1977) used the myenteric plexus of the guinea pig ileum to establish for the first time that opioids were released from nerve terminals.

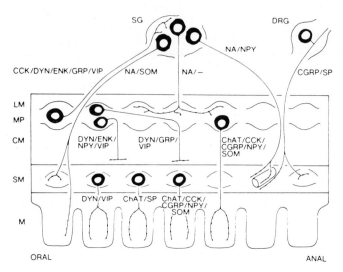

Fig. 6. Schematic diagram of the location and projections of neurons with respect to the coexistence of classical transmitters and peptides with opioid peptides in the enteric nervous system of guinea pigs. Note that DYN and ENK are prominently expressed in combination with other neuropeptides in neurons in the myenteric plexus, whereas DYN is the only opioid produced (along with vasoactive intestinal polypeptide) by neurons in the submucous plexus. Peptide abbreviations as in Tables 1 and 2; *LM*, longitudinal muscle layer; *MP*, myenteric plexus; *CM*, circular muscle layer; *SM*, submucous plexus; *M*, mucosa; *SG*, sympathetic ganglion; *DRG*, dorsal root ganglion. (From Furness and Costa 1987)

The most comprehensive analysis of transmitters in enteric neurons is found in the work on guinea pig of Costa, Furness and their colleagues (Costa et al. 1986; Furness and Costa 1987; see also Schultzberg et al. 1980). In this work they have advanced the concept that "chemical coding" – the combination of coexisting neurotransmitters plus the morphology, connections and location of an enteric neuron – serves to identify functionally unique populations of neurons. Prominent within the scheme is the position of the opioids (Fig. 6). Two opioidergic populations of neurons have been identified in the *myenteric* plexus. One of these produces DYN-ir, ENK-ir, neuropeptide Y-ir, and vasoactive intestinal peptide-ir and projects to nearby circular muscle. The other population produces DYN-ir, gastrin releasing peptide-ir, and vasoactive intestinal polypeptide-ir and projects more anally to the circular layer of muscle (Furness and Costa 1987; see also Vincent et al. 1984). In the *submucous* plexus, 45% of the neurons produce DYN-ir as well as vasoactive intestinal polypeptide-ir and project into the mucosal layer (Furness and Costa 1987).

Several examples of coexistence of opioids and other transmitters have been reported in other species. ENK-ir and substance P-ir coexist in myenteric neurons in cat ileum (Domoto et al. 1984), and a similar coexistence was found in a population of fibers which supply the external muscle of the human gastrointestinal tract (WATTCHOW et al. 1988), where these fibers may have an excitatory function. ENK-ir fibers (some of which also contain bombesin-ir) innervate cell bodies in celiac-superior mesenteric ganglion of rat. They appear to originate both from the gut and from preganglionic neurons in the spinal cord (JÄRVI 1989).

C. Implications

I. Patterns of Expression

Considering the number of instances in which opioid peptides are now known to coexist with classical transmitters and other families of neuropeptides, one is forced to conclude that opioids are unlikely to be the exclusive neurotransmitter produced by any given population of neurons. This conclusion requires that the concept of "opioidergic" neurons be clarified in order to imply correctly the variety of other transmitter substances produced and released by neurons which produce opioids. In this context, it is important to emphasize that the "cocktail" of transmitters produced by "opioidergic" neurons in one region of the nervous system will differ from the cocktail of transmitters produced and released by "opioidergic" neurons in another region, or a homologous "opioidergic" neuron (i.e., from the same circuit) in another species.

Another source of variability in characterizing patterns of coexistence with respect to opioids and other transmitters is the possibility that the expression of at least some transmitter substances may be plastic and respond to developmental, physiological, or pathological cues. For example, during development motoneurons express several neuropeptides, many of which drop to undetectable levels during postnatal life (Ho 1988; VILLAR et al. 1988, 1991; SEROOGY et al. 1991). In addition, the expression of some neuropeptides is dramatically increased from undetectable levels to high levels of expression upon injury to axons (see VILLAR et al. 1989).

Finally, there are many cases in which the coexisting classical transmitters or neuropeptides have not been described for given populations of opioid neurons. Part of the reason for this lack of information is that until recently there have not been immunocytochemical techniques that would allow the localization of some of the classical transmitters such as glutamate, aspartate, and glycine. However, the immunofluorescent method for localizing glutamate was recently applied in combination with immunofluorescent methods for serotonin and substance P and it was found that all three substances coexist in a subpopulation of bulbospinal neurons (NICHOLAS et al. 1992). Thus, it is likely that many patterns and combinations of coexistence of opioids with other transmitters remain to be discovered.

II. Pharmacology and Physiology

Administration of opioid antagonists to normal animals and human beings poses few risks because most basal, physiological states are not disturbed (see JAFFE and MARTIN 1990). For example, even though exogenously applied opioids profoundly elevate nociceptive thresholds, naloxone has only modest effects upon nociceptive thresholds in naive mice (FREDERICKSON et al. 1977). In most attempts to use opioid antagonists as a tool to disclose the physiological effects of endogenous opioids, the effects have been either difficult to observe or modest in magnitude. This suggests either that opioids are not normally released during tonic, physiological activity of nerve pathways which contain them or, alternatively, that they are released as but one of several constituents of the neurotransmitter cocktail produced by the neuron in question, and that an antagonist at opioid receptors is not sufficient to block the effects caused by the cocktail of transmitters released upon depolarization of the neuron. Thus, even though the systems of opioid receptors, when activated in isolation by exogenous opioids, can powerfully affect neuronal activity, it is likely that under physiological circumstances endogenous opioids are coreleased with other transmitters whose actions at least partially mask the effects of opioids.

Acknowledgements. We are grateful to many colleagues who have collaborated in the studies on these topics in our laboratories. We thank Katarina Åman, Waldtraut Hiort, and Jianlin Wang for expert technical assistance. Studies in our laboratories have been supported by grants from the National Institute on Drug Abuse (DA 02148; DA 06299), the Swedish Medical Research Council (04X-2887), and the National Institute of Mental Health (MH 43230) and by the Curtis L. Carlson Visiting Professorship.

References

Abou-Madi L, Pontarotti P, Tramu G, Cupo A, Eybalin M (1987) Coexistence of putative neuroactive substances in lateral olivocochlear neurons of rat and guinea pig. Hear Res 30:135–146

Adachi T, Hisano S, Daikoku S (1985) Intragranular colocalization of immuno-reactive methionine-enkephalin and oxytocin within the nerve terminals in the posterior pituitary. J Histochem Cytochem 33:891–899

Agnati LF, Fuxe K, Locatelli V, Benfenati F, Zini I, Panerai AE, El EMF, Hökfelt T (1982) Neuroanatomical methods for the quantitative evaluation of co-existence of transmitters in nerve cells. Analysis of the ACTH- and beta-endorphin immunoreactive nerve cell bodies of the mediobasal hypothalamus of the rat. J Neurosci Methods 5:203–214

Altschuler RA, Parakkal MH, Fex J (1983) Localization of enkephalin-like immuno-reactivity in acetylcholinesterase-positive cells in the guinea-pig lateral superior olivary complex that project to the cochlea. Neuroscience 9:621–630

Altschuler RA, Fex J, Parakkal MH, Eckenstein F (1984) Colocalization of enkephalin-like and choline acetyltransferase-like immunoreactivities in olivocochlear neurons of the guinea pig. J Histochem Cytochem 32:839–843

Anderson KD, Reiner A (1990) Extensive co-occurrence of substance P and dynorphin in striatal projection neurons: an evolutionarily conserved feature of basal ganglia organization. J Comp Neurol 295:339–369

Armstrong DM, Miller RJ, Beaudet A, Pickel VM (1984) Enkephalin-like immuno-reactivity in rat area postrema: ultrastructural localization and coexistence with serotonin. Brain Res 310:269–278

Aronin N, Difiglia M, Graveland GA, Schwartz WJ, Wu JY (1984) Localization of immunoreactive enkephalins in GABA synthesizing neurons of the rat neostriatum. Brain Res 300:376–380

Arvidsson U, Cullheim S, Ulfhake B, Ramírez V, Dagerlind Å, Luppi P-H, Kitahama K, Jouvet M, Terenius L, Åman K, Hökfelt T (1992) Distribution of enkephalin and its relation to serotonin in cat and monkey spinal cord and brain stem. Synapse (in press)

Augustine GJ, Charlton MP, Smith SJ (1987) Calcium action in synaptic transmitter release. Annu Rev Neurosci 10:633–693

Beauvillain JC, Tramu G, Garaud JC (1984) Coexistence of substances related to enkephalin and somatostatin in granules of the guinea-pig median eminence: demonstration by use of colloidal gold immunocytochemical methods. Brain Res 301:389–393

Bjartell A, Fenger M, Ekman R, Sundler F (1990) Amidated joining peptide in the human pituitary, gut, adrenal gland and bronchial carcinoids. Immunocyto-chemical and immunochemical evidence. Peptides 11:149–161

Bloch B, Bugnon C, Fellmann D, Lenys D (1978) Antigenic determinants of beta-LPH, beta-MSH, alpha-endorphin, ACTH and alpha-MSH revealed by anti-beta-endorphin in neurons of the human infundibular nucleus. C R Acad Sci D (Paris) 287:1019–1022

Bloom F, Battenberg E, Rossier J, Ling N, Guillemin R (1978) Neurons containing beta-endorphin in rat brain exist separately from those containing enkephalin: immunocytochemical studies. Proc Natl Acad Sci USA 75:1591–1595

Bondy CA, Gainer H, Russell JT (1988) Dynorphin A inhibits and naloxone increases the electrically stimulated release of oxytocin but not vasopressin from the terminals of the neural lobe. Endocrinology 122:1321–1327

Brownstein MJ, Saavedra JM, Axelrod J, Carpenter DO (1974) Coexistence of several putative neurotransmitters in single identified neurons of *Aplysia*. Proc Natl Acad Sci USA 71:4662–4665

Burgoyne RD, Morgan A (1990) Evidence for a role of calpactin in calcium-dependent exocytosis. Biochem Soc Trans 18:1101–1104

Ceccatelli S, Eriksson M, Hökfelt T (1989a) Distribution and coexistence of corticotropin releasing factor-, neurotensin-, enkephalin-, cholecystokinin-, galanin- and vasoactive intestinal polypeptide/peptide histidine isoleucine-like peptides in the parvocellular part of the paraventricular nucleus. Neuro-endocrinology 49:309–323

Ceccatelli S, Millhorn DE, Hökfelt T, Goldstein M (1989b) Evidence for the occurrence of an enkephalin-like peptide in adrenaline and noradrenaline neurons of the rat medulla oblongata. Exp Brain Res 74:631–640

Chan-Palay V, Palay S (1984) Coexistence of neuroactive substances in neurons. Wiley, New York

Charnay Y, Leger L, Dray F, Berod A, Jouvet M, Pujol JF, Dubois PM (1982) Evidence for the presence of enkephalin in catecholaminergic neurones of cat locus coeruleus. Neurosci Lett 30:147–151

Charnay Y, Leger L, Dray F, Dubois PM (1984) The co-localization of monoamines and enkephalins in the central nervous system. Ann Endocrinol (Paris) 45:201–206

Chiba T, Masuko S (1987) Synaptic structure of the monoamine and peptide nerve terminals in the intermediolateral nucleus of the guinea pig thoracic spinal cord. J Comp Neurol 262:242–55

Chiba T, Masuko S (1989a) Coexistence of multiple peptides in small intensely fluorescent (SIF) cells of inferior mesenteric ganglion of the guinea pig. Cell Tissue Res 255:523–527

Chiba T, Masuko S (1989b) Coexistence of varying combinations of neuropeptides with 5-hydroxytryptamine in neurons of the raphe pallidus et obscurus projecting to the spinal cord. Neurosci Res 7:13–23

Cortés R, Ceccatelli S, Schalling M, Hökfelt T (1990) Differential effects of intracerebroventricular colchicine administration on the expression of mRNAs for neuropeptides and neurotransmitter enzymes, with special emphasis on galanin: an in situ hybridization study. Synapse 6:369–391

Costa M, Furness JB, Gibbins IL (1986) Chemical coding of enteric neurons. In: Hökfelt T, Fuxe K, Pernow B (eds) Coexistence of neural messengers: a new principle in chemical transmission. Elsevier, Amsterdam, p 217 (Progress in brain research, vol 68)

Guello AC, Priestley JV, Milstein C (1982) Immunocytochemistry with internally labeled monoclonal antibodies. Proc Natl Acad Sci USA 79:665–669

Cummings S, King JS (1990) Coexistence of corticotropin releasing factor and enkephalin in cerebellar afferent systems. Synapse 5:167–174

Cutler DF, Cramer LP (1990) Sorting during transport to the surface of PC12 cells: divergence of synaptic vesicle and secretory granule proteins. J Cell Biol 110: 721–730

Dagerlind Å, Friberg K, Bean AJ, Hökfelt T (1992) Sensitive mRNA detection using unfixed tissue: combined radioactive and non-radioactive in situ hybridization histochemistry. Histochemistry (submitted)

Dahlström A (1968) Effect of colchicine on transport of amine storage granules in sympathetic nerves of rat. Eur J Pharmacol 5:111–113

Dalsgaard CJ, Hökfelt T, Elfvin LG, Terenius L (1982) Enkephalin-containing sympathetic preganglionic neurons projecting to the inferior mesenteric ganglion: evidence from combined retrograde tracing and immunohistochemistry. Neuroscience 7:2039–2050

De Camilli P, Jahn R (1990) Pathways to regulated exocytosis in neurons. Annu Rev Physiol 52:625–645

de Groat WC (1987) Neuropeptides in pelvic afferent pathways. Experientia 43: 801–813

De Potter WP, Coen EP, De Potter RW (1987) Evidence for the coexistence and co-release of Met-enkephalin and noradrenaline from sympathetic nerves of the bovine vas deferens. Neuroscience 20:855–866

Domoto T, Gonda T, Oki M, Yanaihara N (1984) Coexistence of substance P- and methionine5-enkephalin-like immunoreactivity in nerve cells of the myenteric ganglia in the cat ileum. Neurosci Lett 47:9–13

Douglas WW (1968) Stimulus-secretion coupling: the concept and clues from chromaffin and other cells. Br J Pharmacol 34:451–474

Elde RP, Hökfelt T, Johansson O, Terenius L (1976) Immunohistochemical studies using antibodies to leucine-enkephalin: initial observations on the nervous system of the rat. Neuroscience 1:349–351

Erichsen JT, Reiner A, Karten HJ (1982) Co-occurrence of substance P-like and Leu-enkephalin-like immunoreactivities in neurones and fibres of avian nervous system. Nature 295:407–410

Everitt BJ, Meister B, Hökfelt T, Melander T, Terenius L, Rökaeus Å, Theodorsson-Norheim E, Dockray G, Edwardson J, Cuello C, Elde R, Goldstein M, Hemmings H, Ouimet C, Walaas I, Greengard P, Vale W, Weber E, Wu J-Y, Chang K-J (1986) The hypothalamic arcuate nucleus-median eminence complex: immunohistochemistry of transmitters, peptides and DARPP-32 with special reference to coexistence in dopamine neurons. Brain Res Rev 11:97–155

Fallon JH, Ciofi P (1990) Dynorphin-containing neurons. In: Björklund A, Hökfelt T, Kuhar MJ (eds) Neuropeptides in the CNS, part II, edn. Elsevier, Amsterdam, pp 1–130 (Handbook of chemical neuroanatomy, vol 9)

Frederickson RC, Burgis V, Edwards JD (1977) Hyperalgesia induced by naloxone follows diurnal rhythm in responsivity to painful stimuli. Science 198:756–758

Fried G, Terenius L, Hökfelt T, Goldstein M (1985) Evidence for differential localization of noradrenaline and neuropeptide Y in neuronal storage vesicles isolated from rat vas deferens. J Neurosci 5:450–458

Fried G, Terenius L, Brodin E, Efendic S, Dockray G, Fahrenkrug J, Goldstein M, Hökfelt T (1986) Neuropeptide Y, enkephalin and noradrenaline coexist in sympathetic neurons innervating the bovine spleen. Biochemical and immuno-histochemical evidence. Cell Tissue Res 243:495–508

Fried G, Meister B, Wikström M, Terenius L, Goldstein M (1989) Galanin-, neuropeptide Y- and enkephalin-like immunoreactivities in catecholamine-storing paraganglia of the fetal guinea pig and newborn pig. Cell Tissue Res 255:495–504

Furness JB, Costa M (1987) The enteric nervous system. Churchill Livingstone, Edinburgh

Gall C (1984) The distribution of cholecystokinin-like immunoreactivity in the hippocampal formation of the guinea pig: localization in the mossy fibers. Brain Res 306:73–83

Gall C, Lauterborn J, Burks D, Seroogy K (1987) Co-localization of enkephalin and cholecystokinin in discrete areas of rat brain. Brain Res 403:403–408

Garry MG, Miller KE, Seybold VS (1989) Lumbar dorsal root ganglia of the cat: a quantitative study of peptide immunoreactivity and cell size. J Comp Neurol 284:36–47 (erratum in J Comp Neurol 288(4):698)

Gaymann W, Martin R (1987) A re-examination of the localization of immuno-reactive dynorphin(1–8), Leu-enkephalin and Met-enkephalin in the rat neurohypophysis. Neuroscience 20:1069–1080

Gaymann W, Martin R (1989) Immunoreactive galanin-like material in magno-cellular hypothalamo-neurohypophysial neurones of the rat. Cell Tissue Res 255:139–147

Geuze HJ, Slot JW, van der Ley P, Scheffer RC (1981) Use of colloidal gold particles in double-labeling immunoelectron microscopy of ultrathin frozen tissue sections. J Cell Biol 89:653–65

Gibbins IL, Morris JL (1987) Co-existence of neuropeptides in sympathetic, cranial autonomic and sensory neurons innervating the iris of the guinea-pig. J Auton Nerv Syst 21:67–82

Gibbins IL, Furness JB, Costa M (1987) Pathway-specific patterns of the co-existence of substance P, calcitonin gene-related peptide, cholecystokinin and dynorphin in neurons of the dorsal root ganglia of the guinea-pig. Cell Tissue Res 248:417–437

Gilbert RF, Bennett GW, Marsden CA, Emson PC (1981) The effects of 5-hydroxytryptamine-depleting drugs on peptides in the ventral spinal cord. Eur J Pharmacol 76:203–210

Gilbert RF, Emson PC, Hunt SP, Bennett GW, Marsden CA, Sandberg BE, Steinbusch HW, Verhofstad AA (1982) The effects of monoamine neurotoxins on peptides in the rat spinal cord. Neuroscience 7:69–87

Glazer EJ, Basbaum AI (1980) Leucine enkephalin: localization in and axoplasmic transport by sacral parasympathetic preganglionic neurons. Science 208:1479–1481

Glazer EJ, Steinbusch H, Verhofstad A, Basbaum AI (1981) Serotonin neurons in nucleus raphe dorsalis and paragigantocellularis of the cat contain enkephalin. J Physiol (Paris) 77:241–245

Guthrie J, Basbaum AI (1984) Colocalization of immunoreactive proenkephalin and prodynorphin products in medullary neurons of the rat. Neuropeptides 4:437–445

Hamano K, Katayama KY, Kiyama H, Ishimoto I, Manabe R, Tohyama M (1989) Coexistence of enkephalin and somatostatin in the chicken retina. Brain Res 489:254–260

Hancock MB (1986) Two-color immunoperoxidase staining: visualization of anatomic relationships between immunoreactive neural elements. Am J Anat 175:343–352

Harlan RE, Shivers BD, Romano GJ, Howells RD, Pfaff DW (1987) Localization of preproenkephalin mRNA in the rat brain and spinal cord by in situ hybridization. J Comp Neurol 258:159–184

Heym C, Kummer W (1989) Immunohistochemical distribution and colocalization of regulatory peptides in the carotid body. J Electron Microsc Tech 12:331–342

Ho RH (1988) Somatostatin immunoreactive structures in the developing rat spinal cord. Brain Res Bull 21:105–116

Hökfelt T (1968) In vitro studies on central and peripheral monoamine neurons at the ultrastructural level. Z Zellforsch Mikrosk Anat 91:1–74

Hökfelt T, Dahlström A (1971) Effects of two mitosis inhibitors (colchicine and vinblastine) on the distribution and axonal transport of noradrenaline storage particles, studied by fluorescence and electron microscopy. Z Zellforsch Mikrosk Anat 119:460–482

Hökfelt T, Elde R, Johansson O, Terenius L, Stein L (1977a) The distribution of enkephalin-immunoreactive cell bodies in the rat central nervous system. Neurosci Lett 5:25–31

Hökfelt T, Elfvin L-G, Elde R, Schultzberg M, Goldstein M, Luft R (1977b) Occurrence of somatostatin-like immunoreactivity in some peripheral sympathetic noradrenergic neurons. Proc Natl Acad Sci USA 74:3587–3591

Hökfelt T, Ljungdahl Å, Steinbusch H, Verhofstad A, Nilsson G, Brodin E, Pernow B, Goldstein M (1978) Immunohistochemical evidence of substance P-like immunoreactivity in some 5-hydroxytryptamine-containing neurons in the rat central nervous system. Neuroscience 3:517–538

Hökfelt T, Lundberg JM, Schultzberg M, Johansson O, Ljungdahl Å, Rehfeld J (1980) Coexistence of peptides and putative transmitters in neurons. In: Costa E, Trabucchi M (eds) Neural peptides and neuronal communication. Raven, New York, pp 1–23

Hökfelt T, Fuxe K, Pernow B (1986) Coexistence of neuronal messengers: a new principle in chemical transmission. Elsevier, Amsterdam (Progress in brain research, vol 68)

Hökfelt T, Fahrenkrug J, Ju G, Ceccatelli S, Tsuruo Y, Meister B, Mutt V, Rundgren M, Brodin E, Terenius L et al. (1987) Analysis of peptide histidine-isoleucine/vasoactive intestinal polypeptide-immunoreactive neurons in the central nervous system with special reference to their relation to corticotropin releasing factor- and enkephalin-like immunoreactivities in the paraventricular hypothalamic nucleus. Neuroscience 23:827–857

Hökfelt T, Meister B, Melander T, Schalling M, Staines W, Millhorn D, Seroogy K, Tsuruo Y, Holets V, Ceccatelli S, Villar M, Ju G, Freedman J, Olson L, Lindh B, Bartfai T, Fisone G, Le Greves P, Terenius L, Post C, Mollenholt P, Dean J, Goldstein M (1988) Coexistence of multiple neuronal messengers: new aspects on chemical transmission. In: Costa E (ed) Fidia research foundation neuroscience award lectures. Raven, New York, pp 61–113

Hunt SP, Emson PC, Gilbert R, Goldstein M, Kimmell JR (1981) Presence of avian pancreatic polypeptide-like immunoreactivity in catecholamine and methionine-enkephalin-containing neurones within the central nervous system. Neurosci Lett 21:125–130

Iadarola MJ, Brady LS, Draisci G, Dubner R (1988a) Enhancement of dynorphin gene expression in spinal cord following experimental inflammation: stimulus specificity, behavioral parameters and opioid receptor binding. Pain 35:313–326

Iadarola MJ, Douglass J, Civelli O, Naranjo JR (1988b) Differential activation of spinal cord dynorphin and enkephalin neurons during hyperalgesia: evidence using cDNA hybridization. Brain Res 455:205–212

Ibuki T, Okamura H, Miyazaki M, Kimura H, Yanaihara N, Ibata Y (1988) Colocalization of GABA and (Met)enkephalin-Arg6-Gly7-Leu8 in the rat cerebellum. Neurosci Lett 91:131–135

Ichikawa H, Matsuo S, Wakisaka S, Itotagawa T, Kato J, Akai M (1990) Leucine-enkephalin-, neurokinin A- and cholecystokinin-like immunoreactivities in the guinea pig tongue. Arch Oral Biol 35:181–188

Jaffe JH, Martin WR (1990) Opioid analgesics and antagonists. In: Gilman AG, Rall TW, Nies AS, Taylor P (eds) The pharmacological basis of therapeutics, 8th edn. Pergamon, New York, pp 485–521

Järvi R (1989) Localization of bombesin-, neuropeptide Y-, enkephalin- and tyrosine hydroxylase-like immunoreactivities in rat coeliac-superior mesenteric ganglion. Histochemistry 92:231–236

Johansson O, Hökfelt T, Pernow B, Jeffcoate SL, White N, Steinbusch HW, Verhofstad AA, Emson PC, Spindel E (1981) Immunohistochemical support for three putative transmitters in one neuron: coexistence of 5-hydroxytryptamine-, substance P- and thyrotropin releasing hormone-like immunoreactivity in medullary neurons projecting to the spinal cord. Neuroscience 6:1857–1881

Joseph SA, Piekut DT (1986) Dual immunostaining procedure demonstrating neurotransmitter and neuropeptide codistribution in the same brain section. Am J Anat 175:331–342

Ju G, Melander T, Ceccatelli S, Hökfelt T, Frey P (1987) Immunohistochemical evidence for a spinothalamic pathway co-containing cholecystokinin- and galanin-like immunoreactivities in the rat. Neuroscience 20:439–456

Kanagawa Y, Matsuyama T, Wanaka A, Yoneda S, Kimura K, Kamada T, Steinbusch HW, Tohyama M (1986) Coexistence of enkephalin- and serotonin-like substances in single small intensely fluorescent cells of the guinea pig superior cervical ganglion. Brain Res 379:377–379

Katoh S, Hisano S, Kawano H, Kagotani Y, Daikoku S (1988) Light- and electron-microscopic evidence of costoring of immunoreactive enkephalins and substance P in dorsal horn neurons of rat. Cell Tissue Res 253:297–303

Katz B (1969) The release of neural transmitter substances. Liverpool University Press, Liverpool

Kawatani M, Nagel J, de Graat GW (1986) Identification of neuropeptides in pelvic and pudendal nerve afferent pathways to the sacral spinal cord of the cat. J Comp Neurol 249:117–132

Kelley RB (1988) The cell biology of the nerve terminal. Neuron 1:431–438

Khachaturian H, Lewis ME, Schäfer MK-H, Watson SJ (1985a) Anatomy of the CNS opioid systems. Trends Neurosci 8:111–119

Khachaturian H, Lewis ME, Tsou K, Watson SJ (1985b) b-Endorphin, a-MSH, ACTH, and related peptides. In: Björklund A, Hökfelt T (eds) GABA and neuropeptides in the CNS, part I, edn, pp 216–272. Elsevier, Amsterdam (Handbook of chemical neuroanatomy, vol 4)

Kiyama H, Emson PC, Tohyama M (1990) Recent progress in the use of the technique of non-radioactive in situ hybridization histochemistry: new tools for molecular neurobiology. Neurosci Res 9:1–21

Klein RL, Thureson-Klein ÅK (1990) Neuropeptide co-storage and exocytosis by neuronal large dense-cored vesicles: how good is the evidence? In: Osborne NN (ed) Current aspects of the neuroscience. Macmillan, London, pp 219–258

Kondo H, Kuramoto H, Wainer BH, Yanaihara N (1985) Evidence for the co-existence of acetylcholine and enkephalin in the sympathetic preganglionic neurons of rats. Brain Res 335:309–314

Kreutzberg GW (1969) Neuronal dynamics and axonal flow: IV. Blockage of intra-axonal enzyme transport by colchicine. Proc Natl Acad Sci USA 62:722–728

618 highR. ELDE and T. HÖKFELT

Krukoff TL (1987) Coexistence of neuropeptides in sympathetic preganglionic neurons of the cat. Peptides 8:109–112

Lam DM, Li HB, Su YY, Watt CB (1985) The signature hypothesis: co-localizations of neuroactive substances as anatomical probes for circuitry analyses. Vision Res 25:1353–1364

Lang RE, Taugner G, Gaida W, Ganten D, Kraft K, Unger T, Wunderlich I (1982) Evidence against co-storage of enkephalins with noradrenaline in bovine adrenal medullary granules. Eur J Pharmacol 86:117–120

Leboulenger F, Leroux P, Delarue C, Tonon MC, Charnay Y, Dubois PM, Coy DH, Vaudry H (1983a) Co-localization of vasoactive intestinal peptide (VIP) and enkephalins in chromaffin cells of the adrenal gland of amphibia. Stimulation of corticosteroid production by VIP. Life Sci 32:375–383

Leboulenger F, Leroux P, Tonon MC, Coy DH, Vaudry H, Pelletier G (1983b) Coexistence of vasoactive intestinal peptide and enkephalins in the adrenal chromaffin granules of the frog. Neurosci Lett 37:221–225

Léger L, Charnay Y, Dubois PM, Jouvet M (1986) Distribution of enkephalin-immunoreactive cell bodies in relation to serotonin-containing neurons in the raphe nuclei of the cat: immunohistochemical evidence for the coexistence of enkephalins and serotonin in certain cells. Brain Res 362:63–73

Lehtosalo JI, Ylikoski J, Eranko L, Eranko O, Panula P (1984) Immunohistochemical localization of unique enkephalin sequences contained in pre-proenkephalin A in the guinea pig cochlea. Hear Res 16:101–107

Li HB, Watt CB, Lam DM (1985) The coexistence of two neuroactive peptides in a subpopulation of retinal amacrine cells. Brain Res 345:176–180

Li HB, Watt CB, Lam DM (1990) Double-label analyses of somatostatin's coexistence with enkephalin and gamma-aminobutyric acid in amacrine cells of the chicken retina. Brain Res 525:304–309

Livett BG, Day R, Elde RP, Howe PR (1982) Co-storage of enkephalins and adrenaline in the bovine adrenal medulla. Neuroscience 7:1323–1332

Lundberg JM, Hökfelt T (1983) Coexistence of peptides and classical transmitters. Trends Neurosci 6:325–333

Lundberg JM, Hamberger B, Schultzberg M, Hökfelt T, Granberg PO, Efendić S, Terenius L, Goldstein M, Luft R (1979) Enkephalin- and somatostatin-like immunoreactivities in human adrenal medulla and pheochromocytoma. Proc Natl Acad Sci USA 76:4079–4083

Lundberg JM, Fried G, Fahrenkrug J, Holmstedt B, Hökfelt T, Lagercrantz H, Lundgren G, Änggård A (1981) Subcellular fractionation of cat submandibular gland: comparative studies on the distribution of acetylcholine and vasoactive intestinal polypeptide (VIP). Neuroscience 6:1001–1010

Lundberg JM, Hökfelt T, Änggård A, Terenius L, Elde R, Markey K, Goldstein M, Kimmel J (1982) Organizational principles in the peripheral sympathetic nervous system: subdivision by coexisting peptides (somatostatin-, avian pancreatic polypeptide-, and vasoactive intestinal polypeptide-like immunoreactive materials). Proc Natl Acad Sci USA 79:1303–1307

Martin R, Voigt KH (1981) Enkephalins co-exist with oxytocin and vasopressin in nerve terminals of rat neurohypophysis. Nature 289:502–504

Martin R, Geis R, Holl R, Schafer M, Voigt KH (1983) Co-existence of unrelated peptides in oxytocin and vasopressin terminals of rat neurohypophyses: immunoreactive methionine-enkephalin-, leucine-enkephalin- and cholecystokinin-like substances. Neuroscience 8:213–227

McGinty JF, Bloom FE (1983) Double immunostaining reveals distinctions among opioid peptidergic neurons in the medial basal hypothalamus. Brain Res 278:145–153

Meister B, Hökfelt T (1988) Peptide- and transmitter-containing neurons in the mediobasal hypothalamus and their relation to GABAergic systems: possible roles in control of prolactin and growth hormone secretion. Synapse 2:585–605

Meister B, Ceccatelli S, Hökfelt T, Anden NE, Anden M, Theodorsson E (1989) Neurotransmitters, neuropeptides and binding sites in the rat mediobasal hypothalamus: effects of monosodium glutamate (MSG) lesions. Exp Brain Res 76:343–368

Meister B, Cortés R, Villar MJ, Schalling M, Hökfelt T (1990a) Peptides and transmitter enzymes in hypothalamic magnocellular neurons after administration of hyperosmotic stimuli: comparison between messenger RNA and peptide/ protein levels. Cell Tissue Res 260:279–297

Meister B, Villar MJ, Ceccatelli S, Hökfelt T (1990b) Localization of chemical messengers in magnocellular neurons of the hypothalamic supraoptic and paraventricular nuclei: an immunohistochemical study using experimental manipulations. Neuroscience 37:603–633

Meriney SD, Ford MJ, Oliva D, Pilar G (1991) Endogenous opioids modulate neuronal survival in the developing avian ciliary ganglion. J Neurosci 11: 3705–3717

Miller KE, Seybold VS (1987) Comparison of met-enkephalin-, dynorphin A-, and neurotensin-immunoreactive neurons in the cat and rat spinal cords: I. Lumbar cord. J Comp Neurol 255:293–304

Miller KE, Seybold VS (1989) Comparison of met-enkephalin, dynorphin A, and neurotensin immunoreactive neurons in the cat and rat spinal cords: II. Segmental differences in the marginal zone. J Comp Neurol 279:619–628

Millhorn DE, Hökfelt T, Terenius L, Buchan A, Brown JC (1987a) Somatostatin- and enkephalin-like immunoreactivities are frequently colocalized in neurons in the caudal brain stem of rat. Exp Brain Res 67:420–428

Millhorn DE, Seroogy K, Hökfelt T, Schmued LC, Terenius L, Buchan A, Brown JC (1987b) Neurons of the ventral medulla oblongata that contain both somatostatin and enkephalin immunoreactivities project to nucleus tractus solitarii and spinal cord. Brain Res 424:99–108

Millhorn DE, Hökfelt T, Verhofstad AA, Terenius L (1989) Individual cells in the raphe nuclei of the medulla oblongata in rat that contain immunoreactivities for both serotonin and enkephalin project to the spinal cord. Exp Brain Res 75: 536–542

Milner TA, Pickel VM, Reis DJ (1989) Ultrastructural basis for interactions between central opioids and catecholamines: I. Rostral ventrolateral medulla. J Neurosci 9:2114–2130

Mize RR (1989) Enkephalin-like immunoreactivity in the cat superior colliculus: distribution, ultrastructure, and colocalization with GABA. J Comp Neurol 285:133–155

Molander C, Xu Q, Grant G (1984) The cytoarchitectonic organization of the spinal cord in the rat: I. The lower thoracic and lumbosacral cord. J Comp Neurol 230:133–141

Morris JL, Gibbins IL, Furness JB, Costa M, Murphy R (1985) Co-localization of neuropeptide Y, vasoactive intestinal polypeptide and dynorphin in non-noradrenergic axons of the guinea pig uterine artery. Neurosci Lett 62:31–37

Mossberg K, Arvidsson U, Ulfhake B (1990) Computerized quantification of immunofluorescence-labeled axon terminals and analysis of co-localization of neurochemicals in axon terminals with a confocal scanning laser microscope. J Histochem Cytochem 38:179–190

Murakami S, Okamura H, Pelletier G, Ibata Y (1989) Differential colocalization of neuropeptide Y- and methionine-enkephalin-Arg6-Gly7-Leu8-like immuno-reactivity in catecholaminergic neurons in the rat brain stem. J Comp Neurol 281:532–544

Nairn RC (1969) Fluorescent protein tracing. Livingstone, Edinburgh

Nakane PK (1968) Simultaneous localization of multiple tissue antigens using the peroxidase-labeled antibody method: a study on pituitary glands of the rat. J Histochem Cytochem 16:557–560

Navone F, Greengard P, DeCamilli P (1984) Synapsin I in nerve terminals: selective association with small synaptic vesicles. Science 226:1209

Neal CJ, Newman SW (1991) Prodynorphin- and substance P-containing neurons project to the medial preoptic area in the male Syrian hamster brain. Brain Res 546:119–131

Neal CJ, Swann JM, Newman SW (1989) The colocalization of substance P and prodynorphin immunoreactivity in neurons of the medial preoptic area, bed nucleus of the stria terminalis and medial nucleus of the amygdala of the Syrian hamster. Brain Res 496:1–13

Nicholas AP, Pieribone VA, Arvidsson U, Hökfelt T (1992) Serotonin-, substance P- and glutamate/aspartate-like immunoreactivities in medullo-spinal pathways of rat and primate. Neuroscience (in press)

O'Donohue TL, Handelmann GE, Miller RL, Jacobowitz DM (1982) N-acetylation regulates the behavioral activity of alpha-melanotropin in a multineuro-transmitter neuron. Science 215:1125–1127

Okamura H, Murakami S, Yanaihara N, Ibata Y (1989) Coexistence of catecholamine and methionine enkephalin-Arg6-Gly7-Leu8 in neurons of the rat ventrolateral medulla oblongata. Application of combined peptide immunocytochemistry and histofluorescence method in the same vibratome section. Histochemistry 91: 31–34

Osbome NN (1983) Dale's Principle and Communication between Neurones. Pergamon, Oxford, pp

Owman C, Håkanson R, Sundler F (1973) Occurrence and function of amines in endocrine cells producing polypeptide hormones. Fed Proc 32:1785–1791

Pearse AGE (1969) The cytochemistry and ultrastructure of polypeptide hormone producing cells of the APUD series and the embryologic, physiologic and pathologic implications of the concept. J Histochem Cytochem 17:303–313

Pelto-Huikko M, Salminen T, Hervonen A (1985) Localization of enkephalins in adrenaline cells and the nerves innervating adrenaline cells in rat adrenal medulla. Histochemistry 82:377–383

Penny GR, Afsharpour S, Kitai ST (1986) The glutamate decarboxylase-, leucine enkephalin-, methionine enkephalin- and substance P-immunoreactive neurons in the neostriatum of the rat and cat: evidence for partial population overlap. Neuroscience 17:1011–1045

Petrenko AG, Perin MS, Davletov BA, Ushkaryov YA, Geppert M, Südhof TC (1991) Binding of synaptotagmin to the a-latrotoxin receptor implicates both in synaptic vesicle exocytosis. Nature 353:65–68

Petrusz P, Merchenthaler I, Maderdrut JL (1985) Distribution of enkephalin-containing neurons in the central nervous system. In: Björklund A, Hökfelt T (eds) GABA and neuropeptides in the CNS, part I. Elsevier, Amsterdam, pp 273–334 (Handbook of chemical neuroanatomy, vol 4)

Pickel VM (1985) General morphological features of peptidergic neurons. In: Björklund A, Hökfelt T (eds) GABA and neuropeptides in the CNS, part I. Elsevier, Amsterdam, pp 72–92 (Handbook of chemical neuroanatomy, vol 4)

Pilcher WH, Joseph AS (1986) Differential sensitivity of hypothalamic and medullary opiocortin and tyrosine hydroxylase neurons to the neurotoxic effects of monosodium glutamate (MSG). Peptides 7:783–789

Pow DV, Morris JF (1991) Membrane routing during exocytosis and endocytosis in neuroendocrine neurones and endocrine cells: use of colloidal gold particles and immunocytochemical discrimination of membrane compartments. Cell Tissue Res 264:299–316

Pretel S, Piekut D (1990) Coexistence of corticotropin-releasing factor and enkephalin in the paraventricular nucleus of the rat. J Comp Neurol 294: 192–201

Pruss RM, Mezey E, Forman DS, Eiden LE, Hotchkiss AJ, DiMaggio DA, O'Donohue TL (1986) Enkephalin and neuropeptide Y: two colocalized neuropeptides are independently regulated in primary cultures of bovine chromaffin cells. Neuropeptides 7:315–327

Reiner A, Anderson KD (1990) The patterns of neurotransmitter and neuropeptide cooccurrence among striatal projection neurons: conclusions based on recent findings. Brain Res Rev 15:251–265

Rökaeus A, Pruss RM, Eiden LE (1990) Galanin gene expression in chromaffin cells is controlled by calcium and protein kinase signaling pathways. Endocrinology 127:3096–3102

Roth J, Bendayan M, Orci L (1978) Ultrastructural localization of intracellular antigens by the use of protein A-gold complex. J Histochem Cytochem 26: 1074–1081

Ruda MA, Iadarola MJ, Cohen LV, Young W (1988) In situ hybridization histochemistry and immunocytochemistry reveal an increase in spinal dynorphin biosynthesis in a rat model of peripheral inflammation and hyperalgesia. Proc Natl Acad Sci USA 85:622–626

Sasek CA, Elde RP (1986) Coexistence of enkephalin and dynorphin immunoreactivities in neurons in the dorsal gray commissure of the sixth lumbar and first sacral spinal cord segments in rat. Brain Res 381:8–14

Sasek CA, Helke CJ (1989) Enkephalin-immunoreactive neuronal projections from the medulla oblongata to the intermediolateral cell column: relationship to substance P-immunoreactive neurons. J Comp Neurol 287:484–494

Sawchenko PE, Swanson LW (1985) Localization, colocalization, and plasticity of corticotropin-releasing factor immunoreactivity in rat brain. Fed Proc 44: 221–227

Sawchenko PE, Arias C, Bittencourt JC (1990) Inhibin beta, somatostatin, and enkephalin immunoreactivities coexist in caudal medullary neurons that project to the paraventricular nucleus of the hypothalamus. J Comp Neurol 291: 269–280

Schultzberg M, Lundberg JM, Hökfelt T, Terenius L, Brandt J, Elde RP, Goldstein M (1978) Enkephalin-like immunoreactivity in gland cells and nerve terminals of the adrenal medulla. Neuroscience 3:1169–1186

Schultzberg M, Hökfelt T, Terenius L, Elfvin LG, Lundberg JM, Brandt J, Elde RP, Goldstein M (1979) Enkephalin immunoreactive nerve fibres and cell bodies in sympathetic ganglia of the guinea-pig and rat. Neuroscience 4:240–270

Schultzberg M, Hökfelt T, Nilsson G, Terenius L, Rehfeld JF, Brown M, Elde R, Goldstein M, Said S (1980) Distribution of peptide- and catecholamine-containing neurons in the gastro-intestinal tract of rat and guinea-pig: immunohistochemical studies with antisera to substance P, vasoactive intestinal polypeptide, enkephalins, somatostatin, gastrin/cholecystokinin, neurotensin and dopamine beta-hydroxylase. Neuroscience 5:689–744

Schulz R, Wüster M, Simantov R, Snyder S, Herz A (1977) Electrically stimulated release of opiate-like material from the myenteric plexus of the guinea-pig ileum. Eur J Pharmacol 41:347–348

Schwartz EA (1987) Depolarization without calcium can release g-aminobutyric acid from a retinal neuron. Science 238:350–355

Senba E, Yanaihara C, Yanaihara N, Tohyama M (1988) Co-localization of substance P and Met-enkephalin-Arg6-Gly7-Leu8 in the intraspinal neurons of the rat, with special reference to the neurons in the substantia gelatinosa. Brain Res 453:110–116

Seroogy KB, Bayliss DA, Szymeczek CL, Hökfelt T, Millhorn DE (1991) Transient expression of somatostatin messenger RNA and peptide in the hypoglossal nucleus of the neonatal rat. Brain Res Dev Brain Res 60:241–252

Sherman TG, Civelli O, Douglass J, Herbert E, Watson SJ (1986) Coordinate expression of hypothalamic pro-dynorphin and pro-vasopressin mRNAs with osmotic stimulation. Neuroendocrinology 44:222–228

Shimada S, Inagaki S, Kubota Y, Kito S, Shiotani Y, Tohyama M (1987) Co-existence of substance P- and enkephalin-like peptides in single neurons of the rat hypothalamus. Brain Res 425:256–262

Shinoda K, Michigami T, Awano K, Shiotani Y (1988) Analysis of the rat inter-peduncular subnuclei by immunocytochemical double-staining for enkephalin and substance P, with some reference to the coexistence of both peptides. J Comp Neurol 271:243–256

Snyder SH, Bredt DS (1991) Nitric oxide as a neuronal messenger. Trends Pharmacol Sci 12:125–128

Staines WA, Meister B, Melander T, Nagy JI, Hökfelt T (1988) Three-color immunofluorescence histochemistry allowing triple labeling within a single section. J Histochem Cytochem 36:145–151

Südhof TC, Jahn R (1991) Proteins of synaptic vesicles involved in exocytosis and membrane recycling. Neuron 6:665–677

Sugimoto T, Mizuno N (1986) Immunohistochemical demonstration of neurotensin in striatal neurons of the cat, with particular reference to coexistence with enkephalin. Brain Res 398:195–198

Sugimoto T, Mizuno N (1987) Neurotensin in projection neurons of the striatum and nucleus accumbens, with reference to coexistence with enkephalin and GABA: an immunohistochemical study in the cat. J Comp Neurol 257:383–395

Summy-Long JY, Miller DS, Rosella DLM, Hartman RD, Emmert SE (1984) A functional role for opioid peptides in the differential secretion of vasopressin and oxytocin. Brain Res 309:362–366

Tashiro T, Takahashi O, Satoda T, Matsushima R, Mizuno N (1987) Immuno-histochemical demonstration of coexistence of enkephalin- and substance P-like immunoreactivities in axonal components in the lumber segments of cat spinal cord. Brain Res 424:391–395

Thomas L, Betz H (1990) Synaptophysin binds to physophilin, a putative synaptic plasma membrane protein. J Cell Biol 111:2041–2052

Tohyama Y, Senba E, Yamashita T, Kitajiri M, Kuriyama H, Kumazawa T, Ohata K, Tohyama M (1990) Coexistence of calcitonin gene-related peptide and enkephalin in single neurons of the lateral superior olivary nucleus of the guinea pig that project to the cochlea as lateral olivocochlear system. Brain Res 515:312–314

Tramu G, Pillez A, Leonardelli J (1978) An efficient method of antibody elution for the successive or simultaneous localization of two antigens by immunocyto-chemistry. J Histochem Cytochem 26:322–324

Trimble WS, Linial M, Scheller RH (1991) Cellular and molecular biology of the presynaptic nerve terminal. Annu Rev Neurosci 14:93–122

Tsuruo Y, Ceccatelli S, Villar MJ, Hökfelt T, Visser TJ, Terenius L, Goldstein M, Brown JC, Buchan A, Walsh J, Morris M, Sofroniew MV, Verhofstad A (1988) Coexistence of TRH with other neuroactive substances in the rat central nervous system. J Chem Neuroanat 1:235–253

Tuchscherer MM, Seybold VS (1989) A quantitative study of the coexistence of peptides in varicosities within the superficial laminae of the dorsal horn of the rat spinal cord. J Neurosci 9:195–205

Tuchscherer MM, Knox C, Seybold VS (1987) Substance P and cholecystokinin-like immunoreactive varicosities in somatosensory and autonomic regions of the rat spinal cord: a quantitative study of coexistence. J Neurosci 7:3984–3995

Vallarino M, Delbende C, Bunel DT, Ottonello I, Vaudry H (1989) Pro-opiomelanocortin (POMC)-related peptides in the brain of the rainbow trout, *Salmo gairdneri*. Peptides 10:1223–1230

Valtorta F, Tarelli FT, Campanati L, Villa A, Greengard P (1989) Synaptophysin and synapsin I as tools for the study of the exo-endocytotic cycle. Cell Biol Int Rep 13:1023–1038

Verhage M, McMahon HT, Ghijsen WEJM, Boomsma F, Scholten G, Wiegant VM, Nicholls DG (1991) Differential release of amino acids, neuropeptides, and catecholamines from isolated nerve terminals. Neuron 6:517–524

Villar MJ, Huchet M, Hökfelt T, Changeux JP, Fahrenkrug J, Brown JC (1988) Existence and coexistence of calcitonin gene-related peptide, vasoactive intestinal polypeptide- and somatostatin-like immunoreactivities in spinal cord motoneurons of developing embryos and post-hatch chicks. Neurosci Lett 86:114–118

Villar MJ, Cortés R, Theodorsson E, Wiesenfeld HZ, Schalling M, Fahrenkrug J, Emson PC, Hökfelt T (1989) Neuropeptide expression in rat dorsal root ganglion cells and spinal cord after peripheral nerve injury with special reference to galanin. Neuroscience 33:587–604

Villar MJ, Roa M, Huchet M, Changeux JP, Valentino KL, Hökfelt T (1991) Occurrence of neuropeptide K-like immunoreactivity in ventral horn cells of the chicken spinal cord during development. Brain Res 541:149–153

Vincent SR, Dalsgaard CJ, Schultzberg M, Hökfelt T, Christensson I, Terenius L (1984) Dynorphin-immunoreactive neurons in the autonomic nervous system. Neuroscience 11:973–987

Viveros OH, Diliberto EJJ, Daniels AJ (1983) Biochemical and functional evidence for the cosecretion of multiple messengers from single and multiple compartments. Fed Proc 42:2923–2928

Wang YN, Wyatt RJ (1987) Comparative immunohistochemical demonstration of peptide F- and other enkephalin-containing neurons in the enteric nervous system of the rat. Synapse 1:208–213

Watson SJ, Barchas JD, Li CH (1977) β-Lipotropin: localization of cells and axons in rat brain by immunocytochemistry. Proc Natl Acad Sci USA 74:5155–5158

Watson SJ, Akil H, Fischli W, Goldstein A, Zimmerman E, Nilaver G, van Wimersma Griedanus T (1982) Dynorphin and vasopressin: common localization in magnocellular neurons. Science 216:85–87

Watt CB, Su YY, Lam DM (1984) Interactions between enkephalin and GABA in avian retina. Nature 311:761–763

Watt CB, Li T, Lam DM, Wu SM (1988) Quantitative studies of enkephalin's coexistence with gamma-aminobutyric acid, glycine and neurotensin in amacrine cells of the chicken retina. Brain Res 444:366–370

Wattchow DA, Furness JB, Costa M (1988) Distribution and coexistence of peptides in nerve fibers of the external muscle of the human gastrointestinal tract. Gastroenterology 95:32–41

Weihe E, Millan MJ, Leibold A, Nohr D, Herz A (1988) Co-localization of proenkephalin- and prodynorphin-derived opioid peptides in laminae IV/V spinal neurons revealed in arthritic rats. Neurosci Lett 85:187–192

Wessendorf MW (1990) Characterization and use of multi-color fluorescence microscopic techniques. In: Hökfelt T, Björklund A, Wouterlood FG, van den Pol AN (eds) Analysis of neuronal microcircuits and synaptic interactions. Elsevier, Amsterdam, pp 1–45 (Handbook of chemical neuroanatomy, vol 8)

Wessendorf MW, Elde RP (1985) Characterization of an immunofluorescence technique for the demonstration of coexisting neurotransmitters within nerve fibers and terminals. J Histochem Cytochem 33:984–994

Wessendorf MW, Appel NM, Molitor TW, Elde RP (1990) A method for immuno-fluorescent demonstration of three coexisting neurotransmitters in rat brain and spinal cord, using the fluorophores fluorescein, lissamine rhodamine, and 7-amino-4-methylcoumarin-3-acetic acid. J Histochem Cytochem 38:1859–1877

Whitnall MH, Gainer H, Cox BM, Molineaux CJ (1983) Dynorphin-A-(1-8) is contained within vasopressin neurosecretory vesicles in rat pituitary. Science 222:1137–1139

Winkler H, Apps DK, Fischer CR (1986) The molecular function of adrenal chromaffin granules: established facts and unresolved topics. Neuroscience 18:261–290

Wolfe DE, Axelrod J, Potter LT, Richardson KC (1962) Localizing tritiated norepinephrine in sympathetic axons by electron microscope autoradiography. Science 138:440–442

Wolter HJ (1985) α-Melanotropin, β-endorphin and adrenocorticotropin-like immunoreactivities are colocalized within duodenal myenteric plexus perikarya. Brain Res 325:290–293

Wu SM, Lam DM (1988) The coexistence of three neuroactive substances in amacrine cells of the chicken retina. Brain Res 458:195–198

Yoshida M, Taniguchi Y (1988) Projection of pro-opiomelanocortin neurons from the rat arcuate nucleus to the midbrain central gray as demonstrated by double staining with retrograde labeling and immunohistochemistry. Arch Histol Cytol 51:175–183

Young WS III (1990) In situ hybridization histochemistry. In: Hökfelt T, Björklund A, Wouterlood FG, van den Pol AN (eds) Analysis of neuronal microcircuits and synaptic interactions. Elsevier, Amsterdam, pp 481–512 (Handbook of chemical neuroanatomy, vol 8)

Young WS III, Mezey E, Siegel RE (1986) Vasopressin and oxytocin mRNAs in adrenalectomized and Brattleboro rats: analysis of quantitative in situ hybridization histochemistry. Brain Res 387:231–241

Zahm DS, Zaborszky L, Alones VE, Heimer L (1985) Evidence for the coexistence of glutamate decarboxylase and Met-enkephalin immunoreactivities in axon terminals of rat ventral pallidum. Brain Res 325:317–321

Interrelationships of Opioid, Dopaminergic, Cholinergic, and GABAergic Pathways in the Central Nervous System

P.L. WOOD

A. Introduction

It is the purpose of this chapter to give an overview of the complex interactions between endogenous opioid, dopaminergic, cholinergic, and GABAergic pathways in the brain. The effects described involve both acute and long-term adaptive changes as well as reciprocal interactions. Within this complex framework some general principles will evolve; however, as with so many other CNS pathways, there are species differences which require definition to demonstrate the limits of apparent generalizations. While this review will focus on neurochemical indices of CNS functional changes it is pharmacologically induced alterations which will be summarized; therefore, whenever possible studies of both dose-response and time course relationships will be referenced.

B. Cholinergic Systems

I. Introduction

Modulation of cholinergic transmission by opiates and opioid peptides has been an intensive area of investigation based upon the initial observations that, during opiate withdrawal, many of the symptoms of the withdrawal reaction involved cholinergic signs (see also Chap. 6). Subsequent detailed studies have revealed potent regulation of central cholinergic pathways, two of which are discussed here (WOOD et al. 1984a; WOOD and McQUADE 1986). For a review of methods used to assess central cholinergic transmission see CHENEY et al. (1989). The majority of neurochemical studies of these pathways have utilized two methodologies: (1) release of acetycholine (ACh) into perfusion cups placed on the cortical surface and (2) assessment of ACh dynamics via labeling the choline precursor pool with a radioactive or stable isotope (CHENEY et al. 1989).

II. Septohippocampal Cholinergic Pathway

The septohippocampal cholinergic pathway (SHCP) consists of large cell bodies in the medial septum and diagonal band of broca which send their axons, via the fimbria/fornix, to the hippocampus (Fig. 1). This cholinergic pathway is potently depressed, as assessed by decreases in TR_{ACh}, by μ-and δ- but not κ-opioid receptor agonists (Table 1; Cheney et al. 1974; Wood and Stotland 1980). Enhanced release of endogenous enkephalins after treatment with kyotorphin also leads to a naloxone-reversible depression of SHCP function (Rackham et al. 1982). Additionally, the ε-agonist β-endorphin depresses acetylcholine turnover (TR_{ACh}) in the hippocampus (Moroni et al. 1977). The possibility of ε-receptor involvement in these actions requires more detailed study but may involve ε-receptors in the septum (Akil et al. 1980) and the β-endorphin innervation which originates from cell bodies within the hypothalamus (Watson and Barchas 1979; Bloom et al. 1978). The anatomical locus of the μ- and δ-effects also appears to be at the level of the cholinergic cell bodies since the actions of parenteral and intraventricular drug treatments are reproduced by intra-septal injections (Moroni et al. 1977; Wood et al. 1984a,c). This intraseptal locus of action further appears to be transsynaptic in that the actions of opiates are antagonized by the GABA-A antagonist, bicuculline (Wood et al. 1979), indicating that opioid receptor modulation of septal GABAergic interneurons leads to a transsynaptic modulation of SHCP neurons (Fig. 1). These data would support the concept that the majority of inputs to the septum terminate in the lateral septum on GABAergic interneurons, which in turn modulate medial septal cholinergic cell bodies (Costa et al. 1983).

In contrast to μ- and δ-agonists, κ-agonists do not alter SHCP cholinergic function (Wood and Stotland 1980; Wood and Rackham 1981; Wood 1984). Agonist/antagonist analgesics, such as pentazocine and butorphanol, which clearly demonstrate receptor dualism (Martin 1967; Wood et al. 1983a) also do not alter TR_{ACh} in the hippocampus (Wood and Stotland 1980).

With regard to possible receptor isotypes, the μ-receptor type regulating SHCP cholinergic function has been tentatively classified as a μ-1 isoreceptor (Wood 1984), based on correlations between opiate doses for analgesia and depression of cholinergic transmission (Zsilla et al. 1976) and lack of reversal by κ-agonists at doses which express μ-2 antagonism (Wood 1984).

Tonic opioid activity does not appear to be involved in the regulation of the SHCP since TR_{ACh} in this pathway is unaltered by the opiate antagonist naloxone or the enkephalinase inhibitor thiorphan (Wood and McQuade 1986).

III. Nucleus Basalis-Cortical Cholinergic Pathway

The nucleus basalis-cortical cholinergic pathway (NBCP) originates from magnocellular cholinergic cell bodies in the nucleus basalis of Meynart in the basal forebrain and sends long axons to wide fields in the frontal and parietal cerebral cortices (Fig. 1). As with the SHCP, this cholinergic pro-

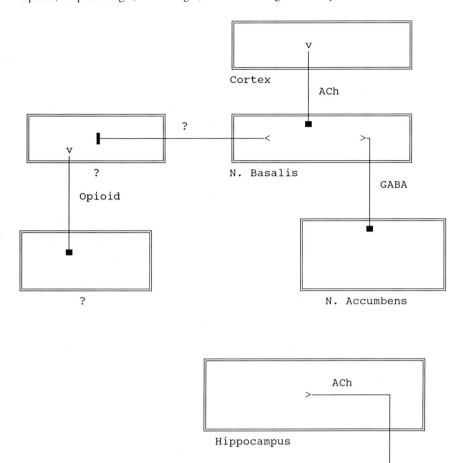

Fig. 1. Anatomical relationships of opioid, GABAergic and cholinergic pathways in the rodent forebrain

jection is depressed, as assessed both by decreases in TR_{ACh} and ACh collected in cortical perfusion cups, by μ- and δ-agonists (Table 1; PEPEU 1973; CHENEY et al. 1974, 1975; JHAMANDAS et al. 1975; MORONI et al. 1977; WOOD and STOTLAND 1980; WOOD et al. 1979, 1984a). In this case, the opioid receptor localization has not been clearly defined; however, local opiate injections and studies of cortical slices have ruled out a role for opioid receptors in the cortex (SZERB 1974; JHAMANDAS et al. 1975) and in the nucleus basalis (WOOD et al. 1984a; WOOD and McQUADE 1986). Indeed, it appears that an afferent to the nucleus basalis, with axons passing through the nucleus parafasicularis of the thalamus, might possess opioid receptor regulation and in turn influence the cholinergic activity of the NBCP (JHAMANDAS and SUTAK 1976; WOOD et al. 1984a). However, a transsynaptic action involving the inhibitory GABAergic nucleus accumbens-nucleus basalis pathway (WOOD and RICHARD 1982b; WOOD 1986; WOOD and McQUADE 1986) could lead to depressed cortical cholinergic function (Fig. 1), since morphine has been demonstrated to increase GABA turnover in the nucleus accumbens (WENZEL and KUSCHINSKY 1990).

κ-Agonists also do not influence TR_{ACh} in the NBCP while agonist/antagonist analgesics depress cholinergic function (WOOD and STOTLAND 1980; WOOD and RACKHAM 1981). These actions are stereospecific and naloxone reversible, but the opioid receptor subtype involved remains to be defined.

The μ-receptor regulating NBCP function has also been tentatively classified as a μ-1 isoreceptor (WOOD 1984; PASTERNAK and WOOD 1986). Partial μ-agonists, such as buprenorphine, depress cholinergic transmission in both the SHCP and NBCP with an inverted U dose-response relationship (WOOD and RACKHAM 1981).

While naloxone has no effect on ACh recovered in cortical perfusions cups (JHAMANDAS and SUTAK 1976) or cortical TR_{ACh} (WOOD and STOTLAND 1980), a transsynaptic modulation of the NBCP is present at a subcortical site as evidenced by greater cortical ACh release induced in rats, by electrical stimulation of the medial thalamus, or by reticular formation, after naloxone treatment (JHAMANDAS and SUTAK 1976). The enkephalinase inhibitor thiorphan does not appear to change the tone of this modulatory input (WOOD and McQUADE 1986).

C. Dopaminergic Pathways

I. Introduction

Previous reviews of the actions of opiates and opioid peptides on dopamine (DA) metabolism (WOOD 1983), of the technical limitations of assessing opioid receptor effects (WOOD 1988), and methods used to assess DA metabolism and release (WOOD and ALTAR 1988) are available for an historical overview of this research area. With regard to the neurochemical indices of dopaminergic function, precursor labeling is used to assess DA synthesis (CHENEY et al. 1975); dihydroxyphenylacetic acid (DOPAC) is used as an index of intraneuronal DA metabolism in dopaminergic nerve endings (WOOD and ALTAR 1988), and 3-methoxytyramine (3-MT), a DA metabolite generated in the synaptic cleft, is used as an index of DA release

Table 1. Actions of opiates and opioid peptides, striatal DOPAC levels, and TR_{ACh} in the parietal cortex and hippocampus[a]

Opiate (mg/kg) or [µg ivt]	TR_{ACh}		Striatal DOPAC
	Parietal cortex	Hippocampus (% of control)	
µ			
Morphine (2)	–	–	158
(16)	65	60	172
(32)	57	44	185
Etorphine (0.002)	70	45	186
Methadone (5)	67	40	199
δ			
DADLE [0.5]	–	–	126
[2]	–	–	147
[10]	60	50	176
[20]	55	19	–
κ			
EKC (4)	100	100	100
(16)	100	100	100
MR-2034 (8)	100	100	100
(16)	100	100	100
Tifluadom (12)	100	100	100
U50488H (16)	100	100	100
Agonist/Antagonists			
Butorphanol (2)	70	100	129
(16)	60	100	153
(64)	61	100	120
Pentazocine (8)	72	100	100
(32)	57	100	164
(64)	59	100	100
Antagonists			
Naloxone (2)	100	100	100
(5)	100	100	100
Zenazocine (0.2)	100	100	100
(2)	100	100	100
(4)	100	100	100

[a] ZSILLA et al. 1976; MORONI et al. 1977; WOOD and STOTLAND 1980; WOOD et al. 1980, 1984a,b; WOOD and McQUADE 1986; WOOD 1984.

(WOOD and ALTAR 1988) as is extracellular DA collected via intracerebral dialysis (WOOD et al. 1987c). In areas of diffuse dopaminergic innervation, like the cortex, 3-MT accumulation after inhibition of monoamine oxidase is a more reliable index of DA release in vivo (WOOD et al. 1987b).

II. Nigrostriatal Pathway

The nigrostriatal pathway consists of dopaminergic cell bodies in the substantia nigra (SN) and ascending axons which terminate throughout the striatum. Within the striatum, μ- and δ-agonists induce stereospecific and naloxone-reversible increases in DA synthesis (Smith et al. 1972; Ahtee and Kaarianen 1973; Cheney et al. 1975; Biggio et al. 1978) and DA metabolism as reflected by increases in DOPAC (Table 1; Wood et al. 1980). In marked contrast, changes in striatal DA release are species and strain specific. In the rat, there is no increase in DA release as reflected by lack of effect of morphine in striatal tissue slices (Kuschinsky and Hornykiewicz 1974); by no change in 3-MT levels, an index of DA release (Wood et al. 1980; Wood 1983; Yonehara and Clouet 1984; Wood and Altar 1988); by no change in 3-MT accumulation after inhibition of monoamine oxidase (Westerink 1978; Wood and Rao 1991); and by no change in the incorporation of radioactive label from [^{3}H]tyrosine into striatal 3-MT (Algeri et al. 1978; Groppetti et al. 1977). These data are all consistent with a lack of effect of opiates and opioid peptides on DA release in the rat striatum; however, a report of small and transient increases in DA collected in rat striatal dialysates after morphine has appeared (Di Chiara and Imperato 1988a). This report requires further confirmation and validation of the monitored electrochemical signal as DA.

In contrast to the rat, opiates and opioid peptides increase DA release in the mouse striatum as reflected by increased motor activity (Kuschinsky and Hornykiewicz 1974; Racagni et al. 1979) and increases in striatal 3-MT (Racagni et al. 1979; Wood and Richard 1982a). Increased DA release has also been demonstrated in the hamster but not the gerbil (Wood 1983).

The actions of opiates on nigrostriatal DA metabolism are complex in that they involve opioid receptor populations on dopaminergic nerve endings in the striatum (Pollard et al. 1977; Racagni et al. 1979; Wood and Richard 1982a), on cell bodies in the SN (Llorens-Cortes et al. 1979), and on the terminals of afferents to the SN (Llorens-Cortes et al. 1979; Gale et al. 1979). In the case of the mouse, where opiates induce striatal DA release, there are apparently none of the opioid receptors present on DA nerve endings in the striatum (Racagni et al. 1979; Wood and Richard 1982a).

As with cholinergic pathways, κ-agonists do not alter nigrostriatal dopamine metabolism or release as assessed by biochemical indices (Wood et al. 1980; Wood 1984). Using striatal dialysis, small decreases in DA release have been observed with parenteral administration of κ-agonists (Di Chiara and Imperato 1988a) and intranigral (pars reticulata) administration of dynorphin A (Reid et al. 1990). However, neither dynorphin (Wood et al. 1987a) nor κ-agonists (Wood et al. 1980; Wood 1983; Beck and Krieglstein 1986) have been shown to alter striatal DOPAC. The physiological significance of the small decreases in striatal DA release after κ-agonists, therefore, remains to be determined.

Agonist/antagonist analgesics are more complicated in that their actions on nigrostriatal DA metabolism are expressed as bell-shaped dose-response

Table 2. Actions of the μ-agonist morphine, the δ-agonist DADLE and the agonist/antagonist butorphanol on striatal DOPAC in rats made tolerant to morphine or butorphanol[a]

Treatment	Naive	Morphine-tolerant	Butorphanol-tolerant
		(DOPAC as % of control)	
Morphine	180	110	168
Butorphanol	165	168	110
DADLE	175	163	139

[a] Wood et al. 1983a.

curves (Wood et al. 1980). This dose-response relationship was shown to be stereospecific and to involve an opioid agonist component at low doses with a further receptor action, at higher doses, reversing the actions of the initial agonist component ("receptor dualism"; Wood et al. 1983b). This inhibitory receptor action remains to be defined as to receptor type but anatomically involves a receptor localization caudal to the striatum since acute transection of the nigrostriatal pathway converts the bell-shaped dose-response curve of agonist/antagonist analgesics into a classical agonist dose-response relationship (Wood et al. 1983b). The agonist portion of the butorphanol dose-response curve is unlikely to involve a μ-receptor since butorphanol still induces DOPAC increases in morphine-tolerant but not in butorphanol-tolerant rats (Wood et al. 1983a). In this experiment the δ-agonist D-Ala2-Leu5-enkephalin (DADLE) still increased striatal DOPAC levels in both morphine- and butorphanol-tolerant rats (Table 2). These data support unique μ- and δ-regulation of nigrostriatal DA neurons and further suggest that butorphanol's actions are independent of both of these receptor types.

Opioid receptor antagonists, such as naloxone, have no effect on DA metabolism, suggesting a lack of tonic opioid transmission on the nigrostrital pathway in vivo (Wood et al. 1980). However, studies with enkephalinase inhibitors have clearly demonstrated increased DA synthesis (Llorens-Cortes and Schwartz 1984), DA metabolism (Wood 1982), and DA release (Dourmap et al. 1990) in the striatum after inhibition of this enzyme, which degrades endogenous enkephalins. These data therefore suggest a phasic modulation of DA transmission by endogenous enkephalinergic pathways (Wood 1982).

The μ-receptor regulating DA metabolism in the nigrostriatal pathway has been tentatively classified as μ-2, based upon lack of reversal by the μ-1-antagonist naloxonazine (Wood and Pasternak 1983) and reversal of μ effects by κ-agonists at μ-2-antagonist doses (Wood et al. 1982, 1983a; Wood 1984).

Table 3. Regional effects of the μ-agonist morphine and the agonist/antagonist butorphanol on DOPAC and 3-MT levels in the rat[a]

Brain region	Morphine		Butorphanol	
	DOPAC	3-MT	DOPAC	3-MT
Striatum	↑	↔	↑	↔
Nucleus accumbens	↑	↑	↑	↑
Olfactory tubercle	↑	↑	↔	↔
Entorhinal cortex	↔	↔	↔	↔
Prefrontal cortex	↑	↑	↔	↔
Pyriform cortex	↑	↑	↔	↔
Cingulate cortex	↑	↑	↔	↔

[a] Westerink 1978; Wood et al. 1980; Iyengar et al. 1987a,b; Wood and Rao 1991.

III. Mesolimbic Pathways

The mesolimbic DA projections from the ventral tegmental area (VTA) to the septum are only modestly modified by high doses of the μ-agonist morphine (Wood 1983) and the enkephalin analog, D-Ala$_2$-Leu$_5$-enkephalinamide (Collu et al. 1980). In contrast, the DA projections from the VTA to the nucleus accumbens are potently modulated by opiates and opioid peptides. These actions of μ- and δ-opioid receptor agonists include increased DA synthesis as monitored by precursor labeling (Carenzi et al. 1975), increased DA metabolism as reflected by increases in DOPAC (Wood 1983), and increased DA release as reflected by increased 3-MT levels (Wood 1983; Wood and Rao 1991), increased 3-MT accumulation after inhibition of monoamine oxidase (Westerink 1978; Wood and Rao 1991), and increased DA in nucleus accumbens dialysates (Di Chiara and Imperato 1988a). The agonist/antagonist butorphanol has also been shown to increase both DA metabolism and release in the rat nucleus accumbens (Table 3) with a typical agonist dose-response curve rather than the bell-shaped dose-response relationship which characterizes the actions of butorphanol in the striatum (Iyengar et al. 1987a).

The actions of β-endorphin on DA metabolism in the nucleus accumbens have also been studied as a result of the β-endorphin innervation of this nucleus (Bloom et al. 1978; Watson et al. 1979) and possible ε-receptors in this region (Akil et al. 1980). Using rats made tolerant to β-endorphin and rats made tolerant to a combination of morphine and DADLE (Table 4), a significant reduction but not an elimination of the effects of β-endorphin was observed (Iyengar et al. 1989). These data suggest that a component of β-endorphin's actions may be independent of μ- and δ-receptors. This conclusion has not been supported by the complete blockade of β-endorphin

Table 4. Actions of morphine, DADLE, and β-endorphin on rat nucleus accumbens DOPAC levels in rats made tolerant to β-endorphin or to a combination of morphine and DADLE[a]

Treatment	Naive	β-endorphin tolerant	Morphine/DADLE tolerant
		(DOPAC as % of control)	
Morphine	166	165	117
β-endorphin	176	138	273
DADLE	168	184	119

[a] IYENGAR et al. 1989.

actions by the potent μ-antagonist D-Pen-Cys-Tyr-D-Trp-Orn-Thr-Pen-Thr-NH$_2$ (SPANAGEL et al. 1990). However, in lieu of a definitive ε-receptor-binding assay, we do not know the affinity of this antagonist for ε-receptors.

It is this opioid receptor augmentation of meso-accumbens DA release which may play a key role in the reward-reinforcing properties of opiates and a number of other drugs which activate this pathway (BOZARTH and WISE 1981, 1984; DI CHIARA and IMPERATO 1988b). In contrast, κ-opiates, which are not reinforcing, decrease DA release in the nucleus accumbens (DI CHIARA and IMPERATO 1988a), an observation supported by κ-dependent decreases in 3-MT in this nucleus (unpublished observations).

In studies of opiate effects on DA metabolism in the olfactory tubercle, μ- and δ-agonists were observed to increase DOPAC levels in a naloxone-reversible manner (IYENGAR et al. 1987b; see also Chap. 56 in part II of this volume). Morphine has also been demonstrated to increase 3-MT accumulation after inhibition of monoamine oxidase, indicating enhanced DA release (WESTERINK 1978). In this pathway, the κ-agonists, MR-2034 and U50488H also increased DOPAC while the κ-agonists tifluadom and ethylketazocine did not; the agonist/antagonist butorphanol was also ineffective in increasing DOPAC in the olfactory tubercle (IYENGAR et al. 1987a). While the actions of U50488H and MR2034 were reversed by naloxone they were not reversed by quadazocine (WOOD et al. 1984b). In toto, these data lead to the suggestion of possible κ-receptor subtypes (IYENGAR et al. 1987b; WOOD and IYENGAR 1986).

IV. Mesocortical Pathways

The VTA also possesses widespread but more disperse projections to different regions of the cerebral cortex. In a regional analysis of the effects of morphine on these projections, both increased DA metabolism (KIM et al. 1986a,b) and increased DA release as assessed by increased 3-MT levels and increased 3-MT accumulation after inhibition of monoamine oxidase (WOOD and RAO 1991) were monitored in the cingulate, pyriform, and prefrontal cortices. No changes in these parameters were detected in the entorhinal cortex. These data indicate that opiates and opioid peptides can also alter cortical function by activation of ascending dopaminergic projections.

The agonist/antagonist butorphanol, in contrast to its augmentation of DA metabolism in the striatum and nucleus accumbens, does not alter DA metabolism in the cingulate, pyriform, prefrontal, or entorhinal cortices (IYENGAR et al. 1987). These data further support a unique receptor action for butorphanol in the striatum, independent of μ- or δ-receptors.

D. GABAergic Pathways

The analysis of drug effects on GABA turnover in the brain has offered a number of technical limitations in that the direct precursor, glutamate, is also contained in neurotransmitter and metabolic pools (WOOD et al. 1988). The approaches which have been most successively utilized include monitoring GABA accumulation after inhibition of GABA transaminase and monitoring the incorporation of precursor label into GABA (reviewed in WOOD and CHENEY 1985). The former method suffers from the limitations of the pharmacological effects of the GABA transaminase inhibitor itself while the precursor approach suffers from the lack of clear definition of the glutamate precursor pool for GABA. This latter problem has been corrected to some extent by making no assumptions about the glutamate precursor pool and using label incorporated into CNS glucose as a reference precursor pool (WOOD et al. 1988).

Using the precursor labeling approach, subcutaneous morphine and intraventricular (i.v.t.) β-endorphin have been shown to decrease the turnover of GABA in the interneuronal pool of the nucleus caudatus (MORONI et al. 1978) while increasing GABA turnover in the GABAergic projections from the caudate to the globus pallidus (MORONI et al. 1978, 1979). These actions were reproduced by intracaudatal drug administration, supporting a locus of action in the nucleus caudatus (MORONI et al. 1979). Parenteral morphine and i.v.t. β-endorphin increased GABA turnover in the substantia nigra, actions not reproduced by intracaudatal drug injections, further suggesting a nigral site of drug action (MORONI et al. 1978, 1979; WENZEL and KUSCHINSKY 1990). Similarly, morphine has been shown to increase GABA turnover in the GABAergic neurons projecting from the substantia nigra, pars reticularis, to the superior colliculus (WOOD and COSI 1987). In marked contrast, the κ-agonist U50488H decreased GABAergic turnover in the superior colliculus (WOOD and COSI 1987). These actions were all naloxone reversible (Table 5) but need more in-depth pharmacological analysis.

Within the nucleus accumbens, morphine also augments GABA turnover (WENZEL and KUSCHINSKY 1990).

Table 5. Actions of opiates on GABA turnover in rat brain regions[a]

Region	Drug (mg/kg)	GABA turnover (% control)
Caudate	Morphine (10)	64
	(20)	59
	(40)	38
Globus pallidus	Morphine (10)	164
	(20)	150
	(40)	307
Substantia nigra	Morphine (10)	179
	(20)	215
	(40)	263
Superior colliculus	Morphine (8)	148
	U50488H (4)	89
	(12)	73
	(24)	75
	Naloxone (2)	100
	U (12) + N (2)	96

[a] Moroni et al. 1978; Wood et al. 1987a.

E. Striatal Opioid Peptide Gene Expression

I. Introduction

The neurochemical analysis of pharmacological effects on central neuropeptide pathways, such as enkephalinergic neurons, possesses some similarities to the investigation of monoamine pathways (Fig. 2) (see also Chap. 24). However, while degradation products may be useful as indices of peptide release, for example, Tyr-Gly-Gly, as an index of enkephalin release (Fig. 2; Llorens-Cortes et al. 1990; Houdi and Van Loon 1990), the analysis of peptide synthesis is more complicated. Initial efforts of precursor labeling of enkephalin proved fruitless as a result of the slow turnover rates of these peptide pools. A more productive approach resulted from the measurement of chronic rather than acute drug effects on steady-state enkephalin levels (Hong et al. 1978) and the quantitation of pre-proenkephalin mRNA (Schwartz and Costa 1986; Höllt 1986). These approaches have been expanded to a large number of other CNS peptides and have yielded valuable information on neuropeptide dynamics and alterations in these dynamics after drug treatments.

II. Met-Enkephalin

The striatum contains both enkephalinergic interneurons and projection neurons to the globus pallidus. Early studies of Met-enkephalin levels

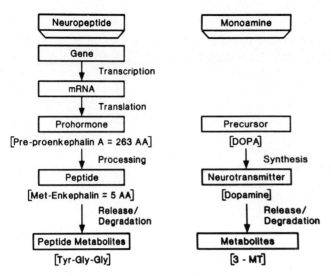

Fig. 2. Comparison of the biosynthetic and degradative steps for CNS monoamines and neuropeptides which can be assessed neurochemically

(Hong et al. 1978) and preproenkephalin mRNA (Mocchetti et al. 1985; Schwartz and Costa 1986) after chronic haloperidol treatment demonstrated that chronic DA receptor blockade enhanced enkephalin biosynthesis in the striatum. Similar results were obtained with depot neuroleptic preparations (Petrack et al. 1990) and with 6-hydroxydopamine lesions of the nigrostriatal dopaminergic pathway (Thal et al. 1983; Li et al. 1990). These increases in striatal Met-enkephalin levels and preproenkephalin mRNA occur with both classical (e.g., haloperidol) and atypical (e.g., clozapine) neuroleptics (Angulo et al. 1990). The increases in Met-enkephalin levels, with chronic neuroleptics, are also paralleled by increases in larger molecular weight precursor forms of Met-enkephalin ("cryptic enkephalin"; Mocchetti et al. 1985; Houdi and Van Loon 1990) and by increased Met-enkephalin release as reflected by increases in the synaptically formed metabolite Tyr-Gly-Gly (Houdi and Van Loon 1990).

Studies with selective D-1- and D-2-receptor antagonists have indicated that the effects of chronic neuroleptic treatment on striatal preproenkephalin mRNA levels are D-1-receptor mediated (Jiang et al. 1990). These studies are all consistent with a tonic inhibitory tone exerted on striatal enkephalinergic neurons by the nigrostriatal dopaminergic pathway.

In contrast, proenkephalin gene expression is tonically augmented by the corticostriatal glutamatergic pathway as evidenced by decreased preproenkephalin mRNA in the striata of decorticate rats (Uhl et al. 1988b). The effects of excitatory amino acid receptor antagonists remain to be tested in this paradigm.

The striatum is also rich in GABAergic interneurons. Potentiation of these neurons with benzodiazepines, GABA transaminase inhibition, and GABA-A agonists results in rapid decreases in striatal Tyr-Gly-Gly, indicating acute decreases in Met-enkephalin release (Llorens-Cortes et al. 1990). These decreases in enkephalin release are temporally followed by decreases in Met-enkephalin levels and preproenkephalin mRNA (Duka et al. 1980; Sivam and Hong 1986; Llorens-Cortes et al. 1990). After chronic treatment (>8 days) both Met-enkephalin and preproenkephalin mRNA are increased (Wuster et al. 1980; Sivam and Hong 1986). These data indicate that acute GABAergic actions lead to decreased enkephalin release and a depression of preproenkephalin gene expression; actions which under chronic conditions adapt as reflected by an augmented expression of preproenkephalin mRNA.

Pharmacological alterations of opioid transmission in the striatum also result in altered enkephalin synthesis in this brain region. Chronic morphine treatment results in decreased preproenkephalin mRNA but no change in Met-enkephalin steady-state levels (Uhl et al. 1988a). For the mirror image, injection of an irreversible opiate antagonist into the striatum (Morris et al. 1988b) or chronic treatment with parenteral naltrexone (Tempel et al. 1990) results in increased Met-enkephalin and preproenkepkalin mRNA levels. These data argue for either feedback changes or an autoregulation of enkephalinergic neurons in the striatum, mediated by μ-receptors.

III. Dynorphin

The dynorphin peptides are contained within striatal neurons which form a feedback pathway to the SN (Vincent et al. 1982) and thereby act to modulate the output of nigral pars reticulta neurons. These striatal projection neurons have been shown to be tonically potentiated by inputs from the dorsal raphe (Morris et al. 1988a). The effects of selective 5-HT receptor antagonists on gene expression in these neurons remain to be investigated.

Similarly, striatal dynorphin-containing neurons appear to be tonically activated by nigrostriatal dopaminergic input since dynorphin and preprodynorphin mRNA are both decreased by 6-hydroxydopamine lesions of this pathway (Li et al. 1990). In this regard, apomorphine (Jiang et al. 1990) and methamphetamine (Hanson et al. 1987) increase dynorphin levels in the striatum; actions which are reversed by D-1- but not D-2-receptor blockade. These data argue for a tonic activation of striatal dynorphin-containing neurons by dopaminergic nigrostriatal neurons impinging on neurons with D-1 receptors.

F. Conclusions

Opioid neurons and their target populations are widespread in the CNS. This anatomical complexity is further elaborated by the three major opioid peptide genes, the multiple opioid peptide products and the multiple opioid receptor systems described for the CNS. Unraveling the physiological significance of these fascinating peptides is therefore extremely complex. However, as described in this chapter, via studying the reciprocal interactions of defined dopaminergic, cholinergic, and GABAergic pathways with opioid neurons, we are establishing a data base of neurochemical data which will help to define the role(s) of different CNS pathways in complex behaviors (Wood and Iyengar 1988; Iyengar and Wood 1989).

References

Ahtee L, Kaariainen I (1973) The effect of narcotic analgesics on the homovanillic acid content of rat nucleus caudatus. Eur J Pharmacol 22:206–208

Akil H, Hewlett WA, Barchas JD, Li CH (1980) Binding of ^{3}H-β-endorphin to rat brain membranes: characterization of opiate receptors and interaction with ACTH. Eur J Pharmacol 64:1–8

Algeri S, Brunello N, Calderini A, Consolazione A (1978) Effect of enkephalins on catecholamine metabolism in rat CNS. Adv Biochem Psychopharmacol 18: 199–210

Angulo JA, Cadet JL, Woolley CS, Suber F, McEwen BS (1990) Effect of chronic typical and atypical neuroleptic treatment on proenkephalin mRNA levels in the striatum and nucleus accumbens of the rat. J Neurochem 54:1889–1894

Beck T, Krieglstein J (1986) The effects of tifluadom and ketazocine on behavior, dopamine turnover in the basal ganglia and local cerebral glucose utilization of rats. Brain Res 381:327–335

Biggio G, Casu M, Corda MG, Di Bello C, Gessa GL (1978) Stimulation of dopamine synthesis in caudate nucleus by intrastriatal enkephalins and antagonism by naloxone. Science 200:552–554

Bloom FE, Rossier J, Batenberg ELF, Bayon A, French E, Hendrickson SJ, Siggins GR, Segal D, Browne R, Ling N, Guillemin R (1978) Beta endorphin: cellular localization, electrophysiological and behavioral effects. Adv Biochem Psychopharmacol 18:89–109

Bozarth MA, Wise RA (1981) Intracranial self-administration of morphine into the ventral tegmental area in rats. Life Sci 28:551–555

Bozarth MA, Wise RA (1984) Anatomically distinct opiate receptor fields mediate reward and physical dependence. Science 244:516–517

Carenzi A, Cheney DL, Costa E, Guidotti A, Racagni G (1975) Actions of opiates, antipsychotics, amphetamine and apomorphine on dopamine receptors in rat striatum: in vivo changes of 3′,5′-cyclic AMP content and acetylcholine turnover rate. Neuropharmacology 14:927–939

Cheney DL, Trabucchi M, Racagni G, Wang C, Costa E (1974) Effects of acute and chronic morphine on regional rat brain acetylcholine turnover rate. Life Sci 15:1977

Cheney DL, Trabucchi M, Racagni G, Wang C, Costa E (1975) An analysis at the synaptic level of the morphine action in striatum and N. accumbens, dopamine and acetylcholine interaction. Life Sci 17:1–8

Cheney DL, Lehmann J, Cosi C, Wood PL (1989) Determination of acetylcholine dynamics. Neuromethods 12:443–495

Collu RE, Stefanini E, Vernaleone F, Marchisio AM, Devoto P, Argiolas A (1980) Biochemical characterization of the dopaminergic innervation of the rat septum. Life Sci 26:1665–1673

Costa E, Panula P, Thompson HK, Cheney DL (1983) The transsynaptic regulation of the septal-hippocampal cholinergic neurons. Life Sci 32:165–179

Di Chiara G, Imperato A (1988a) Opposite effects of mu and kappa opiate agonists on dopamine release in the nucleus accumbens and in the dorsal caudate of freely moving rats. J Pharmacol Exp Ther 244:1067–1080

Di Chiara G, Imperato A (1988b) Drugs abused by humans preferentially increase synaptic dopamine concentrations in the mesolimbic system of freely moving rats. Proc Natl Acad Sci USA 85:5274–5278

Dourmap N, Michael-Titus A, Costentin J (1990) Local enkephalins tonically modulate dopamine release in the striatum: a microdialysis study. Brain Res 524:153–155

Duka T, Wuster M, Herz A (1980) Benzodiazepines modulate striatal enkephalin levels via a GABergic mechanism. Life Sci 26:771–776

Gale K, Moroni F, Kumakura K, Guidotti A (1979) Opiate receptors in substantia nigra: role in the regulation of striatal tyrosine hydroxylase. Neuropharmacology 18:427–430

Groppetti A, Algeri S, Cattabeni F, DiGiulio AM, Galli CL, Ponzio F, Spano PF (1977) Changes in specific activity of dopamine metabolites as evidence of a multiple compartmentation of dopamine in striatal neurons. J Neurochem 28: 193–197

Hanson GR, Merchant KM, Letter AA, Bush L, Gibb JW (1987) Methamphetamine-induced changes in the striatal-nigral dynorphin system: role of D-1 and D-2 receptors. Eur J Pharmacol 144:245–246

Höllt V (1986) Opioid peptide processing and receptor selectivity. Annu Rev Pharmacol Toxicol 26:59–72

Hong JS, Yang H-YT, Fratta W, Costa E (1978) Rat striatal methionine-enkephalin content after chronic treatment with cataleptogenic and noncataleptogenic antischizophrenic drugs. J Pharmacol Exp Ther 205:141–147

Houdi AA, Van Loon GR (1990) Haloperidol-induced increase in striatal concentration of the tripeptide, Tyr-Gly-Gly, provides an index of increased enkephalin release in vivo. J Neurochem 54:1360–1366

Iyengar S, Wood PL (1989) Multiplicity and classification of opioid receptors. In: Szekely JI, Ramabadran K (eds) Opioid peptides, vol 4. CRC Press, Boca Raton, pp 115–132

Iyengar S, Kim HS, Wood PL (1987a) Agonist action of the agonist/antagonist analgesic butorphanol on dopamine metabolism in the nucleus accumbens of the rat. Neurosci Lett 77:226–230

Iyengar S, Kim HS, Wood PL (1987b) Effects of kappa opiate agonists on neurochemical and neuroendocrine indices: evidence for kappa receptor subtypes. Life Sci 39:637–644

Iyengar S, Kim HS, Marien M, McHugh D, Wood PL (1989) Modulation of mesolimbic dopaminergic projections by β-endorphin in the rat. Neuropharmacology 28:123–128

Jhamandas K, Sutak M (1976) Morphine-naloxone interaction in the central cholinergic system: the influence of subcortical lesioning and electrical stimulation. Br J Pharmacol 58:101–107

Jhamandas K, Hron V, Sutak M (1975) Comparative effects of opiate agonists methadone, levorphanol and their isomers on the release of cortical ACH in vivo and in vitro. Can J Physiol Pharmacol 50:57–62

Jiang H-K, McGinty JF, Hong JS (1990) Differential modulation of striatonigral dynorphin and enkephalin by dopamine receptor subtypes. Brain Res 507:57–64

Kim HS, Iyengar S, Wood PL (1986a) Opiate actions of mesocortical dopamine metabolism in the rat. Life Sci 39:2033–2036

Kim HS, Iyengar S, Wood PL (1986b) Reversal of the actions of morphine on mesocortical dopamine metabolism in the rat by the kappa agonist MR-2034:

tentative mu-2 opioid control of mesocortical dopaminergic projections. Life Sci 41:1711–1715

Kuschinsky K, Hornykiewicz O (1974) Effects of morphine on striatal dopamine metabolism: possible mechanism of its opposite effect on locomotor activity in rats and mice. Eur J Pharmacol 26:41–50

Li SJ, Jiang HK, Stachowiak MS, Hudson PM, Owyang V, Nanry K, Tilson HA, Hong JS (1990) Influence of nigrostriatal dopaminergic tone on the biosynthesis of dynorphin and enkephalin in rat striatum. Mol Brain Res 8:219–225

Llorens-Cortes C, Pollard H, Schwartz JC (1979) Localization of opiate receptors in substantia nigra evidence by lesion studies. Neurosci Lett 12:165–170

Llorens-Cortes C, Schwartz J-C (1984) Changes in turnover of cerebral monoamines following inhibition of enkephalin metabolism by thiorphan and bestatin. Eur J Pharmacol 104:369–374

Llorens-Cortes C, Van Amsterdam JGC, Giros B, Quach TT, Schwartz JC (1990) Enkephalin biosynthesis and release in mouse striatum are inhibited by GABA receptor stimulation: compared changes in preproenkephalin mRNA and Tyr-Gly-Gly levels. Mol Brain Res 8:227–233

Martin WR (1967) Opioid antagonists. Pharmacol Rev 19:463–521

Mocchetti I, Schwartz JP, Costa E (1985) Use of mRNA hybridization and radio-immunoassay to study mechanisms of drug-induced accumulation of enkephalins in rat brain structures. Mol Pharmacol 28:86–91

Moroni F, Cheney DL, Costa E (1977) Inhibition of acetylcholine turnover in rat hippocampus by intraseptal injections of β-endorphin and morphine. Naunyn Schmiedebergs Arch Exp Pharmacol 299:149–153

Moroni F, Cheney DL, Peralta E, Costa E (1978) Opiate receptor agonists as modulators of gamma-aminobutyric acid turnover in the nucleus caudatus, globus pallidus and substantia nigra of the rat. J Pharmacol Exp Ther 207:870–877

Moroni F, Peralta E, Cheney DL, Costa E (1979) On the regulation of gamma-aminobutyric acid neurons in caudatus, pallidus and nigra: effects of opioids and dopamine agonists. J Pharmacol Exp Ther 208:190–194

Morris BJ, Reimer S, Hollt V, Herz A (1988a) Regulation of striatal prodynorphin mRNA levels by the raphe-striatal pathway. Mol Brain Res 4:15–22

Morris BJ, Hollt V, Herz A (1988b) Opioid gene expression in rat striatum is modulated via opioid receptors: evidence from localized receptor inactivation. Neurosci Lett 89:80–84

Pasternak GW, Wood PL (1986) Minireview: multiple mu opioid receptors. Life Sci 38:1889–1898

Pepeu G (1973) The release of acetylcholine from the brain: an approach to the study of the central cholinergic mechanisms. Prog Neurobiol 2:259–288

Petrack B, Emmett MR, Rao JT, Kim HS, Wood PL (1990) Increases in rat striatal preproenkephalin mRNA levels following chronic treatment with the depot neuroleptic, haloperidol decanoate. Life Sci 46:687–691

Pollard H, Llorens C, Bonnet JJ, Costentin J, Schwartz JC (1977) Opiate receptors on mesolimbic dopaminergic neurons. Neurosci Lett 7:295–299

Racagni C, Bruno F, Iuliano E, Paoletti R (1979) Differential sensitivity to behavioral and biochemical correlations. J Pharmacol Exp Ther 209:111–116

Rackham A, Wood PL, Hudgin RL (1982) Kyotorphan (tyrosine- arginine): further evidence for indirect opiate receptor activation. Life Sci 30:1337–1342

Reid MS, O'Connor WT, Herrera-Marschitz M, Ungerstedt U (1990) The effects of intranigral GABA and dynorphin A injections on striatal dopamine and GABA release: evidence that dopamine provides inhibitory regulation of striatal GABA neurons via D2 receptors. Brain Res 519:255–260

Schwartz JP, Costa E (1986) Hybridization approaches to the study of neuropeptides. Annu Rev Neurosci 9:277–304

Sivam SP, Hong JS (1986) GABAergic regulation of enkephalin in rat striatum: alterations in Met5-enkephalin, precursor content and preproenkephalin messenger RNA abundance. J Pharmacol Exp Ther 237:326–331

Smith CB, Sheldon MT, Bednarczyk JH, Villarreal JE (1972) Morphine-induced increases in the incorporation of 14C-tyrosine into 14C-dopamine and 14C-norepinephrine in the mouse brain: antagonism by naloxone and tolerance. J Pharmacol Exp Ther 180:547–557

Spanagel R, Herz A, Shippenberg TS (1990) Identification of the opioid receptor types mediating β-endorphin-induced alterations in dopamine release in the nucleus accumbens. Eur J Pharmacol 190:177–184

Szerb J (1974) Lack of effect of morphine in reducing the release of labelled acetylcholine from brain slices stimulated electrically. Eur J Pharmacol 29:192–194

Tempel A, Kessler JA, Zukin RS (1990) Chronic naltrexone treatment increases expression of preproenkephalin and preprotachykinin mRNA in discrete brain regions. J Neurosci 10:741–747

Thal LJ, Sharpless NS, Hirschhorn ID, Horowitz SG, Makman MH (1983) Striatal met-enkephalin increases following nigrostriatal denervation. Biochem Pharmacol 32:3297–3301

Uhl GR, Ryan JP, Schwartz JP (1988a) Morphine alters preproenkephalin gene expression. Brain Res 100:391–397

Uhl GR, Navia B, Douglas J (1988b) Differential expression of preproenkephalin and preprodynorphin mRNAs in striatal neurons: high levels of preproenkephalin expression depend on cerebral cortical afferents. J Neurosci 8:4755–4764

Vincent S, Hokfelt T, Christensson I, Terenius L (1982) Immunohistochemical evidence for a dynorphin immunoreactive striato-nigral pathway. Eur J Pharmacol 85:251–252

Watson SJ, Barchas JD (1979) Anatomy of the endogenous opioid peptides and related substances: the enkephalins, β-endorphin, β-lipotropin and ACTH. In: Beers RF, Bassett EG (eds) Mechanisms of pain and analgesic compounds. Raven, New York, p 227

Wenzel J, Kuschinsky K (1990) Effects of morphine on gamma-aminobutyric acid turnover in the basal gamglia. Possible correlation with its biphasic action on motility. Arzneimittelforschung 40:811–813

Westerink BHC (1978) Effect of centrally acting drugs on regional dopamine metabolism. Adv Biochem Psychopharmacol 19:255–266

Wood PL (1982) Phasic enkephalinergic modulation of nigrostriatal dopamine metabolism: potentiation with enkephalinase inhibitors. Eur J Pharmacol 82:119–120

Wood PL (1983) Opioid regulation of CNS dopaminergic pathways: a review of methodology, receptor types, regional variations and species differences. Peptides 4:595–601

Wood PL (1984) Kappa agonist analgesics: evidence for mu-2 and delta receptor antagonism. Drug Dev Res 4:429–435

Wood PL (1986) Pharmacological evaluation of GABAergic and glutamatergic inputs to the nucleus basalis – cortical and the septal – hippocampal cholinergic projections. Can J Physiol Pharmacol 64:325–328

Wood PL (1988) The significance of multiple CNS opioid receptor types: a review of critical considerations relating to technical details and anatomy in the study of central opioid actions. Peptides 9:49–55

Wood PL, Altar CA (1988) Dopamine release in vivo from nigrostriatal, mesolimbic, and mesocortical neurons: utility of 3-methoxytyramine measurements. Pharmacol Rev 40:163–187

Wood PL, Cheney DL (1985) Gas chromatography-mass fragmentography of amino acids. Neuromethods 3:51–80

Wood PL, Cosi C (1987) Kappa receptor modulation of the nigrocollicular GABA pathway in the rat. Soc Neurosci Abstr 13:402.10

Wood PL, Iyengar S (1986) Kappa isoreceptors: neurochemical and neuroendocrine evidence. NIDA Monogr 71:102–108

Wood PL, Iyengar S (1988) Central actions of opiates and opioid peptides: in vivo evidence for opioid receptor multiplicity. In: Pasternak GW (ed) The opiate receptors. Humana Press, Clifton, pp 307–356

Wood PL, McQuade P (1986) Substantia innominata cortical cholinergic pathway: regulatory afferents. Adv Behav Biol 30:999–1006

Wood PL, Pasternak GW (1983) Specific mu-2 opioid iso-receptor regulation of nigrostriatal neurons: in vivo evidence with naloxonazine. Neurosci Lett 37: 291–293

Wood PL, Rackham A (1981) Actions of kappa, sigma and partial mu narcotic receptor agonists on rat brain acetylcholine turnover. Neurosci Lett 23:75–80

Wood PL, Rao TS (1991) Morphine stimulation of mesolimbic and mesocortical but not nigrostriatal dopamine release in the rat as reflected by changes in 3-methoxytyramine levels. Neuropharmacology 30:399–401

Wood PL, Richard JW (1982a) Morphine and nigrostriatal function in the rat and mouse: the role of nigral and striatal opiate receptors. Neuropharmacology 21:1305–1310

Wood PL, Richard J (1982b) GABAergic regulation of the substantia innominata-cortical cholinergic pathway. Neuropharmacology 21:969–972

Wood PL, Stotland LM (1980) Actions of enkephalin, mu and partial agonist analgesics on acetylcholine turnover in rat brain. Neuropharmacology 19: 975–982

Wood PL, Cheney DL, Costa E (1979) An investigation of whether septal β-aminobutyrate-containing interneurons are involved in the reduction of the turnover rate of acetylcholine elicited by substance P and β-endorphin in the hippocampus. Neuroscience 4:1479–1484

Wood PL, Sotland M, Richard JW, Rackham A (1980) Actions of mu, kappa, sigma, delta, and agonist/antagonist opiates on striatal dopaminergic function. J Pharmacol Exp Ther 215:697–703

Wood PL, Richard JW, Thakur M (1982) Mu opiate isoreceptors: differentiation with kappa agonists. Life Sci 31:2313–2317

Wood PL, Sanschagrin D, Richard JW, Thakur M (1983a) Multiple receptor affinities of kappa and agonist/antagonist analgesics: in vivo assessment. J Pharmacol Exp Ther 226:545–550

Wood PL, McQuade P, Richard JW, Thakur M (1983b) Agonist/antagonist analgesics and nigrostriatal dopamine metabolism in the rat: evidence for receptor dualism. Life Sci 33:759–762

Wood PL, Stotland LM, Racham A (1984a) Opiate receptor regulation of acetylcholine metabolism: role of mu, delta, kappa and sigma receptors. In: Hanin I (ed) Dynamics of neurotransmitter function. Raven, New York, pp 99–107

Wood PL, Pilapil C, Thakur M, Richard JW (1984b) WIN 44,441: a stereospecific and long-acting narcotic antagonist. Pharm Res 1:46–48

Wood PL, McQuade PS, Nair NPV (1984c) GABAergic and opioid regulation of the substantia innominata-cortical cholinergic pathway in the rat. Prog Neuro-psychopharmacol Biol Psychiatry 8:789–792

Wood PL, Kim HS, Cosi C, Iyengar S (1987a) The endogenous kappa agonist, dynorphin (1–13), does not alter basal or morphine-stimulated dopamine metabolism in the nigrostriatal pathway of the rat. Neuropharmacology 26: 1585–1588

Wood PL, Kim HS, Altar CA (1987b) In vivo assessment of dopamine and norepinephrine release in rat neocortex: GC-MF measurement of 3-methoxytyramine (3-MT) and normetanephrine (NMN). J Neurochem 48: 574–579

Wood PL, Kim HS, Marien MR (1987c) Intracerebral dialysis: direct evidence for the utility of 3-MT measurements as an index of dopamine release. Life Sci 41:1–5

Wood PL, Kim HS, Cheney DL, Cosi C, Marien M, Rao TS, Martin LL (1988) Constant infusion of [$^{13}C_6$]glucose: simultaneous measurement of GABA and glutamate turnover in defined rat brain regions of single animals. Neuropharmacology 27:669–676

Wüster M, Duka T, Herz A (1980) Diazepam effects on striatal Met-enkephalin levels following long-term pharmacological manipulations. Neuropharmacology 19:501–505

Yonehara N, Clouet DH (1984) Effects of delta and mu opiopeptides on the turnover and release of dopamine in rat striatum. J Pharmacol Exp Ther 231:38–42

Zsilla G, Cheney DL, Racagni G, Costa E (1976) Correlation between analgesia and the decrease of acetylcholine turover rate in cortex and hippocampus elicited by morphine, meperidine, viminol R2 and azidomorphine. J Pharmacol Exp Ther 199:662–668

CHAPTER 26

Selectivity of Ligands for Opioid Receptors

A.D. CORBETT, S.J. PATERSON, and H.W. KOSTERLITZ

A. Introduction

Since the discovery of the endogenous opioid peptides (HUGHES et al. 1975b), our understanding of the mode of action of opioids has advanced rapidly. It is now known that in mammals the opioid peptides are derived from three precursor molecules, proopiomelanocortin (MAINS et al. 1977; ROBERTS and HERBERT 1977a,b; NAKANISHI et al. 1979), proenkephalin (NODA et al. 1982; GUBLER et al. 1982), and prodynorphin (KAKIDANI et al. 1982; FISCHLI et al. 1982; KILPATRICK et al. 1982). Furthermore, the endogenous opioid peptides interact with three well-defined types of receptor, μ, δ, and κ (see PATERSON et al. 1984).

Notwithstanding the progress in this field, there remain many unsolved problems regarding the physiology and pharmacology of opioids. One of the major barriers to the furtherance of opioid research has been the lack of suitable nonendogenous ligands, particularly antagonists. Such compounds must have high affinity and selectivity for one receptor type and also be resistant to peptidases. The endogenous opioid peptides do not fulfil these criteria since they lack the necessary selectivity (Sect. C) and most are susceptible to breakdown by tissue peptidases (HAMBROOK et al. 1976; McKNIGHT et al. 1983); there are no endogenous antagonists. Consequently, many attempts have been made to develop suitable ligands, both peptides and nonpeptides. It is only now that selective compounds are becoming readily available.

In this chapter we have reviewed the selectivities and affinities of available opioid ligands at μ-, δ-, and κ-opioid-receptors. We have emphasized those highly selective ligands which are available but have also drawn attention to commonly used opioids which do not have the necessary selectivity.

B. Methods Used to Determine the Selectivity of Opioid Compounds

A great variety of in vivo and in vitro methods have been used in the investigation of the actions of opioid ligands and the receptors with which they interact (see also Chaps. 1 and 4). Two in vitro techniques have proven to be of particular value in determining the receptor selectivity of opioids: radioreceptor binding assays in membrane fragments and bioassays in isolated intact tissues. A receptor consists of a recognition site to which a drug binds and the transduction mechanisms which lead to a biological response. Binding assays provide information about the recognition site of a receptor; they can be used to determine the degree of selectivity of an opioid for the different opioid binding sites. Since binding assays do not distinguish between the agonist or antagonist nature of the ligand-receptor interaction, it is necessary to correlate the results obtained in binding assays with those obtained in bioassays. The importance of this approach is emphasized by the findings that a ligand, such as bremazocine, may be an agonist at one type of opioid receptor (κ) and an antagonist at other types (μ and δ) (Sect. D.III.2).

I. Radioreceptor Binding Assays

The characterization of binding sites is usually approached in one of two ways. In the first, the equilibrium dissociation constant (K_D) and the maximum number of binding sites are estimated from saturation experiments. In the second approach, the binding characteristics of unlabeled ligands are determined by their competitive displacement of labeled compounds of known binding characteristics. The theoretical and practical problems associated with the investigation of opioid binding have recently been reviewed by LESLIE (1987).

In this review the selectivities of opioid compounds are expressed as their relative affinities for the three opioid binding sites (PATERSON et al. 1984; KOSTERLITZ 1985). The inhibitory binding constant (K_i) is calculated from the IC$_{50}$ value using the equation $K_i = \text{IC}_{50}/(1 + [L]/K_D)$, where $[L]$ is the concentration of the tritiated ligand and K_D its equilibrium dissociation constant (CHENG and PRUSOFF 1973). If the compound interacts with two binding sites, its selectivity may be expressed as the ratio of the two K_i values. However, if the compound interacts with three or more sites it is more difficult to define selectivity. Since the affinity constant is the reciprocal of the inhibitory binding constant, the selectivity of a compound can be obtained by comparing its affinity at the different binding sites. With opioids, the relative affinities at the three binding sites have been calculated by use of the equation K_i^{-1} at μ, δ, or $\kappa/(K_i^{-1}$ at μ + K_i^{-1} at δ + K_i^{-1} at κ). Although the derived value for the relative affinity has no tangible meaning, since mathematically one cannot add affinities, this representation provides a means of comparing the selectivity of compounds, independent of their affinities. If a compound interacts with only one of the three opioid binding sites, it will have a relative affinity of 1 at that binding site whereas a compound which interacts equally with the three sites will have a relative affinity of 0.33 at each site. The potency of the compound is indicated by the inclusion of its affinity at the preferred site. An alternative method for displaying the selectivity of compounds is to convert the K_i values into pK_i values (log K_i) which are displayed graphically (GOLDSTEIN 1987; GOLDSTEIN and NAIDU 1989). In this representation, the degree of selectivity is proportional to the difference in the pK_i values. Although both methods impart the same information, we feel that the use of relative affinities give a more immediate, if less mathematically rigorous, appreciation of the data.

A selective compound is one which interacts with only one type of binding site under all assay conditions, i.e., has a relative binding affinity of 1. In the absence of such ligands, a compound which in binding assays is at least 100 times more active at its preferred site than at other opioid binding sites may, for practical purposes, be considered to be selective; such a ligand would have a relative affinity >0.98. A compound with lower relative affinities may display a preference for one of the sites but would not be selective.

It is impossible to compare directly binding data obtained in different laboratories because of the variability of the experimental conditions. In this review, the K_i values for a particular compound at μ-, δ-, and κ-sites are those determined in a single laboratory with one species. Where ligands have been investigated in more than one laboratory, the K_i values cited here represent values obtained by the use of the most selective labeling techniques. In most cases the assays have been performed at 25° or 37°C but in a few instances the assays were carried out at 0°C to minimize degradation of peptide opioids.

With the development of the highly selective ligands outlined in this chapter, it has now become possible to label selectively each of the μ-, δ-, and κ-opioid binding sites. The μ-binding sites are labeled with [3H]-[D-Ala^2,MePhe^4,Gly-ol^5]enkephalin (KOSTERLITZ and PATERSON 1981), [3H]-Tyr-Pro-MePhe-D-Pro-NH$_2$ (PL O17; HAWKINS et al. 1987), or [3H]-D-Phe-Cys-Tyr-D-Trp-Orn-Thr-Pen-Thr-NH$_2$ (CTOP; HAWKINS et al. 1989), the δ-binding site with [3H]-[D-Pen^2,D-Pen^5]enkephalin (AKIYAMA et al. 1985; COTTON et al. 1985), [3H]-[D-Ser(O-$tert$-butyl)^2,Leu^5]enkephalyl-Thr (DELAY-GOYET et al. 1988) or [3H]-[D-Pen^2,pClPhe^4,D-Pen^5]enkephalin (VAUGHN et al. 1989), and the κ-sites with [3H]-U-69593 (LAHTI et al. 1985), [3H]-PD117302 (CLARK et al. 1988) or [3H]-CI-977 (BOYLE et al. 1990).

At present there is increasing evidence that there may be subtypes of these three receptors (see Chaps. 4 and 5). However, the possible subtypes are still not well defined in binding assays and so far there is no convincing evidence for receptor subtypes in bioassays.

II. Bioassays

While responses to opioids will have to be tested finally in vivo, the pharmacological effects are often more readily analyzed in excised tissues. Much of our understanding of the heterogeneity of the opioid receptors, even the discovery of the endogenous opioid peptides, is owed to the use of isolated tissue preparations in which neurotransmission is sensitive to inhibition by opioids. In this approach, the relative potencies of opioid agonists are assessed by their ability to inhibit the electrically evoked contractions of isolated tissue preparations from five different species: the contractions of the mouse vas deferens are inhibited by μ-, δ-, and κ-opioid agonists (Hughes et al. 1975a; Hutchinson et al. 1975; Lord et al. 1977; Leslie et al. 1980; Cox and Chavkin 1983), those of the guinea pig myenteric plexus-longitudinal muscle preparation by μ- and κ-agonists (Lord et al. 1977; Leslie et al. 1980; Chavkin et al. 1982), those of the rabbit vas deferens by κ-agonists (Oka et al. 1981), and those of the hamster vas deferens by δ-agonists (McKnight et al. 1984, 1985). The contractions of the rat vas deferens are inhibited mainly, but not exclusively, by μ-agonists (Lemaire et al. 1978; Gillan et al. 1981; Liao et al. 1981). Although it is still a matter of some controversy, it has been proposed that the actions of β-endorphin in the rat vas deferens are mediated by a fourth type of opioid receptor, termed ε (Schulz et al. 1979, 1981; Wüster et al. 1979).

In the investigation of the receptor selectivity of opioid ligands it is necessary to use, wherever possible, bioassay preparations which contain only one type of opioid receptor. Of the bioassay preparations used routinely, the hamster vas deferens and the rabbit vas deferens contain a homogeneous population of opioid receptors. An alternative to the use of selective tissues is the irreversible blockade of a single receptor type. The opioid receptor alkylating agent β-funaltrexamine has been used to block irreversibly μ-opioid receptors in the guinea pig myenteric plexus preparation, giving rise to a tissue containing almost exclusively κ-receptors (Portoghese et al. 1980; Corbett et al. 1985b). Furthermore, the nonselective opioid receptor alkylating agent β-chlornaltrexamine was used to block κ-receptors in the guinea pig myenteric plexus preparation when the μ-receptors were protected by a high concentration of a selective μ-ligand (Portoghese et al. 1979; Goldstein and James 1984; Corbett and Kosterlitz 1986; Traynor et al. 1987).

The unequivocal interpretation of results obtained in pharmacological assays on isolated tissues is difficult unless the opioid compound has complete selectivity for one type of receptor. Many opioids interact with more than one receptor type and most of the bioassay preparations contain a heterogeneous population of opioid receptors. Under these circumstances selective antagonists are essential for defining the types of receptor which mediate the inhibitory actions; selective antagonists are considered in Sect. D.

C. Selectivity of Endogenous Opioid Peptides

In mammals, the endogenous opioid peptides are derived from three precursors, proopiomelanocortin, proenkephalin, or prodynorphin, and a

Table 1. Inhibitory effects (K_i, nM) of proenkephalin-derived peptides on binding at μ-, δ-, and κ-binding sites

Peptide	K_i(nM)			Affinity at		Relative affinity at			Reference
	μ-Site	δ-Site	κ-Site	μ-Site $(K_i,nM)^{-1}$	δ-Site $(K_i,nM)^{-1}$	μ-Site	δ-Site	κ-Site	
[Leu⁵]enkephalin	19	1.2	8210		0.83	0.06	0.94	0	[a]
[Met⁵]enkephalin	9.5	0.91	4442		1.1	0.09	0.91	0	[b]
[Met⁵]enkephalyl-Arg-Phe	3.7	9.4	93	0.27		0.70	0.27	0.03	[c]
[Met⁵]enkephalyl-Arg-Gly-Leu	6.6	4.8	79			0.41	0.56	0.03	[c]
Metorphamide	0.12	2.7	0.25	8.3	0.21	0.66	0.03	0.31	[b]
[Met⁵]enkephalyl-Arg-Arg-Val-NH₂									
BAM 12 [Met⁵]enkephalyl-Arg-Arg-Val-Gly-Arg-Pro-Glu	0.16	1.4	0.41	6.3		0.66	0.08	0.26	[d]
BAM 18 [Met⁵]enkephalyl-Arg-Arg-Val-Gly-Arg-Pro-Glu-Trp-Trp-Met-Asp-Tyr-Gln	0.29	3.2	0.75	3.5		0.68	0.08	0.26	[c]
BAM 22 [Met⁵]enkephalyl-Arg-Arg-Val-Gly-Arg-Pro-Glu-Trp-Trp-Met-Asp-Tyr-Gln-Lys-Arg-Tyr-Gly	0.10	0.66	0.17	10		0.57	0.09	0.34	[d]
Peptide E [Met⁵]enkephalyl-Arg-Arg-Val-Gly-Arg-Pro-Glu-Trp-Trp-Met-Asp-Tyr-Gln-Lys-Arg-Tyr-Gly-Gly-Phe-Met	0.53	1.7	1.1	1.9		0.56	0.17	0.27	[d]
Peptide F [Met⁵]enkephalyl-Lys-Lys-Met-Asp-Glu-Leu-Tyr-Pro-Leu-Glu-Val-Glu-Glu-Glu-Ala-Asn-Gly-Gly-Val-Leu-Gly-Lys-Arg-Tyr-Gly-Gly-Phe-Leu	25	29	78	0.04		0.46	0.39	0.15	[d]

The μ-binding sites were labeled with [³H]-[D-Ala²,MePhe⁴,Gly-ol⁵]enkephalin, the δ-sites with [³H]-[D-Ala²,D-Leu⁵]enkephalin [a,b,c,d] or [³H]-[D-Ala²,D-Leu⁵]enkephalin in the presence of unlabeled Tyr-Pro-MePhe-D-Pro-NH₂ (PL O17) [c], and the κ-sites with [³H]-(−)-bremazocine in the presence of unlabeled [D-Ala²,MePhe⁴,Gly-ol⁵]enkephalin and [D-Ala²,D-Leu⁵]enkephalin [a,b,c,d] or [³H]-ethylketazocine in the presence of unlabeled Tyr-Pro-MePhe-D-Pro-NH₂ (PL O17) and [D-Ser²,L-Leu⁵]enkephalyl-Thr [c]. Assays were performed in homogenates of guinea pig brain at 0°C [a,b,c,d] or 22°C [c].
Relative affinity is K_i^{-1} at μ, δ, or κ/(K_i^{-1} at μ + K_i^{-1} at δ + K_i^{-1} at κ) and was calculated from the data shown.
[a] CORBETT et al. (1982); [b] WEBER et al. (1983); [c] KOSTERLITZ and PATERSON (1985); [d] PATERSON (1986); [e] HURLBUT et al. (1987).

selection has been made of peptides which may be physiologically important. We have also included the two families of opioid peptides found in amphibian skin, dermorphin and the deltorphins, which are unique among peptides synthesized by animal cells in that they contain a D-amino acid (AMICHE et al. 1988, 1989; LAZARUS et al. 1989; KREIL et al. 1989; ERSPAMER et al. 1989).

I. Proenkephalin-Derived Peptides

1. Activity in Binding Assays

The endogenous opioid peptides derived from proenkephalin display marked differences in their relative affinities for the μ-, δ-, and κ-binding sites; none of the ligands has a relative binding affinity which approaches unity at a particular site. The pentapeptides [Met^5]enkephalin and [Leu^5]enkephalin have high affinities for the δ-binding site but lower affinities for the μ-site and negligible affinity for the κ-site; the relative affinities at the δ-site are about 0.90 (Table 1). Extension of [Met^5]enkephalin at the carboxyl-terminus decreases the preference for the δ-binding site. The octapeptide [Met^5]enkephalyl-Arg-Gly-Leu has a reduced relative affinity for the δ-site of 0.56, whereas [Met^5]enkephalyl-Arg-Phe has a preference for the μ-site; both peptides have low κ-affinity.

Extension of [Met^5]enkephalin by the basic amino acids Arg^6-Arg^7 (metorphamide, BAM 12, BAM 18, BAM 22 and peptide E) leads to a different pattern of opioid activity. The binding at the μ-site is preponderant but there is significant κ-binding; there is now only little binding at the δ-site. The affinities at the μ- and κ-binding sites are much greater than those of the other fragments of proenkephalin. Metorphamide has the very high affinity of $8.3 \, \text{n}M^{-1}$ at the μ-site in contrast to [Met^5]enkephalin, which has an affinity of $1.1 \, \text{n}M^{-1}$ at the δ-site. It should be noted that [Met^5]enkephalyl-Arg-Phe has the highest relative affinity for the μ-site but with an affinity of only $0.27 \, \text{n}M^{-1}$.

2. Activity in Bioassays

With the exception of peptide F, the fragments of proenkephalin discussed are rapidly broken down by tissue peptidases. Therefore, the in vitro activity has to be determined in the presence of enzyme inhibitors (MCKNIGHT et al. 1983) and particular care must be taken when interpreting information obtained from in vivo administration.

The results obtained with bioassays (Table 2) are in general agreement with the data obtained from the inhibitory binding assays. [Met^5]enkephalin and [Leu^5]enkephalin are active at the δ-receptors in the vasa deferentia of hamster and mouse but they are almost devoid of activity in the rabbit vas deferens, which has only κ-receptors. [Met^5]enkephalyl-Arg-Phe and

Table 2. Inhibitory effects (IC_{50}, nM) of proenkephalin-derived peptides on the electrically evoked contractions of the guinea pig myenteric plexus-longitudinal muscle (GPI) and the vasa deferentia of the mouse (MVD), hamster (HVD), rabbit, (LVD), and rat (RVD)

Peptide	GPI ($\mu + \kappa$)	MVD ($\mu + \delta + \kappa$)	HVD (δ)	LVD (κ)	RVD (μ)
[Leu^5]enkephalin	36[a]	1.7[a]	54[b]	>10 000[c]	550[a]
[Met^5]enkephalin	6.7[a]	1.5[a]	57[b]	>10 000[c]	260[a]
[Met^5]enkephalyl-Arg-Phe	10[a]	5.3[a]	92[b]	830[d]	396[a]
[Met^5]enkephalyl-Arg-Gly-Leu	35[a]	2.9[a]	80[b]	760[d]	512[a]
Metorphamide	2.5[c]	6.2[c]	800[b]	41[e]	>3 000[c]
BAM 12	128[f]	227[f]	ND	1 800[g]	16 000[d]
BAM 18	1.4[h]	227[h]	ND	ND	ND
BAM 22	0.6[f]	42[f]	ND	3 900[g]	1 200[f]
Peptide E	2.2[f]	50[f]	670[b]	6 100[g]	2 900[f]
Peptide F	294[f]	270[f]	>3000[b]	30 000[g]	3 000[f]

ND, not determined
The Krebs solution contained the following peptidase inhibitors: bestatin (10 μM or 30 μM for the vasa deferentia of the hamster and rabbit), thiorphan (0.3 μM or 10 μM for the vas deferens of the hamster), captopril (10 μM), and L-leucyl-L-leucine (2 mM).
[a] McKnight et al. (1983); [b] McKnight et al. (1985); [c] Corbett et al. (1982); [d] Corbett and Kosterlitz (unpublished observations); [e] Weber et al. (1983); [f] Höllt et al. (1985); [g] Rezvani et al. (1983); [h] Hurlbut et al. (1987).

[Met^5]enkephalyl-Arg-Gly-Leu are also active in the hamster and the mouse vasa deferentia but, unlike the pentapeptides, they have some minor activity in the rabbit vas deferens. The pharmacological profiles of metorphamide and related peptides correlate well with the binding data. They are potent agonists in the guinea pig myenteric plexus, which responds to μ- and κ-agonists, and are less potent in the mouse vas deferens, which contains μ-, δ-, and κ-receptors. It may be important that metorphamide is the only opioid peptide other than those derived from prodynorphin, which shows potent agonist activity at the κ-receptors in the rabbit vas deferens (Table 2).

II. Prodynorphin-Derived Peptides

1. Activity in Binding Assays

The opioid fragments of prodynorphin have [Leu^5]enkephalin at the amino terminus but it is still unclear whether this δ-preferring pentapeptide is processed directly from prodynorphin (see Chap. 17). In binding assays, the prodynorphin peptides have a high affinity for κ-binding sites (Table 3) but they also have affinity for the μ-site and somewhat less for the δ-site. None of the prodynorphin peptides are selective for the κ-site, since their relative

Table 3. Inhibitory effects (K_i, nM) of prodynorphin-derived peptides on binding at μ-, δ-, and κ-binding sites

Peptide	μ-Site	δ-Site	κ-Site	Affinity at κ-Site $(K_i, nM)^{-1}$	Relative affinity at μ-Site	δ-Site	κ-Site	Reference
	K_i(nM)							
Dynorphin A(1–8) [Leu⁵]enkephalyl-Arg-Arg-Ile	3.8	5.0	1.3	0.77	0.22	0.16	0.62	[a]
Dynorphin A [Leu⁵]enkephalyl-Arg-Arg-Ile-Arg-Pro-Lys-Leu-Lys-Trp-Asp-Asn-Gln	0.73	2.4	0.12	8.3	0.14	0.04	0.82	[a]
Dynorphin B [Leu⁵]enkephalyl-Arg-Arg-Gln-Phe-Lys-Val-Val-Thr	0.68	2.9	0.12	8.3	0.15	0.03	0.82	[b]
β-Neoendorphin [Leu⁵]enkephalyl-Arg-Lys-Tyr-Pro	6.9	2.1	1.2	0.83	0.10	0.33	0.57	[b]
α-Neoendorphin [Leu⁵]enkephalyl-Arg-Lys-Tyr-Pro-Lys	1.2	0.57	0.20	5.0	0.11	0.23	0.66	[a]

The μ-binding sites were labeled with $[^3H]$-[D-Ala²,MePhe⁴,Gly-ol⁵]enkephalin, the δ-sites with $[^3H]$-[D-Ala²,D-Leu⁵]enkephalin, and the κ-sites with $[^3H]$-(−)-bremazocine in the presence of unlabeled [D-Ala²,MePhe⁴,Gly-ol⁵]enkephalin and [D-Ala²,D-Leu⁵]enkephalin. Assays were performed in homogenates of guinea pig brain at 0°C. Relative affinity is K_i^{-1} at μ, δ, or κ/(K_i^{-1} at μ + K_i^{-1} at δ + K_i^{-1} at κ) and was calculated from the data shown. [a] Corbett et al. (1982); [b] Paterson et al. (1984).

Table 4. Inhibitory effects (IC$_{50}$,nM) of prodynorphin-derived peptides on the electrically evoked contractions of the guinea pig myenteric plexus-longitudinal muscle (GPI) and the vasa deferentia of the mouse (MVD), hamster (HVD), rabbit (LVD), and rat (RVD)

Peptide	GPI ($\mu + \kappa$)	MVD ($\mu + \delta + \kappa$)	HVD (δ)	LVD (κ)	RVD (μ)
Dynorphin A(1–8)	4.9[a]	9.2[a]	1 040[b]	12[a]	>10 000[a]
Dynorphin A	0.29[a]	0.91[a]	450[b]	3.0[a]	>10 000[a]
Dynorphin B	0.25[c]	2.1[c]	530[b]	4.8[c]	>10 000[d]
β-Neoendorphin	3.3[c]	9.9[c]	244[b]	63[c]	>10 000[e]
α-Neoendorphin	3.0[a]	7.7[a]	168[b]	21[a]	>10 000[a]

ND, not determined.
The Krebs solution contained the following peptidase inhibitors: bestatin (10 μM or 30 μM for the vasa deferentia of the hamster and rabbit), thiorphan (0.3 μM or 10 μM for the vas deferens of the hamster), captopril (10 μM) and L-leucyl-L-leucine (2 mM).
[a] CORBETT et al. (1982); [b] McKNIGHT et al. (1985); [c] PATERSON et al. (1984); [d] CORBETT and KOSTERLITZ (unpublished observations); [e] McKNIGHT et al. (1982).

κ-affinities are <0.83 but both dynorphin A and dynorphin B have high affinity for this site, 8.3 nM^{-1}. Dynorphin A(1–8), α-neoendorphin, and β-neoendorphin have lower affinities for the κ-site with significant affinity for the μ- and δ-sites; their relative affinities at the preferred κ-sites are less than 0.66.

2. Activity in Bioassays

The results of the bioassays confirm those of the binding assays (Table 4). All five peptides depress the electrically evoked contractions of the κ-sensitive rabbit vas deferens, dynorphin A and dynorphin B being particularly effective. They are potent agonists at κ-receptors in the guinea pig myenteric plexus and in the nonselective mouse vas deferens; they are weak agonists at the δ-receptors in the hamster vas deferens. In the vas deferens of the rat none of the fragments of prodynorphin has agonist or antagonist activity.

All of the prodynorphin-derived peptides are subject to enzymatic breakdown.

III. Proopiomelanocortin-Derived Peptides

1. Activity in Binding Assays

β$_h$-Endorphin and β$_p$-endorphin have similar affinities for the μ- and δ-binding sites; they are much less active at the κ-binding site (Table 5). The removal of four amino acids from the carboxyl-terminus of β$_p$-endorphin to

Table 5. Inhibitory effects (K_i, nM) of proopiomelanocortin-derived peptides on binding at μ-, δ-, and κ-binding sites

Peptide	K_i (nM)			Affinity at (K_i, nM)$^{-1}$		Relative affinity at			Reference
	μ-Site	δ-Site	κ-Site	μ-Site	δ-Site	μ-Site	δ-Site	κ-Site	
β$_h$-Endorphin Tyr-Gly-Gly-Phe-Met-Thr-Ser-Glu-Lys-Ser-Gln-Thr-Pro-Leu-Val-Thr-Leu-Phe-Lys-Asn-Ala-Ile-Ile-Lys-Asn-Ala-Tyr-Lys-Lys-Gly-Glu	2.1	2.4	96	0.48		0.53	0.45	0.02	a
β$_p$-Endorphin Tyr-Gly-Gly-Phe-Met-Thr-Ser-Glu-Lys-Ser-Gln-Thr-Pro-Leu-Val-Thr-Leu-Phe-Lys-Asn-Ala-Ile-Val-Lys-Asn-Ala-His-Lys-Lys-Gly-Gln	1.9	1.3	26		0.77	0.40	0.57	0.03	b
β$_p$-Endorphin(1–27) Tyr-Gly-Gly-Phe-Met-Thr-Ser-Glu-Lys-Ser-Gln-Thr-Pro-Leu-Val-Thr-Leu-Phe-Lys-Asn-Ala-Ile-Val-Lys-Asn-Ala-His	3.0	2.4	185		0.42	0.44	0.55	0.01	b
N-Acetyl-β$_h$-Endorphin Ac-Tyr-Gly-Gly-Phe-Met-Thr-Ser-Glu-Lys-Ser-Gln-Thr-Pro-Leu-Val-Thr-Leu-Phe-Lys-Asn-Ala-Ile-Ile-Lys-Asn-Ala-Tyr-Lys-Lys-Gly-Glu	2800	3000	N.D.	0.0004		0.52	0.48	–	c

The μ-binding sites were labeled with [³H]-[D-Ala²,MePhe⁴,Gly-ol⁵]enkephalin [a,b] or [³H]-[D-Ala²,D-Leu⁵]enkephalin and the κ-sites with [³H]-(−)-bremazocine in the presence of unlabeled [D-Ala²,MePhe⁴,Gly-ol⁵]enkephalin and [D-Ala²,D-Leu⁵]enkephalin [a,b].
Assays were performed in homogenates of guinea pig [a,b] or rat [c] brain at 0°C [a,b] or 35°C [c].
Relative affinity is K_i^{-1} at μ, δ, or κ/(K_i^{-1} at μ + K_i^{-1} at δ + K_i^{-1} at κ) and was calculated from the data shown.
[a] KOSTERLITZ and PATERSON (1985); [b] PATERSON (1986); [c] AKIL et al. (1981).

Table 6. Inhibitory effects (IC_{50},nM) of proopiomelanocortin-derived peptides on the electrically evoked contractions of the guinea pig myenteric plexus-longitudinal muscle (GPI) and the vasa deferentia of the mouse (MVD), hamster (HVD), rabbit (LVD), and rat (RVD)

Peptide	GPI ($\mu + \kappa$)	MVD ($\mu + \delta + \kappa$)	HVD (δ)	LVD (κ)	RVD (μ)
β_h-Endorphin	62[a]	40[a]	730[b]	>30 000[c]	19[a]
β_p-Endorphin	60[a]	49[a]	ND	ND	15[a]
β_p-Endorphin(1–27)	74[a]	39[a]	ND	ND	4.6[a]
N-Acetyl-β_h-endorphin	Inactive[d]	Inactive[d]	ND	ND	Inactive[d]

ND, not determined.
The Krebs solution contained the following peptidase inhibitors: bestatin (10 μM or 30 μM for the vasa deferentia of the hamster and rabbit), thiorphan (0.3 μM or 10 μM for the vas deferens of the hamster), captopril (10 μM) and L-leucyl-L-leucine (2 mM).
[a] McKnight et al. (1983); [b] McKnight et al. (1985); [c] McKnight et al. (1982); [d] Schulz et al. (1981).

give β_p-endorphin(1–27) causes a small reduction in affinity for all three sites and the relative μ-affinity is unchanged at about 0.55. N-Acetyl-β_h-endorphin has negligible affinity for any of the opioid binding sites.

2. Activity in Bioassays

In the isolated tissue preparations, β_h-endorphin, β_p-endorphin, and β_p-endorphin(1–27) were equiactive in inhibiting the responses of the guinea pig myenteric plexus and the vasa deferentia of the mouse and the rat (Table 6). β_h-Endorphin was only weakly active in the hamster vas deferens and inactive at the κ-receptors of the rabbit vas deferens.

IV. Dermorphin and Deltorphins

In comparison with the nonselective mammalian opioid peptides, amphibian skin contains opioid peptides which are much more selective (see Chap. 21).

1. Activity in Binding Assays

Dermorphin is a highly selective μ-ligand without significant affinity at the δ- and κ-sites (Table 7). It has a relative μ-affinity of >0.989 and is therefore much more selective than any mammalian peptide.

The deltorphins, deltorphin (dermenkephalin; Mor et al. 1989), [D-Ala²]deltorphin I, and [D-Ala²]deltorphin II, are highly selective for the δ-binding site, having relative binding affinities >0.99 (Table 7). Their μ-affinity is negligible and they are inactive at the κ-sites. [D-Ala²]deltorphin I is particularly potent as its affinity is 6.7 nM^{-1} at the δ-binding site.

Table 7. Inhibitory effects (K_i, nM) of dermorphin and deltorphins on binding at μ-, δ-, and κ-binding sites

Peptide	K_i(nM)			Affinity at (K_i, nM)$^{-1}$		Relative affinity at			Reference
	μ-Site	δ-Site	κ-Site	μ-Site	δ-Site	μ-Site	δ-Site	κ-Site	
Dermorphin Tyr-D-Ala-Phe-Gly-Tyr-Pro-Ser-NH$_2$	0.70	62	>10000	1.4		0.989	0.011	0	a
Deltorphin Tyr-D-Met-Phe-His-Leu-Met-Asp-NH$_2$	1630	2.4	>10000		0.42	0.002	0.998	0	b
[D-Ala^2]deltorphin I Tyr-D-Ala-Phe-Asp-Val-Val-Gly-NH$_2$	3150	0.15	>10000		6.7	<0.001	>0.999	0	b
[D-Ala^2]deltorphin II Tyr-D-Ala-Phe-Glu-Val-Val-Gly-NH$_2$	2450	0.71	>10000		1.4	<0.001	>0.999	0	b

The μ-binding sites were labeled with [³H]-[D-Ala²,MePhe⁴,Gly-ol⁵]enkephalin, the δ-sites with [³H]-[D-Pen²,D-Pen⁵]enkephalin [a] or [³H]-[D-Ala²]deltorphin I [b] and the κ-sites with [³H]-ethylketazocine [a] or [³H]-(−)-bremazocine [b]. Assays were performed in homogenates of rat brain [a,b] or guinea pig cerebellum [a,b] at 24°C [a] or 35°C [b]. Relative affinity is K_i^{-1} at μ, δ, or κ/(K_i^{-1} at μ + K_i^{-1} at δ + K_i^{-1} at κ) and was calculated from the data shown. [a] AMICHE et al. (1988); [b] ERSPAMER et al. (1989).

Table 8. Inhibitory effects (IC_{50},nM) of dermorphin and deltorphins on the electrically evoked contractions of the guinea pig myenteric plexus-longitudinal muscle (GPI) and the vasa deferentia of the mouse (MVD), hamster (HVD), rabbit (LVD), and rat (RVD)

Peptide	GPI ($\mu + \kappa$)	MVD ($\mu + \delta + \kappa$)	HVD (δ)	LVD (κ)	RVD (μ)
Dermorphin	1.4[a]	2.4[a]	>10 000[a]	>1 000[b]	>1 000[b]
Deltorphin	5 000[a]	1.4[a]	13[a]	>1 000[b]	>1 000[b]
[D-Ala²]deltorphin I	>1 500[b]	0.21[b]	ND	>1 000[b]	>1 000[b]
[D-Ala²]deltorphin II	>3 000[b]	0.32[b]	ND	>1 000[b]	>1 000[b]

ND, not determined.
The Krebs solution contained the following peptidase inhibitors for the vas deferens of the hamster: bestatin ($10 \mu M$), amastatin ($10 \mu M$), thiorphan ($10 \mu M$) and captopril ($10 \mu M$).
[a] SAGAN et al. (1991); [b] ERSPAMER et al. (1989).

2. Activity in Bioassays

Dermorphin is a potent agonist in the guinea pig myenteric plexus and is also active in the mouse vas deferens (Table 8). As expected from the absence of κ-binding activity, dermorphin is inactive in the rabbit vas deferens; surprisingly, this μ-preferring peptide is without activity in the rat vas deferens.

The δ-selectivity of the deltorphins is reflected in the bioassays (Table 8). They are almost inactive in the guinea pig myenteric plexus and the rabbit and rat vasa deferentia, which have no δ-receptors. They are highly potent in the mouse vas deferens, which contains μ-, δ-, and κ-receptors. Confirmation of the δ-activity was obtained with antagonists. The activity of the deltorphins in the mouse vas deferens is antagonized by the selective δ-receptor antagonists naltrindole (ERSPAMER et al. 1989) and ICI 174864 (AMICHE et al. 1989) and also by high concentrations of naloxone, $K_e > 75$ nM (ERSPAMER et al. 1989). Unfortunately, the δ-activity of the [D-Ala²] deltorphins has not as yet been assessed in the hamster vas deferens.

D. Selectivity of Nonendogenous Opioid Compounds

As none of the mammalian endogenous opioid peptides are selective ligands or are enzymatically stable, a large number of peptide and nonpeptide analogues have been synthesized. Although morphine has been shown to be present in low concentrations in mammalian tissue and therefore may be an endogenous ligand (DONNERER et al. 1986, 1987; WEITZ et al. 1986, 1987), it has been included in this section because it is not a peptide. In the tables showing the binding selectivities, the compounds have been arranged in order of decreasing selectivity for the site at which they have their

Table 9. Inhibitory effects (K_i,nM) of opioids with a preference for the μ-binding site on binding at μ-, δ-, and κ-binding sites

	μ-Site	δ-Site	κ-Site	Affinity at μ-site $(K_i,nM)^{-1}$	Relative affinity at μ-Site	δ-Site	κ-Site	Reference
	(K_i,nM)							
μ-Agonists								
Ohmefentanyl	0.0079	10	32	127	0.999	0.001	0	a
Tyr-D-Arg-Phe-Lys-NH$_2$	3.6	9000	2140	0.28	0.998	0	0.002	b
Tyr-Pro-MePhe-D-Pro-NH$_2$ (PL 017)	11	7250	16000	0.091	0.998	0.002	0	c
Alfentanyl	39	21200	ND	0.026	0.998	0.002	–	d
Tyr-D-Orn-Phe-Asp-NH$_2$	10	2220	ND	0.10	0.995	0.005	–	e
[D-Ala^2,MePhe^4,Gly-ol^5]enkephalin	1.9	345	6090	0.53	0.994	0.006	0	f
Tyr-Pro-Phe-Pro-NH$_2$	140	23800	39300	0.0071	0.990	0.006	0.004	g
Oxymorphone	0.78	50	137	1.3	0.979	0.015	0.006	g
Morphine	1.8	90	317	0.56	0.975	0.029	0.006	g
[D-Ala^2,MePhe^4,Met(O)ol^5]enkephalin (FK33,824)	1.0	31	1740	1.0*	0.968	0.031	0.001	h
Normorphine	4.0	310	149	0.25	0.962	0.012	0.026	g
Fentanyl	7.0	150	470	0.14	0.94	0.05	0.01	g
Sufentanyl	1.6	23	124	0.63	0.92	0.07	0.01	g
Pethidine	385	4350	5140	0.003	0.86	0.08	0.06	g
Methadone	4.5	15	1630	0.22	0.77	0.23	0	g

μ-Antagonists

Ligand								
D-Phe-Cys-Tyr-D-Trp-Orn-Thr-Pen-Thr-NH₂ (CTOP)	1.7	>1000	>1000	0.59	0.999	<0.001	<0.001	i
Tic-D-Phe-Cys-Tyr-D-Trp-Arg-Thr-Pen-Thr-NH₂ (TCTAP)	1.0	1270	ND	1.0	0.999	0.001	–	j
Cyprodime	9.4	356	176	0.11	0.93	0.02	0.05	k
β-Funaltrexamine*	0.40	18	2.8	2.5	0.86	0.02	0.12	l
Naltrexone	1.1	6.6	8.5	0.91	0.77	0.13	0.10	g
β-Chlornaltrexamine	0.53	6.7	1.4	1.9	0.69	0.05	0.26	h
Naloxone	1.8	23	4.8	0.56	0.69	0.05	0.26	c
(−)-Win 44441	0.67	6.4	0.69	1.5	0.48	0.05	0.47	c

ND, not determined.

* Agonist activity at κ-receptors (see Table 10).

The μ-binding sites were labeled with [³H]-[D-Ala²,MePhe⁴,Gly-ol⁵]enkephalin [a,b,c,d,e,f,g,h,i,k,l] or [³H]-D-Phe-Cys-Tyr-D-Trp-Orn-Pen-Thr-NH₂ [j], the δ-sites with [³H]-[D-Pen²,D-Pen⁵]enkephalin [a,b,c,d,i,j], [³H]-[D-Ser²,L-Leu⁵]enkephalyl-Thr [e], [³H]-[D-Ala²,D-Leu⁵]enkephalin [g] or [³H]-[D-Ala²,D-Leu⁵]enkephalin in the presence of unlabeled [D-Ala²,MePhe⁴,Gly-ol⁵]enkephalin or morphine [f,h,i,k] and the κ-sites with [³H]-U-69593 [b,c,i,k] or either [³H]-(−)-bremazocine [a,f,h,l] or [³H]-(−)ethylketazocine [g] in the presence of unlabeled [D-Ala²,MePhe⁴,Gly-ol⁵]enkephalin and [D-Ala²,D-Leu⁵]enkephalin.

Assays were performed in homogenates of guinea pig [a,b,c,f,g,h,i,l] or rat [d,e,j,k] brain at 0°C [e], 23°C [a] or 25°C [b,c,d,f,g,h,i,j,k,l].

Relative affinity is K_i^{-1} at μ, δ or κ/(K_i^{-1} at μ + K_i^{-1} at δ + K_i^{-1} at κ) and was calculated from the data shown. Tic is tetrahydroisoquinolinecarboxylate. Win 44441 is α-2,5,9-trimethyl-2-(cyclopropyl-3-pentanyl)-2′-hydroxy-6,7-benzomorphan.

[a] GOLDSTEIN and NAIDU (1989); [b] KOSTERLITZ et al. (1990); [c] PATERSON (1991); [d] YEADON and KITCHEN (1988); [e] SCHILLER et al. (1987); [f] CORBETT et al. (1984); [g] MAGNAN et al. (1982); [h] PATERSON (1986); [i] KOSTERLITZ and PATERSON (1990); [j] KAZMIERSKI and PATERSON (1988); [k] PORINI et al. (1990); [l] CORBETT et al. (1985b).

highest affinity (see Chap. 12). The opioids also have been divided into two categories based on their pharmacological activity: agonists and antagonists. The order of the compounds in the bioassay tables is the same as in the corresponding binding tables to permit ready comparison of the two sets of data.

The compounds have been assayed for antagonist actions in each of the five bioassay tissues. The values quoted for the equilibrium dissociation constant (K_e, nM) are those found for antagonism of selective agonists for each receptor type; the μ-agonists used were [D-Ala^2,MePhe^4,Gly-ol^5]enkephalin, Tyr-Pro-MePhe-D-Pro-NH$_2$, morphine, or normorphine; the δ-agonists were [D-Pen^2,D-Pen^5]enkephalin, [D-Thr^2,L-Leu^5]enkephalyl-Thr, or [D-Ala^2,D-Leu^5]enkephalin; and the κ-agonists were U-69593, U-50488, or ethylketazocine.

I. Compounds with a Preference for the μ-Binding Site

1. Activity in Binding Assays

The μ-agonist morphine has a relative affinity for the μ-binding site of 0.975 (Table 9). A number of opioid compounds which are more selective than morphine for the μ-binding site have been developed based on fentanyl. Sufentanyl has the same relative affinities as fentanyl but is more potent. Alfentanyl is considerably more selective for the μ-binding site with a relative affinity of 0.998 but has only a fifth of the potency of fentanyl. Ohmefentanyl, a more recently developed analogue (JIN et al. 1987), combines high μ-selectivity (0.999), with the very high affinity of 127 nM^{-1} being 1000 times more potent than the parent compound fentanyl.

Although [Met^5]enkephalin has a preference for the δ-binding site (Table 1), the stable analogue [D-Ala^2,MePhe^4,Met(O)ol^5]enkephalin (FK 33,824; RÖMER et al. 1977) has a binding pattern similar to that of normorphine and has a relative μ-affinity of 0.968 (Table 9). [D-Ala^2,MePhe^4,Gly-ol^5]enkephalin was developed (HANDA et al. 1981) as a compound which is more selective for the μ-binding site, having a relative affinity of 0.994. Tyr-Pro-Phe-Pro-NH$_2$ (morphiceptin), an opioid peptide derived from β-casein (HENSCHEN et al. 1979), is a highly selective μ-ligand with a relative affinity of 0.990 but a low potency. Of the many analogues of morphiceptin which have been synthesized, Tyr-Pro-MePhe-D-Pro-NH$_2$ (PL 017; CHANG et al. 1983) displays both an increase in potency and selectivity when compared with morphiceptin (Table 9). Similarly, SCHILLER et al. (1987, 1989) have synthesized a number of peptides related to the μ-selective amphibian opioid dermorphin (Table 7). A number of these analogues have a greater selectivity than dermorphin but their affinities are lower. Of these, the tetrapeptide amides Tyr-D-Arg-Phe-Lys-NH$_2$ and Tyr-D-Orn-Phe-Asp-NH$_2$ are the most μ-selective (Table 9).

Table 10. Inhibitory effects (IC_{50}, nM) of opioids with a preference for the μ-binding site on the electrically evoked contractions of the myenteric plexus-longitudinal muscle of the guinea pig (GPI) and the vasa deferentia of the mouse (MVD), hamster (HVD), rabbit (LVD), and rat (RVD)

	GPI ($\mu + \kappa$)	MVD ($\mu + \delta + \kappa$)	HVD (δ)	LVD (κ)	RVD (μ)
μ-Agonists					
Ohmefentanyl	0.15[a]	0.89[a]	ND	149[a]	4.4[a]
Tyr-D-Arg-Phe-Lys-NH$_2$	254[b]	781[b]	ND	ND	ND
Tyr-Pro-MePhe-D-Pro-NH$_2$	34[c]	240[c]	ND	ND	ND
Tyr-D-Orn-Phe-Asp-NH$_2$	36[d]	3 880[d]	ND	ND	ND
[D-Ala^2, MePhe^4, Gly-ol^5] enkephalin	4.5[e]	33[e]	>10 000[f]	>10 000[e]	105[e]
Tyr-Pro-Phe-Pro-NH$_2$	318[c]	4 800[c]	ND	ND	ND
Oxymorphone	12[g]	883[g]	ND	ND	>5 000[g]
Morphine	28[j]	478[ij]	>10 000[f]	>10 000[ij]	>10 000[j]
[D-Ala^2, MePhe^4, Met(O)ol^5] enkephalin	4.7[h]	29[h]	ND	ND	246[h]
Normorphine	73[g]	440[g]	>10 000[f]	ND	2 068[g]
Fentanyl	0.92[g]	26[g]	Inactive[i]	ND	153[g]
Sufentanyl	0.65[g]	1.75[g]	ND	ND	28[g]
Pethidine	1 109[g]	16 000[g]	ND	ND	>20 000[g]
Methadone	22[g]	523[g]	Inactive[ij]	Inactive[ij]	1 650[g]
κ-Agonist					
β-Funaltrexamine*	4.4[k]	190[k]	Inactive[k]	990[k]	Inactive[k]

ND, not determined.

* Antagonist at μ- and δ-receptors (see Table 15).

[a] JIN et al. (1987); [b] SCHILLER et al. (1989); [c] CHANG et al. (1983); [d] SCHILLER et al. (1987); [e] CORBETT et al. (1984); [f] McKNIGHT et al. (1985); [g] MAGNAN et al. (1982); [h] WÜSTER et al. (1979); [i] SHEEHAN et al. (1986); [j] MILLER et al. (1986); [k] CORBETT et al. (1985b).

Naloxone was the first opioid which was an antagonist but had no agonist activity (BLUMBERG et al. 1961). It has highest affinity for the μ-binding site but also has high affinity for the κ-binding site and low affinity for the δ-site (Table 9). It should be noted that the benzomorphan (−)-Win 44441, which is often used as a κ-antagonist, has equal relative affinities at the μ- and κ-binding sites. More recently, the morphinan cyprodime has been synthesized (SCHMIDHAMMER et al. 1989); it has a greater preference than naloxone for the μ-binding site but it is less potent. Furthermore, there are a number of cyclic octapeptides related to somatostatin (PELTON et al. 1986; KAZMIERSKI et al. 1988) which have μ-affinities similar to naloxone but are much more selective. The two most selective compounds, D-Phe-Cys-Tyr-D-Trp-Thr-Orn-Pen-Thr-NH$_2$ (CTOP) and Tic-D-Phe-Cys-Tyr-D-

Trp-Arg-Thr-Pen-Thr-NH$_2$ (TCTAP), have relative μ-affinities of 0.999 (Table 9).

2. Agonist Activity in Bioassays

The compounds classified as μ-agonists in Table 9 are agonists in the guinea pig myenteric plexus preparation and the mouse vas deferens; they are more potent in the myenteric plexus (Table 10). Since the equilibrium dissociation constant (K_e) for antagonism by naloxone is 2–3 nM, these inhibitory effects are due to activation of μ-receptors (Lord et al. 1977; Handa et al. 1981; Chang et al. 1983; Jin et al. 1987; Schiller et al. 1987, 1989). Of the compounds tested in the hamster and rabbit vasa deferentia, only ohmefentanyl had agonist activity in the rabbit. This was unexpected, since in binding assays ohmefentanyl was the most selective μ-ligand.

In the rat vas deferens, most of the compounds are either weak agonists or inactive (Table 10). The two groups of compounds which are potent agonists are the fentanyl derivatives and the two enkephalin analogues. As the agonist effects of these compounds are blocked by low concentrations of naloxone, it was proposed that they probably interact with μ-receptors in this preparation (Gillan et al. 1981). However, the exact nature of the opioid receptors in the rat vas deferens remains unclear.

β-Funaltrexamine (β-FNA) is an agonist in the guinea pig myenteric plexus. This effect is mediated by κ-receptors since a higher concentration of naloxone, 10–30 nM, is required to block this action than is necessary to antagonize μ-agonists (Miller et al. 1986). Furthermore, the agonist potency of β-FNA is not altered after preincubation of the tissue with β-FNA which irreversibly and selectively blocks the μ-receptors (Hayes et al. 1985; Schmidt et al. 1985). β-FNA is a weak agonist at the κ-receptors in the vas deferentia of the mouse and the rabbit but is inactive in the vasa deferentia of the hamster and the rat (Table 10).

3. Antagonist Activity in Bioassays

Naloxone is a potent antagonist in all five assay tissues; it has highest affinity for the μ-receptors with lower affinity for the κ-receptor and lowest affinity for the δ-receptor (Table 15). It has the same affinity for the μ-receptors in the guinea pig ileum and mouse vas deferens but it is a less potent antagonist of μ-ligands in the rat vas deferens. In low concentrations, naloxone can be used as a μ-antagonist but, if the concentrations are raised, it also has antagonist activity at δ- and κ-receptors. To preclude any nonopioid effects when high concentrations of (−)-naloxone are used, (+)-naloxone should also be tested. Naltrexone and (−)-Win 44441 have similar patterns of antagonist activity as found for naloxone but are more potent. In agreement with the results from the binding assays, the morphinan cyprodime is a more selective μ-antagonist than either naloxone or naltrexone but it is much less potent. The highly selective μ-ligands CTOP and TCTAP are μ-antagonists devoid of δ-antagonist activity (Table 15). However, in the guinea pig myenteric plexus, the ratios of the K_e at μ-receptors to the K_e at κ-receptors are similar for CTOP and naloxone. This discrepancy between the selectivity of CTOP in binding assays and bioassays requires further investigation.

II. Compounds with a Preference for the δ-Binding Site

1. Activity in Binding Assays

[Leu^5]enkephalin is a relatively selective δ-ligand (Table 1), but, like most endogenous opioid peptides, it is rapidly degraded by tissue peptidases (HAMBROOK et al. 1976; McKNIGHT et al. 1983). The first analogue resistant to peptidases was [D-Ala^2,D-Leu^5]enkephalin, which has a pattern of activity similar to [Leu^5]enkephalin (Table 11). The hexapeptides [D-Ser^2,L-Leu^5]enkephalyl-Thr (GACEL et al. 1980) and [D-Thr^2,L-Leu^5]enkephalyl-Thr (ZAJAC et al. 1983) have improved selectivity for the δ-binding site (Table 11). Among other [Leu^5]enkephalin analogues which have a pattern of activity little different from [D-Ala^2,D-Leu^5]enkephalin are [D-Ala^2,Ser(OBz)^5]enkephalin (SHI et al. 1981) and the dimers DPE$_2$ and DTE$_{12}$ (SHIMOHIGASHI et al. 1982). The cyclic enkephalin analogues [D-Pen^2,D-Pen^5]enkephalin and [D-Pen^2,L-Pen^5]enkephalin (MOSBERG et al. 1983) have a much improved selectivity for the δ-binding site. The introduction of a halogen atom, e.g., Cl, at position 4, further enhances δ-affinity (Table 11); other halogenated analogues have similar profiles (TOTH et al. 1989).

[^{3}H]-[D-Pen^2,D-Pen^5]enkephalin is less potent in binding assays in homogenates of rat brain than in homogenates of guinea pig brain (COTTON et al. 1985; DELAY-GOYET et al. 1985). This observation led Roques and his coworker to develop a number of linear analogues of [D-Ser^2,L-Leu^5]enkephalyl-Thr which combined improved δ-selectivity with improved potency in the rat (GACEL et al. 1988). The most selective of these compounds are [D-Ser(O-tert-butyl)^2,L-Leu^5]enkephalyl-Thr(O-tert-butyl) and [D-Ser(O-tert-butyl)^2,L-Leu^5]enkephalyl-Thr. Another analogue of [D-Ala^2,L-Leu^5]enkephalin which has enhanced δ-selectivity in binding assays is [D-Ala^2,(2R,3S)-∇^EMePhe^4,L-Leu^5]enkephalin (SHIMOHIGASHI et al. 1987). Although this analogue has a relative δ-affinity of 0.996, its potency is low (Table 11).

The first δ-antagonist to be synthesized was ICI 154129, which is a selective δ-ligand but its affinity for the δ-binding site is only 0.0013 nM^{-1}. The stable analogue ICI 174864 (COTTON et al. 1984) displays a higher δ-selectivity and potency with a relative affinity of 0.991. A major advance has been the development of the nonpeptide δ-antagonist naltrindole

Table 11. The inhibitory effects (K_i, nM) of opioids with a preference for the δ-binding site on binding at μ-, δ-, and κ-binding sites

	μ-Site	δ-Site	κ-Site	Affinity at δ-Site $K_i(nM)^{-1}$	Relative affinity at μ-Site	δ-Site	κ-Site	Reference
	K_i(nM)							
δ-Agonists								
[D-Pen^2,p-ClPhe^4,D-Pen^5]enkephalin	780	1.6	ND	0.63	0.002	0.998	—	a
[D-Ser(O-tert-butyl)^2,L-Leu^5]enkephalyl-Thr(O-tert-butyl)	480	1.7	ND	0.59	0.004	0.996	—	b
[D-Pen^2,D-Pen^5]enkephalin	710	2.7	>15 000	0.37	0.004	0.996	0	c
[D-Pen^2,L-Pen^5]enkephalin	660	2.8	>15 000	0.36	0.004	0.996	0	c
[D-Ala^2,(2R, 3S)-▽^{E}Phe^4, L-Leu^5]enkephalin	3290	13	>10 000	0.077	0.004	0.996	0	d,e
[D-Ser(O-tert-butyl)^2,L-Leu^5]enkephalyl-Thr	370	2.8	ND	0.36	0.007	0.993	—	b
[D-Ser^2,L-Leu^5]enkephalyl-Thr	39	1.8	6040	0.56	0.045	0.955	0	c
[D-Thr^2,L-Leu^5]enkephalyl-Thr	34	2.7	14 500	0.37	0.073	0.927	0	c
[D-Ala^2,D-Leu^5]enkephalin	14	2.1	16 000	0.48	0.13	0.87	0	c
Tyr-D-Ala-Gly-Phe-Leu-NH-(CH$_2$)$_2$-NH-Leu-Phe-Gly-D-Ala-Tyr (DPE$_2$)	5.5	0.66	33	1.5	0.10	0.88	0.02	c
[D-Ala^2,Ser(OBz)^5]enkephalin	12	2.1	11 700	0.48	0.15	0.85	0	c
Tyr-D-Ala-Gly-Phe-NH-(CH$_2$)$_{12}$-NH-Phe-Gly-D-Ala-Tyr (DTE$_{12}$)	38	10	87	0.10	0.19	0.73	0.08	c
δ-Antagonists								
ICI 174864	29 600	190	65 400	0.0052	0.006	0.991	0.003	f
Naltrindole	11	0.12	18	8.3	0.011	0.983	0.006	g
ICI 154129	10 100	780	>50 000	0.0013	0.072	0.928	0	c

ND, not determined.
The μ-binding sites were labeled with [^{3}H]-[D-Ala^2,MePhe^4,Gly-ol^5]enkephalin [b,c,d,f,g] or [^{3}H]-D-Phe-Cys-Tyr-D-Trp-Orn-Thr-Pen-Thr-NH$_2$ [a], the δ-sites with [^{3}H]-[D-Pen^2,D-Pen^5]enkephalin [a,f,g], [^{3}H]-[D-Ser(O-tert-butyl)^2,L-Leu^5]enkephalyl-Thr [b], [^{3}H]-[D-Ala^2,D-Leu^5]enkephalin [d] or [^{3}H]-[D-Ala^2,MePhe^4, Gly-ol^5]enkephalin [c] and the κ-sites with [^{3}H]-U-69593 [f,g] or [^{3}H]-(−)-bremazocine in the presence of unlabeled [D-Ala^2, MePhe^4, Gly-ol^5]enkephalin and [D-Ala^2,D-Leu^5]enkephalin [c,e]. Assays were performed in homogenates of guinea pig [c,e,f] or rat [a,b,d,g] brain at 25°C [a,c,d,e,f,g] or 37°C [b]. Relative affinity is K_i^{-1} at μ, δ or κ/(K_i^{-1} at μ + K_i^{-1} at δ + K_i^{-1} at κ) and was calculated from the data shown. Pen, β,β-dimethylcysteine; Bz, benzoyl; Aib, α-aminoisobutyric acid; ICI 154129, N,N-diallyl-Tyr-Gly-Gly-ψ-(CH$_2$S)-Phe-Leu; ICI 174864, N,N-diallyl-Tyr-Aib-Aib-Phe-Leu.
[a] TOTH et al. (1989); [b] DELAY-GOYET et al. (1988); [c] CORBETT et al. (1984); [d] SHIMOHIGASHI et al. (1987); [e] SHIMOHIGASHI et al. (1988); [f] PATERSON (1991); [g] TAKEMORI et al. (1988).

Table 12. Inhibitory effects (IC$_{50}$, nM) of opioids with a preference for the δ-binding site on the electrically evoked contractions of the myenteric plexus-longitudinal muscle of the guinea pig (GPI) and the vasa deferentia of the mouse (MVD), hamster (HVD), rabbit (LVD), and rat (RVD)

	GPI (μ + κ)	MVD (μ + δ + κ)	HVD (δ)	LVD (κ)	RVD (μ)
δ-Agonists					
[D-Pen^2,p-ClPhe^4,D-Pen^5]enkephalin	8 300[a]	0.89[a]	ND	ND	ND
[D-Ser(O-tert-butyl)^2,L-Leu^5]enkephalyl-Thr(O-tert-butyl)	2 790[b]	0.60[b]	ND	ND	ND
[D-Pen^2,D-Pen^5]enkephalin	2 350[c]	2.8[c]	74[d]	>3 000[c]	>10 000[c]
[D-Pen^2,L-Pen^5]enkephalin	3 000[c]	4.1[c]	81[d]	>3 000[c]	>10 000[c]
[D-Ala^2,(2R,3S)-∇^{E}Phe^4,L-Leu^5]enkephalin	3 700[e]	2000[e]	ND	ND	ND
[D-Ser(O-tert-butyl)^2,L-Leu^5]enkephalyl-Thr	1 800[b]	1.1[b]	ND	ND	ND
[D-Ser^2,L-Leu^5]enkephalyl-Thr	110[c]	0.59[c]	21[d]	>3 000[c]	200[c]
[D-Thr^2,L-Leu^5]enkephalyl-Thr	68[c]	0.41[c]	21[d]	>3 000[c]	400[c]
[D-Ala^2,D-Leu^5]enkephalin	8.9[c]	0.73[c]	21[d]	>3 000[c]	130[c]
Tyr-D-Ala-Gly-Phe-Leu-NH-(CH$_2$)$_2$-NH-Leu-Phe-Gly-D-Ala-Tyr	220[f]	0.40[f]	ND	ND	ND
[D-Ala^2,Ser(OBz)^5]enkephalin	26[c]	1.5[c]	ND	ND	180[c]
Tyr-D-Ala-Gly-Phe-NH-(CH$_2$)$_{12}$-NH-Phe-Gly-D-Ala-Tyr	1 000[f]	38[f]	ND	ND	ND

ND, not determined.
[a] Toth et al. (1989); [b] Gacel et al. (1988); [c] Corbett et al. (1984); [d] McKnight et al. (1985); [e] Shimohigashi et al. (1987); [f] Costa et al. (1985).

Table 13. Inhibitory effects (K_i, nM) of opioids with a preference for the κ-binding site on binding at μ-, δ-, and κ-binding sites

	μ-Site	δ-Site	κ-Site	Affinity at κ-Site	Relative affinity at			Reference
	(K_i, nM)			$(K_i, nM)^{-1}$	μ-Site	δ-Site	κ-Site	
κ-Agonists								
CI-977	100	1040	0.11	9.1	0.001	0	0.999	a
ICI 197067	246	4450	0.17	5.9	0.001	0	0.999	b
U-69593	2350	19700	1.4	0.74	0.001	0	0.999	c
U-50488	435	9200	0.69	1.5	0.002	0	0.998	a
PD 117302	194	5780	0.58	1.7	0.003	0	0.997	c
U-62066	44	4530	0.35	2.9	0.008	0	0.992	a
[D-Pro10]Dynorphin A(1–11)	0.56	2.3	0.029	35	0.05	0.01	0.94	c
Tifluadom	22	290	4.1	0.25	0.15	0.01	0.84	d
(−)-Bremazocine*	0.62	0.78	0.075	13	0.10	0.08	0.82	b
(−)-Ethylketazocine*	1.0	5.5	0.52	1.9	0.32	0.06	0.62	c
Etorphine	1.0	0.56	0.23	4.4	0.14	0.25	0.61	e

Diprenorphine**	0.24		1.0		0.14		7.1		0.30		0.09		0.61 [e]
Mr 2034*	0.66		5.8		0.45		2.2		0.39		0.04		0.57 [e]
κ-Antagonists													
Norbinaltorphimine	14		10		0.34		2.9		0.02		0.03		0.95 [e]
Mr 2266	1.3		2.7		0.28		3.6		0.16		0.08		0.76 [b]
Binaltorphimine	1.3		5.8		0.79		1.3		0.35		0.08		0.57 [f]

* Antagonist activity at μ- and δ-receptors; ** antagonist activity at μ-, δ-, and κ-receptors (see Table 15). The μ-binding sites were labeled with [³H]-[D-Ala²,MePhe⁴,Gly-ol⁵]enkephalin [a,b,c,f], [³H]-[D-Pen²,D-Pen⁵]enkephalin, the δ-sites with [³H]-[D-Pen²,D-Pen⁵]enkephalin [a,b,c,f], [³H]-[D-Ala²,D-Leu⁵]enkephalin [e] or [³H]-[D-Ala²,MePhe⁴,Gly-ol⁵]enkephalin in the presence of unlabeled [D-Ala²,MePhe⁴,Gly-ol⁵]enkephalin [d] and the κ-sites with [³H]-U-69593 [a,b,c,f] or either [³H]-(−)-bromazocine [d] or [³H]-(−)-ethylketazocine [e] in the presence of unlabeled [D-Ala²,MePhe⁴,Gly-ol⁵]enkephalin and [D-Ala²,D-Leu⁵]enkephalin. Assays were performed in homogenates of guinea pig brain at 25°C [a,b,c,d,e] or 37°C [f]. Relative affinity is K_i^{-1} at μ, δ, or κ/(K_i^{-1} at μ + K_i^{-1} at δ + K_i^{-1} at κ) and was calculated from the data shown.

CI-977, (5R)-(5α,7α,8β)-N-methyl-N-[7-(1-pyrrolidinyl)-1-oxaspiro[4,5]dec-8-yl]-4-benzofuranacetamide monohydride; ICI 197067, (2S)-N-[2-(N-methyl-3,4-dichlorophenylacetamido)-3-methylbutyl]pyrrolidine hydrochloride; U-69593, (+)-(5α,7α,8β)-N-methyl-N-[7-(1-pyrrolidinyl)-1-oxaspiro[4,5]dec-8-yl]benzeneacetamide; U-50488, (±)-trans-3,4-dichloro-N-methyl-N-[2-(1-pyrrolidinyl)cyclohexyl]-benzeneacetamide; PD 117302, (±)-trans-N-methyl-N-[2-(1-pyrrolidinyl)cyclohexyl]benzo[b]thiophene-4-acetamide; U-62066, (±)-(5α,7α,8β)-3,4-dichloro-N-methyl-N-[7-(1-pyrrolidinyl)-1-oxaspiro[4,5]dec-8-yl] benzeneacetamide; Mr 2034, (−)-α5,9-dimethyl-2-(L-tetrahydrofurfuryl)-2'-hydroxy-6,7-benzomorphan; Mr 2266, (−)-α5,9-diethyl-2-(3-furylmethyl)-2'-hydroxy-6,7-benzomorphan.

[a] HUNTER et al. (1990); [b] PATERSON (1991); [c] KOSTERLITZ et al. (1990); [d] KOSTERLITZ and PATERSON (1985); [e] MAGNAN et al. (1982); [f] TAKEMORI et al. (1988).

(PORTOGHESE et al. 1988), which has a binding profile similar to that of ICI 174864 but is over 1500 times more potent than the peptide (Table 11).

2. Agonist Activity in Bioassays

In the myenteric plexus preparation, which has no δ-receptors, all compounds with the exception of [D-Ala^2,(2R,3S)-∇^EMePhe^4,L-Leu^5]enkephalin and [D-Ala^2,D-Leu^5]enkephalin are much less potent than in the vasa deferentia of the mouse or the hamster (Table 12). The hamster vas deferens contains only δ-receptors; the agonist activities in the mouse vas deferens, which contains μ-, δ-, and κ-receptors, are also most likely to be at δ-receptors since the K_e value of naloxone is higher than $20\,nM$ (KOSTERLITZ et al. 1980; MOSBERG et al. 1983). In the absence of data in the hamster vas deferens, verification of δ-binding selectivity may be obtained when the ratio of IC$_{50}$ at the μ- and κ-receptors in the myenteric plexus to the IC$_{50}$ in the mouse vas deferens is high, e.g., 1000 or more with [D-Pen^2,p-ClPhe^4,D-Pen^5]enkephalin.

The δ-ligands tested have no agonist action in the rabbit vas deferens. The selective δ-ligands [D-Pen^2,D-Pen^5]enkephalin and [D-Pen^2, L-Pen^5]enkephalin are inactive in the rat vas deferens.

δ-Ligands with low selectivity for the δ-binding site have weak agonist activity in the rat vas deferens (Table 12) which is not blocked by the δ-antagonist ICI 174864 (SHEEHAN et al. 1988); antagonism by naloxone is obtained at a concentration higher that required to block μ-ligands (GILLAN et al. 1981). It may be concluded that the rat vas deferens contains no δ-receptors.

It is of interest that there is no correlation between affinity at the δ-binding site and potency in the mouse vas deferens. In particular, the finding that [D-Ala^2,(2R,3S)-∇^EMePhe^4,L-Leu^5]enkephalin has a very low potency in the vas deferens (IC$_{50}$, 2000 nM) but has a K_i of 13 nM at the δ-binding site, has been interpreted as evidence for subtypes of δ-receptors (SHIMOHIGASHI et al. 1987; VAUGHN et al. 1990). So far, this compound has not been tested for δ-activity on the hamster vas deferens.

3. Antagonist Activity in Bioassays

ICI 174864 is an antagonist at δ-receptors in the mouse and hamster vas deferentia (Table 15). In agreement with its high δ-selectivity in binding assays, ICI 174864 has no antagonist effect at μ- or κ-receptors when the concentrations are 100 greater than that necessary for blocking δ-receptors.

Naltrindole is about 60 times more potent than ICI 174864 at antagonizing δ-ligands in the mouse vas deferens. It is 81 times more potent at δ-receptors than at μ-receptors and 370 times more potent at δ-receptors than at κ-receptors (Table 15).

III. Compounds with a Preference for the κ-Binding Site

1. Activity in Binding Assays

The first near-selective κ-agonist was the benzodiazepine derivative ti-fluadom (RÖMER et al. 1982), which has a relative κ-affinity of 0.84 (Table 13). Since some of the peptides derived from prodynorphin have a relative κ-affinity of up to 0.83 (Table 3), a number of analogues of dynorphin A have been synthesized. Of these, [D-Pro[10]]dynorphin A(1–11) (GAIRIN et al. 1986) is a κ-preferring analogue with a relative affinity of 0.94 and an unusually high affinity of $35\,nM^{-1}$ (Table 13).

The most selective ligands for the κ-binding site are some benzene-acetamide derivatives. The first compound was U-50488 (VON VOIGTLANDER et al. 1983), which was followed by U-62066 (spiradoline) and U-69593 (LAHTI et al. 1985). Related compounds are ICI 197067 (COSTELLO et al. 1988), PD117302 (CLARK et al. 1988), and CI-997 (HUNTER et al. 1990). They are selective κ-ligands with relative affinities of more than 0.99 and potencies varying from 0.74 to 9.1 nM (Table 13).

Binaltorphimine and norbinaltorphimine (PORTOGHESE et al. 1987) are of particular interest. In binding assays binaltorphimine interacts with κ-sites and with μ-sites whereas norbinaltorphimine is a selective κ-ligand with a relative κ-affinity of 0.95 (Table 13). In bioassays these compounds are antagonists (Table 15).

2. Agonist Activity in Bioassays

All compounds, with the exception of diprenorphine, are agonists in the guinea pig myenteric plexus preparation, the rabbit vas deferens, and the mouse vas deferens (Table 14); the available data indicate that they are less potent in the vasa deferentia than in the myenteric plexus. Diprenorphine, on the other hand, has agonist activity only in the guinea pig myenteric plexus. These agonist actions are at κ-receptors (LORD et al. 1977; RÖMER et al. 1980; CORBETT et al. 1986; JIN et al. 1987; COSTELLO et al. 1988; MEECHAM et al. 1989). The compounds have little effect at the δ-receptors in the hamster vas deferens.

It is important to note that Mr 2034, ethylketazocine, diprenorphine, and bremazocine are antagonists at μ-receptors and at δ-receptors although they are agonists at κ-receptors (Table 15).

3. Antagonist Activity in Bioassays

Although Mr 2266 displays a preference for the κ-binding site (Table 13), this κ-selectivity is not reflected in bioassays (Table 14). It is equipotent as an antagonist of κ- and of μ-ligands in the guinea pig myenteric plexus and mouse vas deferens and in the rat vas deferens it is an effective antagonist of

Table 14. Inhibitory effects (IC$_{50}$,nM) of opioids with a preference for the κ-binding site on the electrically evoked contractions of the myenteric plexus-longitudinal muscle of the guinea pig (GPI) and the vasa deferentia of the mouse (MVD), hamster (HVD), rabbit (LVD), and rat (RVD)

	GPI (μ + κ)	MVD (μ + δ + κ)	HVD (δ)	LVD (κ)	RVD (μ)
κ-*Agonists*					
CI-977	0.09[a]	ND	ND	3.3[a]	ND
ICI 197067	0.18[b]	15[b]	ND	ND	ND
U-69593	2.00[c]	ND	>10000[c]	33[c]	>10000[c]
U-50488	16[d]	11[d]	>10000[e]	33[d]	>10000[d]
PD 117302	1.0[a]	ND	ND	58[a]	ND
U-62066	0.88[a]	ND	ND	29[a]	ND
[D-Pro^{10}]dynorphin A(1–11)	3.3[f]	ND	930[f]	12[f]	ND
Tifluadom	0.39[g]	15[g]	>10000[h]	5.7[g]	>10000[g]
(−)-Bremazocine*	0.13[i]	1.98[i]	>10000[e]	4.2[g]	Inactive[i]
(−)-Ethylketazocine*	0.18[i]	4.4[i]	>10000[e]	40[g]	Inactive[j]
Etorphine	0.08[i]	0.40[i]	210[e]	ND	5.0[i]
Diprenorphine**	1.4[j]	>10000[j]	>10000[j]	>10000[j]	>10000[j]
Mr 2034*	0.77[i]	20[i]	>10000[e]	96[g]	Inactive[i]

ND, not determined.
* Antagonist activity at μ- and δ-receptors; ** antagonist activity at μ-, δ-, and κ-receptors (see Table 15).
[a] Hunter et al. (1990); [b] Costello et al. (1988); [c] Corbett et al. (1985a); [d] Jin et al. (1987); [e] McKnight et al. (1985); [f] Gairin et al. (1986); [g] Miller et al. 1986; [h] Miller and Shaw (1985); [i] Magnan et al. (1982); [j] Traynor et al. (1987).

the selective μ-ligand [D-Ala^2,MePhe^4,Gly-ol^5]enkephalin. Mr 2266 is less potent as an antagonist at δ-receptors.

Diprenorphine is an antagonist at all opioid receptors with the exception of the κ-receptors in the guinea pig ileum, where it has agonist activity (Table 15).

Norbinaltorphimine is a more selective κ-antagonist than binaltorphimine as the ratio of the K_e at κ-receptors to the K_e at μ-receptors is 500 for norbinaltorphimine but is only 38 for binaltorphimine (Table 15). As norbinaltorphimine is also a more potent κ-antagonist, both binding assays and bioassays indicate that norbinaltorphimine is a highly potent and selective κ-antagonist. However, the in vivo selectivity of norbinaltorphimine is less than that anticipated from in vitro results (Birch et al. 1987).

Bremazocine, ethylketazocine, and Mr 2034 are antagonists at the δ-receptors in the hamster vas deferens and at the μ-receptors in the rat vas deferens (Table 15). Since these compounds are potent κ-agonists in the mouse vas deferens and the guinea pig ileum, it is difficult to demonstrate their antagonist actions at μ- and δ-receptors in these tissues. As far as bremazocine is concerned, it is possible to determine its μ-antagonist potency in the guinea pig myenteric plexus after irreversible blockade of

Table 15. Antagonist potencies (K_e, nM) of opioids in the myenteric plexus-longitudinal muscle of the guinea pig ileum (GPI) and the vasa deferentia of the mouse (MVD), hamster (HVD), rabbit (LVD), and rat (RVD)

	GPI		MVD			HVD	LVD	RVD
					K_e (nM)			
	μ	κ	μ	δ	κ	δ	κ	μ
Compounds with a preference for the μ-binding site								
μ-Antagonists								
D-Phe-Cys-Tyr-D-Trp-Orn-Thr-Pen-Thr-NH$_2$ (CTOP)	16[a]	444[a]	ND	NA 1μM[b]	ND	ND	ND	ND
Tic-D-Phe-Cys-Tyr-D-Trp-Arg-Thr-Pen-Thr-NH$_2$ (TCTAP)	2.0[b]	ND	ND	NA 1μM[b]	ND	ND	ND	ND
Cyprodime	31[c]	1157[c]	55[c]	6108[c]	1551[c]	ND	ND	62[c]
Naltrexone	0.36[d]	4.4[d]	1.2[e]	12[e]	4.4[e]	ND	9[e]	3.1[e]
Naloxone	1.9[f]	18[f]	1.6[g]	49[h]	16[i]	51[j]	35[e]	7.5[g]
(−)-Win 44441	0.67[k]	2.8[k]	1.4[e]	15[e]	5.5[e]	ND	14[e]	0.5[e]
Compounds with a preference for the δ-binding site								
δ-Antagonists								
ICI 174864	NA 1μM[l]	ND	>5000[e]	17[m]	>5000[e]	44[j]	>10000[e]	ND
Naltrindole	22[n]	100[n]	ND	0.27[n]	ND	ND	ND	ND
ICI 154129	8000[o]	ND	7408[o]	130[m]	>3000[o]	937[p]	ND	ND
16-Methylcyprenorphine	0.65[q]	33[q]	1.8[q]	0.73[q]	60[q]	17[q]	62[q]	2.2[r]

Table 15. *Continued*

	K_e(nM)							
	GPI		MVD			HVD	LVD	RVD
	μ	κ	μ	κ	δ	δ	κ	μ
Compounds with a preference for the κ-binding site								
κ-Agonists								
(−)-Bremazocine	1.6[s]	Ag	ND	Ag	ND	16[j]	Ag	2.7[g]
(−)-Ethylketazocine	ND	Ag	ND	Ag	ND	200[j]	Ag	82[g]
Diprenorphine	0.31[t]	Ag	0.4[e]	0.5[e]	3.6[e]	1.5[t]	1.4[t]	0.20[t]
Mr 2034	ND	Ag	ND	Ag	ND	245[j]	Ag	18[g]
κ-Antagonists								
Norbinaltorphimine	25[u]	0.05[u]	25[u]	0.063[u]	16[u]	25[u]	0.041[u]	40[u]
Mr 2266	1.5[y]	1.3[y]	3.7[e]	2.2[w]	14[w]	20[x]	2.7[w]	3.5[e]
Binaltorphimine	4.6[y]	0.12[z]	13[y]	0.22[y]	3.1[y]	ND	ND	ND
TENA	6.3[k]	0.18[k]	15[k]	7.1[k]	100[k]	ND	ND	ND

ND, not determined; NA, not active. Ag agonist at κ-receptors (see Table 14). The antagonist potencies were determined at μ-receptors against [D-Ala²,MePhe⁴,Gly-ol⁵]enkephalin [a,c,f,g,n,p,r,s,t,v,w,x,y], Tyr-Pro-MePhe-D-Pro-NH₂ [b], normorphine [c,d,l,q,t,u], or morphine [k], at δ-receptors against [D-Pen²,D-Pen⁵]enkephalin [b,h,j,n,w,y], [D-Ala²,D-Leu⁵]enkephalin [c,t,u,x,z], or [D-Thr²,L-Leu⁵]enkephalyl-Thr [e]) and at κ-receptors against U-69 593 [a,f,y], U-50 488 [i,o,v,w,z] or ethylketazocine [c,d,e,k,n,q,t,u]).

TENA is 6β,6′β[ethylenebis(oxyethyleneimino)]bis[17-(cyclopropylmethyl)-4,5α-epoxymorphinan-3,14-diol].

[a] KOSTERLITZ and PATERSON (1990); [b] KRAMER et al. (1989); [c] SCHMIDHAMMER et al. (1989); [d] ARCHER et al. (1985); [e] MILLER et al. (1986); [f] CORBETT et al. (1985a); [g] GILLAN et al. (1981); [h] MOSBERG et al. (1983); [i] COSTELLO et al. (1988); [j] McKNIGHT et al. (1985); [k] PORTOGHESE and TAKEMORI (1985); [l] COHEN et al. (1986); [m] BERZETEI et al. (1987); [n] PORTOGHESE et al. (1988); [o] SHAW et al. (1982); [p] MILLER and SHAW (1985); [q] SMITH (1987); [r] SHEEHAN et al. (1988); [s] CORBETT and KOSTERLITZ (1986); [t] TRAYNOR et al. (1987); [u] BIRCH et al. (1987); [v] JIN et al. (1987); [w] BERZETEI et al. (1988); [x] SHEEHAN et al. (1986); [y] SCHMIDHAMMER and SMITH (1989); [z] PORTOGHESE et al. (1987).

the κ-receptors by preincubation of the tissue with β-chlornaltrexamine (CORBETT and KOSTERLITZ 1986).

References

Akil H, Young E, Watson SJ (1981) Opiate binding properties of naturally occurring N- and C-terminus modified β-endorphins. Peptides 2:289–292

Akiyama K, Gee KW, Mosberg HI, Hruby VJ, Yamamura HI (1985) Characterization of [³H][2-D-penicillamine,5-D-penicillamine]-enkephalin binding to δ opiate receptors in the rat brain and neuroblastoma-glioma hybrid cell line (NG 108–15). Proc Natl Acad Sci USA 82:2543–2547

Amiche M, Sagan S, Mor A, Delfour A, Nicolas P (1988) Characterization of the receptor binding profile of ³H-dermorphin in the rat brain. Int J Pept Protein Res 32:506–511

Amiche M, Sagan S, Mor A, Delfour A, Nicolas P (1989) Dermenkephalin (Tyr-D-Met-Phe-His-Leu-Met-Asp-NH₂): a potent and fully specific agonist for the δ-opioid receptor. Mol Pharmacol 35:774–779

Archer S, Seyed-Mozaffari A, Ward S, Kosterlitz HW, Paterson SJ, McKnight AT, Corbett AD (1985) 10-Ketonaltrexone and 10-ketooxymorphone. J Med Chem 28:974–976

Berzetei IP, Yamamura HI, Duckles SP (1987) Characterization of rabbit ear artery opioid receptors using a δ-selective agonist and antagonist. Eur J Pharmacol 139:61–66

Berzetei IP, Fong A, Yamamura HI, Duckles SP (1988) Characterization of κ-opioid receptors in the rabbit ear artery. Eur J Pharmacol 151:449–455

Birch PJ, Hayes AG, Sheehan MJ, Tyers MB (1987) Norbinaltorphimine: antagonist profile at κ opioid receptors. Eur J Pharmacol 144:405–408

Blumberg H, Dayton HB, George M, Rapaport DN (1961) N-allylnoroxymorphine: a potent narcotic antagonist. Fed Proc 2:311

Boyle SJ, Meecham KG, Hunter JC, Hughes J (1990) [³H]-CI-977: a highly selective ligand for the κ-opioid receptor in both guinea-pig and rat forebrain. Mol Neuropharmacol 1:23–29

Chang KJ, Wei ET, Killian A, Chang JK (1983) Potent morphiceptin analogs: structure activity relationships and morphine-like properties. J Pharmacol Exp Ther 227:403–408

Chavkin C, James IF, Goldstein A (1982) Dynorphin is a specific endogenous ligand of the κ opioid receptor. Science 215:413–415

Cheng Y-C, Prusoff WH (1973) Relationship between the inhibition constant (Kᵢ) and the concentration of inhibitor which causes 50 per cent inhibition (I50) of an enzymatic reaction. Biochem Pharmacol 22:3099–3108

Clark CR, Birchmore B, Sharif NA, Hunter JC, Hill RG, Hughes J (1988) PD117302: a selective agonist for the κ-opioid receptor. Br J Pharmacol 93:618–626

Cohen ML, Shuman RT, Osborne JJ, Gesellchen PD (1986) Opioid agonist activity of ICI 174864 and its carboxypeptidase degradation product, LY 281217. J Pharmacol Exp Ther 238:769–771

Corbett AD, Paterson SJ, McKnight AT, Magnan J, Kosterlitz HW (1982) Dynorphin-(1–8) and dynorphin-(1–9) are ligands for the κ-subtype of opiate receptor. Nature 299:79–81

Corbett AD, Gillan MGC, Kosterlitz HW, McKnight AT, Paterson SJ, Robson LE (1984) Selectivities of opioid peptide analogues as agonists and antagonists at the δ-receptor. Br J Pharmacol 83:271–279

Corbett AD, Gillan MGC, Kosterlitz HW, Paterson SJ (1985a) Binding and pharmacological profile of a highly selective ligand for the κ-opioid receptor – U-69,593. Br J Pharmacol 86:704P

Corbett AD, Kosterlitz HW, McKnight AT, Paterson SJ, Robson LE (1985b) Pre-incubation of the guinea-pig myenteric plexus with β-funaltrexamine: discrepancy between binding assays and bioassays. Br J Pharmacol 85:665–673

Corbett AD, Kosterlitz HW (1986) Bremazocine is an agonist at κ-opioid receptors and an antagonist at μ-opioid receptors in the guinea pig myenteric plexus. Br J Pharmacol 89:245–249

Costa T, Wüster M, Herz A, Shimohigashi Y, Chen H-C, Rodbard D (1985) Receptor binding and biological activity of bivalent enkephalins. Biochem Pharmacol 34:25–30

Costello GF, Main BG, Barlow JJ, Carroll JA, Shaw JS (1988) A novel series of potent and selective agonists at opioid κ-receptors. Eur J Pharmacol 151:475–478

Cotton R, Giles MG, Miller L, Shaw JS, Timms D (1984) ICI 174864: a highly selective antagonist for the opioid δ-receptor. Eur J Pharmacol 97:331–332

Cotton R, Kosterlitz HW, Paterson SJ, Rance MJ, Traynor JR (1985) The use of [^{3}H]-[D-Pen^2,D-Pen^5]enkephalin as a highly selective ligand for the δ-binding site. Br J Pharmacol 84:927–932

Cox BM, Chavkin C (1983) Comparison of dynorphin-selective kappa-receptors in mouse vas deferens and guinea-pig ileum. Mol Pharmacol 23:36–43

Delay-Goyet P, Zajac J-M, Rigaudy P, Foucaud B, Roques BP (1985) Comparative binding properties of linear and cyclic δ-selective enkephalin analogues: [^{3}H]-[D-Thr^2,Leu^5]enkephalyl-Thr^6 and [^{3}H]-[D-Pen^2,D-Pen^5]enkephalin. FEBS Lett 183:439–443

Delay-Goyet P, Seguin C, Gacel G, Roques BP (1988) [^{3}H]-[D-Ser(O-tert-butyl)^2,Leu^5]enkephalyl-Thr^6 and [^{3}H]-[D-Ser(O-tert-butyl)^2,Leu^5]enkephalyl-Thr^6(O-tert-butyl). Two new enkephalin analogs with both a good selectivity and a high affinity towards δ-opioid binding sites. J Biol Chem 263:4124–4130

Donnerer J, Oka K, Brossi A, Rice KC, Spector S (1986) Presence and formation of codeine and morphine in the rat. Proc Natl Acad Sci USA 83:4566–4567

Donnerer J, Cardinale G, Coffey J, Lisak CA, Jardine I, Spector S (1987) Chemical characterization and regulation of endogenous morphine and codeine in the rat. J Pharmacol Exp Ther 242:583–587

Erspamer V, Melchiorri P, Falconieri-Erspamer G, Negri L, Corsi R, Severini C, Barra D, Simmaco M, Kreil G (1989) Deltorphins: a family of naturally occurring peptides with high affinity and selectivity for δ opioid binding sites. Proc Natl Acad Sci USA 86:5188–5192

Fischli W, Goldstein A, Hunkapillar MV, Hood LE (1982) Isolation and amino acid sequence analysis of a 4000 dalton dynorphin from porcine pituitary. Proc Natl Acad Sci USA 79:5435–5437

Gacel G, Fournie-Zaluski MC, Roques BP (1980) Tyr-D-Ser-Gly-Phe-Leu-Thr, a highly selective ligand for δ-opiate receptors. FEBS Lett 118:245–247

Gacel G, Dauge V, Breuze P, Delay-Goyet P, Roques BP (1988) Development of conformationally constrained linear peptides exhibiting a high affinity and pronounced selectivity for δ-opioid receptors. J Med Chem 31:1891–1897

Gairin JE, Jomary C, Prodayrol L, Cros J, Meunier J-C (1986) ^{125}I-DPDYN, monoiodo[D-Pro^{10}]dynorphin(1–11): a highly radioactive and selective probe for the study of kappa opioid receptors. Biochem Biophys Res Commun 134:1142–1150

Gillan MGC, Kosterlitz HW, Magnan J (1981) Unexpected antagonism in the rat vas deferens by benzomorphans which are agonists in other pharmacological tests. Br J Pharmacol 72:13–15

Goldstein A (1987) Binding selectivity profiles for ligands of multiple receptor types: focus on opioid receptors. Trends Neurosci 8:456–459

Goldstein A, James IF (1984) Site-directed alkylation of multiple opioid receptors: II. Pharmacological selectivity. Mol Pharmacol 25:343–348

Goldstein A, Naidu A (1989) Multiple opioid receptors: ligand selectivity profiles and binding site signatures. Mol Pharmacol 36:265–272

Gubler U, Seeberg PH, Hoffman BJ, Gage LP, Udenfriend S (1982) Molecular cloning establishes proenkephalin as precursor of enkephalin-containing peptides. Nature 295:206–208

Hambrook JM, Morgan BA, Rance MJ, Smith CFC (1976) Mode of deactivation of the enkephalins by rat and human plasma and rat brain homogenates. Nature 262:782–783

Handa BK, Lane AC, Lord JAH, Morgan BA, Rance MJ, Smith CFC (1981) Analogues of β-LPH$_{61-64}$ possessing selective agonist activity at μ-opiate receptors. Eur J Pharmacol 70:531–540

Hawkins KN, Morelli M, Gulya K, Chang K-J, Yamamura HI (1987) Autoradiographic localization of [^{3}H][MePhe^3,D-Pro^4] morphiceptin ([^{3}H]PL O17) to μ-opioid receptors in rat brain. Eur J Pharmacol 133:351–352

Hawkins KN, Knapp RJ, Lui GK, Gulya K, Kazmierski W, Wan Y-P, Pelto JT, Hruby VJ, Yamamura HI (1989) [^{3}H]-[D-Phe-Cys-Tyr-D-Trp-Orn-Thr-Pen-Thr-NH$_2$] ([^{3}H]CTOP), a potent and highly selective peptide for μ opioid receptors in rat brain. J Pharmacol Exp Ther 248:73–80

Hayes AG, Sheehan MJ, Tyers MB (1985) Determination of the receptor selectivity of opioid agonists in the guinea-pig ileum and mouse vas deferens using β-FNA. Br J Pharmacol 86:899–904

Henschen A, Lottspeich F, Brantl V, Teschemacher H (1979) Novel opioid peptides derived from casein (β-casomorphins): II. Structure of active components from bovine casein peptone. Hoppe-Seyler's Z Physiol Chem 360:1217–1224

Höllt V, Sanchez-Blasquez P, Garzon J (1985) Multiple opioid ligands and receptors in the control of nociception. Philos Trans R Soc Lond [Biol] 308:299–310

Hughes J, Kosterlitz HW, Leslie FM (1975a) Effect of morphine on adrenergic transmission in the mouse vas deferens. Assessment of agonist and antagonist potencies of narcotic analgesics. Br J Pharmacol 53:371–381

Hughes J, Smith TW, Kosterlitz HW, Fothergill LA, Morgan BA, Morris HR (1975b) Identification of two related peptides from the brain with potent opiate agonist activity. Nature 258:577–579

Hunter JC, Leighton GE, Meecham KG, Boyle S, Horwell DC, Rees DC, Hughes J (1990) CI-977, a novel and selective agonist for the κ-opioid receptor. Br J Pharmacol 101:183–189

Hurlbut DE, Evans CJ, Barchas JD, Leslie FM (1987) Pharmacological properties of a proenkephalin A-derived peptide: BAM 18. Eur J Pharmacol 138:359–366

Hutchinson M, Kosterlitz HW, Leslie FM, Waterfield AA, Terenius L (1975) Assessment in the guinea-pig ileum and mouse vas deferens of benzomorphans which have strong antinociceptive activity but do not substitute for morphine in the dependent monkey. Br J Pharmacol 55:541–546

Jin W, Chen X, Chi Z (1987) The choice of opioid receptor subtype in isolated preparations by ohmefentanyl. Sci Sin 30:176–181

Kakidani H, Furutani Y, Takahashi H, Noda M, Morimoto Y, Hirose T, Asai M, Inayama S, Nakanishi S, Numa S (1982) Cloning and sequence analysis of cDNA for porcine β-neo-endorphin/dynorphin precursor. Nature 298:245–249

Kazmierski W, Wire WS, Lui GK, Knapp RJ, Shook JE, Burks TF, Yamamura H, Hruby VJ (1988) Design and synthesis of somatostatin analogues with topographical properties that lead to highly potent and specific μ opioid receptor antagonists with greatly reduced binding at somatostatin receptors. J Med Chem 31:2170–2177

Kilpatrick DL, Wahlstrom A, Lahm H-W, Blacher R, Udenfriend S (1982) Rimorphin, a unique, naturally occurring [Leu]enkephalin-containing peptide found in association with dynorphin and α-neo-endorphin. Proc Natl Acad Sci USA 79:6480–6483

Kosterlitz HW (1985) Opioid peptides and their receptors. Proc R Soc Lond [Biol] 225:27–40

Kosterlitz HW, Paterson SJ (1981) Tyr-D-Ala-Gly-MePhe-NH(CH₂)₂OH is a selective ligand for the μ-opiate binding site. Br J Pharmacol 73:299P

Kosterlitz HW, Paterson SJ (1985) Types of opioid receptors: relation to antinociception. Philos Trans R Soc Lond [Biol] 308:291–297

Kosterlitz HW, Paterson SJ (1990) D-Phe-Cys-Tyr-D-Trp-Orn-Thr-Pen-Thr-NH₂ is a highly selective μ-ligand with low in vitro antagonist activity. Br J Pharmacol 99:291P

Kosterlitz HW, Lord JAH, Paterson SJ, Waterfield AA (1980) Effect of changes in the structure of enkephalins and of narcotic analgesic drugs on their interaction with μ- and δ-receptors. Br J Pharmacol 68:333–342

Kosterlitz HW, Corbett AD, Paterson SJ (1990) Opioid receptors and their ligands. In: Harris LS (ed) Problems of drug dependence 1989. Natl Inst Drug Abuse Res Monogr Ser 95:159–166

Kramer TH, Shook JE, Kazmierski W, Ayres EA, Wire WS, Hruby VJ, Burks TF (1989) Novel peptidic mu opioid antagonists: pharmacologic characterization in vitro and in vivo. J Pharmacol Exp Ther 249:544–551

Kreil G, Barra D, Simmaco M, Erspamer V, Falconieri-Erspamer G, Negri L, Severini C, Corsi R, Melchiorri P (1989) Deltorphin, a novel amphibian skin peptide with high selectivity and affinity for δ opioid receptors. Eur J Pharmacol 162:123–128

Lahti RA, Mickelson MM, McCall JM, Von Voigtlander (1985) [³H]U-69593, a highly selective ligand for the opioid κ-receptor. Eur J Pharmacol 109:281–284

Lazarus LH, Wilson WE, de Castiglione R, Guglietta A (1989) Dermorphin gene sequence peptide with high affinity and selectivity for δ opioid receptors. J Biol Chem 264:3047

Lemaire S, Magnan J, Regoli D (1978) Rat vas deferens: a specific bioassay for endogenous opioid peptides. Br J Pharmacol 64:327–329

Leslie FM (1987) Methods used in the study of opioids. Pharmacol Rev 39:197–249

Leslie FM, Chavkin C, Cox BM (1980) Opioid binding properties of brain and peripheral tissues: evidence for heterogeneity in opioid ligand binding sites. J Pharmacol Exp Ther 214:395–402

Liao CS, Day AR, Freer RJ (1981) Evidence for a single opioid receptor type in the field stimulated rat vas deferens. Life Sci 29:2617–2622

Lord JAH, Waterfield AA, Hughes J, Kosterlitz HW (1977) Endogenous opioid peptides: multiple agonists and receptors. Nature 267:495–499

Magnan J, Paterson SJ, Tavani A, Kosterlitz HW (1982) The binding spectrum of narcotic analgesic drugs with different agonist and antagonist properties. Naunyn Schmiedebergs Arch Pharmacol 319:197–205

Mains RE, Eipper BA, Ling N (1977) Common precursor to corticotropins and endorphins. Proc Natl Acad Sci USA 74:3014–3018

McKnight AT, Corbett AD, Paterson SJ, Magnan J, Kosterlitz HW (1982) Comparison of in vitro potencies in pharmacological and binding assays after inhibition of peptidases reveals that dynorphin (1–9) is a potent κ-agonist. Life Sci 31:1725–1728

McKnight AT, Corbett AD, Kosterlitz HW (1983) Increase in potencies of opioid peptides after peptidase inhibition. Eur J Pharmacol 86:393–402

McKnight AT, Corbett AD, Marcoli M, Kosterlitz HW (1984) Hamster vas deferens contains δ-opioid receptors. Neuropeptides 5:97–100

McKnight AT, Corbett AD, Marcoli M, Kosterlitz HW (1985) The opioid receptors in the hamster vas deferens are of the δ-type. Neuropharmacology 24:1011–1017

Meecham KJ, Boyle SJ, Hunter JC, Hughes J (1989) An in vitro profile of activity for the (+) and (−) enantiomers of spiradoline and PD117302. Eur J Pharmacol 173:151–157

Miller L, Shaw JS (1985) Characterization of the δ-opioid receptor on the hamster vas deferens. Neuropeptides 6:531–536

Miller L, Shaw JS, Whiting EM (1986) The contribution of intrinsic activity to the actions of opioids in vitro. Br J Pharmacol 87:595–601

Mor A, Delfour A, Sagan S, Amiche M, Pradelles P, Rossier J, Nicolas P (1989) Isolation of dermenkephalin from amphibian skin, a high affinity δ-selective opioid heptapeptide containing a D-amino acid residue. FEBS Lett 255:269–274

Mosberg HI, Hurst R, Hruby VJ, Gee K, Yamamura HI, Galligan JJ, Burks TF (1983) Bis-penicillamine enkephalins possess highly improved specificity towards δ opioid receptors. Proc Natl Acad Sci USA 80:5871–5874

Nakanishi S, Inoue A, Kita T, Nakamura M, Chang ACY, Cohen SM, Numa S (1979) Nucleotide sequence of cloned cDNA for bovine corticotropin-β-lipotropin precursor. Nature 278:423–427

Noda M, Furutani Y, Takahashi H, Toyosato M, Hirose T, Inayama S, Nakanishi S, Numa S (1982) Cloning and sequence analysis of cDNA for bovine preproenkephalin. Nature 295:202–206

Oka T, Negishi K, Suda M, Matsumiya T, Inazu T, Masaaki U (1981) Rabbit vas deferens: a specific bioassay for opioid κ-recptor agonists. Eur J Pharmacol 73:235–236

Paterson SJ (1986) Multiple opioid binding sites and their ligands. PhD thesis, University of Aberdeen

Paterson SJ (1991) Opioid receptors. In: Stone TW (ed) Aspects of Synaptic Transmission: LTP, galanin, opioids, autonomic and 5-HT, vol 1. Taylor and Francis, London, pp 117–140

Paterson SJ, Robson LE, Kosterlitz HW (1984) Opioid receptors. In: Udenfriend S, Meienhoffer J (eds) The peptides: analysis, synthesis and biology, vol 6. Academic, London, pp 147–189

Pelton JT, Gulya K, Hruby VJ, Duckles SJ, Yamamura HI (1986) Somatostatin analogs with affinity for opiate receptors in rat brain binding assays. Peptides 6 (Suppl 1):159–163

Porini G, Petrillo P, Colombo M, Tavani A (1990) In vitro binding profile of cyprodime, a reported mu-opioid antagonist. In: van Ree JM, Mulder AH, Wiegant VM, van Wimersma Greidanus TB (eds) New leads in opioid research. Excerpta Medica, Amsterdam, pp 225–227

Portoghese PS, Takemori AE (1985) TENA, a selective kappa opioid receptor antagonist. Life Sci 36:810–805

Portoghese PS, Larson DL, Jiang JB, Caruso TP, Takemori AE (1979) Synthesis and pharmacological characterization of an alkylating analogue (chlornaltrexamine) of naltrexone with ultra-long lasting narcotic antagonist properties. J Med Chem 22:168–173

Portoghese PS, Larson DL, Sayre DS, Fries DS, Takemori AE (1980) A novel opioid receptor site directed alkylating agent with irreversible narcotic antagonistic and reversible agonistic activities. J Med Chem 26:1341–1343

Portoghese PS, Lipkowski AW, Takemori AE (1987) Binaltorphimine and nor-binaltorphimine, potent and selective κ-opioid receptor antagonists. Life Sci 40:1287–1292

Portoghese PS, Sultana M, Takemori AE (1988) Naltrindole, a highly selective and potent non-peptide δ-opioid receptor antagonist. Eur J Pharmacol 146:185–186

Rezvani A, Höllt V, Way EL (1983) κ-Receptor activities of three opioid peptide families. Life Sci 33 (Suppl 1):271–274

Roberts JL, Herbert E (1977a) Characterization of a common precursor to corticotropin and β-lipotropin: cell-free synthesis of the precursor and identification of corticotropin peptides in the molecule. Proc Natl Acad Sci USA 74:4826–4830

Roberts JL, Herbert E (1977b) Characterization of a common precursor to corticotropin and β-lipotropin: identification of β-lipotropin peptides and their arrangement relative to corticotropin in the precursor synthesized in a cell-free system. Proc Natl Acad Sci USA 74:5300–5304

Römer D, Buscher HH, Hill RC, Pless J, Bauer W, Cardinaux F, Closse A, Hauser D, Huguenin R (1977) A synthetic enkephalin analogue with prolonged parenteral and oral analgesic activity. Nature 268:547–549

Römer D, Buscher H, Hill RC, Maurer R, Petcher TJ, Welle HB, Bakel CCK, Akkerman AM (1980) Bremazocine: a potent, long-acting opiate kappa agonist. Life Sci 27:971–978

Römer D, Buscher H, Hill RC, Maurer R, Petcher TJ, Zeugner H, Benson W, Finner E, Milkowski W, Thies PW (1982) An opioid benzodiazepine. Nature 298:759–760

Sagan S, Corbett AD, Amiche M, Delfour A, Nicolas P, Kosterlitz HW (1991) Opioid activity of dermenkephalin analogues in the guinea-pig myenteric plexus and hamster vas deferens. Br J Pharmacol 104:428–432

Schiller PW, Nguyen TM-D, Maziak LA, Wilkes BC, Lemieux C (1987) Structure-activity relationships of cyclic opioid peptide analogues containing phenylalanine residue in the 3-position. J Med Chem 30:2094–2099

Schiller PW, Nguyen TM-D, Chung NN, Lemieux C (1989) Dermorphin analogues carrying an increased positive charge in their "message" domain display extremely high μ-opioid receptor selectivity. J Med Chem 32:698–703

Schmidhammer H, Smith CFC (1989) A simple and efficient method for the preparation of binaltorphimine and derivatives and determination of their κ-opioid antagonist selectivity. Helv Chim Acta 72:675–677

Schmidhammer H, Burkard WP, Eggstein-Aeppli L, Smith CFC (1989) Synthesis and biological evaluation of 14-alkoxymorphinans: 2. (−)-N-(cyclopropylmethyl)-4, 14-dimethoxymorphinan-6-one, a selective μ opioid receptor antagonist. J Med Chem 32:418–421

Schmidt WK, Tam SW, Shotzberger GS, Smith DH, Clark R, Vernier VG (1985) Nalbuphine. Drug Alcohol Depend 14:339–362

Schulz R, Faase E, Wüster M, Herz A (1979) Selective receptors for β-endorphin in the rat vas deferens. Life Sci 24:843–849

Schulz R, Wüster M, Herz A (1981) Pharmacological characterization of the ε-receptor. J Pharmacol Exp Ther 216:604–606

Shaw JS, Miller L, Turnbull MJ, Gormley JJ, Morley JS (1982) Selective antagonists at the opiate delta-receptor. Life Sci 31:1259–1262

Sheehan MJ, Hayes AG, Tyers MB (1986) Pharmacology of δ-opioid receptors in the hamster vas deferens. Eur J Pharmacol 130:57–64

Sheehan MJ, Hayes AG, Tyers MB (1988) Lack of evidence for ε-opioid receptors in the rat vas deferens. Eur J Pharmacol 154:237–245

Shi P, Niu J, Wu S, Zou G (1981) Enkephalin analogs with extremely high affinity for δ-receptor. Kexue Tongbao 26:750–752

Shimohigashi Y, Costa T, Matsuura S, Chen H-C, Rodbard D (1982) Dimeric enkephalins display affinity and selectivity for the delta opiate receptor. Mol Pharmacol 21:558–563

Shimohigashi Y, Costa T, Pfeiffer A, Herz A, Kimura H, Stammer CH (1987) [E]Phe[4]-enkephalin analogs. Delta receptors in rat brain are different from those in mouse vas deferens. FEBS Lett 222:71–74

Shimohigashi Y, Takano Y, Kamiya H, Costa T, Herz A, Stammer CH (1988) A highly selective ligand for brain δ opiate receptors, a [E]Phe[4]-enkephalin analog, suppresses μ receptor-mediated thermal analgesia by morphine. FEBS Lett 233:289–229

Smith CFC (1987) 16-Me-Cyprenorphine (RX 8008M): a potent opioid antagonist with some δ selectivity. Life Sci 40:267–274

Takemori AE, Begonia YH, Naeseth JS, Portoghese PS (1988) Norbinaltorphimine, a highly selective kappa-opioid antagonist in analgesia and receptor binding assays. J Pharmacol Exp Ther 246:255–258

Toth G, Kramer TH, Knapp R, Lui G, Davis P, Burks TF, Yamamura HI, Hruby VJ (1989) [D-Pen[2],D-Pen[5]]enkephalin analogues with increased affinity and selectivity for δ-opioid receptors. J Med Chem 33:249–253

Traynor JR, Corbett AD, Kosterlitz HW (1987) Diprenorphine has agonist activity at opioid κ-receptors in the myenteric plexus of the guinea-pig ileum. Eur J Pharmacol 137:85–89

Vaughn LK, Knapp RJ, Toth G, Wan Y-P, Hruby VJ, Yamamura HI (1989) A high affinity, highly selective ligand for the delta opioid receptor: [³H]-[D-Pen²,pCl-Phe⁴,D-Pen⁵]enkephalin. Life Sci 45:1001–1008

Vaughn LK, Wire SW, Davis P, Shimohigashi Y, Toth G, Knapp RJ, Hruby VJ, Burks TF, Yamamura HI (1990) Differentiation between rat brain and mouse vas deferens δ-opioid receptors. Eur J Pharmacol 177:99–101

Von Voigtlander PF, Lahti RA, Ludens JH (1983) U-50,488: a selective and structurally novel non-mu (kappa) opioid agonist. J Pharmacol Exp Ther 224:7–12

Weber E, Esch FS, Bohlen P, Paterson SJ, Corbett AD, McKnight AT, Kosterlitz HW, Barchas JD, Evans CJ (1983) Metorphamide: isolation, structure, and biological activity of an amidated opioid octapeptide from bovine brain. Proc Natl Acad Sci USA 80:7362–7366

Weitz CJ, Lowney LI, Faull KF, Feistner G, Goldstein A (1986) Morphine and codeine from mammalian brain. Proc Natl Acad Sci USA 83:9784–9788

Weitz CJ, Faull KF, Goldstein A (1987) Synthesis of the skeleton of the morphine molecule by mammalian liver. Nature 330:674–677

Wüster M, Schulz R, Herz A (1979) Selectivity of opioids towards the μ-, δ-, and ε-opiate receptors. Neurosci Lett 15:193–198

Yeadon M, Kitchen I (1988) Comparative binding of μ and δ selective ligands in whole brain and pons/medulla from rat: affinity profiles of fentanyl derivatives. Neuropharmacology 27:345–348

Zajac JM, Gacel G, Petit F, Dodey P, Rossignol P, Roques B (1983) Deltakephalin, Tyr-D-Thr-Gly-Phe-Leu-Thr: a new highly potent and fully specific agonist for opiate δ-receptors. Biochem Biophys Res Commun 111:390–397

Development of Receptor-Selective Opioid Peptide Analogs as Pharmacologic Tools and as Potential Drugs

P.W. SCHILLER

A. Introduction

Much progress has been made in the elucidation of opioid receptor heterogeneity during the past 15 years. The existence of three major opioid receptor types (μ, δ, κ) (MARTIN et al. 1976; LORD et al. 1977) is now firmly established and there is strong evidence in favor of a fourth receptor type, the ε-receptor (SCHULZ et al. 1979). More recently obtained physiological and receptor binding data led to the proposal of various opioid receptor subtypes (μ_1, μ_2, κ_1, κ_2, κ_3) (reviewed in CLARK et al. 1989). Opioids produce a large variety of well-known central and peripheral effects, including spinal and supraspinal analgesia, tolerance and physical dependence, respiratory depression, euphoria, dysphoria and hallucinations, sedation, appetite suppression and other behavioral effects, control and release of several hormones and neurotransmitters, effects on gastrointestinal motility, hyperthermia/hypothermia, cardiovascular effects, effects on tumor growth, and effects on the immune response. Both for the elucidation of the physiological role(s) of the various receptor classes and for the development of opioid-derived drugs it is of great importance to establish clear-cut correlations between specific opioid receptor types and distinct opioid effects. For this purpose further efforts are needed to develop opioid agonists and antagonists with high selectivity for the various receptor types and subtypes. The fact that morphine displays only limited μ-receptor selectivity is well known and the characterization of the various opioid peptides generated through processing of the three mammalian precursors showed that none of them is very receptor selective (reviewed in HÖLLT 1986). Thus, the enkephalins display only slight preference for δ-receptors over μ-receptors and metorphamide is only moderately μ-selective. The dynorphins preferentially interact with κ-receptors but also bind to μ- and δ-receptors with somewhat lower affinity. β-Endorphin has high affinity for both μ- and δ-receptors and may also interact with a specific receptor of its own, the ε-receptor. The dermorphins display marked but by no means optimal μ-selectivity and the various peptides of the β-casomorphin family are either only moderately μ-selective and/or have relatively low affinity (e.g., morphiceptin). The only naturally occurring opioid peptides with high receptor specificity are the δ-selective deltorphins (ERSPAMER et al. 1989).

Excellent progress has been made in recent years in the development of receptor-selective nonpeptide opioid agonists and antagonists, as described elsewhere in this volume (Chaps. 11, 12). Most of the opioid peptide analogs prepared to date are structurally derived from the enkephalins; however, most interesting analogs of the dermorphins, β-casomorphins, dynorphins, and β-endorphin have also been developed. Major drawbacks of the natural enkephalins, *H*-Tyr-Gly-Gly-Phe-Met(or Leu)-OH, as pharmacologic tools or potential drugs are their susceptibility to rapid enyzmatic degradation, their poor absorption properties, their relative inability to cross the blood-brain barrier, and their lack of sufficient receptor specificity. In an early effort, the stability of the enkephalin molecule against enzymolysis was much improved through substitution of D-alanine in the 2-position of the peptide sequence and through amidation of the C-terminal carboxyl group (PERT et al. 1976). Shortly afterwards, appropriate structural modifications led to enkephalin analogs, such as the Sandoz compound FK33-824 (*H*-Tyr-D-Ala-Gly-MePhe-Met(*O*)-ol) (ROEMER et al. 1977), that were able to produce a long-lasting analgesic effect after systemic administration. Synthetic efforts during the past decade have been mainly aimed at developing opioid peptide analogs with improved receptor selectivity and progress made in this area will be the major topic of this review. The present discussion will be limited to the most selective and the most frequently used opioid peptide analogs and no attempt will be made to write a comprehensive review of the more than 1000 analogs of the enkephalins, β-casomorphins, dermorphins, deltorphins, dynorphins, and β-endorphin that have been synthesized to date. More comprehensive information on structures and activity profiles of opioid peptide analogs is contained in several published review articles (MORLEY 1980; YAMASHIRO and LI 1984; HANSEN and MORGAN 1984; MORLEY and DUTTA 1986; HRUBY and GEHRIG 1989; SCHILLER 1991). The major design strategies that have been used in the development of receptor-selective opioid peptide analogs and that will be discussed in this chapter include:

1. The "classical" approach of substitution, deletion, or addition of natural or artifical (nonproteinogenic) amino acids.
2. Design of bivalent ligands containing two opioid peptide moieties separated by a spacer of appropriate length and simultaneously interacting with two receptor binding sites of the same type.
3. Incorporation of conformational constraints through appropriate peptide cyclizations or substitution of conformationally restricted amino acid analogs.
4. Modification of peptide bonds.

A review of receptor-selective opioid peptide analogs with agonist or reversible antagonist properties will constitute the major part of this chapter. Furthermore, we will discuss a number of selective irreversible opioid receptor ligands that have been obtained through incorporation of chemical (e.g., electrophilic) affinity labels or photoaffinity labels into opioid peptide analogs. The chapter concludes with an examination of the receptor selectivity profiles of opioid peptide analogs that have already been tested in clinical trials or that are of interest as potential future drugs.

B. Determination of Receptor Selectivity

The receptor preference of opioid compounds can be determined and expressed in terms of either receptor binding selectivity or pharmacologic selectivity (JAMES and GOLDSTEIN 1984). Whereas the binding selectivity depends only on the relative affinities for the different receptor types, the pharmacologic selectivity is determined by three parameters – receptor binding affinity, intrinsic activity (efficacy), and receptor reserve – which all may vary among different receptor types.

Opioid receptor binding selectivities are determined by displacement of relatively receptor-selective radioligands from binding sites in rat or guinea pig brain membrane preparations. To determine the binding selectivity ratios as accurately as possible, it is imperative to use the most selective radioligands available in the binding experiments. Since brain membrane preparations contain heterogeneous populations of opioid receptors, the most precise selectivity ratios can be obtained by using membrane preparations that have been enriched in a particular receptor type by means of a selective receptor alkylation/protection procedure (JAMES et al. 1982). Binding selectivity profiles of about 40 opioid ligands have been determined by using the latter method (JAMES and GOLDSTEIN 1984; GOLDSTEIN and NAIDU 1989). Binding competition experiments permit the direct measurement of a compound's IC_{50} for displacing the radioligand. The apparent dissociation constant (K_i) can then be calculated from the determined IC_{50} value and from the dissociation constant and concentration of the radioligand, according to the equation of CHENG and PRUSOFF (1973). Whereas the K_i represents the more correct affinity measure, IC_{50}s only are often indicated in the literature and, accordingly, receptor binding selectivity ratios in the tables of this chapter will be presented either as IC_{50} ratios or as K_i ratios.

Pharmacologic selectivities of opioid compounds can be determined with bioassays based on inhibition of electrically evoked contractions of the guinea pig ileum (GPI), mouse vas deferens (MVD), rat vas deferens (RVD), hamster vas deferens (HVD), and rabbit vas deferens (LVD) (see Chaps. 2, 26). Whereas the HVD and LVD contain quite homogeneous populations of δ- and κ-receptors, respectively, the opioid receptor populations present in the GPI, MVD, and RVD are heterogeneous. In the GPI both μ- and κ-receptors exist and the MVD contains μ- and κ-receptors in addition to the predominant δ-receptors. μ-Receptors and most likely also ε-receptors mediate opioid effects in the RVD. Obviously, the ratios of the

IC$_{50}$ values determined in the most frequently performed GPI and MVD assays are not precise indicators of μ- versus δ-selectivity due to the existing receptor heterogeneity. In particular, relatively low IC$_{50}$(MVD)/IC$_{50}$(GPI) ratios are often observed with highly μ-selective ligands because they interact not only with μ-receptors in the ileum but also with the μ-receptors present in the vas. This is illustrated with the example of morphiceptin, which shows an IC$_{50}$(MVD)/IC$_{50}$(GPI) ratio of only about three, in contrast to the much higher K_i^δ/K_i^μ ratio (~500) obtained in the receptor binding assays.

The assessment of the receptor preferences of the opioid peptide analogs discussed in the present review will be based on receptor binding selectivity ratios rather than on pharmacologic selectivity ratios. The comparison of receptor binding data is of course complicated by the different assay procedures and conditions (radioligands, temperature, ions, etc.) being used in different laboratories. Nevertheless, for the reasons outlined above, receptor binding data permit a more accurate estimate of the selectivity of a ligand with regard to its initial binding to the various types of receptors than it is the case with bioassay data. Agonist potencies obtained in the GPI and MVD assay have been reported for nearly all analogs listed in Tables 1–3, and in the case of peptides with antagonist properties K_e values have been determined with various selective agonists in the in vitro bioassays.

C. Development of μ-, δ-, and κ-Receptor-Selective Opioid Peptide Analogs with Agonist Properties

I. μ-Selective Agonists

Several linear analogs of enkephalin, β-casomorphin, and dermorphin with selectivity for μ-receptors have been obtained through substitution of various natural or artificial amino acids, amino acid deletions, and end group modification or deletion. Opioid peptide dimers and cyclic opioid peptide analogs with high μ-receptor preference have also been developed. The receptor binding profiles of the most important μ-selective opioid peptide analogs with agonist properties that were developed by using these various design strategies are presented in Table 1.

1. Linear Opioid Peptide Analogs

Perhaps the most popular μ-selective enkephalin analog is the pentapeptide *H*-Tyr-D-Ala-Gly-MePhe-Gly-ol (DAGO) (HANDA et al. 1981), which has been tritiated and is often used as a μ-selective radioligand. Enkephalin-related tetrapeptide analogs with very high μ-receptor selectivity are the Lilly compound NMe-Tyr-D-Ala-Gly-*N*(Et)-CH(CH$_2$Ph)-CH$_2$-N(CH$_3$)$_2$

(LY164929) (SHUMAN et al. 1990) and H-Tyr-D-Met(O)-Gly-MePhe-ol (Syndyphalin) (KISO et al. 1981; QUIRION et al. 1982). Both these peptides lack the 5-position residue present in the natural enkephalin sequence and contain an N-alkylated and otherwise modified Phe residue at the C-terminus. Among several C-terminally truncated enkephalin derivatives in which the Phe^4 residue had been replaced by an aliphatic moiety (GACEL et al. 1988a), the analog H-Tyr-D-Ala-Gly-NH-CH$_2$-CH$_2$-CH(CH$_3$)$_2$ (TRIMU 5) turned out to be the most μ-selective one. In a direct comparison under identical binding assay conditions, TRIMU 5 showed a selectivity ratio (K_i^δ/K_i^μ = 102) comparable to that of DAGO (K_i^δ/K_i^μ = 179) but slightly lower μ-receptor affinity.

Unlike the δ-selective enkephalins, the heptapeptide β-casomorphin (H-Tyr-Pro-Phe-Pro-Gly-Pro-Ile-OH), first isolated from an enzymatic casein digest by HENSCHEN et al. (1979), displays moderate μ-selectivity (K_i^δ/K_i^μ = 8.33). Subsequently, the N-terminal tetrapeptide amide of β-casomorphin, also known as morphiceptin, was shown to be considerably more μ-selective than the parent heptapeptide (CHANG et al. 1981). A further improvement in μ-selectivity was observed with the morphiceptin analog H-Tyr-Pro-NMePhe-D-Pro-NH$_2$ (PLO17) (CHANG et al. 1983), which in a direct comparison with DAGO under identical binding assay conditions showed about half the affinity for μ-receptors but a selectivity ratio (K_i^δ/K_i^μ = 1470) somewhat higher than that of DAGO (K_i^δ/K_i^μ = 1050) (SCHILLER et al. 1990a).

In contrast to most other naturally occurring opioid peptides, dermorphin (H-Tyr-D-Ala-Phe-Gly-Tyr-Pro-Ser-NH$_2$) (MONTECUCCHI et al. 1981) contains a D-alanine residue in the 2-position as well as a C-terminal carboxamide group and, therefore, is relatively more resistant to enzymolysis. The natural heptapeptide shows quite high μ-selectivity (Table 1) but is by no means the most selective μ-ligand known, as recently claimed in the literature (SAGAN et al. 1989). Deletion of the C-terminal tripeptide segment in dermorphin resulted in a tetrapeptide, H-Try-D-Ala-Phe-Gly-NH$_2$, with μ-selectivity similar to that of the parent heptapeptide. In comparison with the latter compound, a sevenfold improvement in μ-selectivity was observed with the two tetrapeptide analogs H-Tyr-D-Met(O)-Phe-Gly-OCH$_3$ and H-Try-D-Met(O)-Phe-D-Ala-OCH$_3$, which both were nearly as μ-selective as DAGO but somewhat less potent (MARASTONI et al. 1987). Several dermorphin-(1–4) tetrapeptide analogs with a D-arginine residue substituted in the 2-position have been reported to be potent analgesics (SASAKI et al. 1985). A recently performed receptor binding study showed that one of these analogs, H-Tyr-D-Arg-Phe-Gly-OH, was quite μ-selective (K_i^δ/K_i^μ = 285) (SCHILLER et al., unpublished results). On the basis of a proposal that δ-receptors may be located in a cationic membrane environment from which positively charged ligands would be excluded due to an electrostatic repulsive effect (SCHWYZER 1986), a series of dermorphin-(1–4) tetrapeptide analogs carrying an increasingly higher positive charge

Table 1. Receptor affinities and selectivity ratios of μ-selective opioid peptide analogs (agonists)

Compound	μ-Affinity IC$_{50}^{\mu}$ [nM], K$_i^{\mu}$ [nM]	δ-Affinity IC$_{50}^{\delta}$ [nM], K$_i^{\delta}$ [nM]	Selectivity ratio (δ/μ)[a]	Reference
H-Tyr-D-Ala-Gly-MePhe-Gly-ol (DAGO)	1.29	120	93	HANDA et al. (1981)
	1.22	1280	1050	SCHILLER et al. (1985a, 1990a)
	3.9	700	179	GACEL et al. (1988a)
NMe-Tyr-D-Ala-Gly-N(Et)-CH(CH$_2$-Phe)CH$_2$-N(CH$_3$)$_2$ (LY164929)	0.6	900	1500	SHUMAN et al. (1990)
H-Tyr-D-Met(O)-Gly-MePhe-ol (syndyphalin)	0.29	1250	4310	KISO et al. (1981)
H-Tyr-D-Ala-Gly-NH-CH$_2$-CH$_2$-CH(CH$_3$)$_2$ (TRIMU 5)	10.0	1020	102	QUIRION et al. (1982) GACEL et al. (1988a)
H-Tyr-Pro-MePhe-D-Pro-NH$_2$ (PLO17)	5.5	10000	1820	CHANG et al. (1983)
	2.89	4250	1470	SCHILLER et al. (1990a)
H-Tyr-D-Ala-Phe-Gly-Tyr-Pro-Ser-NH$_2$ (dermorphin)	5.7	210	36.8	MARASTONI et al. (1987)
H-Tyr-D-Arg-Phe-Gly-OH	1.05	359	342	SAGAN et al. (1989)
H-Tyr-D-Arg-Phe-Lys-NH$_2$ (DALDA)	1.70	484	285	SCHILLER et al., unpublished data
	1.69	19200	11400	SCHILLER et al. (1989a)
H-Tyr-D-Ala-Phe-Phe-NH$_2$ (TAPP)	1.53	626	409	SCHILLER et al. (1989a,b)

H-Tyr-D-Ala-1-Nap-1-Nap-NH$_2$	2.88	1180	410	SCHILLER et al. (1989b)
(H-Tyr-D-Ala-Gly-NH-CH$_2$)$_2$ (DTRE)$_2$	0.034	14	412	LUTZ et al. (1985)
H-Tyr-cyclo[-D-A$_2$bu-Gly-Phe-Leu-]	13.8	115	8.33	SCHILLER and DiMaio (1982)
H-Tyr-cyclo[-D-Orn-Gly-Phe-Leu-]	31.4	100	3.81	DiMaio et al. (1982)
H-Tyr-cyclo[-D-Lys-Gly-Phe-Leu-]	5.58	76.4	13.7	SHERMAN et al. (1989)
H-Tyr-cyclo[-D-Glu-Gly-gPhe-D-Leu-]	11.0	389	35.4	BERMAN et al. (1983)
H-Tyr-cyclo[-D-Lys-Glyψ[CSNH]-Phe-Leu-]	4.55	654	144	SHERMAN et al. (1989)
H-Tyr-D-Orn-Phe-Asp-NH$_2$	10.4	2200	212	SCHILLER et al. (1985a)
H-Tyr-D-Cys-Phe-Cys-NH$_2$	11.0	373	33.9	SCHILLER et al. (1987)

[a] IC$_{50}^{\delta}$/IC$_{50}^{\mu}$ or K_i^{δ}/K_i^{μ} ratio.

were recently prepared in an effort to develop highly selective μ-ligands (SCHILLER et al. 1989a). A progressive increase in μ-selectivity as a consequence of a gradual decrease in δ-affinity was indeed observed with the analogs H-Tyr-D-Nva-Phe-Nle-HN$_2$, H-Tyr-D-Arg-Phe-Nle-NH$_2$, and H-Try-D-Arg-Phe-Lys-NH$_2$, which carry a net positive charge of 1+, 2+, and 3+, respectively. The most selective compound was H-Try-D-Arg-Phe-Lys-NH$_2$ ([D-Arg^2, Lys^4]dermorphin-(1–4)-$a$mide; DALDA) which showed a selectivity ratio ($K_i^\delta/K_i^\mu = 11\,400$) more than ten times higher than that of DAGO ($K_i^\delta/K_i^\mu = 1050$) and eight times higher than that of PLO17 ($K_i^\delta/K_i^\mu = 1470$) in a direct comparison under identical binding assay conditions (SCHILLER et al. 1990a) (Table 1). Furthermore, this compound does not have significant affinity for κ-receptors ($K_i^\kappa > 1\,\mu M$). According to these data DALDA appears to be the most selective μ-agonist developed so far and should be useful not only as a research tool in basic opioid pharmacology but also for studying specifically peripheral μ-receptor interactions, because its very polar character should prevent it from crossing the blood-brain barrier.

Evidence has been obtained to indicate that the Phe^4 aromatic ring of the enkephalins may interact with an opioid receptor subsite different from that to which Phe^3 aromatic rings of dermorphin and β-casomorphin bind (SCHILLER et al. 1983). In view of this intriguing possibility it was of interest to prepare dermorphin/enkephalin hybrid peptides that contain a Phe residue in the 3- *and* 4-position. The recently prepared prototype analog H-Tyr-D-Ala-Phe-Phe-NH$_2$ (TAPP) showed high μ-receptor affinity and high μ-selectivity ($K_i^\delta/K_i^\mu = 409$) (SCHILLER et al. 1989a,b). Nitration in the para position of the Phe aromatic rings of TAPP produced an affinity drop in the case of the Phe^3 residue and an affinity increase in the case of the Phe^4 residue (SCHILLER et al. 1989b) as it had also been observed with opioid peptides containing a single Phe residue only in either the 3-position (dermorphin, β-casomorphins) or the 4-position (enkephalins). These results lend further support to the idea that the two Phe aromatic rings in TAPP may indeed interact with two distinct opioid receptor subsites. In contrast to the polar analog DALDA, TAPP is a molecule with a relatively lipophilic character. Bulky, hydrophobic amino acids, such as tryptophan or 1 (or 2)-naphthylalanine (Nap) were substituted in positions 3 and 4 of TAPP in an effort to develop even more lipophilic opioid peptide analogs (SCHILLER et al. 1989b). These analogs retained excellent μ-receptor affinity and high μ-selectivity, as observed, for example, with the tetrapeptide H-Tyr-D-Ala-1-Nap-1-Nap-NH$_2$ ($K_i^\delta/K_i^\mu = 410$) (Table 1).

2. Opioid Peptide Dimers

The development of bivalent ligands containing two opioid peptides linked via their C-terminal carboxyl group through flexible spacers of varying length represents a relatively new strategy for the design of receptor-selective ligands. The rationale for the bivalent ligand approach was based on experimental evidence that opioid receptors might be clustered together on the membrane surface and on the expectation that at a certain spacer length bivalent ligands might simultaneously occupy two distinct receptor binding sites. Entropy considerations predict that in such a situation a bivalent ligand would show considerably higher affinity than a corresponding monovalent ligand. Moreover, it is assumed that the average distance between two μ-binding sites and two δ-binding sites might be different which would permit the development of μ- or δ-selective ligands through variation of the spacer length. Because of their increased molecular size such bivalent ligands are perhaps not so attractive as candidates for peptide drug development, but might represent valuable tools for basic opioid receptor research, since their use might permit a rough estimate of the distance between proximal receptor binding sites. The best example of a μ-selective bivalent opioid peptide ligand is $(H\text{-Tyr-D-Ala-Gly-NH-CH}_2)_2$ $(\text{DTRE})_2$, which showed a K_i^{δ}/K_i^{μ} ratio of 412 in the receptor binding assays (LUTZ et al. 1985) (Table 1), whereas the corresponding monovalent ligand, $H\text{-Tyr-D-Ala-Gly-NH}_2$ (TRE), had much weaker affinity for μ-receptors and was only moderately μ-selective. $(\text{DTRE})_2$ was shown to be about three times less μ-selective than morphiceptin in a direct comparison under identical assay conditions (LUTZ et al. 1985). Evidence in support of the assumption that $(\text{DTRE})_2$ does indeed occupy two distinct μ-binding sites was obtained in further studies with so-called handicapped dimers in which the Tyr[1] residue of one of the two peptide segments was replaced by D-Tyr or Phe and which showed much diminished μ-affinity (SHIMOHIGASHI et al. 1987a). However, because of the shortness of the spacer ($\text{-CH}_2\text{-CH}_2\text{-}$) contained in $(\text{DTRE})_2$ it seems likely that this bivalent ligand may not be able to bridge two separate μ-receptors but rather may simultaneously interact with the binding sites on two putative subunits of the μ-receptor.

3. Cyclic Opioid Peptide Analogs

There is ample experimental evidence indicating that the natural enkephalins are very flexible molecules capable of assuming various different conformations of comparatively low energy (for a review, see SCHILLER 1984). This structural flexibility may be the major reason for the lack of receptor selectivity of these linear pentapeptides and, therefore, it was attempted to develop more selective analogs through incorporation of conformational constraints. The most drastic restriction of the overall conformation can be achieved through appropriate peptide cyclizations. In the case of the enkephalins, various cyclizations via side chains of appropriately substituted amino acid residues were successfully performed. An early example was the cyclic analog $H\text{-Tyr-cyclo[-D-A}_2\text{bu-Gly-Phe-Leu-]}$, which was obtained through substitution of D-α,γ-diaminobutyric acid (A$_2$bu) in position 2 of the [Leu^5]enkephalin sequence and cyclization of the γ-amino group of A$_2$bu to the C-terminal carboxyl group (DiMaio and Schiller 1980). This compound showed high potency at the μ-receptor and considerable μ-receptor selectivity (Schiller and DiMaio 1982) (Table 1). The observation that the corresponding open-chain analog H-Tyr-D-Abu-Gly-Phe-Leu-NH$_2$ (Abu = α-aminobutyric acid) was nonselective represented the first conclusive demonstration that receptor selectivity may indeed result as a consequence of conformational restriction. Homologs of this cyclic prototype analog with varying side chain length in the 2-position, such as H-Tyr-cyclo[-D-Orn-Gly-Phe-Leu-] and H-Tyr-cyclo[-D-Lys-Gly-Phe-Leu-], also displayed high potency and μ-selectivity (DiMaio et al. 1982). The receptor selectivity of some of these cyclic analogs could be further improved through various peptide bond modifications. Thus, the reversal of two peptide bonds in the ring structure of H-Tyr-cyclo[-D-A$_2$bu-Gly-Phe-Leu-] led to a compound, H-Tyr-cyclo[-Glu-Gly-gPhe-D-Leu-] (gPhe denotes the gem diamino equivalent of Phe) which is three times more μ-selective than the cyclic parent peptide (Berman et al. 1983). Similarly, replacement of the peptide bond in the 3- to 4-position of H-Tyr-cyclo[-D-Lys-Gly-Phe-Leu-] with a thioamide moiety produced a compound, H-Tyr-cyclo[-D-Lys-Glyψ[CSNH]Phe-Leu-], showing an approximate tenfold improvement in μ-selectivity (Sherman et al. 1989).

The most selective cyclic opioid peptide analog with agonist properties reported to date is the side chain-to-side chain cyclized dermorphin tetrapeptide analog H-Tyr-D-Orn-Phe-Asp-NH$_2$ (K_i^δ/K_i^μ = 213) (Schiller et al. 1985a). A structurally related cystine-containing analog, H-Tyr-D-Cys-Phe-Cys-NH$_2$, also showed pronounced μ-selectivity (Schiller et al. 1987).

Conformational studies of these various cyclic opioid peptide analogs have not yet led to a consensus concerning a possible unique bioactive conformation at the μ-receptor (for a review, see Schiller and Wilkes 1988). However, these investigations clearly demonstrated that the ring structures in these compounds still retain some structural flexibility and that the various intramolecular hydrogen bonds observed are constantly formed, broken, and reformed, as shown most convincingly in molecular dynamics studies (Mammi et al. 1985). In the case of both H-Tyr-cyclo[-D-A$_2$bu-Gly-Phe-Leu-] and H-Tyr-cyclo[-D-Orn-Gly-Phe-Leu-], the results of both NMR studies and computer simulations indicated the existence of a hydrogen bond which defines a γ-turn centered on Phe^4 (Kessler et al. 1985; Mammi et al. 1985). This interesting observation prompted the design of a peptidomimetic in which one of the peptide bonds in the γ-turn structure of the cyclic parent peptide is replaced by a trans-olefin and the oxygen and hydrogen atoms engaged in the hydrogen bond (C=O H-N) are replaced with an ethylene moiety (Huffman et al. 1989) (Fig. 1). The two diastereomers of the bicyclic compound with either R or S configuration at the chiral center of the γ-turn mimic could be obtained separately and were both found to have very low activity. Possible explanations for the lack of significant activity of this peptidomimetic may be: (1) the γ-turn structure detected in the conformational studies of the monocyclic parent peptide may

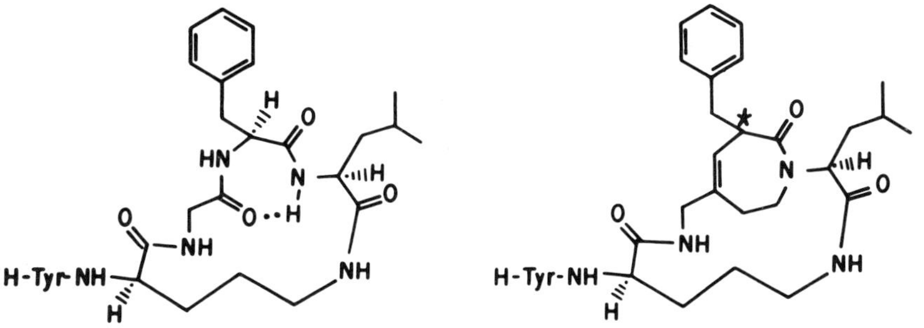

Fig. 1. Structural formulas of the cyclic enkephalin analog H-Tyr-cyclo[-D-Orn-Gly-Phe-Leu-] (*left*) and of a bicylic analog containing a γ-turn mimic (*right*)

not be a structural feature of the bioactive conformation; (2) the Gly^3 carbonyl group which is no longer present in the γ-turn mimic may be important for the interaction with the receptor; and (3) the ethylene bridge introduced in the mimic may interfere with the receptor binding process either due to unfavorable steric interactions or due to the fact that it produces too much rigidity in the molecule. Despite the lack of activity the preparation of this compound represents a conceptually interesting first step toward the goal of developing rationally designed peptidomimetics of enkephalin, and further efforts in this direction will certainly be worthwhile.

A recently performed molecular mechanics study permitted the identification of the lowest energy conformations of the cyclic dermorphin analog H-Tyr-D-Orn-Phe-Asp-NH$_2$ and of nine structurally related cyclic tetrapeptide analogs showing considerable diversity in μ-receptor affinity (WILKES and SCHILLER 1990). The outcome of this conformation-activity study led to the suggestion that a tilted stacking arrangement of the Tyr^1 and Phe^3 aromatic rings may represent an important structural requirement for high μ-receptor affinity of the examined cyclic dermorphin analogs. However, this theoretical analysis also revealed that the exocyclic Tyr^1 residue and the Phe^3 side chain still enjoy considerable orientational freedom and that these moieties also need to be conformationally restricted in order to obtain more definitive insight into the receptor-bound conformation. This was achieved with an analog of H-Tyr-D-Orn-Phe-Glu-NH$_2$ containing 6-hydroxy-2-aminotetralin-2-carboxylic acid (Hat) and 2-aminoindan-2-carboxylic acid (Aic) in place of Tyr^1 and Phe^3, respectively (SCHILLER et al. 1991) (Fig. 2). Interestingly, both diastereomers (I and II) of H-(D or L)-Hat-D-Orn-Aic-Glu-NH$_2$ showed quite high μ-receptor affinity and μ-selectivity (I: $K_i^\mu = 19.8\,\text{n}M$, $K_i^\delta/K_i^\mu = 19.0$; II: $K_i^\mu = 29.8\,\text{n}M$, $K_i^\delta/K_i^\mu = 12.4$). These tricyclic peptides represent the structurally most rigid rationally designed opioid peptidomimetics reported to date, since essentially they contain only two freely rotatable bonds. Molecular dynamics simulations demonstrated the enhanced rigidity of both Hat

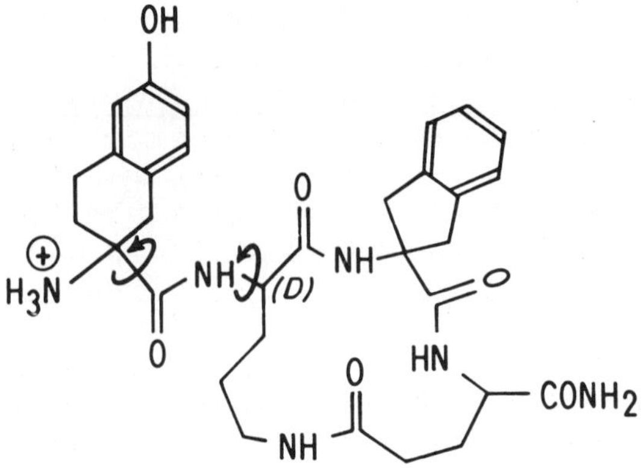

Fig. 2. Structural formula of the opioid peptidomimetic H-Hat-D-Orn-Aic-Glu-NH$_2$

peptides as compared to the parent peptide H-Tyr-D-Orn-Phe-Glu-NH$_2$ and a molecular mechanics study performed with H-Hat-D-Orn-Aic-Glu-NH$_2$ revealed that its lowest energy conformation is characterized by a close proximity between the two aromatic rings, as it was also the case in the lowest energy conformers of H-Try-D-Orn-Phe-Glu-NH$_2$ and H-Try-D-Orn-Phe-Asp-NH$_2$.

II. δ-Selective Agonists

Linear opioid peptides with high δ-selectivity include various enkephalin analogs that have been developed over the years as well as the recently discovered, highly δ-selective deltorphins and their analogs. As in the case of the μ-selective peptide ligands, opioid peptide dimers and cyclic opioid peptide analogs with greatly improved δ-selectivity have also been obtained.

1. Linear Opioid Peptide Analogs

The natural enkephalins display slight preference for δ-receptors over μ-receptors. An early analog, H-Tyr-D-Ala-Gly-Phe-D-Leu-OH (DADLE) (BEDDELL et al. 1977), showed only slightly improved δ-receptor selectivity (Table 2). Nevertheless, DADLE has frequently been used and continues to be used as a "δ-selective" ligand. Substitution of a D-serine residue in the 2-position of [Leu^5]enkephalin and extension of the peptide chain with a threonine residue at the C-terminus led to a further slight improvement in δ-selectivity (GACEL et al. 1980). The resulting hexapeptide analog, H-Tyr-D-Ser-Gly-Phe-Leu-Thr-OH (DSLET), retained quite high affinity for δ-receptors but somewhat reduced μ-receptor affinity, presumably due to an unfavorable interaction of the Ser^2 side chain hydroxyl group with a hydrophobic pocket of the μ-receptor. Replacement of the D-Ser^2 residue with D-threonine produced a compound, H-Tyr-D-Thr-Gly-Phe-Leu-Thr-OH (DTLET), showing a further threefold increase in δ-selectivity (Zajac et al. 1983). On the basis of the rationale that increased bulkiness of the side chains in the 2- and 6-position of DSLET might increase δ-selectivity due to steric interference at the μ-receptor, analogs with a *tert*-butyl group attached to the hydroxyl function of Ser and/or Thr were recently synthesized (Gacel et al. 1988b). Among several prepared compounds, H-Tyr-D-Ser(OtBu)-Gly-Phe-Leu-Thr-OH (DSTBULET) and H-Tyr-D-Ser(OtBu)-Gly-Phe-Leu-Thr(OtBu)-OH (BUBU) were the most δ-selective with K_i^μ/K_i^δ values of 60.9 and 101, respectively. Finally, replacement of the D-Ser(OtBu)^2 residue in BUBU with D-Cys(StBu) has recently been shown to produce a further tenfold improvement in δ-selectivity as a consequence of decreased binding to μ-receptors (Gacel et al. 1990). The latter compound, H-Tyr-D-Cys(StBu)-Gly-Phe-Leu-Thr(OtBu)-OH (BUBUC), showed a K_i^μ/K_i^δ ratio of 1020 and it appears that its δ-selectivity is higher than that of the cyclic enkephalin analog DPDPE (see below) and comparable to that of the deltorphins. In another interesting approach, the Phe^4 residue in [D-Ala^2,Leu^5]enkephalin was replaced with the conformationally restricted phenylalanine analog E-cyclopropylphenylalanine (∇^EPhe) (Shimohigashi et al. 1987b). One of the obtained isomers, H-Tyr-D-Ala-Gly-(2R,3S)-∇^EPhe-Leu-OH, showed quite high δ-selectivity (K_i^μ/K_i^δ = 253).

One of the most exciting developments in the opioid peptide field in recent years has been the isolation of novel, highly δ-selective opioid peptides from frog skin extracts. The heptapeptide H-Tyr-D-Met-Phe-His-Leu-Met-Asp-NH$_2$ was first isolated and characterized by Kreil et al. (1989) and named deltorphin. An alternative name, dermenkephalin, was proposed by Amiche et al. (1989), who also characterized this peptide. Selectivity ratios (K_i^μ/K_i^δ) ranging from 51 to 676 have been reported for deltorphin (Table 2). In a direct comparison with the cyclic enkephalin analog DPDPE (see below) under identical binding assay conditions, deltorphin turned out to be more δ-selective in one study (Erspamer et al. 1989) and less δ-selective in another (Amiche et al. 1989). Very soon after the discovery of deltorphin the further analysis of frog skin extracts led to the isolation of two other heptapeptides, H-Tyr-D-Ala-Phe-Asp-Val-Val-Gly-NH$_2$ ([D-Ala^2]deltorphin I) and H-Tyr-D-Ala-Phe-Glu-Val-Val-Gly-NH$_2$ ([D-Ala^2]deltorphin II), which apparently showed even higher δ-receptor preference than deltorphin, the most selective one being [D-Ala^2]deltorphin I with a reported K_i^μ/K_i^δ ratio of 21 000 (Erspamer et al. 1989). Since the latter two peptides contain the same N-terminal tripeptide segment, H-Tyr-D-Ala-Phe-, as the μ-selective opioid peptide dermorphin, it is obvious that the C-terminal tetrapeptide segment is of crucial importance for the δ-receptor selectivity of [D-Ala^2]deltorphins I and II. [D-Ala^2]deltorphin I has been reported to be nearly 100 times more δ-selective than DPDPE (Erspamer et al. 1989), mostly as a consequence of its much higher δ-

Table 2. Receptor affinities and selectivity ratios of δ-selective opioid peptide analogs (agonists)

Compound	μ-Affinity IC_{50}^{μ} [nM], K_i^{μ} [nM]	δ-Affinity IC_{50}^{δ} [nM], K_i^{δ} [nM]	Selectivity ratio $(\mu/\delta)^a$	Reference
[Leu^5] enkephalin	9.43	2.54	3.71	SCHILLER et al. (1985a)
H-Tyr-D-Ala-Gly-Phe-D-Leu-OH (DADLE)	7.7	2.4	3.20	RIGAUDY et al. (1987)
H-Tyr-D-Ser-Gly-Phe-Leu-Thr-OH (DSLET)	7.59	1.70	4.46	KONDO et al. (1986)
	31.0	4.80	6.46	GACEL et al. (1988b)
H-Tyr-D-Thr-Gly-Phe-Leu-Thr-OH (DTLET)	23.3	1.35	17.3	GACEL et al. (1988b)
H-Tyr-D-Ser(OtBu)-Gly-Phe-Leu-Thr-OH (DSTBULET)	374	6.14	60.9	GACEL et al. (1988b)
H-Tyr-D-Ser(OtBu)-Gly-Phe-Leu-Thr(OtBu)-OH (BUBU)	475	4.68	101	GACEL et al. (1988b)
	480	1.69	280	GACEL et al. (1990)
H-Tyr-D-Cys(StBu)-Gly-Phe-Leu-Thr(OtBu)-OH (BUBUC)	2980	2.90	1020	GACEL et al. (1990)
H-Tyr-D-Met-Phe-His-Leu-Met-Asp-NH$_2$ (deltorphin)	1630	2.41	676	ERSPAMER et al. (1989)
	367	3.15	117	AMICHE et al. (1989)
	267	5.2	51	SAGAN et al. (1989)
H-Tyr-D-Ala-Phe-Asp-Val-Val-Gly-NH$_2$ ([D-Ala^2] deltorphin I)	3150	0.15	21000	ERSPAMER et al. (1989)
	325	2.69	121	SCHILLER et al., unpublished data
H-Tyr-D-Ala-Phe-Glu-Val-Val-Gly-NH$_2$ ([D-Ala^2] deltorphin II)	2450	0.71	3450	ERSPAMER et al. (1989)

Compound					Ratio[a]	Reference
H-Tyr-D-Ala-(D or L)-Atc-Asp-Val-Val-Gly-NH$_2$ (I)		671		5.36	125	Schiller et al., unpublished data
H-Tyr-D-Ala-(D or L)-Atc-Asp-Val-Val-Gly-NH$_2$ (II)		1410		6.52	216	Schiller et al., unpublished data
(*H*-Tyr-D-Ala-Gly-Phe-NH(CH$_2$)$_6$)$_2$ (DTE$_{12}$)	96.3		1.06		90.8	Shimohigashi et al. (1982)
H-Tyr-D-Pen-Gly-Phe-D-Pen-OH (DPDPE)	2240	993	16.2	19.2	138	Mosberg et al. (1983b)
					51.7	Gacel et al. (1987)
	609		5.25		116	Thót et al. (1990)
	7720		6.44		1200	Mosberg et al. (1988)
H-Tyr-D-Pen-Gly-Phe-L-Pen-OH (DPLPE)	3710		10.0		371	Mosberg et al. (1983b)
H-Tyr-D-Pen-Gly-pCl-Phe-D-Pen-OH	901		1.57		80.1	Gacel et al. (1987)
		873		10.9	574	Thót et al. (1990)
H-Tyr-D-Cys-Phe-D-Pen-OH	1210		1.90		637	Mosberg et al. (1988)

[a] $IC_{50}^{\mu}/IC_{50}^{\delta}$ or K_i^{μ}/K_i^{δ} ratio.

receptor affinity. Further binding studies need to be carried out in order to determine more definitively to what extent the selectivity of the deltorphins exceeds that of other δ-ligands. In a direct comparison under identical assay conditions the two diastereomeric analogs H-Tyr-D-Ala-(D or L)-Atc-Asp-Val-Val-Gly-NH$_2$ (Atc = 2-aminotetralin-2-carboxylic acid) both showed δ-receptor affinity and δ-selectivity comparable to that of the parent peptide [D-Ala^2]deltorphin I (Schiller et al. 1990b) (Table 2). As a consequence of the replacement of the Phe^3 residue in [D-Ala^2]deltorphin I with the cyclic phenylalanine analog Atc, these analogs can be expected to be more lipophilic and, possibly, more enzyme resistant than the native parent peptide.

2. Opioid Peptide Dimers

Among various prepared dimeric enkephalin analogs, a compound containing two H-Tyr-D-Ala-Gly-Phe-NH$_2$ segments linked by a 12-methylene bridge (DTE$_{12}$) was the most δ-selective (K_i^μ / K_i^δ = 91), whereas the monomeric tetrapeptide amide was moderately μ-selective (Shimohigashi et al. 1982). Direct comparison showed that DTE$_{12}$ is about five times more δ-selective than DTLET.

3. Cyclic Opioid Peptide Analogs

Cyclic enkephalin analogs containing half-cystine residues in the 2- and 5-position (H-Tyr-D-Cys-Gly-Phe-D(or L)-Cys-X [X = NH$_2$ or OH]) were first synthesized by Sarantakis (1979) and independently by Schiller et al. (1981). Whereas these analogs were relatively nonselective (Schiller et al. 1981, 1985b), substitution of a penicillamine (Pen) residue for Cys in position 2 and/or 5 resulted in compounds with markedly improved δ-selectivity (Mosberg et al. 1982, 1983a,b). The most δ-selective cyclic analogs of this type turned out to be H-Tyr-D-Pen-Gly-Phe-D-Pen-OH (DPDPE) and H-Tyr-D-Pen-Gly-Phe-L-Pen-OH (DPLPE) (Mosberg et al. 1983b) (Table 2). In a recent study Mosberg et al. (1987) conclusively showed that the δ-receptor preference of these two analogs is due to the presence of the bulky *gem* dimethyl groups in the 2-position side chain, which cause more severe steric interference at the μ-receptor than at the δ-receptor. A recent direct comparison showed that the δ-selectivity of DPDPE and DPLPE was higher than that of DTLET and comparable to that of DSTBULET and BUBU (Gacel et al. 1987). However, the δ-affinity of the latter two analogs was somewhat higher than that of the cyclic analogs. Replacement of Phe^4 in DPDPE with p-chlorophenylalanine (pCl-Phe) resulted in a compound, H-Tyr-D-Pen-Gly-pCl-Phe-D-Pen-OH, showing a fivefold improvement in δ-selectivity due to an increase in δ-affinity (Thót et al. 1990). Recently performed conformational studies have not yet led to a consensus with regard to the bioactive conformation of DPDPE at the δ-receptor. Another interesting cyclic peptide with δ-receptor preference is the recently reported analog H-Tyr-D-Cys-Phe-D-Pen-OH (Mosberg et al. 1988), which is structurally derived from the μ-selective tetrapeptide analog H-Tyr-D-Cys-Phe-Cys-NH$_2$ (Schiller et al. 1987) and which in comparison with DPDPE was about half as δ-selective but three times more potent.

III. κ-Selective Agonists

The 17-peptide dynorphin A (H-Tyr-Gly-Gly-Phe-Leu-Arg-Arg-Ile-Arg-Pro-Lys-Leu-Lys-Trp-Asp-Asn-Gln-OH) and the C-terminally truncated fragment dynorphin A-(1–13) display only limited selectivity for κ- versus μ- and δ-receptors. In comparison with dynorphin A-(1–13), the analog [Ala^8]dynorphin A-(1–13) was about four times more κ-selective toward both the μ- and the δ-receptor and slight improvements in κ-selectivity were also observed with the analogs [Trp^8]dynorphin A-(1–13) and [D-Pro^{10}]dynorphin A-(1–13) (Lemaire et al. 1986). The 11-peptide dynorphin A-(1–11) and particularly its analog [D-Pro^{10}]dynorphin A-(1–11) also showed somewhat improved κ-selectivity (Gairin et al. 1984). An interesting new concept in the design of dynorphin analogs was the replacement of the potential amphiphilic β-strand region encompassing residues 7–15 with a segment of alternating Lys and Val residues, resulting in a compound, [Lys^{6,7,9,15}, Val^{8,12,14}, Ser^{16,17}]dynorphin A, with about two to three times higher κ- versus μ- and κ- versus δ-selectivity (Yang and Taylor 1990). Among several cyclic dynorphin analogs that have been prepared, [D-Cys^2,Cys^5]dynorphin A-(1–13) was δ-selective rather than κ-selective (Shearman et al. 1985) and the cyclic lactam analogs [D-Orn^2,Asp^5]dynorphin A-(1–8), [Orn^5,Asp^8]dynorphin A-(1–13), [Orn^5,Asp^{10}]dynorphin A-(1–13) and [Orn^5,Asp^{13}]dynorphin A-(1–13) all turned out to be μ-selective (Schiller et al. 1988). These results indicate that the various performed cyclizations produced overall folded conformations which are not compatible with the conformational requirements of the κ-receptor. A further cystine-bridged analog, [D-Cys^8, D-Cys^{13}]dynorphin A-(1–13)-amide, bound to κ-receptors with quite high affinity but its κ versus μ-selectivity was low (Kawasaki et al. 1990). In conclusion, structure-activity work in the dynorphin area has so far produced compounds showing only a modest improvement in κ-selectivity and further efforts are necessary to obtain highly κ-selective dynorphin analogs.

D. Selective Opioid Peptide Analogs with Antagonist Properties

The most potent and selective μ-antagonists known to date are not derived from opioid peptides but from somatostatin. Maurer et al. (1982) first demonstrated that the somatostatin analog H-D-Phe-Cys-Phe-D-Trp-Lys-Thr-Cys-Thr-ol (SMS-201995) is a potent opioid antagonist with high preference for μ-receptors over δ-receptors. No structural relationships between SMS-201995 and the various opiates and opioid peptides are apparent and the discovery of this antagonist was indeed serendipitous. Subsequently, SMS-201995 served as parent compound for the development of various analogs with further improved μ-antagonist properties. Thus, the compounds *H*-D-Phe-Cys-Tyr-D-Trp-Lys-Thr-Pen-Thr-NH$_2$ (CTP) and *H*-D-Phe-Cys-Tyr-D-Trp-Orn-Thr-Pen-Thr-NH$_2$ (CTOP) were also highly μ-selective opioid antagonists and, in contrast to SMS-201995, showed greatly reduced affinity for the somatostatin receptor (PELTON et al. 1985, 1986). The most selective μ-antagonist reported to date is the heptapeptide *H*-D-Tic-Cys-Tyr-D-Trp-Orn-Thr-Pen-Thr-NH$_2$ (TCTOP) (Tic = tetra-hydroisoquinoline-3-carboxylic acid) which showed an IC$_{50}{}^\delta$/IC$_{50}{}^\mu$ ratio of 11 400 in the receptor binding assays and also bound very poorly to the somatostatin receptor (KAZMIERSKI et al. 1988). Two other somatostatin analogs, *H*-D-Nal-Cys-Tyr-D-Trp-Lys-Val-Cys-Thr-NH$_2$ (Nal = 3-(2-naphthyl)-alanine and *H*-D-Nal-Cys-Tyr-D-Pal-Lys-Val-Cys-Thr-NH$_2$ (Pal = 3-(3-pyridyl)-alanine) also turned out to be opioid antagonists with quite high preference for μ-receptors over δ-receptors (WALKER et al. 1987).

Opioid antagonists with δ-selectivity have been obtained through diallylation of the N-terminal α-amino group of various enkephalin-related peptides. This structural modification in conjunction with replacement of the 3- to 4-position peptide bond with a thiomethylene moiety resulted in a compound, *N,N*-diallyl-Tyr-Gly-Glyψ[CH$_2$S]Phe-Leu-OH (ICI 154129), which showed considerable δ-selectivity (K_i^μ/K_i^δ = 12.9) but poor δ-affinity (SHAW et al. 1982; CORBETT et al. 1984). A conformationally restricted version of this analog, *N,N*-diallyl-Tyr-Aib-Aib-Phe-Leu-OH (ICI 174864) was a moderately potent δ-antagonist in the MVD assay and, in comparison with ICI 154129, showed about four times higher δ-receptor affinity and ten times higher δ-selectivity (K_i^μ/K_i^δ = 128) (COTTON et al. 1984; CORBETT et al. 1984). Replacement of the Gly^2-Gly^3 dipeptide unit with the rigid spacer *p*-aminobenzoic acid (-NH-φ-CO-) resulted in a compound, *N,N*-diallyl-Tyr-*p*-NH-φ-CO-Phe-Leu-OH, which showed about the same δ-antagonist potency and selectivity as ICI 174864 in the MVD assay (THORNBER et al. 1986a). The dimeric ligand (*N,N*-diallyl-Tyr-Gly-Gly-Phe-Leu-NH-CH$_2$)$_2$ was also reported to be a fairly potent and selective δ-antagonist, even though it did not simultaneously interact with two distinct δ-receptor binding sites (THORNBER et al. 1986b).

Efforts to develop κ-selective antagonists through structural modification of dynorphin A so far have not been successful. Three 11-peptide analogs, [D-Trp^{2,8}, D-Pro^{10}]dynorphin A-(1–11), [D-Trp^{5,8}, D-Pro^{10}]dynorphin A-(1–11), and [D-Trp^{2,4,8}, D-Pro^{10}]dynorphin A-(1–11), were weak antagonists of dynorphin A and their κ versus μ-selectivity was low (GAIRIN et al. 1986). The diallylated analogs [*N,N*-diallyl-Tyr^1, D-Pro^{10}]dynorphin A-(1–11), and [*N,N*-diallyl-Tyr^1, Aib^{2,3}, D-Pro^{10}]dynorphin A-(1–11) turned out to be pure but not very selective κ-antagonists (GAIRIN et al. 1988).

E. Irreversible Opioid Receptor Peptide Ligands

Irreversible opioid receptor ligands are needed as tools in either basic opioid pharmacology or in opioid receptor labeling experiments. A number of selective nonpeptide opiates and opioid peptide analogs carrying either a chemical affinity label or a photoaffinity label have been reported. Progress made in the development of affinity-labeled nonpeptide opioids is described elsewhere in this volume (Chap. 12).

I. Chemical Affinity Labels

A chloromethyl ketone derivative of enkephalin, H-Tyr-D-Ala-Gly-Phe-Leu-CH$_2$Cl (DALECK), showed moderate preference for μ-receptors over δ-receptors in rat brain (Table 3) and was used for covalent labeling of opioid receptors (VENN and BARNARD 1981; SZÜCS et al. 1987; NEWMAN and BARNARD 1984). The more recently developed tetrapeptide derivative H-Tyr-D-Ala-Gly-MePhe-CH$_2$Cl (DAMK) is more μ-selective than DALECK and was shown to label irreversibly and selectively high affinity μ-binding sites (BENYHE et al. 1987). Moderate δ-selectivity was observed with the hexapeptide analog [D-Ala^2,Leu^5,Cys^6]enkephalin (DALCE), which binds covalently to δ-receptors, presumably by forming a disulfide bond between its single Cys^6 sulfhydryl group and a sulfhydryl moiety at the binding site.

II. Photoaffinity Labels

A number of receptor-selective photoaffinity labels have been obtained through incorporation of photolabile groups into opioid peptide analogs that display high preference for one or the other of the different receptor types. μ-Selective photoaffinity labels were prepared through replacement of the Phe^4 (or MePhe^4) residue in DAGO, TAPP, or CTP with the corresponding p-azidophenylalanine (Phe(pN$_3$)) derivative or through substitution of p-benzoylphenylalanine (Bpa) in the 4-position of morphiceptin. The resulting analogs, H-Tyr-D-Ala-Gly-MePhe(pN$_3$)-Gly-ol (GARBAY-JAUREGUIBERRY et al. 1984), H-Tyr-D-Ala-Phe-Phe(pN$_3$)-NH$_2$ (SCHILLER et al. 1989b), and H-D-Phe-Cys-Phe(pN$_3$)-D-Trp-Lys-Thr-Pen-Thr-NH$_2$ (LANDIS et al. 1989) retained high μ-selectivity (Table 3), whereas the morphiceptin analog H-Tyr-Pro-Phe-Bpa-NH$_2$ (HERBLIN et al. 1987) was somewhat less selective. Highest μ-selectivity was observed with the Phe(pN$_3$) analog of CTP. However, the TAPP analog H-Tyr-D-Ala-Phe-Phe(pN$_3$)-NH$_2$ was only four times less μ-selective and, since its μ-receptor affinity is 30 times higher than that of the CTP-derived photoaffinity label, may be particularly useful for μ-receptor labeling experiments. The photoaffinity labels derived from DAGO and morphiceptin have already been used for the selective, irreversible labeling of μ-receptors (GARBAY-JAUREGUIBERRY et al. 1984;

Table 3. Receptor affinities and selectivities of irreversible opioid peptide ligands

Compound	μ-Affinity IC_{50}^{μ} [nM]	δ-Affinity IC_{50}^{δ} [nM]	Selectivity $IC_{50}^{\delta}/IC_{50}^{\mu}$	Reference
H-Tyr-D-Ala-Gly-Phe-Leu-CH$_2$Cl (DALECK)	3.5	50	14.3	Venn and Barnard (1981); Szücs et al. (1987)
H-Tyr-D-Ala-Gly-MePhe-CH$_2$Cl (DAMK)	2.0	80	40.0	Benyhe et al. (1987)
H-Tyr-D-Ala-Gly-Phe-Leu-Cys-OH (DALCE)	55	4.1	0.0745	Bowen et al. (1987)
H-Tyr-D-Ala-Gly-MePhe(pN$_3$)-Gly-ol	25.0[a]	3480[a]	136	Garbay-Jaureguiberry et al. (1984)
H-Tyr-D-Ala-Phe-Phe(pN$_3$)-NH$_2$	1.49[a]	159[a]	107	Schiller et al. (1989b)
H-D-Phe-Cys-Phe(pN$_3$)-D-Trp-Lys-Thr-Pen-Thr-NH$_2$	49	20000	408	Landis et al. (1989)
H-Tyr-Pro-Phe-Bpa-NH$_2$	0.268	3.67	13.7	Herblin et al. (1987)
H-Tyr-D-Thr-Gly-Phe(pN$_3$)-Leu-Thr-OH	72.2[a]	1.4[a]	0.0194	Garbay-Jaureguiberry et al. (1984)
H-Tyr-D-Pen-Gly-Phe(pN$_3$)-D-Pen-OH	3615	33	0.00913	Landis et al. (1989)

[a] These numbers represent K_i values.

HERBLIN et al. 1987). Photoaffinity labels with δ-selectivity are the DTLET and DPDPE derivatives H-Tyr-D-Thr-Gly-Phe(pN$_3$)-Leu-Thr-OH (GARBAY-JAUREGUIBERRY et al. 1984) and H-Tyr-D-Pen-Gly-Phe(pN$_3$)-D-Pen-OH (LANDIS et al. 1989). Selective photoaffinity labeling of δ-receptors was achieved with the DTLET derivative.

F. Selective Opioid Peptide Analogs as Drug Candidates

The Sandoz compound FK 33-824 (H-Tyr-D-Ala-Gly-MePhe-Met(O)-ol (ROEMER et al. 1977) and the Eli Lilly compound metkephamid (H-Tyr-D-Ala-Gly-Phe-MeMet-NH$_2$ (FREDERICKSON et al. 1981) are the two best known enkephalin analogs that have undergone quite extensive clinical testing. As indicated in Table 4, FK 33-824 shows only slight preference for μ-receptors over δ-receptors and metkephamid is essentially nonselective toward μ- and δ-receptors. A most important aspect of these two compounds was their demonstrated ability to produce a long-lasting analgesic effect after systemic administration and, therefore, they were considered as promising candidates for drug development. However, FK 33-824 was subsequently shown to produce a number of quite serious side effects (VON GRAFFENRIED et al. 1978) (Table 4) and is no longer pursued clinically as an analgesic candidate. Metkephamid also showed various side effects but was nevertheless further investigated clinically because of the claim that it may exert its analgesic effect through interaction with δ-receptors and that it may produce less physical dependence than morphine (FREDERICKSON et al. 1981). However, this claim was not substantiated by the results of recently performed receptor binding studies (SHUMAN et al. 1990) (Table 4), which indicated that metkephamid has at least as high affinity for μ-receptors as for δ-receptors. Metkephamid was also of potential interest for use in obstetric analgesia, since it was shown not to cross the placental barrier to a significant extent in the pregnant sheep model (FREDERICKSON 1986). However, the compound was finally abandoned as candidate for obstetric analgesia because it also produced a transient hypotensive effect in the particular obstetric population that had been subjected to a clinical trial. A third enkephalin analog, H-Tyr-D-Met-Gly-Phe-Pro-NH$_2$, also turned out to be a potent analgesic but again produced a number of quite serious side effects in a clinical trial (FÖLDES et al. 1983). The various side effects observed with FK 33-824, metkephamid, and H-Tyr-D-Met-Gly-Phe-Pro-NH$_2$ gave rise to a certain discouragement with regard to the potential of opioid peptide analogs as drug candidates. It should be pointed out, however, that at least some of these side effects may be due to the demonstrated lack of receptor selectivity of these three early enkephalin analogs. As illustrated in this review article, more recently developed opioid peptide analogs show much improved receptor selectivity and some of them may have better potential for application in various types of analgesia.

Table 4. Clinical testing of enkephalin analogs

Compound	Selectivity	Analgesia	Side effects	Reference
H-Tyr-D-Ala-Gly-MePhe-Met-ol (FK33-824)	$K_i^\delta / K_i^\mu = 3.4$	Centrally mediated (systemic administration)	Muscle heaviness Chest oppression Anxiety Bowel sound increase Chemosis Whole body flush, etc.	ROEMER et al. (1977) KOSTERLITZ et al. (1980) VON GRAFFENRIED et al. (1978)
H-Tyr-D-Ala-Gly-Phe-MeMet-NH$_2$ (metkephamid)	$IC_{50}^\delta / IC_{50}^\mu = 1.76$	Centrally mediated (systemic administration) Does not cross placental barrier	Heavy sensation in extremities Nasal congestion Emotional detachment Conjunctival injection Hypotension, etc.	SHUMAN et al. (1990) FREDERICKSON et al. (1981) FREDERICKSON (1986)
H-Tyr-D-Met-Gly-Phe-Pro-NH$_2$	$K_i^\delta / K_i^\mu = 6.48$	Centrally mediated (systemic administration)	Heaviness in the limbs Dry mouth Conjunctival injection Emotional detachment Drowsiness, etc.	BAJUSZ et al. (1980) FÖLDES et al. (1983)
H-Tyr-D-Arg-Gly-Phe(pNO$_2$)-Pro-NH$_2$ (BW443C)	Somewhat μ-selective	Peripherally mediated (s.c. administration)	Nasal stuffiness Dry mouth Postural hypotension *No* central effects (sedation, mood change, respiratory depression, etc.)	HARDY et al. (1988) POSNER et al. (1988)

Recently, evidence has been obtained to indicate that opioids may produce peripherally mediated analgesic effects, particularly in hyperalgesic and inflammatory conditions (SMITH et al. 1982; STEIN et al. 1988). Such effects have been demonstrated with opioid compounds that are unable to cross the blood-brain barrier (e.g., N-methyl-morphine) and the underlying mechanism is currently under investigation (see Chap. 34). Peripherally acting analgesics have potential for clinical applications because they will not produce centrally mediated side effects, such as dependence and respiratory depression. Using the mouse writhing test model, HARDY et al. (1988) have been able to demonstrate that the relatively polar and moderately μ-selective enkephalin analog H-Tyr-D-Arg-Gly-Phe(pNO$_2$)-Pro-NH$_2$ (BW443C) was also able to produce peripherally mediated antinociception at a low dose. Preliminary clinical studies indicated that side effects of BW443C given by i.v. infusions were relatively minor (POSNER et al. 1988) (see Table 4) and central activity (sedation, respiratory depression, mood changes, etc.) was not observed. A series of structurally related D-Arg^2-enkephalin analogs (HARDY et al. 1989) and the polar and highly μ-selective dermorphin analog DALDA (H-Tyr-D-Arg-Phe-Lys-NH$_2$) (SCHILLER et al. 1989a, 1990a) have also been reported to exert peripheral analgesic effects which could be antagonized with quaternized opiate antagonists.

Effects of opioid peptides in the gastrointestinal tract might also be exploited for the development of potential drugs. Thus, the somewhat μ-selective enkephalin analog H-Tyr-D-Met(O)-Gly-Phe(pNO$_2$)-Pro-NH$_2$ (BW942C) was shown to be a safe and effective agent for controlling diarrhea after cisplatin administration in cancer patients without causing major side effects (KRIS et al. 1988). Another enkephalin analog, H-Tyr-D-Lys-Gly-Phe-Hctl (Hoe 825) (Hctl = homocysteine-thiolactone), produced a powerful gut-stimulating effect and may have therapeutic potential for the management of paralytic ileus or other gut dysfunctions requiring stimulation of motor activity (GEIGER et al. 1983; BICKEL et al. 1985). Hoe 825 is quite μ-selective ($K_i^\delta/K_i^\mu=37.7$; SCHILLER et al., unpublished data) and showed almost no side effects in a clinical test with healthy volunteers (JIAN et al. 1987).

G. Conclusions

During the past decade extensive synthetic efforts based on various design principles produced a number of opioid peptide analogs with high selectivity for either μ- or δ-receptors. On the other hand, peptide analogs showing high preference for κ-opioid receptors need yet to be developed. The development of opioid peptide analogs with selectivity for the putative μ-, δ-, and κ-receptor subtypes represents an important future challenge. The results of early clinical trials with relatively nonselective enkephalin analogs did not look promising because of a number of serious side effects produced by these compounds. Peptide analogs with high selectivity for distinct opioid receptor types and subtypes can be expected to produce fewer side effects and should be examined in future clinical trials. The development of peptide analogs showing great diversity in the relative lipophilicity/hydrophilicity of their structures offers the possibility of obtaining compounds that may or may not cross certain barriers (blood-brain barrier, placental barrier, etc.) and that may act at either central or distinct peripheral sites as potential therapeutic agents in various clinical situations.

Acknowledgement. The author's work described in this review was supported by operating grants from the Medical Research Council of Canada (MT-5655) and the US National Institute on Drug Abuse (DA-O4443 and DA-O6252).

References

Amiche M, Sagan S, Mor A, Delfour A, Nicolas P (1989) Dermenkephalin (Try-D-Met-Phe-His-Leu-Met-Asp-NH$_2$): a potent and fully specific agonist for the δ opioid receptor. Mol Pharmacol 35:774–779

Bajusz S, Rónai AZ, Székely JI, Miglécz E, Berzétei I (1980) Further enhancement of analgesic activity: enkephalin analogs with terminal guanidino group. FEBS Lett 110:85–87

Beddell CR, Clark RB, Hardy GW, Lowe LA, Ubatuba FB, Vane JR, Wilkinson S, Chang K-J, Cuatrecasas P, Miller RJ (1977) Structural requirements for opioid activity of analogues of the enkephalins. Proc R Soc Lond [Biol] 198:249–265

Benyhe S, Hepp J, Simon J, Borsodi A, Medzihradszky K, Wollemann M (1987) Tyr-D-Ala-Gly-(Me)Phe-chloromethyl ketone: a mu specific affinity label for the opioid receptor. Neuropeptides 9:225–235

Berman JM, Goodman M, Nguyen TM-D, Schiller PW (1983) Cyclic and acyclic partial retro-inverso enkephalins: µ-receptor selective enzyme-resistant analogs. Biochem Biophys Res Commun 115:864–870

Bickel M, Alpermann H-G, Roche M, Schemann M, Ehrlein H-J (1985) Pharmacology of a gut motility stimulating enkephalin analogue. Drug Res 35:1417–1426

Bowen WD, Hellewell SB, Kelemen M, Huey R, Stewart D (1987) Affinity labeling of δ-opiate receptors using [D-Ala^2, Leu^5, Cys^6]enkephalin. J Biol Chem 262:13434–13439

Chang K-J, Killian A, Hazum E, Cuatrecasas P, Chang J-K (1981) Morphiceptin (*H*-Tyr-Pro-Phe-Pro-NH$_2$): a potent and specific agonist for morphine (µ) receptors. Science 212:75–77

Chang K-J, Wei ET, Killian A, Chang K-J (1983) Potent morphiceptin analogs: structure activity relationships and morphine-like activities. J Pharmacol Exp Ther 227:403–408

Cheng YC, Prusoff WH (1973) Relationship between the inhibition constant (K_I) and the concentration of inhibitor which causes 50 per cent inhibition (I_{50}) of an enzymatic reaction. Biochem Pharmacol 22:3099–3102

Clark JA, Liu L, Price M, Hersh B, Edelson M, Pasternak GW (1989) Kappa opiate receptor multiplicity: evidence for two U50,488-sensitive κ_1 subtypes and a novel κ_3 subtype. J Pharmacol Exp Ther 251:461–468

Corbett AD, Gillan MGC, Kosterlitz HW, McKnight AT, Paterson SJ, Robson LE (1984) Selectivities of opioid peptide analogues as agonists and antagonists at the δ-receptor. Br J Pharmacol 83:271–279

Cotton R, Giles MG, Miller L, Shaw JS, Timms D (1984) ICI 174864: a highly selective antagonist for the opioid δ-receptor. Eur J Pharmacol 97:331–332

DiMaio J, Schiller PW (1980) A cyclic enkephalin analog with high in vitro opiate activity. Proc Natl Acad Sci USA 77:7162–7166

DiMaio J, Nguyen TM-D, Lemieux C, Schiller PW (1982) Synthesis and pharmacological characterization in vitro of cyclic enkephalin analogues: effect of conformational constraints on opiate receptor selectivity. J Med Chem 25:1432–1438

Erspamer V, Melchiorri P, Falconieri-Erspamer G, Negri L, Corsi R, Severini C, Barra D, Simmaco M, Kreil G (1989) Deltorphins: a family of naturally occurring peptides with high affinity and selectivity for δ opioid binding sites. Proc Natl Acad Sci USA 86:5188–5192

Földes J, Török K, Székely JI, Borvendég J, Karczag I, Tolna J, Marosfi S, Váradi A, Gara A, Rónai AZ, Szilágyi G (1983) Human tolerability studies with D-Met^2, Pro^5-enkephalinamide. Life Sci 33:769–772

Frederickson RCA (1986) Progress in the potential use of enkephalin analogs. In: Rapaka RS, Hawks RL (eds) Opioid peptides: Molecular pharmacology, biosynthesis, and analysis. Natl Inst Drug Abuse Res Monogr Ser 70:367

Frederickson RCA, Smithwick EL, Shuman R, Bemis KG (1981) Metkephamid, a systemically active analog of methionine enkephalin with potent opioid δ-receptor activity. Science 211:603–604

Gacel G, Fournié-Zaluski MC, Roques BP (1980) Tyr-D-Ser-Gly-Phe-Leu-Thr, a highly preferential ligand for δ-opiate receptors. FEBS Lett 118:245–247

Gacel G, Belleney J, Delay-Goyet P, Seguin C, Morgat J-L, Roques BP (1987) High affinity and improved selectivity for δ opioid receptors exhibited by new linear hexapeptides. In: Theodoropoulos D (ed) Peptides 1986. Proceedings of the 19th European peptide symposium. de Gruyter, Berlin, p 377

Gacel G, Zajac JM, Delay-Goyet P, Daugé V, Roques BP (1988a) Investigation of the structural parameters involved in the μ and δ opioid receptor discrimination of linear enkephalin-related peptides. J Med Chem 31:374–383

Gacel G, Daugé V, Breuzé P, Delay-Goyet P, Roques BP (1988b) Development of conformationally constrained linear peptides exhibiting a high affinity and pronounced selectivity for δ opioid receptors. J Med Chem 31:1891–1897

Gacel G, Fellion E, Baamonde A, Daugé V, Roques BP (1990) Synthesis, biochemical and pharmacological properties of BUBUC, a highly selective and systemically active agonist for in vivo studies of δ opioid receptors. Peptides 11:983–988

Gairin JE, Gouarderes C, Mazarguil H, Alvinerie P, Cros J (1984) [D-Pro^{10}]dynorphin-(1–11) is a highly potent and selective ligand for κ opioid receptors. Eur J Pharmacol 106:457–458

Gairin JE, Mazarguil H, Alvinerie P, Saint-Pierre S, Meunier J-C, Cros J (1986) Synthesis and biological activities of dynorphin A analogues with opioid antagonist properties. J Med Chem 29:1913–1917

Gairin JE, Mazarguil H, Alvinerie P, Botanch C, Cros J, Meunier J-C (1988) N,N-Diallyltyrosyl substitution confers antagonist properties on the κ-selective opioid peptide [D-Pro^{10}]dynorphin A-(1–11). Br J Pharmacol 95:1023–1030

Garbay-Jaureguiberry C, Robichon A, Daugé V, Rossignol P, Roques BP (1984) Highly selective photoaffinity labeling of μ and δ opioid receptors. Proc Natl Acad Sci USA 81:7718–7722

Geiger R, Bickel M, Teetz V, Alpermann H-G (1983) Central and peripheral action of enkephalin analogues. Hoppe Seyler's Z Physiol Chem 364:1555–1562

Goldstein A, Naidu A (1989) Multiple opioid receptors: ligand selectivity profiles and binding site signatures. Mol Pharmacol 36:265–272

Handa BK, Lane AC, Lord JAH, Morgan BA, Rance MJ, Smith CFC (1981) Analogues of β-LPH$^{61-64}$ possessing selective agonist activity at μ-opiate receptors. Eur J Pharmacol 70:531–540

Hansen PE, Morgan BA (1984) Structure-activity relationships in enkephalin peptides. In: Udenfriend S, Meienhofer J (eds) The peptides: analysis, synthesis, biology, vol 6. Academic, Orlando, p 269

Hardy GW, Lowe LA, Sang PY, Simpkin DSA, Wilkinson S, Follenfant RL, Smith
    TW (1988) Peripherally acting enkephalin analogues. 1. Polar pentapeptides.
    J Med Chem 31:960–966
Hardy GW, Lowe LA, Mills G, Sang PW, Simpkin DSA, Follenfant RL, Shankley
    C, Smith TW (1989) Peripherally acting enkephalin analogues. 2. Polar tri- and
    tetrapeptides. J Med Chem 32:1108–1118
Henschen A, Lottspeich F, Brantl V, Teschemacher H (1979) Novel opioid peptides
    derived from casein (β-casomorphins): I. Structure of active components from
    bovine casein peptone. Hoppe-Seyler's Z Physiol Chem 360:1217–1224
Herblin WF, Kauer JC, Tam SW (1987) Photoinactivation of the μ opioid receptor
    using a novel synthetic morphiceptin analog. Eur J Pharmacol 139:273–279
Höllt V (1986) Opioid peptide processing and receptor selectivity. Annu Rev
    Pharmacol Toxicol 26:59–77
Hruby VJ, Gehrig CA (1989) Recent developments in the design of receptor specific
    opioid peptides. Med Res Rev 9:343–401
Huffman WF, Callahan JF, Codd EE, Eggleston DS, Lemieux C, Newlander KA,
    Schiller PW, Takata DT, Walker RF (1989) Mimics of secondary structural
    elements of peptides and proteins. In: Tam J, Kaiser ET (eds) Synthetic
    peptides: approaches to biological problems (UCLA symposia on molecular and
    cellular biology, new series, vol 86). Liss, New York, p 257
James IF, Goldstein A (1984) Site-directed alkylation of multiple opioid receptors.
    I. Binding selectivity. Mol Pharmacol 25:337–342
James IF, Chavkin C, Goldstein A (1982) Preparation of brain membranes
    containing a single type of opioid receptor highly selective for dynorphin. Proc
    Natl Acad Sci USA 79:7570–7574
Jian R, Janssens J, Vantrappen G, Ceccatelli P (1987) Influence of metenkephalin
    analogue on motor activity of the gastrointestinal tract. Gastroenterology
    93:114–120
Kawasaki, AM, Knapp R, Wire WS, Kramer T, Yamamura HI, Burks TF, Hruby
    VJ (1990) Cyclic dynorphin A analogs with high selectivities and potencies at κ
    opioid receptors. In: Rivier JE, Marshall GR (eds) Peptides: chemistry,
    structure, biology. Proceedings of the 11th American peptide symposium.
    ESCOM, Leiden, p 337
Kazmierski W, Wire WS, Lui GK, Knapp RJ, Shook JE, Burks TF, Yamamura HI,
    Hruby VJ (1988) Design and synthesis of somatostatin analogues with
    topographical properties that lead to highly potent and specific μ opioid receptor
    antagonists with greatly reduced binding at somatostatin receptors. J Med Chem
    31:2170–2177
Kessler H, Hölzemann G, Zechel C (1985) Peptide conformations. 33. Con-
    formational analysis of cyclic enkephalin analogs of the type Tyr-cyclo-(-N^ω-
    Xxx-Gly-Phe-Leu-). Int J Pept Protein Res 25:267–279
Kiso Y, Yamaguchi M, Akita T, Moritoki H, Takei M, Nakamura H (1981) Simple
    tripeptide hydroxyalkylamides exhibit surprisingly high and long-lasting opioid
    activities. Naturwissenschaften 68:210–212
Kondo M, Kodama H, Costa T, Shimohigashi Y (1986) Cystamine-enkephalin
    dimer. Int J Pept Protein Res 27:153–159
Kosterlitz HW, Lord JAH, Paterson SJ, Waterfield AA (1980) Effects of changes in
    the structure of enkephalins and of narcotic analgesic drugs on their interactions
    with μ- and δ-receptors. Br J Pharmacol 68:333–342
Kreil G, Barra D, Simmaco M, Erspamer V, Falconieri-Erspamer G, Negri L,
    Severini C, Corsi R, Melchiorri P (1989) Deltorphin, a novel amphibian skin
    peptide with high selectivity and affinity for δ opioid receptors. Eur J Pharmacol
    162:123–128
Kris MG, Gralla RJ, Clark RA, Tyson LB, Groshen S (1988) Control of
    chemotherapy-induced diarrhea with the synthetic enkephalin BW942C: a
    randomized trial with placebo in patients receiving cisplatin. J Clin Oncol
    6:663–668

Landis G, Lui G, Shook JE, Yamamura HI, Burks TF, Hruby VJ (1989) Synthesis of highly μ and δ opioid receptor selective peptides containing a photoaffinity group. J Med Chem 32:638–643

Lemaire S, Lafrance L, Dumont M (1986) Synthesis and bilogical activity of dynorphin-(1–13) and analogs substituted in positions 8 and 10. Int J Pept Protein Res 27:300–305

Lord JAH, Waterfield AA, Hughes J, Kosterlitz HW (1977) Endogenous opioid peptides: multiple agonists and receptors. Nature 267:495–499

Lutz RA, Cruciani RA, Shimohigashi Y, Costa T, Kassis S, Munson PJ, Rodbard D (1985) Increased affinity and selectivity of enkephalin tripeptide (Tyr-D-Ala-Gly) dimers. Eur J Pharmacol 111:257–261

Mammi NJ, Hassan, M, Goodman M (1985) Conformational analysis of a cyclic enkephalin analogue by ^{1}HNMR and computer simulations. J Am Chem Soc 107:4008–4013

Marastoni M, Salvadori S, Balboni G, Borea PA, Marzola G, Tomatis R (1987) Synthesis and activity profiles of new dermorphin-(1–4) peptide analogues. J Med Chem 30:1538–1542

Martin WR, Eades CG, Thompson JA, Huppler RA, Gilbert PE (1976) The effects of morphine- and nalorphine-like drugs in the nondependent and morphine-dependent chronic spinal dog. J Pharmacol Exp Ther 197:517–523

Maurer R, Gaehwiler BH, Buescher HH, Hill RC, Roemer D (1982) Opiate antagonistic properties of an octapeptide somatostatin analog. Proc Natl Acd Sci USA 79:4815–4817

Montecucchi PC, deCastiglione R, Piani S, Gozzini L, Erspamer V (1981) Amino acid composition and sequence of dermorphin, a novel opiate-like peptide from the skin of *Phyllomedusa sauvagei*. Int J Pept Protein Res 17:275–283

Morley JS (1980) Structure-activity relationships of enkephalin-like peptides. Annu Rev Pharmacol Toxicol 20:81–110

Morley JS, Dutta AS (1986) Structure-activity relationships of opioid peptides. In: Rapaka RS, Barnett G, Hawks RL (eds) Opioid peptides: Medicinal chemistry. Natl Inst Drug Abuse Res Monogr Ser 69:42

Mosberg HI, Hurst R, Hruby VJ, Galligan JI, Burks IF, Gee K, Yamamura HI (1982) [D-Pen^2,L-Cys^5]Enkephalinamide and [D-Pen^2,D-Cys^5]enkephalinamide, conformationally constrained cyclic enkephalinamide analogs with δ receptor specificity. Biochem Biophys Res Commun 106:506–512

Mosberg HI, Hurst, R, Hruby VJ, Galligan JJ, Burks TF, Gee K, Yamamura HI (1983a) Conformationally constrained cyclic enkephalin analogs with pronounced delta opioid receptor agonist selectivity. Life Sci 32:2565–2569

Mosberg HI, Hurst R, Hruby VJ, Gee K, Yamamura HI, Galligan JJ, Burks TF (1983b) Bis-penicillamine enkephalins posses highly improved specificity toward δ opioid receptors. Proc Natl Acad Sci USA 80:5871–5874

Mosberg HI, Omnaas JR, Goldstein A (1987) Structural requirements for delta opioid receptor binding. Mol Pharmacol 31:599–602

Mosberg HI, Omnaas JR, Medzihradsky F, Smith GB (1988) Cyclic disulfide- and dithioether-containing opioid tetrapeptides: development of a ligand with high delta opioid receptor selectivity and affinity. Life Sci 43:1013–1020

Newman EL, Barnard EA (1984) Identification of an opioid receptor subunit carrying the μ binding site. Biochemistry 23:5385–5389

Pelton JT, Gulya K, Hruby VJ, Duckles SP, Yamamura HI (1985) Conformationally restricted analogs of somatostatin with high μ-opiate specificity. Proc Natl Acad Sci USA 82:236–239

Pelton JT, Kazmierski W, Gulya K, Yamamura HI, Hruby VJ (1986) Design and synthesis of conformationally constrained somatostatin analogues with high potency and specificity for μ opioid receptors. J Med Chem 29:2370–2375

Pert CB, Pert A, Chang J-K, Fong BTW (1976) (D-Ala^2)-Met-enkephalinamide: a potent, long-lasting synthetic pentapeptide analgesic. Science 194:330–332

Posner J, Dean K, Jeal S, Moody SG, Peck AW, Rutter G, Telekes A (1988) A preliminary study of the pharmacodynamics and pharmacokinetics of a novel enkephalin analogue [Tyr-D-Arg-Gly-Phe(4NO$_2$)-Pro-NH$_2$ (BW443C)] in healthy volunteers. Eur J Clin Pharmacol 34:67–71

Quirion R, Kiso Y, Pert CB (1982) Syndyphalin SD-25: a highly selective ligand for μ opiate receptors. FEBS Lett 141:203–206

Rigaudy P, Garbay-Jaureguiberry C, Jacquemin-Sablon A, LePecq J-B, Roques BP (1987) Synthesis and binding properties to DNA and to opioid receptors of enkephalin-ellipticinium conjugates. Int J Pept Protein Res 30:347–355

Roemer D, Buescher HH, Hill RC, Pless J, Bauer W, Cardinaux F, Closse A, Hauser D, Huguenin R (1977) A synthetic enkephalin analogue with prolonged parenteral and oral analgesic activity. Nature 268:547–549

Sagan S, Amiche M, Delfour A, Mor A, Camus A, Nicolas P (1989) Molecular determinants of receptor affinity and selectivity of the natural Δ-opioid agonist dermenkephalin. J Biol Chem 264:17100–17106

Sarantakis D (1979) Analgesic polypeptide. U S Patent 4,148,786

Sasaki Y, Matsui M, Fujita H, Hosono M, Taguchi M, Suzuki K, Sakurada S, Sato T, Sakurada T, Kisara K (1985) The analgesic activity of D-Arg^2-dermorphin and its N-terminal tetrapeptide analogs after subcutaneous administration in mice. Neuropeptides 5:391–394

Schiller PW (1984) Conformational analysis of enkephalin and conformation-activity relationships. In: Udenfriend S, Meienhofer J (eds) The peptides: analysis, synthesis, biology, vol 6. Academic, Orlando, p 219

Schiller PW (1991) Development of receptor specific opioid peptide analogs. In: Ellis GP, West GB (eds) Progress in medicinal chemistry. Elsevier, Amsterdam, p 301

Schiller PW, DiMaio J (1982) Opiate receptor subclasses differ in their conformational requirements. Nature 297:74–76

Schiller PW, Wilkes BC (1988) Conformational analysis of cyclic opioid peptide analogs. In: Rapaka RS, Dhawan BN (eds) Recent progress in the chemistry and biology of opioid peptides. Natl Inst Drug Abuse Res Monogr Ser 87:60

Schiller PW, Eggimann B, DiMaio J, Lemieux C, Nguyen TM-D (1981) Cyclic enkephalin analogs containing a cystine bridge. Biochem Biophys Res Commun 101:337–343

Schiller PW, Nguyen TM-D, DiMaio J, Lemieux C (1983) Comparison of μ-, δ- and κ-receptor binding sites through pharmacologic evaluation of p-nitrophenyl-alanine analogs of opioid peptides. Life Sci 33:319–322

Schiller PW, Nguyen TM-D, Maziak LA, Lemieux C (1985a) A novel cyclic opioid peptide analog showing high preference for μ-receptors. Biochem Biophys Res Commun 127:558–564

Schiller PW, DiMaio J, Nguyen TM-D (1985b) Activity profiles of conformationally restricted opioid peptide analogs. In: Ovchinnikov YA (ed) Proceedings of the 16th FEBS meeting. VNU Science, Utrecht, p 457

Schiller PW, Nguyen TM-D, Maziak LA, Wilkes BC, Lemieux C (1987) Structure-activity relationships of cyclic opioid peptide analogues containing a phenylalanine residue in the 3-position. J Med Chem 30:2094–2099

Schiller PW, Nguyen TM-D, Lemieux C (1988) Synthesis and opioid activity profiles of cyclic dynorphin analogs. Tetrahedron 44:733–743

Schiller PW, Nguyen TM-D, Chung NN, Lemieux C (1989a) Dermorphin analogues carrying an increased positive net charge in their "message" domain display extremely high μ opioid recptor selectivity. J Med Chem 32:698–703

Schiller PW, Nguyen TM-D, Lemieux C (1989b) New types of opioid peptide analogs showing high μ-receptor selectivity and preference for either central or peripheral sites. In: Jung G, Bayer E (eds) Peptides 1988 Proceedings of the 20th European peptide symposium. DeGruyter, Berlin, p 613

Schiller PW, Nguyen TM-D, Chung NN, Dionne G, Martel R (1990a) Peripheral antinociceptive effect of an extremely μ-selective polar dermorphin analog (DALDA) In: Quirion R, Jhamandas K, Gianoulakis C (eds) The international narcotics research conference (INRC) 1989. Liss, New York, p 53

Schiller PW, Nguyen TM-D, Weltrowska G, Lemieux C, Chung NN (1990b) Development of [D-Ala²]deltorphin I analogs with extraordinary delta receptor selectivity. In: van Ree JM, Mulder AH, Wiegant VM, van Wimersma Greidanus TB (eds) New leads in opioid research. Excerpta Medica, Amsterdam, p 288

Schiller PW, Weltrowska G, Nguyen TM-D, Lemieux C, Chung NN, Wilkes BC (1991) The use of multiple conformational restriction in the development of opioid peptidomimetics. In: Giralt E, Andreu D (eds) Peptides 1990. Proceedings of the 21st European peptide symposium. ESCOM, Leiden, p 621

Schulz R, Fasse E, Wüster M, Herz A (1979) Selective receptors for β-endorphin on the rat vas deferens. Life Sci 24:843–850

Schwyzer R (1986) Molecular mechanism of opioid receptor selection. Biochemistry 25:6335–6342

Shaw JS, Miller L, Turnbull MJ, Gormley JJ, Morley JS (1982) Selective antagonists at the opiate delta receptor. Life Sci 31:1259–1262

Shearman GT, Schultz R, Schiller PW, Herz A (1985) Generalization tests with intraventricularly applied pro-enkephalin B-derived peptides in rats trained to discriminate the opioid kappa receptor agonist ethylketocyclazocine. Psychopharmacology 85:440–443

Sherman DB, Spatola AF, Wire WS, Burks TF, Nguyen TM-D, Schiller PW (1989) Biological activities of cyclic enkephalin pseudopeptides containing thioamides as amide bond replacements. Biochem Biophys Res Commun 162:1126–1132

Shimohigashi Y, Costa T, Chen H-C, Rodbard D (1982) Dimeric tetrapeptide enkephalins display extraordinary selectivity for the δ opiate receptor. Nature 297:333–335

Shimohigashi Y, Ogasawara T, Koshizaka T, Waki M, Kato T, Izumiya N, Kurono M, Yagi K (1987a) Interaction of dimers of inactive enkephalin fragments with μ opiate receptors. Biochem Biophys Res Commun 146:1109–1115

Shimohigashi Y, Costa T, Pfeiffer A, Herz A, Kimura H, Stammer CH (1987b) ∇^EPhe⁴-enkephalin analogs. FEBS Lett 222:71–74

Shuman RT, Hynes MD, Woods JH, Gesellchen P (1990) A highly selective in vitro μ-opioid agonist with atypical in vivo pharmacology. In: Rivier JE, Marshall GR (eds) Peptides: chemistry, structure, biology. Proceedings of the 11th American peptide symposium. ESCOM, Leiden, p 326

Smith TW, Buchan P, Parsons DN, Wilkinson S (1982) Peripheral antinociceptive effects of N-methyl morphine. Life Sci 31:1205–1208

Stein C, Millan MJ, Yassouridis A, Herz A (1988) Antinociceptive effects of μ- and κ-agonists in inflammation are enhanced by a peripheral opioid receptor-specific mechanism. Eur J Pharmacol 155:255–264

Szücs M, Belcheva M, Simon J, Benyhe S, Tóth G, Hepp J, Wollemann M, Medzihradszky K (1987) Covalent labeling of opioid receptors with ³H-D-Ala²-Leu⁵-enkephalin chloromethyl ketone. I. Binding characteristics in rat brain membranes. Life Sci 41:177–184

Thornber CW, Shaw JS, Miller L, Hayward CF, Morley JS, Timms D, Wilkinson A (1986a) New δ-receptor antagonists. In: Holaday JW, Law P-Y, Herz A (eds) Progress in opioid research. Natl Inst Drug Abuse Res Monogr Ser 75:177

Thornber CW, Shaw JS, Miller L, Hayward CF (1986b) Dimeric opioid antagonists. Natl Inst Drug Abuse Res Monogr Ser 75:181

Thót G, Kramer TH, Knapp R, Lui G, Davis P, Burks TF, Yamamura HI, Hruby VJ (1990) [D-Pen², D-Pen⁵]enkephalin analogues with increased affinity and selectivity for δ opioid receptors. J Med Chem 33:249–253

Venn RF, Barnard EA (1981) A potent peptide affinity reagent for the opiate receptor. J Biol Chem 256:1529–1532

Von Graffenried B, del Pozo E, Roubicek J, Krebs E, Poldinger W, Burmeister P, Kerp L (1978) Effects of the synthetic enkephalin analogue FK33-824 in man. Nature 272:729–730

Walker JM, Bowen WD, Atkins SD, Hemstreet MK, Coy DH (1987) μ-Opiate binding and morphine antagonism by octapeptide analogs of somatostatin. Peptides 8:869–875

Wilkes BC, Schiller PW (1990) Conformation-activity relationships of cyclic dermorphin analogues. Biopolymers 29:89–95

Yamashiro D, Li CH (1984) β-Endorphin: structure and activity. In: Udenfriend S, Meienhofer J (eds) The peptides: analysis, synthesis, biology, vol 6. Academic, Orlando, p 191

Yang C-C, Taylor JW (1990) The design, synthesis and biological studies of synthetic peptide models of dynorphin A (1–17). In: Rivier JE, Marshall GR (eds) Peptides: chemistry, structure, biology. Proceedings of the 11th American peptide symposium. ESCOM, Leiden, p 346

Zajac JM, Gacel G, Petit F, Dodey P, Rossignol P, Roques BP (1983) Deltakephalin, Tyr-D-Thr-Gly-Phe-Leu-Thr: a new highly potent and fully specific agonist for opiate δ-receptors. Biochem Biophys Res Commun 111:390–397

CHAPTER 28

Ontogeny of Mammalian Opioid Systems

J.E. PINTAR and R.E.M. SCOTT

A. Introduction

At least two of the three distinct genes encoding peptides with opioid activity are expressed during prenatal development not only in the CNS and endocrine cells, but also in specific peripheral tissues. Although it is not yet known whether any of the opioid peptides derived from these opioid precursors are required for normal development, any prospective action requires not only gene activation, but also appropriate maturation of numerous cellular functions including biosynthesis, posttranslational processing, and regulation of synthesis and secretion. In addition, the cognate receptor(s) for presumptive bioactive peptides must be present and active. In this review, we will synthesize the information available on prenatal expression of all three opioid systems, proopiomelanocortin (POMC), proenkephalin (PENK), and prodynorphin (PDYN), but will focus on differentiation of POMC cells in the rodent pituitary where the most complete information is available. Relevant studies and reviews beyond the scope of this review will be cited as appropriate, and the authors apologize in advance for being unable to cite or discuss in detail all relevant work because of space limitations.

B. Embryological Considerations

Because pituitary POMC cells represent the best-studied opiate precursor population during differentiation, it is important to review the ontogeny of the pituitary especially in light of recent experimental observations that have clarified its origin. It is well known that two distinct pituitary cell types, the corticotroph and melanotroph, express the single functional POMC gene found in most vertebrates. These cell types are found in two distinct regions of the pituitary, the anterior and intermediate lobes, in most vertebrate species. These lobes, in turn, are derived from different parts of the adeno-hypophysis, which includes not only the anterior and intermediate pituitary lobes but also the pars tuberalis (SCHWIND 1928; SVALANDER 1974; IKEDA et al. 1988). The cells comprising the adenohypophysis are derived from an invagination of the oral ectoderm, Rathke's pouch. In both the avian (COULY and LEDOUARIN 1985) and the amphibian (EAGLESON et al. 1986), it has been shown that Rathke's pouch originates from the anterior ventral neural ridge, the most anterior region of the neural fold area that is just rostral to the neural plate. The presumptive pituitary is immediately rostral to the presumptive hypothalamic area, another region characterized by POMC cells, and is transiently separated from it during folding of the embyro. Although these two fetal regions are not the only areas where the POMC gene is activated, these observations suggest that instructive signals initiating POMC expression are particularly abundant in this region. In addition, it has been shown that the interaction between the presumptive posterior lobe (the infundibulum, an outpocketing of the diencephalon) and Rathke's pouch during early development is required for differentiation of the frog intermediate lobe (Hanuoka 1967), although the role and mechanism of this interaction during mammalian pituitary development remains to be determined (Pintar and Lugo 1987).

The regulatory regions of the POMC gene that are necessary and sufficient for anterior and intermediate pituitary expression in vivo have been deduced from transgenic mouse studies (G.D. Hammer et al. 1990) and reside between nucleotides -706 and $+64$; thus these regions likely bind the appropriate transcription factors that elicit POMC expression. An important issue, which is unresolved, is the identity of the molecular mechanisms by which distinct POMC populations express not only POMC but also the cell-type specific sets of distinct genes that are characteristic of the distinct cell phenotypes.

C. Opioid Gene Activation

The onset of POMC transcription has been followed in many tissue types using methods that both measure RNA in tissue extracts and follow mRNA-containing cells by in situ hybridization; these studies have often been accompanied by immunocytochemical studies. Widespread occurrence of PENK mRNA in both neural and nonneural sites has recently been noted, while the expression of dynorphin appears thus far to be limited to its sites of expression in the adult brain.

I. Proopiomelanocortin

1. Brain

The major populations of adult CNS POMC neurons are located in the adult hypothalamic arcuate and solitary nuclei (Khatchaturian et al. 1985a). During rodent development, the first fetal cells to become immunoreactive for POMC peptides appear in the ventral diencephalon at equivalent developmental stages in both the rat (embryonic day (e) 12; Khatchaturian et al. 1983) and mouse (e10.5; Elkabes et al. 1989) at the age when these cells first become postmitotic (KHATCHATURIAN et al. 1985b). This region contains neuronal cell bodies that are the progenitors of the arcuate nucleus (KHATCHATURIAN et al. 1985b). The ontogeny of other POMC neuronal cell groups has not been followed so precisely. The initial site of POMC expression in *Xenopus laevis*, where development of the pituitary gland is quite different, is distinct from rodents. In this species, unlike rodents, cells containing POMC mRNA appear first in the pituitary plate prior to their appearance in the diencephalon (HAYES and LOH 1990).

2. Pituitary

In the rat, levels of both POMC mRNA and the intron A-containing precursor of POMC mRNA have been measured quantitatively from e15 onwards using RNase protection assays with a cRNA probe containing both intron and exon sequences (SCOTT et al. 1990). These data show that the ratios of hnRNA/mRNA are proportionately higher in both POMC populations at all prenatal ages than in the adult. Presumably this reflects the fact that cells that have been differentiated for varying periods are included in each sample, including newly differentiated cells where adult steady-state RNA levels have not been reached (SCOTT et al. 1990). Even with this caveat, however, mRNA levels measured at postnatal ages (SCOTT et al. 1990) generally correlate with peptide levels previously reported (SATO and MAINS 1985). In both cases, anterior lobe (AL) levels at birth are closer to adult levels than intermediate lobe (IL) levels. Combined in situ hybridization/immunocytochemistry studies have been reported for both mouse and rat and indicate that, in both species, POMC mRNA and POMC-related peptides are first detected at different times in anterior and intermediate lobes. In the mouse, POMC mRNA and ACTH immunoreactivity are first seen at e12.5 and are located in the most ventral region of the presumptive anterior lobe, while both POMC mRNA and corresponding peptides are not seen in the developing IL at e14.5; no difference between the onset of mRNA and peptide accumulation was detected (ELKABES et al. 1989). A similar pattern is seen in the rat, where POMC mRNA is first detected at e13 in the ventral aspect of Rathke's pouch, which eventually gives rise to the AL, while POMC mRNA is not seen in IL until e15 (LUGO et al. 1989). IL POMC mRNA and peptide were first detected in a specific midcaudal region of this lobe and subsequently extended in a gradient-like pattern to the rest of the IL. In the rat, a short interval (0.5 days) between POMC mRNA detection and POMC peptide accumulation has been detected. Semiquantitative measurements of in situ labeling showed that POMC mRNA content/cell increases during development and that adult levels are not achieved by birth in either AL or IL populations. Taken together, these results from rodent species provide strong evidence that factors eliciting POMC transcription in these two pituitary cell populations act at distinct times during development.

3. Testis

In the adult testis, most POMC mRNA has a size of about 800–900 nucleotides, which is about 300 nucleotides shorter than pituitary POMC mRNA (Pintar et al. 1984). This characteristic size of the major testicular POMC mRNA species has been observed in mouse testis as early as e17 (Gizang-Ginsberg and Wolgemuth 1987). Prenatal POMC immunoreactive interstitial cells are also detectable in the mouse and peak as a percentage of testicular cells coincident with the prenatal peak of testosterone that occurs just prior to birth. During the first 2 weeks after birth, testicular POMC peptides become undetectable immunocytochemically (Shaha et al. 1984) and POMC mRNA cannot be detected by Northern blot analysis (Gizang-Ginsberg and Wolgemuth 1987). The function, if any, of POMC expression in the fetal testis remains unknown.

4. Placenta

Expression of the POMC gene has been demonstrated in both rat and human placenta. In the rat, expression levels do not change between 2 and 3 weeks of pregnancy (mid- to late gestation in the rat) when normalized to tissue RNA (Chen et al. 1986). Processing of placental POMC is similar to the adult anterior lobe (see below), although some of the ACTH domain is cleaved to α-MSH-sized peptides. β-Endorphin (β-EP) is the predominant opioid peptide that has been detected in human placental extracts and represents about 50% of the β-LPH immunoreactivity (Liotta and Krieger 1980). Parenthetically, corticotrophin-releasing hormone (CRH) is produced by the human placenta in levels that can alter maternal serum circulating ACTH and β-EP levels (Goland et al. 1986) but this additional CRH can apparently be buffered by corresponding increases in a recently described CRH-binding protein that inhibits CRH bioactivity (Potter et al. 1991).

II. Enkephalin

Initial analysis of PENK during development primarily relied on immunocytochemical procedures. Although these studies have been valuable in identifying these cell types prenatally (see Palmer et al. 1982), the extent of PENK precursor processing in the fetus has been relatively unexplored. As a result, some cell types that contain PENK mRNA and/or contain precursor forms that are not recognized by many antisera made to end product peptides may have been overlooked. More recent studies have used in situ hybridization to detect PENK mRNA-containing cells and have described interesting patterns of expression that as yet, however, do not have a functional correlate.

1. Brain (Striatal)

In the adult rat, large amounts of PENK are synthesized in the striatum. The ontogeny of PENK expression in the striatal regions has been studied in detail. A combined in situ hybridization/immunocytochemical analysis showed that PENK mRNA first appears at e16 in the caudal ventrolateral striatum, although immunoreactivity (enk-RGL) was not detected until e17–18 (Tecott et al. 1989). Accumulation of PENK mRNA in different striatal regions accompanied the general birthdates of striatal neurons and did not exhibit a "patchy" appearance characteristic of striatal "striosomes" at any time. A limited in situ analysis of postnatal ages did not detect any evidence of alterations in PENK levels during these stages of development. Northern analysis has, however, suggested that PENK mRNA in the striatum exhibits a biphasic pattern of expression during postnatal ages (Schwartz and Simantov 1988; Rosen and Polakiewicz 1989). PENK mRNA remained constant from e14 to birth, and then increased to a peak at p2 before declining back to embryonic levels. At ~p14 PENK mRNA increased again, reaching adult levels by ~p28. Surprisingly, it appeared that the biphasic nature of mRNA accumulation was not reflected in levels of peptide in the striatum.

2. Glia

Many recent studies have shown that PENK expression is not restricted to neural cells during development. It is, for example, now clear that PENK mRNA and at least the PENK prohormone are present in glia. It was first reported that glial cells in the cerebellum were immunopositive for enkephalin during early postnatal ages (Zagon et al. 1985). Subsequently, cultured embryonic and neonatal astrocytes, identified by glial fibrillary acidic protein (GFAP) immunoreactivity, have been found to contain significant levels of preproenkephalin mRNA (Vilijn et al. 1988; Schwartz and Simantov 1988; Melner et al. 1990) and at least some processed met-enkephalin-arg-phe (met-RF) (Shinoda et al. 1989; Melner et al. 1990). Astrocytes cultured from different areas of the brain contain different levels of PENK mRNA; for example, glia cultured from hypothalamus have higher levels of PENK mRNA than glia from the striatum or cerebellum (Vilijn et al. 1988). It has thus been suggested that PENK-expressing astrocytes may play a role in brain development in vivo and that regional differences among astrocytes may affect this process. It is of interest that blockade of opioid receptors with naloxone enhances neurite outgrowth from explant cultures (Hauser et al. 1989), but direct genetic interference with opioid synthesis in vivo will be necessary to prove a relationship between opioid expression and aspects of neurogenesis. The extent of glial PENK processing in vivo needs to be assessed more directly; the possibility that PENK processing differs among regions should be examined, since PENK mRNA and its translated precursor form, but not PENK-derived peptides, have been detected recently in adult cerebellum (Spruce et al. 1990).

3. Fetal Mesoderm

Cells outside the CNS also express PENK mRNA during development. Adult cardiac myocytes were the first nonendocrine cell type shown to express PENK (Howells et al. 1986) and a broad pattern of PENK expression that is not neuro- or neuroendocrine related has now been documented during fetal rodent development. The present consensus from numerous studies is that PENK mRNA is transiently expressed in numerous mesodermally derived tissues during prenatal and early postnatal development. The most complete study so far (Keshet et al. 1989) detected PENK mRNA by in situ hybridization in numerous nondifferentiated mesodermal cells including the perichondrium, dermis, sclera of the eye, and mesenchyme of the kidney during mid-gestational stages (e15.5). Expression in these tissues dropped to undetectable levels upon terminal differentiation. Other studies have confirmed the developmentally regulated nature of mesodermal PENK expression (Polakiewicz and Rosen 1990; Kew and Kilpatrick 1990), further indicate that PENK mRNA is associated with the polysome fraction and thus actively translated (Kew and Kilpatrick 1990), and provide limited documentation that PENK-related peptides are present (Keshet et al. 1989; Polakiewicz and Rosen 1990). The expression pattern is consistent with possible autocrine or paracrine effects on proliferation, but no direct evidence yet suggests an essential role for this expression.

III. Dynorphin

Cells immunoreactive for dynorphin A in the supraoptic and paraventricular nuclei and the lateral hypothalamic area are born at early times in the rat (e12–e13; Khatchaturian et al. 1985b), although the regulation of PDYN gene expression during ontogeny remains largely unexplored. One report of changes in steady state postnatal levels of dynorphin mRNA in pooled samples of striatum and hypothalamus suggests that concentrations of PDYN mRNA exhibit different developmental profiles in these regions. Thus, for example, PDYN mRNA levels appear to peak in the 1st week after birth and then again after weaning in hypothalamus while, for example, decreasing in the pons and striatum (Rosen and Polakiewicz 1989). In contrast to PENK expression in glial cells (see above), no PDYN mRNA has been detected in cultured neonatal glial cells from any brain regions (Vilijn et al. 1988).

D. Ontogeny of Opioid Precursor Processing

The end points of opioid precursor processing differ among tissues that express the genes for these precursors. It is thus important from developmental, cell biological, and physiological perspectives to determine whether the time at which processing begins is identical to the time at which prohormone synthesis is initiated and whether the processing patterns that are distinctive of specific cell populations in the adult are invariant during development. Since opioid precursor genes are generally present in a single copy, it is expected (but not yet proven) that the tissue-specific differences in processing are regulated by differences in the type and level of processing enzymes themselves. Thus, knowledge of the ontogenetic processing patterns can reveal much about the cell biology of processing and the activation of processing genes. Finally, these analyses can establish which peptides are actually present at different developmental stages and thus which of the functions ascribed to these peptides during ontogeny are at least possible. The posttranslational processing of POMC is the least complex and thus better understood in development than those of the other opioid precursors.

I. Proopiomelanocortin

In the rat, numerous early immunocytochemical studies were carried out prior to the time when the multipeptide structure of the POMC precursor became known (see DUPOUY 1980; see also MULCHAHEY et al. 1987). Therefore, although these studies identified POMC cells, the extent of processing could not be deduced because the ability of antisera to recognize biosynthetic precursors, in addition to end product peptides, was not assessed. Some more recent studies have used antibodies specific for distinct POMC processing end points either immunocytochemically or in conjunction with peptide analysis and have provided evidence for POMC precursor processing at the fetal ages when immunoreactive cells are first detected.

1. Immunocytochemical Analyses

Immunocytochemically, the anterior lobe corticotroph is the first pituitary hormone-containing cell to differentiate (SETALO and NAKANE 1972; NAKANE et al. 1977; WATANABE and DAIKOKU 1979). Immunocytochemically detectable cells are initially detected in the presumptive anterior lobe of the pituitary at ~e14 using antisera against ACTH(1–39) (WATANABE and DAIKOKU 1979) and other POMC-derived peptides (16K fragment, ACTH and β-EP; KHATCHATURIAN et al. 1983). The studies by Khachaturian were the first to suggest that cells with α-MSH like properties are transiently present in the anterior lobe. These des-acetyl-α-MSH-containing cells persist in the rat anterior lobe well into neonatal life (SATO and MAINS 1985) and are also found in the human fetal pituitary (TILDERS et al. 1981).

2. Biochemical Analyses

Biochemical characterization of POMC-derived peptide products in the fetal rat pituitary at early ages (e14–e17) have demonstrated that about 50% of the total molar amount of POMC immunoreactivity is contained in the POMC precursor. The precursor molecules that do undergo processing have ACTH and β-LPH domains that are essentially completely proteolytically cleaved to amidated des-acetyl α-MSH and des-acetyl β-EP (Allen et al. 1984; Pintar et al. 1986). Thus both the endoprotease(s) involved in cleavage and the amidation enzyme (PAM) are active as early as immuno-positive cells are detected. From e18 onwards the anterior and neurointer-mediate lobes have been studied separately at both prenatal (Pintar and Lugo 1987) and postnatal ages (Sato and Mains 1985). In the anterior lobe, there is a gradual shift in ACTH domain processing from the essentially complete cleavage that characterizes early ages to the extremely limited cleavage that characterizes the adult. The basis for this transition is still unknown, but it is possible that developmentally regulated expression of the Kex-related PC1 and PC2 that have recently been identified in rodents (Seidah et al. 1991) may have a role. Since PC2 is expressed predominantly in the adult intermediate lobe, it is possible that this enzyme performs intermediate lobe-specific cleavages and, if transiently expressed in the fetal anterior lobe POMC cells, could account for the processing end points that have been observed. In the neurointermediate lobe, N-acetylated forms of α-MSH and β-EP have been biochemically characterized as early as e21 in the rat although, unlike the adult, significant levels of nonacetylated β-EP are present in the IL at prenatal ages. Further, immunocytochemically detectable N-acetyl-endorphin cells are restricted to the intermediate lobe throughout prenatal development and appear essentially coincidently with β-EP immunoreactive cells during ontogeny (Pintar and Lugo 1987) at the same time α-MSH is first detected biochemically (Loh et al. 1980; Khorram and McCann 1984). Thus both liberation of β-EP and its acetylation arise essentially concurrently during ontogeny, which presumably reflects the coordinated expression of the cognate genes.

II. Dynorphin

The PDYN-related peptides in the pituitary are the only non-POMC opioid system that has been studied to any extent during development. The pro-cessing of dynorphin peptides in the anterior and neural lobes, like POMC peptides, exhibits developmental changes that share some characteristics with the ontogeny of POMC processing. For example, the relative levels of dynorphin immunoreactivity in the pituitary are nearer adult levels in the anterior lobe rather than in the neurointermediate lobe at birth (Seizinger et al. 1984). Further, processing of the dyn (1–32) domain of the PDYN precursor undergoes a developmental switch, with the extent of processing less complete in the neonate than in the adult (Seizinger et al. 1984).

E. Ontogeny of Regulated Release

I. Secretory Granules, Regulators of POMC Secretion and the Portal System

The secretory response of cells containing POMC peptides is primarily regulated by hypothalamic factors (such as CRH) as well as adrenal hormones (such as glucocorticoids) that form an integral part of the hypothalamic-hypophysial-adrenal axis. During development, the onset of basal secretory capability from peptide-producing cells is dependent on the differentiation of the secretory apparatus and formation of secretory granules. Stimulation of secretion requires the onset of expression of those factors that can regulate secretion in conjunction with an effective delivery system, and the ability of opiate cells in the process of differentiation to respond to these regulators during development via functional receptors. Again, the development of the POMC system has been the most thoroughly studied so far.

Corticotrophin-releasing hormone immunoreactivity has been detected as early as e15 in whole brain (RUNDLE and FUNDER 1988), and CRH mRNA-containing cells have been detected at e17 in the hypothalamus using in situ hybridization (GRINO et al. 1989). Maturation of the portal system vasculature is also essential to transmit hypothalamic regulators to pituitary targets, and each time that this system has been reexamined with more sensitive procedures the development of at least a rudimentary portal system has been noted at younger ages. Thus although the capillary loops of the pars externa of the median eminence do not appear until 3–4 days after birth (GLYDON 1957; FINK and SMITH 1971; NEGM 1971), it has been suggested that before this time neurosecretory products from the hypothalamus may reach the pituitary by simple diffusion (WATKINS and CHOY 1979). The finding that neurosecretory endings reach the external median eminence before birth is consistent with an earlier maturation of a rudimentary portal system than previously thought (SZABO and CSANYI 1982).

The presence of secretory granules is generally used as evidence of hormonal activity in these cells (YOSHIDA 1966; SVALANDER 1974; STOECKEL et al. 1979; DUPOUY 1980). In the rat, ultrastructural studies have shown the presence of primordial granules in the anterior lobe at e14 and in the IL at e16, and of mature secretory granules at e15 and e17, respectively (SVALANDER 1974). In the anterior lobe, the location of these granules at the cell periphery, which characterizes adult corticotrophs, begins during fetal stages (HEMMING et al. 1983). These data would suggest that the fetal AL pituitary may be capable of hormonal release as early as e14. However, some hormone production, storage, and release may occur without the formation of granules (DUPOUY 1980). For example, reactive material not associated with secretory granules has been reported (PELLETIER et al. 1977) and, in addition, hormone secretion has been observed from a cultured cell line derived from Rathke's pouch that lacks secretory granules (Bowie et al. 1978; Shiino et al. 1978). Early in vitro studies detected stimulation of steroid secretion from adult rat adrenals after coincubation with late (e21–e22) fetal pituitaries, suggesting that, at this age, whole rat pituitaries were capable of releasing ACTH (Milcovic and Milcovic 1962).

II. Functional Receptors for Secretagogues

Fetal and neonatal POMC peptide release has been studied by bioassay or radioimmunoassay (RIA) from serum or tissue culture media (Schmitt et al. 1981; Dupouy and Chatelain 1984). Whole pituitary glands responded to ovine CRH and argenine-vasopressin by e17, although the response to AVP was much lower than that to CRH (Dupouy and Chatelain 1984). In addition, corticosterone significantly decreased ACTH release at all ages, indicating that functional receptors were present as early as e17. A superfusion system using whole pituitaries detected immunoreactive β-EP release in response to CRH as early as e15 (Hotta et al. 1988). Explant cultures of postnatal day 1 pituitary regions showed regulatory responses similar to those observed in the adult. Thus, CRH and cAMP both stimulated peptide release from AL while the glucocorticoid analogue dexamethasone inhibited CRH-stimulated release, while, in explanted postnatal day 1 intermediate lobes, higher levels of CRH, β-adrenergic agonists, and cAMP all stimulated secretion (Sato and Mains 1986). Inhibition of CRH-stimulated release by glucocorticoids has been demonstrated in fetal sheep and neonatal lamb pituitary cultures and was most pronounced at the earliest ages studied (Durand et al. 1986). In vivo studies in sheep determined ACTH levels utilizing RIAs after injections of CRH or vasopressin or both. These studies, however, did not identify the source of the plasma POMC peptides. It is possible that they could have originated from other sources as described above. In addition, almost all in vitro fetal studies performed thus far have utilized whole pituitaries or cells dispersed from whole pituitaries and no attempt was made to separate anterior from neurointermediate lobes.

The reverse hemolytic plaque assay has also been used to study the ontogeny of release of POMC peptides in response to secretagogues from the fetal pituitary (Pintar and Lugo 1987; Lugo 1989; Lugo and Pintar, submitted). Pituitary AL and IL cells have been studied in order to determine the time when basal release begins, the time of onset of response to physiological regulators, and the nature of the individual cell responses. These studies have shown that AL POMC cells are capable of constitutive release, but not CRH-stimulated release, at e13.5, the time when peptide accumulation is first detected immunocytochemically. CRH-stimulated release was first detected at e15.5 as was the glucocorticoid inhibition of this CRH-stimulated release, indicating the presence of functional CRH and glucocorticoid receptors at this age in AL corticotrophs. Dopaminergic agonists did not appear to inhibit CRH-stimulated release at any age studied during development in the AL. Melanotrophs exhibited basal secretion at e17.5 but did not respond to high concentrations of CRH until e19.5. In contrast to corticotrophs, melanotroph secretion was inhibited by the dopaminergic agonist bromocryptine at the earliest age examined, e17.5. Surprisingly, starting at e17.5 and continuing until p3, preincubation with dexamethasone abolished any response to CRH, and this inhibitory effect persisted through postnatal day 2. Beginning at postnatal day 3, when the dopaminergic influence on the IL commences (Davis et al. 1984), the inhibitory effect of dexamethasone on CRH-stimulated release from melanotrophs was no longer present. These results indicate that glucocorticoids can transiently elicit a biological response in melanotrophs during development.

F. Function

I. Ontogeny of Opioid Receptors

Opioid receptors have been subclassified into three pharmacologically distinct types, μ, δ, and κ (Lord et al. 1977). Ligand binding studies have been the primary method employed in studying opioid receptor development in fetal and neonatal animals. Most studies of opioid receptor ontogeny have involved the rat CNS, and prenatal studies have primarily assayed whole brain homogenates due to small size and the limited amount of material involved. Naloxone was shown to bind to rat whole brain by e15 (Coyle and Pert 1976) and saturation curves indicated that the increase in opioid binding that occurs with age results from increases in the concentration of receptors and not from changes in affinity of the receptor for the ligand (Petrillo et al. 1987). Ligand autoradiographic studies have supplemented these binding data. Naloxone binding has since been detected in the striatum at ~e14 and in the olfactory cortical primordium and the medial septum at e16 (Kent et al. 1982). Autoradiographic studies have also indicated sex differences in localization of opioid receptors using [^{3}H]naloxone during development. In the medial preoptic area there is an increase in opioid receptor density from day 3 to day 10 in the female which is absent in the males (R.P. Hammer 1985).

The use of selective ligands has allowed a comparative study of the ontogeny of μ-, δ-, and κ-receptors, and binding studies have shown a clear pattern of differential ontogeny of these opioid receptor subtypes. Heterogeneity of these opioid receptors has been shown in early postnatal ages and, in rat brain, postnatal development of the μ-, δ-, and κ-opioid binding sites occurs at different rates and is characterized by distinct spatial patterns (Spain et al. 1985; Kornblum et al. 1987). Most notably, the development of the δ-binding sites lags behind that of the μ- and κ-sites and does not reach adult levels until later in development. In addition, the ontogeny of the κ-receptors differs from that of the μ-receptors in that there is a significant increase in μ-receptor density as the rat brain matures, but a much smaller increase in κ-receptor density. Thus the μ-receptors must increase more rapidly during development. κ-Receptor levels are low at birth and have only increased twofold by the 5th postnatal week. κ-Receptors are present in high densities in the forebrain as a streak along the ventrolateral striatum and within the olfactory tubercle and medial accumbuns at birth while the μ-site is present throughout the striatum in addition to the olfactory tubercle and the medial accumbuns. Autoradiographic studies indicate that μ- and κ-receptors appear in the mesencephalon and rostral midbrain near birth while both appear in the thalamus during the 1st week postnatally and increase to adult levels during the following 2 weeks. It appears that in certain regions such as the globus palladus and midbrain tegmentum both μ- and κ-binding sites are present in moderately high densities at early stages of postnatal development, but then decrease to lower adult levels during the first postnatal month. Autoradiographic studies have indicated transient developmental expression of μ-receptors in several brain regions such as the neostriatum and olfactory tubercle. This could be due to dilution of receptor-containing cells by other neuronal processes and proliferating glial cells during development (Kornblum et al. 1987).

The ontogeny of δ-receptor binding is different from the other receptors in that δ-receptors appear at later stages of neuronal development but in an anatomical distribution similar to that of the adult (Petrillo et al. 1987). There are very low numbers of δ-binding sites in brain of neonatal rats, although these sites have agonist affinity similar to adult δ-receptors. δ-Receptor density increases markedly during the third postnatal week and appears in the neostriatum and olfactory tubercle prior to other brain regions. Also, binding in the deep layers of the neocortex appears prior to binding in the superficial level (Kornblum et al. 1987).

The pattern of the relative rates of postnatal development of μ-, δ-, and κ-sites in mouse brain closely resembles that observed in rats (Tavani et al. 1985). However, it has been reported that the concentration of κ-sites in 3-day-old mice was significantly lower than that found in rats of the same age (Petrillo et al. 1987). As in rats, little if any change in affinity of the receptor was detected and development of μ- and κ-binding sites preceded that of δ-sites (Tavani et al. 1985). Studies in lambs demonstrated, as expected from the advanced development at birth, that a more fully mature receptor system is present at birth than in rats and mice (Dunlap et al. 1986). Analysis of the ontogeny of the opioid receptor types in the rat spinal cord indicated that μ- and κ-receptors were expressed prenatally at e15, while δ-receptor binding did not appear until after birth at around p1, with the number of κ-receptor sites predominating throughout development. There is a peak in the number of μ- and κ-sites around birth in the spinal column, unlike the brain, where the receptor subtypes reach maximal levels only in the adult. The adult levels of μ- and κ-receptor sites are lower by as much as 50% than those expressed in the neonatal or early postnatal period. The differences between spinal cord and brain may result from averaging in whole brain membrane receptor density present in specific brain regions. As mentioned above, autoradiographic studies indicate the transient expression of μ-receptors in several specific regions. Finally, the binding properties of p1 κ-sites were found to be similar to those displayed by κ-receptors in adult spinal cord (ATTALI et al. 1990).

II. Putative Role(s) of Opioid Peptides in Developmental Processes

The role that the opioid peptide regions of the three opioid genes have in development has not yet been elucidated, No direct role has been proven, although other regions of the POMC precursor molecule have demonstrated affects on developmental processes. For example, it is well known that ACTH is required for maturation of the adrenal gland, and it has been a long-standing idea that α-MSH-sized peptides can influence fetal growth (SWAAB er al. 1976). For opioid peptides, the most direct role proposed involves modulating neurite extension in the CNS (HAUSER et al. 1989). This idea, however, has still not received definitive experimental support since thus far no effects that can be directly attributed to opioid deprivation have been demonstrated.

G. Prospectus

The precise role, if any, that opioid peptides play in development remains obscure. Reverse genetic approaches (CAPPECHI 1989) now allow null or modified alleles of a specific gene to be exchanged with the normal endogenous sequences in embryonic stem (ES) cells. The modified ES cells can then contribute to the germ-line of chimeric mice and allow the effects of the alteration to be investigated in both the heterozygous and homozygous states and the consequences of the disruption assessed. Interference with opioid binding alters neurite outgrowth in vitro, but a direct role for opioid peptides will require that these effects, like those of α-MSH on growth, result when the portions of the precursor genes that encode opioid peptides be altered and result in developmental defects. Since the pituitary POMC system has been studied more extensively than other brain and peripheral regions where opioid genes are expressed, the types of cell interactions that elicit POMC transcription in anterior and intermediate lobe pituitary populations is likely to be the area where progress is first made in understanding opioid cell differentiation. The recent identification of the relevant promoter sequences needed for tissue-specific expression (G.D. HAMMER et al. 1990) should allow *trans*-acting factors that promote and stabilize POMC expression during development to be isolated and characterized.

References

Allen RG, Pintar JE, Stack J, Kendall JW (1984) Biosynthesis and processing of proopiomelanocortin-derived peptides during fetal pituitary development. Dev Biol 102:43–50

Attali B, Saya D, Vogel Z (1990) Pre- and postnatal development of opiate receptor subtypes in rat spinal cord. Dev Brain Res 53:97–102

Bowie EP, Ishikawa H, Shiino M, Rennels EG (1978) An immunocytochemical study of a rat pituitary multipotential clone. J Histochem Cytochem 26:94–97

Capecchi MR (1989) The new mouse genetics – altering the genome by gene targeting. Trends Gen 5:70–76

Chen C-LC, Chang CC, Kreiger DT, Bardin CW (1986) Expression and regulation of proopiomelanocortin-like gene in ovary and placenta: comparison with the testes. Endocrinology 118:2382–2389

Couly GF, LeDouarin NM (1985) Mapping of the early neural primordium in quail-chick chimeras: I. Developmental relationships between placodes, facial ectoderm, and prosencephalon. Dev Biol 110:422–439

Coyle KT, Pert CB (1976) Ontogenetic development of [^{3}H]naloxone binding in the rat brain. Neuropharmacology 15:555–560

Davis MD, Lichtensteiger W, Schlumpf M, Bruinink A (1984) Early postnatal development of pituitary intermediate lobe control in the rat by dopamine neurons. Neuroendocrinology 39:1–12

Dunlap CE III, Christ GJ, Rose JC (1986) Characterization of opioid receptor binding in adult and fetal sheep brain regions. Dev Brain Res 24:279–285

Dupouy JP (1980) Differentiation of MSH-containing, ACTH-containing and LPH-containing cells in the hypophysis during embryonic and fetal development. Int Rev Cytol 68:197–249

Dupouy JP, Chatelain A (1984) In-vitro effects of corticosterone, synthetic ovine corticotrophin releasing factor and arginine vasopressin on the release of adrenocorticotrophin by fetal rat pituitary glands. J Endocrinol 101:339–344

Durand P, Cathiard A-M, Dacheuxz F, Naaman S, Saez JM (1986) In vitro stimulation and inhibition of adrenocorticotrophin release by pituitary cells from ovine fetuses and lambs. Endocrinology 118:11387–11394

Eagleson GW, Jenks BG, Overbecke AP (1986) The pituitary adrenocorticotropes originate from neural ridge tissue in Xenopus laevis. J Embryol Exp Morphol 95:1–14

Elkabes S, Loh YP, Nieburgs A, Wray S (1989) Prenatal ontogenesis of pro-opiomelanocortin in the mouse central nervous system and pituitary gland: an in situ hybridization and immunocytochemical study. Dev Brain Res 46:85–95

Fink G, Smith GD (1971) Ultrastructural features of the developing hypothalamo-hypophysial axis in the rat. A corrolative study. Z Zellforsch Mikrosk Anat 119:208–226

Gizang-Ginsberg E, Wolgemuth D (1987) Expression of the proopiomelanocortin gene is developmentally regulated and affected by germ cells in the male mouse reproductive system. Proc Natl Acad Sci USA 84:1600–1604

Glydon RSJ (1957) The development of the blood supply of the pituitary in the albino rat, with special reference to the portal vessels. J Anat 91:237–244

Goland RS, Wardlaw SL, Stark RI, Brown LS Jr, Frantz AG (1986) High levels of corticotropin-releasing hormone in human plasma during pregnancy, labour and delivery. J Clin Endocrinol Metab 63:1199–1203

Grino M, Young WS III, Burgunder J-M (1989) Ontogeny of expression of the corticotropin-releasing factor gene in the hypothalamic paraventricular nucleus and of the proopiomelanocortin gene in rat pituitary. Endocrinology 124:60–68

Hammer GD, Fairchild-Harkness V, Low MJ (1990) Pituitary specific and hormonally regulated gene expression directed by the rat proopiomelanocortin promoter in transgenic mice. Mol Endocrinol 4:1689–1697

Hammer RP Jr (1985) Ontogeny of opiate receptors in the rat medial preoptic area: critical periods in regional development. Int J Dev Neurosci 3:541–548

Hanuoka Y (1967) The effects of posterior hypothalectomy upon the growth and metamorphosis of the tadpole of *Rana pipiens*. Gen Comp Endocrinol 8:417–431

Hauser KF, McLaughlin PJ, Zagon IS (1989) Endogenous opioid systems and the regulation of dendritic growth and spine formation. J Comp Neurol 281:13–22

Hayes WP, Loh YP (1990) Correlated onset and patterning of proopiomelanocortin gene expression in embryonic *Xenopus* brain and pituitary. Development 110:747–757

Hemming FJ, Begeot M, Dubois MP, Dubois PM (1983) Ultrastructural identification of corticotropes of the fetal rat. In-vivo and in-vitro immunocytochemistry. Cell Tissue Res 234:427–437

Hotta M, Shibasaki T, Akitsugu M, Imaki T, Demura H, Ohno H, Daikoku S, Benoit R, Ling N, Shizume K (1988) Ontogeny of pituitary responsiveness to corticotropin-releasing hormone in rat. Regul Pept 21:245–252

Howells RD, Kilpatrick DL, Bailey LD, Noe M, Udenfriend S (1986) Proenkephalin mRNA in rat heart. Proc Natl Acad Sci USA 83:1960–1963

Ikeda H, Suzuki J, Sasano N, Niizuma H (1988) The development and morphogenesis of the human pituitary gland. Anat Embryol (Berl) 178:327–336

Kent JL, Pert CB, Herkenham M (1982) Ontogeny of opiate receptors in rat forebrain: visualization by in vitro autoradiography. Dev Brain Res 2:487–504

Keshet E, Polakiewicz D, Itin A, Ornoy A, Rosen H (1989) Proenkephalin A is expressed in mesodermal lineages during organogenesis. EMBO J 8:2917–2923

Kew D, Kilpatrick DL (1990) Widespread organ expression of the rat proenkephalin gene during early postnatal development. Mol Endocrinol 4:337–340

Khachaturian H, Alessi NE, Munfakh N, Watson SJ (1983) Ontogeny of opioid and related peptides in the rat CNS and pituitary: an immunocytochemical study. Life Sci 33:61–64

Khachaturian H, Lewis ME, Schafer MKH, Watson SJ (1985a) Anatomy of the CNS opioid systems. Trends Neurosci 8:111–119

Khachaturian H, Lewis ME, Alessi NE, Watson SJ (1985b) Time of origin peptide-containing neurons in the rat hypothalamus. J Comp Neurol 236:538–546

Khorram O, McCann SM (1984) Pre- and postnatal developmental changes in hypothalamic and pituitary content of α-melanocyte-stimulating hormone and somatostatin in the rat. Biol Neonate 46:80–88

Kornblum HI, Hurlbut DE, Leslie FM (1987) Postnatal development of multiple opioid receptors in rat brain. Dev Brain Res 37:21–41

Liotta AS, Kreiger DT (1980) In vitro biosynthesis and comparative posttranslational processing of immunoreactive precursor corticotropin/β-endorphin by human placental and pituitary cells. Endocrinology 106:1504–1511

Loh YP, Eskay RL, Brownstein M (1980) α-MSH-like peptides in rat brain: identification and changes in level during development. Biochem Biophys Res Comm 94:916–923

Lord JAH, Waterfield AA, Hughes J, Kosterlitz HW (1977) Endogenous opioid peptides: multiple agonists and receptors. Nature 267:495–499

Lugo DI (1989) Proopiomelanocortin gene expression and peptide secretion in the developing rat pituitary gland. PhD thesis, Columbia University

Lugo DI, Roberts JL, Pintar JE (1989) Analysis of proopiomelanocortin gene expression during prenatal development of the rat pituitary gland. Mol Endocrinol 1313–1324

Melner MH, Low KG, Allen RG, Nielson CP, Young SL, Saneto RP (1990) The regulation of proenkephalin expression in a distinct population of glial cells. EMBO J 9:791–796

Milcovic K, Milcovic S (1962) Studies of the pituitary-adrenocortical system in the fetal rat. Endocrinology 71:799–802

Mulchahey JJ, DiBlasio AM, Martin MC, Blumenfeld Z, Jaffe RB (1987) Hormone production and peptide regulation of the human fetal pituitary gland. Endocr Rev 8:406–412

Nakane PR, Setalo G, Mazurkiewicz JE (1977) The origin of ACTH cells in rat anterior pituitary. Ann NY Acad Sci 297:201–204

Negm IM (1971) The vascular blood supply of the pituitary and its development. Acat Anat (Basel) 80:601–619

Palmer MR, Miller RJ, Olson L, Seiger A (1982) Prenatal ontogeny of neurons with enkephalin-like immunoreactivity in the rat central nervous system: an immunohistochemical mapping investigation. Med Biol 60:61–88

Pelletier G, Leclerc R, Labric F, Cote J, Chrétien M, Lis M (1977) Immunohistochemical localization of lipotropic hormone in the pituitary gland. Endocrinology 100:770–776

Petrillo P, Tavani A, Verotta D, Robson LE, Kosterlitz HW (1987) Differential postnatal development of μ- δ- and κ-opioid binding sites in rat brain. Dev Brain Res 31:53–58

Pintar JE, Lugo DI (1987) Proopiomelanocortin gene expression, prohormone processing, and secretion during fetal rat pituitary development. Ann NY Acad Sci 512:318–327

Pintar JE, Schachter BS, Herman AT, Durgerian S, Kreiger DT (1984) Characterization and localization of proopiomelanocortin messenger RNA in the adult rat testes. Science 225:632–634

Polakiewicz RD, Rosen H (1990) Regulated expression of proenkephalin A during ontogenic development of mesenchymal derivative tissues. Mol Cell Biol 10:736–742

Potter E, Behan DP, Fischer WH, Linton EA, Lowry PJ, Vale WW (1991) Cloning and characterization of the cDNAs for human and rat corticotropin releasing factor-binding proteins. Nature 349:423–426

Rosen H, Polakiewicz R (1989) Postnatal expression of opioid genes in rat brain. Dev Brain Res 46:123–129

Rundle SE, Funder JW (1988) Ontogeny of corticotropin-releasing factor and arginine vasopressin in the rat. Neuroendocrinology 47:374–378

Sato SM, Mains RE (1985) Posttranslational processing of proadrenocorticotropin/ endorphin-derived peptides during postnatal development in the rat pituitary. Endocrinology 117:773–786

Sato SM, Mains RE (1986) Regulation of adrenocorticotropin/endorphin-related peptide secretion in neonatal rat pituitary cultures. Endocrinology 119:793–801

Schmitt G, Stoeckel ME, Koch B (1981) Evidence for a possible dopaminergic control of pituitary alpha-MSH during ontogenesis in mice. Neuroendocrinology 33:306–311

Schwartz JP, Simantov R (1988) Developmental expression of proenkephalin mRNA in rat striatum and in striatal cultures. Dev Brain Res 40:311–314

Schwind JL (1928) The development of the hypophysis cerebri of the albino rat. Am J Anat 41:295–319

Scott REM, Autelitano DJ, Lugo DI, Blum M, Roberts JL, Pintar JE (1990) Developmental changes in levels of proopiomelanocortin intron A-containing heterogeneous nuclear RNA and mature messenger RNA in the anterior and neurointermediate lobes of the rat pituitary. Mol Endocrinol 4:812–820

Seidah NG, Markinkiewicz M, Benjannet S, Gaspar L, Beaubien G, Mattei MG, Lazure C, Mbikay M, Chrétien M (1991) Cloning and primary sequence of a mouse candidate prohormone convertase PC1 homologous to PC2, furin, and Kex2: distinct chromosome localization and messenger RNA distribution in brain and pituitary compared to PC2. Mol Endocrinol 5:111–122

Seizinger BR, Liebisch DC, Grimm C, Herz A (1984) Ontogenetic development of the proenkephalin B (=pro-dynorphin) opioid peptide system in the rat pituitary. Neuroendocrinology 39:414–422

Setalo G, Nakane P (1972) Studies on the functional differentiation of cells in fetal anterior pituitary glands of rats with peroxidase labelled antibody method. Anat Rec 172:403–404

Shaha C, Liotta AS, Kreiger DT, Bardin CW (1984) The ontogeny of immunoreactive β-endorphin in fetal, neonatal, and pubertal testes from mouse and human. Endocrinology 114:1584–1591

Shiino M, Ishikawa H, Rennels EG (1978) Accumulation of secretory granules in pituitary clonal cells derived from the epithelium of Rathke's pouch. Cell Tissue Res 186:53–61

Shinoda H, Marini AM, Losi C, Schwartz JP (1989) Brain expression and gene specificity of neuropeptide gene expression in cultured astrocytes. Science 245:415–417

Spain JW, Roth BL, Coscia CJ (1985) Differential ontogeny of multiple opioid receptors (μ, δ, and κ). J Neurosci 5:584–588

Spruce BA, Curtis R, Wilkin GP, Glover DM (1990) A neuropeptide precursor in cerebellum: proenkephalin exists in subpopulations of both neurons and astrocytes. EMBO J 9:1787–1795

Stoeckel ME, Hindelang-Gertner C, Porte A (1979) Embryonic development and secretory differentiation in the pars tuberalis of the mouse hypophysis. Cell Tissue Res 198:465–476

Svalander C (1974) Ultrastructure of the fetal rat adenohypophysis. Acta Endocrinol [Suppl] (Copenh) 188:1–114

Swaab DF, Visser M, Tilders FJH (1976) Stimulation of intra-uterine growth in rat by melanocyte-stimulating hormone. J Endocrinol 70:445–455

Szabo K, Csanyi K (1982) The vascular architecture of the developing pituitary-median eminence complex in the rat. Cell Tissue Res 224:563–577

Tavani A, Robson LE, Kosterltz HW (1985) Differential postnatal development of μ-, δ- and κ-opioid binding sites in mouse brain. Dev Brain Res 23:306–309

Tecott LH, Rubenstein JLR, Paxino G, Evans CJ, Eberwine JH, Valentino KL (1989) Developmental expression of proenkephalin mRNA and peptides in rat striatum. Dev Brain Res 49:75–86

Tilders H, Parker CR, Barnea A, Porter JC (1981) The major immunoreactive melanocyte-stimulating hormone (α-MSH)-like substance found in human fetal pituitary tissue is not MSH but may be desacetyl MSH (adrenocorticotropin$_{1-13}$NH$_2$). J Clin Endocrinol Metab 52:319–323

Vilijn MH, Vaysse PJJ, Zukin RS, Kessler JA (1988) Expression of preproenkephalin mRNA by cultured astrocytes and neurons. Proc Natl Acad Sci USA 85:6551–6555

Watanabe YG, Daikoku S (1979) An immunohistochemical study on the histogenesis of adenohypophysial cells in fetal rats. Dev Biol 68:557–567

Watkins WB, Choy VJ (1979) Maturation of the hypothalamo-neurohypophysial system. Neurophysin, vasopressin and oxytocin in the median eminance of the developing rat brain. Cell Tissue Res 197:337–346

Yoshida Y (1966) Electron microscopy of the anterior pituitary gland under normal and different experimental conditions. Exp Pathol 1:439–454

Zagon IS, Rhodes RE, McLaughlin PJ (1985) Distribution of enkephalin immunoreactivity in germinative cells of developing rat cerebellum. Science 227:1049–1051

Section D: Neurophysiology

CHAPTER 29

Opioids and Sensory Processing in the Central Nervous System

A.W. Duggan and S.M. Fleetwood-Walker

A. Introduction

When considering opioids and sensory systems there are two important questions. The first deals with how opiate drugs relieve pain; the second consideration is how opioid peptides physiologically influence sensory processing. Since pain is a perception, the potential sites at which a drug could act to produce an alteration in its quality or intensity are legion. Much of the research discussed in this section demonstrates that opiates do reduce the amount of information reaching the brain in response to a peripheral stimulus normally perceived as painful. Thus, these experiments lead to the conclusion that opiates produce a diminution in the intensity of perceived pain through a reduction in the transmitted message. If opiates also act in the brain to alter perception to a given message, then this currently seems unamenable to investigation by electrophysiological means. But the possibility remains.

Most research on opiates and sensory information has attempted to explain how these drugs relieve pain in man, but there is considerable evidence that the question is wider than nociception alone. Although much sensory information impinges on consciousness, much does not. Amongst the latter can be listed impulses from muscle spindles, tendons and joints, and that from deep sensors such as the heart and lungs. Indeed some of the undesired effects of opiates on respiration and circulation may result from alterations in the processing of sensory information from such structures. Although much of the discussion which follows will indeed focus on opiates and analgesia, this simply reflects the emphasis of recent research. From space restrictions, this review has had to be limited to sensory processing in the spinal cord, thalamus and cerebral cortex.

B. Opioids and the Spinal Cord

I. Spinal Processing of Nociceptive Information

This has been recently reviewed by several authors (Willis 1982, 1985; Zieglgansberger 1986; Besson and Chaouch 1987) and the reader is

referred to these accounts for a more detailed discussion. A brief out-
line will be given. In the cat and rat peripheral nervous system, noxious,
mechanical, cutaneous stimuli produce impulses in small myelinated (Aδ)
fibres; noxious thermal mechanical and chemical stimuli produce impulses in
unmyelinated fibres (BESSOU and PERL 1969). The central terminals of the
small myelinated fibres are mainly in lamina I of the dorsal horn; the
unmyelinated nociceptors terminate mainly in lamina II, the substantia
gelatinosa (LIGHT and PERL 1977). Both visceral (CERVERO 1985) and deep
somatic (CRAIG and MENSE 1983; CRAIG et al. 1988) nociceptors do not
terminate in the substantia gelatinosa, but rather in lamina I and deeply, in
lamina V. Impulses in nociceptors can be viewed as having three main
destinations: motoneurones, autonomic areas and the areas of the brain
important in the perception of pain. A number of spinal neurones projecting to supraspinal areas are excited by peripheral noxious stimuli. These
include spinomesencephalic neurones, many of which are found in lamina I,
spinothalamic neurones which are found superficially in lamina I, but also
more deeply in laminae V–VII, spinocervical neurones found mainly in
lamina V and spinoreticular neurones (WILLIS 1985). In anaesthetised
animals very few of these neurones are excited exclusively by noxious
peripheral stimuli; most transmit information about a number of sensory modalities. How the brain deals with this plurality of information is
unknown.

Interposed between the central terminals of nociceptors and projecting
neurones are many ill-defined interneurones, but there is evidence that
what is transmitted to the brain is subject to considerable control both
segmentally, intersegmentally and by descending fibres from the brain. Thus
there is a tonic inhibition from the brain stem which affects spinal transmission of a host of afferent information, including nociception (LUNDBERG
1982; DUGGAN and MORTON 1988). Impulses in other afferent fibres may
control spinal transmission of nociceptive information and such control was
the basis of the gate hypothesis of MELZACK and WALL (1965).

II. Systemic Administration of Opiates and the Responses
of Spinal Neurones

If opiates do reduce the nociceptive message transmitted to parts of the
brain important in pain perception, then electrophysiological methods
should be able to identify where the reduction occurs and some of the
mechanisms involved. Early experiments had shown that opiates reduced
spinal reflexes in spinal animals (WIKLER 1950) and, in 1977, YAKSH and
RUDY showed that administering opiates to the surface of the spinal cord
produced regional analgesia. Such observations formed a basis for extended
investigation of the effects of opiates on spinal neurones. Given that opiates
have effects in the spinal cord of spinal animals the first consideration is

whether there is any specificity in the action of these drugs in terms of type of neurone affected, type of afferent pathway affected, or both.

1. Neuronal Types

There are surprisingly little data on cell types affected by opiates. An early study (KITAHATA et al. 1974) found that morphine (2 mg kg^{-1}) had a greater effect in reducing the spontaneous firing of neurones of laminae I and V of the decerebrate spinal cat than that of cells of other laminae. Evoked firing was not studied. There is considerable evidence that opiates influence the firing of motoneurones and this will be discussed subsequently. In the spinal cat, morphine (1–4 mg kg^{-1}) was shown to increase the ventral root evoked firing of Renshaw cells (DUGGAN et al. 1976a). There appear to be no data on the effects of intravenous opiates on identified spinal neurones, such as spinomesencephalic, spinothalamic, 1A inhibitory interneurones, to name but a few.

2. Responses to Peripheral Stimuli

Spinal neurones can be excited or inhibited both from the periphery and from propriospinal and supraspinal sources. Most studies have examined responses to either electrical stimulation of peripheral nerve or to natural stimuli applied to the skin. There are some methodological problems with both of these techniques.

a) Excitation of Dorsal Horn Neurones

In the cat intravenous morphine (0.3–2.0 mg kg^{-1}) (LE BARS et al. 1976a,b; DUGGAN et al. 1980), phenoperidine (0.2 mg kg^{-1}, BESSON et al. 1973) and fentanyl (20–40 μg kg^{-1}, IWATA and SAKAI 1971) depressed the excitation of dorsal horn neurones by electrical stimulation of slowly conducting (Aδ and C) fibres of a peripheral nerve with minimal or no effect on excitation by Aαβ fibres. Systemic naloxone reversed the action of all of these opiates. It was not known in these experiments, if the cells studied were local interneurones or if they projected to supraspinal areas. JURNA and GROSSMAN (1976) studied the excitation of anterolateral tract axons of the cat by electrical stimulation of peripheral nerves and hence of neurones projecting either to the brain or to cephalic spinal segments. Morphine (0.5 mg kg^{-1}) reduced excitation by stimulation of Aδ and C fibres, but not that by Aαβ fibre stimulation. This effect, which is fundamental to much of this review, is shown in Fig. 1. In a similar study in the rat (JURNA and HEINZ 1979), morphine (0.5 mg kg^{-1}), meperidine (1 mg kg^{-1}) and levophanol (0.5 mg kg^{-1}) produced naloxone-reversible reductions in excitation of anterolateral tract axons by impulses in unmyelinated primary afferents.

In subsequent work JURNA (1984) showed differences between the mechanisms involved in opiate depression of activity in ascending axons and

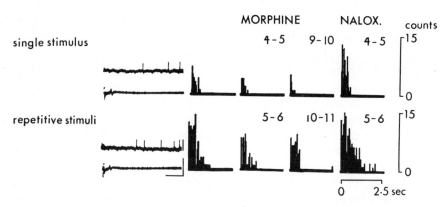

Fig. 1. Depression by morphine, $0.5 \, \text{mg} \, \text{kg}^{-1}$, of the excitation of an anterolateral tract axon of the spinal cat by electrical stimulation of C fibres of the sural nerve. The voltage records to the left show action potentials of the axon (*upper traces*) to single and repetitive stimuli and the potentials simultaneously recorded in the sural nerve (*lower traces*). A C-fibre compound action potential is visible in the latter. The histograms *to the right* represent 12 summed responses. Depression by morphine (most evident 10 min after injection) was rapidly reversed by naloxone $0.05 \, \text{mg} \, \text{kg}^{-1}$. Calibration for voltage records 100 ms and $100 \, \mu\text{V}$ for upper, $500 \, \mu\text{V}$ for lower records. (Reproduced with permission from Jurna and Grossman 1976)

flexor reflexes of the rat. Intravenous morphine ($2.0 \, \text{mg} \, \text{kg}^{-1}$) depressed both phenomena, but aminophylline ($25 \, \text{mg} \, \text{kg}^{-1}$ i.p.) only reversed the depression of spinal reflexes by morphine. Intrathecal administration of the lipid-soluble dibutyryl cyclic adenosine monophosphate enhanced activity in ascending axons, but reduced the flexor reflex. Although these results are difficult to reconcile by a common mechanism, they emphasize that motor and sensory events are differently controlled and that impairment of flexor reflexes is not necessarily to be equated with analgesia. Headley et al. (1987) noted that larger doses of systemic morphine and U50488H were required to depress the firing of neurones of the dorsal horn than those depressing flexor reflexes of the rat.

These studies using electrical stimulation of nerve suggest that opiates preferentially reduce spinal transmission of impulses in small-diameter primary afferents. Such a conclusion needs confirmation using natural peripheral stimuli, since any inhibitory process may depress the asynchronous excitatory postsynaptic potentials (EPSPs) produced in spinal neurones by the relatively large temporal spread of impulses in C fibres, more than with the rapidly rising, near synchronous EPSPs resulting from A fibre electrical activation. Thus the selectivity may be artefactual.

When natural stimuli have been used to excite spinal neurones, opiates have mainly reduced excitation by noxious stimuli, but there have been some dissenting data. In the experiments of Zieglgansberger and Bayerl (1976) the excitation of cat dorsal horn neurones by noxious skin indentation was reduced by morphine $(2\,mg\,kg^{-1})$ and etorphine $(1-10\,\mu g\,kg^{-1})$. The latter drug also partly reduced excitation by light brushing of the skin. Two groups (CALVILLO et al. 1974; TOYOOKA et al. 1977) observed a reduction by morphine and meperidine in the excitation of dorsal horn neurones of the cat by noxious heating of the skin, but the selectivity of this action was not examined. Also in the cat, however, EINSPAHR and PIERCEY (1980) found a non-selective reduction by morphine $(1-2\,mg\,kg^{-1})$ of excitation of dorsal horn neurones by noxious heat to the skin and by movement of hairs. When using noxious heat as a stimulus, the activation of nociceptors is markedly dependent on cutaneous blood flow (DUGGAN and GRIERSMITH 1979a) through effects on the rate of dissipation of heat conducted to the dermis. Although it is still unknown how important this effect is with systemically administered opiates, collectively the data on activation of dorsal horn neurones by both electrical and natural stimuli do indicate a reduction of spinal processing of nociceptive information by opiates. The selectivity of this action, however, remains uncertain since detailed studies on the effects of systemic opiates on the spinal processing of information in the multiple functional types of primary afferents have not been performed.

b) Inhibition of Dorsal Horn Neurones

Some neurones of the dorsal horn are inhibited by noxious heat to the periphery. HARRIS and RYALL (1988) found such inhibition in the rat to be unaffected by a dose of morphine $(2\,mg\,kg^{-1})$, which reduced excitation of other neurones by noxious heat. This result implies either that there are separate populations of primary afferents producing excitation or inhibition and only one is acted upon by opiates, or that a significant part of the effect of morphine is on neural structures beyond transmitter release from primary afferents.

c) Excitation of Motoneurones

Although motoneurones are not normally considered as part of sensory pathways, the transmission of sensory information to motoneurones is subject to modification by opiates. The subject is of importance since inhibition of a motor response such as tail-flick in the rat is commonly equated with analgesia and one conclusion from this section is that opioids can affect pathways to motoneurones and those to the brain differentially. It is not intended to discuss spinal pathways from primary afferents to motoneurones in detail and the reader requiring further information is referred to the reviews of BALDISSERA et al. (1981), BURKE (1985) and SCHOMBURG (1990).

α) *Nociceptive Pathways*. By electrophysiological techniques there is general accord that analgesic doses of opiates depress the firing of motoneurones to peripheral noxious stimuli in spinal animals. This has been shown in the cat (KOLL et al. 1963; BELL and MARTIN 1977), rat (HEADLEY et al. 1987), rabbit (Clarke and Ford 1987), dog (Wikler and Frank 1948; Martin et al. 1964, 1976) and man (Willer 1985). Although behavioural experiments had implied that opiates acting at different receptors had differential effects on reflexes to thermal and mechanical noxious stimuli (Tyers 1980; Schmauss and Yaksh 1984; Millan 1987), experiments measuring the firing of single motoneurones (Parsons and Headley 1989) have shown this distinction to be artefactual. Thus, when peripheral noxious thermal and mechanical stimuli were graded so as to produce equal firing rates in motoneurones of the rat, the κ-opioids, U50488H and tifluadom behaved similarly to the μ-agonist fentanyl, in reducing responses to both types of stimulus. Woolf and Wall (1986) found that doses of morphine of $20\,\text{mg}\,\text{kg}^{-1}$ were required to depress the flexor reflex of the decerebrate spinal rat, but that $0.5\,\text{mg}\,\text{kg}^{-1}$ was sufficient to reduce the facilitation of this reflex produced by brief tetanic stimulation of C fibres of a hind limb nerve. This latter dose, however, was effective in reducing the firing of motoneurones to noxious heating and pricking of the skin in the experiments of Parsons and Headley (1989). It is possible that these natural stimuli involve some facilitation of the type described by Woolf and Wall (1986) and it decays relatively rapidly.

β) *Non-nociceptive Pathways.* Although earlier accounts were optimistic that opiates would be relatively selective in depressing nociceptive reflexes, the collective data now indicate that such optimism was unfounded. Opiates have been found to reduce a number of spinal events. Although monosynaptic reflexes in extensor motoneurones induced by a single stimulus to large-diameter afferents have not been reduced by systemic opiates (Wikler and Frank 1948; Cook and Bonnycastle 1953; Kruglov 1964), analgesic doses of these drugs have reduced such reflexes when elicited by repetitive nerve stimulation (Krivoy et al. 1973; Jurna and Schafer 1965). In addition, Jurna (1966) found that the firing of motoneurones of the decerebrate cat to sustained muscle stretch was reduced by analgesic doses of morphine and meperidine. A single nerve stimulus adequate to excite motoneurones monosynaptically will also excite interneurones (both excitatory and inhibitory), but, even if the latter influence motoneurone excitability, this effect will be too late to alter the amplitude of the monosynaptic reflex. With repetitive stimulation, however, the influence of interneurones activated by the stimulus can be important and administered drugs could influence reflexes through an action on such interneurones.

III. Localized Administration of Opioids

The experiments discussed to here indicate that systemic opiates have effects on spinal neurones, but cannot localize sites of action to discrete neural structures and give only limited information on the possible physiological roles of opioid peptides in the spinal cord. Localization of the action of opioids to fine structures requires administration from micropipettes either by ionophoresis or by pressure ejection. Investigation of the physiological roles of opioid peptides also requires focal administration of ligands specific for known endogenous opioid receptors, and of antagonists acting on these receptors, since endogenous opioids are released from discrete neural structures. In addition, results will be meaningful only when exogenous compounds are administered at sites which are accessed physiologically by erdogenous opioids. A major obstacle to progress in this field has been the non-opioid effects of the available drugs.

1. µ-Receptor-Preferring Ligands

Most early experiments were carried out with morphine, which, while relatively selective for µ-sites, has significant activity at δ-receptors, but minimal activity at κ-sites (KOSTERLITZ et al. 1985). Many large neurones in laminae IV/V of the dorsal horn integrate somatosensory responses (generally reacting to both noxious and innocuous cutaneous stimuli) and these account for most of the neuronal samples described in these studies. When morphine has been applied ionophoretically in the vicinity of such neurones in the cat, several groups have described inhibition of neuronal activity, including spontaneous activity and that evoked by noxious stimuli or by excitatory amino acids (CALVILLO et al. 1974, 1979; ZIEGLGANSBERGER and BAYERL 1976). However, the specificity of inhibition of noxious, as opposed to innocuous stimulus-evoked responses, was not examined and excitatory effects with a lack of modality-specificity have also been described (DOSTROVSKY and POMERANZ 1976; DUGGAN et al. 1976a). Most evidence indicates that these effects of morphine administered near cell bodies of neurones in the lower dorsal horn are neither readily reversible by naloxone, nor show the stereospecificity of levorphanol compared with dextorphan that would be expected of an authentic µ-receptor event. This suggests that the actions of opiates in laminae IV/V may represent a non-specific biophysical phenomenon and accords with the paucity of µ-ligand binding sites found in this location. Supporting this conclusion, a broad range of opioids (and even naloxone) administered ionophoretically was described to produce inhibitions of reticular formation neurones in a rank order quite unrelated to their receptor activity and rarely influenced by opioid antagonists (MORRIS et al. 1984). In addition morphine administration has been reported to elicit bursts of abnormally configured action potentials in dorsal horn neurones (DUGGAN and CURTIS 1972). When morphine has been applied to sites in the superficial dorsal horn (more appropriate in terms of µ-binding site location), a striking specificity has been observed. DUGGAN et al. (1976b, 1977a, 1981) described naloxone-sensitive selective inhibition of nociceptive activity of neurones of laminae IV/V when morphine was ejected from a second microelectrode placed in the superficial dorsal horn in the region of the substantia gelatinosa. If the dorsal electrode was moved closer to the laminae IV/V cells being recorded, the specificity was lost. SASTRY and GOH (1983) also described selective inhibition of nociceptive responses of deeper neurones by morphine and an enkephalin analogue administered in the substantia gelatinosa. More recent studies have been carried out with highly μ-selective opioid peptides. FLEETWOOD-WALKER et al. (1988) found that [D-Ala^2,MePhe^4,Gly-ol^5]enkephalin (DAGO) applied ionophoretically in the region of the substantia gelatinosa just dorsal to cat spinocervical tract neurones had a potent, selective and naloxone-reversible antinociceptive action (see Fig. 2C). In contrast, the peptide was inactive in the proximity of the cell bodies in laminae IV/V (Fig. 2G). Further studies in the rat (where only a single multibarrel electrode can feasibly be used) confirmed the inactivity of this μ-agonist close to laminae IV/V neurones, but revealed a selective, naloxone-reversible antinociceptive influence on lamina I neurones when ejected in superficial laminae (HOPE et al. 1990). Endogenous ligands having a high, but not absolute, affinity for the μ-receptor have given similar results. Metorphamide (WEBER et al. 1983) with 2- and 20-fold more selectivity for μ- than for κ- and δ-sites (KOSTERLITZ et al. 1985) is one such compound. When applied in the substantia gelatinosa, metorphamide reduced noxious thermal responses and C-fibre-evoked respones of deeper neurones in a naloxone-reversible fashion (ZHAO et al. 1986). Although responses to innocuous events were unaltered, metorphamide often reduced spontaneous activity. Among opioid peptides, metorphamide may indeed be the best current candidate for a μ-selective endogenous agonist – should such a substance exist. In addition dermorphin (an amphibian-derived peptide) selectively inhibited

---→

Fig. 2A–H. The effects of opioid ligands, selective for different opioid receptor subtypes (indicated), on the responses of identified spinocervical tract cells. The neurones were located in laminae III–V, and excited by noxious and non-noxious natural stimuli applied to the ipsilateral cutaneous receptive field of the neurone. Responses (increases in firing rate above background) were integrated and expressed as a percentage of the near control responses. These values (mean ± SEM) were plotted against the ionophoretic-ejecting current for each agonist, applied in a standard time sequence. When the opioids were ionophoresed into the region of the substantia gelatinosa (A–C) there was no significant effect by either **A** the κ-agonist dynorphin$_{1-13}$ or **B** the δ-preferring agonists DADL, DSLET or DLPEN, but **C** shows the marked and selective reduction in the noxious thermal responses by the μ-agonist DAGO. This is in marked contrast to the effects seen when the opioids were ionophoresed in close proximity to the cell body (**D,E,F,G**). The κ-preferring agonists dynorphin A$_{1-13}$ **D** and U50488H **E** produced a selective antinociceptive effect, whereas the δ-preferring agonist DADL **F** and the μ-agonist DAGO **G** showed no significant effect. (*indicates significant reduction from control responses, $P < 0.05$ by matched paired t tests on the original data). (Reproduced with permission from FLEETWOOD-WALKER et al. 1988). **H** A schematic diagram showing the main locations of the opioid receptor types within the dorsal horn of the spinal cord, in association with a cutaneous nociceptive pathway

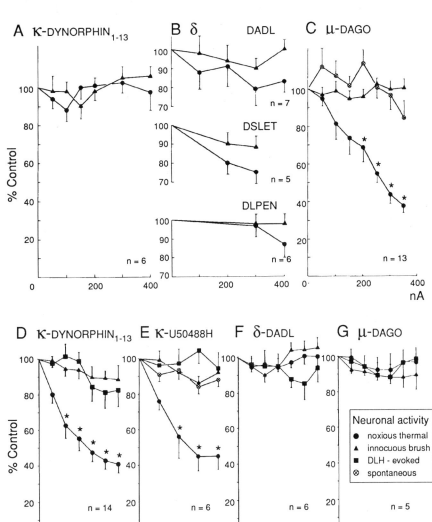

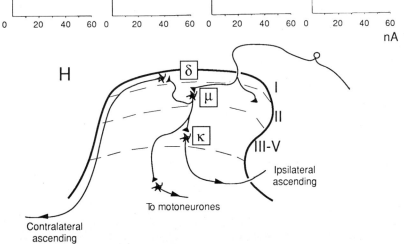

C-fibre-evoked responses in dorsal horn neurones when applied to the spinal cord surface (Sullivan and Dickenson 1988), but its more discrete administration has not been studied.

2. δ-Receptor-Preferring Ligands

The conclusions that can be drawn from local actions of δ-agonists are less clear cut. This is despite the fact that the enkephalins are slightly δ-selective (with significant μ, but little κ-receptor activity; Kosterlitz et al. 1985). The synthesis of highly δ-selective ligands, however, is a relatively recent development. Early experiments showed that when both [Met^5]enkephalinamide and [D-Ala^2,D-Leu^5]enkephalinamide were ejected in the substantia gelatinosa (Duggan et al. 1977b, 1981; Davies and Dray 1978; Sastry and Goh 1983) as with morphine, the nociceptive activation of laminae IV/V neurones was selectively reduced. Depression of spontaneous activity was often seen. Both ionophoretic and systemic naloxone reversed these effects of the opioids, the latter in a dose (0.1 mg kg^{-1}) also adequate to reverse the action of morphine administered in the substantia gelatinosa. Evidence that the action of [Met^5]enkephalin in the superficial dorsal horn may be largely mediated by μ-receptors has been provided from in vitro spinal preparations (Jeftinija 1988). Experiments using more specific δ-ligands have enabled better interpretation of these effects of enkephalins. Thus, when [D-Ala^2,D-Leu^5]enkephalin was applied in the substantia gelatinosa, whilst recording from cat spinocervical tract neurones in laminae IV/V, sensory responses were slightly attenuated in a minority of neurones (Fleetwood-Walker et al. 1988). This is shown in Fig. 2B. However, repeating the experiments with the progressively more δ:μ-selective agonists [D-Ser^2,L-Leu^5]enkephalyl-Thr (DSLET) and [D-Pen^2,L-Pen^5]enkephalin (DLPEN) led to a disappearance of the effect (Fig. 2B). This supports the previous conclusion that the effects of enkephalins in the substantia gelatinosa are mediated predominantly through μ-receptors.

When enkephalins have been administered close to the cell bodies of laminae IV/V or lamina I neurones, however, the results have been quite different. When applied near laminae IV/V cell bodies, both [Met^5]enkephalin and [Met^5]enkephalinamide reduced activity evoked by noxious and innocuous cutaneous stimuli and by L-glutamate (Zleglgansberger and Tulloch 1979; Duggan et al. 1977b). Identified spinothalamic tract neurones reacted similarly (Willcockson et al. 1984, 1986). Although this suggests a direct postsynaptic action on the recorded cell, when recording intracellularly, Zieglgansberger and Tulloch (1979) found no membrane potential or conductance changes that could underly such a phenomenon. In contrast, selective antinociceptive actions of enkephalins applied near deep neurones have also been described (Randic and Miletic 1978; Satoh et al. 1979). These actions of enkephalins were readily reversed by ionophoretic, but incompletely by systemic, naloxone, the latter being given at doses severalfold higher than those needed to block the action of systemic morphine. Since naloxone is in the order of tenfold more potent as a μ- than as a κ- or δ-antagonist (KOSTERLITZ et al. 1985), this result is consistent with a non-μ-mediated effect. Indeed, the μ-agonist DAGO ionophoresed near cat or rat laminae IV/V neurones had no effect (Fig. 2F; FLEETWOOD-WALKER et al. 1988; HOPE et al. 1990). In contrast, κ-agonists displayed prominent influences on responses of these cells (see below), but the minimal activity of enkephalins at κ-sites (around 3 orders of magnitude less than at δ- or μ-sites; KOSTERLITZ et al. 1985) makes it far from certain that κ-receptors mediate the observed effects of the enkephalins and [Met^5]enkephalinamide in laminae IV/V. Ionophoresis of DADL and the highly δ-selective DPDPE in the same experiments was without effect, suggesting that δ-receptors too were not closely involved in enkephalin inhibition of laminae IV–V neurones. However, lamina I cells (some of which were spinomesencephalic and spinothalamic tract cells) were clearly inhibited by DPDPE [and the inhibition was reversed by the δ-selective antagonist ICI 178864 (COTTON et al. 1984)] when applied nearby in the superficial dorsal horn (HOPE et al. 1990). Subpopulations of neurones displayed non-selective inhibition (perhaps a direct postsynaptic influence), selective antinociceptive effects (perhaps an action in substantia gelatinosa), or no effect. Topical application of DPDPE was reported to partially inhibit C-, and not A-fibre-evoked activity of neurones sampled from laminna V through to lamina I of the rat, suggesting a discrete action at δ-receptors at a site interposed between primary afferents and the recorded neurones, perhaps in the substantia gelatinosa (DICKENSON et al. 1987), but studies of this type cannot localise sites of action to spinal laminae. Similar results were recorded with another δ-selective agonist Tyr-D-Ser(OtBu)-Gly-Phe-Leu-Thr (SULLIVAN et al. 1989). It may be that the inhibition of lamina I cells observed by HOPE et al. (1990) underlies the analgesia seen with selective δ-agonists administered intrathecally and that such a confined influence explains the relatively modest potency of the behavioural effects observed (RODRIGUEZ et al. 1986).

3. κ-Receptor-Preferring Ligands

κ-Ligands have not been extensively used in ionophoretic experiments. In the experiments of FLEETWOOD-WALKER et al. (1988), application of the relatively selective κ-agonists dynorphin A$_{1-13}$ and U50488H near laminae IV/V spinocervical tract neurones of cat (but not in the substantia gelatinosa, Fig. 2A) exerted potent, naloxone-sensitive inhibition of responses to noxious stimuli (Fig. 2D,E; FLEETWOOD-WALKER et al. 1988). Both thermal and mechanical noxious stimuli from cutaneous origins were readily suppressed. Similar results were recorded in rat laminae IV/V neurones with local ionophoresis of U50488H, but, when the experiments focused on lamina I neurones, no κ-agonist effects were apparent (HOPE et al. 1990). When the mixed μ/κ-agonist metorphamide was ionophoresed close to laminae IV/V neurones, it also displayed a relatively selective inhibition of nociceptive responses (and also spontaneous activity), but with much less effect on responses to innocuous stimuli (ZHAO et al. 1986). This zonal localization of κ-opioid efficacy to laminae IV/V may well account for the preferential potency of κ-opioids on visceral, rather than cutaneous, nociception since, as discussed earlier, most visceral afferents terminate superficially to and deep to, rather than in, the substantia gelatinosa. Although ionophoretic administration of κ-agonists has uniformly resulted in inhibition, this has not been so with topical administration. Topical application of κ-agonists has resulted in variable excitation and inhibition of neuronal responses to afferent stimulation (HYLDEN et al. 1990; KNOX and DICKENSON 1987), but the effects were either incompletely or not reversed by naloxone. Indeed, κ-agonists can display very pronounced non-opioid effects on motor function (PRZEWLOCKI et al. 1983), neurotoxicity (STEWART and ISAAC 1989) and even apparent attenuation of μ-agonist-elicited antinociception (KNOX and DICKENSON 1987; SCHMAUSS and HERZ 1987), but these actions have not been explained at the electrophysiological level.

These ionophoretic studies clearly indicate that opioid receptors are not randomly distributed in the spinal cord, but that receptor types occur preferentially in restricted areas. This conclusion is supported by autoradiographic studies of ligand binding in the spinal cord.

Early evidence emphasised the binding of opiate-derived ligands to the more superficial parts of the dorsal horn. For example, with in vivo labelling in rats with [3H]diprenorphine, autoradiographic grains were concentrated in a dense band over the marginal zone and substantia gelatinosa (PERT et al. 1975; ATWEH and KUHAR 1977). Diprenorphine, however, has affinity for μ-, δ- and κ-receptors. De-afferentation studies indicated that a proportion of the μ- (and perhaps also δ-) sites were associated with primary afferents (FIELDS et al. 1980). The binding of the selective μ-ligand DAGO, however, was heavily concentrated in laminae I and II with relatively little in deeper laminae (GOUARDERES et al. 1985; MORRIS and HERZ 1987), confirming the conclusion of the ionophoretic experiments.

The distribution of δ- and κ-sites has been studied by using [3H]DADL and [3H]bremazocine in the presence of agents to block overlap labelling of other sites. MORRIS and HERZ (1987) localized δ-ligand binding sites in the rat specifically to lamina I. DASHWOOD et al. (1986) showed the selective ligand [3H]DLPEN bound to deeper as well as superficial layers of the rat dorsal horn, although TRAYNOR et al. (1990) illustrated a relatively restricted superficial distribution. These results, while supporting the potent actions of δ-ligands in lamina I, do suggest that some of the actions of enkephalins on deeper neurones could, in part, involve δ-receptors.

The presence of κ-sites in deep as well as (more prominently) superficial dorsal horn was suggested by results from SLATER and PATEL (1983) and

MORRIS and HERZ (1987) in the rat and GOUARDERES et al. (1986) in man. Non-selective or partially selective ligands in the presence of a screen of μ/δ-blockers were again used. Nevertheless, a relatively consistent picture was developed of a clear presence of κ-sites, not solely restricted to the substantia gelatinosa. In ligand binding studies, the highly κ-selective arylacetamide ligand [^{3}H]U-69593 has revealed in both dog (HUNTER et al. 1989) and rat (ALLERTON et al. 1989) spinal cords small populations of well-characterised κ-receptors. It may be that these sites represent only a subpopulation of κ-receptors, since other distinct κ-subtypes, $κ_2$ and $κ_3$, have been proposed (ATTALI et al. 1982; CLARK et al. 1989). Overall these studies give support to the action of κ-ligands on neurones deep to the substantia gelatinosa, but it does appear surprising that neurones of lamina I were not affected by ionophoretically applied dynorphin and U50488H. Figure 2H illustrates the proposed lamina distribution of opioid receptor sites.

IV. Functional Consequences of Opioid Receptor Activation to Spinal Sensory Processing

Predicting what opiate receptor activation will do to sensory processing requires detailed knowledge of the location of such receptors. There are two main considerations. Firstly, from the viewpoint of single neurones it is important to determine whether the relevant receptors are located on dendrites, cell bodies or fibres making connections with a given neurone. Secondly, the location and function of neurones bearing opiate receptors within sensory pathways of the spinal cord will clearly determine the functional consequences of opioid receptor activation for sensory processing. Our initial discussion will centre on the opioid receptors of the superficial dorsal horn. Within this area three neural elements require consideration as bearing opioid receptors: the terminals of primary afferent fibres, the intrinsic neurones of this area and the terminals of fibres of supraspinal and propriospinal origin. The functional consequences will differ if opioid receptors are located predominantly on one of these structures and hence they will be discussed separately.

1. Opioid Receptors and the Central Terminals of Nociceptors

There is evidence for opiate-binding sites near the spinal terminations of primary afferent fibres (FIELDS et al. 1980). A probable consequence of activation of opiate receptors on primary afferents would be a reduction of transmitter release by a process comparable to presynaptic inhibition of release by γ-aminobutyric acid (GABA).

a) Terminal Excitability

With large-diameter primary afferents, presynaptic inhibition is a process whereby depolarization of a terminal by GABA results in less transmitter release when the terminal is invaded by an action potential (CURTIS et al. 1980). The depolarization can be detected electrophysiologically as a decrease in the threshold for electrical stimulation of the terminal by an adjacent microelectrode. If opioids act similarly to GABA on the central terminals of nociceptors, then ionophoretic administration of these compounds should decrease terminal excitability. This has not been observed. SASTRY (1978, 1979, 1980) found that morphine and [Met^5]enkephalin decreased the excitability of the central terminals of both small myelinated and unmyelinated primary afferents. CARSTENS ct al. (1979b, 1987) found systemic morphine decreased the excitability of unmyelinated primary afferents within the spinal cord. GABA has been shown to depolarize the cell bodies of large-diameter primary afferent neurones, with the inference that receptors at central terminals may also be expressed on cell bodies. Opioids active at μ-, δ- and κ-receptors have been shown to shorten the action potential duration of a proportion of cultured dorsal root ganglion cells of the mouse (WERZ and MACDONALD 1982, 1985; SHEN and CRAIN 1989), when applied in micromolar concentrations. Such an effect, occurring at terminals, might be expected to reduce transmitter release. SHEN and CRAIN (1989), however, showed that nanomolar concentrations of opioid peptides increased the action potential duration of cultured dorsal root ganglion neurones and thus could increase transmitter release at endings and perhaps exert bimodal effects on nociceptive processing. The relevance of these findings to the concentrations attained by analgesic doses of opiates and to the amounts of synaptically released opioid peptides remains uncertain.

b) Release of Tachykinins

The transmitters released from nociceptive primary afferents are not documented with certainty, but considerable evidence points to a role for L-glutamate and a number of neuropeptides (reviewed by DUGGAN and WEIHE 1990). Prominent among the latter is substance P (SP) and a number of techniques have shown that substance P appears in or around the spinal cord with peripheral noxious stimuli (Go and YAKSH 1987; KURAISHI et al. 1983, 1989; BRODIN et al. 1987; DUGGAN et al. 1988). Inhibition of SP has been shown when opioids have been superfused to both slice preparations (JESSELL and IVERSEN 1977; MAUBORGNE et al. 1987; POHL et al. 1989) and to the spinal cord in vivo (YAKSH et al. 1980; Go and YAKSH 1987).

The concentrations of drugs in all of these experiments were high (10^{-3}–$10^{-5} M$). No group has found that systemic analgesic doses of morphine reduce SP release in the dorsal horn. KURAISHI et al. (1983) found that morphine ($10 \, \text{mg kg}^{-1}$) failed to reduce SP release (measured with push-pull cannulae) from noxious mechanical stimulation of the rat, although morphine ($10^{-5} M$) added to the perfusion did reduce release. With antibody microprobes. MORTON et al. (1990) failed to observe any effect of morphine, given in two dose ranges (1–$6 \, \text{mg kg}^{-1}$ and 10–$20 \, \text{mg kg}^{-1}$), on

SP release in the dorsal horn of the cat following noxious mechanical or thermal cutaneous stimulation.

If inhibition of transmitter release from the central terminals of nociceptors is the main mechanism of action of, for example, µ-agonists, it follows that subsequent synaptic events should be reduced by morphine. It also follows that, for sensory processing, transmission of nociceptive information to all subsequent targets, such as areas of the brain important in perception, autonomic areas and motoneurones involved in reflexes would be reduced. As cited previously, however, HARRIS and RYALL (1988) found that doses of morphine reducing excitation of dorsal horn neurones by peripheral nociceptors did not reduce inhibition of other neurones from the same source.

Collectively these findings suggest that high concentrations of opiates can reduce the release of SP from the central terminals of small-diameter primary afferents, but that it has not been shown that this occurs with analgesic doses of morphine. It also has not been shown that a physiological process results in a reduction, by opioid peptides, of neuropeptide release from primary afferents.

2. Receptors on the Somata and Processes of Spinal Neurones

Since only a subpopulation of µ- and δ-sites in the superficial dorsal horn is lost after dorsal rhizotomy (FIELDS et al. 1980; ZAJAC et al. 1989), at least some of the receptors must be present on intrinsic spinal elements. The same is most probably true of κ-receptors.

An opioid could affect the excitability of a neurone postsynaptically by a number of processes which include: (a) acting as a receptor antagonist; (b) hyperpolarizing or depolarizing the membrane either by directly opening ion channels or through intracellular second messengers; or (c) acting as a neuromodulator, i.e. having little effect on membrane conductances per se, but altering the ability of other compounds to do so.

There is no convincing evidence that opioids act as antagonists at receptors for other neuroactive compounds. Indeed, such a mechanism requires that naloxone acts as an agonist. Elsewhere in this volume (NORTH) the membrane effects of opioids are considered at length and an important finding is that many neurones are hyperpolarized by µ- and δ-opioids through activation of a potassium conductance, which involves intracellular G-proteins. Such an action produces inhibition of neuronal activity. Hyperpolarization of spinal neurones by opiates (YOSHIMURA and NORTH 1983) and by [Met^5]enkephalin (MURASE et al. 1982; ZIEGLGAENSBERGER and SUTOR 1983) has been observed in slice preparations, but the difficulties of in vivo recording have prevented confirmation of this under more physiological conditions. Similarly inhibitory actions of κ-opioids, involving attenuation of Ca^{2+} conductances, have been investigated in dissociated immature dorsal root ganglion neurones (WERZ and MACDONALD 1985) and in locus coeruleus slices, resulting in reductions of EPSPs by a presynaptic action (McFadzean 1988), but not in whole animal preparations.

A neuromodulatory action of opiates was originally proposed by Zieglgaensberger and Bayerl (1976). Morphine reduced depolarization of motoneurones by L-glutamate and also reduced the rate of rise of primary afferent induced EPSPs, without altering membrane conductance or membrane potential. A similar effect was described with [Met^5]enkephalin (Zieglgaensberger and Tulloch 1979). The receptor specificity in these experiments was uncertain, however, and more specific ligands appear not to have been subsequently used. These experiments were performed under in vivo conditions using glued assemblies of recording and drug-administering micropipettes. Tissue debris around the drug-administering micropipette can occlude access to the soma of the cell recorded from, whilst allowing access to sites on dendrites where EPSPs are generated. It has been shown that, under such conditions, glycine (a compound known to hyperpolarize motoneurones) can produce large reductions in EPSPs without detectable changes in membrane potential or conductance (Zhao and Duggan 1984).

Can these membrane actions of opioids explain the relatively selective reduction of the nociceptive responses of dorsal horn neurones, when the drugs have been administered ionophoretically? Zieglgaensberger and Bayerl (1976) proposed that an impairment in the rate of rise of EPSPs would have a greater effect on transmission of impulses in C, when compared with A fibres. This may be true with electrical stimulation of nerve, but with natural stimuli such differences in the rate of rise of EPSPs may not occur. Most groups, moreover (including Zieglgaensberger and Tulloch 1979), have not observed any modality-selectivity of opioid peptide inhibition near the bodies of laminae IV/V neurones. For a membrane hyperpolarization to explain selectivity of opioids, anatomical explanations include the receptors being either restricted to interneurones on nociceptive pathways, and hence interposed between primary afferents and the neurones from which recordings have been obtained, or located distally on dendrites and adjacent to synapses receiving nociceptive input either mono- or polysynaptically. A further possibility relates to the convergence of influences on a particular cellular process. Consider, for example, if a nociceptive transmitter (perhaps a tachykinin) were to act on a neurone by attenuating a particular K^+ conductance. If an opioid were to act specifically by promoting opening of the same K^+ channel, it would very efficiently reverse the functional effects of the nociceptive transmitter. In contrast, if a non-nociceptive mechano-receptor afferent were to release glutamate, for example, inducing Na^+ and Ca^{2+} entry, the influence of such a process may be less securely limited by opioids modulating the K^+ channel status of the cell.

3. Receptors and Supraspinal Fibres

Two main questions arise. Firstly do opioids have interactions with the terminals of fibres of supraspinal origin and, secondly, to what extent are the effects of systemic opiates on the spinal cord indirect and result from effects at supraspinal levels on neurones controlling spinal events? The second question will be discussed later.

Several lines of evidence have indicated an interaction between noradrenaline and opioids. Following the initial observation that clonidine suppressed the hyperexcitability of neurones of the locus coeruleus, produced by opiate withdrawal (AGHAJANIAN 1978), a synergism between μ-opioids and compounds acting at α_2-adrenoceptors has been found, both for inhibition of the tail-flick of the rat (SPAULDING et al. 1979) and inhibition of C fibre evoked activity in ascending axons of the rat (WILCOX et al. 1987). The hyperexcitability of laminae IV/V neurones produced by administering naloxone after morphine, in the substantia gelatinosa of the cat, was readily reduced by clonidine (ZHAO and DUGGAN 1987). The membrane basis of these interactions probably lies in a coupling of differing receptors to the same ion channel (Chap. 30). Naloxone has not reduced inhibition by noradrenaline (FLEETWOOD-WALKER et al. 1987; HEADLEY et al. 1978). Interestingly, whilst the α_2-adrenoceptor antagonist idazoxan had no effect on the antinociceptive effect of DAGO (μ) in the substantia gelatinosa, it reliably reversed that of dynorphin A_{1-13} and U50488H in laminae IV–V (FLEETWOOD-WALKER et al. 1988). Analogously, naloxone has not reduced the action of 5-HT (HEADLEY et al. 1978), but the inhibition of tail-flick of the rat produced by intrathecal dynorphin was reduced by prior administration of the neurotoxin 5,6-dihydroxytryptamine (VON VOIGTLANDER et al. 1984). It has been proposed (IGGO et al. 1985) that the relevant κ-receptors are located on tonically active spinal neurones which inhibit monoamine release from descending fibres. Such disinhibition would result in a release of noradrenaline which is known to preferentially reduce the nociceptive responses of deep dorsal horn neurones (HEADLEY et al. 1978). This is unlikely to be a complete explanation of the action of κ-ligands, since κ-receptors were first proposed through the action of ethylketocyclazocine on the spinal cord of chronic spinal dogs where all descending monoamine-containing fibres would have degenerated (MARTIN et al. 1964).

These extended considerations of opioid receptors and neural elements of the dorsal horn permit some conclusions on the functional significance of opioid receptor activation for sensory processing.

It appears that a postsynaptic action of μ-agonists on neurones intrinsic to the substantia gelatinosa is responsible for the selective inhibition of the nociceptive responses of deeper neurones of laminae IV/V. The organisation of neurones within the substantia gelatinosa is not well understood, but it is probable that μ-receptors are located only on defined excitatory pathways. It seems reasonable to propose, however, that the nociceptive activation of many supraspinally projecting neurones of the spinal cord would be reduced by activation of μ-receptors in the substantia gelatinosa and that this is an important component of opiate analgesia. Whether μ-receptor activation in the substantia gelatinosa also impairs transmission of nociceptive (and other) information to motoneurones and autonomic areas cannot be decided, but it is a likely possibility. A preferential action of δ-ligands on neurones of lamina I does seem appropriate for analgesia. Thus, this lamina contains a proportion of spinothalamic and spinomesencephalic neurones and these are proposed as ultimately important in pain perception. Little can be said about δ-receptors and sensory transmission to the ventral horn. It is more difficult to hypothesize on the functional consequences of κ-receptor activation. The zonal localization of κ-effects to deeper laminae of the spinal cord may relate to the usage of κ-agonists with visceral pain, since many visceral afferents terminate superficial to and ventral to, but not in, the substantia gelatinosa. κ-receptors may well also be involved in many processes unrelated to nociception. As will be subsequently discussed, naloxone administration reveals many such events in the spinal cord and the importance of κ- and other opioid receptors in these processes is unknown.

V. Opiates and Descending Inhibition

The preceding sections have shown that systemic opiates impair the spinal transmission of nociceptive information to supraspinal areas and that locally administered opioids also have such an effect. Many supraspinal controls, however, are exerted on spinal neurones and it is probable that systemically administered opiates will influence these controls. Thus when considering the overall effects of systemic opiates on spinal neurones, a distinction needs to be made between direct spinal actions and indirect, supraspinally mediated effects. This field is replete with controversy and some experimental differences need to be pointed out.

Firstly, it may not be correct to assume that supraspinal controls on pathways to motoneurones will necessarily be affected similarly to controls on pathways to areas of the brain important in perception. Elsewhere in this volume (Chap. 31, part II), evidence is presented that the firing of certain raphe neurones can be closely linked to movement of the tail of the rat in response to a noxious stimulus and that altered firing of such neurones following systemic opiates can be correlated to inhibition of tail movement. Although inhibition of tail-flick to a noxious stimulus is commonly described as indicating analgesia, the latter implies a lack of pain perception and this is an assumption. Pharmacological differences between the effects of opiates on pathways to motoneurones and to ascending tracts were previously cited (JURNA 1984).

Several groups have observed inhibition of the nociceptive responses of dorsal horn neurones, when opiates have been microinjected in brain stem sites such as the periaqueductal grey (BENNETT and MAYER 1979; GEBHART et al. 1984; JONES and GEBHART 1988) and the more caudal medulla (TAKAGI et al. 1976; DU et al. 1984). Others (LE BARS et al. 1980; BOUHASSIRA et al. 1988; DICKENSON and LE BARS 1987a,b) found that microinjection of morphine at brain stem sites predominantly enhanced the excitation of dorsal horn neurones by impulses in unmyelinated primary afferents. Given the complexity of the brain stem, these varied results are perhaps not unexpected. Since the relationship between concentrations attained at a site in the brain by systemic administration and those following microinjection are uncertain, it is difficult to relate these results to the question: do systemic analgesic doses of opiates increase supraspinal inhibition of neurones transmitting nociceptive information to the brain? Microinjection of naloxone at supraspinal sites following systemic morphine is more likely to give relevant answers.

In the cat, the responses of many dorsal horn neurones to peripheral noxious stimuli is subject to powerful tonic inhibition from the brain stem (WALL 1967; HANDWERKER et al. 1975; DUGGAN and MORTON 1988). The net inhibition on a particular neurone can be measured by cooling the cephalic spinal cord. Both JURNA and GROSSMAN (1976) and DUGGAN et al. (1980) found that analgesic doses of morphine, far from increasing descending inhibition of the dorsal horn neurones studied, actually decreased it.

A number of investigators have employed intrathecal administration of opiates, in investigating spinal and supraspinal actions of opiates, and these have recently been summarised by ADVOKAT (1988). It is the opinion of the present reviewers that, given the wide distribution of opiate receptors in the brain and the complexity of brain control of spinal events, it is highly likely that analgesic doses of opiates will influence the latter. It has not been convincingly demonstrated, however, that the reduction in spinal transmission of nociceptive information to areas important in pain perception results from an increase in supraspinal inhibition. The evidence is substantial for increased supraspinal inhibition of transmission to motoneurones, following systemic opiates.

VI. Physiological Roles of Opioid Peptides in Sensory Processing

In considering the possible physiological roles of opioid peptides in sensory processing it is evident that most experiments employing electrophysiological methods have centered on pain and hence have examined inhibition of spinal neurones believed to be important in transmission of nociceptive information to the brain. Such experiments, however, have had only limited success in revealing opioidergic inhibition and most evidence for the latter has come from experiments on spinal reflexes or from studying neurones in the ventral horn of the spinal cord. Ideally, when describing a physiological event involving opioid peptides, one would like to state (a) what is released, (b) the receptor(s) acted upon, (c) the physiological alteration in the structure bearing the relevant receptors and (d) the consequences for neural processing. With opioid peptides, in no instance is it possible to give such a complete description.

1. Spinal Release of Opioid Peptides

By a variety of techniques, electrical stimulation of unmyelinated primary afferents has been shown to produce a spinal release of [Met^5]enkephalin (Yaksh and Elde 1981; Le Bars et al. 1987; Cesselin et al. 1989), [Mct^5]enkephalin Lys^6 and [Met^5]enkephalin Arg^6, Phe^7 (Nyberg et al. 1983), [Met^5]enkephalin Arg^{6}Gly^{7}Leu^8 (Iadarola et al. 1986) and dynorphin (Hutchison and Morton 1989; Hutchison et al. 1990), but it has not been possible to relate such release to events in the spinal cord much less to sensory processing. It is important in future research to localise release to discrete laminae or nuclei and this appears feasible with the antibody microprobe (Duggan et al. 1988).

Descriptions of opioid receptors involved in physiological events are still imperfect through lack of specific antagonists which can be administered systemically, topically and microionophoretically. Most experiments have defined naloxone-reversible events and thus permit no firm conclusions on the likely receptors involved. There are relatively few results with the more selective antagonists such as naloxonazine (Pasternak and Wood 1986), β-furaltrexamine (Takemori et al. 1981) and nor-binaltorphimine (Portoghese et al. 1987).

2. Tonic Opioidergic Inhibition

If an inhibition involving opioids is tonically present on a neurone, then an opioid antagonist should alter the basal properties of that neurone.

a) Dorsal Horn

When unidentified neurones of the dorsal horn have been examined in both the cat and rat, however, the effects of naloxone on both basal and evoked responses have been infrequent and inconsistent (Duggan et al. 1977c; Rivot et al. 1979; Henry 1979, 1981; Zieglgansberger and Tulloch 1979; Sinclair et al. 1980; Fitzgerald and Woolf 1980). When ascending axons in the anterolateral funiculus were examined in both rat (Bernatsky et al. 1983) and cat (Duggan et al. 1985), naloxone consistently increased firing to electrical stimulation of peripheral C fibres. Figure 3A (left records) illustrates this action in the cat. Figure 3A (right records) shows that transmission of information in large-diameter muscle afferents to supraspinal areas is not modified by naloxone in the cat. These findings suggest that opioids affect organised systems in specific ways and much research is required to define these systems functionally.

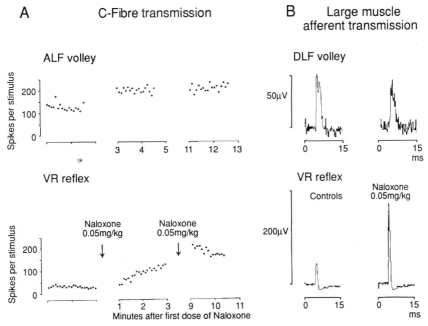

Fig. 3A,B. Differential effects of naloxone (0.5 mg kg^{-1}) on transmission of impulses in primary afferents to ascending spinal tracts and to ventral roots. **A** Each plotted point represents the number of action potentials produced by electrical stimulation of unmyelinated primary afferents of a tibial nerve. *Upper record*, impulses recorded in the ipsilateral first sacral ventral root. *Lower record*, impulses recorded by ball electrodes placed on the contralateral anterolateral spinal fasciculus at a high cervical level. Naloxone increased the responses in both recording situations. **B** Averaged records (*n* = 16) of potentials recorded in ventral roots (*upper records*) and the ipsilateral dorsolateral fasciculus (*lower records*) from electrical stimulation of the combined medial and lateral gastrocnemii nerves of the cat with a stimulus strength 16 times threshold for the fastest conducting fibres. Naloxone increased the ventral root reflex without altering the DLF volleys to the same stimuli. (Reproduced with permission from DUGGAN et al. 1985)

b) Ventral Horn

In the anaesthetised spinal cat, the excitation of motoneurones by sensory afferents is regularly altered by naloxone, a finding which contrasts with studies on neurones of the dorsal horn. Initially this was shown with excitation of motoneurones by peripheral C fibre stimulation (McCLANE and MARTIN 1967; BELL and MARTIN 1977) and is a result readily interpretable in terms of opioid peptides suppressing a nociceptive response. It is shown in Figure 4A (lower records). Subsequently, however, it was shown that, in spinal cats, naloxone (0.1–2.0 mg kg^{-1}) increased monosynaptic reflexes in both flexor and extensor muscles (see Fig. 4B, lower records) and poly-synaptic reflexes to impulses in large-diameter cutaneous afferents (GOLDFARB and HU 1976; DUGGAN et al. 1984). Intracellular recordings showed that, even with single motoneurones, EPSPs from a number of peripheral nerves were all increased by naloxone (MORTON et al. 1982). In the spinal rabbit, CLARKE et al. (1989) have shown that reflexes evoked in a number of muscles, both flexor and extensor, from electrical stimulation of nerves supplying the heel were enhanced by naloxone ($0.005-0.2\,\mathrm{mg\,kg^{-1}}$). In the rat, however, PARSONS and HEADLEY (1988) found no enhancement by naloxone of motoneurone firing to noxious and non-noxious cutaneous stimuli.

Little is known of the mechanisms of the inhibitions reduced by naloxone in spinal cats and rabbits. When sensory fibres are stimulated electrically, a host of inhibitory as well as excitatory processes are activated. With a monosynaptic reflex, however, motoneurone excitation occurs before any inhibition (also activated by the stimulus) can influence motoneurone excitability. Thus, enhanced monosynaptic reflexes following naloxone almost certainly result from block of a tonically present opioidergic inhibition. The opioids could be released near motoneurones or, remotely, to control the activity of interneurones which tonically control motoneurone excitability. ZHAO and DUGGAN (1987) found that administering naloxone near motoneurones failed to increase evoked EPSPs, a result favouring a remote release of opioid peptides. The control may be exerted on GABA-releasing neurones producing tonic presynaptic inhibition on the terminals of primary afferent fibres. Although the inhibition revealed by naloxone is called segmental, it could be a propriospinal control, since spinal cord transection is usually done at the thoracolumbar junction and the reflexes studied were in lower lumbar and upper sacral segments.

It is clear from the effects of naloxone on sensory activation of motoneurones that opioid peptides have roles in the spinal cord which cannot be linked to nociception alone. When considering supraspinal control of spinal neurones, virtually all experiments, however, have been directed at nociception and, by inference, to the perception of pain.

3. Phasic Opioidergic Inhibition

It is perhaps a surprising result that in the cat no spinal inhibition of supraspinal origin has been reduced by naloxone. Thus both CARSTENS et al. (1979a) and DUGGAN and GRIERSMITH (1979b) failed to reduce inhibition of the nociceptive responses of dorsal horn neurones by electrical stimulation of the periaqueductal grey.

In the rat inhibition of the nociceptive responses of dorsal horn neurones by stimulation in the medullary raphe was reduced by naloxone (RIVOT et al. 1979). Also in the rat the inhibition of dorsal horn neurones of lumbar segments by noxious stimuli applied remotely (the diffuse noxious inhibitory control, LE BARS et al. 1979) was reduced by naloxone (LE BARS et al. 1981). Naloxone, however, failed to reduce inhibition in the dorsal horn from electrical stimulation in the periaqueductal grey matter (JURNA 1980). Reduction or an inhibition by naloxone does not necessarily imply a release of opioids in the spinal cord. Alterations in the excitability of neurones adjacent to a brain stem stimulating electrode will alter the effect of a stimulus.

C. Thalamus and Cerebral Cortex

Any pharmacological study of the modification of a perception, such as pain, suffers from an inability to state which of a varied collection of neurophysiological events can necessarily be linked to the altered percept. Changes in the motivational-affective response to pain may well involve limbic areas such as the amygdala, hippocampus and hypothalamus, areas where systemic opiates and opioid peptides have been shown to alter neuronal firing. For the present review, however, considerations have been restricted to the thalamus and cerebral cortex, mainly because of the better-documented involvement of these areas in sensory processing.

I. Thalamus

1. Ventrobasal Nuclei

The thalamus is a large complex area with many nuclear groups and the relationship of these to nociception is not well defined. The ventrobasal group of neurones receives a large afferent input from the medial lemniscus and this information relates to non-noxious mechanical events in skin and muscle. In addition a proportion of spinothalamic tract fibres bearing information on non-noxious and noxious peripheral events terminate in ventrobasal nuclei (LUND and WEBSTER 1967). Local actions of opioids are possible since regions of the ventrobasal thalamus, including the ventroposterolateral nucleus, do contain opioid ligand binding sites. The numbers are low when compared to other parts of the central nervous system and are almost exclusively of the μ-type with few or no δ- and κ-receptors present (MANSOUR et al. 1987). Pro-enkephalin-containing fibres are sparsely represented in ventrobasal thalamic regions and pro-dynorphin-containing fibres appear to be virtually absent (KHACHATURIAN et al. 1985). Although much of the experimental work has been carried out using the rat, in a number of other species including man (QUIRION et al. 1987; MANSOUR et al. 1988), κ-receptors are more strongly represented in many regions, including the thalamus.

There is evidence that transmission of impulses in the rapidly conducting lemniscal pathway appears not to be altered by opiates. Thus excitation of ventrobasal thalamic neurons by peripheral non-noxious stimuli was not altered by analgesic doses of morphine (SINITSIN 1964; HILL and PEPPER 1978; BENOIST et al. 1983).

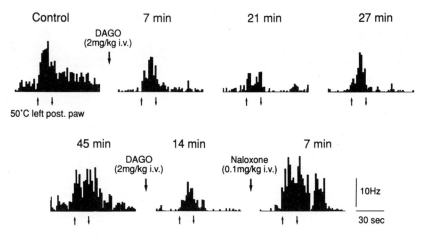

Fig. 4. Effects of an intravenously applied μ-receptor selective opioid DAGO on nociceptive responses of a ventrobasal thalamic neurone. The sample records illustrate the firing frequency of ventrobasal thalamic neurones of the rat and show increases in firing frequency to heating of the left hind (post.) paw. Above each record the time after administration of DAGO or naloxone is indicated. In the lower traces, naloxone was administered 15 min after the second dose of DAGO. (Reproduced by permission from Benoist et al. 1986)

Recent work in the rat has shown that a proportion of ventrobasal thalamic neurones are excited by noxious cutaneous stimuli. Such excitation may occur by spinothalamic pathways. Benoist et al. (1983) found that systemic morphine reduced the nociceptive responses of such neurones and emphasized that the effective doses (ED$_{50}$ of 0.09 mg kg^{-1}) were much lower than those needed to have a similar action on spinal neurones. This effectiveness of low doses of systemic morphine on thalamic neurones of the rat has been observed by other investigators. Thus Hill et al. (1982) compared neurones in or near to the ventrobasal complex with trigeminal neurones and Carlsson et al. (1988) studied neurones of the dorsomedial part of the ventral complex and ascending axons of the spinal cord. In both cases more than four times the dose needed in the thalamus was required at the other site. Such an effect is likely to result from an action of opiates at several sites on the complex polysynaptic pathway from first central synapse to thalamus. Benoist et al. (1986) have shown that systemic administration of opioid peptides such as the μ-agonist DAGO (2.0 mg kg^{-1}) and the δ-ligand DSLET (3 mg kg^{-1}) reduces the nociceptive responses of ventrobasal neurones of the rat. This effect of systemically administered DAGO is shown in Fig. 4. Such a result suggests that some opioid peptides penetrate the blood-brain barrier, at least in part, but the precise sites of action remain uncertain in experiments of this type.

A direct depressant action by morphine on ventrobasal thalamus has not been shown. Indeed one study in the cat found that morphine, administered ionophoretically, excited most of the neurones studied (DUGGAN et al. 1976a). KAYSER and GUILBAUD (1984) have drawn attention to the excitation of a proportion of ventrobasal thalamic neurones of the rat by peripheral noxious stimuli and the remarkable enhancement of such firing with the development of peripheral inflammation such as arthritis. Such enhanced firing also occurred with non-noxious stimulation of the inflamed joint and was reduced by systemic morphine. With inflammation of an area, non-noxious stimulation can be perceived as painful and such allodynia may not be wholly of peripheral origin. Central alterations of sensory processing may occur at several levels of the neuraxis. The ability of opiates and opioid peptides to influence these changes in sensory processing and whether alterations occur in areas such as the thalamus is an important area for future research.

There appear to be no systematic studies of the effects of opioid peptides, specific for different opioid receptors, on neurones of the ventrobasal thalamus or adjacent nuclei. Evidence for tonic activity of opioid peptides has come from the effects of administering naloxone. In normal rats, JURNA (1988) found that intravenous naloxone had mixed effects on the nociceptive responses of neurones adjacent to the ventrobasal complex (nucleus ventralis, pars dorsomedialis). Naloxone, $1 \, mg \, kg^{-1}$, predominantly inhibited responses, but with doses of $5 \, mg \, kg^{-1}$ facilitation and inhibition occurred in equal numbers. In rats with experimental arthritis, KAYSER et al. (1988) found that very low doses of naloxone ($3 \, \mu g \, kg^{-1}$) produced what they termed paradoxical antinociception and also reduced the nociceptive responses of ventrobasal thalamic neurones. This laboratory has also found that higher doses of naloxone ($1-3 \, mg \, kg^{-1}$) produced hyperalgesia in arthritic animals, but no associated studies were made of the firing of ventrobasal thalamic neurones. The results of JURNA (1988) suggest that enhanced nociceptive responses may be observed with the higher doses of naloxone. These so-called paradoxical effects of naloxone have been recently reviewed by KAYSER et al. (1988), who have proposed autoreceptors on the terminals of opioid peptide-releasing neurones. With a complex neuronal network, however, in which tonically active opioid peptide-releasing neurones control the activity of other neurones (including other opioid-releasing neurones), then the effect of a low dose of naloxone is, to a large extent, unpredictable. It depends on the relative numbers of, and tonic activity in, opioid synapses prior to the last one affecting the neurone under study.

2. Medial and Dorsal Thalamic Nuclei

Medial and dorsal to the ventrobasal nuclei lie the intralaminar and dorsal thalamic nuclei which include the centromedian, parafascicularis, and dorsomedial nuclei. Both physiological and anatomical evidence points to a role for these nuclei in processing of nociceptive information (ALBE-FESSARD and Kruger 1962; Bowsher 1957; Kaelber et al. 1975; Woda et al. 1975). Microinjection of opiates in medial thalamic areas of the rat produces analgesia (Yaksh and Rudy 1978). A number of the dorsomedial regions of the thalamus of the rat contain abundant μ-receptors, a moderate population of κ-binding sites and perhaps a small number of δ-sites (Mansour et al. 1987). The distribution is not entirely coincident, however, with those zones proposed as important in nociceptive processing. In the centralis lateralis nucleus, for example [one of the sites of termination of the spinothalamic tract in the rat (Lund and Webster 1967; Boivie 1979)], opioid receptors are notably deficient. Nevertheless there is clearly the potential for opioid-mediated regulation of nociceptive processing at local, if not immediately adjacent, sites. Moderate densities of pro-enkephalin-containing fibres are present in some parts of the dorsomedial thalamus (Khachaturian et al. 1985).

Nakahama et al. (1981) found selective depression by morphine $(1\,mg\,kg^{-1})$ and pentazocine $(2\,mg\,kg^{-1})$ of the nociceptive responses of neurones of the medial thalamic nuclei of the cat. In the rat intravenous morphine $(0.25-1.17\,\mu g\,kg^{-1})$ reduced the nociceptive responses of neurones of the nucleus lateralis anterior (Hill and Pepper 1978).

Ionophoretic studies have observed direct actions of opiates on medial thalamic neurones but the results have not been uniform. In the cat morphine depressed the firing of medial thalamic neurones but naloxone acted similarly, and did not antagonize the action of morphine (Duggan and Hall 1977). In the rat, depression of spontaneous firing has been the predominant effect of morphine administered ionophoretically, but excitation has been reported by most investigators (Hill and Pepper 1978; Reyes-Vazquez and Dafny 1982; Reyes-Vasquez et al. 1989; Prieto-Gomez et al. 1989). Naloxone reversal of any effect of morphine was not seen by Hill and Pepper (1978), who studied neurones of the nucleus lateralis anterior, but reversal of depression by morphine was reported by the other groups cited. Thus, both Reyes-Vasquez et al. (1989) and Prieto-Gomez et al. (1989) found that ionophoretic morphine reduced the nociceptive responses of medial thalamic neurones of the rat.

There are several deficits in knowledge of the way in which opiates and opioid peptides influence thalamic neurones. Significant amongst these is how opioid peptides having high specificity for particular receptors modify the responses of thalamic neurones to peripheral stimuli. In addition, there are no published studies on opiates and neurones of the thalamic nucleus submedius, an area of considerable recent interest to physiologists in relation to nociception (Craig and Burton 1981).

It is not possible to relate the present experimental data to perception of pain, but others have made interesting proposals. Thus Guilbaud (1985) has hypothesised that the responses of neurones of the medial thalamus do not encode the magnitude of a peripheral noxious stimulus accurately and thus may not be primarily concerned with the sensory discriminative aspect of pain. Thus the direct effects of opiates in the medial thalamus may be more relevant to the affective concomitants to pain.

II. Cerebral Cortex

A number of cortical events have been shown to be altered by systemic opiates but in most cases it is uncertain to what extent these changes result from direct actions in the cerebral cortex or result from effects on sub-cortical neurones.

In several species, analgesic doses of morphine have been shown to produce a sleep-like pattern in the cortical electroencephalogram without associated drowsiness in behaviour. This has been shown in the rat (CAHEN and WIKLER 1944; DIMPFEL et al. 1989), cat (NAVARRO and ELLIOTT 1971), dog (WIKLER 1952), rabbit (NAVARRO and ELLIOTT 1971) and man (WIKLER 1954). It is unknown if this behavioural, electrophysiological dissociation is also seen in some of the thalamic nuclei of these species since comparable recordings in conscious animals have not been performed.

Several groups have examined the effects of systemic opiates on cortical evoked potentials but such studies have difficulties in interpretation since responses in the somatosensory cortex to peripheral noxious and non-noxious stimuli are not consistently different (BROMM 1985). The short latency response recorded in the region of the primary somatosensory cortex following electrical stimulation of the sciatic nerve of the anaesthetised cat (SINITSIN 1964) and rat (JURNA et al. 1972; BISCOE et al. 1972) was not reduced by analgesic doses of morphine. In the study of BISCOE et al. (1972) it was noted that etorphine $(2-12\,\mu g\,kg^{-1})$ increased the latency of the first recorded response in a naloxone-reversible manner, an effect that was also observed following pentazocine administration to guinea pigs (MOYANO et al. 1975). Cortical evoked potentials produced by electrical stimulation of the tooth pulp of the dog (CHIN and DOMINO 1961) were not reduced by systemic morphine.

In humans there is evidence that late cortical evoked potentials are reduced by systemic opiates. Large doses of fentanyl $(10\,\mu g\,kg^{-1})$ reduced the late (latency of 150 ms) but not the early (5-ms latency) component of both auditory and large-diameter primary afferent induced cortical evoked potentials (VELASCO et al. 1984). These long latency somatic evoked potentials have been increased by naloxone (BUCHSBAUM et al. 1977; VELASCO et al. 1984). Using a brief laser pulse as a painful stimulus, BROMM (1985) also observed a reduction of late (>150 ms) evoked potentials by systemic morphine.

Events in the visual cortex have been studied for modification by opiates since these drugs have minor effects on visual signal detection performance (ROTHENBURG et al. 1979). WILKINSON and HOSHO (1982) found analgesic doses of morphine increased cortical evoked potentials from electrical stimulation of the optic chiasm of the anaesthetised cat. The significance of this increase is unknown.

An analysis of the effects of opiates on cortical evoked potentials requires differentiation between actions at subcortical sites and direct effects at opiate receptors in the cerebral cortex. The three types of opiate receptor are present in the cerebral cortex of the rat and cat where they demonstrate distinctly different laminar distributions (MANSOUR et al. 1986, 1987; WALKER et al. 1988) but several authors have drawn attention to the prominence of κ-binding sites in the cerebral cortex of several species (QUIRION et al. 1987; HALL et al. 1987; WALKER et al. 1988; HUNTER et al. 1989). Both pro-enkephalin and pro-dynorphin-containing fibres are present in cortical areas (KHACHATURIAN et al. 1985), supporting the possibility of local opioid-mediated influences on nociception at the highest levels.

In the cat consistent naloxone-reversible effects of morphine administered ionophoretically near neurones of the somatosensory cerebral cortex have not been observed (BIOULAC et al. 1975). In the somatosensory cortex of the rat, neurones were predominently inhibited by ionophoretic morphine, an effect that was blocked by naloxone (SATOH et al. 1974). Inhibition has been the predominant effect when enkephalins have been administered near neurones of several areas of the cerebral cortex of the rat (FREDERICKSON and NORRIS 1976; ZIEGLGANSBERGER et al. 1976; PALMER et al. 1978; STREJCKOVA et al. 1985). Intracellular recordings from neurones of rat cortical slices have shown a depression by DADL of depolarization by L-glutamate with no effect on membrane potential (SUTOR and ZIEGLGANSBERGER 1984). In these experiments the effects of dynorphin$_{1-17}$ were very variable. There appears to be no systematic study of the effects of ligands, having high specificity for different opiate receptors, on neurones of the cerebral cortex. It needs to be noted that the many opioids with affinity for κ-receptors have been shown to antagonize excitation by N-methyl-D-aspartate (LODGE et al. 1984). This activity, however, relates better to the binding to sigma sites which these compounds show.

D. Deficits in Knowledge and Prospects for Future Research

To the present reviewers it appears that considerable progress has been made on the first question which we have addressed: how opiate drugs attenuate the perception of pain. Experiments both in the spinal cord and at supraspinal sites indicate that there is a reduction in the transmitted nociceptive message to the brain. It appears that a significant component of morphine analgesia is mediated by activity at μ-opioid receptors in the superficial dorsal horn of the spinal cord. The relative importance of effects on intrinsic neurones of this area, on the central terminals of peripheral nociceptors and on the spinal terminations of supraspinal fibres requires further experimentation.

When comparing the present account with a prior review (DUGGAN and NORTH 1984) it is evident that, while much has been learnt on the consequences of activation of differing opioid receptors in the dorsal horn of the spinal cord, progress in defining the physiological roles of opioid peptides in sensory processing both in the spinal cord and at supraspinal sites has been slow. Indeed in no case is it possible to describe an opioidergic event completely, i.e. what opioid peptide(s) is (are) released by a particular stimulus, what receptors are activated, the neurones bearing the receptors and the functional consequences for sensory processing.

It is as yet unclear which opioid receptor types mediate endogenous actions of opioids released under physiological or experimental conditions, such as stimulation-produced analgesia. Further experiments using newer antagonists with increased pharmacological specificity are required to resolve this question. Much research has examined opioid peptides from the viewpoint of the physiology of receptor types. Under physiological conditions, however, this approach may not represent the real situation. Indeed one of the more puzzling aspects of opioid peptides is the poor receptor selectivity of the endogenous compounds known to be synthesised and suspected of being released. A range of endogenous opioids resulting from the processing of preproenkephalin and preprodynorphin precursors with differing profiles of receptor selectivity are found in the dorsal horn, particularly in the marginal zone and substantia gelatinosa. It is further possible that the enzymatic cleavage patterns occurring in particular cells may differ, so as to provide releasable opioids with somewhat different profiles of activity.

The preproenkephalin products include [Met^5]enkephalin and [Leu^5]enkephalin (both with greater activity at δ- than for μ-sites and little activity at κ-sites; KOSTERLITZ et al. 1985) and also metorphamide, which despite being present only at quite low levels in spinal cord (ZAMIR et al. 1985) is interesting in being a μ/κ-selective agonist (KOSTERLITZ et al. 1985). The pre-prodynorphin derived dynorphins and neo-endorphins [with a range of modest selectivities for κ-sites (KOSTERLITZ et al. 1985)] are also found in the dorsal horn (AKIL, this volume; GOLDSTEIN et al. 1981; FISCHLI et al. 1982; MINAMINO et al. 1981; KANGAWA et al. 1981). It is far from clear that any of these endogenous ligands would act truly selectively in situ, but rather a number of systems may be influenced by the action of individual peptides. It is clear that whilst receptor sites for μ-, δ- and κ-ligands are present in dorsal horn, they are only likely to be of physiological importance if they can be accessed by appropriate agonists. Many of the endogenous opioid peptides are less specific for particular receptors than some of the synthetic analogues now available and it is feasible that the local distribution of receptor sites will determine the predominant action of an opioid. Hypothetically, a somewhat δ-preferring agonist such as [Leu^5]enkephalin could have a μ-mediated action, if only those sites were available to it, and it reached high enough synaptic concentrations. Conversely, even a relatively selective opioid could activate several accessible receptor types to differing degrees, depending on the local receptor distribution. A regulatory physiological system could thus function adequately with marginally selective agonists and thus there is no need to postulate the existence of undiscovered wholly specific agonists for each receptor type.

This brief description highlights what we believe to be one of the most important areas for future research into opioids and sensory processing: the definition of which endogenous compounds are released and which receptors they act upon and what neural structure bear these receptors. The neurophysiological experiments described here provide a neural basis for the pharmacological observations that μ-, δ-, and κ-opioids exert distinct antinociceptive actions particularly at a spinal level. The exact means by which opioids exert their cellular actions (see Chap. 30) and how these actions interact with the controls of transmission of other sensory information are issues that will lead to a more complete understanding of the role of opioids in sensory processing.

Acknowledgements. The preparation of this manuscript owes much to the assistance of A. STIRLING-WHYTE and C. WARWICK. Many colleagues sent reprints and manuscripts for which we are grateful. Our research is supported by the Wellcome Trust and the Medical Research Council.

References

Advokat C (1988) The role of descending inhibition in morphine-induced analgesia. Trends Pharmacol Sci 9:330–334

Aghajanian GK (1978) Tolerance of locus coeruleus neurones to morphine and suppression of withdrawal response by clonidine. Nature 276:186–188

Albe-Fessard D, Kruger L (1962) Duality of unit discharges from cat centrum medianum in response to natural and electrical stimulation. J Neurophysiol 25:3–20

Allerton CA, Smith JAM, Hunter JC, Hill RG, Hughes J (1989) Correlation of ontogeny with function of [^{3}H]U69593 labelled κ opioid binding sites in the rat spinal cord. Brain Res 502:149–157

Attali B, Gouarderes C, Mazarguil H, Audigier Y, Cros J (1982) Evidence for multiple "kappa" binding sites by use of opioid peptides in the guinea-pig lumbo-sacral spinal cord. Neuropeptides 3:53–64

Atweh SF, Kuhar ML (1977) Autoradiographic localization of opiate receptors in rat brain: I. Spinal cord and lower medulla. Brain Res 124:53–67

Baldissera F, Hultborn H, Illert M (1981) Integration in spinal neuronal systems. In: Brooks VB (ed) Handbook of physiology, vol 2: I. Nervous system, motor control, part I. American Physiological Society, Bethesda, pp 509–595

Bell JA, Martin WR (1977) The effect of the narcotic antagonists naloxone, naltrexone and nalorphine on spinal cord C-fiber reflexes evoked by electrical stimulation or radiant heat. Eur J Pharmacol 42:147–154

Bennett GJ, Mayer DJ (1979) Inhibition of spinal cord interneurons by narcotic microinjection and focal electrical stimulation in the periaqueductal central gray matter. Brain Res 172:243–258

Benoist JM, Kayser V, Gautron M, Guilbaud G (1983) Low dose of morphine strongly depresses responses of specific nociceptive neurons in the ventrobasal complex of the rat. Pain 15:333–344

Benoist JM, Kayser V, Gacel G, Zajac JM, Gautron M, Roques B, Guilbaud G (1986) Differential depressive action of two μ and δ opioid ligands on neuronal responses to noxious stimuli in the thalamic ventrobasal complex of rat. Brain Res 398:49–56

Bernatzky G, Doi T, Jurna K (1983) Effects of intrathecally administered pentobarbital and naloxone on the activity evoked in ascending axons of the rat spinal cord by stimulation of afferent A and C fibres. Further evidence for a tonic endorphinergic inhibition in nociception. Naunyn Schmiedebergs Arch Pharmacol 323:211–216

Besson JM, Chaouch A (1987) Peripheral and spinal mechanisms of nociception. Physiol Rev 67:67–186

Besson JM, Wyon-Maillard MC, Benoist C, Conseiller C, Hammann KF (1973) Effects of phenoperidine on lamina V cells in the cat dorsal horn. J Pharmacol Exp Ther 187:239–245

Bessou P, Perl ER (1969) Responses of cutaneous sensory units with unmeylinated fibres to noxious stimuli. J Neurophysiol 32:1025–1043

Bioulac B, Lund JP, Puil E (1975) Morphine excitation in the cerebral cortex. Can J Physiol Pharmacol 53:683–687

Biscoe TJ, Duggan AW, Lodge D (1972) Effect of etorphine, morphine and diprenorphine on neurones of the cerebral cortex and spinal cord of the rat. Br J Pharmacol 46:201–212

Boivie J (1979) An anatomical reinvestigation of the termination of the spinothalamic tract in the monkey. J Comp Neurol 186:343–370

Bouhassira D, Villanueva L, Le Bars D (1988) Intracerebroventricular morphine decreases descending inhibitions acting on lumbar dorsal horn neuronal activities related to pain in the rat. J Pharmacol Exp Ther 247/1:332–342

Bowsher D (1957) Termination of the central pathway in man: the conscious appreciation of pain. Brain 80:606–622

Brodin E, Linderoth B,Gazelius B, Ungerstedt U (1987) In vivo release of substance P in cat dorsal horn studied with microdialysis. Neurosci Lett 76:357–362

Bromm B (1985) Evoked cerebral potential and pain. In: Fields HL et al. (eds) Advances in pain research and therapy, vol 9. Raven, New York, pp 305–329

Buchsbaum MS, Davis GC, Bunney WE Jr (1977) Naloxone alters pain perception and somatosensory evoked potentials in normal subjects. Nature 270:620–622

Burke RE (1985) Integration of sensory information and motor commands in the spinal cord. In: Stein PSG (ed) Motor control: from movement trajectories to neural mechanisms. Society for Neuroscience, Bethesda, pp 44–66

Cahen RL, Wikler A (1944) Effects of morphine on cortical electrical activity of the rat. Yale J Biol Med 16:240–243

Calvillo O, Henry JL, Neuman RS (1974) Effects of morphine and naloxone on dorsal horn neurones in the cat. Can J Physiol Pharmacol 52:1207–1211

Calvillo O, Henry JL, Neuman RS (1979) Actions of narcotic analgesics and antagonists on spinal units responding to natural stimulation in the cat. Can J Physiol Pharmacol 51:652–663

Carlsson K-H, Monzel W, Jurna I (1988) Depression by morphine and the non-opioid analgesic agents, metamizol (dipyrone), lysine acetylsalicylate and paracetamol, of activity in rat thalamus neurones evoked by electrical stimulation of nociceptive afferents. Pain 32:313–326

Carstens E, Klumpp D, Zimmermann M (1979a) The opiate antagonist naloxone does not affect descending inhibition from midbrain of nociceptive spinal neuronal discharges in the cat. Neurosci Lett 11:323–327

Carstens E, Tulloch I, Zieglgansberger W, Zimmermann M (1979b) Presynaptic excitability changes induced by morphine in single cutaneous afferent C and A fibres. Pflugers Archiv Ges Physiol 379:143–147

Carstens E, Gilly H, Schreiber H, Zimmermann M (1987) Effects of midbrain stimulation and iontophoretic application of serotonin, noradrenaline, morphine and GABA on electrical thresholds of afferent C- and A-fibre terminals in cat spinal cord. Neuroscience 21:395–406

Cervero F (1985) Visceral nociception: peripheral and central aspects of visceral nociceptive systems. Philos Trans R Soc Lond [Biol] 308:325–337

Cesselin F, Bourgoin S, Clot AM, Hamon M, Le Bars D (1989) Segmental release of Met-enkephalin-like material from the spinal cord of rats, elicited by noxious thermal stimuli. Brain Res 484:71–77

Chin JH, Domino EF (1961) Effects of morphine on brain potentials evoked by stimulation of the tooth pulp of the dog. J Pharmacol Exp Ther 132:74–86

Clark JA, Liu L, Price M, Hersh B, Edelson M, Pasternak GW (1989) Kappa opiate receptor multiplicity: evidence for two U50,488-sensitive κ_1 subtypes and a novel κ_3 subtype. J Pharmacol Exp Ther 251:461–468

Clarke RW, Ford TW (1987) The contributions of μ, δ, and κ-opioid receptors to the actions of endogenous opioids on spinal reflexes in the rabbit. Br J Pharmacol 91:579–589

Clarke RW, Ford TW, Taylor JS (1989) Activation by high intensity peripheral nerve stimulation of adrenergic and opioidergic inhibition of a spinal reflex in the decerebrated rabbit. Brain Res 505:1–6

Cook L, Bonnycastle DD (1953) An examination of some spinal and ganglionic actions of analgesic materials. J Pharmacol Exp Ther 109:35–44

Cotton R, Giles MG, Miller L, Shaw JS, Timms D (1984) ICI 174864. A highly selective antagonist at the opioid delta receptor. Eur J Pharmacol 97:331–332

Craig AD Jr, Burton H (1981) Spinal and medullary lamina I projection to nucleus submedius in medial thalamus: a possible pain center. J Neurophysiol 45:443–466

Craig AD, Mense S (1983) The distribution of fine afferent fibers from the gastrocnemius soleus muscle in the dorsal horn of the cat as revealed by transport of horseradish peroxidase. Neurosci Lett 41:233–238

Craig AD, Heppelmann, Schaible H-G (1988) The projection of the medial and posterior articular nerves of the cat's knee to the spinal cord. J Comp Neurol 276:279–288

Curtis DR, Bornstein JC, Lodge D (1980) In vivo analysis of GABA receptors on primary afferent terminations in the cat. Brain Res 194:255–258

Dashwood MR, Dickenson AH, Knox R, Roques BP, Sullivan AF (1986) Mu and delta opiate receptors: location and influences on nociceptive transmission in the rat spinal cord. J Physiol (Lond) 376:57P

Davies J, Dray A (1978) Pharmacological and electrophysiological studies of morphine and enkephalin on rat supraspinal neurones and cat spinal neurones. Br J Pharmacol 63:87–96

Dickenson AH, Le Bars D (1987a) Supraspinal morphine and descending inhibitions acting on the dorsal horn of the rat. J Physiol 384:81–107

Dickenson AH, Le Bars D (1987b) Lack of evidence for increased descending inhibition on the dorsal horn of the rat following periaqueductal grey morphine injections. Br J Pharmacol 92:271–280

Dickenson AH, Sullivan AF, Knox R, Zajac J, Roques BP (1987) Opioid receptor subtypes in the rat spinal cord: electrophysiological studies with μ- and δ-opioid receptor agonists in the control of nociception. Brain Res 413:36–44

Dimpfel W, Spuler M, Nickel B (1989) Dose- and time-dependent action of morphine, tramadol and flupirtine as studied by radioelectroencephalography in the freely behaving rat. Neuropsychobiology 20:164–168

Dostrovsky JO, Pomeranz B (1976) Interaction of iontophoretically applied morphine with responses of interneurones in cat spinal cord. Exp Neurol 52:325–338

Du H-J, Kitahata LM, Thalhammer JG, Zimmermann M (1984) Inhibition of nociceptive neuronal responses in the cat's spinal dorsal horn by electrical stimulation and morphine microinjection in nucleus raphe magnus. Pain 19: 249–257

Duggan AW, Curtis DR (1972) Morphine and the synaptic activation of Renshaw cells. Neuropharmacology 11:189–196

Duggan AW, Griersmith BT (1979a) Methylxanthine, adenosine 3′,5′-cyclic monophosphate and the spinal transmission of nociceptive information. Br J Pharmacol 67:51–57

Duggan AW, Griersmith BT (1979b) Inhibition of the spinal transmission of nociceptive information by supraspinal stimulation in the cat. Pain 6:149–161

Duggan AW, Hall JG (1977) Morphine, naloxone and the responses of medial thalamic neurones of the cat. Brain Res 122:49–57

Duggan AW, Morton CR (1988) Tonic descending inhibition and spinal nociceptive transmission. In: Fields HL, Besson J-M (eds) Progress in brain research, vol 77. Elsevier, Amsterdam, pp 193–207

Duggan AW, North RA (1984) Electrophysiology of opioids. Pharmacol Rev 35:219–281

Duggan AW, Weihe E (1990) Central transmission of impulses in nociceptors: events in the superficial dorsal horn. In: Basbaum AI, Besson J-M (eds) Towards a new pharmacotherapy of pain. Wiley, New York, pp 35–68

Duggan AW, Davies J, Hall JG (1976a) Effects of opiate agonists and antagonists on central neurons of the cat. J Pharmacol Exp Ther 196:107–120

Duggan AW, Hall JG, Headley PM (1976b) Morphine, enkephalin and the substantia gelatinosa. Nature 264:456–458

Duggan AW, Hall JG, Headley PM (1977a) Suppression of transmission of nociceptive impulses by morphine: selective effects of morphine administered in the region of the substantia gelatinosa. Br J Pharmacol 61:65–76

Duggan AW, Hall JG, Headley PM (1977b) Enkephalins and dorsal horn neurones of the cat: effects on responses to noxious and innocuous skin stimuli. Br J Pharmacol 61:399–408

Duggan AW, Hall JG, Headley PM, Griersmith BT (1977c) The effect of naloxone on the excitation of dorsal horn of the cat by noxious and non-noxious cutaneous stimuli. Brain Res 138:185–189

Duggan AW, Griersmith BT, North RA (1980) Morphine and surpaspinal inhibition of neurones: evidence that morphine decreases tonic descending inhibition in the anaesthetized cat. Br J Pharmacol 69:461–466

Duggan AW, Johnson SM, Morton CR (1981) Differing distributions of receptors for morphine and Met[5]-enkephalinamide in the dorsal horn of the cat. Brain Res 229:379–387

Duggan AW, Morton CR, Johnson SM, Zhao ZQ (1984) Opioid antagonists and spinal reflexes in the anaesthetized cat. Brain Res 297:33–40

Duggan AW, Hall JG, Foong FW, Zhao ZQ (1985) A differential effect of naloxone on transmission of impulses in primary afferents to ventral roots and ascending spinal tracts. Brain Res 344:316–321

Duggan AW, Hendry IA, Morton CR, Hutchison WD, Zhao ZQ (1988) Cutaneous stimuli releasing immunoreactive substance P in the dorsal horn of the cat. Brain Res 451:261–273

Einspahr FJ, Piercey MF (1980) Morphine depresses dorsal horn neuron responses to controlled noxious and non-noxious cutaneous stimulation. J Pharmacol Exp Ther 213:456–461

Fields HL, Emson PC, Leigh BK, Gilbert RFT, Iversen LL (1980) Multiple opiate receptor sites on primary afferent fibres. Nature 284:351–353

Fischli W, Goldstein A, Hunkapiller MW, Hood LE (1982) Isolation and amino acid sequence analysis of 4,000-dalton dynorphin from porcine pituitary. Proc Natl Acad Sci USA 79:5435–5437

Fitzgerald M, Woolf CJ (1980) The stereospecific effect of naloxone on rat dorsal horn neurones: inhibition in superficial laminae and excitation in deeper laminae. Pain 9:293–306

Fleetwood-Walker SM, Hope PJ, Mitchell R, Molony V (1987) Is there an inter-
    action between opioid and noradrenergic antinociceptive mechanisms in dorsal
    horn? Neurosci. Lett [Suppl] 29:S41
Fleetwood-Walker SM, Hope PJ, Mitchell R, El-Yassir N, Molony V (1988) The
    influence of opioid receptor subtypes on the processing of nociceptive inputs in
    the spinal dorsal horn of the cat. Brain Res 451:213–226
Frederickson RCA, Norris FH (1976) Enkephalin-induced depression of single
    neurons in brain areas with opiate receptors – antagonism by naloxone. Science
    194:440–442
Gebhart GF, Sandkuhler J, Thalhammer JG, Zimmermann M (1984) Inhibition in
    spinal cord of nociceptive information by electrical stimulation and morphine
    microinjection at identical sites in midbrain of the cat. J Neurophysiol 51:75–89
Go VLW, Yaksh TL (1987) Release of substance P from the cat spinal cord. J
    Physiol (Lond) 391:141–167
Goldfarb J, Hu TW (1976) Enhancement of reflexes by naloxone in spinal cats.
    Neuropharmacology 15:785–792
Goldstein A, Fischli W, Lowney LI, Hunkapiller M, Hood L (1981) Porcine
    pituitary dynorphin: complete amino acid sequence of the biologically active
    heptadecapeptide. Proc Natl Acad Sci USA 78:7219–7223
Gouarderes C, Cros J, Quirion R (1985) Autoradiographic localisation of μ, δ and κ
    opioid receptor binding sites in rat and guinea pig spinal cord. Neuropeptides
    6:331–342
Gouarderes C, Kopp N, Cros J, Quirion R (1986) Kappa opioid receptors in human
    lumbo-sacral spinal cord. Brain Res Bull 16:355–361
Guilbaud G (1985) Thalamic nociceptive systems. Philos Trans R Soc Lond [Biol]
    308/1136:339–345
Hall MD, Smith JAM, Hunter JC, Hill RG, Hughes J (1987) Evidence for kappa
    opioid receptor sub-types in the guinea-pig cortex. Soc Neurosci Abstr 13:136
Handwerker HO, Iggo A, Zimmermann M (1975) Segmental and supraspinal actions
    on dorsal horn neurones responding to noxious and non-noxious skin stimuli.
    Pain 1:147–165
Harris NC, Ryall RW (1988) Opiates distinguish spinal excitation from inhibition
    evoked by noxious heat stimuli in the rat: relevance to theories of analgesia. Br
    J Pharmacol 94:185–191
Headley PM, Duggan AW, Griersmith BT (1978) Selective reduction by
    noradrenaline and 5-hydroxytryptamine of nociceptive responses of cat dorsal
    horn neurones. Brain Res 145:185–189
Headley PM, Parsons CG, West DC (1987) Opioid receptor-mediated effects on
    spinal responses to controlled noxious natural peripheral stimuli: technical
    considerations. In: Schmidt RF, Schaible H-G, Vahle-Hinz C (eds) Fine afferent
    nerve fibres and pain. VCH, Weinheim, pp 227–235
Henry JL (1979) Naloxone excites nociceptive units in the lumbar dorsal horn of the
    spinal cat. Neuroscience 4:1485–1491
Henry JL (1981) Diurnal variation in excitation of dorsal horn units by naloxone in
    the spinal cat suggests a circulating opioid factor. Neuroscience 6:1935–1942
Hill RG, Pepper CM (1978) The depression of thalamic nociceptive neurones by D-
    Ala^2,D-leu^5-enkephalin. Eur J Pharmacol 47:223–225
Hill RG, Salt TE, Pepper CM (1982) A comparison of the effectiveness of intra-
    venous morphine at attenuating the nociceptive responses of medullary dorsal
    horn and thalamic neurones. Life Sci 33:2331–2334
Hope PJ, Fleetwood-Walker SM, Mitchell R (1990) Distinct antinociceptive actions
    mediated by different opioid receptors in the region of lamina I and laminae
    III–V of the dorsal horn of the rat. Br J Pharmacol 101:477–483
Hunter JC, Birchmore B, Woodruff R, Hughes J (1989) Kappa opioid binding sites
    in the dog cerebral cortex and spinal cord. Neuroscience 31/3:735–743
Hutchison WD, Morton CR, Terenius L (1990) Dynorphin A: in vivo release in the
    spinal cord of the cat. Brain Res 532:299–306

Hylden JLK, Nahin RL, Traub RJ, Dubner R (1990) Effects of spinal kappa-opioid agonists on the responsiveness of nociceptive superficial dorsal horn neurons. Pain 44:187–193

Iadarola MJ, Tang J, Costa E, Yang H-YT (1986) Analgesic activity and release of [met^5]enkephalin-arg^6-gly^7-leu^8 from rat spinal cord in vivo. Eur J Pharmacol 121:39–48

Iggo A, Steedman WM, Fleetwood-Walker SM (1985) Spinal processing: anatomy and physiology of spinal nociceptive mechanisms. Philos Trans R Soc Lond [Biol] 308:235–252

Iwata M, Sakai Y (1971) The effects of fentanyl upon the spinal interneurones activated by Aα afferent fibres of the cutaneous nerve of the cat. Jpn J Pharmacol 21:413–416

Jeftinija S (1988) Enkephalins modulate excitatory synaptic transmission in the superficial dorsal horn by acting at mu-opioid receptor sites. Brain Res 460:260–268

Jessell TM, Iversen LL (1977) Opiate analgesics inhibit substance P release from rat trigeminal nucleus. Nature 268:549–551

Jones SL, Gebhart GF (1988) Inhibition of spinal nociceptive transmission from the midbrain, pons and medulla in the rat: activation of descending inhibition by morphine, glutamate and electrical stimulation. Brain Res 460:281–296

Jurna I (1966) Inhibition of the effect of repetitive stimulation on spinal motoneurones of the cat by morphine and pethidine. Int J Neuropharmacol 5:117–123

Jurna I (1980) Effect of stimulation in the periaqueductal grey matter on activity in ascending axons of the rat spinal cord: selective inhibition of activity evoked by afferent Aα and C fibre stimulation and failure of naloxone to reduce inhibition. Brain Res 196:33–42

Jurna I (1984) Cyclic nucleotides and aminophyline produce different effects on nociceptive motor and sensory responses in the rat spinal cord. Naunyn Schmiedebergs Arch Pharmacol 327:23–30

Jurna I (1988) Dose-dependent inhibition by naloxone of nociceptive activity evoked in the rat thalamus. Pain 35:349–354

Jurna I, Grossman W (1976) The effect of morphine on the activity evoked in ventrolateral tract axons of the cat spinal cord. Exp Brain Res 24:473–484

Jurna I, Heinz G (1979) Differential effects of morphine and opioid analgesics on A and C fibre-evoked activity in ascending axons of the rat spinal cord. Brain Res 171:573–576

Jurna I, Schafer H (1965) Depression of post tetanic potentiation in the spinal cord by morphine and pethidine. Experientia 21:226–227

Jurna I, Schlue WR, Tamm U (1972) The effect of morphine on primary somatosensory evoked respones in the rat cerebral cortex. Neuropharmacology 11:409–415

Kaelber WW, Mitchell CL, Yormat AJ, Afifi AK, Lorens SA (1975) Centrum medianum-parafascicularis lesions and reactivity to noxious and non-noxious stimuli. Exp Neurol 46:282–290

Kangawa K, Minamino N, Chino N, Sakakibara S, Matsuo H (1981) The complete amino acid sequence of alpha-neo-endorphin. Biochem Biophys Res Commun 99:871–878

Kayser V, Guilbaud G (1984) Further evidence or changes in the responsiveness of somatosensory neurones in arthritic rats: a study of the posterior intralaminar region of the thalamus. Brain Res 323:144–147

Kayser V, Benoist JM, Neil A, Gautron M, Guilbaud G (1988) Behavioural and electrophysiological studies on the paradoxical antinociceptive effects of an extremely low dose of naloxone in an animal model of acute and localized inflammation. Exp Brain Res 73:402–410

Khachaturian H, Lewis ME, Schafer MKH, Watson SJ (1985) Anatomy of the CNS opioid systems. Trends Neurosci 8:111–119

Kitahata LM, Kosaka Y, Taub A, Bonikos K, Hoffert M (1974) Lamina-specific suppression of dorsal horn unit activity by morphine sulfate. Anesthesiology 41:39–48

Knox RJ, Dickenson AH (1987) Effects of selective and non-selective κ-opioid receptor agonists on cutaneous C-fibre-evoked responses of rat dorsal horn neurones. Brain Res 415:21–29

Koll W, Haase J, Block G, Muhlberg B (1963) The predilective section of small doses of morphine on nociceptive spinal reflexes of low spinal cats. Int J Neuropharmacol 2:57–65

Kosterlitz HW, Corbett AD, Gillan MGC, McKnight AT, Paterson SJ, Robson LE (1985) Recent developments in the bioassy of opioids. Regul Pept [Suppl] 4:1–7

Krivoy W, Kroeger D, Zimmermann E (1973) Actions of morphine on the segmental reflex of the decerebrate spinal cat. Br J Pharmacol 47:457–464

Kruglov NA (1964) Effect of morphine group analgesics on the central inhibitory mechanisms. Int J Neuropharmacol 3:197–203

Kuraishi Y, Hirota N, Sugimoto M, Satoh M, Takagi H (1983) Effects of morphine on noxious stimuli-induced release of substance P from rabbit dorsal horn in vivo. Life Sci 33 (Suppl 1):693–696

Kuraishi Y, Hirota N, Sato Y, Hanashima N, Takagi H, Satoh M (1989) Stimulus specificity of peripherally evoked substance P release from the rabbit dorsal horn in situ. Neuroscience 30:241–250

Le Bars D, Menetrey D, Besson JM (1976a) Effects of morphine upon the lamina V type cells activities in the dorsal horn of the decerebrate cat. Brain Res 113: 293–310

Le Bars D, Guilbaud G, Jurna I, Besson JM (1976b) Differential effects of morphine on responses of dorsal horn lamina V type cells elicited by A and C fibre stimulation in the spinal cat. Brain Res 115:518–524

Le Bars D, Dickenson AH, Besson JM (1979) Diffuse noxious inhibitory controls (DNIC). Lack of effect on non-convergent neurones, supraspinal involvement and theoretical implications. Pain 6:305–327

Le Bars D, Dickenson AH, Besson JM (1980) Microinjection of morphine within nucleus raphe magnus and dorsal horn neurone activities related to nociception in the rat. Brain Res 189:467–481

Le Bars D, Chitour D, Kraus E, Dickenson AH, Besson JM (1981) Effect of naloxone upon diffuse noxious inhibitory controls (DNIC) in the rat. Brain Res 204:387–402

Le Bars D, Bourgoin S, Clot AM, Hamon M, Cesselin F (1987) Noxious mechnical stimuli increase the release of Met-enkephalin-like material heterosegmentally in the rat spinal cord. Brain Res 402:188–192

Light AR, Perl ER (1977) Differential termination of large diameter and small diameter primary afferent fibres in the spinal dorsal gray matter as indicated by labelling with horseradish peroxidase. Neurosci Lett 6:59–63

Lodge D, Berry SC, Church J, Martin D, McGhee A, Lai H-M, Thomson AM (1984) Isomers of cyclazine as excitatory amino acid antagonists. Neuropeptides 15:245–248

Lund RD, Webster KE (1967) Thalamic afferents from the spinal cord and trigeminal nuclei. J Comp Neurol 130:313–328

Lundberg A (1982) Inhibitory control from the brain stem of transmission from primary afferents to motoneurones, primary afferent terminals and ascending pathways. In: Sjolund B, Bjorklund (eds) Brain stem control of spinal mechanisms. Elsevier, Amsterdam, pp 179–224

Mansour A, Khachaturian H, Lewis ME, Akil H, Watson SJ (1987) Auto-radiographic differentiation of μ, δ and κ opioid receptors in the rat forebrain and midbrain. J Neurosci 7:2445–2464

Mansour A, Lewis ME, Khachaturian H, Akil H, Watson SJ (1986) Pharmacological and anatomical evidence of selective μ, δ and κ opioid receptor binding in rat brain. Brain Res 399:69–79

Mansour A, Khachaturian H, Lewis ME, Akil H, Watson SJ (1988) Anatomy of CNS opioid receptors. Trends Neurosci 11:308–314

Martin WR, Eades CG, Fraser HF, Wikler A (1964) Use of hindlimb reflexes of the chronic spinal dog for comparing analgesics. J Pharmacol Exp Ther 144:8–11

Martin WR, Eades CG, Thompson JA, Huppler RE, Gilbert PE (1976) The effects of morphine and nalorphine-like drugs in the non-dependent and morphine-dependent chronic spinal dog. J Pharmacol Exp Ther 197:517–532

Mauborgne A, Lutz O, Legrand JC, Hamon M, Cesselin F (1987) Opposite effects of μ and δ opioid receptor agonists on the in vitro release of substance P-like material from the rat spinal cord. J Neurochem 48:529–537

McClane TK, Martin WR (1967) Effects of morphine, nalorphine, cyclazocine and naloxone on the flexor reflex. Int J Neuropharmacol 6:89–98

McFadzean I (1988) The ionic mechanisms underlying opioid actions. Neuropeptides 11/4:173–180

Melzack R, Wall PD (1965) Pain mechanisms: a new theory. Science 150:971–979

Millan MJ (1987) Multiple opioid systems and pain. Pain 27:303–347

Minamino N, Kangawa K, Chino N, Sakakibara S, Matsuo H (1981) Beta-neo-endorphin, a new hypothalamic "big" leu-enkephalin of porcine origin: its purification and the complete amino acid sequence. Biochem Biophys Res Commun 99:864–870

Morris BR, Herz A (1987) Distinct distribution of opioid receptor types in rat lumbar spinal cord. Naunyn Schmiedebergs Arch Pharmacol 336:240–243

Morris R, Cahusac PMB, Hill RG (1984) The effects of microiontophoretically-applied opioids and opiate antagonists on nociceptive responses of neurones of the caudal reticular formation in the rat. Neuropharmacology 23/5:497–504

Morton CD, Hutchison WD, Duggan AW, Hendry IA (1990) Morphine and substance P release in the spinal cord. Exp Brain Res 82:89–96

Morton CR, Zhao ZQ, Duggan AW (1982) A function of opioid peptides in the spinal cord of the cat: intracellular studies of motoneurones during naloxone administration. Neuropeptides 3:83–90

Moyano RS, Kayser D, Grall Y, Hernandez A, Ruiz S, Paeille C (1975) Effect of pentazocine on the evoked potentials recorded in the primary somesthetic cortical ares of guinea pigs. Brain Res 88:475–481

Murase K, Nedeljkov TV, Randic M (1982) The actions of neuropeptides on dorsal horn neurons in the rat spinal cord preparation: an intracellular study. Brain Res 234:170–176

Nakahama H, Shima K, Aya K, Kisara K, Skaurada S (1981) Antinociceptive action of morphine and pentazocine on unit activity in the nucleus centralis lateralis, nucleus ventralis lateralis and nearby structures of the cat. Pain 10:47–56

Navarro G, Elliott HW (1971) The effects of morphine, morphinine and thebaine on the EEG and behaviour of rabbits and cats. Neuropharmacology 10:367–377

Nyberg F, Yaksh TL, Terenius L (1983) Opioid activity released from cat spinal cord by sciatic nerve stimulation. Life Sci 33(Suppl 1):17–20

Palmer MR, Morris DH, Taylor DA, Stewart JM, Hoffer BJ (1978) Electro-physiological effects of enkephalin analogs in rat cortex. Life Sci 23:851–860

Parsons CG, Headley PM (1988) What doses of intravenous naloxone differentiate between mu and kappa opioid effects on spinal nociceptive reflexes in the rat? Adv Biosci 75:471–474

Parsons CG, Headley PM (1989) On the selectivity of intravenous mu- and kappa-opioids between nociceptive and non-nociceptive reflexes in the spinalized rat. Br J Pharmacol 98:544–551

Pasternak CW, Wood PJ (1986) Multiple mu opiate receptors. Life Sci 38:1889–1898

Pert CB, Kuhar MJ, Snyder SH (1975) Autoradiographic localization of the opiate receptor in rat brain. Life Sci 16:1849–1854

Pohl M, Mauborgne A, Bourgoin S, Benoliel JJ, Hamon M, Cesselin F (1989) Neonatal capsaicin treatment abolishes the modulations by opioids of substance P release from rat spinal cord slices. Neurosci Lett 96:102–107

Portoghese PS, Lipkowski AW, Takemori AE (1987) Binaltorphimine and nor-binaltorphimine, potent and selective κ-opioid receptor antagonists. Life Sci 40:1287–1292

Prieto-Gomez B, Dafny N, Reyes-Vazquez C (1989) Dorsal raphe stimulation, 5-HT and morphine microiontophoresis effects on noxious and non noxious identified neurons in the medial thalamus of the rat. Brain Res Bull 22:937–943

Przewlocki R, Shearman GT, Herz A (1983) Mixed opioid/non-opioid effects of dynorphin and dynorphin related peptides after their intrathecal injection in rats. Neuropeptides 3:233–240

Quirion R, Pilapil C, Magnan J (1987) Localisation of κ opioid receptor binding sites in human forebrain using [³H]U69593: comparison with [³H]bremazocine. Cell Mol Biol 7:303–307

Randic M, Miletic V (1978) Depressant actions of methionine-enkephalin and somatostatin in cat dorsal horn neurones activated by noxious stimuli. Brain Res 152:196–202

Reyes-Vazquez C, Dafny N (1982) Response characteristics of thalamic neurons to microiontophoretically applied morphine. Neuropharmacology 21:733–738

Reyes-Vazquez C, Qiao J-T, Dafny N (1989) Nociceptive responses in nucleus parafascicularis thalami are modulated by dorsal raphe stimulation and microiontophoretic application of morphine and serotonin. Brain Res Bull 23:405–411

Rivot JP, Chaouch A, Besson JM (1979) The influence of naloxone on the C fiber response of dorsal horn neurons and their inhibitory control by raphe magnus stimulation. Brain Res 176:355–364

Rodriguez RE, Leighton G, Hill RG, Hughes J (1986) In vivo evidence for spinal delta opiate receptor operated antinociception. Neuropeptides 8:221–241

Rothenburg S, Peck EA, Schottenfeld S, Betley GE, Altman JL (1979) Methadone depression of visual signal detection performance. Pharmacol Biochem Behav 11:521–527

Sastry BR (1978) Morphine and met-enkephalin effects of sural Aδ afferent terminal excitability. Eur J Pharmacol 50:269–276

Sastry BR (1979) Presynaptic effects of morphine and methionine enkephalin in feline spinal cord. Neuropharmacology 18:367–375

Sastry BR (1980) Potentiation of presynaptic inhibition of nociceptive pathways as a mechanism for analgesia. Can J Physiol Pharmacol 58:97–100

Sastry BR, Goh JW (1983) Actions of morphine and met-enkepalinamide on nociceptor drive neurones in substantia gelatinosa and deeper dorsal horn. Neuropharmacology 22:119–122

Satoh M, Zieglgansberger W, Fries W, Herz A (1974) Opiate agonist-antagonist interaction at cortical neurones of naive and tolerant dependent rats. Brain Res 82:378–382

Satoh M, Kawajiri S-I, Ukai Y, Yamamoto M (1979) Selective and non-selective inhibition by enkephalins and noradrenaline of nociceptive response of lamina V type neurons in the spinal dorsal horn of the rabbit. Brain Res 177:384–387

Schmauss C, Herz A (1987) Intrathecally-administered dynorphin(1–17) modulates morphine-induced antinociception differently in morphine-naive and morphine-tolerant rats. Eur J Pharmacol 135:429–431

Schmauss C, Yaksh TL (1984) In vivo studies on spinal opiate receptor systems mediating antinociception: II. Pharmacological profiles suggesting a differential association of mu, delta and kappa receptors with visceral, chemical and cutaneous thermal stimuli in the rat. J Pharmacol Exp Ther 228:1–12

Schomburg ED (1990) Spinal sensorimotor systems and their supraspinal control. Neurosci Res 7:265–340

Shen K, Crain SM (1989) Dual opioid modulation of the action potential duration of mouse dorsal root ganglion neurons in culture. Brain Res 491:227–242

Sinclair JG, Fox RE, Mokha SS, Iggo A (1980) The effect of naloxone on the inhibition of nociceptor driven neurones in the cat spinal cord. QJ Exp Physiol 65:181–188

Sinitsin LN (1964) Effect of morphine and other analgesics on brain evoked potentials. Int J Neuropharmacol 3:321–326

Slater P, Patel S (1983) Autoradiographic localisation of opiate κ-receptors in the rat spinal cord. Eur J Pharmacol 92:159–160

Spaulding TC, Fielding S, Venafro JJ, Lal H (1979) Antinociceptive activity of clonidine and its potentiation of morphine analgesia. Eur J Pharmacol 58:19–25

Stewart P, Isaac L (1989) Localization of dynorphin-induced neurotoxicity in rat spinal cord. Life Sci 44:1505–1514

Strejckova A, Jakoubek B, Kraus M, Mares P (1985) Changes in the activity of rat cortical and hippocampal neurones after the iontophoretic administration of beta-endorphin, glutamate and GABA. Physiol Bohemoslov 34:567–573

Sullivan AF, Dickenson AH (1988) Electrophysiological studies on the spinal effects of dermorphin, an endogenous μ-opioid agonist. Brain Res 461:182–185

Sullivan AF, Dickenson AH, Roques BP (1989) δ-opioid mediated inhibitions of acute and prolonged noxious-evoked respones in rat dorsal horn neurones. Br J Pharmacol 98:1039–1049

Sutor B, Zieglgänsberger W (1984) Actions of D-ala$_2$-D-leu$_5$-enkephalin and dynorphin A (1–17) on neocortical neurons in vitro. Neuropeptides 5:241–244

Takagi H, Doi T, Akaike A (1976) Microinjection of morphine into the medial part of the bulbar reticular formation in rabbit and rat: inhibitory effects on lamina V cells of spinal corsal horn and behavioral analgesia. In: Kosterlitz HW (ed) Opiates and endogenous opioid peptides. Elsevier, Amsterdam, pp 191–198

Takemori AE, Larson DL, Portoghese PS (1981) The irreversible narcotic antagonistic and reversible agonistic properties of the fumarate methyl ester derivative of naltrexone. Eur J Pharmacol 70:445–451

Toyooka H, Hanoaka K, Ohtani M, Yamashita M, Taub A, Kitahata LM (1977) Suppressive effect of morphine on single-unit activity of cells in Rexed lamina VII. Anesthesiology 47:513–517

Traynor JR, Hunter JC, Rodriguez RE, Hill RG, Hughes J (1990) δ-opioid receptor binding sites in rodent spinal cord. Br J Pharmacol 100/2:319–323

Tyers MB (1980) A classification of opiate receptors that mediate antinociception in animals. Br J Pharmacol 69:503–512

Velasco M, Velasco F, Castaneda R, Sanchez R (1984) Effects of fentanyl and naloxone on human somatic and auditory-evoked potential components. Neuropharmacology 23:359–366

Von Voigtlander PF, Lewis RA, Neff GL (1984) Kappa opioid analgesia is dependent on serotonergic mechanisms. J Pharmacol Exp Ther 231:270–274

Walker JM, Bowen WD, Thompson LA, Frascella J, Lehmkuhle S, Hughes HC (1988) Distribution of opiate receptors within visual structures of the cat brain. Exp Brain Res 73:523–532

Wall PD (1967) The laminar organization of dorsal horn and effects of descending impulses. J Physiol (Lond) 188:403–423

Weber E, Esch FS, Bohlen P, Corbett AD, McKnight AT, Kosterlitz HW, Barchas JD, Evans CJ (1983) Metorphamide: isolation, structure and biologic activity of an amidated opioid octapeptide from bovine brain. Proc Natl Acad Sci USA 80:7362–7366

Werz MA, Macdonald RL (1982) Heterogeneous sensitivity of cultured dorsal root ganglion neurones to opioid peptides selective for μ- and δ-opiate receptors. Nature 299:730–733

Werz MA, Macdonald RL (1985) Dynorphin and neoendorphin peptides decrease dorsal root ganglion neuron calcium-dependent action potential duration. J Pharmacol Exp Ther 234:49–56

Wikler A (1950) Sites and mechanisms of action of morphine and related drugs in the central nervous system. Pharmacol Rev 2:435–461

Wikler A (1952) Pharmacologic dissociation of behavior and EEG "sleep patterns" in dogs: morphine, N-allylnormorphine and atropine. Proc Soc Exp Biol Med 79:261–265

Wikler A (1954) Clinical and electroencephalographic studies on the effects of mescaline, N-allylnormorphine and morphine in man. J Nerv Ment Dis 120: 157–175

Wikler A, Frank K (1948) Hindlimb reflexes of chronic spinal dogs during cycles of addiction to morphine and methadone. J Pharmacol Exp Ther 94:382–400

Wilcox GL, Carlsson K-H, Jochim A, Jurna I (1987) Mutual potentiation of antinociceptive effects of morphine and clonidine on motor and sensory responses in rat spinal cord. Brain Res 405:84–93

Wilkinson DM, Hosko MJ (1982) Selective augmentation of visual pathways by morphine in α-chloralose-anaesthetized cats. Exp Neurol 77:519–533

Willcockson WS, Chung JM, Hori Y, Lee KH, Willis WD (1984) Effects of iontophoretically released peptides on primate spinothalamic tract cells. J Neurosci 4:741–750

Willcockson WS, Kim J, Shin HK, Chung JM, Willis WD (1986) Actions of opioids on primate spinothalamic neurons. J Neurosci 6:2509–2520

Willer JC (1985) Studies on pain. Effects of morphine on a spinal nociceptive flexion reflex and related pain sensation in man. Brain Res 331/1:105–114

Willis WD (1982) Mechanisms of medial brain-stem stimulation-induced inhibition in spinothalamic neurons. In: Sjolund B, Bjorklund A (eds) Brain stem control of spinal mechanisms. Elsevier, Amsterdam, pp 411–438

Willis WD (1985) Nociceptive pathways: anatomy and physiology of nociceptive ascending pathways. Philos Trans R Soc Lond [Biol] 308:253–268

Willis WD, Coggeshall RE (1978) Sensory mechanisms of the spinal cord. Plean, New York

Woda A, Azexad J, Guilbaud G, Besson JM (1975) Etude microphysiologique des projections thalamiques de la pulpe dentaire chez le chat. Brain Res 89:193–213

Woolf CJ, Wall PD (1986) Morphine-sensitive and morphine-insensitive actions of C-fibre input on the rat spinal cord. Neurosci Lett 64:221–225

Yaksh TL, Elde RP (1981) Factors governing release of methionine enkephalin-like immunoreactivity from mesencephalon and spinal cord of the cat in vivo. J Neurophysiol 46:1056–1075

Yaksh TL, Rudy TA (1977) Studies on the direct spinal action of narcotics in the production of analgesia in the rat. J Pharmacol Exp Ther 202:411–418

Yaksh TL, Rudy TA (1978) Narcotic analgesics: CNS sites and mechanisms of action as revealed by intracerebral injection techniques. Pain 4:299–360

Yaksh TL, Jessell TM, Gamse R, Mudge AW, Leeman SE (1980) Intrathecal morphine inhibits substance P release from mammalian spinal cord in vivo. Nature 286:155–157

Yoshimura M, North RA (1983) Substantia gelatinosa neurones hyperpolarised in vitro by enkephalin. Nature 305:529–530

Zajac JM, Lombard MC, Peschanski M, Besson JM, Roques BP (1989) Autoradiographic study of mu and delta opioid binding sites and neutral endopeptidase-24.11 in rat after dorsal rhizotomy. Brain Res 477:400–403

Zamir N, Weber E, Palkovits M, Brownstein MJ (1985) Distribution of immuno-reactive metorphamide (adrenorphin) in discrete regions of the rat brain: comparison with Met-enkephalin-Arg^6-Gly^7-Leu^8. Brain Res 361:193–199

Zhao ZQ, Duggan AW (1984) Microelectrophoretic administration of naloxone near motoneurones fails to reproduce the effects of systemic naloxone in anaesthetized cats. Neurosci Lett 45:305–310

Zhao ZQ, Duggan AW (1987) Clonidine and the hyper-responsiveness of dorsal horn neurones following morphine withdrawal in the spinal cat. Neuro-pharmacology 26:1499–1502

Zhao ZQ, Morton CR, Hall JG, Duggan AW (1986) The selective effects of metorphamide on dorsal horn neurones of the cat spinal cord. Neuropeptides 8:327–334

Zieglgänsberger W (1986) Central control of nociception. In: Mountcastle VB, Bloom FE, Geiger SR (eds) Handbook of physiology – the nervous system IV. Williams and Wilkins, Baltimore, pp 581–645

Zieglgänsberger W, Bayerl H (1976) The mechanisms of inhibition of neuronal activity by opiates in the spinal cord of the cat. Brain Res 115:111–128

Zieglgänsberger W, Sutor B (1983) Responses of substantia gelatinosa neurones to putative neurotransmitters in an in vitro preparation of the adult rat spinal cord. Brain Res 279:316–320

Zieglgänsberger W, Tulloch IF (1979) The effects of methionine and leucine enkephalin on spinal neurones of the cat. Brain Res 167:53–64

Zieglgänsberger W, Fry JP, Herz A, Moroder L, Wunsch E (1976) Enkephalin induced inhibition of cortical neurones and the lack of this effect in morphine tolerant/dependent rats. Brain Res 115:160–164

CHAPTER 30

Opioid Actions on Membrane Ion Channels

R.A. NORTH

A. Introduction

Drugs, hormones, and neurotransmitters can open and close ion channels by several molecular mechanisms. First, the transmitter receptor might itself comprise the ion channel: examples are the nicotinic acetylcholine (ACh) receptors, the glutamate receptors, γ-aminobutyric acid (GABA$_A$) receptors, 5-hydroxytryptamine (5-HT$_3$) receptors, and adenosine 5'-triphosphate (ATP P$_{2x}$) receptors (NORTH 1989a). In this case, the channel is named for the transmitter that causes it to open whereas other channels are usually named for the ions that pass through them. The movement of ions through such ligand-gated channels has immediate electrical consequences and may have secondary metabolic consequences; for example, significant entry of calcium ions through the channel may activate intracellular enzymes.

Second, the transmitter receptor might belong to the family that couples directly to a guanosine 5'-triphosphate (GTP)-binding protein (G protein). Binding of agonist induces a conformational change in the G protein as a result of which guanosine diphosphate dissociates from the α-subunit and GTP associates in its place. Thus activated, the α-subunit separates from the β- and γ-subunits, and is free to interact directly with other nearby molecules, which include enzymes, transporters, and ion channels (BROWN and BIRNBAUMER 1990). The α-subunit itself has GTPase activity; as bound GTP is hydrolyzed the subunit becomes inactivated. Ion channels can be directly influenced by the binding of activated G protein, or they may be affected consequentially by the products of enzyme activation or inhibition, through phosphorylation or changes in channel gene transcription.

Third, the receptor may itself be an enzyme, with a ligand-binding site on the cell exterior and a catalytic domain exposed to the cytoplasm; examples include the atrial naturetic factor receptor that functions as guanylyl cyclase, and many growth factor receptors that are tyrosine kinases. Clearly, ion channels may also be an eventual target of signaling processes initiated through such receptors.

Experiments in which the time course of drug action is measured can be helpful to distinguish among these types of action. In the first case, the channel opens within less than a millisecond of agonist binding. Agonists acting through the second mechanism, in which receptor and channel are relatively close to each other within the membrane, bring about their effects with a time to onset of tens of milliseconds, and a duration typically of 0.5–2 s. Agonists that bring about channel phosphorylation more usually act in the time frame of seconds to minutes, while actions that result from changes in gene transcription would be expected to take several hours (KACZMAREK and LEVITAN 1987).

Information regarding the structure of the receptor protein is particularly useful for the assignment of receptors to the above classes because different members of the same family of receptors have common structural motifs. This information is not yet available for the opioid receptors. Therefore, inferences must be made by careful comparison of the actions of opioids on ion channels with the actions of other transmitters acting through receptor-channel transduction pathways that are more fully understood. This principle should be borne in mind as the actions of opioids are presented in the subsequent sections.

B. Calcium Channels

I. Types of Calcium Channels

Calcium ions can enter cells through cation nonselective channels (e.g., nicotinic ACh receptors, P_{2x} receptors, and glutamate receptors of the N-methyl-D-aspartate class); indeed, such channels often have a higher permeability to calcium than to sodium, but the relatively low concentration of calcium normally present outside the cell means that calcium carries a tiny fraction of the inward current (e.g., DECKER and DANI 1990; WESTBROOK and JAHR 1989). Calcium ions can also enter cells through voltage-independent, or background, channels; this has been particularly studied in lymphocytes (YOUNG et al. 1988). However, the most abundant types of calcium channels found in nerve cells are calcium channels that are opened by membrane depolarization (TSIEN 1983).

Voltage-dependent calcium channels are often divided into three groups depending on the magnitude of the unitary current observed when the channel opens and barium ions pass through it (NOWYCKY et al. 1985; TSIEN 1983; HESS 1990). Conductances of large (L $\simeq$ 25 pS), intermediate (N $\simeq$ 13 pS), and small (T $\simeq$ 8 pS) amplitudes are observed in the same or different cells. Further distinguishing criteria are that T channels open when the membrane is depolarized to about −50 mV from a relatively hyperpolarized potential; current through these channels is thus thought to underlie the "low-voltage-activated" (LVA) current previously described (CARBONE and LUX 1984). T channels open only transiently at the onset of a maintained depolarization. L channels are activated by strong depolarization (typically to about −10 mV) from normal resting potentials (−50 to −70 mV); these channels are more likely to open in the presence of agonist dihydropyridines such as Bay K 8644 and their opening is impaired by antagonists such as nitrendipine. Current through these channels contributes to the "high-voltage activated" (HVA) current recorded from intact cells. N channels are activated by similar depolarizations from the resting potential but are insensitive to dihydropyridine drugs. It was earlier suggested that the opening of N channels declines when the depolarization is continued for tens or hundreds of milliseconds, whereas current through L channels does not; it is now realized that this is too variable a property to be useful in channel classification. The molecular structure of one type of L channel is known, and the main, pore-forming α_1-subunit shows considerable homology to voltage-dependent sodium and potassium channels (CATTERALL 1988).

II. μ-Receptors

Activation of μ-receptors reduces voltage-dependent calcium currents in differentiated SH-SY5Y cells, a clonal cell line derived from a human neuroblastoma (SEWARD et al. 1991). μ-Receptor selectivity was shown by the effectiveness of Tyr-D-Ala-Gly-MePhe-Gly-ol (DAMGO; EC_{50} about 10 nM) and the failure of ICI174864 [N,N-bisallyl-Tyr-D-Ala-Aib-Aib-Phe-Leu-OH; Aib = aminoisobutyrate)] to block the action of DAMGO. The inhibition of the current was maximal within 1–2 min, was maintained during applications of up to 20 min, and reversed readily when agonist application was discontinued. Maximal inhibition (46%) was produced by 300 nM DAMGO. The calcium current in these cells is also inhibited by agonists selective for δ-receptors (see below).

The calcium current in dorsal root ganglion cells dissociated from adult rats is also inhibited by agonists acting at μ-receptors (DAMGO, morphine; SCHROEDER et al. 1991). In this case, the somewhat κ-selective agonist U50488H (*trans*-(±)-3,4-dichloro-N-methyl-[2-(1-pyrrolidinyl)cyclohexyl] benzeneacetamide methane sulfonate) and dynorphin were effective too, although some cells responded more strongly to μ-agonists and others more strongly to κ-agonists. Involvement of μ-receptors was confirmed by the effectiveness of β-funaltrexamine to block irreversibly the action of DAMGO but not that of U50488H. DPDPE (Tyr-D-Pen-Gly-Phe-D-Pen) (10 μM) was not effective.

III. δ-Receptors

Guinea pig submucous plexus neurons express δ-receptors, and their activation results in calcium conductance decrease (Fig. 1) (SURPRENANT et al. 1990; SHEN et al. 1990). The inhibition of calcium currents was observed with [Met^5]enkephalin and DPDPE though not with dynorphin (100 nM) or DAMGO (1 μM). The action of [Met^5]enkephalin was blocked by ICI174864. These findings on the submucous plexus neurons are noteworthy in three respects. First, these are the only cells in which opiates have been

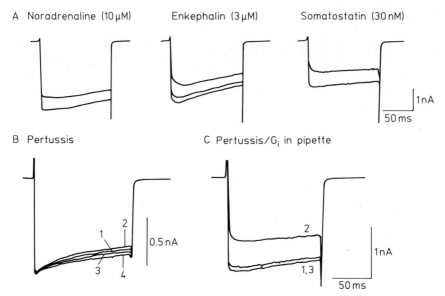

A Noradrenaline (10 µM)   Enkephalin (3 µM)   Somatostatin (30 nM)

B Pertussis   C Pertussis/G$_i$ in pipette

Fig. 1A–C. Opioids inhibit calcium currents. Recordings are from submucous plexus neurons dissociated from adult guinea pigs; external solution contained 2.5 or 5 mM calcium and tetrodotoxin (1 µM) to block sodium currents. **A** Noradrenaline, [Met^5]enkephalin, and somatostatin each inhibit the current in the same neuron. Records are membrane currents evoked by a depolarizing voltage pulse from the holding potential of −70 mV to 10 mV. Each set of traces are currents recorded before, during (the smaller current), and after application of the agonist. Noradrenaline was applied 8 min after beginning whole-cell recording; [Met^5]enkephalin was applied 10 min after washout of noradrenaline, and somatostatin was applied 10 min after washout of [Met^5]enkephalin. **B** inhibition of calcium current by agonists is blocked by pertussis toxin. Superimposed traces show currents evoked in control solution (*1*), in [Met^5]enkephalin, 3 µM (*2*), in noradrenaline, 30 µM (*3*), and in somatostatin, 30 nM (*4*). These normally supramaximal concentrations of agonist were ineffective on this cell that had been pretreated with pertussis toxin (40 ng/ml) for 18 h. **C** Opioid action is restored by G protein. Whole-cell recording was made from a neuron that had been pretreated with pertussis toxin (10 µg/ml for 5 h); the pipette contained G$_i$ purified from pig heart. The control trace was recorded 5 min after breaking into the cell interior; [Met^5]enkephalin (1 µM) applied soon after reversibly inhibited the calcium current, as in control cells (**A**). (Adapted from SURPRENANT et al. 1990)

shown *both* to decrease calcium currents *and* to increase potassium conductance (see below). Second, measurement of current through single calcium channels showed that the calcium channels affected were of the N-type (8–12 pS conductance). Third, the observation of the action of [Met^5]enkephalin when applied to the outer surface of excised patches of membrane indicates that no freely diffusible second messenger is required for the transduction between receptor and channel.

IV. κ-Receptors

The original suggestion that κ-agonists inhibit voltage-dependent calcium currents came from observations of the duration of action potentials in mouse cultured dorsal root ganglion cells (see below). Subsequent voltage-clamp recordings show conclusively that the selective agonist dynorphin inhibits the calcium current in these neurons (GROSS and MACDONALD 1987; MACDONALD and WERZ 1986; GROSS et al. 1990). Others have reported similar though less complete results in which dynorphin inhibited calcium currents in spinal cord (SAH 1990) and dorsal root ganglia (BEAN 1989) cultured from rat.

V. Unclassified Receptors

Opiates inhibit calcium currents in NG108-15 cells (TSUNOO et al. 1986; SHIMAHARA and ICARD-LIEPKALNS 1987; HESCHELER et al. 1987; BROWN et al. 1989); results with selective agonists have not been reported, but δ-receptors are abundant on these cells.

VI. Experiments on Action Potential Duration

Effects of opioids on calcium currents have sometimes been inferred from measurements of action potential duration. These experiments are carried out in the presence of extracellular tetraethylammonium or barium, or intracellular caesium, to reduce voltage-dependent potassium currents. The action potentials are therefore considerably prolonged relative to the duration under physiological conditions. Under these circumstances, administration of agents that are known to reduce calcium entry through voltage-dependent channels (such as cadmium or cobalt) reduce the duration of the action potential. When opioids reduce the duration of the action potential they may also do so by reducing calcium currents. However, such an interpretation must be regarded with circumspection. The action potential eventually repolarizes, even though many voltage-dependent potassium channels are blocked, and this repolarization results from outward current flowing through residual unblocked potassium channels. Thus, any action of opioids to increase the conductance of such residual potassium channels could result in a reduction in the action potential duration. A further difficulty with experiments of this kind is that the action potential duration is critically dependent on the membrane potential from which it is evoked, a reflection of the degree of inactivation of calcium and potassium conductances at the initiation of the depolarization; this also complicates quantitative studies of agonist action.

Notwithstanding the above limitations, the method has provided initial information on ionic mechanism and very useful information on receptor type. Calcium currents in chick dorsal root ganglion cells are inhibited by

[Met⁵]enkephalin (MUDGE et al. 1979). WERZ and MACDONALD (1985; MACDONALD and WERZ 1986) showed that subpopulations of mouse dorsal root ganglion cells express κ-receptors, activation of which reduces the duration of action potentials prolonged by internal caesium. Essentially similar results have been reported by the group of Crain (CRAIN and SHEN 1990; CHALAZONITIS and CRAIN 1986).

Adult mammalian neurons in vitro are similarly affected. CHERUBINI and NORTH (1985) showed this for neurons of the guinea pig myenteric plexus, using U50488H and β-FNA as κ-selective agonists, and HIGASHI et al. (1982) showed this for rabbit nodose ganglion cells, using morphine as the agonist. An interesting observation made both by HIGASHI et al. (1982) and by CRAIN and colleagues (SHEN and CRAIN 1989; CRAIN and SHEN 1990) is that concentrations of morphine or D-Ala-D-Leu-enkephalin that are too low to cause action potential shortening actually cause action potential prolongation. Evidence was presented that this effect results from an intracellular transduction mechanism distinct from that from responsible for action potential shortening.

VII. Type of Calcium Current Inhibited

In only one study has the calcium current reduced by opioids been identified at the single channel level (SHEN et al. 1990). In this case, the current affected was clearly of the N type, having a unit conductance of about 10 pS and being activated by depolarizations from about −70 mV to 0 mV. This identification of the single channel is in good agreement with the results of recording the calcium current from the entire neuron; submucous plexus neurons have no detectable low-voltage activated current (T component) or dihydropyridine-sensitive current (L component) (SURPRENANT et al. 1990).

Other investigators have tried to identify the type of calcium channel affected on the basis of whole-cell currents. Thus, in rat dorsal root ganglion cells and in SH-SY5Y neuroblastoma cells the current was classed as N-like by respect of the potential at which it activated and insensitivity to dihydropyridines (SCHROEDER et al. 1990, 1991; SEWARD and HENDERSON 1990). A rather less satisfactory way to classify the current (see HESS 1990) is on the basis of whether or not it declines during a maintained depolarization; in mouse cultured dorsal root ganglion cells dynorphin reduces predominantly the inactivating or N component of the high-voltage activated current (GROSS and MACDONALD 1987).

VIII. Mechanism of Opioid Action

1. Role of G Proteins

Precisely how activation of opioid receptors results in inhibition of calcium currents is not known. The first step is undoubtedly activation of a G protein. Whole-cell recordings made with electrodes that contain non-hydrolyzable derivatives of GTP [such as GTP-γ-S (guanosine 5'-γ-thiophosphate)] show that the inhibitory action of the opioids becomes irreversible (BROWN et al. 1989; SURPRENANT et al. 1990), as expected when α-subunit is not able to hydrolyze the bound GTP. In other cases, introduction of GTP-γ-S into the cell interior reduces the current directly even in the absence of external opioids (e.g., HESCHELER et al. 1987; DOLPHIN and SCOTT 1989).

The action of opioids can be entirely blocked by pretreatment with pertussis toxin in all cases in which the experiment was attempted (NG108-15 cells: HESCHELER et al. 1987; BROWN et al. 1989; mouse dorsal root ganglia: SHEN and CRAIN 1989; guinea pig submucous plexus neurons: SURPRENANT et al. 1990; SH-SYS5 cells: SEWARD et al. 1991). In NG108-15 cells they can also be blocked by preinjecting the cells with antibodies against G_o though not G_i (MCFADZEAN et al. 1989). This last result is in general agreement with the earlier work of HESCHELER et al. (1987), who found that G_o is more effective than G_i to reconstitute the inhibitory action of opioids in cells in which this had been lost by prior treatment with pertussis toxin. SURPRENANT et al. (1990) found that both G_o and G_i could restore the opioid action in submucous neurons previously treated with pertussis toxin (Fig. 1).

The above experiments speak directly to the involvement of a pertussis toxin-sensitive G portein in mediating the inhibitory effects of opioids on calcium currents. A pertussis toxin-sensitive G protein is also involved in the inhibition of adenylyl cyclase by opioid agonists, but several studies suggest that this action is not related to the inhibition of calcium current (HESCHELER et al. 1987; SEWARD et al. 1991). Actually, the catalytic subunit of cyclic adenosine 3',5'-monophosphate (cAMP) dependent protein kinase (A-kinase) increases calcium current in mouse dorsal root ganglion cells, and makes the current more sensitive to the inhibitory action of dynorphin (GROSS et al. 1990).

Evidence has been presented that the action potential broadening effect of very low concentrations of DAMGO ($1-10\,\mathrm{n}M$) that is found in cultures of mouse dorsal root ganglia results from an increase in cAMP levels. Intracellular dialysis with a peptide inhibitor of protein kinase A completely blocked the spike-broadening effect but did not alter the reduction in spike duration seen with higher opioid concentrations (CHEN et al. 1988).

2. Time Course of Agonist Action

The time course of opioid action to inhibit voltage-dependent calcium currents has not been studied in any detail. However, noradrenaline and δ-receptor agonists decrease the same calcium current in guinea pig submucous plexus neurons; noradrenaline reduces the current within 200 ms of its application to the neuron surface (SURPRENANT et al. 1990). A similarly brief latency to the action of noradrenaline was reported by BEAN (1989) for dorsal root ganglion cells.

3. Single Channel Studies

The finding that opioids remain effective to reduce calcium current opening in excised membrane patches strongly suggests that a diffusible second messenger (such as cAMP) is not required (SHEN et al. 1990). There is now a growing consensus that activated G protein might bind directly to the voltage-dependent calcium channel, and thereby reduce the probability that it opens during membrane depolarization (BROWN and BIRNBAUMER 1990); reconstitution of the individual proteins in artificial membranes or heterologous cells will probably be required to resolve this question.

4. Voltage Dependence of Agonist Action?

It has been suggested that transmitters such as opioids might inhibit calcium currents by changing their voltage-dependence (BEAN 1989). It is envisaged that voltage-dependent N-type channels can exist in two states; in one state they are fully opened by depolarizations from the resting potential to about 0 mV but in the other state depolarizations to much more positive potentials are required to open the channels. In this case, transmitters such as opioids might simply switch a population of channels from the first state to the second state, from which they could not open with the usual depolarizations to about 0 mV. The model is attractive because it provides an apparent explanation for the finding that opioids and other transmitters reduce the initial peak of the calcium current more than they reduce the later sustained current component; the slower activation of the calcium current in the presence of a transmitter may reflect the time required for channels to pass from the second state back to the first state, from which they can then open. The model predicts that agonists should be without effect on calcium currents at very positive potentials. This has been reported by BEAN (1989) and SEWARD et al. (1991) but, to the contrary, no voltage dependence to the agonist action was found by SURPRENANT et al. (1990), MCFADZEAN and DOCHERTY 1989, SAH (1990), SCHROEDER et al. (1991), or GROSS and MACDONALD (1987) even at potentials so positive that the calcium current was reversed.

IX. Other Receptors That Reduce Calcium Currents

The action of opioids to inhibit neuronal calcium currents is shared by many other receptors (Fig. 1). These all belong to a subgroup of the larger family of G protein coupled receptors and include adenosine A_1, muscarinic M_2, $GABA_B$, 5-HT_{1A}, somatostatin, galanin, neuropeptide Y, dopamine D_2, and noradrenaline α_2 (see SAH 1990; NORTH 1989). In several cases, one or more other agonists have been shown to inhibit calcium currents in the same neuron that is affected by an opioid (e.g., noradrenaline and opioid in NG108-15 cells: BROWN et al. 1989; McFADZEAN and DOCHERTY 1989; enkephalin and somatostatin in NG108-15 cells: TSUNOO et al. 1986; noradrenaline, δ-opioids, and somatostatin in guinea pig submucous plexus neurons: SURPRENANT et al. 1990) (Fig. 1).

X. Calcium Current Inhibition and Presynaptic Inhibition

It has been widely held that a reduction in voltage-dependent calcium currents at the nerve terminal could underlie the presynaptic inhibition of transmitter release observed with opioids (NORTH and WILLIAMS 1983). This is an attractive possibility but there are a number of observations that make it unlikely. First, a striking feature of the inhibition by opioids (and other agonists) of calcium currents is that it is partial, rarely exceeding 50%. Even several agonists applied together cannot reduce the current more than a maximal concentration of one agonist applied alone, or more than intracellular application of GTP-γ-S (SURPRENANT et al. 1990). Thus, there is a component of the calcium current that is insensitive to opioids and other agonists acting through G proteins. Indeed, in guinea pig submucous plexus, somatostatin, [Met^5]enkephalin, and noradrenaline all reduce calcium currents, but only noradrenaline causes any presynaptic inhibition (SHEN and SURPRENANT 1990). These observations present difficulties for theories that implicate inhibition of calcium current in presynaptic inhibition because opioids generally completely block the release of neurotransmitters evoked by electrical stimulation. Second, presynaptic inhibition by receptors in this family has often been found to be insensitive to pertussis toxin, even in conditions where the reduction of calcium current is blocked (e.g., SURPRENANT et al. 1990). Third, it is increasingly realized that G protein can play a role in transmitter secretion that is quite independent of ion channels; in other words the need to invoke actions on ion channels has partly disappeared (ULLRICH and WOLLHEIM 1988).

C. Potassium Channels

I. Types of Potassium Channels

Potassium channels can be classified according to what opens or closes them. Some are primarily affected by membrane potential (voltage-dependent potassium channels) and others are primarily affected by the binding of internal ligands; some are clearly intermediate, being opened by both voltage and intracellular messengers (RUDY 1988). Voltage-dependent potassium channels are of two main functional types, those that remain open during a maintained depolarization (often called delayed rectifier channels) and those that close despite the maintained depolarization (transient or A currents). The molecular structure of voltage-dependent channels is now known; the channels appear to be formed by the oligomerization of four subunits, each of which is homologous to one of the four internal repeats of the voltage-dependent sodium or calcium channel α-subunit (CATTERALL 1988). Channels that are primarily gated by ligands include channels opened by binding of G proteins (BROWN and BIRNBAUMER 1990), channels closed by binding of internal ATP (ASHCROFT 1988), and channels that are opened by an increase in intracellular calcium concentration (LATORRE et al. 1989).

A significant body of literature testifies to the direct inhibitory action of opioids on single vertebrate neurons (reviewed by DUGGAN and NORTH 1984). Where excitation occurs (olfactory bulb, hippocampus, ventral tegmental area), it results from inhibition of inhibitory interneurons (NICOLL et al. 1980; MADISON and NICOLL 1988; JOHNSON and NORTH 1990). Where it has been studied in detail, with measurements of ion reversal potentials, the inhibition has been found to result from an increase in membrane potassium conductance. In less detailed studies, membrane hyperpolarization has been recorded and involvement of a potassium conductance has been inferred from supporting evidence such as demonstration of a membrane resistance decrease, or reduction of the opioid effect by potassium channel blockers.

II. μ-Receptors

Increase in potassium conductance by opioids acting at μ-receptors has been shown for guinea pig myenteric plexus (NORTH and TONINI 1977; NORTH et al. 1979), locus ceruleus (PEPPER and HENDERSON 1980), arcuate hypothalamic nucleus (LOOSE et al. 1990; KELLY et al. 1990; LOOSE and KELLY 1990), paraventricular and supraoptic hypothalamic nuclei (WUARIN and DUDEK 1990; WUARIN et al. 1988), and secondary neurons of raphe magnus (PAN et al. 1990), and for rat locus ceruleus (WILLIAMS et al. 1982; NORTH and WILLIAMS 1985; WILLIAMS and NORTH 1984) (Fig. 2), nucleus parabrachialis (CHRISTIE and NORTH 1988), substantia gelatinosa of the spinal cord (YOSHIMURA and NORTH 1983), secondary (nondopamine) neurons of the substantia nigra pars compacta (LACEY et al. 1989) and ventral tegmental area (JOHNSON and NORTH 1990), inhibitory interneurons of the hippocampus (MADISON and NICOLL 1988), dorsal motor nucleus of the vagus (DUAN et al. 1990), and secondary neurons of the raphe magnus (PAN et al. 1990). In most of these cases, involvement of μ-receptors is inferred from the effectiveness of DAMGO coupled with lack of action of DPDPE, although in a number of cases the dissociation constant for naloxone has been measured by Schild analysis and found to be close to that expected for μ-receptors (LORD et al. 1977) (Fig. 2).

III. δ-Receptors

Increase in potassium conductance results from δ-receptor activation in neurons of the guinea pig submucous plexus (MIHARA and NORTH 1986) (Fig.

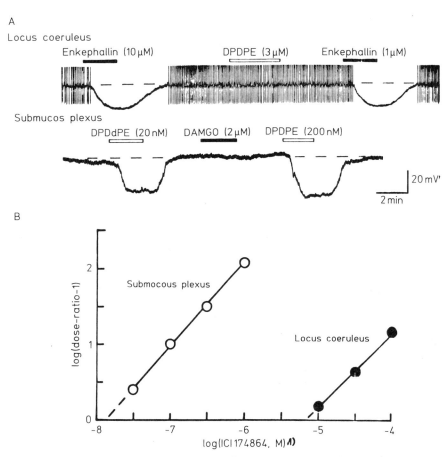

Fig. 2A,B. Hyperpolarizations of different neurons through μ- and δ-receptors. **A** Intracellular recordings from neurons in rat locus ceruleus and guinea pig submucous plexus. DPDPE (20 nM) causes a large hyperpolarization in the submucous plexus but a 100-fold higher concentration is without effect in the locus ceruleus. Conversely, DAMGO (2 μM) has no effect in the submucous plexus but causes large hyperpolarizations in the locus ceruleus (not shown). Vertical deflections on upper record are spontaneously occurring action potentials, full amplitude not shown. The slower rate of onset and offset of drug action in the locus ceruleus reflects the diffusion barriers in the brain slice compared with isolated submucous ganglia. **B** Schild analysis confirms that submucous plexus neurons express δ-receptors and locus ceruleus neurons express μ-receptors. The two Schild plots are derived from two neurons, one in each tissue. In each case, several concentrations of [Met⁵]enkephalin were applied, in the absence and then in the presence of three or four concentrations of ICI 174864. The hyperpolarizations were measured and the dose ratios computed. In each tissue, ICI 174864 acted as a competitive antagonist, but the estimates of the dissociation equilibrium constants differed by more than 300-fold. [Adapted from NORTH et al. (1987) and NORTH (1986)]

2). DAMGO is ineffective on these neurons at concentrations up to $10\,\mu M$ (NORTH et al. 1987), whereas DPDPE is active at nM concentrations (Fig. 2). The dissociation constants for naloxone and for ICI174864 also indicate that a δ-receptor is responsible for the potassium conductance increase and resulting hyperpolarization (Fig. 2).

IV. Other Receptors

Agonists selective for κ-receptors have not been shown to increase membrane potassium conductance. It would be surprising if activation of κ-receptors did not result in potassium conductance increase in some cells, in view of the evidence that agonists at other receptors in this family (e.g., somatostatin, $GABA_B$, D_2, α_2, $5\text{-}HT_{1A}$, μ, δ) have been shown to affect *both* calcium currents and potassium currents.

V. Experiments on Action Potential Duration

The duration of the action potential of mouse dorsal root ganglion neurons in culture is reduced by opioids selective for μ- and κ-receptors; however, in contrast to κ-agonists, these effects are not seen when intracellular caesium is used to reduce outward potassium currents. It is inferred from these experiments that the μ- and δ-opioids act by increasing the voltage-dependent potassium conductance that contributes to action potential repolarization (WERZ and MACDONALD 1983).

VI. Hyperpolarization and Inhibition of Firing

DUGGAN and NORTH (1984) reviewed the extensive literature on the inhibitory actions of opioids in different regions of the nervous system. Such inhibition in vivo could result from a direct hyperpolarization of the cell, or from a reduction in excitatory input to the cell. Recording in vitro can often distinguish between these possibilities. Thus, direct hyperpolarizing actions of opioid peptides have been reported in circumstances where the ionic mechanism has not been determined. These include the dorsal roots of the frog isolated spinal cord (EVANS and HILL 1978; NICOLL 1982), rat dorsal horn neurons (MURASE et al. 1982; JEFTINIJA 1988), and frog sympathetic ganglia (WOUTERS and VAN DER BERCKEN 1979).

VII. Type of Potassium Current Increased

The most detailed account of the properties of the potassium conductance increased by opioids comes from studies in the rat locus ceruleus and guinea pig submucous plexus (NORTH and WILLIAMS 1985; NORTH et al. 1987; WILLIAMS et al. 1988). The conductance has the property of becoming larger as the membrane is hyperpolarized (inward rectification). For example, the conductance increase in a typical locus ceruleus neuron is 6 nS at the resting potential (about -60 mV) and 11 nS at -120 mV. When opioids open these potassium channels, outward current flows; this hyperpolarizes the membrane. The hyperpolarization increases the effectiveness of the opioids to open further potassium channels. In other words, this property of the conductance tends to amplify the opioid action on the membrane potential. A conductance having basically similar properties is increased by δ-agonists in guinea pig submucous plexus neurons (NORTH et al. 1987).

There are other features of the opioid-activated potassium conductance, in both rat locus ceruleus and guinea pig submucous plexus, that provide useful information about the underlying channels. The conductance increased by the agonists is not obviously time dependent; the current develops within a few milliseconds when the membrane potential is changed. The inward rectification of the conductance is blocked by barium ($10 \mu M - 1$ mM), caesium (2 mM), and rubidium (1–2 mM); rubidium permeates in addition to preventing inward rectification. These properties are strikingly similar to potassium currents in a wide range of cells that show inward rectification in the absence of any agonist (see refs. in WILLIAMS et al. 1988). The conductance is relatively insensitive to tetraethylammonium and not affected by apamin (NORTH and WILLIAMS 1985; NORTH et al. 1987).

The properties of single channels opened by opioids have been reported for the rat locus ceruleus (cell-attached configuration; MIYAKE et al. 1989) and for the guinea pig submucous plexus (excised outside-out configuration) (SHEN et al. 1990). Tight-seal recordings were made from dissociated locus ceruleus neurons using microelectrodes that contained 140 mM potassium chloride. Unitary potassium currents were observed that had a conductance of about 5 pS, but only if the recording pipette contained an opioid agonist (usually DAMGO). The probability of opening of the channels was greater when higher DAMGO concentrations were used. The unitary conductance of the channel and the mean open time are similar to those first reported for the channels opened by ACh acting at muscarinic receptors in the heart (SAKMANN et al. 1983).

Outside-out membrane patches pulled from guinea pig submucous plexus neurons show unitary activity of several different potassium channels (SHEN et al. 1990). In equal potassium concentrations, these can be grouped by amplitude into large (about 250 pS), intermediate (about 150 pS), and small (20–60 pS). Application of [Met[5]]enkephalin to the exposed outer surface of such patches increases the activity of all channels in the patch (Fig. 3). The conductance and open probability of these channels is not strongly voltage-dependent indicating that they are resting or background channels that contribute to the resting potential of the cell.

WIMPEY and CHAVKIN (1990) have recently found that a quite different potassium conductance is increased by opioids. Neurons dissociated from the hippocampus showed two different types of response to opioids. A small population of cells showed an outward current that was generally similar

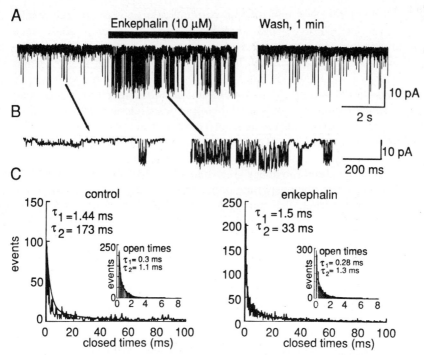

Fig. 3A–C. Single potassium channels opened by opioids. Single-channel recordings were made from excised outside-out patches of membrane from a guinea pig submucous plexus neuron. **A** Unitary currents at $-50\,\mathrm{mV}$ are inward (both inside and outside faces of the membrane were exposed to $150\,\mathrm{m}M$ potassium). Two channels are active (about 50 and 250 pS). [Met^5]enkephalin ($10\,\mu M$) was applied to the extracellular surface of the patch during the time indicated by the bar. It caused a marked increase in the probability of opening of both potassium channels which reversed when the application was discontinued. **B** Channel openings from record A at a higher recording speed. **C** Results from another similar experiment in which a single channel was active in the patch (43 pS). The distribution of open times (*insets*) were well fitted by two exponentials, and these were not affected by [Met^5]enkephalin. [Met^5]enkephalin acts by reducing the longer of the two closed states, thus increasing the proportion of time that the channel spends open. (Unpublished observations)

in its properties to the inwardly rectifying current described above. The majority of neurons, however, show no effect of opioids at the resting potential of the cell, but an increase in the outward current evoked by membrane depolarization. The effect of the opioids was rendered irreversible by allowing GTP-γ-S to diffuse into the cell interior. This increase in a delayed rectifier provides a possible explanation for the observations described above on dorsal root ganglion cells, where opioids reduce the duration of the action potential, because delayed rectifier potassium currents are usually responsible for action potential repolarization.

Table 1. Summary of tissues in which opioids have been shown to increase potassium conductance or to hyperpolarize the membrane

Tissue	Receptor	Reference
Guinea pig		
Myenteric plexus	?	NORTH and TONINI 1977
	?	NORTH et al. 1979
Submucous plexus	δ	MIHARA and NORTH 1986; SHEN et al. 1990
Locus ceruleus	?	PEPPER and HENDERSON 1980
Arcuate nucleus	μ	LOOSE et al. 1990; KELLY et al. 1990 LOOSE and KELLY 1990
Paraventricular and suprapoptic nuclei	μ	WUARIN and DUDEK 1990; WUARIN et al. 1988
Raphe magnus secondary cells	μ	PAN et al. 1990
Rat		
Locus ceruleus	μ	WILLIAMS et al. 1982; NORTH and WILLIAMS 1985; WILLIAMS and NORTH 1984; MIYAKE et al. 1989
Nucleus parabrachialis	μ	CHRISTIE and NORTH 1988
Substantia gelatinosa	?	YOSHIMURA and NORTH 1983; MURASE et al. 1982
Substantia nigra secondary neurons	μ	LACEY et al. 1989
Ventral tegmental area inhibitory cells	μ	JOHNSON and NORTH 1990
Hippocampus CA1 inhibitory cells	?	MADISON and NICOLL 1988
Dorsal motor nucleus of vagus	?	DUAN et al. 1990
Raphe magnus secondary cells	μ	PAN et al. 1990
Frog		
Dorsal root of spinal cord	?	EVANS and HILL 1978; NICOLL 1982
Sympathetic ganglion	?	WOUTERS and VAN DER BERCKEN 1979

VIII. Mechanism of Opioid Action

1. Role of G Proteins

Compelling evidence shows that opioid receptors couple to potassium channels through G proteins. First, intracellular GTP-γ-S renders the opioid actions irreversible (NORTH et al. 1987; TATSUMI et al. 1990; WIMPEY and CHAVKIN 1990). Second, pretreatment with pertussis toxin prevents opioids from increasing the potassium conductance. This has been shown by treating rats with pertussis toxin in vivo (AGHAJANIAN and WANG 1986), by exposing tissues to the toxin in vitro (TATSUMI et al. 1990), and by applying the toxin directly to the cell interior with whole-cell recording pipettes (TATSUMI et al. 1990). Furthermore, when recordings are made from neurons previously exposed to pertussis toxin, the coupling between opioid receptor and potass-

ium channel can be restored by including purified G proteins in the recording pipette (TATSUMI et al. 1990). No obvious differences were observed
between the ability of G_o (cow brain) or G_i (pig heart) to reconstitute the
opioid action.

Opioid agonists have been known to inhibit adenylyl cyclase activity for
many years (KLEE and NIRENBERG 1974; COLLIER and ROY 1974). This has
also been shown in the rat locus ceruleus (DUMAN et al. 1988; RASMUSSEN
et al. 1990). It was therefore possible that the increase in potassium conductance resulted from a reduction in intracellular cAMP levels. Considerable evidence exists against this. KARRAS and NORTH (1979) found that the
inhibition of firing of myenteric neurons (which was known to result from a
potassium conductance increase) was unaffected by several procedures likely
to increase intracellular cyclic AMP. Opioid induced potassium currents in
the locus ceruleus and submucous plexus are unaffected by forskolin or
$N^6,O^{2'}$-dibutyryl adenosine $3',5'$-monophosphate (NORTH and WILLIAMS
1985; NORTH et al. 1987).

2. Time Course of Action

When [Met^5]enkephalin is applied briefly (for less than 10 ms) to the surface
of a submucous plexus neuron isolated from the guinea pig, the outward
potassium current develops with a latency of at least 50 ms; this latency
has a high temperature dependence (Q_{10} about 4) (MIHARA and NORTH,
unpublished observations) (Fig. 4). More complete studies have been
carried out for the hyperpolarizing action of noradrenaline, which acts
through α_2-receptors to open the same set of potassium channels in these
cells (SURPRENANT and NORTH 1988; NORTH 1989b). In this case, the minimum latency to the onset of noradrenaline action is also 30–50 ms: control
experiments indicate that diffusion of noradrenaline to the cell surface
accounts for not more than about 1 ms. These experiments exclude the
possibility that opioids (or noradrenaline) are opening a ligand-gated potassium channel.

3. Single Channel Studies

The cell-attached recordings from dissociated locus ceruleus (MIYAKE et al.
1989) indicate that no freely diffusible second messenger intervenes between
μ-receptor and potassium channel. Similarly, the persistence of the
response to opioids in excised outside-out patches from submucous plexus
(SHEN et al. 1990) also shows that the only molecule other than ions
required in the intracellular solution is GTP (Fig. 3). Both these studies
indicate that any other cellular processes involved in coupling receptor to
channel must be delimited to the small patch of membrane enclosed in the
tip of the patch clamp electrode.

These results can be interpreted together with a body of work showing
that purified G proteins increase the probability of opening of potassium

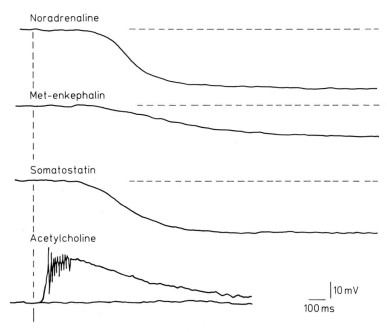

Fig. 4. Latency to onset of opioid-induced hyperpolarization. Intracellular recordings were made from guinea pig submucous plexus neurons. The agonists were applied at the time indicated by the *vertical broken line*. The depolarizing response to acetylcholine occurred after a latency of 20–30 ms; it evoked many action potentials (full amplitude not reproduced). Hyperpolarizing responses to the other agonists all began after a latency of more than 200 ms. Agonists applied by bringing the tip of a glass pipette close to the neuron, and ejecting agonist by a brief pulse of pressure [Noradrenaline (100 μM) 140 kPa for 20 ms; [Met[5]]enkephalin (100 μM) 140 kPa for 30 ms; somatostatin (100 μM) 30 ms, 280 kPa; acetylcholine (100 μM) 70 kPa, 5 ms]. (MIHARA and NORTH, unpublished observations)

channels when applied directly to the inner surface of excised membrane patches (VAN DONGEN et al. 1988; see BROWN and BIRNBAUMER 1990). There is imperfect correlation between the properties of the single channels opened by G proteins applied to the inside of membrane patches from hippocampal neurons (VAN DONGEN et al. 1988) and those opened by opioids applied to the outside of excised patches from submucous plexus neurons; this might result from differences in the conditions used in the two experiments. Both experiments clearly show that activity of several distinct resting, voltage-independent potassium channels can be influenced by G proteins, and by opioids acting through G proteins. Thus, there seems to be no species of potassium channel that is uniquely opened by opioid action; rather several distinct potassium channels can be accessed by the activated G protein.

IX. Other Receptors That Increase Potassium Conductance

The increase in potassium conductance produced by opioids is shared by several other agonists (see NORTH 1989b). In many cases, several receptors are expressed on the same cells, and their activation increases the same conductance (e.g., α_2-adrenoceptors and μ-receptors in rat locus ceruleus: NORTH and WILLIAMS 1985; α_2, somatostatin, and δ-receptors in guinea pig submucous plexus: MIHARA et al. 1987; muscarinic M_2, $GABA_B$, and μ-receptors in rat nucleus parabrachialis: CHRISTIE and NORTH 1988). Furthermore, in excised patches of membrane from guinea pig submucous plexus neurons somatostatin, noradrenaline, and enkephalin each increase the probability of opening of the same single potassium channel. These results show that opioid receptors belong to an extended family of G protein coupled membrane receptors that result in potassium channel opening.

X. Potassium Conductance Increase and Presynaptic Inhibition

Transmitter release from nerves requires depolarization of the terminal and calcium entry through voltage-dependent calcium channels. The period of time for which the terminal is depolarized, the action potential duration, is a critical determinant of the amount of calcium that enters and the amount of transmitter that is released (AUGUSTINE 1990). Two ways in which opioids might inhibit transmitter release are a reduced calcium entry or an increased potassium current leading to earlier repolarization and a shorter action potential. Opioids inhibit noradrenaline release in brain (MONTEL et al. 1975). NAKAMURA et al. (1982) showed that morphine reduced the excitability of the terminal regions of noradrenergic axons arising in the locus ceruleus; the likely reason for a reduced excitability is a membrane hyperpolarization and/or conductance increase. Because the cell bodies of those noradrenergic axons were hyperpolarized by opioids, NORTH and WILLIAMS (1983) proposed that a potassium conductance increase occurring at the nerve terminal could result in a reduction of transmitter release, by reducing the action potential duration.

There are problems with this hypothesis. First, the interpretation depends on the inwardly rectifying potassium conductance contributing to action potential repolarization; this seems unlikely because the conductance is smaller at positive potentials. This problem disappears if opioids are increasing a delayed rectifier type of conductance (WIMPEY and CHAVKIN 1990) because that would be expected to reduce action potential duration. However, an increase in a delayed rectifier would probably not decrease excitability. Second, opioids also inhibit the release of transmitter evoked by solutions containing high potassium concentrations in the presence of tetrodotoxin. BUG et al. (1986) used intracellular recording combined with measurements of [^{3}H]noradrenaline release and showed that a large increase in potassium conductance by opioids could indeed contribute to the inhibition of transmitter release evoked by 35 or 60 mM potassium. However, those studies do not exclude the possibility that the inhibition of release is quite unrelated to an action on potassium channels.

D. Other Ion Channels

The inhibition of firing of neurons in vivo that is generally observed when opioids are applied (see DUGGAN and NORTH 1984) has also been attributed to a reduced excitatory synaptic input. This could be because less excitatory transmitter is released or, conceivably, because the transmitter (usually glutamic acid) has less effect on the postsynaptic cell. This second possibility has been championed by Zieglgänsberger and colleagues (ZIEGLGÄNSBERGER and BAYERL 1976), on the basis of the finding that the initial rate of rise of the excitatory postsynaptic potential is reduced by opioids. However, experiments in vitro have failed to show any effect of opioids on the depolarizations of neurons evoked by glutamic acid, even though reductions in the amplitude of excitatory synaptic potentials have been widely reported (spinal cord/dorsal root ganglion cultures from mouse: MACDONALD and NELSON 1978; rat striatum: JIANG and NORTH 1989; rat locus ceruleus: McFADZEAN et al. 1987). The presynaptic actions of opioids to inhibit the release of excitatory transmitters referred to above seem likely to account for the reduction in the EPSP amplitude observed in vivo. An alternative explanation (DUGGAN and NORTH 1984), that the EPSP is reduced because the synaptic current is shunted by a potassium condutance increase occurring on neuronal dendrites undetected by electrodes in the cell soma, has not been tested experimentally.

E. Changes in Tolerance and Dependence

The long-term actions of opioids at the cellular level have recently been reviewed (JOHNSON and FLEMING 1989); there is little information at the level of ion channels. CRAIN et al. (1988) found that Tyr-D-Ala-Gly-Gly-D-Leu (DADLE) lost its usual action to reduce the action potential duration in cultures of mouse dorsal root ganglion cells that had been chronically exposed to an opioid agonist. Instead, acute application of DADLE now prolonged rather than shortened the spike; this action potential broadening effect is also found in nontolerant cultures, but at much lower agonist concentrations than required to shorten the spike (SHEN and CRAIN 1989; CRAIN and SHEN 1990).

Recordings of membrane current from the rat locus ceruleus show that tolerance develops when the rats are treated chronically with morphine (ANDRADE et al. 1983; CHRISTIE et al. 1987). Intracellular recordings were made from locus ceruleus cells in brain slices removed from rats pretreated for several days with increasing amounts of morphine (CHRISTIE et al. 1987). The basic properties of the neurons appeared to be grossly normal, and the potassium current response to agonists acting at α_2-receptors was unaffected. Normorphine was less effective at increasing the potassium conductance in neurons from morphine-treated rats than in control cells taken from un-treated rats. Tolerance was apparent from a rightward shift in the con-centration-response curve, combined with a decrease in the maximum current. The maximum current response to DAMGO was unaffected, although there was a rightward shift in the dose-response curve. The effects of chronically treating the rat with morphine were not different from the effects of tissue taken from a normal rat and treating it with β-funaltrex-amine – a reduction in the maximum response for partial agonists (such as normorphine) and a simple rightward shift for full agonists. It was concluded from these experiments that chronic morphine treatment either reduced the number of opioid receptors on the surface of the locus ceruleus neuron, or impaired the coupling to G proteins. The cAMP system has been implicated in the long-term actions of opioids in the locus ceruleus (DUMAN et al. 1988; GUITART and NESTLER 1989), but it remains unclear how this is reflected at the level of the ion channel.

F. Concluding Remarks

The experimental work reviewed indicates that there is no unique ion channel associated with the action of opioids. Opening of potassium channels and closing of calcium channels have been described in cells from many regions of the nervous system. Receptor types are not uniquely associated with a given ion channel. Both μ- and δ-receptors couple with potassium channels in various cells, and μ-, δ-, and κ-can all couple with calcium channels. In some cases, single cells express more than one receptor type. Both potassium channel opening and calcium channel closing can result from activating on receptor type on the same cell. The opening of membrane potassium channels and the resulting hyperpolarization seem likely to underlie the inhibition of nerve cells that opioids cause throughout the nervous system. In some regions (e.g., hippocampus, ventral tegmental area) the cells inhibited are local interneurons and this leads to excitation of the principal output neurons by reducing the inhibitory influence of the interneurons.

The coupling of opioid receptors to ion channels is shared by other receptors. Opioid and other receptors can couple to the same individual channel, as in a small patch of membrane excised from the cell surface. Different cells express different combinations of receptors together with opioid receptors; they include α_2-adrenoceptors and somatostatin, GABA$_B$, and muscarinic M$_2$ receptors. This convergence of receptors onto the same channel accounts for the observation that agonists at these receptors commonly share overlapping pharmacological profiles in intact animals. The finding that the molecular mechanism by which opioid receptors couple to ion channels is very similar to that used by, for example, α_2- and M_2-receptors strongly implies that the opioid receptors are close structural relatives of those receptors.

Acknowledgements. Work in the author's laboratory is supported by grants from the US Department of Health and Human Services DA03160, DA03161 and MH40416. I thank Dr. A. Surprenant for comments on the manuscript and for providing Fig. 3 and Catherine Epp for help in preparing the manuscript.

References

Aghajanian GK, Wang YY (1986) Pertussis toxin blocks the outward currents evoked by opiate and α_2 agonists in locus coeruleus. Brain Res 371:390–394

Andrade R, Van der Maalen CP, Aghajanian GK (1983) Morphine tolerance and dependence in the locus coeruleus: single cell studies in brain slices. Eur J Pharmacol 91:161–169

Ashcroft FM (1988) Adenosine 5'-triphosphate-sensitive potassium channels. Annu Rev Neurosci 11:97–118

Augustine GJ (1990) Regulation of transmitter release at the squid giant synapse by presynaptic delayed rectifer potassium channel. J Physiol (Lond) 431:343–364

Bean BP (1989) Neurotransmitter inhibition of neuronal calcium currents by changes in channel voltage dependence. Nature 340:153–156

Brown AM, Birnbaumer L (1990) Ionic channels and their regulation by G protein subunits. Annu Rev Physiol 52:197–213

Brown DA, Docherty RJ, McFadzean I (1989) Calcium channels in vertebrate neurons: experiments on a neuroblastoma hybrid model. Ann NY Acad Sci 560:358–372

Bug W, Williams JT, North RA (1986) Membrane potential measured during potassium evoked noradrenaline release from rat brain neurons: effects of normorphine. J Neurochem 47:652–655

Carbone E, Lux HD (1984) A low voltage-activated fully inactivating Ca channel in vertebrate sensory neurones. Nature 310:501–502

Catterall WA (1988) Structure and function of voltage-sensitive ion channels. Science 242:50–61

Chalazonitis A, Crain SM (1986) Maturation of opioid sensitivity of fetal mouse dorsal root ganglion neruon perikarya in organotypic cultures: regulation by spinal cord. Neuroscience 17:1181–1198

Chen G-G, Chalazonitis A, Shen K-F, Crain SM (1988) Inhibitor of cyclic AMP-dependent protein kinase blocks opioid-induced prolongation of the action potential of mouse sensory ganglion neurons in dissociated cell cultures. Brain Res 462:372–377

Cherubini E, North RA (1985) μ and κ opioids inhibit transmitter release by different mechanisms. Proc Natl Acad Sci USA 82:1860–1863

Christie MJ, North RA (1988) Agonists at μ opioid, M_2 muscarinic and $GABA_B$ receptors increase the same potassium conductance in rat lateral parabrachial neurones. Br J Pharmacol 95:896–902

Christie MJ, Williams JT, North RA (1987) Cellular mechanisms of opioid tolerance: studies in single brain neurons. Mol Pharmacol 32:633–638

Collier HOJ, Roy AC (1974) Morphine-like drugs inhibit the stimulation by E prostaglandins of cyclic AMP formation by rat brain homogenates. Nature 248:24–27

Crain SM, Shen K-F (1990) Opioids can evoke direct receptor-mediated excitatory effects on sensory neurons. Trends Pharmacol Sci 11:77–81

Crain SM, Shen K-F, Chalazonitis A (1988) Opioids excite rather than inhibit sensory neurons after chronic opioid exposure of spinal cord-ganglion cultures. Brain Res 455:99–109

Decker ER, Dani JA (1990) Calcium permeability of the nicotinic acetylcholine receptor: the single channel calcium influx is significant. J Neurosci 10:3413–3421

Dolphin AC, Scott RH (1989) Modulation of Ca^{2+}-channel currents in sensory neurons by pertussis toxin-sensitive G-proteins. Ann NY Acad Sci 560:387–390

Duan S, Shimizu N, Fukuda A, Hori T, Oomura Y (1990) Hyperpolarizing action of enkephalin on neurons in the dorsal motor nucleus of the vagus, in vitro. Brain Res Bull 25:551–559

Duggan AW, North RA (1984) Electrophysiology of opioids. Pharmacol Rev 35:219–281

Duman RS, Tallman JF, Nestler EJ (1988) Acute and chronic opiate regulation of adenylate cyclase in brain: specific effects in locus coeruleus. J Pharmacol Exp Ther 246:1033–1039

Evans RH, Hill RG (1978) Effects of exitatory and inhibitory peptides on isolated spinal cord preparations. In: Ryall RW, Kelly JS (eds) Iontophoresis and transmitter mechanisms in the mammalian central nervous system. Elsevier, Amsterdam, p 101

Gross RA, Macdonald RL (1987) Dynorphin A selectively reduces a large transient (N-type) calcium current of mouse dorsal root ganglion neurons in cell culture. Proc Natl Acad Sci USA 84:5469–5473

Gross RA, Moises HC, Uhler MD, Macdonald RL (1990) Dynorphin A and cAMP dependent protein kinase independently regulate neuronal calcium currents. Proc Natl Acad Sci USA 87:7025–7029

Guitart X, Nestler EJ (1989) Identification of morphine and cyclic AMP regulated phosphoproteins (MARPPs) in the locus coeruleus and other regions of the rat brain: regulation by acute and chronic morphine. J Neurosci 9:4371–4387

Hescheler J, Rosenthal W, Trautwein W, Schultz G (1987) The GTP-binding protein, G_o, regulates neuronal calcium channels. Nature 325:445–447

Hess P (1990) Calcium channels in vertebrate cells. Annu Rev Neurosci 13:337–356

Higashi H, Shinnick Gallagher P, Gallagher JP (1982) Morphine enchances and depresses Ca-dependent responses in visceral primary afferent neurons. Brain Res 251:186–191

Jeftinija S (1988) Enkephalins modulate excitatory synaptic transmission in the superficial dorsal horn by acting at μ-opioid receptor sites. Brain Res 460:260–268

Jiang Z-G, North RA (1992) Pre- and post-synaptic inhibition by opioids in rat striatum. J Neurosci 12:356–361

Johnson SM, Fleming WW (1989) Mechanisms of cellular adaptive sensitivity changes: applications to opioid tolerance and dependence. Pharmacol Rev 41:435–488

Johnson SW, North RA (1992) Opioids excite dopamine neurons by hyperpolarization of local interneurons. J Neurosci 12:483–488

Kaczmarek LK, Levitan IB (1987) Neuromodulation. Oxford University Press, Oxford

Karras PJ, North RA (1979) Inhibition of neuronal firing by opiates: evidence against the involvement of cyclic nucleotides. Br J Pharmacol 65:647–652

Kelly MJ, Loose MD, Ronnekleiv OK (1990) Opioids hyperpolarize β-endorphin neurons via μ-receptor activation of a potassium conductance. Neuroendocrinology 52:268–275

Klee WA, Nirenberg M (1974) A neuroblastoma × glioma hybrid cell line with morphine receptors. Proc Natl Acad Sci USA 71:3474–3477

Lacey MG, Mercuri NB, North RA (1989) Two cells types in rat substantia nigra zona compacta distinguished by membrane properties. J Neurosci 9:1233–1241

Latorre R, Oberhauser A, Labarca P, Alvarez O (1989) Varieties of calcium-activated potassium channels. Annu Rev Physiol 51:385–399

Loose MD, Kelly MJ (1990) Opioids act at μ-receptors to hyperpolarize arcuate neurons via an inwardly rectifying potassium conductance. Brain Res 513: 15–23

Loose MD, Ronnekleiv OK, Kelly MJ (1990) Membrane properties and response to opioids of identified dopamine neurons in the guinea pig hypothalamus. J Neurosci 10:3627–3634

Lord JAH, Waterfield AA, Hughes J, Kosterlitz HW (1977) Endogenous opioid peptides: multiple agonists and receptors. Nature 267:495–499

Macdonald RL, Nelson PG (1978) Specific opiate induced depression of transmitter release from dorsal root ganglion cells in culture. Science 199:1449–1451

Macdonald RL, Werz MA (1986) Dynorphin A decreases voltage-dependent calcium conductance of dorsal root ganglion neurons. J Physiol (Lond) 377:237–249

McFadzean I, Docherty RJ (1989) Noradrenaline and enkephalin-induced inhibition of voltage-sensitive calcium current in NG108-15 hybrid cells: transduction mechanisms. Eur J Neurosci 1:141–147

McFadzean I, Lacey MG, Hill RG, Henderson G (1987) Kappa opioid receptor activation depresses excitatory synaptic input to rat locus coeruleus neurons in vitro. Neuroscience 20:231–239

McFadzean I, Mullaney I, Brown DA, Milligan G (1989) Antibodies to the GTP binding protein, G_o, antagonize noradrenaline-induced calcium current inhibition in NG108-15. Neurone 3:177–182

Madison DV, Nicoll RA (1988) Enkephalin hyperpolarizes interneurons in the rat hippocampus. J Physiol (Lond) 398: 123–130

Mihara S, North RA (1986) Opioids increase potassium conductance in guinea-pig submucous neurones by activating δ receptors. Br J Pharmacol 88:315–322

Mihara S, North RA, Surprenant A (1987) Somatostatin increase an inwardly rectifying potassium conductance in guinea-pig submucous plexus neurones. J Physiol (Lond) 390:335–355

Montel H, Starke K, Taube HD (1975) Influence of morphine and naloxone on the release of noradrenaline from rat cerebllar cortex slices. Naunyn Schmiedebergs Arch Pharmacol 288:427–433

Mudge AW, Leeman SE, Fischbach GD (1979) Enkephalin inhibits release of substance P from sensory neurons in culture and decreases action potential duration. Proc Natl Acad Sci USA 76:526–530

Murase K, Nedeljkov V, Randic M (1982) The actions of neuropeptides on dorsal horn neurons in the rat spinal cord preparation: an intracellular study. Brain Res 234:170–176

Nakamura S, Tepper JM, Young SJ, Ling N, Groves PM (1982) Noradrenergic terminal excitability: effects of opioids. Neurosci Lett 30:57–62

Nicoll RA (1982) Responses of central neurones to opiates and opioid peptides. In: Costa E, Trabucchi M (eds) Regulatory peptides: from molecular biology to function. Raven, New York, p 337

Nicoll RA, Alger BE, Jahr CE (1980) Enkephalin blocks inhibitory pathways in the vertebrate CNS. Nature 287:22–25

North RA (1989a) Neurotransmitters and their receptors: from the clone to the clinic. Semin Neurosci 1:81–90

North RA (1989b) Drug receptors and the inhibtion of nerve cells. Br J Pharmacol 98:13–28

North RA, Tonini M (1977) The mechanism of action of narcotic analgesics in the guinea-pig ileum. Br J Pharmacol 61:541–549

North RA, Williams JT (1983) How do opiates inhibit transmitter release? Trends Neurosci 6:337–339

North RA, Williams JT (1985) On the potassium conductance increased by opioids in rat locus coeruleus neurones. J Physiol (Lond) 364:265–280

North RA, Williams JT, Surprenant A, Christie MJ (1987) μ and δ opioid receptors both belong to a family of receptors which couple to a potassium conductance. Proc Natl Acad Sci USA 84:5487–5491

Nowycky MC, Fox AP, Tsien RW (1985) Three types of neuronal calcium channel with different calcium agonist sensitivity. Nature 316:440–443

Pan ZZ, Williams JT, Osborne PB (1990) Opioid actions on single nucleus raphe magnus neurons from rat and guinea pig in vitro. J Physiol (Lond) 427:519–532

Pepper CM, Henderson G (1980) Opiates and opioid peptides hyperpolarize locus coeruleus neurones in vitro. Science 209:394–396

Rasmussen K, Beitner-Johnson DB, Krystal JH, Aghajanian GK, Nestler EJ (1990) Opiate withdrawal and the rat locus coeruleus: behavioral, electrophysiological, and biochemical correlates. J Neurosci 10:2308–2317

Rudy B (1988) Diversity and ubiquity of K channels. Neuroscience 25:729–749

Sah DWY (1990) Neurotransmitter modulation of calcium current in rat spinal cord neurons. J Neurosci 10:136–141

Sakmann B, Noma A, Trautwein W (1983) Acetylcholine activation of single muscarinic K channels in isolated pacemaker cells of the mammalian heart. Nature 303:250–253

Schroeder JE, Fischbach PS, Mamo M, McCleskey EW (1990) Two components of high-threshold Ca^{2+} current inactivate by different mechanisms. Neurone 5:445–452

Schroeder JE, Fischbach PS, Zheng D, McCleskey EW (1991) Activation of mu opioid receptors inhibits transient high and low threshold Ca^{++} currents, but spares a sustained current. Neuron 6:13–20

Seward EP, Henderson G (1990) Characterization of two components of the N-like, high-threshold-activated calcium channel current in differentiated SH-SY5Y cells. Pflugers Arch 417:223–230

Seward E, Hammond C, Henderson G (1991) μ-opioid receptor-mediated inhibition of the N-type calcium channel current. Proc Roy Soc (Lond) B 244:129–135

Shen K-F, Crain SM (1989) Dual opioid modulation of the action potential duration of mouse dorsal root ganglion neurons in culture. Brain Res 491:227–242

Shen K-Z, Surprenant A (1990) Mechanisms underlying presynaptic inhibition through α_2-adrenoceptors in guinea pig submucosal neurones. J Physiol (Lond) 431:609–628

Shen K-Z, North RA, Surprenant A (1992) Potassium channels opened by noradrenaline and other transmitters in excised membrane patches of guinea-pig submucosal neurones. J Physiol (Lond) 445:581–599

Shimahara T, Icard-Liepkalns C (1987) Activation of enkephalin receptors reduces calcium conductance in neuroblastoma cells. Brain Res 415:357–361

Surprenant A, North RA (1988) Mechanism of synaptic inhibtion by noradrenaline acting at α_2-adrenoceptors. Proc R Soc Lond [Biol] 234:85–114

Surprenant A, Shen K-Z, North RA, Tatsumi H (1990) Inhibition of calcium currents by noradrenaline, somatostatin and opioids in guinea-pig submucosal neurones. J Physiol (Lond) 431:585–608

Tatsumi H, Costa M, Schimerlik M, North RA (1990) Potassium conductance increased by noradrenaline, opioids, somatostatin and G-proteins: whole-cell recording from guinea pig submucous neurons. J Neurosci 10:1675–1682

Tsien RW (1983) Calcium channels in excitable membranes. Annu Rev Physiol 45:341–358

Tsunoo A, Yoshii M, Narahashi T (1986) Block of calcium channels by enkephalin and somatostatin in neuroblastoma-glioma hybrid NG108-15 cells. Proc Natl Acad Sci USA 83:9832–9836

Ullrich S, Wollheim CB (1988) GTP-dependent inhibition of insulin secretion by epinephrine in permeabilized RINm5F cells. J Biol Chem 263:8615–8620

van Dongen AMJ, Codina J, Olate J, Mattera R, Joho R, Birnbaumer L, Brown AM (1988) Newly identified brain potassium channels gated by the guanine nucleotide binding protein G_o. Science 242:1433–1437

Werz MA, Macdonald RL (1983) Opioid peptides selective for mu and delta opiate receptors reduce calcium-dependent action potential duration by increasing potassium conductance. Neurosci Lett 42:173–178

Werz MA, Macdonald RL (1985) Dynorphin and neoendorphin peptides decrease dorsal root ganglion neurons calcium-dependent action potential duration. J Pharmacol Exp Ther 234:49–56

Westbrook GL, Jahr CE (1989) Glutamate receptors in excitatory transmission. Semin Neurosci 1:103–114

Williams JT, North RA (1984) Opiate-receptor interactions on single locus coeruleus neurones. Mol Pharmacol 26:489–497

Williams JT, Egan TM, North RA (1982) Enkephalin opens potassium channels in mammalian central neurones. Nature 299:74–76

Williams JT, North RA, Tokimasa T (1988) Inward rectification of resting and opiate-activated potassium currents in rat locus coeruleus neurons. J Neurosci 8:4299–4306

Wimpey TL, Chavkin C (1991) Opioids activate both an inward rectifier and a novel voltage-gated potassium conductance in the hippocampal formation. Neuron 6:281–289

Wouters W, Van der Bercken J (1979) Hyperpolarization and depression of slow synaptic inhibition in frog sympathetic ganglion. Nature 277:53–54

Wuarin J-P, Dudek FE (1990) Direct effects of an opioid peptide selective for μ-receptors: intracellular recordings in the paraventricular and supraoptic nuclei of the guinea-pig. Neuroscience 36:291–298

Wuarin J-P, Dubois-Dauphin M, Raggenbass M, Dreifuss JJ (1988) Effect of opioid peptides on the paraventricular nucleus of the guinea pig hypothalamus is mediated by μ-type receptors. Brain Res 445:289–296

Young W, Chen J, Jung F, Gardner P (1988) Dihydropyridine Bay K 8644 activates T lymphocyte calcium-permeable channels. Mol Pharmacol 34:239–244

Yoshimura M, North RA (1983) Substantia gelatinosa neurones in vitro hyperpolarized by enkephalin. Nature 305:529–530

Zieglgänsberger W, Bayerl H (1976) The mechanism of inhibition of neuronal activity by opiates in the spinal cord of the cat. Brain Res 115:111–128

Subject Index